ONLINE CONTENT

The following supplemental content is available online at expertconsult.com

ASSESSMENT TOOL

DIGITAL VISUAL DIAGNOSIS IN PEDIATRICS
Assessing Infant Development
Teaching and Review Module
© University of Pittsburgh

VIDEOS

1   NON-SEIZURE NEUROLOGIC SYMPTOMS
Athetosis
Breath-holding Spell
Dystonia
Hemifacial Spasms
Infantile Shudders
Rett Syndrome
Sydenham Chorea

2   RESPIRATORY DISORDERS
Anterior Tracheal Compression
Bronchial Stenosis
Laryngomalacia
Obstructive Apnea
Vocal Cord Dysfunction Paradoxical Movement

3   SEIZURES
Absence
Atonic Seizures
Complex Partial Seizures
Extensor Infantile Spasms
Flexor Infantile Spasms
Gelastic Seizures
Generalized Tonic-Clonic Seizures
Juvenile Myoclonic Epilepsy
Non-Epileptiform Seizure

Zitelli and Davis' ATLAS OF
PEDIATRIC PHYSICAL DIAGNOSIS

Sixth Edition

Zitelli and Davis'
ATLAS OF
PEDIATRIC
PHYSICAL
DIAGNOSIS

Basil J. Zitelli, MD
PROFESSOR OF PEDIATRICS
UNIVERSITY OF PITTSBURGH SCHOOL OF MEDICINE
DIRECTOR
THE PAUL C. GAFFNEY DIAGNOSTIC REFERRAL SERVICE
CHILDREN'S HOSPITAL OF PITTSBURGH OF UPMC
PITTSBURGH, PENNSYLVANIA

Sara C. McIntire, MD
PROFESSOR OF PEDIATRICS
UNIVERSITY OF PITTSBURGH SCHOOL OF MEDICINE
ADVISORY DEAN
OFFICE OF STUDENT AFFAIRS
CHILDREN'S HOSPITAL OF PITTSBURGH OF UPMC
PITTSBURGH, PENNSYLVANIA

Andrew J. Nowalk, MD, PhD
ASSISTANT PROFESSOR OF PEDIATRICS
UNIVERSITY OF PITTSBURGH SCHOOL OF MEDICINE
PEDIATRIC INFECTIOUS DISEASE
CHILDREN'S HOSPITAL OF PITTSBURGH OF UPMC
PITTSBURGH, PENNSYLVANIA

SAUNDERS

ELSEVIER

ELSEVIER
SAUNDERS

1600 John F. Kennedy Blvd.
Ste 1800
Philadelphia, PA 19103-2899

ZITELLI AND DAVIS' ATLAS OF PEDIATRIC PHYSICAL DIAGNOSIS   ISBN: 978-0-323-07932-7

Copyright © 2012 by Saunders, an imprint of Elsevier Inc.
Copyright © 2007, 2002, 1997, 1992, 1987 by Mosby, an affiliate of Elsevier Inc.

Notices

Knowledge and best practice in this field are constantly changing. As new research and experience broaden our understanding, changes in research methods, professional practices, or medical treatment may become necessary.

Practitioners and researchers must always rely on their own experience and knowledge in evaluating and using any information, methods, compounds, or experiments described herein. In using such information or methods they should be mindful of their own safety and the safety of others, including parties for whom they have a professional responsibility.

With respect to any drug or pharmaceutical products identified, readers are advised to check the most current information provided (i) on procedures featured or (ii) by the manufacturer of each product to be administered, to verify the recommended dose or formula, the method and duration of administration, and contraindications. It is the responsibility of practitioners, relying on their own experience and knowledge of their patients, to make diagnoses, to determine dosages and the best treatment for each individual patient, and to take all appropriate safety precautions.

To the fullest extent of the law, neither the Publisher nor the authors, contributors, or editors, assume any liability for any injury and/or damage to persons or property as a matter of products liability, negligence or otherwise, or from any use or operation of any methods, products, instructions, or ideas contained in the material herein.

Library of Congress Cataloging-in-Publication Data
Zitelli and Davis' atlas of pediatric physical diagnosis.—6th ed. / [edited by] Basil J. Zitelli, Sara McIntire, Andrew J. Nowalk.
      p. ; cm.
   Atlas of pediatric physical diagnosis
   Rev. ed. of: Atlas of pediatric physical diagnosis / [edited by] Basil J. Zitelli, Holly W. Davis. c2007.
   Includes bibliographical references and index.
   ISBN 978-0-323-07932-7 (hardcover : alk. paper)
   I. Zitelli, Basil J. (Basil John), 1946- II. McIntire, Sara. III. Nowalk, Andrew J. IV. Atlas of pediatric physical diagnosis. V. Title: Atlas of pediatric physical diagnosis.
   [DNLM: 1. Diagnosis—Atlases. 2. Child. 3. Infant. 4. Physical Examination—Atlases. WS 17]
   LC classification not assigned
   618.92'00754—dc23   2011053495

Acquisitions Editors: Judith Fletcher, Stefanie Jewell-Thomas
Developmental Editor: Joanie Milnes
Publishing Services Manager: Patricia Tannian
Senior Project Manager: Linda Van Pelt
Design Direction: Ellen Zanolle

Printed in China

Last digit is the print number: 9 8 7 6 5 4 3 2 1

To our parents, who were our first teachers:
Hannah L. Zitelli and Patsy A. Zitelli
Thomas P. Nowalk and Lourdes W. Nowalk
George M. McIntire and Charlotte M. McIntire

To my wife, Suzanne, and my children,
Matthew, Daniel, Benjamin, and Anne Zitelli

To my wife, Amy Brinkos, and my children,
James, Max, and Peter Nowalk

To my brother, John, and my children,
Frances and Madeline Marcelle

To those exceptional teachers we have had, whose
dedication, enthusiasm, and creativity helped make the
acquisition, application, and sharing of knowledge more
fun than hard work and who inspired us not only to
perform to the best of our ability but also to
become teachers as well as physicians:

Henry Furrie, Paul C. Gaffney, MD, William H. Zinkham, MD,
J.R. Zuberbuhler, MD, Crystie Halsted, MD,
Ronald Lemire, MD, J. Carlton Gartner Jr., MD,
William I. Cohen, MD

To our residents and students, whose eagerness to learn
and to put their knowledge to use keeps us learning
actively and makes teaching so rewarding

CONTRIBUTORS

Vivek Allada, MD
Associate Professor of Pediatrics
University of Pittsburgh School of Medicine
Clinical Director
Pediatric Cardiology
Heart Center
Children's Hospital of Pittsburgh of UPMC
Pittsburgh, Pennsylvania

Georgianne Arnold, MD
Professor of Pediatrics
University of Pittsburgh School of Medicine
Children's Hospital of Pittsburgh of UPMC
Pittsburgh, Pennsylvania

Jennifer Arnold, MD, MSc
Assistant Professor of Pediatrics
Division of Perinatal-Neonatal Medicine
Medical Director
Pediatric Simulation
Texas Children's Hospital
Houston, Texas

Heather Baumhardt, BS, DDS
Clinical Assistant Professor
University of Pittsburgh School of Dental Medicine
Pediatric Dentistry
Children's Hospital of Pittsburgh of UPMC
Pittsburgh, Pennsylvania

Lee B. Beerman, MD
Professor of Pediatrics
University of Pittsburgh School of Medicine
Division of Pediatric Cardiology
Children's Hospital of Pittsburgh of UPMC
Pittsburgh, Pennsylvania

Mark F. Bellinger, MD
Visiting Professor of Urology
Urology
University of Pittsburgh School of Medicine
Attending Urologist
Urology
Children's Hospital of Pittsburgh of UPMC
Pittsburgh, Pennsylvania

Albert W. Biglan, MD
Formerly Adjunct Professor of Ophthalmology
Children's Hospital of Pittsburgh of UPMC
Pittsburgh, Pennsylvania

Debra L. Bogen, MD
Associate Professor of Pediatrics and Psychiatry
University of Pittsburgh School of Medicine
Division of General Academic Pediatrics
Children's Hospital of Pittsburgh of UPMC
Pittsburgh, Pennsylvania

Beverly S. Brozanski, MD
Professor of Pediatrics
University of Pittsburgh School of Medicine
Clinical Director
Neonatal Intensive Care
Children's Hospital of Pittsburgh of UPMC
Pittsburgh, Pennsylvania

Mary M. Carrasco, MD, MPH
Associate Clinical Professor of Pediatrics
University of Pittsburgh School of Medicine
Director
International and Community Health
Pittsburgh Mercy Health System
Pittsburgh, Pennsylvania

Diego Chaves-Gnecco, MD, MPH
Assistant Professor of Pediatrics
University of Pittsburgh School of Medicine
SALUD PARA NIÑOS Program Director and Founder
Developmental-Behavioral Pediatrics
Children's Hospital of Pittsburgh of UPMC
Pittsburgh, Pennsylvania

Wassim Chemaitilly, MD
Assistant Professor of Pediatrics
Division Director
Pediatric Endocrinology
St. Jude Children's Research Hospital
Memphis, Tennessee

Kenneth P. Cheng, MD
Children's Hospital of Pittsburgh of UPMC
Pittsburgh
Pediatric Ophthalmology and Adult Strabismus
Wexford, Pennsylvania

David H. Chi, MD
Assistant Professor
University of Pittsburgh School of Medicine
Director
Hearing Center
Division of Pediatric Otolaryngology
Children's Hospital of Pittsburgh of UPMC
Pittsburgh, Pennsylvania

Bernard A. Cohen, MD
Professor of Dermatology and Pediatrics
Director
Cutaneous Laser Center
Johns Hopkins University School of Medicine
Baltimore, Maryland

James D. Cooper, MD
Assistant Professor of Pediatrics
University of Pittsburgh School of Medicine
Pediatric Hematology/Oncology/BMT
Children's Hospital of Pittsburgh of UPMC
Pittsburgh, Pennsylvania

Alene D'Alesio, DMD
Clinical Assistant Professor
Pediatric Dentistry
Children's Hospital of Pittsburgh of UPMC
Pittsburgh, Pennsylvania

Katherine P. Davenport, MD
Joseph E. Robert, Jr. Research Fellow
Sheikh Zayed Institute for Pediatric Surgical Innovation
Children's National Medical Center
Washington, District of Columbia

Holly W. Davis, MD
Associate Professor of Pediatrics, Emeritus
University of Pittsburgh School of Medicine
Children's Hospital of Pittsburgh of UPMC
Pittsburgh, Pennsylvania

Vincent F. Deeney, MD
Associate Professor
Department of Orthopaedics
Residency Program Director
Orthopaedic Surgery
University of Pittsburgh Medical Center
Pittsburgh, Pennsylvania

Demetrius Ellis, MD
Professor of Pediatrics and Nephrology
University of Pittsburgh School of Medicine
Children's Hospital of Pittsburgh of UPMC
Pittsburgh, Pennsylvania

Oscar Escobar, MD
Assistant Professor of Pediatrics
University of Pittsburgh School of Medicine
Pediatric Endocrinology, Diabetes and Metabolism
Children's Hospital of Pittsburgh of UPMC
Pittsburgh, Pennsylvania

Heidi M. Feldman, MD, PhD
Ballinger-Swindells Professor
Pediatrics
Stanford University School of Medicine
Stanford, California

Jonathan D. Finder, MD
Professor of Pediatrics
University of Pittsburgh School of Medicine
Clinical Director
Pediatric Pulmonary Medicine
Children's Hospital of Pittsburgh of UPMC
Pittsburgh, Pennsylvania

Robin P. Gehris, MD
Chief
Pediatric Dermatologic Surgery
Dermatology
Children's Hospital of Pittsburgh of UPMC
Pittsburgh, Pennsylvania

Todd Green, MD
Assistant Professor of Pediatrics
University of Pittsburgh School of Medicine
Allergy and Immunology
Children's Hospital of Pittsburgh of UPMC
Pittsburgh, Pennsylvania

Dena Hofkosh, MD
Professor of Pediatrics
University of Pittsburgh School of Medicine
Developmental-Behavioral Pediatrics
Children's Hospital of Pittsburgh of UPMC
Pittsburgh, Pennsylvania

Timothy D. Kane, MD, FACS
Associate Professor of Surgery and Pediatrics
George Washington University School of Medicine
Associate Chief of Clinical Affairs
Pediatric Surgery
Sheikh Zayed Institute for Pediatric Surgical Innovation
Children's National Medical Center
Washington, District of Columbia

Sunhee Kim, MD
Assistant Professor
University of Pittsburgh School of Medicine
Diagnostic Radiology
Children's Hospital of Pittsburgh of UPMC
Pittsburgh, Pennsylvania

Jacqueline Kreutzer, MD, FACC, FSCAI
Associate Professor of Pediatrics
University of Pittsburgh School of Medicine
Department of Pediatrics
University of Pittsburgh
Director
Cardiac Catheterization Laboratory
Pediatric Cardiology
Children's Hospital of Pittsburgh of UPMC
Pittsburgh, Pennsylvania

Alexander Y. Lin, MD
Clinical Instructor
University of Pittsburgh School of Medicine
Craniofacial and Pediatric Plastic Surgery Fellow
Division of Pediatric Plastic Surgery
Children's Hospital of Pittsburgh of UPMC
Division of Plastic Surgery
University of Pittsburgh Medical Center
Pittsburgh, Pennsylvania

Joseph E. Losee, MD, FACS, FAAP
Professor of Surgery and Pediatrics
University of Pittsburgh School of Medicine
Chief
Division of Pediatric Plastic Surgery
Children's Hospital of Pittsburgh of UPMC
Pittsburgh, Pennsylvania

Andrew MacGinnitie, MD, PhD
Assistant Professor of Pediatrics
Harvard Medical School
Associate Clinical Director
Division of Immunology
Children's Hospital of Boston
Boston, Massachusetts

David H. MacKibben, DMD, MDS
Formerly Clinical Associate Professor of Pediatric Dentistry
University of Pittsburgh School of Dental Medicine
Dental Services
Children's Hospital of Pittsburgh of UPMC
Pittsburgh, Pennsylvania

Suneeta Madan-Khetarpal, MD
Associate Professor of Pediatrics
University of Pittsburgh School of Medicine
Division of Medical Genetics
Department of Pediatrics
Children's Hospital of Pittsburgh of UPMC
Pittsburgh, Pennsylvania

Brian Martin, DMD
Clinical Assistant Professor
University of Pittsburgh School of Dental Medicine
Chief
Division of Pediatric Dentistry
Children's Hospital of Pittsburgh of UPMC
Pittsburgh, Pennsylvania

Sara C. McIntire, MD
Professor of Pediatrics
University of Pittsburgh School of Medicine
Advisory Dean
Office of Student Affairs
Children's Hospital of Pittsburgh of UPMC
Pittsburgh, Pennsylvania

Marian G. Michaels, MD, MPH
Professor of Pediatrics and Surgery
University of Pittsburgh School of Medicine
Pediatric Infectious Diseases
University of Pittsburgh School of Medicine
Pittsburgh, Pennsylvania

Yosuke Miyashita, MD, MPH
Assistant Professor of Pediatrics
University of Pittsburgh School of Medicine
Children's Hospital of Pittsburgh of UPMC
Pittsburgh, Pennsylvania

Morey S. Moreland[†]
William F. and Jean W. Donaldson Professor of
  Orthopedic Surgery
University of Pittsburgh School of Medicine
Division of Pediatric Orthopedics
Children's Hospital of Pittsburgh of UPMC
Pittsburgh, Pennsylvania

Pamela J. Murray, MD, MPH
Professor and Vice Chair
Pediatrics
West Virginia University School of Medicine
Morgantown, West Virginia

Mamoun N. Nazif, DDS, MDS
Formerly Clinical Professor of Pediatric Dentistry
University of Pittsburgh School of Dental Medicine
Formerly Staff
Children's Hospital of Pittsburgh
Pittsburgh, Pennsylvania

David Nash, MD
Clinical Assistant Professor of Pediatrics
University of Pittsburgh School of Medicine
Director
Outreach Allergy and Immunology
Division of Pulmonary Medicine, Allergy and Immunology
Department of Pediatrics
Children's Hospital of Pittsburgh of UPMC
Pittsburgh, Pennsylvania

Andrew J. Nowalk, MD, PhD
Assistant Professor of Pediatrics
University of Pittsburgh School of Medicine
Pediatric Infectious Disease
Children's Hospital of Pittsburgh of UPMC
Pittsburgh, Pennsylvania

Melissa M. Riley, MD
Neonatology Fellow
University of Pittsburgh School of Medicine
Division of Newborn Medicine
Children's Hospital of Pittsburgh of UPMC and Magee
  Womens Hospital of UPMC
Pittsburgh, Pennsylvania

A. Kim Ritchey, MD
Professor of Pediatrics
University of Pittsburgh School of Medicine
Chief
Pediatric Hematology/Oncology
Vice Chair for Clinical Affairs
Children's Hospital of Pittsburgh of UPMC
Pittsburgh, Pennsylvania

Paul Rosen, MD, MPH, MMM
Division of Pediatric Rheumatology
Department of Pediatrics
The Nemours/Alfred I. duPont Hospital for Children
Wilmington, Delaware

Jeffrey A. Rudolph, MD
Assistant Professor of Pediatrics
University of Pittsburgh School of Medicine
Division of Pediatric Gastroenterology
Children's Hospital of Pittsburgh of UPMC
Pittsburgh, Pennsylvania

Vera Sperling, MD
Clinical Assistant Professor
University of Pittsburgh School of Medicine
Department of Radiology
Children's Hospital of Pittsburgh of UPMC
Pittsburgh, Pennsylvania

David Stukus, MD
Assistant Professor of Pediatrics
Division of Infectious Diseases, Allergy and Immunology
Nationwide Children's Hospital
Columbus, Ohio

Gina S. Sucato, MD, MPH
Assistant Professor of Pediatrics
University of Pittsburgh School of Medicine
Division of Adolescent Medicine
Children's Hospital of Pittsburgh of UPMC
Pittsburgh, Pennsylvania

[†]*Deceased.*

Sameh Tadros, MD, MSc
Clinical Assistant Professor
University of Pittsburgh School of Medicine
Department of Radiology
Children's Hospital of Pittsburgh of UPMC
Pittsburgh, Pennsylvania

Jean M. Tersak, MD
Assistant Professor of Pediatrics
University of Pittsburgh School of Medicine
Division of Pediatric Hematology/Oncology and Blood and
  Marrow Transplantation
Children's Hospital of Pittsburgh of UPMC
Pittsburgh, Pennsylvania

Kathryn Torok, MD
Assistant Professor of Pediatrics
University of Pittsburgh School of Medicine
Division of Pediatric Rheumatology
Children's Hospital of Pittsburgh of UPMC
Pittsburgh, Pennsylvania

Rajiv Varma, MD
Clinical Associate Professor
Clinical Director
Division of Pediatric Neurology
University of Pittsburgh School of Medicine
Children's Hospital of Pittsburgh of UPMC
Pittsburgh, Pennsylvania

W. Timothy Ward, MD
Professor
Orthopaedic Surgery
University of Pittsburgh School of Medicine
Chief
Pediatric Orthopaedics
Department of Orthopaedic Surgery
Children's Hospital of Pittsburgh of UPMC
Pittsburgh, Pennsylvania

Daniel J. Weiner, MD
Assistant Professor of Pediatrics
Pediatrics
University of Pittsburgh School of Medicine
Co-Director
Antonio J. and Janet Palumbo Cystic Fibrosis Center
Medical Director
Pulmonary Function Laboratory
Children's Hospital of Pittsburgh of UPMC
Pittsburgh, Pennsylvania

Henry B. Wessel, MD
Formerly Clinical Associate Professor of Pediatrics and Child
  Neurology
University of Pittsburgh School of Medicine
Formerly Director
MDA Clinic
Children's Hospital of Pittsburgh of UPMC
Pittsburgh, Pennsylvania

Shelley D. Williams, MD
Associate Professor of Pediatrics and Neurology
University of Pittsburgh School of Medicine
Division of Child Neurology
Children's Hospital of Pittsburgh of UPMC
Pittsburgh, Pennsylvania

Selma F. Witchel, MD
Associate Professor of Pediatrics
Pediatric Endocrinology, Diabetes and Metabolism
University of Pittsburgh School of Medicine
Children's Hospital of Pittsburgh of UPMC
Pittsburgh, Pennsylvania

Robert F. Yellon, MD
Professor of Otolaryngology
University of Pittsburgh School of Medicine
Co-Director
Division of Pediatric Otolaryngology
Director
ENT Clinic Services
Children's Hospital of Pittsburgh of UPMC
Pittsburgh, Pennsylvania

Basil J. Zitelli, MD
Professor of Pediatrics
University of Pittsburgh School of Medicine
Director
The Paul C. Gaffney Diagnostic Referral Service
Children's Hospital of Pittsburgh of UPMC
Pittsburgh, Pennsylvania

FOREWORD

Ralph Major pointed out that physical diagnosis is the bridge between the abstraction called *disease* described in medical books and the reality called *patients with diseases*, who are in front of us. History and physical examination are the fundamental tools of that physical diagnosis. Our ears, eyes, hands, and nose are the tools used in physical diagnosis, and they are readily available. All modern instruments, starting with the stethoscope, are an extension of our sensory system.

Advances in the scientific aspects of medicine have given us tools that help us see parts of the body we could never see, listen to sounds we will never be able to hear, and touch and manipulate inaccessible parts of the body. These technologic advances have contributed enormously to the welfare of our patients. They have also come with a cost, as all new technologies do. Technology has created a barrier between the doctor and the patient. Patients feel that barrier.

Enamored with the technologic advances, patients tend to think that laboratory tests and imaging studies make the diagnosis, not the physician. Physicians in training also are not as skilled in physical examination as physicians of earlier generations. There is a great need to train physicians how to perform a proper physical examination. This atlas of pediatric physical diagnosis, edited by Doctors Zitelli and Davis and, recently, Doctors Nowalk and McIntire, has been filling this need for several years.

This unique compendium of pediatric conditions helps refocus the attention of physicians, the novice and the experienced, on observing patients. It is a visual encyclopedia of both common and uncommon diseases of children. Using excellent photographs, the authors show important and classic physical findings and also proper techniques to use to elicit these findings.

Having used this book for several years, I know that it is user friendly and fun to browse. It is deceptively simple considering the depth and the breadth of subjects covered. With the addition of new sections on genetic diagnosis and the role of imaging studies in physical diagnosis, this book is a "must" for all medical school libraries, pediatrics departments, and teaching clinics.

Browse, read, or study as you please. And enjoy learning.

Balu Athreya, MD
Professor Emeritus of Pediatrics
Perelman School of Medicine
University of Pennsylvania
Clinical Emeritus Professor of Pediatrics
Jefferson Medical College
Thomas Jefferson University
Philadelphia, Pennsylvania
Teaching Consultant
Nemours/Alfred I. duPont Hospital for Children
Wilmington, Delaware

PREFACE

For many disorders, visual recognition remains the key factor in making a correct diagnosis. The experienced clinician who has seen a wide spectrum of disorders carries a wealth of information for diagnosis and teaching. In a time in which use of technology may erode clinical skills, reinforcing the value of a complete history and careful physical examination grows more important.

This book was envisioned by teachers and was developed to aid students, residents, nurses, and practitioners who care for children in the recognition and diagnosis of pediatric disorders. Our goal is to broaden the visual experience of the student and the clinician through rapid visual examination or review of laboratory tests and imaging studies.

The enthusiastic response to the previous editions of the *Atlas of Pediatric Physical Diagnosis* led us to believe that a sixth edition was not only possible but also necessary. Many readers offered helpful suggestions for photographs and topics to be included. Every chapter has been reviewed, revised, and updated. Additional contributors have provided greater depth and dimension. Some chapters have been entirely rewritten,

and a new chapter regarding pediatric radiologic diagnosis has been added. Although new information, including imaging and diagnostic techniques, has been incorporated, we continue to emphasize the key role of the physical examination in each chapter. The book is by no means encyclopedic but rather presents an overview of clinical disorders that lend themselves to visual diagnosis. The accompanying text deliberately emphasizes pertinent historical factors, examination techniques, visual findings, and diagnostic methods rather than therapy. We firmly believe that a careful history and physical examination provide the foundation for any clinical assessment. We have attempted to select disorders that are common or important and, when relevant, to describe the spectrum of clinical findings. It is our hope that this book continues to serve as a useful and practical reference for anyone who cares for children.

Basil J. Zitelli, MD
Sara C. McIntire, MD
Andrew J. Nowalk, MD, PhD

ACKNOWLEDGMENTS

The *Atlas of Pediatric Physical Diagnosis* results from the untiring efforts of many dedicated people who contributed not only to the current edition but also to all previous editions. Although each chapter has been reviewed, and some have been totally rewritten by new and continuing authors, each chapter is in some way built on the foundation of previous editions. All contributors from the first edition onward have left their mark, and their contributions continue to be felt. We remain in their debt.

Many people at Children's Hospital of Pittsburgh have contributed in countless ways to this book. First and foremost, we appreciate the generosity of our patients and their families, who graciously allowed us to photograph them for the education of those who care for children. Secretaries, radiology technicians, file clerks, librarians, medical media staff, and many unnamed colleagues who provided constructive criticism all have given freely of themselves to help us. We could not have succeeded without them. We thank them all for their tireless work, expertise, and unflagging support.

It is impossible to underestimate the work and effort that Dr. Holly Davis has provided in the birth and development of this book through five editions. Her vision, hard work, and contributions both as an editor and as an author have been invaluable and in large part have been responsible for the success of the book. We cannot thank her enough for her work. Holly has graciously agreed to stay on as a contributor to the Child Abuse and Neglect chapter for this edition.

Our colleagues at Elsevier have been patient, understanding, and accommodating in guiding us through the publication process. Special thanks go to Judy Fletcher, Joanie Milnes, Linda Van Pelt, and other staff who worked countless hours in design, layout, and production of the final product.

Finally, we thank the many thousands of readers who have found the previous editions of the *Atlas of Pediatric Physical Diagnosis* useful, for their praise, support, and suggestions. We hope that their suggestions and our efforts have resulted in an improved work that benefits them and their patients.

Basil J. Zitelli, MD

Sara C. McIntire, MD

Andrew J. Nowalk, MD, PhD

CONTENTS

GENETIC DISORDERS AND DYSMORPHIC CONDITIONS

Suneeta Madan-Khetarpal | Georgianne Arnold

The field of pediatric genetics and dysmorphology is complex, interesting, and rapidly evolving. Our knowledge base is gleaned from the careful observations of master clinicians and scientists who recognized clinical characteristics and patterns of malformation in individuals with genetic, teratogenic, developmental, and metabolic problems. They have provided us with a framework for the investigation of patients from clinical and laboratory perspectives. In addition to classic cytogenetics, molecular cytogenetics methods have been increasingly incorporated in clinical settings and have greatly assisted evaluation, enabling far greater understanding of the molecular and physiologic basis of these disorders, and have greatly increased the rate of diagnosis of children with genetic and metabolic disorders. However, even with the availability of an ever-widening array of confirmatory tests, clinical evaluation of patients remains an essential component of the complete assessment of children and adults with genetic diseases and dysmorphic conditions. This stems from the fact that careful evaluation can substantially reduce the number of differential diagnostic possibilities and, thereby, the number of diagnostic tests and the total expense.

Visual identification of dysmorphic features, baseline anthropometrics combined with serial measurements with recognition of patterns of malformation and behavioral phenotypes, remains an integral part of the diagnostic algorithm. As in pediatrics in general, genetic disorders should be investigated on the basis of a careful history, with a family pedigree and a thorough physical examination including evaluation for the presence of major and minor anomalies, and thoughtful laboratory testing. This chapter is designed to present clinicians who care for children with background on the general principles of genetics and dysmorphology, as well as updated information about important advances in our field. Although not exhaustive, it provides a framework for the broad categories of genetic diseases and discusses an approach to the evaluation of the dysmorphic child. Definitions and examples of the types of disorders resulting in genetic and/or congenital anomalies in children are described, including malformations, deformations, disruptions, associations, and sequences. We include examples of disorders inherited through classic mendelian inheritance patterns, including single-gene mutations, such as Marfan syndrome, Rett syndrome, Smith-Lemli-Opitz syndrome, and Conradi-Hünermann syndrome as well as examples of nonmendelian disorders such as teratogenic exposures in utero and disruptions or deformations of previously normal fetal structures. New etiologic mechanisms of diseases such as imprinting abnormalities and expansions of trinucleotide repeats in nuclear deoxyribonucleic acid (DNA) are presented. Last, a newly evolving area of genetics, the investigation of disorders of mitochondrial DNA and/or mitochondrial function, is discussed.

COMMON CHROMOSOMAL DISORDERS

General Principles

The Nature of Chromosomes

Productive insights gleaned from the results of the completed Human Genome Project have dramatically changed some of our understanding of how the human genome functions. However, it is important to introduce to the reader our current understanding of the subject matter. Human hereditary factors are located in *genes* (the *genome*). Approximately 10% are genes that encode proteins that are assembled to form tissue structures or to form enzymes that catalyze chemical reactions within cells. The other 90% have functions that are currently not clear (see also The Nature of Genes and Single-gene Disorders, later). The genes are composed of DNA and are stored in intranuclear cell organelles called *chromosomes*. Each chromosome contains one linear DNA molecule folded over onto itself several times, as well as ribonucleic acid (RNA) and proteins. Because all genes exist in pairs, all chromosomes must likewise exist in pairs. The members of each pair of genes are called *alleles,* and the members of each pair of chromosomes are known as *homologues.* The conventional depiction of the constitution of homologues in the nucleus is called the cell's *karyotype* (Fig. 1-1). If at any gene locus the alleles are identical, that gene locus is *homozygous.* If the alleles are not identical, the gene locus is *heterozygous.*

Except for gametes, normal human cells contain 23 pairs of chromosomes, 46 in all. One of these pairs is concerned in part with inducing the primary sex of the embryonic gonads. These sex chromosomes are called the *X and Y chromosomes*, and they are not genetically homologous except in a few areas. Women have two X chromosomes, whereas men have an X and a Y chromosome. The remaining 22 pairs are called *autosomes* and they determine non–sex-related (somatic) characteristics.

During most of a cell's life cycle, chromosomes are diffusely spread throughout the nucleus and cannot be identified by morphologic means. Only when the cell divides does chromosome morphology become apparent (Fig. 1-2). The in vitro life cycle and the cellular division, or *mitosis*, of a somatic cell are illustrated in Figures 1-3 and 1-4, respectively. The life cycle and divisions, or *meiosis*, of a germ cell are much more complex and are not suitable for ordinary clinical evaluation.

Any somatic cell that can divide in tissue culture can be used for chromosomal (cytogenetic) analyses. The most convenient tissue source is peripheral blood, from which lymphocytes can be stimulated to divide during 2 or 3 days of incubation in tissue culture medium. Fibroblasts obtained from skin remain a frequently used alternative when peripheral

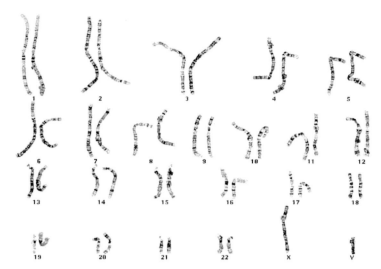

Figure 1-1   Photomicrographs show that this is a G-banded male karyotype. (A female would have two X chromosomes and no Y chromosome.) The horizontal banding produced by the Giemsa staining technique allows for precise identification of homologous chromosomes. *(Courtesy Urvashi Surti, PhD, Pittsburgh Cytogenetics Laboratory.)*

blood lymphocytes are not clinically suitable, but fibroblasts require an incubation period of 4 to 6 weeks. After death, lung tissue is the best tissue to culture for chromosomal analyses, although the process also requires a 4- to 6-week incubation period. Alternatively, skin fibroblasts are frequently obtained postmortem for various enzymatic and cytogenetic analyses, which may be used to confirm a clinical diagnosis. When a treatment decision requires urgency, preliminary

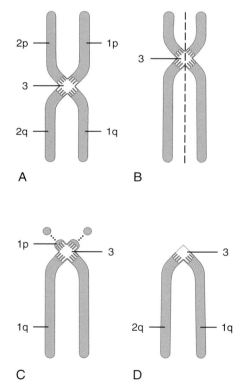

Figure 1-2   Morphology of a chromosome during metaphase. **A,** Metacentric chromosome with centromere (3) in the middle. **B,** Submetacentric chromosome with centromere off-center. **C,** Acrocentric chromosome with centromere near one end. **D,** Telocentric chromosome (not found in humans) with centromere at one end. The DNA of the chromosome has replicated to form two chromatids: *1p* and *1q* represent one complete chromatid, *2p* and *2q* the other complete chromatid (*p* refers to the short arm and *q* refers to the long arm). The chromosome will then divide longitudinally, as shown in **(B).**

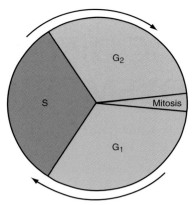

Figure 1-3   The in vitro life cycle of a somatic cell. Interphase lasts 21 hours and can be divided into the following three stages: G_1 (7 hours)—cell performs its tasks; S (7 hours)—DNA replicates; G_2 (7 hours)—cell prepares to divide. Then mitosis occurs.

chromosomal evaluation can be made within 4 to 24 hours by using uncultured bone marrow aspirate. Oftentimes the karyotype is supplemented within 48 to 72 hours by a molecular cytogenetics technique, either interphase or metaphase fluorescence in situ hybridization (FISH), using rapid culturing and diagnostic techniques. More recently, conventional cytogenetics is being substituted by high-resolution molecular karyotyping using microarray-based comparative genomic hybridization (array-CGH). Array-CGH enables copy number changes at high resolution. This is implemented in the clinical setting and is being recommended as the first step in the investigation of patients with developmental delays, mental retardation, and multiple congenital anomalies. FISH and other molecular techniques are now used primarily to confirm the imbalances detected by array-CGH. This is an ever-evolving area, and pediatric clinicians are advised to discuss clinical and laboratory investigations with clinical geneticists and/or laboratory directors before the initiation of tissue sampling to ensure the most productive use of samples and rapid testing methods.

Aneuploidy

Aneuploidy refers to an abnormality in chromosome number, in humans a chromosome number different from an even multiple of 23 (the haploid number) (Fig. 1-5). In aneuploidy

Figure 1-4   Mitosis lasts about 1 hour, during which time the cell divides. **A,** Interphase cell at the end of G_2. **B,** Prophase: replicated DNA condenses and is visible. **C,** Metaphase: 46 duplicated chromosomes align randomly on the spindle and can be photographed for karyotyping. **D,** Anaphase: chromosomes divide longitudinally, and half of each one moves to the opposite pole of the cell. **E,** Telophase: cell wall divides. **F** and **G,** Interphase at G_1: two daughter cells, each with 46 chromosomes.

Figure 1-5 Karyotype of a patient with trisomy 13 demonstrates aneuploidy. Note the extra chromosome 13, causing the cell to have 47 instead of 46 chromosomes. *(Courtesy Urvashi Surti, PhD, Pittsburgh Cytogenetics Laboratory.)*

there are typically 45 or 47 chromosomes instead of the usual 46. Rarely, multiples of the X or Y chromosome result in individuals with 48 or 49 chromosomes. *Double aneuploidy,* the simultaneous occurrence of two nondisjunctional events, has been described in the literature. In the liveborn, it usually involves one autosome and one sex chromosome. Double autosomal trisomy has been found repeatedly in spontaneous abortion but has not been demonstrated in a liveborn infant.

If aneuploidy occurs in a gamete as a result of an error of chromosomal division (nondisjunction or anaphase lag) during meiosis, all cells are affected in the fertilized embryo. With subsequent pregnancies, the risk for another chromosomal abnormality in the offspring is increased approximately 1% to 2% overall, in addition to the general background risk of abnormalities. The couple would be at risk for aneuploidy states of many types, not just the particular aneuploidy in their affected child. We are not yet aware of the underlying mechanism for the increased risk; however, families may benefit from an understanding of the possibilities for prenatal diagnosis in their individual case and may want to be referred for

genetic counseling before the conception of another child (Fig. 1-6, *A-C*).

Mosaic Aneuploidy States. *Mosaicism,* the presence of two or more genetically different cell lines within an individual, can result from an error in division during either meiosis or mitosis. In one possible scenario aneuploidy originates during meiotic division (i.e., before conception). In such cases the fetus starts out with an aneuploid chromosomal number and, subsequently, a division error occurs, resulting in the formation of another cell line that is chromosomally normal. In other cases of mosaicism the one-celled embryo (zygote) is chromosomally normal and a division error occurs after fertilization, during mitosis of an embryonic somatic cell, resulting in aneuploidy. Most individuals with mosaicism have only two or three different lines of embryonic cells. It requires considerable laboratory investigation to distinguish the meiotic or mitotic types. Generally speaking, parents are given a 1% to 2% recurrence risk because of the possibility of mosaicism present in a parental gonad, which is not identifiable in usual tissue sample analyses (Fig. 1-7).

Hypomelanosis of Ito is characterized by marbleized or mottled areas of hypopigmented whorls of skin along the Blaschko lines and is of heterogeneous etiology. Individuals with hypomelanosis of Ito can have multiple congenital anomalies, dysmorphic features, variable mental retardation, and other neurologic findings. Karyotyping from skin lesions will reveal mosaic abnormality of chromosomes from normal or hypopigmented and hyperpigmented regions. Balanced and unbalanced chromosome aberrations and uniparental disomy may be encountered (Fig. 1-8).

Abnormalities of Chromosome Structure

Chromosomes can be normal in number (diploid) but still be abnormal in structure. Inversions (Fig. 1-9), deletions (Fig. 1-10), and translocations (Fig. 1-11) of genetic material are examples of structural chromosomal abnormalities. These can arise as new (sporadic) mutations in the egg or sperm from which the embryo was formed, in which case the parents' recurrence risk for another child with a chromosomal abnormality is again 1% to 2%. However, the abnormality may also be inherited from a phenotypically normal parent who is a "carrier" of a structural chromosomal abnormality (Fig. 1-12). About 1

Figure 1-6 A female, 3 years and 8 months old, with double aneuploidy: aneuploidy depicted by cytogenetic studies. Karyotype and FISH studies show predominantly 47XXX; some 47XXX also have an extra 21 (48XXX+21). The patient has some features of Down syndrome. Note the up-slanted palpebral fissures **(A),** low-set ears **(B),** and unilateral simian crease **(C).** An echocardiogram showed a patent foramen ovale. The patient is receiving behavioral and speech therapy; she is not toilet trained and has an individualized education program (IEP) in preschool. Triple X females are tall and mosaic Down syndrome is similar to full Down syndrome but with a much milder phenotype. Her weight was in the 95th percentile, her height in the 80th, and occipital–frontal circumference (OFC) in the 20th.

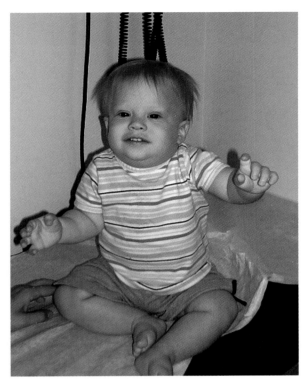

Figure 1-7 A 1-year-old with facies suggestive of Down syndrome. Note the facies and short fifth fingers and clinodactyly. The muscle tone and growth parameters were normal. Cytogenetics studies showed 2% of the cells with 47,XY+21; interphase fluorescence in situ hybridization (FISH) studies with an extra cell count showed trisomy 21 in 1.3% of 523 peripheral lymphocytes analyzed.

Figure 1-8 Hypomelanosis of Ito. Karyotype at birth was normal: 46,XX. At 4 months of age characteristic streaks and whorls of hyper- and hypopigmentation of the skin were noted. A higher cell-count karyotype showed mosaicism for trisomy 14.

Figure 1-10 Deletion *(arrow)* of the p arm of chromosome 5 (cri du chat syndrome). *(Courtesy Urvashi Surti, PhD, Pittsburgh Cytogenetics Laboratory.)*

Figure 1-11 Unbalanced translocation. The additional DNA was translocated onto the q arm of chromosome 5. The abnormality was inherited from a normal carrier father (see Figure 1-12) with a balanced reciprocal translocation between the q arms of chromosome 3 and chromosome 5. The patient died of multiple birth defects and in essence had a partial trisomy of the distal portion of the q arm of chromosome 3.

Figure 1-9 Pericentric inversion *(arrow)* of chromosome 13.

Figure 1-12 A "balanced" reciprocal translocation from chromosomes 3 to 5 in a normal man (the father of the chromosomally defective newborn whose karyotype is shown in Figure 1-11).

in 520 normal individuals carries a balanced but structurally abnormal set of chromosomes, called a *chromosome transloca-tion*. The term *balanced*, for the purposes of this chapter, means that on cytogenetic analysis the structural abnormality does not appear to have resulted in any net loss or gain of genetic material. If the apparently balanced chromosomal abnormality has been transmitted by other members of the family who are apparently phenotypically normal, it is considered a familial balanced translocation. Data suggest that a small percentage of individuals with apparently "balanced" translocations are actually mildly affected clinically by variable degrees of cognitive and physical deficits (Warburton, 1991). Thus high-resolution chromosome analyses and molecular cytogenetics techniques, such as array-CGH, are warranted in these instances including, as needed, in situ hybridization techniques using DNA probes to completely characterize the location of the chromosome breakpoints and to determine on a molecular level whether any genetic material is missing. Molecular studies for imprinting effects may also be warranted.

A frequent way in which families with apparently balanced chromosome translocations present for evaluation occurs when a child is born with structural malformations and on karyotyping is found to have an unbalanced chromosome translocation. This may have occurred de novo in the child's chromosomes only or may be due to a previously undiagnosed familial balanced chromosomal translocation in a parent. Parental karyotypes are used to distinguish the etiology and are crucial in providing accurate genetic counseling regarding future pregnancies for that couple.

Incidence of Chromosomal Abnormalities

Data from Hook (1992) suggest that upward of 50% of human conceptions terminate in a spontaneous abortion. Most of these miscarriages occur so early during gestation that the pregnancy is never recognized. The earlier the abortion occurs, the more likely it is that the miscarried embryo had a chromosomal abnormality. Of recognized first-trimester abortuses, 50% are chromosomally abnormal, compared with 5% of later embryos. Among the chromosomally abnormal abortuses, the most frequent abnormalities are triploidy (69 chromosomes), trisomy 16, and 45,X (Turner syndrome) (Table 1-1). Generally speaking, triploidy and trisomy 16 are not compatible with life and are only occasionally seen among liveborn infants. Despite

the fact that Turner syndrome is relatively common among liveborn infants, the majority of conceptuses with 45,X also abort spontaneously. The incidence of chromosomal abnormalities among liveborn infants in general is about 6 in 1000. Among a group including both stillborn infants and infants who die in the immediate perinatal period, the number is increased to approximately 50 in 1000.

When to Suspect a Chromosomal Abnormality

Chromosomal abnormalities of either number or structure are likely to have a detrimental effect on the phenotype of an affected individual. Aneuploidy of an autosome, or nonsex chromosome, generally significantly impairs physical and cognitive development. However, aneuploidy of a sex chromosome may have little or no apparent effect on the phenotype. One should look for clustering of abnormalities in family members to suggest a problem, although their absence does not rule out a chromosomal abnormality.

Carriers of an inherited or a de novo reciprocal translocation are usually genetically balanced and are subsequently normal. However, their conceptuses are likely to be genetically unbalanced and may abort spontaneously or be born with major congenital anomalies. A history of unexplained infertility, multiple spontaneous abortions (three or more), and particularly of a previous birth to the couple or to a close relative of a child with dysmorphic findings and/or major anomalies may be an indication that one of the parents carries a balanced chromosomal translocation or rearrangement. A chromosome study on the couple is thus indicated, and if translocation is found, they should seek antenatal genetic counseling. This may also be advisable for extended family members.

A normal person who carries a balanced reciprocal translocation can commonly produce six chromosomal types of gamete. On fertilization, these gamete types can result in several possible fertilized embryos: a normal conceptus, a carrier conceptus like the normal carrier parent, two types of immediately lethal conceptus resulting from gross chromosomal imbalances (i.e., too much or too little DNA), or two types of abnormal conceptus caused by lesser chromosomal imbalances. Whether the latter two types abort spontaneously or come to term as liveborns cannot be predicted in advance solely on theoretical grounds. Therefore genetic counseling in such situations depends somewhat on analysis of what has occurred within the individual family and in other families with similar rearrangements. Rarely, other types of chromosomal imbalances are found in conceptuses of such carrier parents.

Experience suggests the following: If a carrier has already produced a chromosomally unbalanced liveborn child, then it is apparent that it is possible for this to occur again in future pregnancies, and the risk that the translocation carrier might have another chromosomally unbalanced liveborn infant can be as high as 20%. However, if the translocation carrier parent has produced either only healthy liveborn infants or spontaneous miscarriages, then it is less likely that the chromosomally unbalanced gametes are viable. Consequently, that person's risk for producing a chromosomally unbalanced liveborn is only about 4%. Last, if a couple of whom one spouse is a carrier has not yet experienced any pregnancies, their risk for a chromosomally abnormal liveborn is estimated to be about 10%.

NEW TECHNOLOGIES

Fluorescence in Situ Hybridization

FISH is a laboratory technology that has revolutionized the diagnostic capabilities of clinical cytogenetic laboratories. In this technique a DNA probe is tagged with a label

Table 1-1	Occurrence of Chromosomal Abnormalities
Among Spontaneous Abortuses	**Incidence (%)**
Overall incidence	32.0
First trimester	52.0
After first trimester	5.8
Type of abnormality seen in spontaneous abortions	
Trisomy 16	
Other trisomies	
Triploidy	
45,X	
Miscellaneous	
Among Liveborns	**No. of Cases per 1000**
Overall incidence	6.20
Abnormality of autosomes	4.19 (males and females)
Trisomies	
Balanced rearrangements	
Unbalanced rearrangements	
Abnormality of sex chromosomes	2.03 (males and females)
In males: XXY, XYY, mosaics	
In females: 45,X (0.08), XXX, mosaics (1.43)	

About one quarter of all conceptuses are chromosomally abnormal. About 50 in 1000 stillborns have a chromosomal abnormality.

that fluoresces when viewed under a special microscope. A cocktail of many repetitive DNA probes blanketing a specific chromosome from end to end can be obtained. This is called a FISH "paint." Using special microscope filters, a clinician can simultaneously FISH paint a slide with probes fluorescing in two or three different colors. FISH paints specific for all chromosomes are available.

Some of the well-recognized syndromes described initially by FISH probes for chromosome microdeletion syndromes include the following:

- Angelman syndrome: del 15q11-13
- Prader-Willi syndrome: del 15q11-13
- Cri du chat syndrome: del 5p15.2
- DiGeorge sequence/velocardiofacial syndrome: del 22q11.2
- Miller-Dieker/lissencephaly syndromes: del 17p13.3
- Williams syndrome: del 7q11.23
- Smith-Magenis syndrome: del 17p11.2
- Wolf-Hirschhorn syndrome: del 4p16.3
- Severe X-linked ichthyosis: del Xp22.3
- 1p36 deletion syndrome
- 1q21.1 deletion syndrome
- 16p13.11 deletion
- Phelan-McDermid syndrome: del 22q13.3

See Figures 1-13 and 1-14 for details on Prader-Willi/Angelman syndrome and Wolf-Hirschhorn syndrome.

Array-based Technology: Microarray for Evaluation of Copy Number Variation

In addition to classic cytogenetics, molecular cytogenetic methods are being incorporated in clinical settings at an increased rate. More recently, conventional cytogenetics is being substituted with high-resolution molecular karyotyping using microarray-based comparative genomic hybridization (array-CGH). Array-CGH analyses are proficient in detecting imbalances in the genome and enable detection of copy-number changes at high resolution. This technique has been implemented by the American College of Medical Genetics (ACMG) as the first step in the investigation of patients with developmental delays, mental retardation, multiple congenital

abnormalities, and autism spectrum disorders and has the highest diagnostic yield, up to approximately 15% to 28%. This is much higher than the diagnostic yield of G-banded karyotypes (on the order of 3%), excluding Down syndrome and other recognizable chromosomal syndrome (Miller et al, 2010). In addition, molecular cytogenetic techniques, such as array-CGH, have demonstrated that approximately 20% of apparently balanced chromosome translocations, de novo or familial, have gain or loss of genetic material at the breakpoints. Therefore, molecular cytogenetic studies are warranted because they completely characterize the location of the chromosome breakpoints and potentially identify additional genetic material that may be duplicated or deleted that would not otherwise be detected by the traditional cytogenetic methods. FISH and other molecular techniques are now used primarily to confirm the imbalances detected by array-CGH. With microarray testing, many new microdeletion and microduplication syndromes have emerged (e.g., deletion 1p36, deletion 1q21.1, and deletion 16p13.11 syndromes) (Fig. 1-15; and see e-Figs. 1-1 through 1-3).

Single-nucleotide polymorphism (SNP) arrays are being used in clinical settings and allow genome-wide copy-number analysis. The copy-number changes may provide insight into abnormalities such as segmental and uniparental disomy by revealing "copy number-neutral" areas of continuous homozygosity that can give rise to disease, congenital anomalies, and/or cognitive impairment. SNP arrays may be helpful in identifying translocated segments in uniparental disomy and in looking for imprinting effects of the chromosomal regions.

Molecular karyotyping and single nucleotide polymorphism (SNP) arrays are ultimately more cost-effective tests and have been extremely useful to clinicians in identifying necessary medical surveillance and treatment options, and they provide information on recurrence risks and prenatal options for families.

The impact of these newer methodologies continues to emerge, but their usefulness in providing information key to clinical prognosis is clearly becoming evident.

Array-CGH has been increasingly used for genetic testing of individuals with idiopathic mental retardation, developmental delay, autism spectrum disorders, and multiple

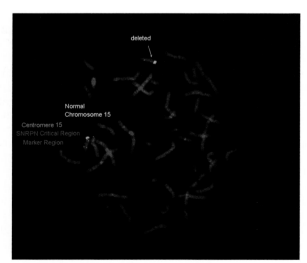

Figure 1-13 4',6'-Diamidino-2-phenylindole (DAPI)–counterstained metaphase and interphase images showing a duplication of the Prader-Willi/Angelman (D15S10 locus) critical region *(red)*. The chromosome 15 centromere is used as a control *(green)*. Adjacent to the centromere in red is the normal pattern for D15S10. SNRPN, small nuclear ribonucleoprotein-associated polypeptide N. *(Courtesy Urvashi Surti, PhD, Pittsburgh Cytogenetics Laboratory.)*

Figure 1-14 Metaphase chromosomes showing a deletion of the Wolf-Hirschhorn syndrome (WHS) critical region *(red)*. A chromosome 4 centromere *(4CEP)* probe is used as a control, shown here in *green*. Absence of the red probe signal on one chromosome 4 *(arrow)* indicates a deletion of the WHS region at 4p16.3. *(Courtesy Urvashi Surti, PhD, Pittsburgh Cytogenetics Laboratory.)*

Table 1-2	Some Syndromes Identifiable with Fluorescence in Situ Hybridization Probes	
Syndrome	**Major Findings**	**Comments**
Cri du chat (deletion 5p15.2)	Microcephaly, round face, down-slanting palpebral fissures, epicanthal folds, hypertelorism, catlike cry in infancy	
Isolated lissencephaly	Lissencephaly (incomplete development of brain with smooth surface)	Approximately 30% have deletion 17p13.3
Miller-Dieker phenotype with lissencephaly	Microcephaly, lissencephaly, variable high forehead, vertical furrowing of central forehead, low-set ears, small nose with anteverted nostrils, congenital heart disease, poor feeding	Deletion 17p13.3 in vast majority
Deletion 22q11.2	Phenotypes: • Velocardiofacial syndrome • DiGeorge sequence • Some cases of Opitz syndrome • Conotruncal type of congenital heart disease (in an infant with dysmorphic features)	Appears to be a common deletion and should be considered in the differential diagnosis of children with multiple anomalies even if the features are not classic to any one phenotype
Wolf-Hirschhorn (deletion 4p16.3)	Moderate to severe cognitive impairment, hypertelorism, preauricular pit or tag, broad nasal bridge, micrognathia, cleft palate, short philtrum, growth deficiency	
Smith-Magenis (deletion 17p11.2)	Brachycephaly, flat facies, broad nasal bridge, short stature	Self-hugging behaviors, sleep disturbances

congenital anomalies. By combining the array-CGH technique with classic cytogenetic and confirmatory FISH and appropriate molecular analyses, we are also able not only to identify cryptic genomic alterations but also to further analyze gross genomic alterations including marker chromosome or other rearrangements identified by the classic cytogenetic analysis.

In cases of disorders with several etiologic mechanisms such as Angelman syndrome, the absence of a deletion does not mean the child does not have the condition. An alternative mechanism, such as an imprinting center defect or uniparental disomy, may be the cause and would require methylation studies for detection.

Figure 1-15 An 8-year-old with del22q.11 and 1p31.1 microdeletion. Patient is short in stature; has a right aortic arch, sacral dimple, left cryptorchidism, and global developmental and significant cognitive and speech delays; and is not toilet trained. He had undergone surgical repair of the palate for velopharyngeal incompetence. Note the low-set, cupped, and posteriorly rotated ears and hypoplastic alae nasi. DiGeorge syndrome was diagnosed in utero by prenatal fluorescence in situ hybridization (FISH) on amniocytes: 46, XY, ish del(22) (q11.2q11.2) (TUPLE1–) was confirmed at 6 years of age by oligonucleotide arrays. In addition, 1p31.1 microdeletion was detected and maternally inherited.

DiGeorge sequence is discussed in Chapter 4, Williams syndrome is discussed in Chapter 5, and Angelman and Prader-Willi syndromes are covered later in this chapter. The remaining syndromes are outlined briefly in Table 1-2 and in Figure 1-16, *A-D*; Figure 1-17; and Figure 1-18.

APPROACH TO THE EVALUATION OF A DYSMORPHIC CHILD

Approximately 2% to 3% of liveborn infants have an observable structural abnormality. This number rises to about 4% to 5% by the time the child is old enough to attend school. Structural differences can be determined to be either major or minor in character (Table 1-3, and Figs. 1-19 and 1-20). Major structural anomalies have functional significance. Examples are polydactyly, colobomas of the iris (see Chapter 19, Fig. 19-69), meningomyelocele, and cleft lip. Minor anomalies are usually of cosmetic importance only. Examples are epicanthal folds of the eyes, single transverse palmar creases, and supernumerary nipples. The incidence of isolated major anomalies in the general newborn population is approximately 1%, and the incidence of minor anomalies is approximately 14%. Both are more common in premature newborns.

The probability of an infant having a major anomaly increases with the number of minor anomalies found. Thus all children with multiple minor anomalies warrant a careful clinical assessment in order to find potentially significant occult major anomalies. Once an anomaly is identified, assessing its significance begins with a determination of whether the anomaly in question is a single localized error in morphogenesis or one component of a multiple malformation syndrome. An understanding of the pathophysiologic mechanisms

Table 1-3	Examples of Congenital Anomalies	
Category	**Major**	**Minor**
Craniofacial	Choanal atresia	Plagiocephaly Flat occiput
Eyes	Coloboma of iris	Epicanthal folds
Ears	Microtia	Preauricular pit
Hands	Polydactyly Absent thumbs	Single transverse palmar crease Clinodactyly

Figure 1-16   A-D, Williams syndrome in four different patients: hallmark features include supravalvular aortic stenosis, hypercalcemia, friendly personality, connective tissue abnormalities, and characteristic facies. Note the periorbital fullness, epicanthal folds, prominent lips, long philtrum, and stellate lacy iris pattern. All cases with clinical features were confirmed on fluorescence in situ hybridization (FISH) alone or microarrays.

Figure 1-17   Metaphase image showing a deletion of the Williams critical region *(red)*. Chromosome 7q31 probe *(green)* is used as a control. Absence of the red probe signal on one chromosome 7 *(arrow)* indicates a deletion of the elastin (ELN) locus at 7q11.23. *(Courtesy Urvashi Surti, PhD, Pittsburgh Cytogenetics Laboratory.)*

Figure 1-18   X-linked steroid sulfatase deficiency. A 14-year-old patient presented with joint laxity, struggles in school, and microcephaly. The karyotype was normal. Note the ichthyosis; the patient's brother was not evaluated but was reported to have ichthyosis, attention-deficit/hyperactivity disorder (ADHD), and seizures. Deletion of the steroid sulfatase (STS) gene from the Xp22.31 region was confirmed by oligonucleotide arrays.

Figure 1-19 Clinical photographs show several minor anomalies seen at birth. **A,** Preauricular skin tag. **B,** Clinodactyly of the fifth finger. **C,** Macroglossia. **D,** Microretrognathia. *(Courtesy Christine L. Williams, MD.)*

Figure 1-20 Clinical photographs show several major anomalies seen at birth. **A,** Encephalocele. **B,** Cleft lip and palate. **C,** Meningomyelocele. **D,** Ectrodactyly (previously termed lobster-claw deformity). **E,** Polydactyly (postaxial). **F,** Bilateral clubfoot. **G,** Hypospadias. **H,** Fused labia with enlarged clitoris. **I,** Imperforate anus. *(Courtesy Christine L. Williams, MD.)*

that produce structural abnormalities or differences provides an opportunity to define the types of structural abnormalities seen. This also assists the process of identifying the etiology and arriving at a specific diagnosis, which then can be useful in determining the prognosis and estimating the risk of recurrence of a similar problem in future pregnancies.

Definitions of the classifications of structural anomalies aid in communication between clinicians and in the process of evaluation and are summarized from Jones (2006):

Malformation: A malformation is an abnormality of embryonic morphogenesis of tissue. It usually results from genetic, chromosomal, or teratogenic influences, but it can be of multifactorial etiology. Malformations are divided into two main categories: those that constitute a single primary defect in development and those that represent a single component of a multiple malformation syndrome. A *multiple malformation syndrome* can be defined as one having several observed structural defects in development involving multiple organ systems that share the same known or presumed etiology. Malformations often require surgical intervention.

Deformation: A deformation represents an alteration (often molding) of an intrinsically normal tissue caused by exposure to unusual extrinsic forces. A classic example is clubfoot, which may be the result of uterine constraint from crowding associated with a multiple gestation. A more severe example is the compressed facial features ("Potter facies") of a child exposed to severe uterine constraint associated with oligohydramnios, due to renal agenesis (see Chapter 13, Fig. 13-38). The vast majority of deformations respond to medical therapy alone and have a relatively good prognosis in contrast to malformations, which frequently require surgical intervention.

Disruption: A disruption represents a breakdown of normally formed tissue; the breakdown may be the result of vascular accidents or exposure to adverse mechanical forces that are usually more severe than those that produce deformation. A classic example is the combination of clefting, constriction bands, and limb reduction defects associated with the presence of amniotic bands (see Chapter 2, Fig. 2-46). The earlier these vascular accidents or abnormal forces occur during embryogenesis, the more severe the resulting defects (Fig. 1-21).

Dysplasia: Dysplasia is characterized by abnormal organization of cells within tissue, which usually has a genetic basis. An example is achondroplasia, the most frequent form of skeletal dysplasia.

(*Note:* Each of the preceding categories can have a sequence [see below] associated with it.)

Figure 1-21   Amniotic band syndrome; note the constriction ring at the ankle and amputation of the toes, a sequela to the amniotic bands.

Sequence: The term *sequence* refers to a recognizable pattern of multiple anomalies that occurs when a single problem in morphogenesis cascades, resulting in secondary and tertiary errors in morphogenesis and a corresponding series of structural alterations. A classic example is the Robin malformation or Pierre Robin sequence, in which the single primary malformation is microretrognathia (see Chapter 23, Fig. 23-63). The resulting glossoptosis, or posterior placement of the tongue in the oropharynx, interferes with normal palatal closure if the lingual displacement occurs before 9 weeks' gestation. The resulting cleft palate is U-shaped, rather than having the V shape that is usually seen in classic cleft palate, a finding that aids in recognition.

Association: An association is a pattern of malformations that occurs together too frequently to be due to random chance alone, but for which no specific etiology is yet recognized.

The approach to the evaluation of a child with a dysmorphologic abnormality is similar to a careful diagnostic evaluation of most pediatric problems, starting with a complete history and careful physical examination. In obtaining these it is helpful to remember that there are six broad etiologic categories to be considered in the differential diagnosis: a known syndrome, an unknown syndrome, a chromosomal abnormality, a teratogen, a congenital infection, and a maternal disease and/or placental abnormalities.

The history should include the following:
- Course of the pregnancy, complications including possible infections or environmental exposures, medications/substance abuse
- Prior pregnancies, spontaneous abortions, stillborns, or infant/child deaths for this couple
- Labor/delivery/perinatal problems
- Past medical history
- Growth and development
- Meticulous family history with family tree going back three generations and including the following:
  - Familial traits and growth characteristics
  - Familial physical or developmental disorders
  - Spontaneous abortions, stillborns, infant/child deaths in extended family

The physical examination entails the following:
- Thorough general examination
- A search for major and/or minor anomalies
- Neurodevelopmental assessment

In addition, focused examination of immediate family members for physical characteristics and growth parameters and review of family photo albums may be helpful.

Determining how the child fits into the norms for growth and development for the general population, for the family's ethnic group(s), and for the extended family is important. One continuing challenge is to determine whether the norms for the family are truly in the normal range for the general population and ethnic background or, in fact, constitute variability of a genetic trait present in its severe expression in the child or family member seen for evaluation.

The identification of a recognizable pattern of both major and minor anomalies provides the clinical dysmorphologist with a diagnosis, or a short list of differential diagnostic possibilities. Thus the detection of major and minor anomalies is critical in the diagnostic process. Identification of specific and unusual malformations that are uncommon and occur in only a few syndromes can be especially helpful. For example, finding that a child has long palpebral fissure length and pronounced fingertip fat pad size in combination with the pattern of anomalies typical of the Kabuki syndrome makes it extremely likely that the diagnosis is the Kabuki syndrome. Training in dysmorphology emphasizes the recognition of key components in patterns of malformation, as well as the specific findings useful in distinguishing syndromes with similarities from one another. Texts that outline currently recognized patterns of malformations can be helpful in assisting the clinician in the identification of specific features that can rule a diagnosis in or out. Commercial computer-based programs exist for syndrome identification; however, these are often more effectively used by experts in the field because of the complexity of terminology and the need for exacting descriptions of the anomalies present in a given child.

A chromosome study should be performed on each child with a syndrome of congenital anomalies. Such a study may establish or confirm the diagnosis of a chromosomal disorder and its hereditary potential and may possibly help map the chromosomal location of genes for those syndromes known to be simple mendelian disorders.

Abnormalities of Autosomes

Down Syndrome

The worldwide incidence of Down syndrome among liveborns is approximately 1 in 660, with 45% of affected individuals born to women older than 35 years of age. The incidence of Down syndrome among conceptuses is far greater than among liveborns because the majority of Down syndrome fetuses spontaneously abort.

No single physical stigma of Down syndrome exists; rather, the clinical diagnosis rests on finding a recognizable constellation of clinical characteristics including a combination of major and minor anomalies (Fig. 1-22).

The most frequent features are up-slanting palpebral fissures and small external ears (by length). Several major anomalies are commonly associated with Down syndrome. Congenital heart disease is found in 45% of cases, particularly atrioventricularis communis and ventricular septal defects. Hence all newborns with Down syndrome should undergo cardiac evaluation with echocardiogram. About 5% have a gastrointestinal anomaly, most commonly duodenal atresia or Hirschsprung's disease. An increased incidence of thyroid disorders also exists, particularly of the autoimmune type. Thus regular testing of thyroid function is recommended. Acute and neonatal leukemias occur 15 to 20 times more frequently in people with Down syndrome than in the general population. In newborns, much of this is represented by transient leukemoid reactions, with complete remission being the most frequent outcome. Quantitative abnormalities are found in many enzyme systems. People with Down syndrome are shorter than family members and the general population and have premature graying of hair. As adults, most males are infertile, but females may reproduce

Figure 1-22 Down syndrome. These clinical photographs show several minor anomalies associated with this disorder. **A,** Characteristic facial features with up-slanting palpebral fissures, epicanthal folds, and flat nasal bridge. **B,** Brushfield spots. **C,** Bridged palmar crease, seen in some affected infants. Two transverse palmar creases are connected by a diagonal line. **D,** Wide space between first and second toes. **E,** Short fifth finger. **F,** Small ears and flat occiput.

and can have children who will also have Down syndrome approximately one third of the time.

Minor anomalies include brachycephaly; inner epicanthal folds; Brushfield spots; flat nasal bridge; a small mouth with protruding tongue that fissures with age; a short neck with redundant skin folds; single transverse palmar (simian) creases; clinodactyly of the fifth fingers, with single digital crease caused by hypoplasia of the middle phalanx; and wide spacing between the first and second toes. The number of such anomalies varies in any particular case.

With rare exceptions, individuals with Down syndrome are cognitively impaired. The degree of impairment varies, with intelligence quotients (IQs) ranging from 20 to 80. Most individuals function in the mild to moderate range of developmental delay. The advent of individualized programs of early intervention therapy, education, and sporting activities has resulted in much improved outcomes and individuals who are much more likely to function at the maximum of their developmental capabilities. Autopsy analyses of brains from individuals with Down syndrome have revealed the neuropathologic changes of Alzheimer's disease in 100% of those older than 40 years. Nevertheless, only about 25% of older individuals with Down syndrome exhibit clinical manifestations of Alzheimer's disease. The reason for the clinical–pathologic discordance is not known. However, there does tend to be a progressive loss of cognitive functioning after the fourth decade of life. Longevity, although less than that of the general population, has steadily increased over the years. Individuals with Down syndrome who do not have congenital heart disease may expect to live well into their 60s. The principal causes of death in children with Down syndrome are infection, congenital heart disease, and malignancy.

The etiology of Down syndrome is trisomy 21, the presence of an extra chromosome 21 either as a simple trisomy or as part of a chromosome 21 fused with another chromosome. These fused chromosomes are often robertsonian translocation chromosomes or isochromosomes. Cases of mosaicism, in which trisomy 21 cell lines coexist with cell lines with the standard 46 chromosomes, exist as well and may range in phenotype from normal to that typical of complete trisomy 21. An association between trisomy 21 and advanced maternal age is clear (Table 1-4).

About 5% of Down syndrome cases represent a centric fusion translocation between the long arm of a chromosome 21 and those of a 13, 14, 15, 21, or 22 acrocentric chromosome. Of these, about one third are inherited from a clinically normal, balanced carrier parent; in the remaining two thirds the translocation is new in the affected child. Chromosome studies should therefore be performed on the parents and appropriate family members of an individual with translocation Down syndrome. If a parent carries a 21/21 translocation, all liveborns will have Down syndrome; for the remaining 21/centric fusion translocations, the empiric recurrence risk for a Down syndrome liveborn is less than 2% if the father is the carrier and roughly 15% if the mother is the carrier. The parents of

children with trisomy 21 may benefit from genetic counseling to determine their individual risk of having another child with Down syndrome or with other chromosomal abnormalities in future pregnancies.

Trisomy 13

Trisomy 13 is a relatively rare (1 in 5000) genetic condition caused by the presence of additional chromosome material from all or a large part of chromosome 13. The vast majority of embryos with classic trisomy for a complete 13th chromosome abort spontaneously, but approximately 5% survive to be liveborn. They have a severe, recognizable pattern of malformation that allows clinicians to suspect this etiology immediately (Fig. 1-23). The hallmark features are defects of forebrain development related to those seen in holoprosencephaly, aplasia cutis congenita, polydactyly (most frequently of the postaxial type), and narrow hyperconvex nails. A broader listing of features is outlined in Table 1-5, which can be useful in comparing the features frequently seen in infants with trisomy 13 with those seen in trisomy 18. As with many syndromes, trisomy 13 and trisomy 18 share structural abnormalities; however, they usually are distinguishable on the basis of the pattern of anomalies present. Liveborn infants with trisomy 13 represent those who have the least severe structural abnormalities of major organs. Of these, about 5% survive the first 6 months of life. Thus discussions with parents about surgical interventions must take into account the small possibility of long-term survival and require sensitivity to the needs of the child and family.

Milder chromosome abnormalities involving extra material determined to originate from chromosome 13 must be identified and distinguished from classic trisomy 13 because the clinical phenotype and prognosis may be different and, in some cases, less severe. Children with mosaicism, that is, with a normal cell line and a trisomy 13 cell line, as well as those with trisomy of part of chromosome 13, can be identified by chromosome analysis. Careful laboratory investigation must be carried out to identify the exact chromosomal abnormality. The advent of FISH technology has dramatically increased the ability of laboratory specialists to characterize chromosome

Table 1-5	Physical Abnormalities and Frequencies of Occurrence in Trisomy 13 and Trisomy 18 Syndromes	
Abnormality	**Trisomy 13**	**Trisomy 18**
Severe developmental retardation	††††	††††
Approximately 90% die within first year	††††	††††
Cryptorchidism in males	††††	††††
Low-set, malformed ears	††††	††††
Multiple major congenital anomalies	††††	††††
Prominent occiput	†	††††
Cleft lip and/or palate	†††	†
Micrognathia	††	†††
Microphthalmos	†††	††
Coloboma of iris	†††	†
Short sternum	†	†††
Rocker-bottom feet	††	†††
Congenital heart disease	††	††††
Scalp defects	†††	†
Flexion deformities of fingers	††	††††
Polydactyly	†††	†
Hypoplasia of nails	††	†††
Hypertonia in infancy	†	†††
Apneic spells in infancy	†††	†
Midline brain defects	†††	†
Horseshoe kidneys	†	†††

Symbols: Relative frequency of occurrence ranges from †††† (usual) to † (rare).

Table 1-4	Maternal Age–Specific Risk for Trisomy 21 at Live Birth	
Maternal Age (yr)		**Prevalence at Live Birth**
25		1/1350
30		1/890
35		1/355
40		1/97
45		1/23

Figure 1-23 Several physical manifestations of trisomy 13. **A,** Facies showing midline defect. **B,** Clenched hand with overlapping fingers. **C,** Postaxial polydactyly. **D,** Equinovarus deformity. **E,** Typical punched-out scalp lesions of aplasia cutis congenita. (**A,** Courtesy T. Kelly, MD, University of Virginia Medical Center, Charlottesville; **B** to **E,** courtesy Kenneth Garver, MD, Pittsburgh, Pa.)

rearrangements, with the goal being to identify the exact breakpoints of the chromosomes involved in the rearrangements. Molecular studies then may be possible to determine any potential impact of the rearrangement on individual genes and their products. This information is extremely helpful to clinicians in determining prognosis and in providing more realistic information when discussing treatment options. Rarely, children who have the recognizable pattern of clinical features of trisomy 13 have normal chromosomes. If a geneticist/dysmorphologist is not already involved, a consultation is warranted to aid in diagnosis and prognosis counseling and to determine any recurrence risks for the parents in future pregnancies.

Trisomy 18

The chromosomal disorder trisomy 18 occurs in approximately 3 in 10,000 newborns, and females are more likely to be liveborn. Affected infants are small for gestational age and have a frail appearance, and the face tends to appear petite relative to the rest of the craniofacial contour (Fig. 1-24, *A*). They also have a recognizable pattern of malformation, but in these infants hallmark features—clenched hands with overlapping fingers (see Fig. 1-24, *B*), short sternum, and "low arch" fingerprint patterns—are minor anomalies. Major anomalies, especially congenital heart disease, are generally present as well and are the source of significant morbidity and mortality. Other common findings include a prominent occiput, low-set and structurally abnormal ears, micrognathia, and rocker-bottom feet (see Fig. 1-24, *C*). See Table 1-5 for a broader listing of clinical features that can be useful in distinguishing trisomy 18 from trisomy 13, which shares many of the same structural abnormalities.

Trisomy 18 was previously thought to be almost invariably fatal in the neonatal period; however, more recent data suggest that a small percentage of children can live longer, and that between 5% and 10% will be alive at their first birthday. Survivors are more frequently female and have less severe structural abnormalities of major organs than most affected infants. Even with optimal neonatal, pediatric, and surgical management and excellent home-based care, children with classic trisomy 18 often "fail to thrive" and have significant developmental and cognitive impairments. Discussions with parents about interventions must take into account the slim possibility of long-term survival and require sensitivity to the needs of the child and family. Great care must be taken in providing a balanced picture to the family when discussing treatment options.

Chromosome analysis allows clinicians to evaluate the etiology of the trisomy and can help determine prognosis. Results can demonstrate classic trisomy 18 due to a complete extra chromosome 18, mosaicism for trisomy 18, or a complex chromosome abnormality involving one or more chromosomes. Children with chromosomal rearrangements that result in partial rather than complete trisomy 18 may have a milder clinical outcome. Trisomy limited to the short arm of chromosome 18 is associated with a significantly milder prognosis, whereas trisomy of the entire long arm of chromosome 18 may be indistinguishable from an individual with classic trisomy 18. An infant with smaller areas of trisomy for the long arm of chromosome 18 may show some, but not all, of the features of classic trisomy 18. Thus chromosomal study of each child is essential.

If a complex chromosome rearrangement is identified in a child, further parental chromosome studies are indicated.

Figure 1-24   Several physical manifestations of trisomy 18. **A,** Typical profile reveals prominent occiput and low-set, posteriorly rotated malformed auricles. **B,** Clenched hand showing typical pattern of overlapping fingers. **C,** Rocker-bottom feet. *(Courtesy Kenneth Garver, MD, Pittsburgh, Pa.)*

Chromosome analysis of the parents will determine whether the rearrangement is new in the child (de novo) or is the result of a familial balanced translocation. Full characterization of the extent of a chromosome rearrangement also allows clinicians to provide more accurate information regarding prognosis, treatment options, and recurrence risk to the family. If a familial balanced translocation is present in one of the parents, other family members may benefit from genetic counseling to discuss recurrence risk and the availability of prenatal diagnosis for future pregnancies.

It has been our experience that parent support organizations can be extremely helpful to family members in the long process of adjustment to having a child with a chromosome problem. If the child dies, these groups can be helpful as a resource to the parents because of the similarity of their collective experience and can assist them in the grieving and healing process. They can also be a source of ongoing support and information to parents of a child with trisomy 13 or trisomy 18 who may live but who will face major medical and developmental challenges due to the chromosomal abnormality.

Abnormalities of Sex Chromosomes

Turner Syndrome

Turner syndrome is one of the three most common chromosomal abnormalities found in early spontaneous abortions. The phenotype is female. About 1 in 2000 liveborn females has Turner syndrome. Primary amenorrhea, sterility, sparse pubic and axillary hair, underdeveloped breasts, and short stature ($4\frac{1}{2}$ to 5 ft) are the usual manifestations. Other external physical features may include webbing of the neck; cubitus valgus; a low-set posterior hairline; a shield chest with widely spaced nipples; and malformed, often protruding, ears (Fig. 1-25, *A-E*). Internally, renal anomalies may be present along

with congenital heart disease, particularly bicuspid aortic valve (in 30% of cases) and coarctation of the aorta (in 10% of cases). Affected women have an infantile uterus, and their ovaries consist only of strands of fibrous connective tissue. Newborns often have lymphedema of the feet and/or hands (Fig. 1-25, *D* and *E*), which can reappear briefly during adolescence. Mental development is usually normal. Schooling and behavioral problems seem to be the same as in age-matched control subjects, although difficulty with spatial orientation such as map reading may be a problem. The classic physical findings of Turner syndrome may be absent, or the abnormalities may be so minimal in the newborn that the diagnosis is missed. The first indication may be unexplained short stature in later childhood or failure to develop secondary sex characteristics by late adolescence. Thus a chromosome study is indicated as part of the diagnostic workup of adolescent girls with these complaints.

The karyotype in the majority of individuals with Turner syndrome is 45,X. Most often, the missing sex chromosome is paternally derived, so the risk of Turner syndrome does not increase with maternal or paternal age. Another 15% of individuals with Turner syndrome are mosaics (XO/XX, XO/XX/XXX, or XO/XY). The physical stigmata may be less marked in mosaics, some of whom may be fertile. If an XY cell line is present, the intraabdominal gonads should be removed because they are prone to malignant change. The remaining cases of Turner syndrome have 46 chromosomes including one normal plus one structurally abnormal X. The latter may have a short (p) arm deletion or may be an isochromosome duplication of the long (q) arm of the X chromosome; usually it is paternally derived. Cases of Turner syndrome with one normal and one abnormal X chromosome are more likely to have other, more serious major anomalies including cognitive deficits. A structurally abnormal X chromosome may lead to abnormal X inactivation resulting in a deleterious dosage

Figure 1-25   Clinical photographs show several physical manifestations associated with Turner syndrome. **A,** In this newborn a webbed neck with low hairline, shield chest with widespread nipples, abnormal ears, and micrognathia are seen. **B,** The low-set posterior hairline can be better appreciated in this older child who also has protruding ears. **C,** In this frontal view mild webbing of the neck and small widely spaced nipples are evident, along with a midline scar from prior cardiac surgery. The ears are low set and prominent, protruding forward. **D** and **E,** The newborn shown in **(A)** also had prominent lymphedema of the hands and feet.

effect for X-linked genes. Karyotypes such as 46,XYp- or 46,Xi(Yq) result in a female with Turner syndrome.

Moreover, loss of the short arm of an X chromosome results in full-blown Turner syndrome; deletion of the long arm usually produces only streak (fibrous) gonads with consequent sterility, amenorrhea, and infantile secondary sex characteristics without the other somatic stigmata of Turner syndrome. If the diagnosis is clinically suspected, a chromosome study should be ordered. Should the affected child be 45,X or a mosaic, the parental risk for recurrence of a chromosomally abnormal liveborn is 1% to 2% but may be higher if a parent carries a structurally abnormal X chromosome.

Antenatal diagnosis of chromosomally abnormal fetuses should be discussed with the parents, and the relatively good prognosis for Turner syndrome liveborns should not be overlooked. Girls with Turner syndrome should receive appropriate hormone therapy during adolescence to enable development of secondary sex characteristics and stimulate menses. Rarely, 45,X women with Turner syndrome have been fertile for a limited number of years.

Klinefelter Syndrome

One in 500 newborn boys has Klinefelter syndrome. The physical stigmata are subtle and usually not obvious until puberty, at which time the normal onset of spermatogenesis is blocked by the presence of two X chromosomes. Consequently the germ cells die, the seminiferous tubules become hyalinized and scarred, and the testes become small. Testosterone levels are below normal adult male levels, although the level varies from case to case (the average being about half as much as normal). Hence there is a wide range in degree of virilization. At one extreme is the man with a small penis and gynecomastia (Fig. 1-26); at the opposite extreme is the virile mesomorph with a normal penis. Scoliosis may develop during adolescence. The average full-scale IQ of men with Klinefelter syndrome is 98, which is about the same as the general population. Behavioral problems may be more common than in the population at large, however.

The karyotype in Klinefelter syndrome is XXY in 80% of cases and mosaic (XY/XXY) in the other 20%. Rarely the latter type may be fertile. About 60% of cases reflect a chromosome error in oogenesis, and in 40% an error in spermatogenesis. The risk of having an affected child increases with maternal age. Males with more than two X chromosomes (XXXY, XXXXY) are usually cognitively impaired and are more likely to have skeletal and other major congenital anomalies such as cleft palate, congenital heart disease (particularly a patent ductus arteriosus), and microcephaly. The parents' recurrence risk for another chromosomally abnormal liveborn is 1% to 2%; antenatal diagnosis with subsequent pregnancies is possible.

Figure 1-26   Clinical photographs show several physical manifestations of Klinefelter syndrome. **A,** Relatively narrow shoulders, increased carrying angle of arms, female distribution of pubic hair, and normal penis but with small scrotum due to small testicular size. **B,** Small testes and penis. **C,** Gynecomastia. (**B,** *Courtesy Peter Lee, MD, Hershey Medical Center, Hershey, Pa;* **C,** *from Gardner LI, editor:* Endocrine and genetic diseases of childhood, *ed 2, Philadelphia, 1975, WB Saunders.)*

XXX and XYY

Triple X females have a karyotype result of 47,XXX. The incidence is approximately 1 in 1000 liveborn females. Affected individuals have no characteristic abnormal physical features. Although usually within the normal range of intelligence, their IQ scores may be lower than those of their normal siblings, delays in development of motor skills and coordination are common, and approximately 60% require some special education classes. Behavioral problems occur in approximately 30% and are usually mild. XXX women are fertile, and their children are usually chromosomally normal.

XYY males have a karyotype result of 47,XYY. The incidence is 1 in 840 liveborn males. They tend to be tall in comparison with their own family members, but generally their phenotypic appearance is normal. As for 47,XXX females, their IQ is usually within the normal range but may be lower than that of siblings. Affected boys often come to medical attention because of problems with fine motor coordination, speech disorders, and learning disabilities. Early reports raised concerns about significant behavioral problems; however, long-term prospective studies now suggest that these boys do not have any greater incidence of problem behaviors than the general population.

The risk of recurrence for a couple with a child with an XXX or XYY karyotype depends on many factors including the parents' own karyotype results and advancing maternal age. Therefore it is recommended that they be referred for individualized genetic counseling when considering future pregnancies.

MOLECULAR CYTOGENETIC SYNDROMES

Advances in molecular genetics have provided new insights into the genetic pathogenesis of several syndromes often associated with specific cytogenetic abnormalities.

Fragile X Syndrome

It has long been recognized that there is a significant excess of males in moderately to severely mentally retarded populations. Much of this inordinate male representation is the result of altered X-linked recessive genes. These may represent new mutations or inheritance of the abnormal gene from normal heterozygous (carrier) mothers. About 1 in 150 individuals, usually male, has some form of X-linked mental retardation. Of these it is estimated that between 30% and 50% have fragile X syndrome.

In 1969 Herbert Lubs noted in short-term lymphocyte cultures the in vitro cytogenetic marker now called *fragile X*. However, its clinical significance was not realized until a 1977 report by G. R. Sutherland in Australia. Under tissue culture conditions that starve the cell of its ability to synthesize thymidylic acid, a chromosome break at Xq27, the distal part of the long arm of the X chromosome (Fig. 1-27), is visible in cells of individuals clinically affected with fragile X syndrome. By pedigree analysis, about 1 in 4000 males has the fragile X gene.

Fragile X syndrome is the first recognized example of a *trinucleotide* repeat disorder. The gene involved, located at Xq27.3, is called *FMR1* and is active in brain cells and sperm. At the start of the gene is the DNA trinucleotide CGG, which in the general population is normally repeated about 5 to 50 times (the average being 30). The presence of from 55 to 200 CGG repeats is considered a fragile X *premutation*. Individuals with a premutation appear clinically normal. The finding of more than 200 linear CGG repeats is considered a *full mutation* and in males results in fragile X syndrome. In females with more than 200 linear CGG repeats, there are clinical effects in 50% and apparently little or no effect in 50%. The explanation for this disparity in females most likely is the phenomenon known as *X chromosome inactivation* (Fig. 1-28).

Figure 1-27 Fragile X chromosome marker in lymphocyte culture. Partial metaphase plate shows the chromosome break at Xq27 *(arrow)* characteristic of fragile X syndrome (solid Giemsa stain).

Table 1-6	Relative Risk of Maternal Transmission of a Fragile X Premutation to Her Offspring as a Full Mutation
Number of CGG Repeats in Mother's Premutation	**Risk of Expansion to Full Mutation in Offspring (%)**
55-59	3.7
60-69	5.3
70-79	31.1
80-89	57.8
90-99	80.1
100-109	100
110-119	98.1
120-129	97.2

From Saul RA, Tarleton JC: *FMR1*-related disorders. GeneReviews [Internet]. Seattle (WA): University of Washington, Seattle; 1993-1998 [updated June 16, 2011]. Available from www.genetests.org.

Premutations and, in females, random X inactivation explain the lack of penetrance of the fragile X gene.

No cases of new mutations for these *FMR1* gene CGG trinucleotide expansions or repeats have been found. That is, all such expansions are inherited from a parent. A man with a premutation passes it on to all of his daughters as a premutation. Men with a full mutation generally do not reproduce. Men with premutations, however, do not have affected sons, because they give their Y chromosome to all of their male offspring.

Women heterozygous for either a premutation or full mutation have a 50% chance of passing it on to each child as follows: If she has a full mutation, she passes it on as a full mutation in most instances; if she has a premutation, she passes it on to her child as either a premutation or expanded into a full mutation, depending on the size of her own premutation. As the number of repeats in the premutation increases, the greater the likelihood that her premutation will expand to a full mutation in her offspring. The relative risk is shown in Table 1-6.

Males affected with fragile X syndrome have cognitive impairment, ranging from severe to borderline in degree. The majority have an IQ between 20 and 49, and the remainder fall in the 50 to borderline IQ range. Furthermore, IQ may decline with age. The majority have speech delay, short attention span, hyperactivity, persistence of mouthing objects, and poor motor coordination. Many exhibit a variety of disordered behaviors including disciplinary problems, temper tantrums, poor eye contact, perseverative speech, hand flapping, avoidance of socialization, and rocking. Physical stigmata may include long, wide, or protruding ears; long face; a prominent jaw; flattened nasal bridge; "velvety" skin; hyperextensible joints; and mitral valve prolapse. Relative macrocephaly is more likely than microcephaly. Macroorchidism is found in most mature males.

Approximately 50% of females affected with full-mutation fragile X are clinically normal. The 50% who are affected

Figure 1-28 Functional behavior of the X chromosome in XX females. **A,** Somatic and premeiotic germ cells. Implantation occurs 5 days after conception, at which time in each female cell either X^M or X^P is randomly genetically inactivated and remains so in each of the cell's descendants. Because the process is random, by determining the proportion of cells with an inactive X^M or inactive X^P in each of a large population of women, a gaussian population distribution of women is generated. That is, most women in the population will have an approximate 50:50 mix of cells, in which each cell expresses either X^M or X^P. However, some women will by chance have more cells with an inactive X^M and vice versa. **B,** Meiotic germ cells. When a female germ cell enters first prophase of meiosis, X inactivation is abolished; both X chromosomes become genetically active through fertilization and continue so until embryonic uterine implantation. Then, as in **(A),** random X inactivation in XX females occurs all over again.

X-CHROMOSOME INACTIVATION

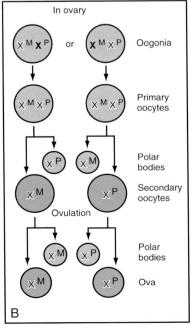

usually have lesser degrees of cognitive impairment than males; about 35% fall in the 20 to 49 IQ range and the remainder fall in the 50 to borderline range. However, learning disabilities, mood disorders, schizoid personality, and significant disturbances in affect, socialization, and communication are common. The physical features often seen in males with fragile X syndrome are less common in females.

Laboratory testing for fragile X mutations is done by molecular genetic techniques. The standard molecular genetic test is Southern blot analysis of DNA extracted from cells, usually in blood. Another molecular genetic technique, polymerase chain reaction (PCR) analysis of DNA, can be done with less blood. These techniques can also be applied to fetal cells for the purpose of antenatal diagnosis. However, if the fetus is a female with a full mutation, it is impossible to predict with certainty whether the child will be clinically affected with fragile X syndrome after birth because of the influence of X inactivation.

Rarely, an individual may seem to have a mild form of fragile X syndrome but tests are negative using these molecular genetic laboratory techniques. Another fragile X gene site (FRAXE) distal to the fragile X gene on Xq is associated with mild mental retardation and a positive fragile X cytogenetic laboratory test.

The number of known trinucleotide expansion disorders is increasing. Three other examples are Huntington disease, caused by a CAG trinucleotide expansion in its gene at the end of chromosome 4p; myotonic dystrophy, resulting from a CTG expansion in its gene on chromosome 19q; and spinobulbar muscular atrophy caused by a CAG expansion in its gene on the proximal part of chromosome Xq.

DISORDERS OF IMPRINTING (EPIGENETIC PHENOMENA): PRADER-WILLI AND ANGELMAN SYNDROMES

Etiologic Mechanisms

Prader-Willi and Angelman syndromes are disorders that derive from abnormalities of imprinted genes. The concept of *imprinting* refers to the fact that the function of certain genes is dependent on their parental origin: maternal versus paternal. This appears particularly true of the 15q11-q13 region of chromosome 15, a region that contains several imprinted genes that, when abnormal, result in recognizable constellations of physical and behavioral problems.

Mechanisms that can produce the Prader-Willi phenotype include the following:

1. A chromosome deletion of 15q11-q13 including the Prader-Willi critical region of the paternally derived chromosome 15 (majority of cases)

2. A structural chromosome abnormality involving the Prader-Willi critical region of 15q11-q13 (translocation, etc.)

3. Maternal uniparental disomy (UPD) in which the child has two maternally derived chromosome 15s and no paternally contributed chromosome 15 (25% of cases). *Note:* The association of UPD with older maternal age suggests that in these cases the fetus may originally have had trisomy 15 but that owing to a phenomenon known as *trisomic rescue,* one of the three chromosome 15s was lost, returning the fetus to the normal chromosome number. If the "lost" chromosome was paternally derived, then UPD-derived Prader-Willi results.

4. Mutations of imprinting control center genes (1% of cases)

The critical region of chromosome 15 for Angelman syndrome is located adjacent to the Prader-Willi critical region. However, when deletion of the Angelman critical region is causative, it is the maternally derived chromosome that is deleted. The six currently identified etiologic mechanisms of Angelman syndrome include the following:

1. A large chromosome deletion of 15q11-q13 including the Angelman critical region of the maternally derived chromosome 15 (68% of cases)

2. A structural chromosome abnormality involving the Angelman critical region of 15q11-q13 (translocation, etc.)

3. Paternal UPD of chromosome 15 (7% of cases)

4. Mutations of imprinting control center genes (3% of cases)

5. Mutations of the ubiquitin-protein ligase gene (*UBE3A*) (11% of cases)

6. Classic phenotype, with no identifiable etiologic mechanisms but a positive family history of other affected individuals (11% of cases)

Note: Mechanisms 4, 5, and 6 account for approximately 25% of cases of Angelman syndrome.

Because of etiologic variability and complexity of the diagnostic process, families of children suspected of having either of these disorders should be referred for genetic evaluation and diagnostic testing to ensure the most accurate determination of etiologic mechanism, and therefore, of recurrence risk.

Current diagnostic testing for these disorders includes the following:

1. Karyotype with high-resolution cytogenetic technology

2. Methylation studies, which determine whether genes within the 15q11-q13 critical region are functional

3. Appropriate oligoarrays that cover and encompass SNRPN (small nuclear ribonucleoprotein-associated polypeptide N) for Prader-Willi syndrome and D15S10 for Angelman syndrome

4. In some cases of Angelman syndrome, direct analysis of the *UBE3A* gene

Clinical Findings in Prader-Willi Syndrome

Newborns affected with Prader-Willi syndrome usually are markedly hypotonic and often have a history of decreased fetal movement in utero and breech fetal position. Although birth is usually at term, birth weights tend to be below 3000 g. In neonates, in addition to hypotonia, poor sucking and swallowing are common and predispose to choking episodes that can cause respiratory problems. Although the baby's cry may be weak and Moro and deep tendon reflexes are often decreased, the neurologic evaluation is otherwise unremarkable. Subsequently motor development is delayed, speech even more so, and most patients have cognitive impairment in the mild to moderate range. Hypotonia abates over the first 2 to 3 years, and patients develop an insatiable appetite that rapidly results in morbid obesity. The distribution of excess fat is particularly prominent over the lower trunk, buttocks, and proximal limb. Although the facies are not particularly dysmorphic, they are similar in most Prader-Willi patients. The bifrontal diameter is narrow, the eyes are often described as "almond shaped," and strabismus is not unusual. Hypopigmentation is common, the patient usually having blond to light brown hair, blue eyes, and sun-sensitive fair skin. Picking of skin sores can become a problem. Hands and feet are noticeably small from birth, and the stature of the older child and adult is short. The penis and testes are hypoplastic in males with Prader-Willi syndrome, although the penile size can be enlarged by testosterone therapy. If the testes are cryptorchid, surgical correction should be attempted. Menarche in females is delayed or absent, and menses, when present, are sparse and irregular. Gonadotropic hormone levels are reduced in both sexes. Infertility is the rule, but there are two known exceptions.

Of particular concern in older children with Prader-Willi syndrome are problems of emotional lability and extreme temper tantrums. These conditions and the overeating often can be partly ameliorated by intensive inpatient behavioral modification programs followed by longitudinal parental support and follow-up in the home. Interestingly, despite a normal basal metabolic rate, weight reduction requires significantly more severe caloric restriction in these patients than in normal persons. Diabetes mellitus can develop in the older child, and its incidence is correlated with the severity of obesity. Although it tends to be insulin resistant, the condition responds well to treatment with oral hypoglycemic agents. Life expectancy can be shortened by cardiorespiratory complications related to the extreme obesity (pickwickian syndrome).

Clinical Findings in Angelman Syndrome

Angelman syndrome, first recognized in 1956, has an incidence of 1 in 15,000 to 1 in 20,000 live births. Except for the tendency to have hypopigmentation, the clinical phenotypes of Prader-Willi and Angelman syndromes are quite different. The latter have severe cognitive deficits; speech is impaired or absent; and inappropriate paroxysms of laughter are common. Physical features include microbrachycephaly, maxillary hypoplasia, large mouth, prognathism, and short stature (in adults). The gait is ataxic, with toe-walking and jerky arm movements. Akinetic or major motor seizures are common. Although survival to adulthood is possible, to date only one patient with Angelman syndrome has been known to reproduce.

Note: Some other examples of imprinting disorders are Beckwith-Wiedemann syndrome (Fig. 1-29, *A-C*).and Russell-Silver syndrome.

THE NATURE OF GENES AND SINGLE-GENE DISORDERS

A gene consists of a sequence of DNA that contains the code for production of a "functional product" along with sequences that ensure "proper expression" of the gene. Its product may be an RNA molecule or a polypeptide chain or protein that ultimately becomes a structural component of a cell or tissue, or of an enzyme. The latter may catalyze a step in formation or modification of another product, a step in cell metabolism, or one of a number of steps involved in the breakdown or degradation of molecules that are no longer necessary. "Proper expression" includes production of the product at the right time, in the needed amount, in the correct cell type and ensures its transport to its proper site of biologic action.

Approximately 30,000 genes are arranged in linear fashion on the chromosomes, all having their own specific locus. Genes range in length from about 1000 to hundreds of thousands of bases in length (any of which can be subject to mutation). Coding sequences for a gene's product, termed *exons,* vary in length and are not continuous but occur in sections with noncoding sequences, termed *introns,* interspersed between them. Exons are further subdivided into triplets of bases, termed *codons,* each of which encodes a specific amino acid within the polypeptide product. Because there are 64 possible triplet combinations of the 4 nucleotide bases (adenine, guanidine, thymine, and cytosine) and 20 amino acids, most amino acids have more than one codon that can specify them, the exceptions being methionine and tryptophan, which have only one specific codon each. In addition, three triplets encode stop codons in the messenger RNA (mRNA) that signal the termination of mRNA translation.

The process of going from DNA code to polypeptide product has many steps and begins with *transcription,* during which the DNA of the gene serves as a template for the formation of an mRNA molecule. RNA synthetase, proteins called *transcription factors,* and regulatory elements all participate in this process, which is initiated and concluded by DNA sequences that signal where to start and stop transcription. After this, both ends of the mRNA molecule undergo modification. Thereafter, the introns are excised and the exons spliced together. Then the mRNA is transported to the rough endoplasmic reticulum within the cytoplasm, where it attaches to

Figure 1-29 **A,** Beckwith-Wiedemann syndrome. Note the macrosomia, macroglossia, and asymmetry with hemihypertrophy and omphalocele and/or umbilical hernia. Craniofacial features also include unusual ear creases. **B,** At 3 months of age; note the macroglossia, right facial prominence, and ear creases. **C,** At 27 months of age; note the resolving umbilical hernia. The elevated α-fetoprotein (AFP) levels from infancy have normalized. The patient has nephromegaly, and is under surveillance for the detection of embryonal tumors by serum AFP and abdominal and renal sonograms every 4 months. Chromosomes were normal male complement, 46,XY. The abnormal methylation pattern of the *LIT1* gene at the 11p15 region confirmed the clinical diagnosis of Beckwith-Wiedemann syndrome.

ribosomes, and the process of *translation* from mRNA template to polypeptide chain begins. During translation transfer RNA (tRNA) molecules, each of which is specifically designed to attach to a particular amino acid, find their target moieties and bring them into position at the correct time over a codon on the mRNA that specifies for their particular amino acid.

After assembly, the polypeptide chain is released from its template and then may be subject to *posttranslational modification*. Steps may include folding, bonding into a three-dimensional conformation, being combined with another or other polypeptide chains as part of a protein complex, being split into smaller segments, and addition of phosphate or carbohydrate moieties. Thereafter, it is transported to its site of action via directional terminal sequences, which are then cleaved from the finished product. Mutation of a gene encoding the polypeptide product or for any molecule used at any step along the entire process can adversely influence the end product.

A single-gene mutation produces a permanent change in a gene's DNA sequence and may involve anywhere from one to several thousands of nucleotides. Most appear to affect only one to a few to several base pairs via substitution of one base for another or by deletion or insertion of one or more bases.

Some mutations have no effect on phenotype or cell function. One example is a base substitution within a codon for an amino acid that changes it to another codon specifying the same amino acid. Still other mutations have no adverse effect but rather encode normal variations in human characteristics (e.g., eye or hair color). Other mutations do have adverse effects and are causative in disease. Examples of these include *missense* mutations, in which a base substitution changes a codon specific for one amino acid into one specifying another; *frameshift* mutations, in which a deletion or insertion is not an exact multiple of three bases, and thereby shifts the reading frame for transcription (and later translation) from that point on; and *nonsense* mutations, in which a base substitution changes a codon for an amino acid into one specifying one of the three possible stop codons in mRNA, thereby stopping translation prematurely.

A single-gene disorder is the result of a mutation altering the DNA sequence within a single gene on one (dominant) or both (recessive) of a pair of chromosomes. Correspondingly, this change may result in alteration of the amount of the gene's product, failure to produce the product at all, and/or compromise of its functional integrity. The greater the degree of functional loss, the more severe the clinical manifestations of the disorder and often the earlier their onset. Figures 1-30 through 1-33 are representative of single-gene disorders.

Mutation(s) of gene(s) within the nuclear genome are also recognized as mendelian disorders. The occurrence and/or recurrence are in fixed proportions (Mendel's laws). These disorders are compiled in a catalog, the Online Mendelian Inheritance in Man (OMIM; http://www.ncbi.nlm.nih.gov/omim), which is a great resource. Phenotype–genotype correlations are unfolded by detailed clinical evaluation, recognition at a clinical level, and confirmation by molecular diagnostics confirming the genotype.

Pedigree analyses are usually helpful. Autosomal, X-linked, recessive, and dominant patterns are recognized. Gene penetrance, disease expressivity, genetic (locus) heterogeneity, and allelic heterogeneity are some of the well-recognized complexities characterizing mendelian disorders.

The family of disorders known as *osteogenesis imperfecta* (OI; see also Chapter 21) provides a good example of the effects of mutations that alter the precursors of a structural protein, type I collagen. Collagen is a triple helix made up of two pro-α1 chains and one pro-α2 chain. The latter are composed of hundreds of amino acid triplet repeats, with glycine (the smallest amino acid) being the first member of each triplet and forming the apex of each bend in the helical structure. A base substitution in a codon specifying glycine at any one of the hundreds of such points along either the *COL1A1* gene (on band 17q21) or the *COL1A2* gene (on band 7q22.1) may result in the production of an unstable mRNA molecule that is degraded in the nucleus, or in the production of structurally abnormal pro-α1 or pro-α2 chains. The assembly of these may be slowed; they may be subject to excessive posttranslational modification, may be unstable and subject to degradation, or may have difficulty conforming and associating with other prochains to form the triple helix. The earlier the altered mRNA codon appears in the translation process, the more abnormal is the resulting prochain structure, and the greater is the degree of compromise of collagen strength and function within connective tissues. Also, because there are two pro-α1 chains for each pro-α2 chain, mutations in the *COL1A1* gene are more likely to be deleterious. These types of mutations, which result in the synthesis of structurally abnormal products, are the basis for clinical abnormalities found in types II to IV OI.

In type I OI, the causative mutations in the *COL1A1* gene (often nonsense or splicing mutations) usually result in the production of mRNA that is so abnormal it is degraded before it can leave the nucleus and be translated, or in the synthesis of a prochain that is unstable and degraded. Hence the mutant gene is unexpressed, that is, a *null mutation*. The end result of this is that the patient can make only 50% of the expected amount of type I collagen, although all of the product is structurally normal. Being the mildest form of OI, it demonstrates the fact that in many cases of mutations involving genes that encode structural polypeptides or proteins, it can be better to have no gene product than to have an abnormal one.

The phenomenon of excessive posttranslational modification of a structurally abnormal gene product is also seen in some types of Ehlers-Danlos syndrome (see Ehlers-Danlos Syndrome, later).

When the gene product is an enzyme or a component of an enzyme, this results in interruption of its step in a chain of reactions that may be involved in the formation or modification of a product, a step in cell metabolism, or in the degradation of molecules no longer needed by the cell. The missed step results in a build-up of substrate from the step preceding the one in which the affected enzyme acts. In some instances this accumulated substrate can be toxic, as in phenylketonuria. In others, ever-expanding storage of substrate can adversely affect cell function, as in the lysosomal storage diseases.

Connective Tissue Disorders of Genetic Origin

See Table 1-7 for examples of some connective tissue disorders of genetic origin.

Marfan Syndrome

Marfan syndrome is a genetic disorder of connective tissue that is inherited as an autosomal dominant trait, although approximately 25% to 30% of cases represent new mutations. The site of the genetic abnormality or mutation is the fibrillin gene *(FBN1)* located at band 15q21.1 on chromosome 15. As a result, the molecular structure of the protein fibrillin, an intrinsic component of connective tissue, is abnormal. Clinical consequences are most notable in the musculoskeletal, cardiovascular, and ocular systems and in the dura. Approximately 70% of cases are familial. Classic phenotypic findings include arachnodactyly (Fig. 1-34, A and B); joint hyperextensibility due to ligamentous laxity (see Chapter 5, Fig. 5-8, B); tall stature with long, thin extremities; a decreased

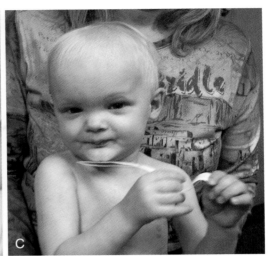

Figure 1-30 Classic presentation for features of X-linked recessive hypohidrotic ectodermal dysplasia at 1 to 20 months of age. At 1 month the infant was admitted to "rule out sepsis" with high fever, but all the workup was negative. **A,** Note the thin, sparse, fine hair. **B,** Severe hypodontia and anterior conical teeth. **C,** Low nasal bridge, periorbital wrinkling, full forehead, prominent lips, and prominent supraorbital ridges. DNA analysis of the *EDA1* gene at the Xq12 region showed the missense mutation and confirmed the clinical diagnosis. The mother and her maternal female relatives have variable and milder clinical features.

upper-to-lower segment ratio; an arm span that exceeds height; and moderate to severe pectus excavatum or carinatum (Fig. 1-34, *C*). Pes planus and thoracolumbar kyphoscoliosis are other common skeletal features (Fig. 1-34, *D*). A defect in the suspensory ligaments of the eye is responsible for subluxation of the lens (seen in 50% to 60% by age 10 years), which is usually displaced in an upward direction. Myopia and astigmatism are common, and affected individuals are also at risk for developing glaucoma, cataracts, and retinal detachment in adulthood. Mitral valve prolapse (MVP) may progress to mitral insufficiency (at times associated with arrhythmias). Of great concern is progressive aneurysmal dilatation of the ascending aorta and, less commonly, the thoracic or abdominal aorta. The latter is the major source of morbidity and mortality because it can result in acute dissection and death. Dural ectasia in the lumbosacral region, assessed by computed tomography (CT) or magnetic resonance imaging (MRI) of the spine, is observed in 65% of cases. The presence of a high arched palate is common. The incidence of hernias, both inguinal and femoral, is increased, and patients often have striae of the skin in unusual places such as the shoulder. Although most Marfan individuals are of normal intelligence, an occasional patient may have learning disabilities.

The disorder is currently diagnosed primarily on clinical grounds. In addition, family history and multiorgan manifestations are variable and may have age-dependent expressivity.

All the manifestations of this condition are classified as either major or minor diagnostic criteria. The diagnostic criteria for Marfan syndrome (first established in Berlin; Beighton et al, 1988) were revised as the Ghent criteria (De Paepe et al, 1996). These have continued to be revised and the most recent revised Ghent diagnostic criteria were established in 2010 (Loeys et al, 2010). The diagnostic criteria are based on cardiovascular, ocular, and skeletal features, the presence of a dural ectasia, and family history. These revisions have placed an increasing emphasis on the cardinal features of Marfan syndrome. Because it takes time for a number of the major abnormalities to develop or to become clinically evident, a firm diagnosis is generally impossible in early childhood, especially in the absence of a positive family history. The molecular testing of an individual who clinically meets the diagnostic criteria for Marfan syndrome is not usually necessary. Molecular testing is being used more frequently in children with an emerging clinical phenotype, especially in the absence of family history. The recurrence risk for affected individuals to their offspring is 50%.

When the diagnosis of Marfan syndrome is strongly suspected or confirmed, patients should be monitored closely during growth spurts for signs of onset and progression of kyphoscoliosis; in addition they should undergo regular ophthalmologic evaluations, and have regular echocardiograms and electrocardiograms. When aortic dilatation is detected,

Figure 1-31 Incontinentia pigmenti syndrome. **A-C,** At 7 weeks of age this patient manifested erythema, and blisters on the trunk and extremities. Hyperkeratotic lesions have already started. This X-linked dominant condition is lethal in males. One third of the patients have psychomotor delays, microcephaly, and seizures, which were not observed in this patient. Mutation(s) in the *NEMO* gene at Xq28 are encountered in the majority of patients. By 5 months of age the rash was already resolving. **D,** Rash replaced with hyperpigmentation on the trunk and pale hairless patches or streaks subsequently on the lower limbs. Patient was confirmed to have intragenic microdeletion of the *NEMO* gene, involving exons 4 through 10.

Figure 1-32 A girl, 3 years and 3 months old, with macrocephaly, macrosomia, and PDD-NOS (pervasive developmental disorder, not otherwise specified). A missense mutation was found in the *PTEN* gene.

Figure 1-33 A 4-month-old male with classic features of Treacher Collins syndrome. Note the down-slanted palpebral fissures, malar hypoplasia, malformed auricle, and mandibular hypoplasia. The mutation was identified as a single sequence variation (Nt2897insC) in the *TCOF1* gene in the 5q31 region that introduces a premature stop codon.

Table 1-7	Differentials for Connective Tissue Disorders	
Diagnosis	**Inheritance**	**Molecular Basis**
Stickler syndrome	AD	*COL2A1* gene
		COL11A1 gene
		COL11A2 gene
		COL9A1 gene
EDS type IV	AD	*COL3A1* gene
EDS type VI	AR	*PLOD1* gene
Beals contractural arachnodactyly	AD	*FBN2* gene
Homocysteinemia	AR	Defect in cobalamin synthesis
Arterial tortuosity syndrome	AR	*SLC2A10* gene
MASS phenotype	AD	*FBN1* gene
Loeys-Dietz syndrome	AD	*TGFBR1* gene
		TGFBR2 gene
Familial aortic aneurysm	AD	*ACTA2* gene
		MYH11 gene
Klinefelter syndrome (47,XXY) or triple X syndrome (47, XXX)	Chromosomal	Chromosomal
Fragile X syndrome	X-linked	*FMR1* gene
Shprintzen-Goldberg syndrome		Unknown

AD, autosomal dominant; AR, autosomal recessive; EDS, Ehlers-Danlos syndrome; MASS, **m**itral valve prolapse, **m**yopia, borderline and non-progressive **a**ortic enlargement, and nonspecific **s**kin and **s**keletal findings that overlap with those seen in Marfan syndrome.

administration of β-blockers can slow progression by decreasing blood pressure and the force of myocardial contractions. Subacute bacterial endocarditis (SBE) prophylaxis may or may not be indicated for patients with evidence of cardiovascular involvement. Patients also should be cautioned to avoid weight lifting and contact sports.

The differential diagnosis of Marfan syndrome includes Loeys-Dietz syndrome; Beals congenital contractural arachnodactyly (Figs. 1-35 through 1-39); homocystinuria; the MASS phenotype (MASS being an acronym for MVP, borderline non-progressive aortic dilatation, striae and marfanoid skeletal features, without ocular findings); familial ectopia lentis; Klinefelter syndrome (47,XXY), triple X syndrome (47,XXX), and many syndromes characterized by joint hypermobility such as Stickler syndrome and Ehlers-Danlos syndrome types IV and VI; familial thoracic aortic aneurysm and aortic dissection (TAAD); neuromuscular disorders; fragile X syndrome; and some of the rare dysmorphologic entities such as Shprintzen-Goldberg syndrome.

Loeys-Dietz syndrome is a more aggressive connective tissue disorder than Marfan syndrome; it is characterized by craniofacial, cutaneous, and skeletal manifestations along with vascular manifestations; and aneurysms and dissection of the aorta (in the root, thoracic, and/or abdominal regions) and cerebral vessels. Tortuosity of blood vessels and heart defects, involving the bicuspid aortic valves and atrial septal defects, may be observed. Translucent skin and organ rupture, specifically in postpartum females, have been reported. Mutations in transforming growth factor-β receptor type 1 (*TGFBR1*) and *TGFBR2* result in Loeys-Dietz syndrome. Research in the area of therapy has found TGF-β to be involved in the formation of aortic aneurysms. Losartan, an angiotensin II type 1 receptor blocker, inhibited TGF-β in a mouse model of Marfan syndrome (as shown by H.C. Dietz; Habashi et al, 2011), leading to inhibition of aortic growth. These results are promising; treatment of patients with Marfan syndrome may reduce aortic enlargement. At present, double-blind studies are being conducted in adults and pediatric patients to look into treatment with losartan (Fig. 1-40).

Ehlers-Danlos Syndrome

Ehlers-Danlos syndrome (EDS) is composed of a group of inherited connective tissue disorders, the major features of which consist of hyperextensibility and fragility of the skin and ligamentous laxity with secondary joint hypermobility. Each type stems from a defect in synthesis of type I, III, or V collagen, resulting in decreased tensile strength of connective tissues. Previously divided into types I to XI, it has been reclassified into six major subgroups on the basis of their predominant clinical features; mode of inheritance; and, when known, underlying defect. Table 1-8 presents these along with their estimated incidence. Given limitations of space, we focus on the clinical features of the four most common types.

Ehlers-Danlos Syndrome: Classic Type

In the classic form of EDS (previously known as subtypes I and II), cutaneous manifestations are especially prominent, although they may have a wide spectrum of severity. Skin hyperextensibility is prominent (Fig. 1-41, *A*); the texture is smooth and "velvety"; and the skin is abnormally fragile, with easy bruising and tearing. Wound healing is impaired and slower than average, often resulting in the formation of unusually wide atrophic scars that have a thin papery quality, sometimes likened to cigarette paper (see Fig. 1-41, *B*).

When these children incur lacerations necessitating wound closure, use of glue or tape is preferable to sutures because the latter tend to tear away from the fragile skin. Staples are better tolerated for closure of operative incisions, and postoperatively development of incisional hernias is not uncommon.

Two features unique to this type are the tendency to form pseudotumors under scars located over bony prominences and to develop subcutaneous fatty tumors over the forearms and shins.

Table 1-8	Classification of Types of Ehlers-Danlos Syndrome			
Type	**Former Type**	**Mode of Inheritance**	**Approximate Incidence**	**Underlying Abnormality**
Classic	I and II	AD	1 per 20,000-40,000	Abnormal electrophoretic mobility of pro-α1 and pro-α2 chains of type V collagen
Hypermobility	III	AD	1 per 10,000-15,000	No specific biochemical defect identified
Vascular	IV	AD	1 per 100,000-200,000	Mutation in *COL3A1* gene resulting in structurally abnormal pro-α1 chain of type III collagen, posttranslational overmodification, thermal instability, or increased sensitivity to proteases
Kyphoscoliotic	VI	AD	Rare	Deficiency of the collagen-modifying enzyme lysylhydroxylase
Arthrochalasia	VIIA and VIIB	AD	Very rare	Mutations resulting in deficient processing of amino-terminal ends of pro-α1 or pro-α2 chains of type I collagen
Dermatosparaxis	VIC	AR	Very rare	Deficiency of procollagen 1 amino-terminal peptidase

AD, autosomal dominant; AR, autosomal recessive.

Figure 1-34   Marfan syndrome. **A** and **B,** This young man has prominent arachnodactyly of both fingers and toes. Note the clubbing due to associated cardiopulmonary problems and the flattening of the arch of his foot. He also has severe pectus carinatum **(C)** and significant kyphosis and joint contractures **(D)**. Also note his long arms.

Figure 1-35   An adult female presented during the first trimester of pregnancy with a long-standing diagnosis of Marfan syndrome. On clinical evaluation, she had hypertelorism, low-set ears, and bifid uvula. Arachnodactyly, kyphoscoliosis, and marfanoid habitus were encountered. Cardiology evaluation was consistent, with an echocardiogram showing dilatation at the aortic root (with aortic sinus measurement of approximately 4.5 cm) and mitral valve prolapse. Cardiac surgery immediately after delivery was recommended. DNA tests confirmed Loeys-Dietz syndrome due to mutation in the *TGFBR1* gene. *FBN1* and *TGFBR2* analyses were normal.

Figure 1-36   Infant with Loeys-Dietz syndrome at 3 months of age. Note the retromicrognathia, hypertelorism, low-set ears, and failure to thrive.

Figure 1-37   The mother has clinical features of Loeys-Dietz syndrome. She has a pathogenic mutation in the *TGFBR1* gene. Her infant son, seen here at 5 months of age, is clinically affected and already has a dilated aorta. His mother had undergone valve-sparing aortic root repair on an emergent basis, due to possible dissection complicated by right coronary artery injury and bypass procedure.

Figure 1-38   **A-C,** Beals contractural arachnodactyly. Note the crumpled ears, arachnodactyly, and joint contractures. The patient was confirmed to have a missense mutation in the fibrillin II gene *(FBN2)*.

Figure 1-39   Beals syndrome variant. This child was found to have an abnormality of fibrillin-2 secretion in fibroblasts. **A,** She was tall and had arachnodactyly with contractures. **B,** Her broad forehead and hypertelorism are physical features that help distinguish her case from classic Beals syndrome and Marfan syndrome.

Effects of Losartan on AT1 Signaling

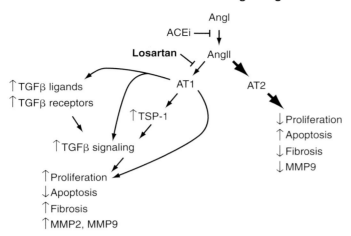

Figure 1-40 Diagram of events mediated by AT1 signaling. ACEi, angiotensin-converting enzyme inhibitor; AngI and AngII, angiotensins I and II; AT1 and AT2, angiotensin II subtypes 1 and 2 receptors; MMP2 and MMP9, matrix metalloproteinases 2 and 9; TGFβ, transforming growth factor-β; TSP-1, thrombospondin-1.

Although usually not as severe as in the hypermobility type, ligamentous laxity and joint hypermobility also are features (see Fig. 1-41, *C* and *D*) and predispose to sprains, subluxations, and dislocations, and to early onset of chronic musculoskeletal pain.

Hypotonia and gross motor delays are seen in some infants and young children with this type of EDS.

Ehlers-Danlos Syndrome: Hypermobility Type

In hypermobility-type EDS, the most common type, ligamentous laxity and attendant joint hypermobility are the major source of symptomatology. All joints, large and small, are affected, and patients are prone to frequent and recurrent subluxations and dislocations, especially of the patella, shoulder, and temporomandibular joints. Chronic limb and joint pain due to the excessive pull placed on periarticular structures, and to dislocations, develops early on and can become increasingly debilitating over time.

Cutaneous manifestations vary widely in severity and include a smooth "velvety" texture, hyperextensibility, and easy bruisability.

Ehlers-Danlos Syndrome: Vascular Type

Vascular-type EDS is the most serious form of EDS because fragility of vascular and visceral tissues accompanies cutaneous and joint abnormalities. Many affected children are born with clubfeet, and they tend to have rather characteristic facial features that include prominent eyes and sunken cheeks (due to decreased subcutaneous facial fat), a thin nose, small chin, and lobeless external ears. Scalp hair is sparse in some.

The skin is thin and appears translucent, giving prominence to the underlying venous pattern, especially over the chest and abdomen. Easy bruisability and skin fragility are significant features, and postoperative wound dehiscence is not unusual. Premature aging of the skin over the distal extremities and early development of varicose veins are also seen. Joint hypermobility is present but is limited to the small joints of the fingers and toes.

Figure 1-41 Ehlers-Danlos syndrome—classic type. **A,** Note the marked hyperextensibility of the skin over this child's arm. **B,** These widened atrophic scars have the thin papery texture that is characteristic of Ehlers-Danlos syndrome. **C** and **D,** Hyperextensibility of the joints of the elbow and fingers is seen as well.

As noted earlier, the feature that makes this type of EDS so serious clinically is the fragility of the walls of medium-size arteries, the intestines, and the uterus. This predisposes to wall rupture with potentially catastrophic results. Arterial and intestinal ruptures are heralded by sudden onset of severe abdominal and/or flank pain, which is promptly followed by signs of shock. Risk of uterine rupture is greatest intrapartum and is associated with significant hemorrhage. Other reported problems include pneumothoraces and development of arteriovenous fistulas.

Because the major complications of this form of EDS tend to occur in the third or fourth decade, exact diagnosis in early childhood can be difficult in patients without a positive family history or in those whose other clinical findings are subtle.

Ehlers-Danlos Syndrome: Kyphoscoliosis Type

Newborns with the kyphoscoliosis form of EDS tend to have severe hypotonia with delayed gross motor development and congenital scoliosis, which is progressive. Some patients develop a marfanoid body habitus with growth. Generalized ligamentous laxity and joint hypermobility may be so severe that the ability to ambulate is lost in the teens or twenties. Osteopenia is seen radiographically, perhaps partly from disuse.

Other features include easy bruisability, skin fragility, and formation of atrophic scars. In contrast to other forms of EDS, children with this type have scleral fragility, which places them at risk for globe rupture following even minor trauma. High myopia and microcornea are seen in some.

Diagnosis

The diagnosis of EDS should be suspected in children who present with unusually distensible skin, especially when atrophic scars are seen, and in those with unusual degrees of joint hypermobility who suffer recurrent joint dislocations. The presence of skin hyperextensibility is best tested over the volar forearm by grasping the skin and pulling until resistance is felt. Evidence of significant joint hypermobility includes the following:

- Ability to touch palms to the floor on forward bending
- Hyperextensibility of knees and elbows greater than 10 degrees
- Ability to appose thumb to the volar forearm
- Passive dorsiflexion of the fifth fingers past 90 degrees

Finding these and other clinical features described earlier in a child with a positive family history is especially helpful. With the exception of the kyphoscoliotic type, for which a urine test is available, confirmatory diagnostic tests usually require skin biopsy.

Depending on type, differential diagnostic considerations may include Marfan syndrome and cutis laxa. Easy bruisability can be mistaken for child abuse.

Osteogenesis Imperfecta

Osteogenesis imperfecta (OI) is a family of genetic connective tissue disorders characterized predominantly by brittle bones. The vast majority of patients have OI type I, II, III, or IV, all of which involve mutations in the *COL1A1* gene and/or *COL1A2* gene that either reduce the amount or alter the structure of type I collagen. A description of some of the many causative mutations and their structural consequences is presented in an earlier section (The Nature of Genes and Single-gene Disorders). Clinical features are presented in Chapter 21. Other, rarer forms of OI include types V through VIII. Of these, OI type V is an autosomal dominant disorder, and OI type VII is autosomal recessive; the mode of inheritance of OI type VI

Figure 1-42 Clinical features suggestive of type III osteogenesis imperfecta (OI); collagen screen results on skin fibroblasts are consistent with type III or type IV OI. The patient would not consider DNA diagnosis. He is wheelchair bound but lives independently.

is unclear, but patients with OI type VI have rhizomelic shortening of the limbs.

Figures 1-42 through 1-44 show examples of defects in collagen synthesis.

ASSOCIATIONS

As noted earlier, an *association* is a pattern of malformations that occurs together too often to be the result of chance alone, but for which no specific cause has yet been identified. This results in a spectrum of anomalies with a wide and variable clinical spectrum.

FAVA (Facio-Auriculo-Vertebral-Anomalies) Spectra

FAVA encompasses a spectrum of hemifacial microsomia and Goldenhar syndromes resulting from developmental defects of the first and second branchial arches. Varied facial defects observed include hypoplasia of the maxilla and/or mandible, a lateral cleft at the angle of the mouth resulting in macrostomia, microtia and preauricular tags and/or pits, deafness, and tongue and palatal involvement with abnormal functioning of the palate.

Vertebral defects are predominantly in the cervical region, observed as a short neck and/or torticollis. Radiologic imaging is able to decipher underlying hemivertebrae and hypoplasia of the vertebrae in the cervical region but may involve the thoracic and lumbar regions. Microphthalmia and/or epibulbar, eyelid coloboma are observed as infrequent features. Congenital heart defects include ventricular septal defect, tetralogy of Fallot, and coarctation of the aorta. Renal defects are occasional features and may present as ectopic, fused kidney or renal agenesis as well as multicystic dysplastic kidney. Ureteral aberrations may be associated as well. CNS involvement is an occasional feature. Intelligence is usually preserved but may be compromised in association with microphthalmia and CNS anomalies. Genetic delineation of etiology is at a research level and clinical cases are not confirmed by mutation analyses. FAVA may overlap with clinical findings of VATER association (see later) and branchio-oto-renal syndrome, also known as Melnick-Fraser syndrome.

Figure 1-44 A grandfather and granddaughter with Stickler syndrome type II. Grandfather has high myopia and status post–unilateral retinal detachment. Grandfather was confirmed to have a frameshift mutation in the collagen II gene, confirming Stickler syndrome type II. The mutation was confirmed in his 5-year-old granddaughter; note the early-onset high myopia and midface hypoplasia. She also had generalized joint laxity. She had surgery for cleft palate and is under surveillance by audiology for conductive hearing loss.

Figure 1-43 Stickler syndrome: short stature, early-onset myopia, midface hypoplasia, submucous cleft palate, sensorineural hearing loss, mild skeletal dysplasia, and joint pain. A missense mutation in the *COL2A1* gene confirmed the clinical diagnosis and is consistent with type I Stickler syndrome.

CHARGE Association

CHARGE is an acronym for a nonrandom association of features including *c*oloboma of the retina, less commonly the iris; *h*eart abnormalities; *a*tresia of the choanae; *r*etarded growth and mental development; *g*enital hypoplasia in males; and *e*ar anomalies that can include deafness. The minimal diagnostic criteria should include abnormalities in four of the six categories, at least one of which must be coloboma or choanal atresia. Cleft lip and/or palate and renal abnormalities are sometimes found. The association includes congenital heart disease, particularly abnormalities of the aortic arch, right

subclavian artery, or ventricular septal defect; agenesis or hypoplasia of the thymus with decreased T-cell production and impaired cell-mediated immunity; partial or less often complete absence of the parathyroid glands, manifest by hypocalcemia and neonatal tetany; and often a facies characterized by wide-spaced, slightly down-slanting palpebral fissures, anteverted nares, a short philtrum, and small, dysmorphic ears (Fig. 1-45). Infants with CHARGE association often die early as a result of their congenital anomalies, but many survive to adulthood. Although developmental delay exists, the IQ range is broad (<30 to 80).

CHARGE has been found to be related to mutations in the *CHD7* gene located on chromosome 8q12. In the neonate, CHARGE association must be differentiated from other chromosomal disorders, such as deletion 22q11.2 or trisomy 13 or 18, and from the more benign nonchromosomal VATER association. When the DiGeorge sequence is present in patients

Figure 1-45 CHARGE association. **A,** Note the short palpebral fissures and ptosis; low-set, dysplastic ears; and small chin. Choanal atresia necessitated tracheotomy. **B,** Another example of an infant with CHARGE association has clinical features that include a prominent forehead, hypertelorism, narrow palpebral fissures, hypoplasia of the right naris, low-set ears, and a cupid's-bow mouth. (**A,** Courtesy W. Tunnessen, MD. **B,** Courtesy Timothy McBride, MD, Fairfax, Va.)

Figure 1-46 This child with VATER association **(A)** has facial features that are not dysmorphic, but he has preaxial polydactyly of the thumb **(B)**, which was associated with radial dysplasia.

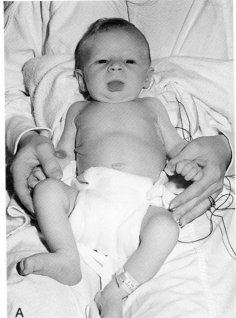

with CHARGE association, a small interstitial deletion of chromosome 22 at q11 is occasionally found with high-resolution cytogenetic techniques and FISH DNA probe.

The etiology of CHARGE association is most likely heterogeneous. Although most cases are sporadic, instances of affected siblings and an affected parent and offspring have been reported. The risk of recurrence must be determined after genetic evaluation and ranges from 4% to 6% to as high as 50%.

VATER Association

VATER is another acronym for a nonrandom association of *v*ertebral and *a*nal anomalies, *t*racheoesophageal fistula with *e*sophageal atresia, and *r*adial and/or renal abnormalities. Most affected newborns have anomalies in all five categories. The acronym can be expanded to VACTERL to include *c*ongenital heart disease (particularly ventricular septal defect) and, less often, other *l*imb defects. Vertebral anomalies include hemivertebrae and sacral abnormalities. Limb deformities consist of ray abnormalities such as radial aplasia or hypoplasia, abnormal thumbs, preaxial polydactyly, and syndactyly (Fig. 1-46). Renal abnormalities include unilateral agenesis and less commonly ectopic or horseshoe kidney. The etiology of VATER association is unknown. Virtually all cases are sporadic. Detection of an abnormal karyotype rules out this disorder. The prognosis for growth and development in newborns who survive infancy is good. Most have normal intelligence and eventually achieve normal stature. Consequently, to make optimal management decisions, it is important to distinguish VATER syndrome from more dire chromosomal abnormalities (such as trisomy 18) or nonchromosomal disorders (such as CHARGE association).

For the purpose of genetic counseling, VATER association must also be differentiated from Townes-Brocks syndrome, an autosomal dominant, simple mendelian genetic disorder with features representing a combination of the findings observed for FAVA and VATER associations. However, in Townes-Brocks syndrome there is often a positive family history of autosomal dominant inheritance of ear, thumb, and anal abnormalities, whereas vertebral anomalies and tracheoesophageal fistula are

unusual. The prognosis for growth and development in patients with Townes-Brocks syndrome is good. However, the risk for recurrence of Townes-Brocks syndrome with a positive family history may be up to 50%, whereas for VATER association the risk may be less than 2%. Antenatal diagnosis for both conditions depends on detecting structural anomalies in the fetus by high-resolution ultrasound.

Other disorders in the list of differential diagnostic possibilities include Fanconi anemia and Holt-Oram syndrome (see Chapter 5, Fig. 5-7). Once chromosome studies are completed and found to be normal, when other disorders are deemed less likely, and a child has the pattern of malformation characteristic of the VATER association, the diagnosis (which remains one of exclusion) can be made.

RECOGNIZABLE MULTIPLE MALFORMATION SYNDROMES

De Lange, Cornelia de Lange, or Brachmann– de Lange Syndrome

De Lange syndrome is characterized by intrauterine growth retardation, persistent postnatal failure to thrive, moderate to severe cognitive impairment, and microcephaly with a flat occiput and low hairline. Facial features are quite distinctive and include long eyelashes; a fine, almost "brushed-on" appearance of the arch to the eyebrows; occasional synophrys due to hirsutism; small nose with anteverted nostrils; long philtrum; downturned upper lip with cupid's-bow shape; and micrognathia (Fig. 1-47, *A* and *B*). Extremities are notable for small hands and feet, and varying abnormalities can include proximally placed thumbs (Fig. 1-47, *C*), flexion contractures of the elbows, hypoplastic limbs, and even overt phocomelia. Hirsutism is generalized and distinctive, and cutis marmorata is a frequent feature. In males, hypospadias with cryptorchidism is common, and females may have a bicornuate uterus. Most affected adults are quite short in stature.

In general, most cases are believed to be the result of new autosomal dominant mutations, and mutations in the *NIPBL* gene on chromosome 5p13 have been identified as responsible

Figure 1-47 Cornelia de Lange syndrome. **A** and **B,** Facial features seen in an infant and an older child include finely arched heavy eyebrows, long eyelashes, small upturned nose, long smooth philtrum, and cupid's-bow mouth. **C,** Small hands, hypoplastic proximally placed thumb, and short fifth finger with mild clinodactyly are examples of commonly associated extremity anomalies. (**A** and **C,** Courtesy A. H. Urbach, MD, Children's Hospital of Pittsburgh, Pittsburgh, Pa.)

for approximately 50% of cases of classic De Lange syndrome. In evaluating cases, careful physical examination of family members must be performed to determine recurrence risks for individual families. Clearly, this disorder can be so mild in expression that many cases may go unrecognized. Families have been identified with severely affected children whose parents have been determined to be subtly affected. In those families autosomal dominant inheritance would apply, with a 50% recurrence risk for any affected individual to have a child with the same disorder. If parents are not thought to be affected, the recurrence risk has been shown to range from 1% to 5%. A few individuals have somewhat similar features, most notably synophrys, and have been found to have an abnormality of the short arm of chromosome 3; thus careful high-resolution chromosome studies are indicated, with particular attention to chromosome 3.

Noonan Syndrome

Noonan syndrome is an autosomal dominant, simple mendelian genetic disorder that shares a number of clinical features with 45,X (Turner syndrome). The disorder has been found to be associated with mutations in the *PTPN11* gene on chromosome 12q24.1 (in 50% of classic cases) and in the *KRAS* gene on chromosome 12p12.1 in 5% to 10% of the cases that are negative for the *PTPN11* mutation. Thus a chromosome study should be performed on any individual in whom this diagnosis

is suspected. It is relatively common and thought to be present in 1 in 1000 to 1 in 2500 individuals. Like many other autosomal dominant disorders, it is seen in both males and females and there is significant variability in clinical expression. Hence careful examination of close relatives of an index case may identify other affected individuals within the extended family, which is helpful when attempting to determine recurrence risks, as that risk would be 50% for offspring of an affected individual. In cases in which the child is considered to be the first in the family with Noonan syndrome, the empiric recurrence risk to apparently unaffected parents is 5%.

The pattern of malformations in Noonan syndrome is characterized by webbing of the neck, sternal abnormalities, pulmonic stenosis, and cryptorchidism in males. Facial characteristics include widely spaced eyes with down-slanting palpebral fissures, ptosis, and retrognathia (see Chapter 5, Fig. 5-9). Ears are often low-set and can be posteriorly rotated. Hair can be coarse and curly, and the posterior hairline is often low. Sternal abnormalities include both pectus excavatum and carinatum, and often there are differences in the number of sternal ossification centers. Many have congenital heart disease with pulmonary valvular stenosis being the most common, followed by septal hypertrophy or defects. Hypertrophic cardiomyopathy is found in approximately 20% and can be sufficiently severe as to necessitate cardiac transplantation. Coagulation abnormalities are found in approximately one third of cases.

Puberty can be delayed in individuals with Noonan syndrome. Cryptorchidism, when present in males, can result in sterility. Females are fertile. Stature is often less than the third percentile, but head circumference and intelligence are usually normal.

Several recognizable patterns of malformation share features in common with Noonan syndrome. Cardio-facio-cutaneous syndrome has additional features suggesting abnormal development of tissues derived from ectoderm, and affected individuals usually have significant CNS abnormalities. The phenotypic features of Noonan syndrome and neurofibromatosis type I may overlap (Watson syndrome). In the Costello syndrome, macrocephaly; coarse facial features; papillomas in the oral, nasal, and anal areas; cutis laxa; and cognitive impairments are seen in addition to findings shared with Noonan syndrome. Genetic heterogeneity is encountered; at least 10 gene loci are involved for the Noonan syndrome and allied disorders, that is, Noonan, cardio-facio-cutaneous, and Costello syndromes. Molecular testing at the clinical level is currently available for *PTPN11* at 12q24.1, *RAF1* at 3p25, *SOS1* at 2p22-p21, *KRAS* at 12p12.1, *HRAS* at 11p15.5, *BRAF* at 7q34, *MEK1* at 15q21, *MEK2* at 7q32, *NRAS* at 1p13.2, and *SHOC2* at 10q25 (Fig. 1-48). Refinement of molecular techniques has enabled the simultaneous analyses of all the genes in a single diagnostic test known as the "Noonan Chip," currently offered by some laboratories. Watson syndrome is characterized by mutation of the neurofibromatosis gene but also shows phenotypic overlap with Noonan syndrome. In addition to short stature, pulmonic stenosis, café au lait spots, and cognitive disabilities, freckling and neurofibromas are also observed.

Kabuki syndrome, characterized by physical growth and psychomotor delays in association with skeletal, cardiac, and craniofacial features, may have an overlapping phenotype with Noonan spectrum disorders. Exome sequencing has identified mutation(s) in the *MLL2* gene at 12q12-14 among patients with Kabuki syndrome (Ng et al, 2010).

Figure 1-49 Noonan syndrome. Note the down-slanting palpebral fissures, ptosis, and low-set posteriorly rotated ears. Patient has bilateral simian creases and underwent cardiac surgeries for severe pulmonic stenosis and atrial septal defect. She has short stature, developmental delays, alternating esotropia, optic nerve cupping, and unilateral pelvicaliectasis. A missense mutation in exon 3 of the *PTPN11* gene resulted in the classic features of Noonan syndrome.

The differential diagnosis also includes several well-known teratogenic exposures including fetal hydantoin syndrome and fetal alcohol syndrome (see Fig. 1-53). Hence careful dysmorphologic assessment of all individuals suspected of having Noonan syndrome is indicated before making a final diagnosis.

Patients with Noonan, LEOPARD, cardio-facio-cutaneous, or Costello syndrome (Figs. 1-49 through 1-52, respectively) are demonstrated by pathogenetic pathways. Interaction of the

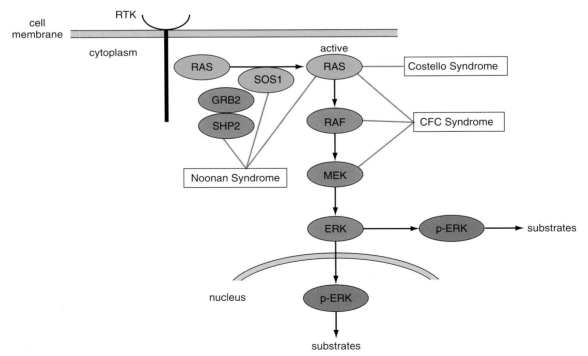

Figure 1-48 The mitogen-activated protein kinase (MAPK) signaling cascade, also known as the RAF/MEK/ERK signaling cascade. Germline mutations that affect components of the RAS-MAPK pathway are involved in the pathogenesis of Noonan syndrome and allied disorders (Noonan phenotype with overlapping features: CFC, LEOPARD, Costello and neurofibromatosis-1). CFC, cardio-facio-cutaneous syndrome; ERK, extracellular signal–regulated kinase; GRB2, growth factor receptor-bound protein 2; MEK, MAPK/ERK kinase; p-ERK, phosphorylated ERK; PTPN11, protein tyrosine phosphate, non-receptor type 11; RAF, murine sarcoma viral oncogene; RAS, rat sarcoma viral oncogene; RTK, receptor tyrosine kinase; SHC, signaling and transforming protein containing src homology 2 and 3, SH2 and SH3 domains; SHP2, src homology region 2-domain phosphatase 2; SOS1, son of sevenless 1. *(Courtesy of Partners Health Care, Laboratory for Molecular Medicine, Harvard Medical School.)*

Figure 1-50 A 10-year-old girl with LEOPARD syndrome. LEOPARD is an acronym for the cardinal features: **l**entigines, **E**CG conduction abnormalities, **o**cular hypertelorism, **p**ulmonic stenosis, **a**bnormal genitalia, **r**etardation of growth, sensorineural **d**eafness. Not all features need to be present to be diagnosed with LEOPARD syndrome.

Figure 1-52 Costello syndrome. Note the macrocephaly, curly sparse hair, short neck, and hypotonia. The patient had a tracheostomy and is gastrostomy tube dependent, and has had global delays with some communication by sign language at 4 years of age. Skin was very lax and soft and a somewhat darker color for the family. A mutation in exon 2 of the *HRAS* gene was classic for Costello syndrome.

many respective gene(s) at the genetic level results in clinical overlap among these entities of "Noonan syndrome and allied disorders." These are therefore an excellent example of locus or genetic heterogeneity. Allelic heterogeneity is observed among classic Noonan phenotype and LEOPARD syndrome clinical picture (see Fig. 1-49).

PATTERNS OF MALFORMATION ASSOCIATED WITH IN UTERO TERATOGEN EXPOSURE

Fetal Alcohol Syndrome

The effect of exposure to significant levels of serum alcohol during gestation results in a pattern of microcephaly, prenatal and postnatal growth deficiency, short palpebral fissures, long

smooth philtrum, and a thin upper lip (Fig. 1-53). Other features include a short nose and hypoplasia of the nails and distal phalanges (particularly the fifth toes). On occasion, affected infants have eyelid ptosis, epicanthal folds, strabismus, small raised hemangiomas, cervical vertebral abnormalities, and congenital heart disease.

Newborns with fetal alcohol syndrome are small for gestational age and have poor catch-up growth postnatally. They may have increased or decreased muscle tone and can be irritable and tremulous. Most older children tend to be thin and hyperactive, and more than 80% have some delay in development, especially fine motor function.

The diagnosis of fetal alcohol syndrome should be reserved for those infants who have a history of in utero exposure to

Figure 1-51 Cardio-facio-cutaneous syndrome. The patient underwent surgical repair of ventricular septal defect and pulmonic stenosis during infancy. Presented at 8 years of age with short stature while receiving growth hormone injections, seizures, and intellectual disabilities. Patient has optic nerve hypoplasia, relative macrocephaly, curly hair, deep palmar creases, and prominent finger pads. Note the prominent forehead, hypertelorism, ptosis, and low-set posterior rotation of ears. The patient carried a clinical diagnosis of Noonan syndrome and tested negative for *PTPN11*, *SOS1*, *RAF1*, and *KRAS* genes. Noonan Chip analysis confirmed the missense pathogenic mutation in the *BRAF* gene, consistent with cardio-facio-cutaneous syndrome.

Figure 1-53 Fetal alcohol syndrome. Note the short palpebral fissure length, mild ptosis, and long simple philtrum.

large amounts of alcohol and who have the characteristic physical features of the disorder. The past practice of labeling children with developmental disorders who do not have the clinical stigmata as having fetal alcohol effects should be abandoned.

Although there may be no absolutely safe level of maternal alcohol consumption throughout pregnancy (particularly in the first trimester), the risk of teratogenesis increases dramatically with increasing degrees of maternal ethanol consumption. Major evidence of fetal alcohol syndrome is observed in 30% to 50% of offspring of mothers who are chronic severe alcoholics, whereas more subtle effects result from ingestion of lesser quantities of alcohol. The risk to the fetus of occasional maternal alcoholic binges is not clear, but such drinking is best avoided. Why some babies are affected and others are not, despite equivalent degrees of maternal alcoholism, is also unclear.

Other examples of teratogen-induced disorders include fetal hydantoin syndrome and fetal retinoic acid (Accutane) embryopathy.

GENETIC DISORDERS OF METABOLISM

Inborn errors of metabolism encompass a wide range of inherited disorders. These include disorders of intermediary metabolism, disorders of organelle function (lysosomal, peroxisomal, or mitochondrial), disorders of cholesterol biosynthesis, disorders of protein glycosylation, disorders of metals, disorders of transport, and others. Although most are enzyme deficiencies that are inherited in an autosomal recessive pattern, various forms in inheritance (dominant, recessive, X-linked, and maternal) are found with metabolic disorders. This brief review is limited to some of the more common metabolic disorders and should be supplemented with a more detailed text on metabolic disorders as needed.

Disorders of Intermediary Metabolism

Intermediary metabolism involves conversion of the nutrients *protein, carbohydrate,* and *fat* into energy (Fig. 1-54). The common endpoint in the metabolism of all three nutrients passes through the Krebs cycle, and then through the electron transport chain where oxidative phosphorylation occurs, consuming oxygen and yielding ATP. A substantial number of errors of intermediary metabolism are detected by expanded *newborn screening,* but some are not detectable or can be missed in some cases.

The *feed–fast cycle* refers to changing patterns of metabolism depending on available energy sources. After eating, the body uses circulating fuels, which are fairly quickly depleted postprandially. The body then largely relies on stored glycogen until these stores are exhausted (approximately 4 to 8 hours, depending on age and clinical circumstances). After glycogen stores are exhausted protein catabolism and fatty acid oxidation become the most important energy sources, and gluconeogenesis is required to support glucose stores. Thus, disorders of glycogen metabolism tend to present after a short fasting interval. However, most disorders of protein or fatty acid oxidation metabolism tend to present after a longer fasting period, after normal glycogen stores are depleted.

Disorders of Protein Metabolism

Proteins are broken down into their basic components, amino acids. *Essential amino acids* cannot be synthesized by the body and must be consumed in the diet. Amino acids can be used to support tissue growth or maintenance, can be

Common Pathways of Intermediary Metabolism

PDH – pyruvate dehydrogenase
PC – pyruvate carboxylase

Figure 1-54 The conversion of protein, carbohydrate, and fat into energy. PDH, pyruvate dehydrogenase; PC, pyruvate carboxylase; R-2 and R-4, fatty acids shortened by successive two-carbon units, the result of β-oxidation.

Table 1-9	Common Findings in Disorders of Protein Metabolism

Disorder	Common Findings
Phenylketonuria	Untreated: MR, eczema, mousy odor, fair coloring Treated: Minimal to mild tremor, executive function deficits
Homocystinuria	Untreated: Variable MR, ectopia lentis, marfanoid habitus, vascular thromboses Treated: Variable persistent vascular issues
MSUD	Untreated: Ketosis, acidosis, coma, death, MR, maple syrup odor, some late onset with intermittent symptoms Treated: Intermittent ketosis/acidosis during intercurrent illnesses, variable developmental delay to normal cognition
Organic acidemia (MMA, PA, IVA)	Untreated: Ketosis, acidosis, death, neutropenia, hyperammonemia, hypotonia, some late onset with failure to thrive, hypotonia Treated: Intermittent ketoacidosis during intercurrent illnesses, metabolic strokes, low to normal tone, delay to normal cognition
Urea cycle defect	Untreated: Hyperammonemia, coma, death, hyperreflexia, MR, variable acidosis, some late onset with intermittent symptoms Treated: Intermittent hyperammonemia with intercurrent illnesses, variable developmental delay to normal cognition

IVA, isovaleric acidemia; MMA, methylmalonic acidemia; MR, mental retardation; MSUD, maple syrup urine disease; PA, propionic acidemia.

converted into other amino acids *(transamination),* can be excreted in the urine, or can be catabolized for energy (see Fig. 1-54). Some characteristic physical findings of protein metabolism disorders are noted in Table 1-9.

Protein Metabolism: Transamination Disorders

Phenylketonuria. A common disorder of transamination is *phenylketonuria* (PKU), in which the transamination of phenylalanine to tyrosine is impaired. PKU is a relatively common autosomal recessive disorder of protein metabolism (affecting 1 in 10,000 to 1 in 15,000), and is most commonly diagnosed by newborn screening. Affected patients follow a diet restricted in phenylalanine (containing just enough natural protein from fruits, vegetables, and limited starches to meet essential phenylalanine needs for growth and maintenance), supplemented with a medical food "formula" containing tyrosine and other essential amino acids and nutrients, and specially formulated low-phenylalanine foods. If untreated, the disorder results in mental retardation, eczematous skin changes, a "mousy" odor, and other changes. Well-treated patients may have mild tremor, but physical examination is otherwise normal. Although cognitive outcomes are normal in most diet-adherent patients, some patients experience mild to moderate difficulties with executive functioning (attention, organization, and working memory). When a woman with PKU is pregnant, she must follow her diet especially carefully to prevent mental retardation and birth defects (particularly defects of the heart and esophagus) in her fetus.

Most PKU is due to a defect in the enzyme phenylalanine hydroxylase. A small proportion of patients with PKU have normal phenylalanine hydroxylase enzyme but have a defect in synthesis or recycling of the enzyme's biopterin cofactor. Because this biopterin cofactor is shared with two other enzymes (tyrosine hydroxylase [a precursor of dopamine, epinephrine, and norepinephrine] and tryptophan hydroxylase [a precursor of serotonin]), patients with biopterin defects have neurotransmitter deficits in addition to PKU. These patients require supplementation with biopterin and/or neurotransmitter replacements in addition to a phenylalanine-restricted diet, and the neurologic outcome is not always normal.

Homocystinuria. Homocysteine is an intermediate in the multistep metabolism of methionine to cysteine. In *homocystinuria,* the metabolism of homocysteine is blocked at the level of the enzyme cystathionine β-synthase. When untreated, in addition to developmental delays, physical findings include various degrees of ectopia lentis; a marfanoid habitus; and, by young adulthood, vascular thromboses (see Table 1-9). Homocystinuria is most commonly diagnosed by newborn screening (by detection of elevated methionine), but the sensitivity of the screen is not complete. Homocystinuria may be present in older children and adults who were born before this disorder was added to the current newborn screening panel. Rarer forms of homocystinuria exist caused by failure to return homocysteine back into methionine, typically due to defects in vitamin B_{12} metabolism.

Maple Syrup Urine Disease. The branched-chain amino acids (valine, leucine, and isoleucine) share a common initial step in catabolism, catalyzed by branched-chain keto acid decarboxylase. A genetic defect in this enzyme leads to *maple syrup urine disease* (MSUD), named because of the characteristic odor of the urine. Affected individuals develop elevations of these three branched-chain amino acids resulting in ketosis and, if untreated, acidosis, coma, and death. Physical examination may identify the odor of maple syrup in cerumen and concentrated urine. The patient may exhibit varying degrees of spasticity or developmental delay, especially if late or poorly treated (see Table 1-9). Elevated leucine levels are intoxicating, and can chronically impair learning and social interactions when poorly controlled. Patients must follow a diet restricted in these three essential amino acids, supplemented with other essential amino acids and nutrients. The most important component of dietary treatment is the prevention of stressful fasting, as this would lead to the increased catabolism of amino acids for energy and thus increased formation of toxic metabolites. Milder variants are known to exist with symptoms including altered mental status or ketosis during intercurrent illnesses. MSUD is most commonly diagnosed by newborn screening, but the sensitivity of screening for milder or intermittent variants is not known, and an infant may already be symptomatic before the screening results are available.

Protein Metabolism: Urea Cycle Disorders

Amino acids are further catabolized by deamination. The amino group is removed and forms ammonia, and the residual carbon skeleton is an organic acid, typically metabolized in the Krebs cycle (see Fig. 1-54). Ammonia is toxic when accumulated, and is normally detoxified in the urea cycle. Metabolic errors are well described in each enzymatic step of the urea cycle. Affected infants classically present with hyperammonemic coma in the neonatal period, typically progressing through poor feeding, respiratory alkalosis, decreasing mental status, vomiting, and neurologic irritability to coma (see Table 1-9). The presence of unexplained respiratory alkalosis or neurologic irritability including hyperreflexia, increased startle, or clonus in an infant with depressed mental status should always prompt a search for an inborn error of metabolism (although these findings will eventually be blunted as coma deepens). Acidosis (rarely even ketoacidosis) may develop as the infant's clinical status deteriorates. Any patient of any age undergoing a lumbar puncture for otherwise unexplained mental status changes should have their plasma ammonia level checked. Analysis of plasma amino acids and orotic acid is key in helping to define the specific urea cycle defect, and additional information on this is available in textbooks dedicated to metabolic disorders.

A significant percentage of patients with urea cycle defects can present later in life with failure to thrive, developmental delays, friable hair (trichorrhexis nodosa, in argininosuccinate lyase deficiency), or in some cases acutely with hyperammonemia during intercurrent illnesses or weaning from breast milk to formula (which is higher in protein). Some patients have presented in adulthood during profound metabolic stress (such as after bariatric surgery or childbirth); thus age is no barrier to diagnosis. Treatment involves careful titration of protein intake to meet requirements for growth and maintenance without providing excess, with supplementation of essential urea cycle intermediates (citrulline or arginine, as determined by the position of the enzymatic block), and with drugs that complex with glutamine or glycine to form urine-soluble nitrogen complexes and provide an alternative excretion pathway for nitrogen. It is particularly important to provide alternative energy intake during fasting to prevent the catabolism of amino acids for energy and the release of ammonia.

Protein Metabolism: Organic Acidemias

Once the ammonia is removed from an amino acid, the remaining carbon skeleton is an *organic acid*. Most organic acids are catabolized to specific Krebs cycle intermediates (see Fig. 1-54). Various errors in catabolism lead to specific organic acid disorders.

Propionic Acidemia and Methylmalonic Acidemia. The most common series of errors is in the catabolism of the carbon skeletons of *v*aline, *o*dd-chain fatty acids, *m*ethionine, *i*soleucine, and *t*hreonine (VOMIT), which pass through propionyl-CoA, methylmalonyl-CoA, and then succinyl-CoA (a Krebs cycle intermediate). Inborn errors of propionyl-CoA carboxylase lead to *propionic acidemia,* and errors of methylmalonyl-CoA mutase lead to *methylmalonic acidemia.* These can present in the neonatal period with acute ketoacidosis, hyperammonemia, and bone marrow suppression (from secondary inhibition of the urea cycle and bone marrow) or at a later age with acute symptoms during an intercurrent illness, or at any time with chronic failure to thrive, hypotonia, or developmental delay. Physical examination is most remarkable for central hypotonia, often with hyperreflexia (see Table 1-9). Patient management includes careful titration of dietary protein to meet the needs for the essential amino acids valine, methionine, isoleucine, and threonine, supplemented with other essential amino acids and nutrients. Alternative forms of calorie supplementation are important during fasting/intercurrent illnesses to prevent protein catabolism.

Disorders of Leucine Catabolism. A number of other organic acidemias are relatively common, including *isovaleric acidemia,* an inborn error in the catabolism of leucine (a complete review of which is beyond the scope of this chapter). The incidence of this disorder on newborn screening is somewhat higher than expected. Expanded newborn screening also has identified an unexpectedly high incidence of *3-methylcrotonyl-CoA carboxylase deficiency,* another inborn error of leucine catabolism. Previously believed to be associated with developmental delays, failure to thrive, and other problems, the clinical significance of this disorder is now unclear. Most organic acidemias are detectable by newborn screening, although the sensitivity for late-onset or milder forms is not yet known.

Disorders of Carbohydrate Metabolism

The basic unit of carbohydrate metabolism is *glucose*. Glucose is metabolized for energy through glycolysis. Complex carbohydrates and alternative carbohydrates (such as galactose or fructose) are converted to glucose or glycolytic intermediates for catabolism. Some of the common disorders of carbohydrate metabolism are listed in Table 1-10.

Carbohydrate Metabolism: Glycogen Metabolism

When carbohydrate intake exceeds immediate need, glucose is stored as *glycogen,* predominantly in the liver. During the interprandial fast, glycogen is used preferentially to meet energy needs by converting it back to glucose. After glycogen stores are exhausted, protein and fat catabolism are enhanced.

Glycogen Storage Disease Type 0. In the case of *glycogen storage disease (GSD) type 0,* glycogen cannot be made. Patients typically have postprandial hyperglycemia and interprandial hypoglycemia, but no other specific physical findings. The liver is not enlarged because glycogen is not stored. In some cases the interprandial hyperglycemia can be mild or overlooked, and the disorder manifests as hypoglycemia during fasting or intercurrent illness.

Other Forms of Glycogen Storage Disease. Other forms of glycogen storage disease affect glycogen metabolism in the liver or muscle. The most common forms of liver glycogen storage disease are types I, III, VI, and IX, in which glycogen can be stored in the liver but not efficiently returned to glucose. The patient most commonly develops hepatomegaly (from stored glycogen), and interprandial hypoglycemia begins within a few hours of eating, when circulating fuels are exhausted. The patient may also manifest "cherubic" cheeks from glycogen storage. Other findings can include elevations in triglycerides, uric acid, and lactate. There are a number of

Table 1-10	Common Findings in Disorders of Carbohydrate Metabolism
Disorder	**Findings**
GSD 0	Postprandial hyperglycemia, interprandial hypoglycemia
GSD I	Interprandial hypoglycemia, hepatomegaly, "cherub" cheeks, neutropenia (type 1b), elevated uric acid, lactate
GSD II	Pompe's disease, cardiomyopathy (infantile form), progressive skeletal and respiratory weakness, elevated CK
GSD III	Hypoglycemia, hepatomegaly, variable myopathy, disorder of glycogen debranching
GSD IV	Hepatomegaly, cirrhosis, disorder of glycogen branching
GSD VI and IX	Hepatomegaly with variable mild hypoglycemia, variable myopathy
Fructose-1,6-bisphosphatase deficiency	Hypoglycemia with prolonged fast/intercurrent illness, may be fructose sensitive, urine organic acids may reveal keto-lactic acidosis with elevated glycerol
Galactosemia	Untreated: Hepatomegaly, cataracts, failure to thrive, liver dysfunction, MR Treated: Variable cognitive deficits
Hereditary fructose intolerance	With fructose ingestion: Hypoglycemia, hypophosphatemia, shock Untreated: Chronic liver disease and failure to thrive

CK, creatine kinase; GSD, glycogen storage disease; MR, mental retardation.

enzymes involved in the formation, branching, debranching, and catabolism of glycogen, and various subtypes of glycogen storage disease are associated with defects in the various enzymatic steps. Some glycogen disorders present predominantly in muscle with weakness, rhabdomyolysis, and other predominantly muscle findings but not significant hypoglycemia. Infantile-onset Pompe's disease (glycogen storage disease type II) presents with progressive weakness in the skeletal and respiratory muscles as well as cardiomyopathy. The electrocardiogram demonstrates a characteristic high-voltage pattern. Some patients with residual enzyme protein respond to enzyme replacement therapy.

Carbohydrate Metabolism: Defects in Glycolysis, Gluconeogenesis, and Metabolism of Other Carbohydrates

Glycolysis, the process of metabolizing glucose to pyruvate, does not have commonly associated inborn errors of metabolism. However, in some cases alternative carbohydrates (such as galactose or fructose) have impaired conversion into a glycolytic substrate.

Galactosemia. Patients who are unable to metabolize galactose have *galactosemia*. After ingestion of galactose (one of the sugars in lactose), patients can present in infancy with hepatomegaly, liver disease, gram-negative sepsis, cataracts, or later with failure to thrive and excretion of galactose (a reducing substance) in the urine. Treatment includes exclusion of galactose from the diet.

Hereditary Fructose Intolerance. Patients with *hereditary fructose intolerance* are unable to metabolize fructose (a common fruit sugar and one of the components of sucrose). They can present with acute decompensation with hypoglycemia and hypophosphatemia from fructose ingestion, but can also present chronically with failure to thrive and liver disease.

Gluconeogenesis. The reverse of glycolysis (*gluconeogenesis*, the production of glucose from distal metabolic substrates) can be impaired by metabolic errors. *Fructose-1,6-bisphosphatase deficiency* is a gluconeogenic enzyme deficiency that results in fasting hypoglycemia. Patients typically tolerate an interprandial fast because glycogen metabolism is intact, but are at risk for hypoglycemia after glycogen stores are exhausted. Most patients present in infancy during an intercurrent illness with hypoglycemia and varying degrees of elevated ketones, lactate, and glycerol.

Other defects in gluconeogenesis as well as ketone synthesis and use disorders are described in more detailed texts.

Defects of Fatty Acid Oxidation

Fatty acid oxidation is a significant source of energy after liver glycogen stores are exhausted. Fatty acids are essentially chains of carbon atoms. β-Oxidation of fatty acids up to 18 carbons in length takes place in the mitochondria. One cycle of β-oxidation removes two carbons from the fat, releasing the two-carbon piece as *acetyl-CoA* (a primary substrate for the Krebs cycle), which also can be converted to a *ketone body* that can be exported to more distal tissues for energy (see Fig. 1-54). The shortened fatty acid undergoes successive cycles of oxidation removing two-carbon units at a time until it is fully metabolized. The enzymes used in fatty acid oxidation change as the fatty acid becomes successively shorter. Absence of ketosis in a patient older than 3 months of age who has hypoglycemia or is undergoing a stressful fast should raise concern for a possible fatty acid oxidation defect. Some of the most common defects of fatty acid oxidation are listed in Table 1-11.

Table 1-11	Common Findings in Fatty Acid Oxidation Disorders
Disorder	**Findings**
Carnitine uptake disorder	Cardiomyopathy, variable weakness, sudden death
CPT I	Infantile onset: Hypoglycemia, acidosis Later onset: Fasting intolerance, exercise intolerance
CPT II	Infantile onset: Hypoglycemia, acidosis Later onset: Fasting or exercise intolerance, rhabdomyolysis
SCAD deficiency	Possible hypotonia, developmental delay, neurologic abnormalities. Phenotype now in question
MCAD deficiency	Potentially fatal hypoglycemia with prolonged fasting
VLCAD deficiency	Infantile onset: Cardiomyopathy, juvenile onset: fasting intolerance Later onset: Exercise intolerance
LCHAD deficiency	Hypoglycemia, rhabdomyolysis, pigmentary retinopathy, fasting intolerance

CPT I and CPT II, carnitine palmitoyltransferase I and II; LCHAD, long-chain 3-hydroxyacyl-CoA dehydrogenase; MCAD, medium-chain acyl-CoA dehydrogenase; SCAD, short-chain acyl-CoA dehydrogenase; VLCAD, very long–chain acyl-CoA dehydrogenase.

Defects of Fatty Acid Oxidation: Carnitine Disorders

Defects of Fatty Acid Transport: Carnitine Uptake Disorder and CPT I, CACT, and CPT II Deficiency. *Long-chain fatty acids* (that is, those having approximately 12 to 18 carbons) must first esterify carnitine in order to pass through the mitochondrial membrane for oxidation. Patients with *carnitine uptake disorder* have impaired transport of carnitine and develop profound carnitine deficiency. Symptoms can include cardiomyopathy, weakness, or simply sudden death. Plasma carnitine levels are very low while urine carnitine is generally elevated. Patients with a *deficiency of carnitine palmitoyltransferase I* (CPT I) are unable to esterify fatty acids to carnitine. The fatty acids are thus unable to penetrate the mitochondria for oxidation. The disorder has variable presentation, including life-threatening neonatal hypoglycemia and acidosis, or later onset fasting or exercise intolerance/rhabdomyolysis. Biochemically, the patient has low levels of acylcarnitines in the plasma. Defects in the *carnitine-acylcarnitine translocase* (CACT) enzyme (which carries fatty acylcarnitines across the mitochondrial membrane) are rare but reported and can be life-threatening; they often resemble CPT II deficiency. Patients with defects in *carnitine palmitoyltransferase II* (CPT II) are unable to release the carnitine from the fatty acid after it has passed inside the mitochondria. Like CPT I deficiency, it has variable severity and can present at any age. Biochemically, patients have elevated acylcarnitines in the plasma. Most carnitine disorders are now diagnosed by newborn screening (by measurement of acylcarnitines), and more mildly affected patients often do not appear ill in the newborn period but still require follow-up and treatment. Carnitine is not required for medium- and short-chain fatty acids to penetrate the mitochondria, and thus patients with severe carnitine disorders may benefit from dietary restriction of long-chain fat and supplementation with medium-chain fat.

Defects of Fatty Acid Oxidation: Acyl-CoA Dehydrogenase Deficiencies

VLCAD, MCAD, SCAD, and LCHAD Deficiency. Inside the mitochondria, the β-oxidation process progressively removes two carbon atoms, forming ketones or acetyl-CoA (see Fig. 1-54). Many of the enzymes in this process have chain length specificity, preferring fats that are long chain (12 to 18 carbons), medium chain (6 to 10 carbons), or short chain. The first step of β-oxidation is performed by an acyl-CoA dehydrogenase with chain length specificity. Deficits in the long-chain enzyme (*very long–chain acyl-CoA dehydrogenase deficiency,* also known as VLCAD or ACADVL deficiency) present with variable severity, from neonatal cardiomyopathy, to later onset fasting or exercise intolerance. Genotype–phenotype correlations between residual enzyme activity and severity are emerging. Treatment includes supplementation with medium-chain fat and prevention of fasting. Defects in the medium-chain enzyme (*medium-chain acyl-CoA dehydrogenase deficiency,* also known as MCAD or ACADM deficiency) are among the most common metabolic disorders (approximately 1 in 15,000 births). Affected patients most commonly present in the toddler period with potentially fatal hypoketotic hypoglycemia or Reye's syndrome–like symptoms during fasting associated with an intercurrent illness. Treatment is primarily by prevention of fasting, although some patients require carnitine supplementation. Defects in the short-chain enzyme (*short-chain acyl-CoA dehydrogenase deficiency,* also known as SCAD or ACADS deficiency) were originally believed to cause hypotonia, hypoglycemia, and developmental abnormalities. However, the clinical significance of this disorder is now in question. Defects are also described in the third step of β-oxidation, another acyl-CoA dehydrogenase enzyme with chain length specificity. The most common enzyme deficiency at this step is *long-chain 3-hydroxyacyl-CoA dehydrogenase (LCHAD) deficiency.* This disorder can also have variable presentation from early hypoketotic hypoglycemia to later fasting or exercise intolerance. More severely affected patients demonstrate a pigmentary retinopathy and episodes of rhabdomyolysis. An increased incidence of HELLP syndrome is reported in pregnant mothers carrying an affected fetus. Some patients have a deficiency of a trifunctional protein that results in defects in multiple steps of the long-chain fatty acid oxidation pathway.

Most disorders of fatty acid oxidation are now detected on newborn screening. However, some infants experience significant morbidity or mortality quickly (early presentation), before the newborn screening results are available. Thus, this group of disorders should always be considered in ill neonates.

Organelle Dysfunction

Important metabolic processes take place in various organelles. These include the *peroxisomes,* the *lysosomes,* and the *mitochondria* (Tables 1-12 through 1-14). Defects in each of these organelles are considered.

Table 1-12 | Common Findings in Peroxisomal Diseases

Disorder	Findings
Zellweger syndrome	Hepatomegaly, profound hypotonia, Down syndrome–like facies, liver dysfunction
Neonatal adrenoleukodystrophy; infantile Refsum disease	Developmental delay, hearing loss, vision impairment, liver dysfunction, coagulopathy, hypotonia of decreasing severity; often slowly progressive
RCDP	Rhizomelia, chondrodysplasia punctata, profound growth failure, and MR
Adrenoleukodystrophy	Developmental regression, progressive leukodystrophy; later onset with demyelination or Addison disease
Adult Refsum disease	Retinitis pigmentosa, ataxia, ichthyosis, and anosmia

MR, mental retardation; RCDP, rhizomelic chondrodysplasia punctata.

Table 1-13 | Classification of Lysosomal Storage Disorders

Disorder Class	Underlying Defect
Mucopolysaccharidoses	Defective metabolism of glycosaminoglycans
Sphingolipidoses and sulfatidoses	Defective degradation of sphingolipids and their components
Glycogen storage diseases	Defective degradation of glycogen
Oligosaccharidoses	Defective degradation of the glycan portion of glycoproteins
Mucolipidoses	Defective degradation of acid mucopolysaccharides, sphingolipids, and/or glycolipids
Defects in degradation or transport of cholesterol, cholesterol esters and other complex lipids	
Lysosomal transport and trafficking defects	

Peroxisomal Disorders

A number of metabolic processes take place in the peroxisome, including the oxidation of very long–chain fats (greater than 20 carbons), metabolism of phytanic acid (present in food), initiation of plasmalogen formation (the most abundant phospholipid in myelin), peroxidation/detoxification,

Table 1-14 | Common Mitochondrial Syndromes

Symptom Complex	Findings	Pathology
MERRF	Mitochondrial encephalopathy, ragged red fibers	tRNA^{Lys}
MELAS	Myoclonic epilepsy, lactic acidosis, stroke-like episodes	>15 mutations described; the most common involves tRNA^{Leu}
NARP	Neuropathy, ataxia, retinitis pigmentosa, ± Leigh disease	Point mutations in mitochondrial component of complex V
MNGIE	Myo-neuro-gastrointestinal disorder and encephalopathy	Nuclear mutation in thymidine phosphorylase; impairs mitochondrial DNA repair mechanisms
LHON	Leber hereditary optic neuropathy	Mutations in mitochondrial component of complex I
Pearson syndrome	Bone marrow–pancreas dysfunction, infantile onset; survivors may develop Kearns-Sayre syndrome	Multiple mitochondrial DNA deletions
Kearns-Sayre syndrome	Ptosis, pigmentary retinopathy, cardiac conduction defects, ataxia, diabetes, CPEO	Multiple mitochondrial DNA deletions
Diabetes-deafness	Type 2 diabetes, hearing loss	Mitochondrial tRNA^{Leu}
Aminoglycoside toxicity	Ototoxicity from aminoglycoside antibiotics	Mitochondrial ribosomal DNA mutations
Leigh disease	Necrotizing changes in basal ganglia and midbrain, hypotonia, failure to thrive, loss of respiratory centers; phenotype caused by numerous underlying energy disorders	Defects in nuclear or mitochondrial genes in complexes I, II, and IV; PDH; PC; NARP; and others

CPEO, chronic progressive external ophthalmoplegia; NARP, neuropathy, ataxia, and retinitis pigmentosa; PC, pyruvate carboxylase; PDH, pyruvate dehydrogenase.

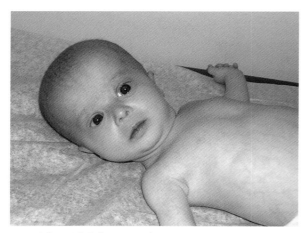

Figure 1-55   Infant with Zellweger syndrome. Note the hypotonia, failure to thrive, and large forehead.

and other processes. Peroxisomal diseases fall into two major categories: those that interfere with assembly of the peroxisome itself (thus affecting all enzyme functions), and those that affect a single enzyme.

Disorders of Peroxisome Biogenesis

A number of mutations in 12 different peroxisome assembly (*PEX*) genes have been identified, leading to a continuum of phenotypes. The most severe of these disorders is *Zellweger syndrome* (Fig. 1-55). Infants with Zellweger syndrome (cerebrohepatorenal syndrome) typically have dysmorphic features often suggestive of Down syndrome, hepatomegaly with liver dysfunction, and profound hypotonia (see Table 1-12). The disorder is typically fatal in infancy or early childhood. *Neonatal adrenal leukodystrophy* and *infantile Refsum disease* are less severe phenotypes. They present with variable severity of developmental delay, hearing loss, vision impairment, liver dysfunction, coagulopathy, and hypotonia and may be slowly progressive (see Table 1-12). Mutations in *PEX7* can lead to a unique phenotype of proximal limb shortening (rhizomelia), chondrodysplasia punctata, and profound growth failure and mental retardation, known as *rhizomelic chondrodysplasia punctata* (RCDP).

Single-Gene Disorders

Numerous disorders of single genes that act in the peroxisome have been described. One of the most common is *X-linked adrenoleukodystrophy*. This disorder predominantly affects males and presents in the first decade of life as a progressive leukodystrophy, or in adulthood as a demyelinating disorder *(adrenomyeloneuropathy)* or *Addison's disease.* The movie "Lorenzo's Oil" increased public recognition of this disorder and the quest for a treatment. Treatment with dietary very long–chain fatty acid restriction and supplementation with erucic acid and oleic acid ("Lorenzo's oil") may be of some benefit in limiting progression if given presymptomatically. Another single-gene disorder, *adult Refsum disease* (ARD), presents with retinitis pigmentosa, ataxia, ichthyosis, and anosmia, and is caused by a defect in the metabolism of phytanic acid.

Diagnosis

Most peroxisomal assembly or single-gene disorders can be diagnosed by evaluating plasma *very long–chain fatty acids,* preferably supplementing testing with red cell plasmalogens, phytanic acid, pipecolic acid, or pristanic acid. (*Note:* Phytanic acid is derived from the diet, and thus young infants or those on elemental diets may have falsely normal levels). It is

important to note that in some single-gene disorders, including RCDP and ARD, very long–chain fatty acid levels may be normal. However, plasmalogens are abnormal in RCDP, and phytanic acid is elevated in ARD. Thus, it is reasonable to test for at least two peroxisomal metabolites when searching for these disorders. DNA analysis is available for a number of peroxisome biogenesis or single-gene disorders.

Lysosomal Disorders

Lysosomes are membrane-bound cytoplasmic organelles that serve as the digestive or recycling plants of cells, their major purposes being to break down cellular waste products and debris and to degrade macromolecules that are no longer needed into smaller components. They perform this function with an array of hydrolytic enzymes that degrade their target molecules in a stepwise fashion. Once the process of degradation is completed, the residual material is transported to the cytoplasm for recycling (as new molecular building blocks) or to the cell membrane for removal. A mutation that results in malfunction of a lysosomal enzyme leads to accumulation of substrate, resulting in the term *storage disorder*. Over time the volume of the stored undegraded substrate increases, progressively distending the lysosome, and ultimately this impairs cell function.

Disorders of Trafficking or Single Lysosomal Enzymes

After translocation and posttranslational modifications, lysosomal enzymes are targeted to the lysosome by specific target sequences. Defects in enzyme trafficking to the lysosome, or in single lysosomal enzymes, result in lysosomal storage disorders. Disorders are classified according to the nature of the accumulated material. More than 40 lysosomal disorders have been described, their unifying characteristic being a failure to degrade a specific component of cellular waste. Defects are classified as defects of degradation of mucopolysaccharides, oligosaccharides, sphingolipidoses, mucolipidoses, and others (see Table 1-13). Stored lysosomal material in tissues can result in coarsening of facial features, hepatomegaly, splenomegaly, bone deformities (dysostosis multiplex), leukodystrophy, and other features. Among the most severe lysosomal disorders is *I-cell disease,* in which many lysosomal enzymes lack the proper sequence for targeting to the lysosome, such that certain lysosomal enzymes are elevated in plasma but are not present within the lysosome. This disorder has a very early prenatal or early infantile onset and is associated with early mortality.

Mucopolysaccharidoses

The *mucopolysaccharidoses* are among the best known lysosomal storage disorders. They are a group of disorders of degradation of glycosaminoglycans, long chains of repeating disaccharide units that are synthesized by connective tissue cells as structural components of connective tissue, bone, cartilage, synovial fluid, skin, cornea, and the reticuloendothelial system. Seven major types have been identified, some with multiple subtypes. Hurler syndrome (type IH) is the prototypical disorders (Fig. 1-56). In the most severe form, onset is between 6 and 24 months with growth retardation, coarse facial features, hepatosplenomegaly, dysostosis multiplex, cardiac valve disease, and other findings. Enzyme replacement therapy can help temporize treatment, but the only significant treatment for infantile onset disease is by bone marrow transplantation, which stabilizes the disorder but does not improve bony abnormalities. Progressively less severe forms include Hurler-Scheie and Scheie syndromes, with increasing residual enzyme activity and decreasing CNS and systemic involvement. Enzyme replacement therapy provides long-term benefits, although bone and joint disease remain

Figure 1-56 Hurler syndrome. **A,** The coarsening of facial features characteristic of this disorder includes prominence of the forehead, a flattened nasal bridge, a short broad nose, and widening of the lips. Features appear puffy due to thickening of the skin. **B,** Progressive joint stiffness and contractures lead to clawing of the hand.

prominent and heart valve damage can continue to progress. Morquio syndrome is associated with sparing of cognition, but presents with typical bony dysplasia (Fig. 1-57).

Diagnosis

Diagnosis of lysosomal disorders typically begins with clinical suspicion, often with assay of urinary mucopolysaccharides or oligosaccharides, specific plasma or fibroblast enzyme assays, or DNA studies depending on the suspected disorder. A complete discussion of all of the mucopolysaccharidoses, oligosaccharidoses, sphingolipidoses, and mucolipidoses is beyond the scope of this chapter but is available in texts dedicated to metabolic disorders.

Figure 1-57 A 5-year-old boy with Morquio syndrome. Urine testing for mucopolysaccharidosis (MPS) showed elevated keratan sulfate.

Disorders of Energy Metabolism: Mitochondrial Disorders

The mitochondria are the sites of *energy metabolism*. Numerous disorders of energy metabolism are described, with their underlying pathology as insufficient availability of energy to tissues. Thus, the tissues and organs most affected by mitochondrial dysfunction are those with high energy demands, particularly neural, muscular, and ocular.

Mitochondria are membrane-bound cytoplasmic organelles that, in essence, serve as the power plants of cells. Because all of one's mitochondria are derived from those present in the oocyte (those of the sperm having been destroyed on fertilization), all mitochondrial DNA (mtDNA) is inherited from one's mother. However, most proteins that act in the mitochondria are nuclear in origin; they are transported into the mitochondria, where they carry out their intended function. Thus most "mitochondrial" disorders actually follow a mendelian pattern of inheritance. However, as each mitochondrion also contains its own separate genome with a maternally inherited, unique DNA code (including 13 genes that function in oxidative phosphorylation as well as its own transfer RNA and replication mechanism), a few mitochondrial disorders have maternal, not nuclear, inheritance.

Lactic Acidosis

Under ordinary circumstances, *pyruvate* enters the Krebs cycle either through conversion to acetyl-CoA by *pyruvate dehydrogenase* (PDH), or through conversion to oxaloacetate by *pyruvate carboxylase* (PC) (see Fig. 1-54). The NADH created in the Krebs cycle is then passed to the electron transport chain for *oxidative phosphorylation* and the production of ATP. The metabolism of 1 molecule of glucose creates a net of 36 ATP molecules. When oxidative phosphorylation is insufficient to meet the body's energy needs, pyruvate is diverted to *lactate,* a conversion that results in a net of only two ATP. *Lactic acidosis* occurs when lactate builds up, and is most commonly secondary to shock, hypoxia, or exercise beyond the body's aerobic capacity. Secondary lactic acidosis can also be caused by tissue hypoxia secondary to use of a tourniquet or excessive crying, or from prolonged storage of room temperature blood samples in a Vacutainer. Secondary elevation of lactate from poor conditions of specimen drawing or handling can lead to invasive and unnecessary testing and procedures, and can be avoided by use of free-flowing or arterial specimens, avoiding multiple draw attempts, and rapid transport of the immediately iced specimen to the laboratory. Pyruvate can also be converted into the amino acid *alanine*. The presence of elevated alanine indicated by plasma or serum amino acid analysis, and/or the presence of elevated lactate or pyruvate on urine organic acid analysis, is suggestive of chronic lactic acidosis even if a plasma lactate measurement is within normal limits.

In some cases, lactic acidosis is not secondary to external factors, but is caused by a primary disorder of energy production. Disorders of primary lactic acidosis usually occur in the metabolism of pyruvate, the Krebs cycle, or during oxidative phosphorylation, and are often referred to broadly as *mitochondrial disorders*.

Disorders of Pyruvate Metabolism

Pyruvate Dehydrogenase Deficiency

Pyruvate is converted to acetyl-CoA by the enzyme *pyruvate dehydrogenase complex* (PDH or PDC) (see Fig. 1-54). PDH is composed of at least four proteins: E1α, E1β, E2, and E3. Defects are most common in the E1α component. The gene encoding this enzyme component is X-linked, but defects in the enzyme are commonly inherited in an autosomal dominant pattern, and thus the number of affected girls with de novo mutations is nearly equal to the number of affected boys; female gender should therefore not rule out this diagnosis. PDH deficiency results in a wide range of effects of varying severity, in some cases manifesting as ataxia and seizures or mild to moderate developmental delay. However, more severe forms can present with lactic acidosis and structural abnormalities of the CNS attributable to prenatal cellular death from energy deficiency, ranging from agenesis of the corpus callosum to profound hydrocephalus.

Pyruvate Carboxylase Deficiency

Pyruvate carboxylase (PC) deficiency can present with mild to severe keto-lactic acidosis, hyperammonemia, and other problems, and can be fatal in early life, or can present more chronically with intermittent keto-lactic acidosis during fasting. Either PDH or PC deficiency (as well as other oxidative phosphorylation disorders) can present as Leigh's disease, a phenotype of progressive cystic degeneration of the basal ganglia and the respiratory centers that reflects profound impairment of energy production in the brain. Infants with profound disorders of pyruvate metabolism sometimes have nonspecific dysmorphic features such as a long philtrum and tented upper lip, probably due to facial hypotonia.

Disorders of the Krebs Cycle

Primary disorders of the *Krebs cycle* are rare, but are typically associated with specific findings on urine organic acid analysis. The presence of small to modest amounts of Krebs cycle intermediates on urine organic acid analysis can be normal in the first year of life. The presence of large elevations or persistent excretion of Krebs cycle intermediates in the urine can signal a disorder of oxidative phosphorylation.

Disorders of Oxidative Phosphorylation

Oxidative phosphorylation (also known as the *electron transport chain*) refers to the process of production of energy (ATP). It takes place in the mitochondria using both nuclearly and mitochondrially encoded enzymes. The enzymatic functions are grouped into complexes. Complex I is composed of more than 40 different enzymes, of which 7 are mitochondrially encoded. Although the vast majority of proteins in other complexes are also nuclearly encoded, mitochondrially encoded proteins are also present in complex III (one), complex IV (three), and complex V (two). A number of defects in the various complexes, both nuclear or mitochondrially encoded, present with a variety of symptoms including developmental delay, failure to thrive, myopathy, hypotonia, ptosis, ophthalmoplegia, hepatopathy, encephalopathy, nephropathy, pigmentary retinopathy, and/or Leigh's disease.

Nuclear Mutations

Most mitochondrial disorders are due to mutations in nuclearly encoded proteins, and are inherited in a mendelian pattern. DNA testing is available for many of these disorders, particularly for complex I and IV deficiency and for various gene mutations responsible for Leigh's disease.

There are also some nuclear genes involved in mitochondrial replication that lead to aberrant mitochondrial replication and/or mitochondrial depletion (e.g., Alpers' syndrome, caused by defects in the gene encoding DNA polymerase subunit γ [PolG1], which results in mitochondrial depletion and is associated with liver disease and cerebral degeneration).

The *TAZ* gene is an X-linked gene encoding cardiolipin, a component of the inner mitochondrial membrane. Mutations in *TAZ* cause Barth syndrome, an X-linked disorder causing infantile cardioskeletal myopathy (commonly non-compaction) and neutropenia.

Mitochondrial Point Mutations

Mutations in the mitochondrial genome are also a cause of mitochondrial dysfunction and are maternally inherited. These mutations can occur in any of the 13 mitochondrial genes involved in oxidative phosphorylation, or can also occur in the transfer RNA, ribosomal RNA, or replicative machinery. Note that whereas each cell contains only one nucleus housing two copies of the genome, each cell also contains multiple mitochondria, and each mitochondrion contains multiple copies of the mitochondrial genome; because of this, nuclear and mitochondrial inheritance patterns are different. Thus individuals can have multiple copies of both wild-type and mutated mitochondrial genomes coexisting in a single mitochondrion or in a single cell; this is known as *heteroplasmy*. There is a *threshold effect* at which point the number of mutated mitochondria becomes sufficient to affect the function of the cell, tissue, or organ. It is therefore possible for syndromic mitochondrial mutations to be maternally inherited in multiple family members, but symptomatic only in those in whom the threshold is reached.

Mitochondrial point mutations can present with variable severity. In adults they often appear in recognizable syndrome patterns. In children they may follow a specific phenotype, but can also be multisystemic and less predictable. One example of a recognizable phenotype is *MELAS syndrome* (mitochondrial myopathy, encephalopathy, lactic acidosis and stroke-like episodes), most commonly due to a specific point mutation in the mitochondrial transfer RNA for leucine (tRNA^{Leu}; see Table 1-14). Other common mitochondrial syndromes associated with point mutations are listed in Table 1-14 as well. In contrast to vascular strokes, strokes due to mitochondrial disease do not typically follow a watershed pattern. Instead, they represent cell death from energy failure rather than blood flow abnormalities. Metabolic strokes can occur anywhere in the brain, although the highest energy-requiring parts of the brain (such as the basal ganglia) are common locations.

Evaluation of a Patient with Suspected Mitochondrial Disease

Traditionally, a patient suspected of having a mitochondrial disease undergoes biopsy of an apparently affected organ (typically muscle) for analysis of the oxidative phosphorylation complexes. However, the expanding availability of testing for mutations in nuclear and mitochondrial genes has created an evolving testing strategy. A testing algorithm can be linked from the Mitochondrial Medicine Society website (http://www.mitosoc.org/blogs/diagnosis), with the full algorithm currently available at the Baylor College of Medicine Medical Genetics Laboratories website (http://www.bcm.edu/geneticlabs/; under "Resources" tab). In some cases, diagnosis can be reached on the basis of guided testing of blood samples, sparing patients an invasive biopsy.

Other Inborn Errors of Metabolism

A number of other inborn errors of metabolism have been identified. These include disorders of metal metabolism (e.g., Menkes disease, Wilson's disease, and others), transport defects (e.g., cystinuria, Hartnup disease), disorders of protein glycosylation (CDG; see below), disorders of cholesterol biosynthesis/sterol metabolism (e.g., Smith-Lemli-Opitz syndrome and others), disorders of biotin and other vitamins, disorders of purines and pyrimidines (e.g., Lesch-Nyhan syndrome), and others.

Menkes Disease

Menkes disease is one disorder of metal metabolism. Failure to absorb copper in the intestine leads to systemic copper deficiency and impairment of copper-dependent mitochondrial enzymes. The disorder is X-linked (the *ATP7A* gene on the long arm of the X chromosome), and thus most affected patients are male. The disorder most commonly presents in infancy with loss of milestones, seizures, mental retardation, tortuous cerebral arteries, sagging facial skin, and weakened bones with fractures that may raise concern for child abuse until the proper diagnosis is made. Hair is coarse and sparse, classically referred to as "kinky." The life span is greatly shortened, to only a few years. Parenteral copper administered to presymptomatic boys may improve outcome, but seems of minimal to no benefit once symptoms have developed (Fig. 1-58).

Congenital Disorders of Glycosylation

Congenital disorders of glycosylation (CDG) are a group of disorders resulting in abnormal posttranslational glycosylation of proteins. To date more than 15 subtypes have been described, each corresponding to an enzymatic step in the protein glycosylation pathway. The most common is CDG type Ia. Typical features include abnormal fat pads on the pubis and over the buttocks, inverted nipples, strabismus, cerebellar atrophy, and failure to thrive. Fatal systemic disease including liver disease can be seen in some cases; others tend to develop ataxia and stroke-like episodes with age. Other subtypes can present with varying features including protein-losing enteropathy, dysmorphic features, and various multisystem presentations. Diagnosis is achieved by noting an abnormal ferritin isoelectric focusing pattern (caused by abnormalities in posttranslational sialic acid residues). This disorder is likely underappreciated and should be considered in any case of multisystem genetic symptoms (Fig. 1-59).

Disorders of Sterol Metabolism

A number of disorders are now associated with various defects in the biosynthesis of cholesterol. Many of these were first described as dysmorphic syndromes before the underlying biochemical abnormality was identified. The prototype disorder is *Smith-Lemli-Opitz syndrome.*

Infants with Smith-Lemli-Opitz syndrome have a defect in the *sonic hedgehog* gene (Fig. 1-60). This gene is involved in limb formation and cholesterol biosynthesis. The biochemical error is a block in the final step of cholesterol formation, with deficiency of cholesterol and accumulation of the precursor 7-dehydrocholesterol. Typical dysmorphic features include upturned nose, low-set ears, and characteristic clenched hands. Affected patients typically have syndactyly of the second and third toes, and can have polydactyly, presumably a direct effect of the gene defect. Some phenotypic findings, such as undervirilization of males, are attributable to cholesterol deficiency causing deficiency of cholesterol-based steroid

Figure 1-58 **A** and **B,** Menkes syndrome associated with seizures, hypotonia, hypopigmentation, global delays, and low serum copper and ceruloplasmin levels. DNA testing showed a splicing defect in the *ATP7A* gene at Xq13.3 region, confirming the clinical finding.

Figure 1-59   **A,** Inverted nipples and **B,** unusual fat distribution on the buttocks seen in some patients with congenital disorders of glycosylation.

hormones. In some cases CNS findings improve with cholesterol supplementation.

There are a number of other disorders in other steps in cholesterol biosynthesis that have various physical and developmental findings. X-linked dominant chondrodysplasia punctata *(Conradi-Hünermann-Happle syndrome)* is believed lethal in males and is associated with mutations in sterol isomerase (emopamil-binding protein; EBP) in females. This results in elevated levels of 8-dehydrocholesterol and 8(9)-cholesterol. Findings include chondrodysplasia punctata, asymmetric limb shortening, scoliosis, and scaly erythematous rash along the

Figure 1-61   Patient with methylmalonic acidemia; note the prominent, simple ears; hypotonia; and midfacial hypoplasia.

lines of Blaschko in infancy that can change into ichthyosis, scarring alopecia, and pigmentary abnormalities.

Inborn Errors of Metabolism and Dysmorphic Features

Some metabolic disorders, particularly CDG and sterol biosynthesis disorders, were originally described as dysmorphic syndromes before the biochemical defect underlying the disorder was understood. The presence of dysmorphic features does not necessarily rule out an underlying metabolic error. As previously noted, infants with Zellweger syndrome often have facial and tone characteristics suggestive of Down syndrome (although the hepatomegaly and other features are distinguishing). Chondrodysplasia punctata can have various metabolic causes, including peroxisomal (severe rhizomelic form with failure to thrive and systemic disease) or sterol (X-linked dominant chondrodysplasia punctata). Children with organic acidemias and children with disorders of energy metabolism are often reported to have "mitochondrial facies" including nonspecific features possibly caused by poor muscle tone such as midfacial hypotonia and prominent ears (Fig. 1-61). Patients with a variety of lysosomal storage diseases often are described as having "coarse" facial features, likely attributable to cellular accumulation of lysosomal material. New research is adding to the list of dysmorphic syndromes having an underlying metabolic etiology, and clearly the presence of dysmorphic features should not necessarily rule out a metabolic disorder.

NEWBORN SCREENING FOR GENETIC DISORDERS

Newborn screening began in the mid-1960s for phenylketonuria when an inexpensive test became available (Robert Guthrie's bacterial inhibition assay, performed with a few drops of

Figure 1-60   Smith-Lemli-Opitz syndrome. **A,** Note the anteverted nostrils, low-set ears, small chin, and clenched hand. **B,** Hypospadias, cryptorchidism, or ambiguous genitalia as shown here may also be seen. *(Courtesy W. Tunnessen, MD.)*

Table 1-15	Secretary's Advisory Committee on Heritable Diseases of Newborns and Children Recommended Uniform Screening Panel: Primary and Secondary Target Disorders

Core Conditions	Secondary Conditions
Propionic acidemia	Methylmalonic acidemia with homocystinuria (Cbl C, D)
Methylmalonic acidemia and cobalamin A, B	Malonic acidemia
Isovaleric acidemia	Isobutyrylglycinuria
3-MCC deficiency	2-Methylbutyrylglycinuria
3-Hydroxy-3-methylglutaric (HMG) aciduria	3-Methylglutaconic aciduria
	2-Methyl-3-hydroxybutyric aciduria
β-Ketothiolase deficiency	Short-chain acyl-CoA dehydrogenase deficiency
Glutaric acidemia type I	
Carnitic uptake/transporter defect	Medium/short-chain L-3-hydroxyacyl-CoA dehydrogenase deficiency
Medium-chain acyl-CoA dehydrogenase deficiency	Glutaric acidemia type II
Very long–chain acyl-CoA dehydrogenase deficiency	Medium-chain ketoacyl-CoA thiolase deficiency
Long-chain L-3 hydroxyacyl-CoA dehydrogenase deficiency	2,4-Dienoyl-CoA reductase deficiency
Trifunctional protein deficiency	Carnitine palmitoyltransferase type I deficiency
Argininosuccinic aciduria	Carnitine palmitoyltransferase type II deficiency
Citrullinemia type I	
Maple syrup urine disease	Carnitine acylcarnitine translocase deficiency
Homocystinuria	Argininemia
Classic phenylketonuria	Citrullinemia type II
Tyrosinemia type I	Hypermethioninemia
Primary congenital hypothyroidism	Benign hyperphenylalaninemia
Congenital adrenal hyperplasia	Biopterin defect in cofactor synthesis
Sickle cell disease	Biopterin defect in cofactor regeneration
Sickle-beta thalassemia	
Sickle-C disease	Tyrosinemia type II
Biotinidase deficiency	Tyrosinemia type III
Critical cyanotic congenital heart disease	Other hemoglobinopathies
	Galactoepimerase deficiency
Cystic fibrosis	Galactokinase deficiency
Classic galactosemia	T-cell–related lymphocyte deficiencies
Hearing loss	
Severe combined immunodeficiencies	

Note 1: For an updated list see http://www.hrsa.gov/advisorycommittees/mchbadvisory/heritabledisorders/recommendedpanel/index.html.

Note 2: Primary care physicians, other pediatric subspecialties, and family practitioners can access the algorithms for the responsibilities as well as immediate management by following the AAP policy statement on newborn screening (2008). Newborn Screening Authoring Committee: Newborn screening expands: recommendations for pediatricians and medical homes—implications for the system. *Pediatrics* 121:192-217, 2008.

Note 3: A reference that the clinicians may find helpful for newborn screening is *Contemporary Pediatrics*, 28:38-47, 2011.

blood on filter paper), and it was demonstrated that early detection and treatment were a cost-effective way to prevent mental retardation. Thyroid testing and other disorders were added over the years. Newborn screening for common genetic and metabolic diseases has been revolutionized by the development of *tandem mass spectrometry*. This technique, requiring only a dried blood spot from the newborn, provides an inexpensive mechanism by which to test for a much larger range of inherited metabolic disorders. In the United States, newborn screening is conducted and regulated by the individual states, and some states now screen for more than 50 disorders.

Disorders detectable by newborn screening include inborn errors of metabolism, hemoglobinopathies, cystic fibrosis, acquired immune deficiency, severe combined immunodeficiency, hearing loss, hypothyroidism, and congenital adrenal hyperplasia. The American College of Medical Genetics has published information sheets for physicians on these disorders (available at the website http://www.acmg.net/AM/Template.cfm?Section=NBS_ACT_Sheets_and_Algorithms_Table&Template=/CM/HTMLDisplay.cfm&ContentID=5072).

This site provides information about the disorders and recommended diagnostic testing.

The technical ability to diagnose genetic and metabolic disorders by newborn screening has outpaced our understanding of the natural history and optimal treatment of some of these disorders. In 2003 the Secretary of Health convened the Secretary's Advisory Committee on Heritable Disorders in Newborns and Children to develop advisory guidelines for newborn screening. The committee developed a list of primary target disorders based on evidence-based guidelines, as well as a list of secondary disorders, which are routinely detectable as part of the testing process for primary target diseases (Table 1-15). New disorders are added to the primary target list after an evidence-based review process. At present, states are not obligated to follow the committee's guidelines.

It is important to remember that newborn screening is a screening program, not a diagnostic program. Not all inborn errors of metabolism are detectable by newborn screening (e.g., some urea cycle defects), and as a screening program it does not have 100% sensitivity. Thus no disorder should be considered "ruled out" in a symptomatic child because of a normal newborn screen result. Screen-positive infants are referred for diagnostic testing. Some cases require a repeat screen, but in some cases results are sufficiently concerning as to prompt a call to the nearest expert referral center and/or the child's primary care provider for emergency evaluation.

ACKNOWLEDGMENTS

The authors thank members of the medical genetics staff who worked tirelessly to help accumulate the clinical pictures; and the families who graciously consented to allow photographs to be taken to advance teaching and education.

References

Beighton P, de Paepe A, Danks D, et al: International nosology of heritable disorders of connective tissue, Berlin, 1986, *Am J Med Genet* 29:581–594, 1988.

De Paepe A, Devereux RB, Dietz HC, et al: Revised diagnostic criteria for the Marfan syndrome, *Am J Med Genet* 62:417–426, 1996.

Habashi JP, Doyle JJ, Holm TM, et al: Angiotensin II type 2 receptor signaling attenuates aortic aneurysm in mice through ERK antagonism, *Science* 332, 361–365, 2011.

Loeys BL, Dietz HC, Braverman AC, et al: The revised Ghent nosology for the Marfan syndrome, *J Med Genet* 47:476–485, 2010.

Miller DT, Adam MP, Aradhya S, et al: Consensus statement: chromosomal microarray is a first-tier clinical diagnostic test for individuals with developmental disabilities or congenital anomalies, *Am J Hum Genet* 86:749–764, 2010.

Ng SB, Bigham AW, Buckingham KJ, et al: Exome sequencing identifies *MLL2* mutations as a cause of Kabuki syndrome, *Nat Genet* 42:790–793, 2010.

Warburton D: De novo balanced chromosome rearrangements and extra marker chromosomes identified at prenatal diagnosis: clinical significance and distribution of breakpoints, *Am J Hum Genet* 49:995–1013, 1991.

Bibliography

Ballif BC, Theisen A, McDonald-McGinn DM, et al: Identification of a previously unrecognized microdeletion syndrome of 16q11.2q12.2, *Clin Genet* 74:469–475, 2008.

Bejjani BA, Saleki R, Ballif BC, et al: Use of targeted array-based CGH for the clinical diagnosis of chromosomal imbalance: is less more? *Am J Med Genet A* 134:259–267, 2005.

Buyse ML, editor: *Birth defects encyclopedia*, Cambridge, Mass, 1990, Blackwell Scientific.

Cooley WC, Graham JM: Down syndrome—an update and review for the primary pediatrician, *Clin Pediatr* 30:233–253, 1991.

Duker AL Ballif BC, Bawle EV, et al: Paternally inherited microdeletion at 15q11.2 confirms a significant role for the SNORD116 C/D box snoRNA cluster in Prader-Willi syndrome, *Eur J Hum Genet* 18:1196–1201, 2010.

Epstein CJ: Down syndrome (trisomy 21). In Scriber CR, Beaudet AL, Sly WS, et al, editors: *The metabolic and molecular basis of inherited disease*, ed 8, New York, 2001, McGraw-Hill, pp 1223–1256.

Francke U: Prader-Willi syndrome: chromosomal and gene aberrations, *Growth Genet Horm* 10:4–7, 1994.

Gorlin RJ, Cohen MM Jr, Hennekam RCM: *Syndromes of the head and neck*, ed 4, New York, 2001, Oxford University Press.

Graham JM Jr: *Smith's recognizable patterns of human deformation*, ed 2, Philadelphia, 1988, WB Saunders.

Hook EB: Chromosome abnormalities: prevalence, risks, and recurrence. In Brock BJH, Rodeck CH, Ferguson-Smith MA, editors: *Prenatal diagnosis and screening*, New York, 1992, Churchill Livingstone, pp 351–392.

Johns DR: Mitochondrial DNA and disease, *N Engl J Med* 333:638–644, 1995.

Jones KL: *Smith's recognizable patterns of human malformation*, ed 6, Philadelphia, 2006, Elsevier Saunders.

Lubs HA: A marker X chromosome, *Am J Hum Genet* 21:231–244, 1969.

Manning M, Hudgins L: Array-based technology and recommendations for utilization in medical genetics practice for detection of chromosome abnormalities, *Genet Med* 12:742–745, 2010.

Nussbaum RL, McInnes RR, Willard HF: *Thompson and Thompson genetics in medicine*, ed 6, Philadelphia, 2004, WB Saunders.

Online Mendelian Inheritance in Man (OMIM): McKusick-Nathans Institute for Genetic Medicine, Johns Hopkins University (Baltimore, Md) and National Center for Biotechnology Information, National Library of Medicine (Bethesda, Md), 2000. Available from http://www.ncbi.nlm.nih.gov/omim/

Patton MA: Noonan syndrome: a review, *Growth Genet Horm* 10:1–3, 1994.

Robinson BH: Lactic acidemia: disorders of pyruvate carboxylase and pyruvate dehydrogenase. In Scriber CR, Beaudet AL, Sly WS, et al, editors: *The metabolic and molecular basis of inherited disease*, ed 8, New York, 2001, McGraw-Hill, pp 2275–2295.

Ryan AK, Goodship JA, Wilson DI, et al: Spectrum of clinical features associated with interstitial chromosome 22q11 deletions: a European collaborative study, *J Med Genet* 34:798–804, 1997.

Shepard TH, Lemire RJ: *Catalog of teratogenic agents*, ed 11, Baltimore, 2004, Johns Hopkins University Press.

Stalker HJ, Williams CA: Genetic counseling in Angelman syndrome: the challenges of multiple causes, *Am J Med Genet* 77:54–59, 1998.

Stevenson RE, Hall JG, Goodman RM, editors: *Human malformations and related anomalies*, ed 2. New York, Oxford University Press, 2006.

Sutherland GR: Fragile sites on human chromosomes: demonstration of their dependence on the type of tissue culture medium, *Science* 197:265–266, 1977.

Sutherland GR, Gecz J, Mulley JC: Fragile X syndrome and other causes of X-linked mental handicap. In Rimoin DL, O'Connor JM, Pyeritz RE, et al, editors: *Emery and Rimoin's principles and practice of medical genetics*, ed 5, Philadelphia, 2006, Churchill Livingstone, pp 2801–2826.

Trask BJ: Fluorescence in situ hybridization, *Trends Genet* 7:149–154, 1991.

Wenger SL, Steele MW, Boone LY, et al: "Balanced" karyotypes in six abnormal offspring of balanced reciprocal translocation normal carrier parents, *Am J Med Genet* 55:47–52, 1995.

Willard HF, Ferguson-Smith MA, Goodfellow PN, et al: Chromosomes and autosomes. In Scriver CR, Beaudet AL, Sly WS, et al, editors: *The metabolic and molecular bases of inherited disease*, New York, 1995, McGraw-Hill.

Wincent J, Anderlid BM, Lagerberg M, et al: High-resolution molecular karyotyping in patients with developmental delay and/or multiple congenital anomalies in a clinical setting, *Clin Genet* 79:147–157, 2011.

General Metabolic References

Fernandes J, Saudubray J-M, van den Berghe G, et al: *Inborn metabolic diseases, diagnosis and treatment*, ed 4, Heidelberg, 2006, Springer Medizin Verlag.

GeneTests: Medical Genetics Information Resource (database online): © University of Washington, Seattle. 1993-2011. Available from www.genetests.org

Lysosomal Disease Program: Educational resource for people dealing with lysosomal storage disorders (LSDs). © 2009 Massachusetts General Hospital. Available from www.mghlysosomal.org

Mayo Clinic Health Information Site (official website of the Mayo Clinic): © 1998-2011 Mayo Foundation for Medical Education and Research. Available from www.mayoclinic.com

National Institute of Neurological Disorders and Stroke (NINDS), National Institutes of Health (NIH): Online resource for disorders of the brain and nervous system. Available from www.ninds.nih.gov

Nyhan WL, Barshoop BA, Ozand PT: *Atlas of metabolic diseases*, ed 2, New York, 2005, Oxford University Press.

Scriver CR, Beaudet AL, Sly WS, et al, editors: *Metabolic and molecular bases of inherited disease*, ed 8. Available from www.ommbid.com. New York, 2004, McGraw-Hill.

NEONATOLOGY

2

Beverly S. Brozanski | Melissa M. Riley | Debra L. Bogen

GENERAL TECHNIQUES OF PHYSICAL EXAMINATION

Assessment of the Newborn

The purposes of the routine newborn assessment are to determine the infant's gestational age, document normal growth and development for a given gestational age, uncover signs of birth-related trauma or congenital anomalies, and evaluate the overall health and condition of the infant. The assessment begins with the establishment of a historical database. Information may be obtained from antenatal, labor, delivery, and postpartum records and a brief interview with the parents (Fig. 2-1). The aim of this data gathering is to assess the fetal and neonatal responses to pregnancy, labor, and delivery; to estimate the risk for hereditary or congenital diseases; and to identify the potential for future difficulties by reviewing the family's social history and observing maternal–infant interactions. This background is recorded in the infant's medical record and serves as a guide to the subsequent physical examination (Table 2-1).

Whenever possible, it is preferable that the newborn be examined in the presence of one or both parents to reassure them regarding normal variations and to discuss any abnormal findings. The baby should remain at least partially clothed through as much of the examination as possible, although a complete and thorough examination is imperative. The examiner's hands should be warm to minimize the chance that the infant will become uncomfortable because of heat loss.

Observation must be done before the quiet infant is disturbed by the examination. By visual inspection the clinician can assess skin and facies; general tonus and symmetry of movement; respiratory rate, retractions, and color; and abdominal contour. Auscultation of the heart and lungs should be done before more stressful portions of the examination, which are likely to make the infant fussy. Allowing the infant to suck on a gloved finger can help quiet the infant and permit assessment of sucking strength and palate integrity. Lifting the infant under the arms (Fig. 2-2) and gently rocking him or her (such that the head swings toward and away from the examiner) is usually calming. This maneuver also induces a reflexive opening of the eyes, which assists the ophthalmologic examination. Sucking also induces eye opening. Such maneuvers may be necessary to convince the examiner that the patient does not have a congenital cataract or an intraorbital mass (see Chapter 19) requiring prompt intervention.

When the abdomen is examined, it often helps to gently flex the hip on the side being examined because this relaxes the abdominal muscles. Most structures in the abdomen are smaller (pyloric olive), softer (liver), more superficial (spleen tip), or deeper (kidneys) than expected. The use of any part of the hand other than the fingertips should be discouraged because maximal sensitivity is essential.

Careful evaluation of the hip joints is a crucial part of each newborn examination because identification and early treatment of congenital dislocation can prevent later disability. Although asymmetry of the buttocks and skin creases or asymmetry of femoral length can be clues to dislocation, the performance of at least one of a number of active motion tests is essential. The Ortolani maneuver involves placing the third or fourth finger over the greater trochanter and the thumb on the medial aspect of the thighs (Fig. 2-3). The thighs are first adducted to try to dislocate a dislocatable hip and then abducted with the fingers pushing toward the midline and the thumbs away from midline to relocate a dislocated hip. A definite "clunk" can be felt and often heard if the femoral head has been dislocated and then moves back into the acetabulum. Often, higher-pitched clicks and snaps that represent nothing more than tendons passing over bone or cartilage can be heard and felt.

Assessment of Gestational Age

One of the unique considerations in the examination of the newborn is the assessment of gestational age. Accurate determination should be the first part of any newborn examination because this provides the context for the remainder of the evaluation. No differential diagnosis of newborn disease can be made without knowing whether the patient is premature or full term and whether he or she is small, large, or appropriate for gestational age. Although an accurate menstrual and pregnancy history usually provides firm evidence of gestational age, there are many cases in which data such as the date of the last menses and the date of the onset of fetal movement are unavailable or unreliable.

Many investigators have developed examination criteria, both morphologic and neurologic, for the assessment of gestational age. Although these criteria are generally useful because of the ordered patterns of fetal development, the clinician cannot rely on any single feature or even small group of features to develop at the same rate in all infants. In fact, assessment of paired structures, such as ears, may reveal slightly different degrees of maturation from one side to the other. Thus all of the available methods involve numerous physical and neurologic items and have, at best, a 2-week range of error.

Although morphologic criteria tend to be uninfluenced by events occurring around the time of delivery, neurologic findings may be unreliable in the presence of a number of conditions including depression secondary to medication, asphyxia, seizures, metabolic diseases, infections, and severe respiratory distress. Even morphologic criteria may be inaccurate if the infant is born with severe edema or growth retardation or side effects from maternal drug use. Such factors must be considered in estimating gestational age.

The Ballard assessment for gestational age determination of newborns uses six morphologic and six neurologic criteria

45

Figure 2-1   Antenatal assessments. This infant has a normal sonographic appearance at 12 weeks' gestation. Knowledge of the results of in utero evaluations may assist in the provision of appropriate antenatal and postnatal care. *(Courtesy Lyndon Hill, MD, Pittsburgh.)*

to estimate gestational age on the basis of an examination performed at 12 to 24 hours of life (Fig. 2-4). Individual findings are scored on a scale of 0 to 5, and the total score is compared with the chart shown in Figure 2-4.

Physical Maturity

One of the most striking differences among newborns of various gestational ages is the quality of the skin. The chemical nature of skin changes during intrauterine development, with a gradual decrease in water content and a thickening of the keratin layer. Very premature infants (24 to 28 weeks) have nearly translucent, paper-thin skin (Fig. 2-5) that is easily abraded. A diffuse red hue and a prominent venous pattern are characteristic. At term, the skin no longer appears thin, and the general color is a pale pink. Some superficial peeling and cracking around the ankles and wrists may be visible. Postterm infants (42 to 44 weeks) often have more diffuse peeling and cracking of the skin because the outermost layers are sloughed (Fig. 2-6).

Figure 2-2   Examination techniques. Holding an infant under the arms and gently rocking calms the infant and reflexively induces eye opening.

Figure 2-3   Ortolani maneuver. The proper hand positioning for this maneuver is demonstrated. Abducting the femur produces a palpable "clunk" in the infant with congenital hip dislocation.

Table 2-1	Newborn Historical Database

Antenatal Record

Maternal age

Maternal medical history

Obstetric history

   Number of previous pregnancies

   Number of term/preterm deliveries

   Outcomes of previous pregnancies

Estimations of gestational age

Antenatal ultrasound or fetal surveillance results (if available)

Complications of pregnancy

Adequacy of antenatal care

Labor and Delivery Record

Date and time of delivery

Duration of labor

Time of the rupture of membranes

Complications or abnormalities of labor

Method of delivery or type of anesthesia

Placental weight and morphologic condition

Birth weight

Need for resuscitation and Apgar scores

Maternal blood type

Postpartum Record

Maternal postpartum complications

Newborn vital sign records

Nursing documentation of the activity and condition of the infant

   On admission to the nursery

   Since admission to the nursery

Abnormal physical findings noted by the nursing staff

Feeding, voiding, and stool history

Observations of maternal–infant interactions

Parental Interview

Parental perceptions of

   Pregnancy

   Labor

   Delivery

History of parental and family illnesses

Health status and growth and development of siblings and other family members

Degree of education, preparation, and planning for newborn care

Available social support systems

Medical follow-up plans

Physical maturity

	0	1	2	3	4	5
Skin	Gelatinous, red, transparent	Smooth, pink, visible veins	Superficial peeling and/or rash, few veins	Cracking, pale area, rare veins	Parchment, deep cracking no vessels	Leathery, cracked, wrinkled
Lanugo	None	Abundant	Thinning	Bald areas	Mostly bald	
Plantar creases	No crease	Faint red marks	Anterior transverse crease only	Creases anterior two thirds	Creases cover entire sole	
Breast	Barely perceptible	Flat areola, no bud	Stippled areola, 1–2 mm bud	Raised areola, 3–4 mm bud	Full areola, 5–10 mm bud	
Ear	Pinna flat, stays folded	Slightly curved pinna, soft, slow recoil	Well-curved pinna, soft but ready recoil	Formed and firm with instant recoil	Thick cartilage, ear stiff	
Genitals: male	Scrotum empty, no rugae		Testes descending, few rugae	Testes down, good rugae	Testes pendulous, deep rugae	
Genitals: female	Prominent clitoris and labia minora		Majora and minora equally prominent	Majora large, minora small	Clitoris and minora completely covered	

Maturity rating

Score	Weeks
5	26
10	28
15	30
20	32
25	34
30	36
35	38
40	40
45	42
50	44

Neuromuscular maturity

Figure 2-4 Gestational age assessment. The six morphologic and six neurologic criteria, in aggregate, yield an estimation of gestational age. *(From Ballard J, Novak KK, Driver M: A simplified score of assessment of fetal maturation of newly born infants.* J Pediatr *95:769-774, 1979.)*

Figure 2-5   Premature skin. This premature infant demonstrates translucent, paper-thin skin with a prominent venous pattern.

Figure 2-7   Lanugo. This fine body hair resembling peach fuzz is present on infants of 24 to 32 weeks' gestation.

The general quality of scalp hair changes during development from rather fine, thin hair (24 to 28 weeks) to coarser, thicker hair (term). Racial differences in hair quality can make this change difficult to assess. A second type of hair, known as lanugo, appears and disappears during development. Lanugo is fine body hair that resembles peach fuzz. It is absent before weeks 20 to 22, becomes diffuse until weeks 30 to 32, and then begins to thin. Assessment of the presence and extent of lanugo is best accomplished by observing the back tangentially (Fig. 2-7).

Transverse creases begin to appear on the anterior portion of the soles of the feet at approximately 32 weeks (Fig. 2-8). By 36 weeks the anterior two thirds of the sole is covered with creases. For adequate assessment of this feature, it is necessary to stretch the skin over the sole gently to distinguish wrinkling from true creases. Infants with congenital neurologic dysfunction involving the lower extremities and infants with pedal edema may lack normal creases.

Breast tissue, which is responsive to maternal hormonal influences, shows progressive increase in size as gestational age advances. Infants born at younger than 28 weeks' gestation have barely perceptible breast tissue (see Fig. 2-5). With advancing age, breast tissue increases in size (see Fig. 2-6) and, occasionally, a term infant has active glandular secretions, which resolve spontaneously. Breast tissue can remain palpable for 2 to 3 months.

Cartilaginous development proceeds in an orderly manner during gestation and can be assessed by examination of the external ear. Although the normal incurving of the upper pinnae begins at 33 to 34 weeks and is complete at term, it is more reliable to assess the extent of cartilage in the pinnae by feeling its edge and folding the ear (Fig. 2-9). Until approximately 32 weeks, there is only minimal recoil of a folded ear, but by term there is instant recoil.

The appearance of the genitalia can be used to assess gestational age. In a boy the testes descend into the scrotum during the last month of gestation, but they are often palpable in the inguinal canal by 28 to 30 weeks. The appearance of rugae on the scrotum parallels testicular migration, appearing first on the anterior scrotum at 36 weeks and covering the entire scrotal sac by 40 weeks. Absence of testicular descent alters the appearance of the scrotum at term. Clearly, congenital cryptorchidism complicates this evaluation. In a girl the

Figure 2-6   Post-term skin. Peeling and cracking of the skin are characteristics of the infant delivered after 42 weeks' gestation.

Figure 2-8   Sole creases. Transverse sole creases cover approximately half the sole in this infant, indicating a gestational age of approximately 34 weeks.

Figure 2-11 General posture. The typical, marked flexor posture of the term infant.

Figure 2-9 Ear cartilage. The lack of cartilage and the easy foldability (lack of recoil) are evident in the ear of this premature infant at 26 weeks.

labia majora tend to be overshadowed by the clitoris and labia minora until 34 to 36 weeks (Fig. 2-10). In cases of fetal malnutrition, lack of subcutaneous fat, which should normally be present in the latter part of gestation, can interfere with assessment of the female genitalia.

Neuromuscular Maturity

Numerous neurologic tests and observations can be used to assess gestational age. Most examiners use the tests that seem to best cover the various facets of neurologic function including range of motion, tone, reflexes, and posture. None is particularly reliable in the presence of illness, and the entire neurologic examination is best done between 12 and 24 hours after birth to allow recovery from the stress of delivery.

The resting supine posture of infants changes with advancing gestational age. The mature infant exhibits a marked flexor posture of the extremities compared with the extensor posture of the premature infant (Fig. 2-11).

Tests for flexion angles assess a combination of muscle tone, ligament and tendon laxity, as well as flexion–extension development. The inexperienced examiner usually assumes

that the very premature infant is the most flexible, but observation of flexion angles demonstrates that this is false. The square-window test of the wrist (Fig. 2-12) is performed by gently flexing the hand on the wrist and assessing the resultant angle. The wrists of babies younger than approximately 32 weeks can be flexed only to 45 to 90 degrees, whereas the wrists of term infants undergo full flexion. Sometime between birth and adulthood this flexion ability is lost. Examination of the flexion of the knees reveals a different pattern of development, with decreasing flexibility as gestational age increases. The knee is completely flexed (Fig. 2-13, *A*) and the thigh is stabilized against the stomach. The leg is extended by raising the foot (Fig. 2-13, *B*). Gentleness is *essential* in these evaluations because any result can be achieved if the examiner applies undue force.

Examination of arm recoil can assess active tone and reflex responsiveness. In this maneuver the supine infant's forearms are fully flexed for 5 seconds, extended by pulling on the hands, and then released. As gestational age increases, the flexion response is more pronounced.

The resting tone of the upper extremities can be assessed by eliciting the scarf sign. Gentle traction of the upper extremities across the chest in a rostral direction ("placing a scarf on the infant") while examining the position of the elbow reveals

Figure 2-10 Premature female genitalia. Prominence of the labia minora in a premature female infant at 28 weeks.

Figure 2-12 Square-window test. The position for assessing the square window is shown. The 45-degree angle seen between the palm and forearm is consistent with a gestational age of 30 to 32 weeks.

Figure 2-13   Knee flexion. The position for assessing knee flexion is shown **(A)**. The foot is elevated to assess the popliteal angle. Note the decreased knee flexibility of this term infant **(B)**.

a decreasing displacement of the elbow as gestational age increases (Fig. 2-14).

In a similar manner the resting tone of the lower extremities can be assessed by the heel-to-ear maneuver. With the baby on its back and the pelvis flat, a foot is moved as near to the ipsilateral ear as possible without exerting undue force. Very premature infants can easily touch their heels to their ears (Fig. 2-15). This becomes somewhat more difficult after 30 weeks and impossible by week 34 of gestation.

Primitive Reflexes

Normal newborns exhibit a large number of easily elicited primitive reflexes that are often altered or absent in the infant with neurologic impairment. These reflexes may be transiently depressed in the infant who has experienced difficulty in achieving the transition between intrauterine and extrauterine existence. The persistent absence or asymmetry of one or more of these reflexes may be a clue to the potential presence of neuromuscular abnormalities requiring further investigation (see Chapter 3).

The rooting reflex may be elicited by lightly stimulating the infant's cheek and observing the reflexive attempts to bring the stimulating object to the mouth. The sucking reflex is activated by placing an object in the infant's mouth and observing the sucking movements. In the grasp reflex (Figs. 2-16 and 2-17), transverse stimulation of the midpalm (without touching the back of the hand) or midsole leads to flexion of the digits or toes around the examiner's fingers.

The Moro reflex (Fig. 2-18, *A* and *B*) evaluates vestibular maturation and the relationship between flexor and extensor tone. Elicitation of the reflex involves a short (10 cm), sudden drop of the head when the infant is supine. The full response involves extension of the arms, "fanning" of the fingers, and then upper extremity flexion followed by a cry. An incomplete but identifiable reflex becomes apparent at approximately 32 weeks' gestation, and by 38 weeks it is essentially complete. Very immature infants demonstrate extension of the arms and fingers but do not show true flexion or make a sustained cry. Marked asymmetry of response may be associated with focal neurologic impairment.

Figure 2-14   Scarf sign. The elbow cannot be drawn, with gentle traction on the upper extremity, across this term infant's chest **(A).** This is in contrast to the marked flexibility of a preterm infant of 29 weeks' gestation **(B).**

Figure 2-15 Heel-to-ear maneuver. The position for assessing the heel-to-ear maneuver is demonstrated. The degree of extension seen is consistent with a 28- to 30-week infant.

Figure 2-17 Grasp reflex (sole). Transverse stimulation of the midsole triggers a grasp by the infant.

Galant's infantile reflex is a truncal incurvation reflex. It can be elicited by holding the infant in ventral suspension and stroking from shoulder to hip along one side of the spine. The infant will contract the abdominal musculature and laterally flex toward the stimulated side. Lack of the Galant reflex may indicate a spinal cord lesion.

These reflexes and a host of other less commonly used reflexes are termed *primitive* because they are present at or shortly after birth and normally disappear after the first few months of life. Just as their absence may indicate neurologic impairment at birth, their abnormal persistence may also be a cause for concern and further evaluation.

Abnormalities of Growth

Intrauterine growth restriction (IUGR), a deviation in the expected fetal growth pattern, complicates up to 8% of all pregnancies, and is associated with an increase in perinatal morbidity and mortality. Infants with IUGR may appear long and thin and often have an obvious loss of subcutaneous tissue, which is best seen as redundant skin folds over the buttocks, thighs, and knees. The etiology of IUGR is multifactorial and includes fetal, placental, or maternal factors that inhibit normal fetal growth. The conditions for IUGR and SGA (small for gestational age) are related but not synonymous. The diagnosis of SGA is based on population norms and includes infants who weigh less than a predetermined cutoff value (Fig. 2-19). There is no universal agreement on the definition of the SGA or LGA (large for gestational age) infant.

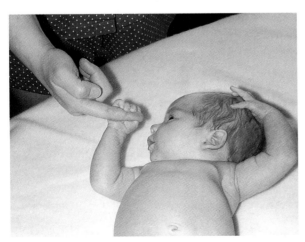

Figure 2-16 Grasp reflex (palm). Transverse stimulation of the midpalm leads to a grasp by the infant.

Similarly, appropriate for gestational age (AGA) infants have growth parameters within 2 standard deviations of the mean, or between the 10th and 90th percentiles, or between the 3rd and 97th percentiles.

The relationship among weight, length, and head circumference can be useful in understanding the etiology of the small size (see Fig. 2-19). By comparing length or head circumference percentiles with the weight percentile at any given gestational age, the clinician can detect growth retardation even if the actual weight still falls within 2 standard deviations of normal. Conditions that affect growth during the third trimester of pregnancy, such as preeclampsia, tend to interfere with the normal acquisition of fatty tissue while sparing brain growth (and thus head circumference) and linear growth. These newborns have an asymmetrical form of growth retardation (Fig. 2-20). Often postmature infants (>42 weeks) have some decrease in weight compared with length or head circumference. Problems beginning earlier than the third trimester tend to produce generalized growth retardation because head circumference, weight, and length are affected to equivalent degrees. Historically, infants with symmetrical IUGR have higher rates of chromosomal disorders, dysmorphic syndromes, and congenital infection and are associated with higher rates of prematurity and neonatal mortality. In very premature infants, global decreases in growth often complicate assessment of gestational age because the tools are rather limited in babies born at 24 to 28 weeks' gestation. A thorough investigation should be undertaken in any unexplained instance of growth retardation.

Multiple-gestation pregnancies often produce newborns that are premature and symmetrically small. Fetal growth decreases as the number of fetuses increases. Although multiple factors interfere with growth in these pregnancies, uterine constraint appears to occur when the combined fetal size approximates 3 kg. Size discordance (>10% difference in weight) between identical twins occurs because their placentas can share vascular connections, resulting in overperfusion of one twin and underperfusion with subsequent growth restriction of the other. Discordance may also occur in dizygotic twins (Fig. 2-21) if one has placental insufficiency. Rarely, only one twin will be afflicted with a chromosomal abnormality or congenital infection.

Newborns that are large for gestational age (LGA) are often the products of pregnancies in diabetic or "prediabetic" mothers. The effect is usually noted during the third trimester, with infants at term who weigh more than 4 kg (8 lb 13 oz). Weight is the most affected parameter, but length and head circumference are often increased as well. Infants of diabetic

Figure 2-18 Moro reflex. **A,** To elicit the reflex, the head is supported and allowed to drop to the level of the bed. The initial extension response to vestibular stimulation is shown in **(B).** The complete response includes secondary flexion and cry.

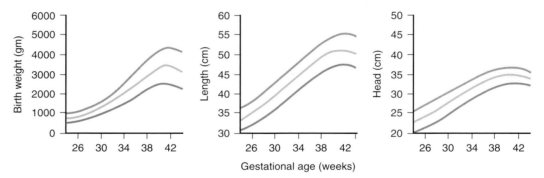

Gestational age (weeks)

Figure 2-19 The mean (±2 standard deviations) weight, length, and head circumference for infants born at various gestational ages. Infants above or below the curves are considered too large or too small for gestational age, respectively. *(From Usher R, McLean F: Intrauterine growth of live-born Caucasian infants at sea level: standards obtained from measurements in 7 dimensions of infants born between 25 and 44 weeks of gestation,* J Pediatr *74:901-910, 1969.)*

Figure 2-20 Intrauterine growth retardation. This term baby weighed only 1.7 kg. The head appears disproportionately large for the thin, wasted body. This resulted from placental insufficiency late in pregnancy. Hypoglycemia may be a complication. *(Courtesy TALC, Institute of Child Health, Bethesda, Md.)*

Figure 2-21 Discordant twins. This is a pair of markedly discordant dizygotic twins. Disturbed placentation accounted for the marked reduction in size of the smaller twin.

Figure 2-22 Large-for-gestational-age infant. This infant of a diabetic mother weighed 5 kg at birth and exhibits the typical rounded facies.

Figure 2-24 Circumvallate placenta. Extension of villous tissue exists beyond the chorionic surface, with a well-defined hyalinized fold at the edge of the chorionic plate.

mothers are often identifiable by macrosomia, round facies (Fig. 2-22), and sometimes plethora and hirsutism (especially of the pinnae). Maternal hyperglycemia causes glycogen deposition in the newborn, resulting in visceromegaly, most notable in the liver and heart. Although babies weighing more than 8 pounds are more likely to be from diabetic pregnancies, a significant number of large full-term newborns are the product of normal pregnancies. Nevertheless, all LGA infants should be routinely screened for hypoglycemia and their mothers investigated for the possibility of undiagnosed diabetes mellitus.

Two fairly unusual syndromes can also cause excessive size: (1) cerebral gigantism, or Sotos syndrome, with macrosomia, macrocephaly, large hands and feet, poor coordination, and variable mental deficiency; and (2) Beckwith-Wiedemann syndrome with macrosomia, macroglossia, omphalocele, linear ear fissures, and neonatal hypoglycemia (see Chapter 9).

Placenta

Careful examination of the placenta can aid in the diagnosis and treatment of many conditions and diseases. Unfortunately, the placenta has been relegated to the afterbirth and is often immediately discarded without knowing the condition of the offspring. After the membranes and cord are trimmed, the normal ratio of fetal-to-placental weight is approximately 4.7 : 1. The configuration, color, condition of the membranes, insertion of the cord, and condition of the fetal and maternal surfaces are all relevant.

The insertion of the umbilical cord into the placenta, which can be central, eccentric, marginal, or velamentous, can be important in understanding unexplained asphyxia or blood loss. In a velamentous insertion (Fig. 2-23), the cord is inserted into the membranes rather than into the placental disk, leaving the umbilical vessels unprotected for a variable distance. These vessels are more prone to rupture, with resultant fetal hemorrhage (vasa previa).

At times, placentation itself is abnormal. In a circumvallate placenta (Fig. 2-24), the villous tissue projects beyond the chorionic surface, with a hyalinized fold at the edge of the chorionic plate. This type of placentation may cause antepartum bleeding, premature labor, and increased perinatal mortality.

Premature placental separation (abruptio placentae) can lead to an accumulation of blood behind the placenta (Fig. 2-25). Although the bleeding is usually of maternal origin, rare fetal blood loss may also occur. Large abruptions may lead to poor growth, fetal asphyxia, or even death. Distinguishing a true abruption, in which an adherent clot compresses the maternal surface, from the nonadherent collection of blood that forms on normal placental separation is important.

Placental infarctions (Fig. 2-26) tend to occur along the margin of the placenta, can vary in color from red to yellowish white, and are most common in pregnancies complicated by hypertension. Small placental infarcts (<30% of placental volume) are usually of little significance. However, large central infarcts can reduce the placental surface available for fetal oxygenation and nutrition and can result in aberrations in fetal growth.

Chorioamnionitis (Fig. 2-27), or inflammation of the fetal membranes, is an immediate clue to potential neonatal infection. On gross examination the membranes lack their normal sheen and translucency, appearing gray or yellow. Inflammation, confirmable by microscopic examination, can also be

Figure 2-23 Velamentous cord insertion. The umbilical cord is inserted into the amniotic membranes rather than into the placental disk. This leaves the umbilical vessels relatively unprotected and predisposes them to rupture.

Figure 2-25 Abruptio placentae. Examination of this placenta reveals a small abruption site, with an adherent blood clot along the margin.

Figure 2-26 Infarcted placenta. A massive placental infarction making up the majority of the villous surface is shown. Such an extensive infarction compromises fetal nutrition and oxygenation.

Figure 2-28 Amnion nodosum. The fetal surface of this placenta from a pregnancy with oligohydramnios demonstrates multiple nodules consistent with amnion nodosum. This finding suggests a strong possibility of renal agenesis or dysgenesis.

found in the fetal vessels of the chorionic plate and umbilical cord.

In pregnancies in which the quantity of amniotic fluid is decreased (oligohydramnios), examination of the amnion may also reveal shiny, gray, flat nodules known as *amnion nodosum* (Fig. 2-28). The presence of these nodules can be an immediate indication of renal dysfunction or renal agenesis in the newborn (or the newborn may have normal renal function). Because such infants may also have hypoplastic lungs and dysmorphic features (such as occurs in Potter syndrome), early diagnosis can be helpful to the physician and family.

In multiple-gestation deliveries, a careful placental evaluation is crucial to determine chorion number and to distinguish between monozygotic and dizygotic twins. The major distinction to be made is whether there is a single chorion, or outer layer of the fetal membranes. When twins with a single chorion are present in a single amniotic cavity (Fig. 2-29), monozygosity is ensured. For all practical purposes, a single chorion that bridges two amniotic sacs is also evidence of monozygotic twins. In this instance it is essential to examine the membranes at the site of connection of the two amniotic sacs. When two chorions and two amnions (or a total of four membranes at their interface) are present (Fig. 2-30), twins may be monozygotic or dizygotic. Approximately 36% of monozygotic twins are dichorionic. Monochorionic (MC) twin placentas, developed for a singleton pregnancy, may not adapt to the demands of twin circulations. The majority of MC twin placentas have connecting vessels, which account for the higher rates of complications.

BIRTH TRAUMA

In the majority of cases a newborn is relatively unscathed by the birth process. However, sometimes transient and permanent stigmata of birth trauma are evident. Prompt identification of such injuries is important for good management and can also prevent inappropriate speculation, diagnostic testing, and treatment.

Caput Succedaneum

Normal transit of the fetal head through the birth canal induces molding of the skull and scalp edema, especially if labor is prolonged. The edema, which can be massive, is known as a *caput succedaneum* (Fig. 2-31). Much of this edema is present at birth and tends to overlie the occipital bones and portions of the parietal bones bilaterally. In some cases, bruising of the scalp may also be present (especially if a vacuum extractor was used). The presence of a caput requires no therapy, and spontaneous resolution within a few days is the rule. Distinguishing caput from a subgaleal (subaponeurotic) hematoma, a rare but serious complication of delivery, is important. A subgaleal hematoma is a collection of blood within scalp tissues extending beneath the epicranial aponeurosis. Palpation of a large caput succedaneum reveals firm, nonpitting swelling. In contrast, the cranial swelling of subgaleal bleeding is boggy due to the palpation of clotted blood just beneath the

Figure 2-27 Chorioamnionitis. This is a placental specimen from a pregnancy with documented amniotic fluid infection. The surface of the membranes is opaque and shows yellowish discoloration.

Figure 2-29 Monochorionic, monoamniotic placenta. Examination of this placenta from monozygotic twins reveals no dividing membranes, thus ensuring monozygosity.

Figure 2-30   Dichorionic, diamniotic placenta. The presence of two amniotic sacs and separate chorions in this twin placenta precludes determination of zygosity.

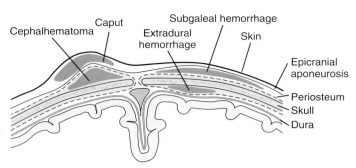

Figure 2-32   Sites of extracranial (and extradural) hemorrhages in the newborn. Schematic diagram of the important tissue planes from skin to dura. *(Modified from Pape KE, Wigglesworth JS:* Haemorrhage, ischaemia and the perinatal brain, *Philadelphia, JB Lippincott, 1979.)*

epicranial aponeurosis (Fig. 2-32). The collection of blood in this potential space can be quite large, and these infants must be monitored for signs of hypovolemia. Serial examinations, which can include measurement of head circumference and hematocrit, are important to identify ongoing blood loss.

Cephalhematoma

Often, confusion arises between the diagnosis of a caput and that of a cephalhematoma. The latter is a localized collection of blood beneath the periosteum of one of the calvarial bones; it may be bilateral, but is most often unilateral (Fig. 2-33). It is distinguished from a caput by the fact that its borders are limited by suture lines, usually those surrounding the parietal bones (see Fig. 2-32). However, diagnosis can be difficult in the immediate newborn period, when there may be overlying scalp edema. On palpation, the border may feel elevated and the center depressed. Most patients have an uncomplicated course of slow resolution over one or more months, although calcification may occur. On occasion, these infants may develop jaundice from the breakdown and resorption of the large hematoma. Underlying hairline skull fractures occur with some regularity but are rarely of clinical significance. The exception is the uncommon development of a leptomeningeal cyst. Radiologic investigation for an underlying depressed fracture is indicated in infants whose histories suggest significant trauma and those having depressed levels of consciousness *or* neurologic abnormalities on examination. Infection is another potentially serious but rare complication, which is

more likely when the integrity of the overlying skin is broken.

Clavicle Fracture

Fracture of a clavicle can occur during delivery when the infant is large, in breech position, or if there is fetal distress requiring rapid extraction. If undisplaced, the fracture may not be painful, and the infant may be asymptomatic (Fig. 2-34). The diagnosis may be suspected by palpation of crepitus or an asymmetrical Moro reflex. If there is pain or discomfort with routine handling, the fracture can be treated by immobilization of the ipsilateral limb and shoulder with the elbow flexed 90 degrees. Immobilization can be discontinued when a callus is palpable at 8 to 10 days. Many nondisplaced clavicle fractures are not diagnosed until the first newborn outpatient follow-up visit, when a large, firm callus may be palpated along the clavicle. If the child has an otherwise normal physical and neurologic examination at this time, a radiograph is not indicated. Radiographs would be indicated to help differentiate whether decreased arm movement is secondary to pain (clavicle fracture) or nerve injury (Erb's palsy).

Meconium Staining

Meconium is noted in the amniotic fluid in as many as 10% of deliveries. The meconium may have been recently expelled or may have been present in the amniotic fluid for hours or days. Because the timing of the passage of meconium may

Figure 2-31   Caput succedaneum. This infant has significant scalp edema as a result of compression during transit through the birth canal. The edema crosses suture lines.

Figure 2-33   Cephalhematoma. In this infant with bilateral cephalhematomas, the midline sagittal suture remained palpable, confirming the subperiosteal location of the hematomas.

Figure 2-34 Clavicle fracture. This infant had a palpable mass over the right clavicle immediately after delivery. Note the discontinuity of the right clavicle.

Figure 2-36 Bruising. This severe bruising of the perineum was the result of a difficult breech labor and delivery.

have significance for the diagnosis of fetal distress, it is useful to examine infants for the presence of meconium staining. It takes at least 4 to 6 hours of contact before staining of the umbilicus, skin, and nails occurs (Fig. 2-35). Often, the meconium-stained infant is postmature and has diffuse peeling of the skin and a shriveled, stained umbilical cord.

Bruises and Petechiae

Superficial bruising can occur when delivery is difficult. This is relatively common with breech presentations (Fig. 2-36) and can include swelling and discoloration of the labia or scrotum (to be distinguished from an incarcerated inguinal hernia). When bruises are extensive, significant secondary jaundice may develop as the extravasated blood is broken down and resorbed. In an infant in whom a nuchal cord is found at delivery, the presence of diffuse petechiae around the head and neck is common and does not warrant further investigation. In addition, petechiae found on the presenting body part are normal. The appearance of new bruises or petechiae

after delivery should alert the physician and nurse to the possibility of a bleeding disorder or infection.

Fat Necrosis

Many infants delivered with the aid of forceps show forceps marks after delivery. These marks tend to fade over 24 to 48 hours. On occasion, a well-circumscribed, firm nodule with purplish discoloration may appear at the site of a forceps mark. This may represent fat necrosis (Fig. 2-37) and resolves spontaneously over weeks to months. The phenomenon may also occur at other sites of trauma. Affected infants may develop symptomatic hypercalcemia.

Nasal Deformities

Abnormalities of the nose are common after delivery, the majority consisting of transient flattening or twisting induced during transit through the birth canal. Less than 1% of nasal deformities are due to actual dislocations of the triangular cartilage of the nasal septum. These can be differentiated from

Figure 2-35 Meconium staining. The marked discoloration of this infant's fingernails resulted from long-standing meconium staining of the amniotic fluid before delivery.

Figure 2-37 Fat necrosis. This discolored nodular lesion on the cheek is characteristic of subcutaneous necrosis of fat secondary to forceps trauma.

Figure 2-38   Nasal deformity. This infant incurred dislocation of the triangular cartilage of the nasal septum during delivery. Inspection of the nose reveals deviation of the septum to the right and asymmetry of the nares **(A).** When the septum is manually moved toward the midline, the asymmetry persists, confirming the dislocation **(B).**

positional deformities by manually moving the septum to the midline and observing the resultant shape of the nares. In a true dislocation, marked asymmetry of the nares persists (Fig. 2-38). Returning the septum to its proper position can be accomplished in the nursery with the guidance of an otolaryngologist. Failure to recognize and treat dislocation may lead to permanent deformity.

Peripheral Nerve Damage

Injury to the peripheral nervous system, especially the facial and brachial nerves, is one of the more common serious occurrences related to birth. Unilateral facial nerve palsy is the most common peripheral nerve injury, with an incidence as high as 1.4 per 1000 live births. Injury can result from direct trauma from forceps or from compression of the nerve against the sacral promontory while the head is in the birth canal. With pronounced nerve injury, there is decreased facial movement and forehead wrinkling on the side of the palsy, eyelid elevation, and flattening of the nasolabial folds and corner of the mouth (Fig. 2-39). Crying accentuates the findings, with the most obvious sign being asymmetrical movement of the mouth. The side that appears to droop when crying is the normal side. The differential diagnosis includes Möbius syndrome (usually bilateral) and absence of the depressor anguli oris muscle, which may be associated with cardiac anomalies. The latter condition is distinguishable from facial nerve palsy by the absence of involvement of the forehead, eyelid, or nasolabial area. The prognosis for facial nerve palsies is excellent, and recovery usually occurs within the first month. In the meantime, prevention of corneal drying is essential. Surgery is reserved for cases in which clear-cut severing of the facial nerve has occurred. Referral should be made if there is no improvement after 2 to 3 months.

The incidence of brachial plexus trauma with current obstetric management is approximately 0.7 per 1000 live births. The mechanism of injury in most instances is traction on the plexus during delivery. Although lesions have classically been divided into those affecting upper spinal segments (Erb's palsy) and those affecting lower segments (Klumpke's palsy), the distinction may not be clear-cut in some cases. Injury to the C5 and C6 fibers is most often identified by the child's arm hanging limply adducted and internally rotated at the shoulder and extended and pronated at the elbow (Fig. 2-40, *A*). Injury affecting the lower segments of C7 and T1 rarely occurs in isolation, causing weakness of the wrist and hand, and ultimately leads to a claw-hand deformity (Fig. 2-40, *B* and *C*). There may be sensory loss along the ulnar side of the hand and forearm in the distribution of the T1 dermatome. If the T1 root is affected with interruption of the sympathetic innervation at that level, Horner's syndrome may be apparent. Appropriate deep-tendon reflexes are absent. It may be difficult to confirm sensory deficit, and autonomic fibers are often intact. Diagnosis is made clinically, but electromyography may be indicated to assess the severity of the injury and to determine the prognosis in patients not showing improvement after 6 to 8 weeks. Treatment should be deferred for at least 7 to 10 days; then specific physical therapy and splinting should be undertaken. Most infants with brachial plexus palsies demonstrate complete recovery in the first few months of life. Earlier recovery suggests better long-term prognosis.

CONGENITAL ANOMALIES

Innumerable congenital anomalies, many of a minor nature, can be noted at birth. Although any single minor malformation may be of little medical consequence, the identification

Figure 2-39   Facial nerve palsy. This infant incurred injury to the right facial nerve, resulting in loss of the nasolabial fold on the affected side and asymmetrical movement of the mouth. The side of the mouth that appears to droop is the normal side.

Figure 2-40   Brachial plexus injury. **A,** Traction injury to C5, C6, and C7 spinal cord segments produced this (Erb) palsy. This infant demonstrates the characteristic posture of the limply adducted and internally rotated arm. **B** and **C,** Infant with Klumpke palsy involving the lower segments of C7 and T1. Note the different posture of the arm compared with the Erb palsy, and the claw-hand deformity. (**B** and **C,** *Courtesy Dr. Michael Painter, Children's Hospital of Pittsburgh.*)

of three or more in a single infant may be a clue to more serious errors of morphogenesis. A careful family history including examination of the parents and siblings can often place these malformations in proper perspective.

Hands and Feet

The majority of minor external anomalies involve the hands, feet, and head. One of the more common abnormalities of digitation, especially in African-American infants, is the presence of a supernumerary digit (Fig. 2-41), which is most often located lateral to the fifth digit on the hand or foot. This condition is distinguishable from true polydactyly because of the small pedicle that attaches the extra digit to the fifth digit. The supernumerary digit may have a fingernail but often lacks bones. Although usually of no consequence, a supernumerary digit has, on occasion, been associated with major central nervous system (CNS) malformations. Removal may be accomplished by applying a ligature around the pedicle (assuming that it is thin and lacks palpable bony tissue) as close as possible to the surface of the fifth digit and allowing for the extra digit to fall off naturally. This usually takes approximately 1 week. Care should be taken to observe for infection.

True polydactyly (duplication of digits) may also be seen (Fig. 2-42). It is most common on the feet but can also occur on the hands. A family history of this anomaly may exist, or it may occur in association with other, more serious patterns of malformation. Although removal is not required, it may be indicated cosmetically.

Syndactyly, fusion of the soft tissues between digits, is relatively common (Fig. 2-43). Once again, a family history can be helpful to determine association with other anomalies. Surgical correction of the syndactylism is usually postponed until 3 years of age unless there is a synchondrosis (cartilaginous union) or synostosis (bony union) that may interfere with growth.

Palmar creases occur as a consequence of flexion of the thickened skin of the hand in the first trimester. Alterations in folding of the palmar plane may be affected by the slope of the third, fourth, and fifth metacarpal–phalangeal joints or relative shortness of the palm. A single, unilateral, midposition plane of flexion, *single palmar crease,* is found in 4% of the population (bilateral in 1% of the population).

External Ear

Careful morphologic examination of the external ear may reveal a number of minor anomalies. One of the more common is the presence of preauricular skin tags located anterior to the tragus (Fig. 2-44). These tags may be unilateral or bilateral and represent remnants of the first branchial arch. Although often of little consequence, they may be seen in serious malformations of branchial arch development involving multiple structures of the head and neck. Surgical removal may be indicated for cosmetic purposes.

A second, often overlooked malformation is the presence of ear pits or congenital aural fistulas located anterior to the tragus (Fig. 2-45). These may be familial, occur twice as often

Figure 2-41   Supernumerary digit. This is the common position for a sixth digit. The thin pedicle distinguishes this anomaly from true polydactyly.

Figure 2-42   Polydactyly. True bilateral polydactyly of the fifth toe is seen in this infant.

Figure 2-43 Syndactyly. This child demonstrates bilateral fusion of the soft tissue between the first and second toes.

Figure 2-45 Aural fistula. A pronounced congenital ear pit is seen anterior to the tragus. Its only significance is that it may become infected.

in girls, and are more common in African Americans. They are of little consequence beyond the fact that they may become infected.

Oral Clefts

Cleft lip and palate are among the most common facial anomalies (Fig. 2-46). These defects represent failure of lip fusion (at 35 days of gestation) and, in some cases, subsequent failure of closure of the palatal shelves (at 8 to 9 weeks of gestation). Although many cases occur spontaneously, others appear to be inherited, and in a minority of instances the defect is one manifestation of a chromosomal disorder. Adequate assessment necessitates careful examination of all structures of the head and neck and their relationship to each other. For example, cleft palate may be coupled with mandibular hypoplasia (Pierre Robin sequence), resulting in significant respiratory obstruction. Because of associated eustachian tube dysfunction, otitis media is an almost invariable complication of cleft palate. Specialized feeding techniques are often necessary for these infants. Even in the absence of an overt cleft, palpation and visualization of the palate and uvula should be routine because clefts of the soft palate (associated with a bifid uvula and a midline notch at the posterior border of the hard palate) can lead to later speech problems (see Chapters 22 and 23).

Midline Defects

Although major malformations of the spinal column, such as myelomeningocele, are readily identifiable (see Chapter 15), diagnostic differentiation between two other midline

defects—pilonidal sinuses and congenital dermal sinuses of the lumbar and sacral spine—can be difficult. A pilonidal sinus tends to be located over the sacrum (Fig. 2-47). The surface opening is usually larger than that of a dermal sinus, but the tract rarely extends into the spinal canal; therefore although infection can occur, CNS extension is unlikely. A congenital dermal sinus is usually located over the lower lumbar region, with a sinus tract that can extend farther down the spinal column. The external orifice may be a small dimple or an easily visible opening surrounded by hair. Recognition is important because there may be an underlying spinal dysraphism, and infection of the tract can extend to the CNS. These abnormalities can herald an occult tethered spinal cord, which may occur with minimal or no neurologic signs. Failure to recognize the possible association of these cutaneous abnormalities with an occult tethered cord could result in later neurologic abnormalities including foot and lower extremity deformities, decreased sensation, weakness, abnormal gait, and bladder dysfunction. Diagnosis can be made by ultrasound, optimally in the newborn period because the acoustic window becomes smaller as the child grows (Fig. 2-48).

Figure 2-46 Cleft lip. A prominent bilateral cleft lip with a complete cleft palate is seen in an infant with trisomy 13. The cleft extends from the soft to the hard palate, exposing the nasal cavity.

Figure 2-44 Ear tags. Multiple preauricular skin tags were seen as an isolated finding in this patient.

Figure 2-47 Pilonidal sinus. This midline sinus overlying the sacrum did not extend to the spinal cord.

Figure 2-49 Localized ectodermal dysplasia. An extensive punched-out area lacking all normal dermal elements is seen in the midline of the scalp of this child with trisomy 13.

Another form of midline defect may occur over the posterior parietal scalp and consists of a localized area of ectodermal dysplasia (Fig. 2-49). This lesion appears "punched out" and lacks all normal dermal elements. It may be associated with chromosomal anomalies, especially trisomy 13, but may be present in otherwise normal infants. Similar lesions, often located on the extremities, should be distinguished from those on the scalp because they often represent a dermatologic defect known as *cutis aplasia*.

Skin

Complete examination of the newborn's entire skin surface is essential. Quality of the neonate's skin can be an indicator of gestational age (see Figs. 2-5 and 2-6). Skin anomalies evident in the newborn period are quite common. These conditions include transient and spontaneously resolving rashes and more permanent variations (see Chapter 8).

Jaundice is a yellow hue of the skin and mucous membranes (Fig. 2-50) and is a cause for concern if noted within the first 24 hours of life. The color is a result of deposited bilirubin, an end product of heme catabolism that occurs in the normal newborn at an increased rate due to decreased red blood cell survival in the neonatal period. Bilirubin can also concentrate and deposit in the brain, leading to neuronal injury and the devastating condition of kernicterus. Physiologic elevation occurs in newborns with a peak at about 3 days. Premature neonates have a delayed and more severe bilirubin peak at 5 days due to delayed maturation of the hepatic uridine diphosphate-glucuronosyltransferase (the enzyme controlling bilirubin conjugation to allow for its excretion). It is routine for newborns to be screened for hyperbilirubinemia before discharge from the hospital. Common risk factors for hyperbilirubinemia include breast-feeding, low birth weight, ABO incompatibility, and cephalhematoma.

Congenital Hip Dislocation

Congenital hip dislocation occurs six times more frequently in females than in males, with an overall incidence of 1.5 in 1000 live births. Associated factors include breech presentation, oligohydramnios, and first-born infants. The pathologic anatomy involves superior capsular laxity and a shallow acetabulum due to limited concentric contact with the femoral head. The key diagnostic sign on physical examination of the newborn is hip instability with the capacity for hip dislocation and subsequent relocation. Only one hip should be examined

Figure 2-48 Transducer is centered in the midline in the sagittal plane over the lower lumbar spine. The lumbar spinal cord *(arrowheads)* extends into the sacral portion of the spinal canal and is dorsally displaced. The conus terminates at the approximate level of S2. CSF, cerebrospinal fluid; vb, vertebral body. *(Courtesy A'Delbert Bowen, MD, Children's Hospital of Pittsburgh.)*

Figure 2-50 Scleral icterus. The yellow hue of a jaundiced newborn may be evident in the sclera, as in this newborn.

Figure 2-51 Coronal flexion images with the transducer over the posterolateral aspect of the hip joint, centered on the femoral head (FH). **A,** Normal cartilaginous femoral head is shown well-seated in the acetabulum *(arrowheads).* **B,** Congenital dislocation with the femoral head markedly subluxed laterally and the invagination of fatty tissue (pulvinar) that occupies the space between the femoral head and the acetabulum *(arrowheads). (Courtesy A'Delbert Bowen, MD, Children's Hospital of Pittsburgh.)*

at a time. Examining both hips simultaneously may impair proprioception such that soft tissue "clicks," due to movement of fascia over the greater trochanter, may be mistaken for the dull "clunk" of dislocation. In experienced hands the diagnosis can easily be confirmed by ultrasonography, which is a sensitive procedure for detecting hip dysplasia (Fig. 2-51) in the immediate newborn period. Screening ultrasound, however, should not be performed before 2 weeks of life because physiologic laxity of the ligaments may result in a high false-positive rate. Ideally, orthopedic consultation for treatment should be obtained within the first 6 months of life.

Amniotic Bands

A number of serious structural deformations can result from early in utero amniotic rupture and subsequent bandline compression or amputation. The band-induced abnormalities generally affect the limbs, digits, and craniofacial structures (Fig. 2-52). This phenomenon is usually sporadic.

Umbilical Hernia

An umbilical hernia is a common finding, especially in African-American infants (Fig. 2-53). The incidence of this defect of the central fascia beneath the umbilicus is also higher in premature infants and those with congenital thyroid deficiency. Distinguishing between this relatively benign fascial defect and the more serious defects of the somites that form the peritoneal, muscular, and ectodermal layers of the abdominal wall underlying the umbilicus, resulting in an omphalocele, is important. In the latter condition, a portion of the intestine is located outside the abdominal wall (see Chapter 17). When large, the distinction is obvious, but in its mildest form, an omphalocele resembles a fixed hernia of the umbilicus. True umbilical hernias usually require no therapy, and spontaneous resolution occurs within the first few years of life. Those that remain after the age of 3 years can be surgically repaired. Attempts to reduce the hernia with tape or coins are ineffective and may result in side effects such as adhesive reaction/allergy. Incarceration is rare.

Figure 2-52 Amniotic bands. A lower extremity amniotic band caused amputation of the toes and constriction around the lower leg.

Figure 2-53 Umbilical hernia. This prominent umbilical hernia was noted at birth in an otherwise normal African-American infant.

Scrotal Swelling

Swelling of the scrotum in the neonate is relatively common, especially in breech deliveries. Although the differential diagnosis includes hematomas, infections, testicular torsion, and tumors, the majority of cases are attributable to hydroceles or fluid accumulation in the tunica vaginalis. Palpation reveals an extremely smooth, firm, egg-shaped mass that brightly transilluminates (Fig. 2-54). When the hydrocele is noncommunicating, the clinician can often palpate above the mass with the thumb and finger and feel a normal spermatic cord. The testicle may be difficult to palpate but is usually visible on transillumination. With inguinal hernias, the prolapsed intestine may transilluminate as well, but it usually presents visible septa under high-intensity light. Furthermore, on palpation there is significant thickening of the spermatic cord. Although a hydrocele may persist for months, the majority resolve spontaneously. There is a high association with inguinal hernias, especially in hydroceles that persist. In such cases the spermatic cord is often noticeably thickened. Given the association with hernias, the possibility of bowel incarceration should be kept in mind. Surgical repair is indicated when a hydrocele persists for more than 6 months or when it is associated with findings suggestive of an inguinal hernia such as a communicating hydrocele. These hydroceles will randomly appear to become smaller and larger over time. (See Chapter 17 for a more detailed discussion of inguinal hernias.)

RESPIRATORY DISTRESS

The differential diagnosis and subsequent management of the infant with respiratory distress are the most frequent challenges encountered by the practitioner of newborn medicine. Problems posed by prematurity, the failure of the necessary transition to extrauterine existence, infectious complications, metabolic derangements, and various congenital and acquired abnormalities of the cardiopulmonary system may all lead to a similar presentation in the newborn period.

Infants with respiratory distress may present with tachypnea or cyanosis (Fig. 2-55), or both, and varying degrees of

Figure 2-55 Cyanosis. This critically ill infant exhibits cyanosis and poor skin perfusion.

a triad of signs, which include *grunting, flaring,* and *retractions (GFR)*. *Grunting* is a characteristic involuntary guttural expiratory sound made by infants as they exhale against a closed glottis in an attempt to maintain expiratory lung volume. *Flaring* refers to the reflexive opening of the nares during inspiration (Fig. 2-56). *Retractions* are the result of increased respiratory effort with high negative intrathoracic pressures leading to an inward collapse of the relatively compliant chest wall of the newborn during inspiration (Fig. 2-57).

Classic respiratory distress syndrome (RDS) is caused by a combination of lung immaturity secondary to preterm delivery and surfactant deficiency. The radiographic findings (Fig. 2-58) in such infants consist of a ground-glass appearance (small airway and alveolar atelectasis) and "air bronchograms" (an outline of the large airways superimposed on the relatively airless lung parenchyma). Infants with RDS usually need supplemental oxygen therapy and surfactant replacement and often require mechanical ventilatory assistance.

Most infants with RDS recover without sequelae. However, a small proportion develops a chronic lung condition known as *bronchopulmonary dysplasia*. Histologically, this condition is characterized by varying degrees of inflammation and fibrosis (Fig. 2-59). The chest x-ray studies of such infants exhibit areas of hyperinflation alternating with atelectasis (Fig. 2-60).

The most common cause of respiratory distress in term infants is transient tachypnea of the newborn (TTN). Thought to be related to the delayed removal of fetal lung fluid, this condition is more common in infants born by cesarean section.

Figure 2-54 Scrotal swelling. This infant demonstrates a unilateral hydrocele that was noted at birth. Transillumination was consistent with the diagnosis.

Figure 2-56 Flaring. Reflexive widening of the nares may be seen in infants with respiratory distress.

Figure 2-57 Retractions. The inward collapse of the lower anterior chest wall can be seen in this premature infant with respiratory distress syndrome.

Figure 2-59 Bronchopulmonary dysplasia. Histologic features include inflammation and fibrosis.

Radiographic findings may include streaky perihilar shadows caused by dilated lymphatics or visible fluid densities within the intralobar fissures (Fig. 2-61), or both. As its name implies, TTN resolves over time, usually with minimal supportive care.

Unfortunately for the clinician, the early clinical and radiographic findings in infants with potentially life-threatening congenital pneumonias may mimic those seen in RDS or TTN (Fig. 2-62). This diagnostic uncertainty leads to early treatment with antibiotics until bacterial cultures, serial chest radiographs, and clinical improvements reassure the practitioner that the discontinuation of such antibiotics is warranted.

Meconium aspiration elicits an inflammatory response within the lungs and may also present as respiratory distress. The radiographic findings consist of irregularly distributed areas of hyperaeration and consolidation throughout the lung parenchyma (Fig. 2-63).

Congenital heart disease (see Chapter 5) and various anomalies of the thoracic cavity or lungs (see Chapter 16) also commonly manifest in the newborn with signs of respiratory distress and should be included in the differential diagnosis. Pulmonary air leak syndromes such as pneumothorax (Fig. 2-64; and see Fig. 17-46) and pneumomediastinum (Fig. 2-65) are among the more common complications.

HYPOTHERMIA

The newly born infant is dependent on the environment as well as its own skin to maintain thermoregulation. Newborns should be placed in a warm environment such as a radiant warmer or on the mother's chest and dried immediately after birth to prevent heat loss. Swaddling and a warm room temperature are basic considerations. An additional heat source such as an incubator may be required in preterm infants.

Purposeful hypothermia may be induced in the infant who suffers from an event of hypoxic–ischemic encephalopathy. Cooling the infant to a core temperature of 33.5°C to 34.5°C for 72 hours reduces the outcome of death and long-term severe neurodevelopmental sequelae.

NEWBORN STOOLS

An infant's first few bowel movements consist of accumulated intestinal cells, bile, and proteinaceous material formed during intestinal development. The material, termed *meconium* (Fig. 2-66), is a sticky, greenish black product mirroring the shape of the fetal intestine. When passed into the amniotic fluid before delivery, it can, if aspirated into the lung, cause an inflammatory pneumonitis. Early passage of meconium is generally precipitated by fetal distress or asphyxia. Failure to pass meconium in the first 2 days of life may indicate intestinal obstruction resulting from stenosis, atresia, or Hirschsprung's disease. The possibility of cystic fibrosis with a meconium ileus should also be considered. In premature infants, failure to pass meconium may reflect meconium plug syndrome (small left colon syndrome), which appears to be a disorder of maturation of intestinal motility. In most cases a

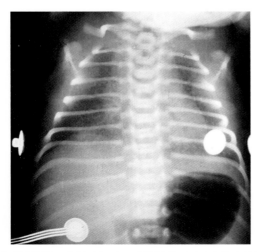

Figure 2-58 Respiratory distress syndrome. Note the ground-glass appearance and the presence of air bronchograms.

Figure 2-60 Bronchopulmonary dysplasia. Note the alternating areas of hyperinflation and atelectasis.

Figure 2-61   Transient tachypnea of the newborn. Radiograph reveals a number of streaky perihilar densities and a visible fluid density in the right major fissure.

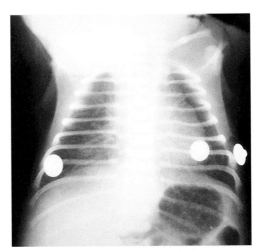

Figure 2-62   Congenital pneumonia. Cultures from the lungs of this infant were positive for group B streptococci. Note the similarity to Figure 2-61, with streaky perihilar densities and visible fluid density in the right major fissure.

Figure 2-63   Meconium aspiration. The radiograph reveals irregularly distributed areas of hyperaeration and consolidation.

Figure 2-64   Tension pneumothorax. Note the shift of the mediastinum, flattening of the diaphragm, and widening of the intercostal spaces. Also note the umbilical central lines, nasogastric tube, and endotracheal tube.

Figure 2-65   Pneumomediastinum. A central collection of air in the mediastinum. Note the support lines and tubes in place.

Figure 2-66   Meconium. A typical sticky, greenish black meconium stool consists of accumulated intestinal cells, bile, and proteinaceous material formed during intestinal development.

Figure 2-67 Transitional stool. At 2 to 3 days after delivery, stools become greenish brown and may contain some milk curds.

Figure 2-69 Formula stool. Infants fed commercial formulas typically have darker, firmer stools than breast-fed infants.

Gastrografin enema leads to prompt passage of meconium without recurrence.

By the third day of life, stools change in character and become known as *transitional* stools (Fig. 2-67). They are greenish brown to yellowish brown, are less sticky than meconium, and may contain some milk curds. In some infants who are fed generous quantities of milk during the first few days, the stool may have an increased liquid component that contains undigested sugar. This diarrheal stool resolves with moderation in the quantity of feeding, because it is caused by the osmotic effect of undigested lactose.

After the third to fourth day, the quality and frequency of stool are often functions of the type of milk ingested. Breast-fed infants have stools that are yellow to golden, mild smelling, and vary from pasty to watery in consistency (Fig. 2-68). Infants fed commercial formulas have pale yellow to light brown stools that are firm and somewhat more offensive in odor (Fig. 2-69). A wide range of normal stool frequency exists in formula-fed neonates. Many infants have a stool after each feeding for the first several weeks, which is due to an active gastrocolic reflex; other infants may have one stool every few days. Breast-fed infants should have at least six stools per day by the third day of life, and this should persist for the first few weeks of life. Infrequent passage of stool in the breast-fed infant is a sign of inadequate feeding in the first weeks of life.

A careful history, with emphasis on an infant's stool pattern, feeding history, and any parental attempts (laxatives, rectal manipulation) to induce bowel movements, can be extremely important. Normal weight gain in the presence of true diarrhea is unusual. Difficulty passing stools (straining, crying, decreased frequency) may reflect local irritation from anal fissure formation rather than true constipation. Constipation is defined by hard pellet stools rather than frequency. The use of a topical lubricant and stool softeners can be recommended to resolve constipation. Failure of such measures suggests the possibility of a significant pathologic condition (see Chapter 17).

ABDOMINAL DISTENTION

A neonate's abdomen is naturally rounded due to poor muscle tone. An excessive protuberance can indicate pathology. As previously discussed, eliciting a thorough stooling history can help differentiate the etiology of abdominal distention. The differential diagnosis includes functional and anatomic obstructions, infection, organomegaly, and masses. The abdomen should be examined while the infant is quiet, with avoidance of examination immediately after a feeding. Radiographic studies such as ultrasound (pre- and postnatal) and abdominal plain films are helpful diagnostic aids. In addition, water-soluble contrast enemas and abdominal computerized tomography scans may be necessary to differentiate an etiology. Surgical consultation may be warranted (see Chapter 17 for further discussion).

BREAST-FEEDING

Human breast milk is the optimal food for almost all infants. The American Academy of Pediatrics and the World Health Organization recommend that infants be fed human milk exclusively for the first 6 months of life and that breast-feeding be continued with the addition of complementary foods until at least age 1 or 2 years, respectively. Human milk provides both immediate and long-term benefits to infants, mothers, and society. The Agency for Healthcare Research and Quality commissioned a systematic review of the literature regarding the benefits and risks of breast-feeding for infants and children in the developed world. Study findings regarding risk reduction afforded breast-fed children compared with formula-fed infants are summarized in Table 2-2. Women who breast-feed have less postpartum bleeding, more rapid involution of the gravid uterus, and reduced risk of type 2 diabetes mellitus, ovarian cancer, and breast cancer. Societal benefits include health care savings due to fewer office visits and hospitalizations, less absenteeism from work, and ecologic benefits.

Figure 2-68 Breast-milk stool. The stools of breast-fed infants are usually yellow, soft, and mild-smelling and typically have the consistency of pea soup. Breast milk stools can also be watery.

Table 2-2	Summary of Findings from 2007 AHRQ Report: Breast-feeding and Maternal and Infant Health Outcomes in Developed Countries

Infants and Children	% Lowered Risk
Lower respiratory tract infections	72
Gastrointestinal infections	64
Otitis media	50
Atopic dermatitis	42
Asthma	27-40
Diabetes type 1	19-27
Diabetes type 2	39
Obesity	7-27
SIDS	36
Childhood leukemias	15-19

AHRQ, Agency for Healthcare Research and Quality.
From Ip S, Chung M, Raman G, et al: *Breastfeeding and maternal and infant health outcomes in developed countries.* Evidence Report/Technology Assessment No. 153 (Prepared by Tufts-New England Medical Center Evidence-based Practice Center, under Contract No. 290-02-0022). AHRQ Publication No. 07-E007. Rockville, Md, 2007, AHRQ.

Breast milk is biologically complex, species specific, and serves both as a source of nutrition and immunologic support for the developing infant. It contains hundreds of bioactive substances including entire white blood cells (e.g., macrophages, T cells, B cells, and neutrophils), proteins such as immunoglobulins (IgA, IgD, IgG, and IgM) and immune-modulating factors (e.g., lactoferrin, lysozyme, and lactoperoxidase), hormones (e.g., thyrotropin-releasing hormone, thyroxine, cortisol, and insulin-like growth factor-1), growth factors (e.g., epidermal growth factor, and human-milk growth factors I, II, and III), enzymes, and cholesterol. These bioactive agents, which are not found in commercially prepared human milk substitutes, augment the infant's immature immune system. Human milk changes during feedings and across time in order to meet the changing nutritional and immunologic needs of infants.

In 2007, 75% of women in the United States initiated breast-feeding, but only 43% were still feeding their infant any breast milk at 6 months and 22% at 12 months compared with the Healthy People 2020 (HP2020) national public health objectives of 75%, 50%, and 25%, respectively. The HP2020 goals for exclusive breast-feeding are that 60% of women will still be exclusively breast-feeding until 3 months and 25% until 6 months; unfortunately, rates of exclusive breast-feeding remain significantly below these recommendations at 33% and 13%, respectively.

Health care providers play an important role in a woman's decision to breast-feed and can also have a significant impact on a woman's success with breast-feeding. Therefore it is important that health care providers know the benefits of breast-feeding, the normal patterns of feeding, elimination, and growth, and be able to assist a woman with latch, positioning, and commonly encountered breast-feeding problems.

Research has shown that women usually choose an infant feeding method before or in the first trimester of pregnancy but that their health care provider's opinions can affect this decision. Therefore, the American College of Obstetricians and Gynecologists and other organizations strongly encourage health care providers to discuss the benefits of breast-feeding in the early reproductive years and reinforce it again early in pregnancy. The benefits of breast-feeding can be discussed in multiple settings, such as school-based education, family planning and obstetric clinics, prenatal visits, and public health campaigns. Women's infant feeding intentions before delivery are the strongest predictor of their actual infant feeding behavior.

Health care providers can help a mother–baby dyad succeed at breast-feeding by providing both clinical expertise and emotional support. The role of the pediatric health care provider in supporting breast-feeding begins either at the prenatal visit or in the newborn nursery. The pediatric health care provider should obtain maternal and birth histories, observe a breast-feeding, and provide appropriate education.

Pregnancy and Breast Development

The human breast is not fully developed until pregnancy. During the first trimester of pregnancy, the ductal system of the breast expands and branches under the influence of estrogen. Nearing the second trimester, the milk-producing cells (acini) begin to accumulate a substance similar to colostrum. Prolactin and placental lactogen support the production of colostrum. During the third trimester, the ductal system of the breast continues to expand and dilate and fill with colostrum. After birth, with the rapid decline in progesterone that occurs with removal of the placenta, milk production begins under the influence of prolactin. The changes in the internal structure of the breast are usually accompanied by external changes as well. Most women experience an increase in breast size, a darkening of the areola, and increased prominence of the Montgomery glands. These breast changes are reassuring that the woman's body is preparing for lactation.

Women who do not experience these breast changes should be closely monitored after delivery for breast-feeding problems, especially inadequate milk supply. Although rare, some women may have insufficient glandular tissue (Fig. 2-70, *A* and *B*) that is associated with insufficient milk supply.

Breast size is not associated with breast-feeding success. Breast reduction surgery can negatively affect a woman's ability to exclusively breast-feed her infant because of disruption of nerves and milk ducts. However, newer surgical techniques result in fewer problems and therefore women who have had breast reduction surgery should be encouraged to try breast-feeding. Augmentation does not usually impact breast-feeding success, although excessively large implants can worsen engorgement. Women who have had breast surgery should be monitored closely in the first few weeks after delivery for evidence of low milk supply and inadequate infant weight gain.

Contraindications to Breast-Feeding

There are few absolute contraindications to breast-feeding. In the developed world, women with HIV/AIDS or human T-lymphotropic virus (HTLV) should not breast-feed. Mothers with active tuberculosis can express their milk and have someone else feed the baby until she has initiated treatment and is no longer considered contagious. Women with herpes simplex infections of the breast should not feed the infant on the side with the herpes lesions; however, they can be fed from the uninfected side as long as the lesions are covered. The American Academy of Pediatrics (AAP) *Red Book* is an excellent source of detailed information about infectious diseases and breast-feeding.

Infants with classic galactosemia should not be breast-fed because human milk contains high levels of lactose. Infants with other forms of galactosemia, tyrosinemia, and phenylketonuria may be partially breast-fed, but this should be determined on an individual basis along with the metabolism/genetics specialist caring for the infant.

Most, but not all, medications are safe for women to take during lactation. The National Library of Medicine website, LactMed, is free and available on the Internet and is an excellent source of information; in addition, it is continuously

Figure 2-70 Insufficient breast glandular tissue. Tubular breast shape, little to no breast enlargement, and little areolar darkening with pregnancy may indicate insufficient glandular tissue. There is often a family history of inadequate milk supply. Women with this condition may benefit from a referral to a lactation consultant. **A,** A 26-hour postpartum woman with tubular-shaped breasts without any fullness. **B,** A woman with insufficient glandular tissue and significantly different breast size who has insufficient milk supply. *(Courtesy Susan Costanza, RN, IBCLC, Rochester General Hospital, Rochester, NY.)*

updated. The AAP breast-feeding policy indicates that tobacco use is not a contraindication to breast-feeding. However, women who smoke tobacco should be encouraged to smoke outside and to decrease cigarette use or preferably to stop smoking. Women who smoke should be counseled to do so after feedings to minimize the transfer of nicotine into breast milk. Women who use illicit drugs should be counseled not to breast-feed. Women prescribed methadone or buprenorphine for the treatment of opiate addiction should be encouraged to breast-feed if they remain adherent to their drug treatment program and do not have any other contraindication to breast-feeding.

Breast-feeding Evaluation

Pediatric health care providers should be comfortable observing and assisting women with breast-feeding, especially during the neonatal period, the first health maintenance examination, and when problems arise such as poor weight gain or painful nursing. A thorough evaluation includes a history, examination of the mother's breasts, observation of the latch and positioning, and assessment of milk transfer. Some health care providers may find it more comfortable to perform the physical examination of the maternal breast with a chaperone, as is done with examinations of the genitalia.

History

The history should be appropriate for the visit. At the neonatal and first postpartum visits it should include pregnancy and birth history, frequency, duration and pattern of nursing,

frequency of voids, frequency and character of stools, weight change, jaundice, pain with nursing, and maternal concerns. The AAP's *Breastfeeding Handbook for Physicians*, Chapter 8 ("Maintenance of Breastfeeding—The Infant") provides key points to support maintenance of breast-feeding for each pediatric visit from birth to 12 months.

Breast Examination

If a woman is having difficulty latching the baby in the neonatal period or if she complains of pain at any time, her breasts should be examined. For latching problems, it is important to determine whether a woman has flat or inverted nipples. Nipple inspection alone does not answer this question and the pinch test must be performed (Fig. 2-71). The nipple

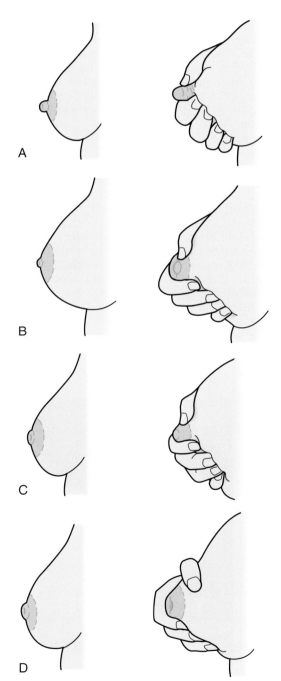

Figure 2-71 Nipple evaluation with the pinch test. **A,** Protracting normal nipple. **B,** Moderate to severe retraction. **C,** Inverted-appearing nipple, which, when compressed using the pinch test, either inverts farther inward or protracts forward. **D,** True inversion: nipple inverts further using pinch test. *(Reprinted with permission from Riordan J, Auerbach K, editors:* Breastfeeding and human lactation, *ed 2, Sudbury, Mass, 1999, Jones & Bartlett, p. 99. Available at www.jbpub.com)*

is normally everted if the nipple protrudes when the areola is compressed, inverted when it retracts toward the breast when the areola is compressed, and flat when it neither protrudes nor retracts. Although flat or inverted nipples may make it more difficult for the infant to latch in the first few days, women with flat or inverted nipples should not be discouraged about breast-feeding because in many cases of flat and inverted nipples, babies latch without difficulty. However, if an infant has difficulty latching, the mother–infant dyad should be seen within the first day of birth by someone experienced in lactation support. The adhesions that cause the nipple to flatten or invert can usually be broken. Having the mother use a manual or electric breast pump for a few minutes before the baby latches to draw out the nipple can do this. Another option is to use a nipple shield (Fig. 2-72) for a short time to allow the baby to latch more easily. If a nipple shield is offered, it should be done under the supervision of someone experienced in lactation support because it is not intended for long-term use. Flat and inverted nipples usually improve with nursing. The use of breast shells during pregnancy has not been shown to improve flat and inverted nipples. Prepregnancy use of shells may undermine a woman's confidence in her ability to nurse her infant and thus may impede successful breast-feeding.

Latch

A key factor in the success of breast-feeding is an appropriate latch (Fig. 2-73, A and B) because it affects both milk supply and comfort. When a baby is properly latched on the breast, the baby's mouth is wide open, with the angle between the baby's upper and lower lips nearly 180 degrees. The upper and lower lips should be everted, with the baby's lips as far back on the areola as possible and the nipple in the back of the baby's mouth. Because of the wide variability in the size of babies' mouths and mothers' nipples and areolas, the amount of areola visible during an effective latch is highly variable. When the infant lets go of the breast, the nipple should not be flattened; it should remain round. A flattened nipple is a sign that the baby's mouth is not opened wide enough during the feeding. When the latch is inadequate (Fig. 2-74), the mother may experience discomfort and the baby may not be able to empty the breast effectively and efficiently. Some women experience normal discomfort just as the baby latches on that resolves in less than a minute. However, if a woman experiences persistent pain with breast-feeding she should unlatch the baby from the breast by inserting a finger into the corner of the baby's mouth and between the gums and gently pressing down toward the baby's chin. The baby should then be repositioned and a proper latch attempted again. If the pain continues, the mother–baby dyad should be observed during a feeding by a person experienced in breast-feeding assessment. An inadequate latch can result in nipple trauma (Fig. 2-75, A and B) and, over time, can compromise milk supply.

Holding Positions and Latch

Optimally, all babies should be placed skin-to-skin on the mother's chest during the first hour of life, when they are wide awake from the adrenaline surge that occurs at the time of delivery. Placing the baby on the mother's chest facilitates early initiation of breast-feeding. Skin-to-skin care improves infant temperature regulation, decreases infant cortisol levels (an indicator of stress), is associated with longer duration of breast-feeding, and supports mother-infant attachment. The four main breast-feeding positions for the newborn are the football (Fig. 2-76, A and B), cross-cradle (Fig. 2-77), classic cradle (Fig. 2-78), and side-lying (Fig. 2-79) positions. Each nursing mother should find the positions that are comfortable for her. Pillows and foot rests can be used to increase comfort. Pillows can be used to raise the baby to the level of the mother's breast for optimal support. In all the positions, it is helpful to support the baby so that he or she feels secure, without a sense of falling. The angle between the baby's neck and chin should be about 90 degrees. The midline of the chin should be aligned with the center of the chest, thus placing the baby's head, neck, and anterior chest in alignment for ease in swallowing.

To initiate the latch, the mother can touch her nipple to the baby's upper lip. This stimulates the baby to open the mouth and lower and extend the tongue. When the baby opens

Figure 2-72   A, A preterm infant is breast-feeding with nipple shield in place. Nipple shields can be used for preterm or term infants who have difficulty with latch for a variety of reasons, such as maternal flat or inverted nipples and engorgement. They are not intended for long-term use and should be used under the supervision of a person well trained in lactation support. **B,** A preterm infant is full and satisfied after breast-feeding with a nipple shield in place. The nipple shield has multiple fenestrations, so the milk comes out as it does from the mother's nipple.

Figure 2-73 **A** and **B,** Good latch. A good latch is characterized by a wide-open mouth, everted lips, and high position on the mother's areola. The angle between the baby's two lips should be close to 180 degrees. *(Courtesy Susan Costanza, RN, IBCLC, Rochester General Hospital, Rochester, NY.)*

Figure 2-74 Inadequate latch is characterized by a partially closed mouth with the angle between the baby's lips less than 90 degrees, often with the lips near the base of the mother's nipple. *(Courtesy Susan Costanza, RN, IBCLC, Rochester General Hospital, Rochester, NY.)*

Figure 2-75 **A** and **B,** Cracked, abraded, bruised nipples and areola. These result from improper latch and positioning. An experienced clinician should assess the mother's technique for holding and latching the baby. *(Courtesy Susan Costanza, RN, IBCLC, Rochester General Hospital, Rochester, NY.)*

Figure 2-76   A and **B,** Football position. This position is especially good for women with large breasts, women who have had a cesarean section, and new mothers because it allows good visualization of the latch and good head control. It is also the position of choice for twins. *(Courtesy Susan Costanza, RN, IBCLC, Rochester General Hospital, Rochester, NY.)*

widely, the mother should place the baby's open mouth past the nipple and as far back onto the areola as possible with the nipple aimed toward the hard palate. The baby's chin and lower lip should make first contact with the breast. Many women have to hold their breast as the baby initially latches. Either the C hold, with the thumb on top of the breast and the other four fingers below, or the scissor hold, with the thumb and index finger on top of the breast and the other three fingers below, can be used. With either hold, the fingers should be off the areola so that they do not interfere with the latch. After the baby is well latched, some women may be able to release the hold on the breast. For women with large breasts, a rolled washcloth can be placed under the breast for support so that the breast doesn't have to be held for the entire feeding.

In all feeding positions, it is essential that the mother be comfortable. This means she should have adequate back, arm/shoulder, and hand support. To minimize the need for a mother to hold her breast throughout the feeding, it is ideal to align the baby's mouth where the breast lays naturally. Line up the tip of the baby's nose with where the mother's nipple lays naturally. When the baby opens the mouth wide, the nipple should slip just under the baby's upper lip. This achieves the asymmetrical latch, which is often more comfortable for women. An asymmetrical latch is one in which the nipple is not in the middle of the baby's mouth but rather is placed just under the infant's upper lip. In this position, more of the mother's areola is visible above the infant's upper lip than below the infant's lower lip (Fig. 2-80).

Football Hold (see Fig. 2-76, *A* and *B*)

The football hold is especially good for women with large breasts and women who have had a cesarean section and cannot tolerate abdominal pressure. Because it allows good visualization of the latch and good head control, it is also an excellent position for premature infants and for new mothers. The mother holds the baby in the same arm as the breast she intends to feed from. The heel of the mother's hand should rest approximately between the baby's scapulae, and her thumb and index finger should be placed on the baby's mastoid processes. The baby's back should rest on the mother's forearm or on a support such as a pillow placed at the level of the breast. The baby's head should be tipped back just slightly. The mother takes her opposite hand and grasps the breast behind the areola. A pillow can be placed under the mother's arm for her support. Depending on the size of the mother's breasts and the length of her arms, the baby may be facing the ceiling or be turned on the side with the baby's abdomen in contact with the mother's ribs. Women with large breasts should place the infant along the side of the breast to avoid the weight of the breast being placed on the infant's chest. The baby's nose, chin, and midchest should be aligned and the neck slightly extended.

Cross-Cradle (see Fig. 2-77)

The cross-cradle is an excellent position because it allows good visualization of the latch and provides firm head control for the neonate. When the baby is several weeks old and has

Figure 2-77   Cross-cradle position. This is an excellent position to use with the young infant because it allows good visualization of the latch and provides firm head control of the neonate. The mother's hand is under the baby's neck. The baby's chin but not the nose is in the mother's breast. More of the areola is covered by the lower lip than by the upper lip, which is characteristic of a normal, asymmetrical latch. *(Courtesy J. Newman, MD, FRCPC, Hospital for Sick Children, Toronto.)*

Figure 2-78   Cradle position. The cradle position is easier to use when the baby has developed a modicum of head control but can also be used in the newborn if the mother finds it comfortable. The infant's nose, chin, and chest are aligned, and the mother and baby are belly-to-belly. *(Courtesy Susan Costanza, RN, IBCLC, Rochester General Hospital, Rochester, NY.)*

Figure 2-79 Side-lying position. This is suitable for mothers who have had a cesarean section, are tired, have a sore perineum, or have a sleepy baby and for nighttime feeding. The mother and baby are belly to belly, and the baby is held on the side by the mother's hand. A receiving blanket can be rolled up and placed behind the infant's back to hold the baby in the position if the mother prefers. (Courtesy Susan Costanza, RN, IBCLC, Rochester General Hospital, Rochester, NY.)

Figure 2-80 Asymmetrical latch. The positioning of the baby's upper lip just above the mother's nipple provides a comfortable latch for many women who experience discomfort with nursing.

Figure 2-81 Plugged milk pores. Plugged milk pores at the end of the nipple cause acute pain with breast-feeding. This should be treated by unroofing the pore with a needle held horizontal to the tip of the nipple. Pain relief is instant when milk is released from the duct. (Courtesy Susan Costanza, RN, IBCLC, Rochester General Hospital, Rochester, NY.)

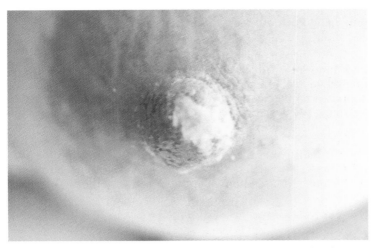

Figure 2-79 Side-lying position. This is suitable for mothers who have had a cesarean section, are tired, have a sore perineum, or have a sleepy baby and for nighttime feeding. The mother and baby are belly to belly, and the baby is held on the side by the mother's hand. A receiving blanket can be rolled up and placed behind the infant's back to hold the baby in the position if the mother prefers. *(Courtesy Susan Costanza, RN, IBCLC, Rochester General Hospital, Rochester, NY.)*

developed a good latch and improved head control, many women transition to the classic cradle hold. In the cross-cradle position, the baby is held by the mother in the arm opposite to the breast she intends the baby to feed from. The baby is turned belly to belly with the mother so that the umbilicus and knees are touching the mother's abdomen. The baby's nose, chin, and midchest are aligned, and the neck is slightly extended. The heel of the mother's hand should rest approximately between the baby's scapulae, and her thumb and index finger should be placed on the baby's mastoid processes. The mother's forearm should rest along the baby's spine, and the baby's bottom should be firmly tucked under the mother's elbow and upper arm, with the baby's head tipped back slightly. When the baby is well latched, the mother may be able to release her hold of the breast and use her arm for additional support of the baby.

Classic Cradle (see Fig. 2-78)

The classic cradle position is easier to use when the baby has developed a modicum of head control, but it can also be used with a newborn if the woman finds it comfortable. The classic cradle has the baby's head in the bend of the mother's arm on the same side as the breast she is offering. The baby's umbilicus and knees should be facing the mother's abdomen. The mother can use her other hand to hold her breast behind the areola to guide it to the baby's mouth.

Figure 2-80 Asymmetrical latch. The positioning of the baby's upper lip just above the mother's nipple provides a comfortable latch for many women who experience discomfort with nursing.

Side-lying Position (see Fig. 2-79)

The side-lying position is good for mothers who have had a cesarean section, have a sore perineum, or are tired; and at nighttime after breast-feeding is well established. It may be helpful to place a pillow behind the mother's low back for support and between her legs if desired for comfort. A rolled receiving blanket can be placed behind the infant to keep the baby in a side-lying position. The mother may initially need assistance in getting her baby latched in this position if she has limited agility after delivery, and because she may not be able to completely visualize the latch. The baby should be turned so that the infant's abdomen is touching the mother's abdomen.

Breast Problems

Engorgement

Engorgement is painful breast fullness caused by vascular congestion, edema, or milk accumulation in the breast tissue. It may be mild to severe and most commonly occurs 2 to 7 days after delivery. Engorgement can be prevented in many cases by encouraging frequent feedings (10 to 12 per day) and proper latch. Despite these preventive efforts, engorgement still occurs and physicians must recognize the signs and symptoms promptly. The signs are firm, sometimes lumpy, tender breasts with increased vascular markings in the face of a maternal sense of fullness to the point of discomfort. If not relieved, engorgement can make it difficult for the baby to latch, may result in decreased milk production, and can contribute to the development of mastitis. Treatment involves frequent emptying of the breasts and symptomatic care. Infants should be nursed frequently, or milk should be expressed manually or with a pump. Warm compresses to soften the breast tissue and manual expression of milk before putting the baby to the breast may make it easier for the baby to latch properly. Cool compresses after feedings may help to decrease vascular congestion.

Sore, Bruised, or Cracked Nipples (see Fig. 2-75, *A* and *B*)

Sore, bruised, or cracked nipples can occur when a baby is not latched properly. The pain caused by these conditions is the reason why many mothers become discouraged and stop breast-feeding. Improper latch, usually too close to the nipple, is the leading cause of sore nipples. Mothers should not be told to grin and bear the pain. They should be promptly referred to an experienced clinician to assess the latch and positioning. Milk pores at the end of the nipple can become plugged (Fig. 2-81), causing acute pain with breast-feeding.

Figure 2-81 Plugged milk pores. Plugged milk pores at the end of the nipple cause acute pain with breast-feeding. This should be treated by unroofing the pore with a needle held horizontal to the tip of the nipple. Pain relief is instant when milk is released from the duct. *(Courtesy Susan Costanza, RN, IBCLC, Rochester General Hospital, Rochester, NY.)*

Figure 2-82 *Candida* infection. Fungal infection of the breast to this degree is uncommon, but more subtle presentations are common. Women with candidal infection of the breast complain of burning or stabbing pain during or after breast-feeding. Most often the mother's breast appears normal or slightly red, but the breast-feeding baby has oral or diaper candidiasis. In this case both mother and baby should be treated. *(Courtesy J. Newman, MD, FRCPC, Hospital for Sick Children, Toronto.)*

Figure 2-83 Thrush. Yeast infection of the infant's mouth can cause the infant to feed poorly, and may also transfer to the mother's breast. It is imperative that breast-feeding infants identified with yeast infection be treated immediately along with the mother.

This should be treated by unroofing the pore with a needle held horizontal to the tip of the nipple. Pain relief is instant when milk is released from the duct.

Yeast Infections (see Fig. 2-82)

Yeast infections of the mother's breast and baby's oropharynx or diaper area are common after the first week or two of life. The signs of thrush in the baby include white plaques on the gingiva and tongue that do not wipe off and are present before and after feeding (Fig. 2-83). Babies may pull on and off the breast when they have thrush, likely due to mouth soreness. Mothers may experience a variety of symptoms from yeast infection of the breast including sharp, stabbing, or burning pain during and after feeding, as well as red, cracked, and sore nipples. If a breast-fed baby has thrush, both mother and baby should be treated even if the mother is asymptomatic at the time of the visit. A number of treatment options exist. The first line of treatment is usually to treat the mother with a topical antifungal agent applied to the nipple and areola after each feeding, and the baby with 1 mL of oral nystatin solution (100,000 IU/mL) four times a day. Treatment should be continued for several days after both are without obvious lesions. The second option is to treat both mother and baby with 0.5% to 1% topical gentian violet once daily for no more than 3

days. Prolonged use can result in mouth ulcers. Combined therapy can be used. For example, the gentian violet may be applied once in the office; treatment at home is continued with antifungal agents. Last, both mother and infant can be treated with oral fluconazole for 10 to 14 days if they are not responding to the other treatments or in the case of recurrent infections. As with all cases of thrush, all artificial nipples should be properly cleaned every day.

Impetigo (see Fig. 2-84, A and B)

Impetigo can also occur on the breast. It should be treated with an oral antibiotic (e.g., cephalexin or appropriate coverage for methicillin-resistant *Staphylococcus aureus* [MRSA], depending on skin isolates in the health care provider's area) if widespread or with a topical antibiotic (e.g., mupirocin) if fairly localized.

Mastitis (see Fig. 2-85)

Mastitis is a bacterial infection of the breast. It can result from blocked ducts or from ascending infection due to cracked nipples. Mastitis presents as acute onset of fever, chills, and extreme breast tenderness over an area of induration and firmness, usually on one breast. This is not a reason to cease breast-feeding. In fact, the treatment includes frequent emptying of the breast, oral antibiotics to cover penicillin-resistant staphylococcal and streptococcal species (e.g., first-generation cephalosporin or dicloxacillin), analgesics, rest, and adequate fluid intake. However, mastitis can progress to breast abscess

Figure 2-84 Impetigo of the breast before treatment **(A)** and after treatment **(B)** with an oral antibiotic. The mother experienced pain with and without nursing. *(Courtesy Nancy G. Powers, MD, Medical Director of Lactation Services, Wesley Medical Center, Wichita, Kan.)*

Figure 2-85 Mastitis, an infection of the breast, often presents as acute onset of fever, chills, and extreme breast tenderness over an area of induration and firmness. This is not a reason to cease breast-feeding. In fact, the treatment includes frequent emptying of the breast and oral antibiotics to cover both staphylococcal and streptococcal species. *(Courtesy J. Newman, MD, FRCPC, Hospital for Sick Children, Toronto.)*

Figure 2-87 Blanching of the nipple just after feeding, due to vasospasm. Mothers describe the pain of vasospasm as burning that begins after the feeding is over, possibly lasting several minutes or more, after which the nipple returns to its normal color; the pain may then become throbbing.

(Fig. 2-86), which requires incision and drainage and antibiotics. This can often be done on an outpatient basis with close follow-up. In the case of an abscess, milk should be expressed and discarded from the affected side until no longer draining and the baby fed only from the unaffected side. Many women report a decrease in milk supply on the side impacted by mastitis or abscess.

Vasospasm: Blanching of the Nipple (see Fig. 2-87)

Some women experience pain just after breast-feeding. If they notice that the nipple turns white just after feeding, they may be experiencing vasospasm of the nipple. Women often describe it as a burning sensation. The causes may include temperature change, inadequate latch, yeast infection, or other causes of nipple trauma. The most important treatment is to address the underlying cause, such as a too-shallow latch. Even when the underlying cause is corrected, the vasospasm may take longer to resolve. A simple first approach is to apply a heating pad or warm compress after feedings. If the vasospasm persists after the underlying cause is treated, the mother should be referred to a breast-feeding expert. They may recommend vitamin B_6 or nifedipine; these treatments, based on anecdotal experiences, have not been well studied.

Assessing Milk Transfer

Many women are concerned that their baby is not getting enough to eat, especially in the first few days when they have colostrum. It is essential to educate mothers about normal

Figure 2-86 Breast abscess is a localized breast infection that requires incision and drainage and treatment with an antibiotic to cover staphylococcal and streptococcal infection. It can occur as a complication of inadequately treated mastitis. *(Courtesy J. Newman, MD, FRCPC, Hospital for Sick Children, Toronto.)*

eating patterns and how to assess whether her infant is getting enough to eat without having to measure it. In the first 1 to 2 days of life, a mother usually produces only about 30 mL of colostrum. Despite the small volume, that is all a newborn needs. Colostrum is extremely high in protein. Parents should be instructed to monitor the following indicators of adequate intake: elimination patterns, weight changes, breast changes, and frequency and duration of feedings.

Elimination

Infants should have increasing numbers of voids and stools with each day. By day 3 of life, babies should have at least four or five voids and transitional stools a few times per day. By day 4 to 5, babies should have more than five voids per day and transitional to yellow stools at least four or five times per day. By day 6 of life, babies should have at least six to eight voids per day and at least four loose to watery yellow stools per day.

Weight Changes

Infants usually lose weight for 2 to 3 days after birth, plateau for a day, and then begin to regain. Infants who are successfully breast-feeding should return to birth weight by no later than 10 days of age. Infants who are still losing weight after 4 days should be assessed by someone with expertise in lactation. Babies should not lose more than 8% from birth weight in the first 3 to 4 days of life. Excessive weight loss is the sign of a breast-feeding problem.

Breast Changes

When a mother senses that her breasts are fuller, heavier, and warmer, this is a sign that the volume of milk she is producing is increasing. This occurs as early as 36 hours in women with previous breast-feeding experience and as late as days 5 to 7 for primiparous women and women with complications or prolonged labor. After a woman notices this change in her breasts, babies should no longer lose weight and should begin to gain at least 20 to 30 g/day. A mother should notice that her breast feels full and heavy before the baby nurses and softer after the baby is finished.

Frequency and Duration of Feedings

For the first 24 to 48 hours after birth, a baby's nursing frequency is highly variable. After that, most babies nurse 10 to 12 times per day (Table 2-3). The baby should be satisfied after the feeding and be content and often asleep. If the baby is not meeting these assessment goals, the mother should seek professional assistance with breast-feeding. According to the American Academy of Pediatrics, all breast-feeding infants should be assessed within 48 to 72 hours of hospital discharge.

Table 2-3	Assessing Milk Transfer			
	Day 0	**Days 1-2**	**Days 3-4**	**Days 5-6**
Voids	≥1	≥2-3	≥4-6	≥6-8
Stools				
Number	≥1	≥1-2	≥2-3	≥3-4
Color	Meconium	Meconium	Transitional	Yellow/seedy
Weight compared with birth weight*	—	≤5% loss	≤8% loss	Should start regaining
Number of feedings per day	4-8	8-12	8-12	8-12

*If an infant is not back to birth weight by 10 days, this is a red flag for breast-feeding difficulties; mother and infant should be referred to a health care provider expert in lactation support.

Table 2-4	Categorization of Types of Ankyloglossia (Tongue-Tie)		
Type	**Attachment under Tongue**	**Attachment to Floor of Mouth**	**Comments**
I*	Tip of tongue	In front of alveolar ridge	Heart-shaped tongue with superior movement
II	2-4 mm behind tip of tongue	Just behind alveolar ridge	
III	Midtongue	Middle of floor of mouth	Tight and inelastic
IV	Base of tongue	Floor of mouth	Thick, shiny, not very elastic

*See Figure 2-88.

Ankyloglossia (tongue-tie) has been recognized since ancient times as a potential problem with breast-feeding. Tongue-tie is a condition in which the lingual frenulum limits the range of motion of the tongue (Fig. 2-88). Normal range of motion of the tongue is demonstrated if the tongue can be extended outside the mouth and to the roof of the mouth without forming a cleft and the lips can easily be licked by the tip of the tongue. Tongue movement forward and up toward the roof of the mouth is essential for successful transfer of milk in breast-feeding. Infants with limited anterior or superior movement of the tongue can have an ineffective latch and cause maternal pain during feedings. In general, tongue-ties are categorized into four types based on the location of the attachment of the frenulum to the underside of the tongue and the floor of the mouth (Table 2-4).

One method used to assess the impact of the frenulum is the Hazelbaker Assessment Tool. Hazelbaker scores consistent with significant ankyloglossia correlate with difficulty in latching for the infant and maternal complaints of sore nipples (Table 2-5).

Premature Infants

Among the many benefits to providing human breast milk to premature infants are decreased risk of perinatal infections and necrotizing enterocolitis, shorter hospital stays, and improved developmental outcomes. Mothers of premature or ill infants should be counseled about the benefits of human breast milk for the health of their infants so that they can make an informed decision. Women who chose to breast-feed their preterm or ill infants in the NICU require support and education. It is important to create a breast-feeding supportive environment in the NICU. This includes allowing flexible visiting hours to encourage breast-feeding, as well as knowledgeable and supportive staff.

Women who choose to provide expressed milk while waiting to breast-feed their infant should be shown how to hand express colostrum or be given access to a hospital-grade double-sided electric breast pump (Fig. 2-89) and instructed in how to use it within a few hours of delivery. Hand

Table 2-5	Hazelbaker Assessment Tool for Lingual Frenulum Function: 1998 Version
Appearance Items	**Function Items**

Appearance of tongue when lifted
  2: Round *or* square
  1: Slight cleft in tip apparent
  0: Heart-shaped
 	
Elasticity of frenulum
  2: Very elastic (excellent)
  1: Moderately elastic
  0: Little *or* no elasticity
 	
Length of lingual frenulum when tongue lifted
  2: More than 1 cm *or* embedded in tongue
  1: 1 cm
  0: Less than 1 cm
 	
Attachment of lingual frenulum to tongue
  2: Posterior to tip
  1: At tip
  0: Notched tip
 	
Attachment of lingual frenulum to inferior alveolar ridge
  2: Attached to floor of mouth *or* well below ridge
  1: Attached just below ridge
  0: Attached at ridge
	Lateralization
	  2: Complete
	  1: Body of tongue but not tongue tip
	  0: None
	
	Lift of tongue
	  2: Tip to midmouth
	  1: Only edges to midmouth
	  0: Tip stays at alveolar ridge or rises to mid-mouth only with jaw closure
	
	Extension of tongue
	  2: Tip over lower lip
	  1: Tip over lower gum only
	  0: Neither of above, *or* anterior or mid-tongue humps
	
	Spread of anterior tongue
	  2: Complete
	  1: Moderate *or* partial
	  0: Little *or* none
	
	Cupping
	  2: Entire edge, firm cup
	  1: Side edges only, moderate cup
	  0: Poor *or* no cup
	
	Peristalsis
	  2: Complete, anterior to posterior (originates at the tip)
	  1: Partial: originating posterior to tip
	  0: None *or* reverse peristalsis
	
	Snapback
	  2: None
	  1: Periodic
	  0: Frequent *or* with each suck

Note: 14 = perfect score (regardless of Appearance Item score); 11 = acceptable if Appearance Item score is 10; <11 = function impaired. Frenotomy should be considered if management fails. Frenotomy is necessary if Appearance Item score is less than 8.

From Amir LH, James JP, Donath SM: Reliability of the Hazelbaker Assessment Tool for lingual frenulum function, *Int Breastfeed J* 1:3, 2006.

Figure 2-88 Ankyloglossia (tongue-tie). In this case the lingual frenulum is attached too near the tip of the tongue. Infants with tongue-tie have limited anterior or superior movement of the tongue, leading to an ineffective latch and causing maternal pain during breast-feeding.

Figure 2-89 Double pumping of the breasts. This is the most efficient and effective way for women to maintain a milk supply when they are unable to breast-feed directly. The pump should initially be set at the minimal setting and gradually increased to a level of comfort for the mother. *(Courtesy Susan Costanza, RN, IBCLC, Rochester General Hospital, Rochester, NY.)*

expression is ideal for the first 1 to 2 days, while only small volumes of colostrum (early milk) are available at each feeding. Hand expression videos are available on the Internet (*http://newborns.stanford.edu/Breastfeeding/HandExpression.html*). In the first few days of pumping, only small amounts of yellow to white colostrum are expressed, as little as a teaspoon per pumping. This is normal. On occasion, the early milk looks rusty or bloody, dubbed the "rusty pipe syndrome" (Fig. 2-90); this is also normal and can be used without concern. However, if the rusty milk continues for more than 1 week, the mother should be referred for further evaluation.

Mothers should be instructed to express their milk at least every 2 to 3 hours during the day and at least once during the night. The volume of milk expressed should increase 3 to 5 days after delivery. Stresses can definitely delay and

decrease milk production, a common problem for mothers with a baby in the neonatal intensive care unit (NICU). Women should be encouraged to keep pumping. Pumped milk should be frozen in small volumes and thawed as needed. The milk should have the date on the label so that the first bottles into the freezer are the first to be used to avoid spoilage and because the milk composition changes over time. Before babies are put to the breast, they can be placed in kangaroo care (i.e., placed on the mother's chest in skin-to-skin contact) to encourage bonding and to begin movement toward breast-feeding.

A baby who is ready to bottle-feed is also ready to breast-feed. Premature babies fed at the breast have on average a lower heart rate, lower respiratory rate, and higher pulse oximetry measurement compared with bottle-fed infants. Babies are usually ready to breast-feed when they are physically stable, display a rhythmic suck–swallow–breath pattern (usually at about 34 weeks), and demonstrate feeding reflexes (rooting, sucking, gagging, and coughing).

A natural progression toward breast-feeding is to start with skin-to-skin contact (kangaroo mother care). When the baby is displaying the rooting reflex, have the mother empty her breasts and then allow the baby to nuzzle and latch onto a breast. When the baby is ready to take milk from the breast, have the mother pump milk until her let-down milk flow slows, and then offer the baby her breast. The first few times a mother offers her baby the breast, she should be observed and supported. If there is concern that the baby is not getting enough milk at the breast or that the infant requires fortified breast milk or formula, there are several options. First, the baby should be weighed on a gram scale (at least twice to ensure accuracy) before the feeding, wearing a clean diaper and the clothes to be worn during the feeding. The baby is then fed and reweighed two more times without a change of diaper or clothes after feeding. The difference between the average postfeed weight and the prefeed weight is the amount (in grams) of breast milk consumed; from this the volume may be calculated. If the baby has not taken "enough," the baby can then be fed by an alternative feeding method to supplement, such as by cup feeding (Fig. 2-91), finger feeding (Fig. 2-92), or gavage. Second, a supplemental nursing system (SNS) (Fig. 2-93, *A* and *B*) filled with expressed breast milk, fortified breast milk, or appropriate formula can be attached to the breast so that the baby receives both breast milk and the supplement. The tip of the tubing must be placed about

Figure 2-90 Rusty pipe syndrome. Rusty or brown, bloody-appearing early milk. This uncommon finding usually occurs in primiparous women early in lactogenesis. They experience painless breast-feeding, and the nipples are not cracked and bleeding. The etiology is uncertain, but the condition may be caused by internal bleeding due to edema and engorgement. This milk is safe and can be used without concern. *(Courtesy Susan Costanza, RN, IBCLC, Rochester General Hospital, NY.)*

Figure 2-91 Cup feeding is an alternative feeding method for infants. A small medicine cup or one designed specifically for this purpose can be used. The cup is placed at the margin of the infant's lower lip and tipped gently toward the mouth. The infant should extrude the tongue and assist feeding by lapping the milk as small amounts are poured between the lower lip and gum. Cup feeding is widely used in underdeveloped countries when mothers are unable to feed their infants from the breast. *(Courtesy Susan Costanza, RN, IBCLC, Rochester General Hospital, Rochester, NY.)*

Figure 2-92   Finger feeding is an alternative method for feeding infants. The largest finger that is convenient for the feeder should be used. The finger used should be held flat and placed far back in the infant's mouth so that the infant's tongue is forward and curved around the sides of the finger. A 5-French, 36-inch feeding tube is convenient because the thin caliber provides a slow flow rate and the length allows some flexibility with positioning. Among the available alternative feeding methods, finger feeding has the added benefit of training the infant with a weak or immature suck to suck in a similar fashion as during breast-feeding. The one drawback to finger feeding is that it is relatively slow. *(Courtesy J. Newman, MD, FRCPC, Hospital for Sick Children, Toronto.)*

one quarter inch past the end of the mother's nipple so that it remains in the back of the oropharynx as the nipple is lengthened in the infant's mouth. The reasons to progress directly to the breast from gavage feeding are multiple. Bottle-feeding and breast-feeding require the use of different oral muscles and sucking mechanics. Premature babies may get used to bottle-feeding and may not breast-feed well as a result. Therefore it is ideal to feed infants by alternative feeding methods when a mother is not available to breast-feed.

Finger feeding is inexpensive and mimics breast-feeding well but is also time consuming. Finger feeding may be accomplished with a 5-French, 36-inch feeding tube. One end of the feeding tube is placed into a bottle of breast milk or supplement, and the other end is placed in a clean (gloved if not the parent) hand with the tip about one quarter of an inch past the end of the index finger. As the baby draws the finger into the back of the mouth and begins to suck, the milk is drawn up into the feeding tube. Finger feeding also helps prepare the baby to suck properly at the breast with a rounded tongue, and milk is provided deep into the baby's mouth.

Cup feeding is another alternative feeding method. The milk can be dispensed from a small medicine cup. The cup is placed near the baby's lower lip so that the milk can be lapped up. It can also be slowly poured between the lower lip and gums. A variety of cups are made specifically to cup-feed infants, such as the Foley cup and Haberman feeder. This method of feeding is more time efficient than finger feeding and usually is used when the mother is not available to feed the baby herself.

Most infants can transition to full feeds at the breast exclusively by 36 to 40 weeks. However, the transition to full breast-feeding should begin as soon as possible. Now that infants are discharged well before term, pediatricians, family practitioners, and lactation consultants in the outpatient setting often provide this education and support. Advice should be individualized to each mother–baby dyad. A general approach is to have the mother dual-pump with a high-grade electric pump every time she offers the baby milk other than at the breast, including if she is using an SNS to provide the supplement. At first the mother may need to pump after every feeding, especially if the baby has not yet reached term, has a weak suck, or is a sleepy baby. This will help to match her milk supply and her baby's increasing needs. Every few days, she can increase the number of feedings at the breast without supplement. The baby's stool and urine output should be monitored to ensure adequate intake, and the baby's weight should be monitored to ensure adequate growth during the transition.

Late Preterm Infants (35 to 37 Weeks)

Late preterm infants are often treated as term infants, but they are at high risk for breast-feeding problems. They may look as though they are feeding well, but they have weaker and less sustained suck patterns than term infants. They are at increased risk for excessive weight loss, hyperbilirubinemia, and rehospitalization. It is essential that health care providers remain vigilant and monitor late preterm infants closely. Mothers of late preterm infants should be instructed to wake infants at least 10 times each 24 hours to feed, and to monitor output and weight loss and jaundice. If the baby does not feed effectively, mothers should be instructed to express their milk and feed it to the infant in order to maintain her milk supply until the baby is able to obtain all milk from the breast directly.

Significant and long-lasting health benefits are associated with breast-feeding both for the individual mother–baby dyad

Figure 2-93   **A** and **B,** Supplemental nursing system (SNS). An SNS allows a baby to receive additional nutrients while still breast-feeding and thus provides stimulation to the breast. It does not interfere with breast-feeding technique and latch. The tip of the SNS tubing should protrude past the end of the nipple by about one quarter of an inch. *(Courtesy Susan Costanza, RN, IBCLC, Rochester General Hospital, Rochester, NY.)*

and society. Breast-feeding is the ideal way to feed babies; however, it is not always easy. Mothers must receive adequate support in order to breast-feed successfully. This support and education are most certainly within the role of the pediatric health care provider. Excellent references including textbooks, journals, websites, books, printed materials, and videos are devoted to breast-feeding for those interested in more in-depth information.

Resources

Academy of Breastfeeding Medicine: Breastfeeding protocols for health professionals. Available from http://www.bfmed.org/Resources/Protocols.aspx

Drugs and Lactation Database (LactMed): Website for information about medications and breast-feeding. Available from http://toxnet.nlm.nih.gov/cgi-bin/sis/htmlgen?LACT

Wellstart International: Breastfeeding curriculum [free]. Available from http://www.wellstart.org

DEVELOPMENTAL– BEHAVIORAL PEDIATRICS

3

Heidi M. Feldman | Diego Chaves-Gnecco | Dena Hofkosh

Pediatricians need to be able to distinguish normal development and individual differences from delayed or atypical patterns of development and behavior. Once developmental or behavioral delays have been identified, the pediatrician conducts a diagnostic workup, initiates management, refers to appropriate services, counsels families, and coordinates care. The goal of this chapter is to review the developmental–behavioral issues faced in routine pediatric practice. In the first half, the fundamental principles of development are applied to each major domain of functioning. Within each domain, discussion centers on the major developmental milestones, methods of assessment, signs of developmental variation, and approaches to children who show developmental delays or deviant patterns. In the second half, several developmental disorders are described including definitions, diagnostic criteria, and the role of physical examination in evaluation, physical findings, and prognosis.

PRINCIPLES OF NORMAL DEVELOPMENT

Development is commonly discussed in terms of domains of function. Gross motor skills refer to the use of the large muscles of the body; fine motor skills refer to the use of small muscles of the hands; cognition means the use of higher mental processes including thinking, memory, and learning; language refers to the comprehension and production of meaningful symbolic communication; and social and emotional functioning refers to emotional reactions to events and interactions with others. Within each domain, skills are acquired in a predictable sequence, although there is wide variation in the age of acquisition of specific milestones. Domains of development are interdependent. Cognitive abilities in infancy cannot readily be distinguished from sensorimotor functioning. Similarly, mature social functioning depends on competent language abilities. Early reflex patterns and congenital sensory and motor capabilities are the building blocks of higher-order skills.

In general, the development of a child is considered to occur in cephalocaudal and centrifugal directions, that is, from head to toe (the child holds his or her head up before being able to sit or stand up) and from proximal to distal (the child has rudimentary whole-hand grasp before developing a fine pincer grasp). Also, the development of a child is considered to occur according to the general principle of dependence to independence (from no mobility to rolling, sitting, creeping, crawling, cruising, and walking) and in response of to stimuli (from generalized reflexes to discrete voluntary actions).

To watch some video examples of normal child development (6, 9, 12, and 18 mo of age) from "Digital Visual Diagnosis in Pediatrics: Assessing Infant Development," log on to the online edition of the *Atlas of Pediatric Physical Diagnosis*, 6th edition, Chapter 3: Developmental–Behavioral Pediatrics. This educational tool consists of both a teaching module and a practice review module.

DEVELOPMENTAL ASSESSMENT

Developmental Surveillance

A central component of health maintenance is the prompt identification of developmental problems and the promotion of development. *Developmental surveillance* refers to the longitudinal, continuous process by which physicians and other professionals use all available clinical tools to determine a child's developmental status, to evaluate his or her developmental progress over time, and to identify children who may be at risk for disorders. Surveillance requires that physicians elicit and appropriately attend to parental concerns at each visit, review teacher and day-care provider concerns, obtain a developmental history, make observations of current development and behavior, perform a physical examination, review screening tests, and use other assessment techniques. Frequent routine assessments promote a longitudinal view of the child and allow parental concerns to be addressed in a timely manner. A formal developmental assessment can be arranged if there are severe or persistent concerns. Parental concerns must be addressed at each visit; parents are accurate reporters of current developmental status and their concerns are sensitive indicators of delays or atypical patterns of development.

Developmental Screening

The physician's ability to identify children with developmental delays and disorders is improved by the appropriate use of validated screening tools (Table 3-1). The tools have been designed to be used with unselected groups of children, ideally as part of routine developmental surveillance at a few selected health maintenance visits, such as the 9-, 18-, 24-, and 36-month visits. The use of these screening tests is not appropriate in populations at risk; such patients require comprehensive assessment. The sensitivity and specificity of these instruments range from 0.70 to 0.90. The clinician's judgment is required in interpretation of test results, particularly of measures that rely on parental report. Children who are developing normally may fail a screening test because of shyness, unfamiliarity with the examiner or the materials, or other factors unrelated to developmental competence. In most cases, a positive screen should be followed by a comprehensive assessment of development and should not be ignored. Screening tests can be used to confirm parental concerns but are not appropriate for diagnosing the nature of the problem. If parental concerns persist despite negative findings, a full evaluation is advisable because of the limited sensitivity of the tests and the importance of attending to parental concerns. To ensure that the performance is representative of the child's ability, screening tests should be performed when the child is physically well, is familiar with the setting and with the examiner, and under minimal stress. Examples of familiar settings include the child's home for infants, toddlers, and younger

Table 3-1	Validated Developmental Screening Tests			
	NAME OF TEST			
	Ages and Stages	**Child Development Inventories**	**Denver II**	**Parents' Evaluation of Developmental Status (PEDS)**
Parent time	10-20 min	30 min	0	5 min
Provider time	1-5 min	10 min	20 min	2 min
Age range covered	4 mo-5 yr	15 mo-6 yr	2 wk-6 yr	0-8 yr

For further information and characteristics of these validated developmental screening tests, consult Resources, preceding the Bibliography at the end of this chapter.

children; the child's preschool becomes another familiar setting for children 3 years of age and older.

GROSS MOTOR DEVELOPMENT

Early Reflex Patterns ("Primitive Reflexes")

At birth, a neonate's movements consist of alternating flexions and extensions that usually are symmetrical and vary in strength with the infant's state of alertness. In addition, involuntary "primitive" reflexes can be elicited; they indicate that the patterns of movement requiring the integrated activity of multiple muscle groups are present even at birth. The intact newborn sucks and grasps reflexively; these are motor patterns that are programmed into the organism to enhance survival. The presence of primitive reflexes in the newborn and the disappearance (integration) of these reflexes in a predictable sequence as the infant matures are indications of typical motor development reflecting many developmental and neural factors, such as underlying myelination of higher cortical pathways that allow for voluntary control of movement. Persistence of primitive reflexes beyond the typical age suggests abnormal myelination of the higher inhibitory pathways as seen in children with pre- or perinatal hypoxic–ischemic brain injury.

Perhaps the best known of these reflex patterns is the Moro response, or startle reflex. This reflex can occur spontaneously after a loud noise, but typically it is elicited during the course of physical examination by an abrupt extension of the infant's neck. The response consists of symmetrical abduction and extension of the arms with extension of the trunk (Fig. 3-1) followed by adduction of the upper extremities, as in an embrace, and frequently is accompanied by crying (Fig. 3-2). The Moro reflex gradually disappears by 4 months of age, associated with the development of cortical functioning. In children up to 4 months of age, the Moro response can be used to evaluate the integrity of the central nervous system and to detect peripheral problems, such as congenital muscu-

loskeletal abnormalities or neural plexus injuries; an asymmetrical response may indicate unilateral weakness.

Another early reflex pattern is called the *asymmetrical tonic neck reflex (ATNR)* (Fig. 3-3, *A* and *B*). A newborn's limb motions are strongly influenced by head position. If the head is directed to one side, either by passive turning or by inducing the baby to follow an object to that side, tone in the extensor muscles increases on that side and in the flexor muscles on the opposite side. This response may not be seen immediately after birth, when the newborn has high flexor tone throughout the body, but it usually appears by 2 to 4 weeks of age. The ATNR allows the baby to sight along the arm to the hand and is considered one of the first steps in the coordination of vision and reaching. This reflex disappears by 4 to 6 months of age, to allow for the development of voluntary reaching.

With the emergence of voluntary control from higher cortical centers, muscular flexion and extension become balanced. Primitive reflexes are replaced by reactions that allow children to maintain a stable posture, even if they are rapidly moved or jolted. A timetable listing the expected emergence and disappearance of primitive reflexes and the protective equilibrium responses is presented in Table 3-2.

Antigravity Muscular Control

Muscle control develops in an organized fashion, from head to toe, or in a cephalocaudal progression—head control followed by reaching, followed by sitting, followed by standing—reflecting neuronal myelination in a typical sequence.

Head Control

The infant's earliest control task is to maintain a stable posture against the influence of gravity. Neck flexors allow head control against gravity when a child is pulled from the supine to the sitting position. Neonates show minimal control of the neck flexors, holding their heads upright only briefly when supported in a sitting position. When an infant is pulled to a sitting position, the head lags behind the arms and shoulders

Figure 3-1 First phase of the Moro response. Symmetrical abduction and extension of the extremities follow a loud noise or an abrupt change in the infant's head position.

Figure 3-2 Second phase of the Moro response. Symmetrical adduction and flexion of the extremities, accompanied by crying.

Figure 3-3 **A** and **B,** Asymmetrical tonic neck reflex (ATNR). Flexion of the arm and leg on the occipital side and extension on the chin side create the "fencer position."

(Fig. 3-4, *A*). By 4 months of age the child is able to support his head, and his head moves along with his shoulders when he is pulled to a sitting position (Fig. 3-4, *B*). At 5 to 6 months of age the infant anticipates the direction of movement of the pull-to-sit maneuver and flexes the neck before the shoulders begin to lift (Fig. 3-4, *C*).

Trunk Control and Sitting

In the prone position a newborn remains in a tightly flexed position and can simply turn the face from side to side along the bed sheets. Progressive control of the shoulders and upper trunk in the first few months of life, plus a decrease in flexor tone, enables the young infant to hold the chest off the bed with the weight supported on the forearms by about 4 months (Fig. 3-5). Evolution of trunk control down the thoracic spine can also be observed with the infant in a sitting position (Fig. 3-6). As control reaches the lumbar area, the lumbar lordotic curve can be seen when the child is standing (Fig. 3-7).

Automatic Reactions: Equilibrium and Protective Reactions

Equilibrium and protective reactions are automatic, reflexive patterns that also emerge in a cephalocaudal sequence. *Head righting* refers to the infant's ability to keep the head vertical despite a tilt of the body. A 4-month-old infant typically demonstrates this ability in vertical suspension when gently swayed from side to side. As control moves downward, protective equilibrium responses can be elicited in a sitting infant by abruptly but gently pushing the infant's center of gravity past the midline in one of the horizontal planes. This is the lateral protective reaction, which involves increased trunk flexor tone toward the force and an outreached hand and limb away from the force; it usually emerges by 6 months of age, and is required for the development of stable, independent sitting (Fig. 3-8). At 10 months the child develops the forward protective or parachute reaction, an outstretching of both arms and legs when the body is abruptly moved head first in a downward direction (Fig. 3-9). The forward protective (parachute) reaction is a programmed reflex that protects the head if the child falls from standing or walking and is generally seen just before these motor skills develop.

Development of Locomotion

Gross motor milestones can also be described in terms of locomotion (Table 3-3). Prone-to-supine (front to back) rolling may be accomplished by 3 to 4 months of age, after the child gains sufficient control of shoulder and upper trunk musculature to prop up on the arms. Supine-to-prone (back to front) rolling requires control of the lumbar spine and hip region, as well as the upper trunk; this is usually present by 5 to 6 months of age. Since the introduction of Back to Sleep (recommended supine sleeping to prevent sudden infant death syndrome), prone-to-supine rolling may appear later, at 5 to 6 months, because the child has had little experience in the prone position; it may actually occur later than supine-to-prone rolling, demonstrating the impact of experience on gross motor skills. Creeping (also called commando or army crawling), accomplished at 5 to 6 months of age (Fig. 3-10, *A*), involves coordinated pulling with upper arms and passive dragging of the legs, akin to a soldier trying to keep the body low to the ground. By 6 to 9 months of age, as voluntary control moves to the hips and legs, the child is capable of getting up on the hands and knees, assuming a quadruped position, and crawling (Fig. 3-10, *B*). The next developmental

Table 3-2	Primitive Reflexes and Protective Equilibrium Responses	
Reflex	**Appearance***	**Disappearance***
Moro	Birth	4 mo
Hand grasp	Birth	3 mo
Crossed adductor	Birth	7 mo
Toe grasp	Birth	8-15 mo
ATNR	2 wk	6 mo
Head righting	4-6 mo	Persists voluntarily
Protective equilibrium	4-6 mo	Persists voluntarily
Parachute	8-9 mo	Persists voluntarily

ATNR, asymmetrical tonic neck reflex.

*Different sources may vary on the precise timing of the appearance and disappearance of these primitive and equilibrium responses.

Figure 3-4   Development of head control on the pull-to-sit maneuver. **A,** At 1 month of age the head lags after the shoulders. **B,** By 4 months of age the child is able to support his head, and his head moves along with his shoulders. **C,** At 5 to 6 months the child anticipates the movement and raises the head before the shoulders.

Figure 3-5   Development of posture in the prone position. **A,** The newborn lies tightly flexed with the pelvis high and the knees under the abdomen. **B,** At 2 months of age, the infant extends the hips and pulls the shoulders up slightly. **C,** At 3 to 4 months, the infant keeps the pelvis flat and lifts the head and shoulders.

Figure 3-6 Development of sitting posture. **A,** At 1 to 2 months of age the head is held up intermittently, but trunk control is lacking. **B,** At 2 to 3 months of age the infant raises the head and shoulders well but lacks control of the thoracolumbar area. **C,** At 3 to 4 months, support in the lumbar area is required to sit. **D,** At 5 to 6 months the infant holds the head erect and the spine straight.

Figure 3-7 Standing. By 1 year of age, the lordotic curve, exaggerated here by a diaper, is evident.

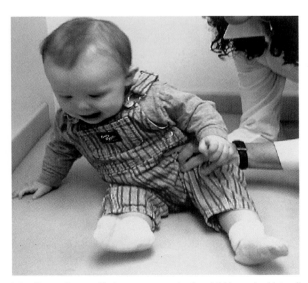

Figure 3-8 Protective equilibrium response. As the child is pushed laterally by the examiner, he flexes his trunk toward the force to regain his center of gravity while one arm extends to protect against falling (lateral propping).

Figure 3-9   Parachute response. As the examiner allows the child to free fall in ventral suspension, the child's extremities extend symmetrically to distribute his weight over a broader and more stable base on landing.

Table 3-3	Early Gross Motor Milestones in the Normal Child

Task	Age Range*
Sits alone momentarily	4-8 mo
Rolls back to stomach	4-10 mo
Sits steadily	5-9 mo
Gets to sitting	6-11 mo
Pulls to standing	6-12 mo
Stands alone	9-16 mo
Walks three steps alone	9-17 mo

*Wide ranges in the attainment of these gross motor milestones in healthy children are the rule rather than the exception.

From Bayley N: *Bayley Scales of Infant Development,* ed 2, San Antonio, Tex, 1993, Psychological Corporation/Harcourt Brace.

milestone is supported standing. By 9 to 10 months of age, many children like to demonstrate this new skill by holding on to a parent or by walking independently while holding on to furniture. This is called *cruising* (Fig. 3-10, *C*). Increased control to the feet and disappearance of the plantar grasp reflex allow the child to walk independently. Walking three steps alone occurs at a median age of about 12 months, with a range of 9 to 17 months of age (Fig. 3-10, *D*).

Development of Complex Gross Motor Patterns

Further progress in gross motor skills continues throughout childhood. The developmental sequence beyond walking incorporates improved balance and coordination and progressive narrowing of the base of support. The sequence of

milestones is as follows: running, jumping on two feet, balancing on one foot, hopping, and skipping. The child simultaneously learns to use muscle groups in timed sequences. By 13½ months the child walks well, and by 36 months he or she can balance on one foot for 1 second. Most children can hop by age 4. They can throw a ball overhand by 22½ months, but catching develops later, at almost 5 years.

GROSS MOTOR ASSESSMENT DURING HEALTH MAINTENANCE VISITS

Evaluation of gross motor skills can begin when the pediatrician enters the office for a well-child visit. The typical 2-month-old infant is cradled in the parent's arms; the 4-month-old has enough strength to support her back when held inside her

Figure 3-10   Development of locomotion. **A,** *Creeping* implies that the belly is still on the floor. **B,** *Crawling* refers to mobility with the child on the hands and knees (quadruped position). **C,** *Cruising* refers to standing with two-handed support on stationary objects before moving with steps. **D,** Early free walking.

Figure 3-11 A 4-month-old has enough strength to support her back when held under her arms by her father's hands but not enough strength to sit on her own.

Table 3-4	Potential Causes of Delayed Gross Motor Development	
Global Developmental Delay	**Motor Dysfunction**	**Motor Intact but Otherwise Restricted**
Genetic syndromes and chromosomal abnormalities	Central nervous system damage— kernicterus, birth injury, neonatal stroke, trauma, prolonged seizures, metabolic insult, infection	Congenital malformations—bony or soft tissue defects
Brain morphologic abnormalities		Diminished energy supply—chronic illness, severe malnutrition
Endocrine deficiencies— hypothyroidism, prolonged hypoglycemia	Spinal cord dysfunction— Werdnig-Hoffmann disease, myelomeningocele, polio	Environmental deprivation—casted, non–weight bearing
Congenital infections		Familial and genetic endowment—slower myelination
Neurodegenerative diseases	Peripheral nerve dysfunction— brachial plexus injury, heritable neuropathies	Sensory deficits— blindness
Idiopathic intellectual disability		Temperamental effects—low activity level, slow to try new tasks
	Motor end-plate dysfunction— myasthenia gravis	Trauma—child abuse
	Muscular disorders— muscular dystrophies	
	Other—benign congenital hypotonia	

arms by her father's hands but not enough strength to sit on her own (Fig. 3-11); the 6-month-old child is sitting with minimal support on the parent's lap or on the examination table next to the parent; the 12-month-old is cruising or toddling through the room. Although there is a wide age range in the onset and duration of each stage, the 6-month-old infant who lacks head control on the pull-to-sit maneuver, who cannot clear the table surface with the chest by supporting weight on the arms when prone, who shows no head righting, or who has persistent primitive reflexes such as a complete Moro response or ATNR is at sufficient variance from peers to warrant evaluation for a possible neuromuscular disorder. In addition, when gross motor delays are found in association with verbal and social delays, asymmetrical use of one limb or one side of the body, or loss of previously attained milestones, diagnostic evaluation is indicated.

Evaluation of the older infant or toddler who has mastered walking can occur in the course of the physical and neurologic evaluation. Many children enjoy showing off their abilities to jump, balance on one foot, hop, and skip. Some pediatricians use gross motor testing to establish rapport at the outset of a physical examination. However, because an aroused preschooler may not cooperate with a sedentary evaluation of heart or ears, many pediatricians hold off on motor evaluation until the conclusion of the examination.

At the discovery of delayed or atypical development, the pediatrician's first task is to develop a differential diagnosis and a plan to establish the specific diagnosis. Potential causes of delayed gross motor development are listed in Table 3-4. Another equally important task is to recommend a treatment program. Early intervention programs and/or physical therapy should be actively considered for children with motor difficulties during infancy through preschool. Adaptive physical education programs are available for older children with mild problems that do not seriously impair function.

FINE MOTOR DEVELOPMENT

Involuntary Grasp

At birth the neonate's fingers and thumb are typically tightly fisted. A newborn grasps reliably and reflexively at any object placed in the palm (Fig. 3-12) and cannot release the grasp. Because of this reflex, the newborn's range of upper extremity motion is functionally limited. Normal development leads to acquisition of a voluntary grasp.

Voluntary Grasp

The reflexive palmar grasp gradually disappears at about 1 month of age. From that point, the infant gains control of fine motor skills in an orderly progression. In the second or third month of life, the infant initially brings both hands together for midline hand play (Fig. 3-13). Shortly after that, the baby begins to swipe at objects held in or near the midline (Fig. 3-14). It is through swiping that the infant increases the exploratory range and fine-tunes the small muscles of the wrist, hand, and fingers.

Improvements in fine motor control increase sensory input from the hands and permit greater hand manipulation through space. By 2 to 3 months of age, the hands are no longer tightly fisted, and the infant may begin sucking on a thumb or individual digit rather than the entire fist for self-comfort. A 3-month-old is usually able to hold an object in either hand

Figure 3-12 Reflex hand grasp. A newborn reflexively grasps at a finger placed in the palm.

Figure 3-13   Midline hand play. A 2-month-old infant brings the hands together at the midline.

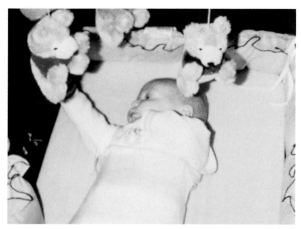

Figure 3-14   Reaching and swiping. A 3-month-old infant uses his entire upper extremity as a unit in interacting with the toy.

if it is placed there, although the ability to grasp voluntarily or to release that object is limited. At approximately 4 to 5 months of age, infants begin to use their hands as entire units to draw objects toward them. Neither the hand nor the thumb functions independently at this point and, consequently, the child uses the hand like a rake.

Next, the child develops the ability to bend the fingers against the palm (palmar grasp), squeeze objects, and obtain them independently for closer inspection. Differentiation of the parts of the hand develops in association with differentiation of the two hands. Between 5 and 7 months of age, the infant can use hands independently to transfer objects across the midline. Further differentiation of the plane of movement of the thumb allows it to adduct as the fingers squeeze against the palm in a radial palmar or whole-hand grasp. With time, the thumb moves from adduction to opposition. The site of pressure of the thumb against the fingers moves away from the palm and toward the fingertips, in what is called an *inferior pincer* or *radial digital grasp,* seen around 9 months of age (Fig. 3-15). By 10 months of age, differentiated use of the fingers allows the child to explore the details of an object.

Between 9 and 12 months of age, the fine pincer grasp develops, allowing opposition of the tip of the thumb and the index finger (see Fig. 3-15). This milestone enables the precise prehension of tiny objects (Fig. 3-16). The infant uses this skill in tasks such as self-feeding and exploration of small objects.

By 1 year, the infant can position the hand in space to achieve vertical or horizontal orientation before grasping or releasing an object.

Development of Complex Fine Motor Skills

Early in the second year of life the young child uses the grasp to master tools and to manipulate objects in new ways. Dropping and throwing, stacking, and putting objects in and out of receptacles become favorite pastimes. Mastery of the cup and spoon supplement or replace finger feeding as a more efficient and less messy means of eating (Fig. 3-17).

Advancements in fine motor planning and control can be demonstrated through the child's ability to stack small cubes. After children master stacking, they show consistent patterns of improvement in reproducing structures that they have watched the examiner assemble (Fig. 3-18). The child's ability to copy a variety of drawings also improves during this period.

Fine Motor Evaluation and Testing

Fine motor testing can be incorporated readily into a physical examination and may uncover problems with vision, neuromuscular control, or perception, in addition to difficulties with attention or cooperation. The 4-month-old child usually can be encouraged to grasp a small toy or tongue depressor. By 6

6 Months Rake	7 Months Inferior-scissors grasp	8 Months Scissors grasp	9 Months Inferior-pincer grasp	10 Months Pincer grasp	12 Months Fine pincer grasp
Thumb adducted, proximal and distal thumb joints flexed, fingers extended	Raking object into palm with flexed fingers and proximal and distal thumb joints flexed	Between thumb and side of curled index finger, distal thumb joint slightly flexed, proximal thumb joint extended	Between ventral surfaces of thumb and index finger, proximal and distal thumb joints extended, beginning opposition	Between distal pads of thumb and index finger, proximal thumb joint extended, distal thumb joint slightly flexed, thumb opposed to index finger	Between fingertips or fingernails, distal thumb joint flexed, proximal thumb joint slightly flexed

Figure 3-15   Development of prehension. *(Modified from Erhardt RP: Developmental hand dysfunction: theory, assessment, treatment, ed 2, San Antonio, Tex, The Psychological Corporation, 1994. Copyright © 1982, 1989, 1994 by Rhoda P. Erhardt. All rights reserved.)*

Figure 3-16   Fine pincer grasp. A 12-month-old child lifts a pill.

to 9 months of age, two tongue depressors should be offered, one for each hand, because the child can operate the hands independently. At 9 to 12 months the child spontaneously points with an isolated index finger or picks up small objects with a fine pincer grasp. Children younger than 18 months of age generally use both hands equally well. Therefore the child who develops consistent handedness with neglect of the other limb before that time should have a neurodevelopmental assessment. The child who has not developed use of the thumb and pincer grasp by 18 months of age deserves further evaluation, as does the child who is unable to copy vertical or horizontal lines by age 3 years or circles by age 4 years.

Fine motor activities can be engaging and nonthreatening to the preschool and school-age child; these activities allow the physician to make valuable observations and to establish rapport. The physician can routinely request that the child use the waiting time or the period of history-taking to draw a self-portrait. These drawings provide a wealth of information not only on the child's capacities for fine motor control but also on cognitive development and social and emotional functioning. A quick method for analyzing the age level of a drawing is to count the number of features in the drawing. The child receives one point for each of the following features: two eyes, two ears, a nose, a mouth, hair, two arms, two legs, two hands, two feet, a neck, and a trunk. Each point converts to the value of $\frac{1}{4}$ year added to a base age of 3 (Fig. 3-19). Screening tests and standardized measures, such as the *Beery-Buktenica Developmental Test of Visual–Motor Integration*, fifth edition, can also be used to assess fine motor skills.

Children with brain damage are at particular risk for problems with perceptual–fine motor integration, even in the absence of visual problems and with minimal involvement of the upper extremities (Fig. 3-20).

Fine motor skills figure prominently in self-care activities. The child who lacks the dexterity to complete simple daily

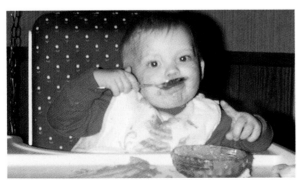

Figure 3-17   Independent feeding. A 15-month-old child employs fine motor skills to use a spoon independently.

activities such as zipping, buttoning, or cutting with a knife may lack the self-esteem that accompanies independent self-care. Furthermore, children who continually depend on parents or teachers may be viewed by peers; teachers; or, perhaps most damagingly, by themselves as less mature. In the school-age child, inefficient fine motor skills can have a significant impact on the ability to write legibly or to compete with peers in timed tasks, even if the child has sound academic and conceptual skills. Occupational therapy and special education may enhance fine motor skills and emotional development in these children.

COGNITIVE DEVELOPMENT

Early Sensory Processing

Innate sensory capabilities serve as the building blocks of cognitive development. Even at birth the healthy neonate responds to visual and auditory stimuli. These responses, like the primitive reflexes, take the form of integrated patterns of activity.

The visual acuity of the full-term infant is estimated to fall between 20/200 and 20/400 and improves rapidly over the first year of life. Even at birth, it is possible to get the full-term newborn to fix on faces 9 to 12 inches from the face and to track objects horizontally at least 30 degrees (Fig. 3-21). Some neonates, if assessed when calm and fully alert, can track objects 180 degrees across the visual field. Newborns also respond to sound, typically quieting in response to a human voice, rattles, or music. In the first days of life, many infants turn to the source of sound and search for it with their eyes. These maneuvers, found on the Brazelton Neonatal Behavioral Assessment Scale, are useful in demonstrating neurobehavioral characteristics of newborns.

Examination must take place at optimal times, when the infant is alert; if the infant is drowsy or agitated, the ability to track visually or to search for sounds is compromised. If, when assessed under optimal circumstances and when fully alert, infants do not demonstrate horizontal tracking of objects, do not look at the toys or people with whom they are involved, or hold their heads in unusual positions, the physician should recommend prompt evaluation for abnormal visual perception or central nervous system development.

Development of Sensorimotor Intelligence

During the first 2 years of life, the sensorimotor period of development, the young child's cognitive abilities can be surmised only through use of the senses and through the physical manipulation of objects. The nature of an infant's thinking is assessed through concrete interaction with the environment. During this period, the child develops an understanding of the concept of object permanence, the ability to recognize that an object exists even when it cannot be seen, heard, or felt. Simultaneously, the child develops an understanding of cause-and-effect relationships. Progress in the child's development of these concepts is an important prerequisite to the development of pure mental activity, reflected in the ability to use symbols and language.

Early progress in the development of object permanence is indicated by the infant's continued though brief gaze at the site where a familiar toy or face has disappeared. At this point, children also repeat actions that they have discovered will produce interesting results. Between 4 and 8 months of age, infants become interested in changes in the position and appearance of toys. They can track an object visually through a vertical fall (Fig. 3-22) and search for a partially hidden toy. They also begin to vary the means of creating interesting

FINE MOTOR TASKS

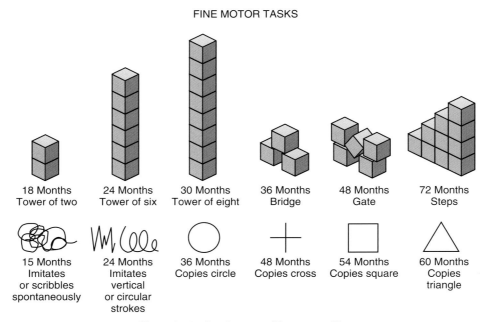

18 Months
Tower of two

24 Months
Tower of six

30 Months
Tower of eight

36 Months
Bridge

48 Months
Gate

72 Months
Steps

15 Months
Imitates
or scribbles
spontaneously

24 Months
Imitates
vertical
or circular
strokes

36 Months
Copies circle

48 Months
Copies cross

54 Months
Copies square

60 Months
Copies
triangle

Figure 3-18   Development of fine motor skills.

effects. In these early months the baby's play consists of exploring toys to gain information about their physical characteristics. Activities such as mouthing, shaking, and banging can provide sensory input about an object beyond its visual features. However, when mouthing of toys persists as the predominant mode of exploration after 12 to 18 months of age, assessment of cognitive function is warranted.

At approximately 9 to 12 months of age, infants can locate objects that have been completely hidden (Fig. 3-23). Not surprisingly, peek-a-boo becomes a favorite pastime at this point. Later, the infant can crawl away from the mother and recall where to return to find her.

As children near 1 year of age, interest in toys extends beyond physical properties (e.g., color, texture). These children may begin to demonstrate their awareness that different objects have different purposes. For example, a child might touch a comb to the hair in a meaningful nonpretend action, typical of the 9- to 12-month age range. Beyond 1 year of age, children begin to vary their behavior to create novel effects. They no longer need to be shown how to work dials or knobs, nor do they need to hit something by accident to discover the interesting effect that will result.

By 18 months of age, children can deduce the location of an object even if they have not seen it hidden from view. They can maintain mental images of desired objects and develop plans for obtaining them. The child's understanding of causality also advances; cause-and-effect relationships no longer need to be direct to be appreciated (Fig. 3-24). These developments herald the beginning of a new stage in cognitive development, that of symbolic thinking. They also indicate that distraction may not succeed in drawing a child away from a desired object; a direct request is required.

Figure 3-19   Development of skill at drawing a person. **A,** This drawing by a 4-year-old child includes five features: eyes, nose, mouth, hair, and legs. To calculate an age equivalent, the child earns ¼ year for each of the five features, added to a base age of 3 years. This drawing has an age equivalent of 4¼ years. **B,** A drawing by the same child at age 5 years. Note the inclusion of ears and arms, as well as improvements in proportion. This drawing has an age equivalent of 4¾ years.

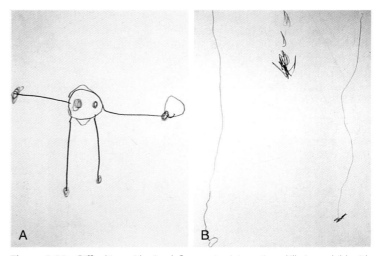

Figure 3-20   Difficulties with visual–fine motor integration skills in a child with cerebral palsy. **A,** Drawing by a bright 4-year-old who was born prematurely but showed no developmental delays. Note the inclusion of seven features: eyes, hair, mouth, arms, hands, legs, and feet. The age equivalent for this drawing is 4¾ years. **B,** Drawing by a 4-year-old child with spastic diplegia. Difficulties in organization appear related to visuomotor integration skills rather than to problems with fine motor skills.

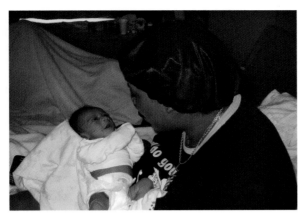

Figure 3-21 Early social skills. A newborn within an hour of birth fixates on the face of the mother.

Figure 3-22 Early object permanence. A 6-month-old infant was able to track his toy through a vertical fall and to search for it on the floor even after his gaze had been interrupted.

Development of Symbolic Capabilities

In the second year of life the child demonstrates mental activity independent of sensory processing or motor manipulation. For example, the child observes a television superhero performing a rescue mission and hours later reenacts the scene with careful precision. Clearly, the child has a mental image of the event and uses it to generate the delayed imitation.

As children develop the capacity for pure mental activity, they use objects to represent other objects or ideas. Genuine pretending begins; the child engages in playful representation of commonplace activities, using objects for their actual purpose but accompanied by exaggerated sounds or gestures. Pretend actions are combined into a series of events. For example, the child may hold a phone to the ear and then to a doll's ear or may feed a teddy bear and then put the bear to bed.

The next stage in development allows the child to plan pretend activities in anticipation of the play theme to come, combining many steps into the play. Preparing for play indicates an advance in pretending beyond that of improvising with the objects at hand. For example, the child might be seen preparing the play area or searching for needed objects and announcing what the objects are meant to represent.

Development of Logical Thinking

The preschool child has well-developed capabilities for mental representation and symbolic thinking. However, the dominance of sensory input, limited life experience, and a lack of formal education lead to a unique and charming logic during this period. Preschoolers often assume that all objects are alive like themselves. A car and a tricycle, for example, may be seen as alive, perhaps because they are capable of movement. Similarly, children claim that the moon follows them on an evening walk.

The logic of the preschooler is in large part influenced by the appearance of objects. Because an airplane appears to become smaller as it takes off, the preschooler may assume that all the people on the plane become smaller as well. Piaget

Figure 3-23 Object permanence. **A** and **B,** An 11-month-old child can locate a small, hidden object even if no part of it remains visible. In doing so, he is demonstrating his understanding that objects are permanent.

Figure 3-24 Mature means–end reasoning. A 15-month-old child turns the key of the music box atop the mobile to make it play. The child's understanding has advanced beyond that of direct causality, such as pulling a toy to bring it closer.

demonstrated that preschoolers seem to think that number and quantity vary with appearance (Fig. 3-25). Under certain circumstances a 4-year-old child may show understanding that a quantity remains invariant unless something is added or subtracted. That same child, however, may insist that two rows of pennies are different in number simply because of a compelling visual difference between them.

The immature logic of the preschooler is gradually replaced by conventional logic and wisdom. School-age children follow logic akin to adult reasoning, at least when the stimuli are concrete. Faced with the same question about the pennies, they readily acknowledge that the two rows have the same number regardless of their visual appearance (see Fig. 3-25). They also know that the airplane just looks smaller because it has moved farther from the viewer, and they giggle at the suggestion that the people on the plane have shrunk. Their logical limitations become obvious when they must reason about the hypothetical or the abstract.

Figure 3-25 Experimental design to demonstrate preoperational logic. The 3- or 4-year-old child agrees that the two rows in **A** have the same number of pennies. After seeing the pennies moved into the configuration in **B,** the child claims that the top row has more because it is longer.

Adolescents, particularly those with the benefits of formal education, tend to extend logical principles to increasingly diverse problems. They can generate multiple logical possibilities systematically when faced with scientific experiments, and they can also consider hypothetical problems. These principles of reasoning are applied not only to schoolwork but also to social situations.

Assessing Cognitive Development

The pediatric office assessment of cognitive ability in the preverbal child is best accomplished by observation of play. The pediatrician can induce the infant to look for a hidden toy or to play a game of peek-a-boo; the infant's anticipation of reappearance indicates the development of the concept of object permanence. Similarly, the toddler's ability to play with a toy telephone indicates the emergence of symbolic thought. Beyond the toddler stage the physician typically relies on conversation and language ability to assess levels of cognitive skill. Screening tests are particularly useful for determining whether cognitive and language skills are within the normal range. Children with language delays may need a formal nonverbal assessment of cognitive abilities by a psychologist.

For the parents, a delay in a child's attainment of a well-known milestone may create tremendous fear about ultimate learning potential. In many cases, such parental concerns are put to rest at that time when the physician determines that the child's learning to date is age-appropriate. If a child does show delays in cognitive development, the physician should generate a differential diagnosis (Table 3-5) from knowledge

Table 3-5	Potentially Remediable Disorders Associated with Developmental Delay
Findings Sometimes Present on History or Examination	**Possible Disorder**
Decreased vision or hearing	Specific sensory deficits
Staring spells, motor automatism	Seizure disorders
Lethargy, ataxia	Overmedication with anticonvulsants
Myxedema, delayed return on DTRs, thick skin and tongue, sparse hair, constipation, increased sleep, coarse voice, short stature, goiter	Hypothyroidism
Irritability, cold sweats, tremor, loss of consciousness	Hypoglycemia
Unexplained bruises in various stages, failure to thrive	Child abuse and neglect
Short stature, weight below third percentile	Malnutrition or systemic illness producing failure to thrive
Poor purposeful attending in multiple settings	ADHD
No specific findings	Environmental deprivation
Anemia	Iron deficiency or lead exposure
Absent venous pulsations or papilledema on funduscopic examination, morning vomiting, headaches, brisk DTRs in lower extremities	Increased intracranial pressure
Vomiting, irritability and seizures, failure to thrive	Some inborn errors of metabolism (e.g., methylmalonic acidemia)
Hepatomegaly, jaundice, hypotonia, susceptibility to infection, cataracts	Galactosemia
Fair hair, blue eyes, "mousy" odor to urine	Phenylketonuria
Ongoing evidence of active or progressive disease	Chronic infection, inflammatory disease, malignancies

ADHD, attention-deficit/hyperactivity disorder; DTR, deep tendon reflex.

of the child's level of functioning in multiple domains, history, and physical examination.

Parents should be given information about their child's delay as early as possible. Pediatricians serve a critical role in referring children to early intervention or special education programs and in monitoring their progress. Active communication between the providers of early intervention and the physician assists a comprehensive and cohesive approach.

Physicians frequently need the consultation of colleagues in psychology and education to assess the cognitive abilities of their older preschool and school-age patients. A number of methods have been devised for formal assessment of mental achievement, and almost all parents are familiar with the terms *intelligence quotient* or *IQ*. Although not a means of comprehensively assessing all mental capabilities, normal IQ scores are (albeit imperfect) predictors of which children will have the attention, social skills, motivation, and intelligence to perform well in school. Low IQ scores may reflect a child's poor ability to grasp new concepts, or they may indicate poor purposeful attending behaviors, as seen in depression or in attention-deficit/hyperactivity disorder (ADHD). Low scores may also reflect poor social adjustment or limitations in test-taking capabilities, such as sitting in a chair at a table and applying maximal effort to a task requested by an unfamiliar authority figure. Frequently, low scores result from a combination of difficulties in several areas.

If children with sensory or motor impairments are tested with instruments normalized on able-bodied children, they often obtain low scores. Different assessment techniques have been devised to circumvent specific disabilities while obtaining information about a child's cognitive abilities; these are typically administered by psychologists, child development specialists, or special educators (Table 3-6).

Assessment of a child's abilities to learn must go beyond standardized IQ tests. For example, some children who can score in the normal range on IQ tests are unable to learn to read. A diversified and individualized assessment process should precede any educational recommendation. The pediatrician, in the role of advocate, should ensure that assessments include information about the child's strengths and weaknesses because educational planning should involve attention to all aspects of the child's abilities. Moreover, the pediatrician

can encourage families to maintain an active, decision-making role in their children's education.

LANGUAGE DEVELOPMENT

Early Skills in Speech Perception and Production

The use of language is the ability to generate and understand reproducible sounds or gestures that are recognized by others as representative of concepts. Language development begins slowly and subtly in the first year of life. Language skills are subdivided into two realms: receptive skills—the ability to comprehend communication, and expressive skills—the ability to produce communication.

Neonates demonstrate skills that are useful in the eventual development of receptive language abilities. Even before birth, fetuses detect sounds and show preferences for some sounds over others. At birth, the newborn is particularly attuned to the human voice and may turn toward a parent who is gently whispering. Children remain interested in sounds as they grow older and turn voluntarily toward the source of a sound by 3 to 4 months of age (Fig. 3-26).

Children can also differentiate speech sounds, even close to birth. Experimental paradigms, using the fact that an infant's heart rate and sucking patterns change when they encounter new environmental stimuli, suggest that infants as young as 1 month of age can differentiate such similar speech sounds as /ba/ and /pa/. Frequent exposure to the native language alters speech perception such that by late infancy it becomes difficult for children to differentiate sounds that are not meaningful distinctions in their own language.

By 2 to 3 months of age, children begin to *coo* or make musical sounds spontaneously. This is the first step toward the development of expressive verbal language. Even in the early stages, children can establish reciprocal patterns, similar to the rhythm of conversation.

By about 6 months of age, children place consonant sounds with vowel sounds, creating what is known as *babble*. In this period the infant says "ma-ma" or "da-da" without necessarily referring to the loving parent. By 9 to 12 months of age, children integrate babble with intonational patterns consistent with the parent's speech. This is called *jargon*.

Later Development

In the second half of the first year the child develops early skills in true receptive language. Milestones are listed in Table 3-7. By 6 months of age, children reliably respond to their

Table 3-6	Tests Used in the Assessment of Cognitive Development	
Type of Scale	**Test(s) Used**	**Age Range**
Standard intelligence scales	Stanford-Binet Intelligence Scales-IV	2-adult
	Wechsler Intelligence Scale for Children-IV	6-16 yr
Nonverbal intelligence scale	Leiter International Performance Scale-R	2-18 yr
Infant development tests	Bayley Scales of Infant Development-III	0-3½ yr
	Gesell Developmental Schedules	0-5 yr
Developmental scale for the visually impaired	Reynell-Zinkin Developmental Scales for Young Children with Visual Impairments	0-5 yr
Adaptive behavior	Vineland Adaptive Behavior Scales-II	0-18 yr
	Adaptive Behavior Assessment System-II	0-21 yr

Figure 3-26 Localizing sound. A 3-month-old infant responds to interesting sounds by looking in the direction of the sound.

Table 3-7	Receptive and Expressive Language Milestones

Age Range	Receptive Response	Expressive Response
0-1½ mo	Startles or widens eyes in response to sound	Shows variation in crying (hunger, pain)
1½-4 mo	Quiets in response to voice, blinks eyes in response to sound	Makes musical sounds; coos; participates in reciprocal exchange
4-9 mo	Turns head toward sound; responds with raised arms when parent says "up" and reaches for child; responds appropriately to friendly or angry voices	Babbles; repeats self-initiated sounds
9-12 mo	Listens selectively to familiar words; begins to respond to "no"; responds to verbal routine such as wave bye-bye or clap; turns in response to own name	Uses symbolic gestures and jargon; repeats parent-initiated sounds
12-18 mo	Points to three body parts (eyes, nose, mouth); understands up to 50 words; recognizes common objects by name (dog, cat, bottle, ball, book); follows one-step commands accompanied by gestures ("give me the doll," "hug your bear," "open your mouth")	Uses words to express needs; learns 20 to 50 words by 18 mo; uses words inconsistently and mixed with jargon, echolalia, or both
18 mo-2 yr	Points to pictures when asked "show me"; understands *soon, in, on,* and *under;* begins to distinguish *you* from *me;* can formulate negative judgments (a pear is not a cookie)	Uses telegraphic two-word sentences ("go bye-bye," "up daddy," "want cookie")
30 mo	Follows two-step commands; can identify objects by use	Uses jargon and echolalia infrequently; makes average sentence of 2½ words; adjectives and adverbs appear; begins to ask questions, asks adults to repeat actions ("do it again")
3 yr	Knows several colors; knows what we do when we are hungry, thirsty, or sleepy; is aware of past and future; understands *today* and *not today*	Uses pronouns and plurals; can tell stories that begin to be understood; uses negative ("I can't," "I won't"); verbalizes toilet needs; can tell full name, age, and gender; forms sentences of three or four words
3½ yr	Can answer such questions as "do you have a doggie?," "which is the boy?," and "what toys do you have?"; understands *little, funny,* and *secret*	Can relate experiences in sequential order; can recite a nursery rhyme; can ask permission
4 yr	Understands same versus different; follows three-step commands; completes opposite analogies (a brother is a boy, a sister is a …); understands why we have houses, stoves, and umbrellas	Tells a story; uses past tense; counts to 3; names primary colors; enjoys rhyming nonsense words, enjoys exaggerations; asks many questions a day
5 yr	Understands what we do with eyes and ears; understands differences in texture (hard, soft, smooth); understands *if, when,* and *why;* identifies words in terms of use; begins to understand left and right	Indicates "I don't know"; indicates *funny,* and *surprise;* can define in terms of use; asks definition of specific words; makes serious inquiries ("how does this work?" and "what does it mean?"); uses mature sentence structure and form

names, and at about 9 months, they can follow verbal routines, such as waving bye-bye or showing how big they are. At about the same age, they also learn that pointing shares the focus of attention. The young infant looks at the point, whereas the older infant looks at the object to which the point is directed.

Receptive language can be demonstrated as children follow increasingly complex commands. For example, children will understand one-step commands such as "throw the ball" by approximately 1 year of age. The labeling of commonplace items in pictures is slightly more complex and begins after 1 year of age. The ability to choose between two pictures when asked "show me the …" should be consistent between 18 and 24 months of age.

By 2½ years of age, receptive language skills have advanced beyond the understanding of simple labels. The child is able to identify objects by their use. Continued advances in receptive language occur during the preschool years and are highly susceptible to environmental stimulation or deprivation.

Expressive language skills (see Table 3-7) lag behind receptive skills in the first year of life. But even before word production begins, a child's gestures have communicative intent. Many 9- to 10-month-olds can communicate that their juice or cereal is "all gone" by placing their hands palms up, at shoulder height. Even older children gesture to make themselves understood because gross and fine motor skills develop faster than the oropharyngeal muscle skills used in articulation.

Expressive language at first develops slowly. The child's first meaningful words are produced around the first birthday. Over the next 6 months the child may master only 20 to 50 more words. These early words come and go from the child's vocabulary and may be idiosyncratic child-forms. After 18 to 24 months, word usage increases rapidly, standard forms replace baby talk, and word combinations begin.

The child's earliest two-word sentences typically contain important content words but lack prepositions, articles, and verb-tense markings. This two-word phase has been called *telegraphic speech* because, like a telegram, the child leaves out nonessential articles and prepositions. Once the child is capable of three- and four-word utterances, length limitations do not appear to be a significant barrier. By age 3 the child has developed complex language with the use of pronouns and prepositions. The child develops the ability to ask questions. At age 2½ years they usually ask "what?" and by age 3 years they most frequently ask "why?" The child also can use negation within a sentence. By age 5 the child uses all parts of speech, as well as clauses and complex sentences.

The rate of language development appears to be associated with both biologic and environmental factors. About half or more of children with first-degree relatives with language and speech delays also show delays. The amount of child-directed speech in the environment is a good predictor of the rate of development for vocabulary and grammar. For this reason, health supervision of infants and toddlers should encourage parents to speak or read to their children.

Table 3-8	Phonemes and Intelligibility	
Age (yr)*	Sounds Mastered	Percent Intelligibility (to a Stranger)
2	—	50
3	14 vowels and *p, b, m*	75
4	10 vowel blends and *n, ng, w, h, t, d, k, g*	100
5	*f, v, y, th, l, wh*	100
6	*r, s, z, ch, j, sh, zh,* and consonant blends	100

*The ages presented here are general guidelines because authorities differ regarding the specific ages associated with articulation and intelligibility.

Mastering Intelligibility and Fluency

Sounds required in language are mastered at different rates. Children who are attempting to say words containing sounds they cannot yet produce have a variety of choices on how to proceed: by omission of the difficult sound (*ba* for bottle), by substitution of a different sound (*fum* for thumb), or by distortion (*goyl* for girl). The information presented in Table 3-8 provides an estimate of when mastery of particular sounds, along with estimates of overall intelligibility, might be expected.

Assessing Language Development

In the early stages of prelinguistic and linguistic development, direct assessment by the pediatrician may be difficult. Children are likely to remain quiet in new situations, especially in the office where they received an injection. It is usually easy to engage a normally developing child of age 3 in conversations. Before that age the physician may need to rely on parental report. Standardized parent reports are available for office use, and parental reports contribute to the assessment of language in screening tests.

The differential diagnosis for delayed expressive language development includes impaired hearing, global developmental delay or intellectual disability, environmental deprivation, autism, emotional maladjustment, or specific language impairment. Keeping this in mind, worrisome clinical situations include the 4- to 6-month-old infant who fails to coo responsively, the 9- to 10-month-old child who does not babble or whose cooing and babbling have diminished, and the 18-month-old child whose repertoire of words includes only *mama* or *dada*. Beyond 18 months a convenient rule of thumb is that children 2 years of age should use two-word utterances, at least half of which should be intelligible. By 3 years of age, children should use phrases of three or more words, three-quarters of which should be intelligible. Children who fail to achieve these developmental milestones should undergo evaluation for hearing loss, as well as for cognitive and emotional impairment.

Families often attribute language delays in their youngster to superficial and easily remediable physiologic or social factors. "Being tongue-tied," for example, in most cases is not an explanation for delayed speech. However, it may be the effect rather than the cause because in some children the frenulum of the tongue may be tight due to not being sufficiently exercised by early verbal practice. Similarly, children rarely delay language because "they don't need it." Children have tremendous motivation to improve their verbal skills, even if they have older siblings who speak for them. For children who want a particular food, for example, a point toward the cupboard door will not specify precisely what is wanted. The parents must offer the items one at a time and await acceptance or rejection. The use of a verbal label will allow the child to meet needs efficiently.

Delays in the development of intelligibility might include any of the following:

1. Lack of intelligible speech by age 3
2. Frequent omission of initial consonants after age 4
3. Continued substitution of easy sounds for more difficult ones after age 5
4. Persistent articulation errors after age 7

If any of these delays persist for 6 months or more, a referral should be initiated.

During the period in which articulation and vocabulary are being mastered, speech dysfluencies are common. Noticeable stuttering or rapid speech beyond age 4 should prompt further attention. The problems of nasality, inaudibility, and unusual pitch sometimes may be helped by a speech pathologist. Furthermore, children of any age who are embarrassed by their speech are appropriate candidates for referral.

Therapy for speech and language disorders helps improve the communication skills of children with language delays and problems of intelligibility. A child whose unusual language pattern is destined to be outgrown will not suffer from monitoring by a communication disorders specialist; the child whose language impairment will not be outgrown has much to lose when help is delayed.

SOCIAL DEVELOPMENT

Early Capabilities: Social Responsivity

The earliest social task of newborns is to establish a mutually satisfying relationship with their caregivers. Neonates begin this process by fixing visually on faces in preference to other sights, a skill that is evident during the first few days of life (see Fig. 3-21). The responsive smile develops soon thereafter (Fig. 3-27). The social smile is another innate behavior, although it may not appear until 4 to 6 weeks of life. Smiling appears in infants from all cultures at about the same time. Infants with visual impairment who cannot appreciate a smile on the faces of their caregivers nonetheless smile at ages comparable with sighted children.

Development of Attachment

During the first 6 months of life, infants are rather indiscriminate in their social behavior, smiling and later laughing with anyone willing to play. Infants develop a sense that their

Figure 3-27　Early smiling. A 19-day-old infant smiles for her parents.

parents exist when out of sight sooner than they learn inanimate objects are permanent. By 6 to 8 months of age, children protest when their parents leave the room. As infants begin to recognize faces of familiar caregivers, they may squirm and cling in the company of unfamiliar people, exhibiting stranger awareness. The severity of the reaction varies with the infant's temperament and with previous experiences. Extreme reactions, known as *stranger anxiety,* may occur in children who have not had routine care from alternative caregivers. Pediatricians are advised to refrain from holding the 9- to 12-month-old child at the well-child visit. A child who remains playful and calm while securely in the parent's arms may quickly fret or cry even if gently removed from that security.

By 1 year of age, most children have experienced periods of separation from a parent, whether it be for minutes or hours. Infants who have developed a secure attachment to their parents show signs of recognition and pleasure when they are reunited with them. While progressing in gross motor development, the child initiates separation by walking away independently and exploring at greater distances from parents. Typically, infants return regularly for some verbal encouragement, eye contact, or hugging and then venture farther. In contrast, infants who have not developed secure attachments may show indifference, ambivalence, or disorganization at reunion with their parents. Their exploration of the environment during the toddler years is limited. These children are at risk for troubled social relationships as they become older.

Development of Social Play

Infants and young toddlers tend to line up and engage in similar activities simultaneously. This pattern is called *parallel play.* Although parents often expect their young toddlers to interact or share with peers, success in this age group is unusual. Sharing for a young toddler involves showing or handing a prized toy to another child, only to take it back within seconds.

By 2 years of age, with the development of symbolic capabilities in cognitive development, children begin to pretend. They will seek to engage their parents in activities that satisfy their growing curiosity. They enjoy reading with caregivers and having their labeling questions answered.

Near 3 years of age, children begin to include one another in their pretending games, taking on roles that become progressively more realistic and interactive. The young preschooler is especially interested in imitating the parent of the same gender but shows no preference for same- or opposite-gender playmates.

The child's abilities to share are shaped by social experiences. Children who attend day care may share successfully at an earlier age than children raised at home (Fig. 3-28).

Although it can be achieved through consistent experience, taking turns is also a challenge for the preschooler who possesses a limited concept of time. Impulse control is just developing in the preschool years. Active goals for this age group include learning to gain the cooperation of one's peers, learning to communicate ideas to new friends, and learning to handle conflicts.

By 4 to 5 years of age, peer interactions grow increasingly cooperative and complicated; pretend play involves themes requiring greater feats of imagination and experience, such as trips or parties. Older preschoolers enjoy helping with household tasks and frequently are more interested in participating in gender-specific activities than they were at an earlier age. This interest may relate to cognitive and social development. As children understand that they are in the same category as their same-gender parent, they become interested in the implications of category membership. Strict adherence to the rules of category membership reflects the concrete and inflexible thinking of the preschooler.

Preschoolers do not often play games with rules. Rules are seen as variable, to be made and broken at the discretion of the players. For example, getting through a board game with preschoolers who decide not to follow the rules, once they discover that the rules are not working in their favor, is often a challenge.

Children become capable of playing by rules when they reach school age. With superior logical capabilities, they realize that rules are invariant and must be followed regardless of the personal implications. As they progress through the elementary-school years, board games and sports become preferred activities for groups of peers.

Development of Sense of Self

Self-awareness and independence develop gradually throughout life. The earliest indications of an emerging identity occur at 6 to 9 months of age, when infants display interest in their own mirror images. Some 7- to 8-month-olds may prefer to grab cups and spoons rather than accept passive roles in eating. These infants may resist pressure to do something that they would prefer not to do (e.g., fussing to stand when placed in a sitting position).

Beyond 1 year of age, toddlers rapidly expand their sense of self. They explore their environment with ease, and they are increasingly able to function independently. They can feed themselves with a cup and spoon, and they have clear ideas about what they want. Children at 1 to 2 years of age also enjoy their own accomplishments and can clap for their own successes (Fig. 3-29).

An emerging sense of self and the thrust for independence make discipline of the toddler a challenge. Parents may need

Figure 3-28 *Sharing.* Two-year-old children with day-care experience share a special treat.

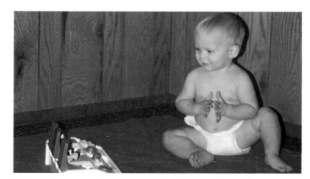

Figure 3-29 Mastery smile. A 15-month-old boy demonstrates that toddlers beyond 1 year of age can take pride in their own accomplishments. This child is applauding his own success at having made the puppets appear.

help in viewing their child's refusals to eat, nap, or be washed as positive steps toward increased independence. They may also need support in setting limits on the child's behaviors.

As the child reaches 2 to 3 years of age, increased independence in verbal abilities, increased awareness of body sensations, and modest skills in donning and doffing clothing combine with the child's desire to imitate adults and to gain parental approval. This combination of accomplishments allows toilet training to begin. In fact, these developmental milestones mentioned may be viewed as readiness signs. The pediatrician can review them with families at the 15- or 18-month visit so that parents can time their toilet-training efforts to the child's developmental rate and style. Children differ substantially in their interest in achieving bladder and bowel control, and parents may benefit from counseling to maintain a relaxed approach.

In other areas as well, children need support in their attempts to initiate and control their own activities. Toward this end, parents can be encouraged to allow their child to practice emerging self-care skills, such as zipping or buttoning a coat, even when the practice costs precious time in a rushed schedule. Should the child become frustrated or disappointed, a response of empathy is likely to soothe more effectively than a response of reason because rational reasoning is limited during this preoperational cognitive period.

By mid- to late elementary school, cognitive development has progressed toward abstract and hypothetical thinking such that children are able to reflect self-consciously about themselves and others. First- or second-graders struggle to understand the causes of conflict or their emotional reactions to it. Older elementary-school children and adolescents are able to analyze situations, reasons, and reactions. They begin to understand their own motivations and the environmental triggers of their responses.

Throughout childhood the desire to grow up is in continued conflict with the desire to remain a child. The young preschooler is just beginning to address this issue. Families frequently report that a child's accomplishments in socioemotional functioning backslide when unexpected stresses challenge household equilibrium or when the child becomes ill. As a result, temporary regressions to earlier levels of functioning may occur in some children. Importantly, parents must learn to view these lapses as expected components of development rather than as intentional lapses on the part of the child. However, if the regression is prolonged and significant, the physician may initiate an evaluation of the child's emotional status.

During elementary-school years, at least in Western cultures, the child's self-image is strongly influenced by success or failure in school. Not only do difficulties with learning put additional pressures on the child, but they also may damage the child's sense of self-worth. Parents and teachers of children with learning problems should be especially willing to praise the child for effort, accomplishments, and good behavior. Physicians should be particularly sensitive to the higher risk of emotional and behavioral problems in children with learning difficulties so that they can make timely referrals to colleagues in the mental health professions.

Evaluation of Social Development

Subtle indicators of social and emotional development can be observed in the course of a routine pediatric visit. The physician has the opportunity to note not only the way the infant behaves but also the style of parental caregiving and the nature of the parent–child relationship. The young infant typically shows social responsiveness to both the parent and the pediatrician, although at 9 months of age, there is a definite preference for the familiar parent. Also at this age, particularly in times of stress, the infant turns to the parent for support and comfort. Children of limited responsiveness, who avoid physical contact, avert their gaze, or in other ways fail to contribute to a mutually satisfying reciprocal exchange are of concern. Of equal concern are parents who are harsh, unresponsive, or threatening in response to the infant's needs.

Given the nature of social development, the assessment of possible problems must rely largely on history. Parents tend to be frank and open about the nature of their relationship with their child if questions are asked in a direct and nonjudgmental way. Difficulties in social development may relate to constitutional and temperamental characteristics of the child, as well as to philosophy and practices of the parent. By remembering the bidirectional nature of causality in social development, the physician can avoid slipping into criticisms or judgments.

The older preschool or school-age child may be able to give, independently, direct information about social development. For example, the child may be able to name special friends and the activities enjoyed with those friends. Young preschoolers might name both boys and girls and list rough-and-tumble or fantasy play as favorite activities. Older preschoolers might name same-gender friends but similar activities. School-age children might add board games and sports to their list of activities.

VARIATIONS IN DEVELOPMENTAL PATTERNS

The presence or absence of a single skill at a particular age is rarely sufficient to determine developmental status. Developmental progress is highly dependent on multiple factors: the general health of the child, opportunities for learning, temperamental characteristics, willingness to try new experiences, genetic endowments, coordination and strength, and socioeconomic factors. If delays occur in more than one domain, persist over time, or both, they are considered significant. The challenge for the pediatrician is to differentiate individual variation from deviation and disorder.

Sometimes the parents raise developmental concerns. These concerns must be addressed freely and openly. Parents are rarely comforted by superficial evaluation and pat reassurance, and although prudent waiting may serve some families well, it may arouse anxiety and anger in others. If a comprehensive evaluation of a given problem is beyond the capabilities of the pediatrician, early referral should be considered.

Evaluation of developmental problems proceeds in the same manner as evaluation of other medical concerns: history, physical examination (including neurologic and developmental evaluation), and laboratory testing. Important in establishing a diagnosis is consideration of the pattern of development across all domains. For example, findings of hypotonia and selective problems in gross motor skills along with normal development in cognition, language, and social skills suggest a neuromuscular disorder or benign congenital hypotonia. In contrast, hypotonia with global developmental delay suggests a central nervous system problem. Differentiating delayed skills from deviant skill patterns is also important. For example, because even neonates can make good eye contact with their caregivers, the toddler who avoids eye contact is showing deviancy rather than delay. The combination of delays or deviances in social behavior and delayed language development is suggestive of an autism spectrum disorder.

Cerebral Palsy

The term *cerebral palsy* (CP) refers to a group of disorders in movement and posture appearing in infancy or early childhood and attributed to nonprogressive disturbances that occurred in the developing fetal or infant brain. The type of cerebral palsy varies according to the location of the injured area. Injury may occur before birth, during labor and delivery, or after birth, up through the preschool years. Although some affected patients may have a history of perinatal complications, the majority do not. In 20% to 30% of cases, no etiology can be established. The key to making the diagnosis is to establish that motor problems are not progressive. Regression of motor skills suggests a different set of diagnostic possibilities including surgically treatable lesions of the brain or spinal cord or inherited neurodegenerative diseases.

CP is classified according to resting tone and what limbs are involved. *Spastic CP* is typically due to injuries to the cortex or pyramidal tract and accounts for approximately 80% of cases. *Spasticity* is defined as a velocity-dependent increase in tone; when the limb is moved quickly there is a catch or resistance to movement. Spasticity also includes hyperreflexia and may be accompanied by clonus and persistence of primitive reflexes. *Extrapyramidal* or *dyskinetic CP* is characterized by abnormal involuntary movements. Rarely, cerebral palsy is manifested as hypotonia, often involving the trunk, and associated with hyperreflexia and persistent primitive reflexes. Categorization of cerebral palsy adds the location of the findings to the predominant findings:

- *Spastic hemiplegia:* Spasticity predominantly affecting one side of the body, usually with upper extremity spasticity more pronounced than lower extremity spasticity
- *Spastic diplegia:* Spasticity predominantly affecting the lower extremities more than the upper extremities
- *Spastic quadriplegia:* Spasticity of all four extremities
- *Athetoid CP, choreoathetoid CP, and dystonic CP:* Abnormal movements often accompanied by hypertonicity

Physical Examination

A diagnosis of cerebral palsy and a determination of its subtype can be established through physical examination. However, physical findings over the first year of life are highly variable and nonspecific. Early signs may include decreased passive tone in the presence of brisk deep tendon reflexes (DTRs) without concomitant weakness. Early problems with sucking and swallowing may predate evidence of motor delays.

The definitive diagnosis of cerebral palsy should be made after 1 year of age in a child born at term, and at 15 to 18 months of age in a child born prematurely, because the early findings may change. The diagnosis is based on abnormal strength, tone posture, and hand use of the upper extremity and strength and tone in the lower extremities. Strength can be assessed by indirect measures, such as by determining the child's ability to push off from a bed, to support his body weight on his legs, and to lift his arms and legs.

Abnormalities of Tone

Because damage to the central nervous system prevents the inhibition and balance of the inherent tone of the muscles, abnormalities of tone are particularly significant in the diagnosis of cerebral palsy. After initial hypotonia, a child may develop increased tone between 12 and 18 months of age, showing clearly rigid or spastic hypertonia by age 2.

The child who demonstrates increased extensor tone beginning in early infancy is also at risk for cerebral palsy. Under normal circumstances, infants younger than 3 months of age, when supported ventrally, maintain their head in slight flexion with the trunk mildly convex (Fig. 3-30, *A*). However, with exaggerated tone in the antigravity muscle group, the infant may elevate the head above the horizontally level trunk (Fig. 3-30, *B*). Similarly, the unknowing parents may be pleased by their child's apparent precocious development of head control when the child is prone or rolls belly-to-back in the first 2 months of life, when in fact both of these findings suggest excessive extensor posturing.

Further evidence of abnormally increased tone is found when the supine child is pulled to an upright position and extends at the hips and knees, coming to stand on pointed toes rather than ending up in the appropriate sitting posture. This child, when placed in vertical suspension, will not right the head as expected and will later scissor the lower extremities as a result of hypertonia of the leg adductors and internal rotators (Fig. 3-31). Parents may find it difficult to position these infants for diapering and feeding; knowledge of the Marie-Foix maneuver, used to break up excessive extension in the lower extremities (Fig. 3-32), will help them.

Abnormalities in Development of Primitive Reflexes and Equilibrium Responses

Abnormal persistence of primitive reflexes is helpful in making a diagnosis of cerebral palsy. Damage to the central nervous system prevents high levels of control from superseding and

Figure 3-30   Ventral suspension. **A,** This infant's posture is normal for a 1- to 3-month-old child held in ventral suspension. The head, hips, and knees are flexed. **B,** For a child 4 months of age or older held in ventral suspension with normal posture, the head, hips, and knees may be extended. This finding is abnormal in a child younger than 3 months of age.

Figure 3-31 Scissoring. Excessive pull of the hip adductors and internal rotators in this child of 3 years results in his legs crossing in a scissor-like pattern while he is supported in vertical suspension.

inhibiting the influence of the early reflexes. Thus obligate or persistent primitive reflexes are signs of cerebral palsy. For example, in the normal variant of the ATNR, the infant can move out of the posture if the gaze is directed to the other side of the body. In an obligate ATNR, however, the infant remains in the fencer position until the head is passively moved. This finding is not normal in a child of any age and is highly suggestive of the static encephalopathy and motor deficit characterizing cerebral palsy.

Also strongly suggestive of cerebral palsy is the nonobligate ATNR that persists beyond 6 months of age. This is one possible explanation for a consistent preference in a 6- to 12-month-old child to sleep or lie with the head turned in a particular direction. Similarly, persistence of the Moro response beyond 6 months of age is associated with cerebral palsy, as is a lack of development of lateral protective equilibrium reactions by 7 to 8 months or of the parachute reaction by 10 months of age.

Figure 3-32 Marie-Foix maneuver. By flexing the child's toes, the therapist can reduce extensor tone enough to obtain abduction of the hip and knee flexion in this child with spastic quadriplegia.

Figure 3-33 Asymmetrical Moro response. Note that one hand is fisted and the other is open. This child warrants a neurologic examination and close follow-up.

Subtypes of Cerebral Palsy

Hemiparesis

Hemiparesis is caused by asymmetrical damage to the motor control areas of the central nervous system. In children with hemiparesis, functional discrepancies often predate asymmetrical changes in tone or reflexes. The upper extremities may be affected more severely than the lower extremities. Asymmetrical use of the upper or lower extremities is rare during the first 4 months of life. When seen in the resting state or when elicited with the ATNR or the Moro response (Fig. 3-33), it is more likely related to lower motor neuron disease than to cerebral injury. At 4 to 6 months, during the development of early reaching and grasping, signs of hemiparesis include the presence of one hand that is fisted, the arm getting caught beneath the body when the child tries to prop up on the elbows or hands, and evidence that the arm is not used in simple tasks. Increased resistance to supination at the wrist, limited flopping of one wrist when the upper extremities are gently shaken, or extra beats of unilateral clonus at the ankle are other clues.

Later, during the first year of life, abnormal findings include a failure to develop the protective response of lateral propping or the development of an asymmetrical parachute response. In addition, crawling may be uneven, with propulsion coming from one side while the opposite arm and leg are dragged behind.

Children with hemiparesis may have difficulty in compensating for their lack of protective responses, their uneven strength, and poor balance. Walking is typically delayed until 2 to 3 years of age. In mildly affected children, walking may be almost normal, but when asked to run, the child may show posturing of the upper extremity in flexion and internal rotation. Usually, the lower limb rotates internally and the foot may be held in equinus, making it functionally longer on the swing-through part of the gait. To clear the foot from the floor, the child compensates by swinging the leg farther out in abduction or by circumducting the affected side. These patterns, in some cases, also can be observed in standing (Fig. 3-34).

Children with hemiparesis may neglect the visual field on their affected side. Parents should position their infant so that visual stimulation is provided to the intact visual field. Another consideration is that of abnormal bony stresses caused by asymmetrical muscle strength. Unequal spinal stresses predispose children with hemiparesis to scoliosis, especially during growth spurts.

Spastic Diplegia and Quadriplegia

Spastic diplegia implies dysfunction of the lower extremities, with normal or limited involvement of the upper extremities. Spastic quadriplegia implies dysfunction of the upper and

Figure 3-34   Note the arm held in flexion and internal rotation and the leg circumducted on the involved side in this child with hemiplegic cerebral palsy.

lower extremities. The child with spasticity may have presenting symptoms that include delayed sitting, crawling, or walking or toe-walking (Fig. 3-35). In the supine position, children with spastic diplegia may keep their lower extremities in the "frog" position, with the hips and knees flexed and the hips externally rotated. In the erect position the child may internally rotate and adduct the legs, leading to scissoring (see Fig. 3-31). The ankles assume the equinus position. Children with spastic diplegia who learn to walk often show persistent toe-walking in the presence of brisk DTRs, limited range of ankle motion, Babinski reflexes, and a normally proportioned muscle mass.

The differential diagnosis of toe-walking includes the muscular dystrophies, tethered spinal cord and spinal tumors, peripheral neuropathies, and fixed bony deformities of the

Figure 3-35   Toe-walking. A 4-year-old child with cerebral palsy cruises on furniture. Notice that the child is crouched because of hamstring tightness and is toe-walking because of gastrocnemius tightness.

feet. Unilateral or asymmetrical toe-walking may indicate leg-length discrepancy or a dislocated hip as an isolated finding or in conjunction with spasticity.

Athetoid or Ataxic Cerebral Palsy

Children with athetoid or ataxic cerebral palsy tend to be hypotonic and normoreflexic in infancy with delayed motor milestones. Between 1 and 2 years of age, hypotonia may be replaced by spasticity, and involuntary movements may appear. Exaggerated tone and dyskinetic movements reach maximal intensity around age 3. Athetoid cerebral palsy has been associated with damage to the basal ganglia caused by bilirubin encephalopathy (kernicterus) or hypoxic–ischemic injury.

Hypotonic Cerebral Palsy

Some hypotonic infants with exaggerated reflexes do not progress to hypertonicity. The child with hypotonic cerebral palsy usually exhibits severe motor and intellectual disability. The prognosis for independent functioning is quite poor. Hypotonic cerebral palsy must be differentiated from benign congenital hypotonia, an isolated disorder of tone, which spares other developmental areas.

Associated Findings with Cerebral Palsy

Up to 75% of children with diplegia or quadriplegia have strabismus (see Chapter 19). Refractive errors are found in 25% to 50% of children with cerebral palsy. Clumsiness because of motor imbalance of the lower extremities may be exaggerated by altered depth perception resulting from impaired visual function. Ophthalmologic referral for phorias and tropias that persist beyond 4 months of age is important to prevent amblyopia.

Hearing loss is also associated with cerebral palsy. Although clinical evaluation may suggest hearing loss, a definitive diagnosis requires an audiologic assessment. Brainstem auditory responses can be obtained to assess hearing capabilities in infants younger than 6 months of age and in older children unable to perform in conventional or conditioned play audiometry because of motor or intellectual problems.

Approximately 50% of children with cerebral palsy have cognitive impairment or intellectual disability. Learning disabilities and attentional weaknesses are more prevalent in this population than in the general population. Furthermore, behavioral problems may develop as a result of the frustration encountered in trying to adjust to motor disabilities.

Prognosis

Overall, the ability of individuals with cerebral palsy to live and work independently depends on the severity of the motor disability and associated cognitive impairments. If a child is 4 years of age or older and has not achieved sitting balance, independent walking with or without crutches is rarely possible. A child 2 to 4 years of age who cannot sit and has persistent primitive reflexes is also unlikely to walk.

Because cerebral palsy affects multiple systems, children with the disorder are best served by an interdisciplinary team including not only medical professionals but also social workers, psychologists, occupational and physical therapists, speech and communication therapists, and educational and vocational specialists. In many cases, children require educational support for physical and intellectual problems. They may also require behavioral management training or pharmacologic intervention for attentional weaknesses. Some of the behavioral problems can be prevented by matching developmental expectations to the child's functional capacities. These children and their families benefit enormously from the support of a primary care physician who offers routine health care maintenance, diagnostic and preventive procedures such as referrals to audiology and ophthalmology specialists, and advice and counseling on the interpretation of team evaluations.

Intellectual Disability (Previously Called Mental Retardation)

In 2007, the American Association on Mental Retardation changed its name to the American Association on Intellectual and Developmental Disabilities and urged the use of the term *intellectual disability* rather than *mental retardation* to refer to a disability characterized by significant limitations both in intellectual functioning (reasoning, learning, problem solving) and in adaptive behavior that arises before age 18 years. In October 2010, President Obama signed S. 2781, also called Rosa's Law. This law requires that the terms *mental retardation* and *mentally retarded individual* be changed, in all federal law, to *intellectual disability* and *individual with an intellectual disability,* respectively. This bill was originally introduced by Senator Barbara Mikulski of Maryland. She named the bill "Rosa's Law" after a young woman in her state who successfully advocated for the elimination of the phrase "mentally retarded" in all state law.

Limitations in intellectual functioning is generally defined as scores on standardized intelligence (IQ) tests that are two or more standard deviations below age-group norms; *adaptive behaviors* refers to the broad areas of conceptual, social, and practical functioning such as learning, communication, self-care, community participation (e.g., riding public transportation, engaging in recreation, voting), and social interactions.

Intellectual disability cannot be diagnosed until the child is old enough to take a standardized IQ test (generally at least 3 to 4 years old). Before that time, a child with delays in two or more domains of development may be described as having global developmental delay; some of these children will later be diagnosed with an intellectual disability. The ability to predict intellectual performance and academic achievement from developmental testing during infancy is quite limited. Only in children falling far behind age expectations should one anticipate permanent intellectual disability. If an infant shows delayed cognitive development, the parents' reasonable concerns can be met with a referral to an early intervention program to increase the probability of improvements over time.

As children with early developmental delays approach school age, particularly if they have had optimal educational support, the ability to predict later difficulties improves. The rate of developmental progress during the preschool years is often a good predictor of later intellectual performance. After initial cognitive developmental delays, if a child can achieve 6 months' progress in 6 months, the prognosis for normal intellectual capacity is good. However, if the child achieves, for example, 4 months' progress in 6 months, the rate of development is 67% of the expected rate and the prognosis for later normal intellectual functioning is poor. By the time a child is 6 to 7 years of age, limitations as measured on an IQ test typically characterize the individual's abilities throughout life. At that point, the term *intellectual disability* replaces *global developmental delay* because the probability that the delay will resolve is very low.

Physical Examination

Physical examination can be helpful in determining the cause of intellectual disability. Most children with intellectual disability are classified in the mild range. These children often have a normal physical examination, with no apparent evidence of major or minor malformations. In contrast to children with severe intellectual disability, who are more readily identified, children with mild intellectual disability are likely to have normal motor milestones and delays only in adaptive areas such as self-care, language acquisition, or play. The detection of disability in these mildly affected youngsters may not occur until the child experiences school performance difficulties.

The average IQ of parents of children with mild intellectual disability is lower than the population norm. Thus many of these parents also show limitations in intellectual abilities. For this reason the etiology of mild intellectual disability is generally believed to be multifactorial, including multiple genetic contributions and limited social enrichment.

The more significant the degree of intellectual disability, the more likely that a specific etiologic factor will be found. Children who score in the moderate, severe, or profound ranges are likely to have congenital malformations of the central nervous system, severe neurologic insults in the prenatal or perinatal period, an inherited disorder, or another specific diagnosis. A systematic approach to the physical examination may reveal clues to the nature of the underlying disorder.

Growth Pattern and Vital Signs

Aberrant growth patterns may be associated with developmental delays and intellectual disabilities. Obesity appears as part of a number of syndromes associated with intellectual disability, such as Laurence-Moon syndrome and Prader-Willi syndrome (see Chapter 1). Children who are exceptionally large may have cerebral gigantism (Sotos syndrome). Small-for-date infants deserve close study for evidence of anomalies or infection; they are also at risk for abnormal development. Extreme to moderate short stature, with or without skeletal dysplasia, is associated with many dysmorphic syndromes that include intellectual disability as an associated finding. Growth curves have been prepared for children with various genetic and chromosomal disorders such as Down syndrome because they tend to be shorter than the general population (Fig. 3-36). However, if children are shorter than expected even for the population of children with the disorder, or if children fail to maintain their own rate of growth after following a percentile, then endocrine function abnormalities such as hypothyroidism should be investigated.

Skin Findings

Hemangiomas, multiple café-au-lait spots, and sebaceous adenomas may be evidence of an underlying neurocutaneous abnormality, thereby providing a constitutional basis for a developmental delay. Neurofibromatosis (type 1) and tuberous sclerosis, both examples of neurocutaneous disorders, are inherited as autosomal dominant, although there is a high rate of spontaneous mutation. If these disorders are diagnosed or suspected, examination of the immediate family is warranted (see Chapter 15). Hirsutism occurs in fetal alcohol (see Chapter 1) and fetal hydantoin syndromes. Abnormal fingernail formation can signal teratogenic influences or ectodermal dysplasias (see Chapter 20).

Cranial Abnormalities

Head circumference as a reflection of brain growth provides an obvious clue to the cause of intellectual disability. Undergrowth of the cranium may indicate central nervous system damage or dysgenesis, and overgrowth may indicate hydrocephalus or megalencephaly. Abnormal skull shape may indicate that the underlying nervous system has undergone unusual physical stresses.

Transillumination aids in the diagnosis of porencephalic cysts or of other structural defects in young infants. The presence of an intracranial bruit may indicate an arteriovenous malformation, although such bruits are sometimes heard in

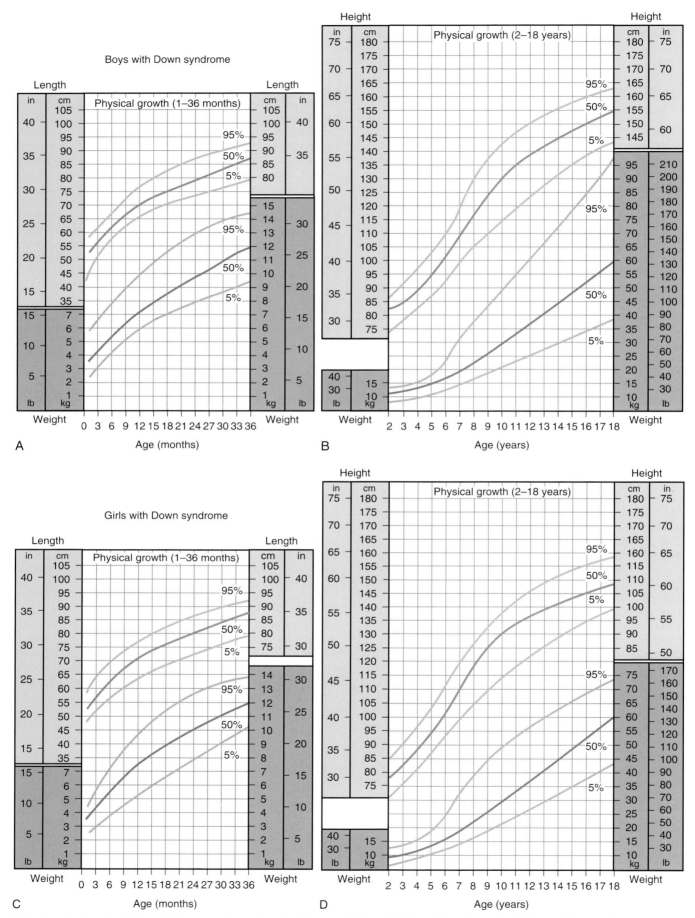

Figure 3-36   Growth charts for children with Down syndrome. *(From Cronk C, Crocker AC, Pueschel SM, et al: Growth charts for children with Down syndrome: 1 month to 18 years of age, Pediatrics 81:102, 1988.)*

Figure 3-37 Down syndrome. Note the upslanting palpebral fissures, flat nasal bridge, epicanthal folds, small ears, and small hands.

normal infants. Even in the absence of these signs, children with moderate, severe, and profound intellectual disability may warrant an imaging study of the central nervous system because of the high incidence of identifiable abnormalities.

Facial Abnormalities

The presence of certain facial characteristics may suggest a specific etiology of intellectual disability. Minor malformations (which include hypotelorism or hypertelorism; epicanthal folds; colobomas; and auricles that are large, abnormally formed, or set low in comparison with the plane of the eyes) are rare in the general population. In isolation, one dysmorphic feature may be insignificant. However, the presence of three or more of these features correlates highly with a major malformation, often of the heart, kidney, or brain. Patterns of dysmorphic features may suggest a specific diagnosis such as a genetic syndrome, chromosomal abnormality, or prenatal exposure. For example, flat facies, upturned palpebral fissures, epicanthal folds, single palmar creases, and clinodactyly are associated with trisomy 21 (Down syndrome) (Fig. 3-37). Likewise, a lengthened philtrum, a thin vermilion border, and microcephaly are clinical features of fetal alcohol syndrome.

Some of these unusual features themselves are clues to the etiology of the intellectual disability or are the result of abnormal functioning, even in prenatal life. For example, aberrant patterning of scalp hair may indicate abnormal cerebral morphology. The pattern of hair growth is affected by pressures from the developing brain on the overlying scalp in early gestation. The absence of a posterior hair whorl or the presence of multiple hair whorls suggests abnormal prenatal brain growth. Small palpebral fissures also result from abnormal brain growth; the eye is an extension of the brain, and small eyes are suggestive of abnormal early brain development. Similarly, a high-arched palate may be secondary to abnormal motor activity of the tongue in utero, suggesting a prenatal origin of motor problems.

Other Physical Abnormalities

Hepatosplenomegaly in the neonatal period may suggest congenital infection or in childhood may indicate a heritable storage disease affecting central nervous system and developmental functioning. Large testes are found in youngsters with fragile X syndrome, whereas hypogonadism is a concomitant of the Prader-Willi syndrome. This syndrome is associated with an abnormality on chromosome 15 (see Chapter 1).

Changes in the long bones of the limbs may show evidence of congenital infection; disproportionate bone length may suggest metabolic disorders such as homocystinuria or the osteochondrodysplasias. Errant toe proportions or changed crease patterns on the hands or soles of the feet may suggest early morphogenetic changes associated with certain defined syndromes. Lethargic or pale children may prompt an examination for iron deficiency or lead intoxication, which also may contribute to subnormal intellectual progress.

The American Academy of Neurology has reviewed the evidence for diagnostic testing in the evaluation of children with global developmental delay and suggests that genetic testing, even in the absence of dysmorphic features, be performed. The highest yield cytogenetic study is a microarray, which should be supplemented with molecular testing for fragile X syndrome. The history and physical examination guide further diagnostic studies including neuroimaging, electroencephalogram (EEG), and metabolic testing. Visual and audiologic assessments are recommended in the evaluation of children with global developmental delay/intellectual disability.

Prognosis

Approximately 3% of children are classified as intellectually disabled at some point in their lives. In a society that prizes intellectual accomplishment, the identification of a child's cognitive delays is upsetting for a family. Findings of unusual features in any aspect of the physical examination may help provide an explanation for abnormal or delayed cognitive development. In evaluating the cause of developmental delay, the greatest need, beyond that of assessing the possibility of remediation, is that of providing the parents with appropriate genetic, behavioral, and educational counseling. Evidence that a child's lack of developmental progress is related to constitutional factors can help relieve parents of guilt feelings.

In the past, physicians have often underestimated the capabilities of children with intellectual disability. Similarly, families often interpret a diagnosis of intellectual disability to mean that their child will make no further developmental progress. Estimates of functional abilities for children who are classified as intellectually disabled are variable. Children with mild intellectual disability (IQ scores 2 to 3 standard deviations below the mean [69 to 55]) can learn to read and write and to do simple mathematics. As adults, they often live independently and hold jobs. The extent of their disability is most prominent during the school years or during times of life crisis beyond school age. Children with moderate intellectual disability (IQ scores 3 to 4 standard deviations below the mean [54 to 40]) will generally learn to read and write only to a first- or second-grade level. Nonetheless, their abilities in language, self-care, and adaptation skills may allow them to live and work in semi-independent settings, with support and supervision as needed. Children with severe and profound intellectual disability (4 to 6 standard deviations below the mean [39 to 24 and below]) require substantial lifelong support.

The benefits of early intervention are maximized by early identification. Careful documentation of the child's opportunities for interaction with parents, other children, and stimulating environments helps in determining the type and degree of intervention necessary. The importance of careful screening of infant and preschool development by informed health professionals and of close collaboration between physicians and early intervention personnel cannot be overemphasized.

Figure 3-38   Child with autism looking at her own image rather than at the objects or person in the room; no interest in social interactions and/or pretend play activity.

Figure 3-40   Child with autism with hand flapping.

Autism Spectrum Disorder

Autism spectrum disorder (ASD) is the term for a category of neurodevelopmental disabilities of varying severity characterized by deficits in social interaction and communication as well as restricted interests and repetitive behaviors. According to the *Diagnostic and Statistical Manual of Mental Disorders,* fourth edition, the spectrum includes autistic disorder (AD; autism); Asperger disorder; childhood disintegrative disorder; and pervasive developmental disorder, not otherwise specified (PDD-NOS). All of these disorders are characterized by deficits in social interaction and communication as well as restricted interests and repetitive behaviors. All children with ASD have deficits in nonverbal and verbal communication used for social interaction, limited social reciprocity, and difficulty developing and maintaining peer relationships as expected for their developmental level (Fig. 3-38). Qualitative impairment in social interactions includes abnormal nonverbal behaviors, such as limited eye-to-eye gaze and unusual facial expressions (Fig. 3-39). The severity of language deficits varies from total lack of language to difficulty in initiating and sustaining conversation. Interests and behaviors are repetitive and restricted and may include unusual sensory behaviors, stereotyped motor or verbal behaviors, excessive adherence to routines and ritualized patterns of behavior, narrow and unusual interests, and repetitive hand movements, such as hand flapping (Fig. 3-40). Individuals with Asperger disorder are generally at the milder end of the spectrum with impaired social relationships and obsessive interests in a single topic or object. The major difference between children with autistic disorder (including children with high-functioning autism) and Asperger disorder is that in the latter there is a history of language developmental milestones being achieved on time (Table 3-9). At the more severe end of the spectrum are individuals with autism who generally have extremely limited social interaction, limited language, and intellectual impairment (Table 3-10 and Fig. 3-41). The term *high-functioning autism* has been reserved for children with all the diagnostic characteristics of ASD including deficits in communication, but with high scores in their IQ testing.

Autistic spectrum disorders present in two distinct patterns. Most children show abnormal social and communicative behaviors starting in early infancy. Parents often report that these children have low tone when held, fail to look at the human face, and do not turn toward the human voice. Some children demonstrate seemingly normal development in infancy and then, often in the second year of life, show regression of social and communicative skills, such as loss of early vocabulary and growing disinterest in social interaction. The nature of the presentation is not associated with severity of symptoms or long-term prognosis.

Surveillance and Screening for ASD

The American Academy of Pediatrics has developed a screening and surveillance algorithm to facilitate early identification of children with ASD. Surveillance includes family history to

Figure 3-39   Autism is characterized by qualitative impairment in social interactions, such as limited eye-to-eye gaze and unusual facial expressions. *(From Phelps R, Feldman HM: The laying on of hands: the physical examination in developmental and behavioral assessment. In Carey WB, Crocker AC, Elias ER, et al, editors:* Developmental–behavioral pediatrics, *ed 4, Philadelphia, 2009, Elsevier, Chapter 76, Figure 76-2.)*

Table 3-9	Difference in Diagnostic Criteria between Autistic Disorder and Asperger Disorder
Autistic Disorder	**Asperger Disorder**
Deficits in social interaction	Deficits in social interaction
Restricted interests and repetitive behaviors	Restricted interests and repetitive behaviors
Deficits in communication	Language developmental milestones achieved on time

ascertain genetic risk, open-ended questions to elicit parental concerns, as well as age-specific questions about social and emotional developmental milestones such as responsiveness to human voice, eye contact, shared attention, imitation, and pretend play. The following "red flags" require immediate evaluation:

- No babbling or pointing or other gesture by 12 months
- No single words by 16 months
- No two-word spontaneous (not echolalic) phrases by 24 months
- Loss of language or social skills at any age

Standardized autism-specific screening tools have been developed and should be used for all children, at least at the 18- and 24-month visits, in addition to the comprehensive screening tools recommended at the younger ages. The Modified Checklist for Autism in Toddlers (M-CHAT) is available at no cost for use in the office setting and can be downloaded from the American Academy of Pediatrics website (www.aap.org). A positive screen on the parent questionnaire should be followed by a specific interview. The positive impact of early therapeutic interventions for children with ASD should motivate the pediatrician to arrange for comprehensive evaluation and intervention if the screening test and interview are positive or when parents and pediatricians are concerned.

Physical Examination

Children with ASD generally have a completely normal physical and neurologic examination. Increased head circumference in the preschool period is associated with a diagnosis of autism, with or without intellectual disability, suggesting that the neurologic basis of autism may include overabundant growth of neurons and synapses or failure of normal processes of pruning of synapses.

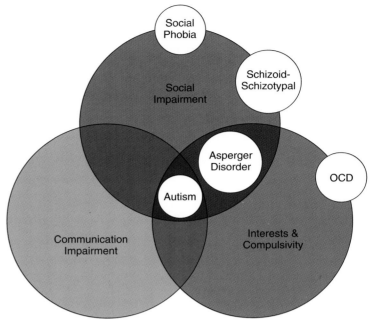

Three Core Dimensions of Autism Spectrum Disorder

Figure 3-41 Core deficits among those with and without autism spectrum disorders (ASDs). *(From Hollander et al: CNS Spectrums 3:22-26, 33-39, 1998.)*

Autism has been associated with other conditions including fragile X syndrome, Rett syndrome, and tuberous sclerosis. Therefore the physical examination of children with abnormal social and communicative development should include the following: a survey for dysmorphic features, such as long face, prominent jaw, and large or protuberant ears;

Table 3-10	Degrees of Autism Spectrum Disorders		
	Mild Autism	**Moderate Autism**	**Severe Autism**
Social interactions	• Unusual or idiosyncratic eye-to-eye gaze, facial expression, body posture • May affiliate with peers but lacks full understanding of social rules • Limited reciprocity in social interaction; insistence on own interests	• Eye-to-eye gaze on own terms and restricted facial expressions • Limited affiliation with peers and poor understanding of social rules • Rare reciprocity though may share enjoyment with family or close friends	• Marked impairment in eye-to-eye gaze, facial expressions • No affiliation with peers and no appreciation of social interaction • Lack of spontaneous seeking to share enjoyment, interests with anyone
Communication	• Unusual features in development of spoken language, such as poor intonation, frequent use of frozen forms • Limited ability to initiate or sustain conversation; poor topic maintenance • Make-believe or social imitative play limited to areas of keen interest	• Obvious delay in the development of spoken language • Marked impairment in initiating and sustaining conversation • Frequent reliance on echolalia and meaningless jargon • Limited spontaneous make-believe or social imitative play appropriate to developmental level	• Total lack of the development of spoken language • No conversational language despite occasional use of words in self-talk • Lack of spontaneous make-believe play or social imitative play appropriate to developmental level
Restricted repetitive and stereotyped patterns of behavior, interests, and activities	• Encompassing preoccupation with one or more interest that is abnormal in either intensity or focus • Inflexible adherence to specific, nonfunctional routines or rituals • Occasional stereotyped and repetitive motor mannerisms	• Encompassing preoccupation with one or more stereotyped and restricted patterns of interest that are abnormal in either intensity or focus • Inflexible adherence to specific, nonfunctional routines or rituals • Frequent stereotyped and repetitive motor mannerisms	• Inflexible adherence to specific, nonfunctional routines or rituals • Frequent stereotyped and repetitive motor mannerisms • Persistent preoccupation with parts of objects

measurement of head circumference to document relative macrocephaly or microcephaly; the evaluation of facial, truncal, and extremity tone; and careful skin examination for hypopigmented lesions.

ASD is a syndrome with many known causes. There is a strong genetic contribution that warrants genetic testing in children, particularly those with intellectual disability (or if intellectual disability cannot be excluded); if there is a family history of fragile X syndrome, undiagnosed intellectual disability, or other family members with autism; or if dysmorphic features are present. Genome microarray is more sensitive than high-resolution chromosome studies and is the genetic test recommended in the evaluation of children with ASD. DNA analysis for fragile X syndrome is also recommended. Other specific findings may require additional laboratory tests, such as genetic tests for tuberous sclerosis in children with hypopigmented skin lesions. Identifying a specific genetic cause is relevant to counseling about recurrence risk in a family and prognosis for the individual.

Selective metabolic testing should be initiated by the presence of suggestive clinical and physical findings such as the following: evidence of lethargy, cyclic vomiting, or early seizures; presence of dysmorphic or coarse features; evidence of intellectual disability or if intellectual disability cannot be ruled out; or if occurrence or adequacy of newborn screening is questionable.

There is no clinical evidence to support the role of routine clinical neuroimaging in the diagnostic evaluation of autism, even in the presence of megalencephaly. However, the *PTEN* gene is associated with autism and macrocephaly.

There is inadequate supporting evidence for hair analysis, celiac antibodies, allergy testing (particularly food allergies for gluten, casein, *Candida,* and other molds), immunologic or neurochemical abnormalities, micronutrients such as vitamin levels, intestinal permeability studies, stool analysis, urinary peptides, mitochondrial disorders (including lactate and pyruvate levels), thyroid function tests, or erythrocyte glutathione peroxidase studies in the diagnosis of ASD.

Children with autistic spectrum disorders are at increased risk of seizure disorders, and unusual movements or lapses in consciousness should prompt evaluation with an electroencephalogram, but there is inadequate evidence to recommend an electroencephalogram study in all individuals with autism. Indications for an adequate sleep-deprived electroencephalogram with appropriate sampling of slow-wave sleep include clinical seizures or suspicion of subclinical seizures and a history of regression (clinically significant loss of social and communicative function) at any age, but especially in toddlers and preschoolers.

Prognosis

Children with ASD benefit substantially from intense early intervention services designed to improve their social interactions and communication skills. Some children with such interventions may be able to attend regular education settings without special services by school age. Therefore prompt referral for early intervention and advocacy for intensive programming is appropriate for toddlers and preschoolers on the autistic spectrum. No definitive treatments are currently available for autistic spectrum disorders. Educational and behavioral interventions address the core characteristics. Medication is often used to manage associated findings, such as inattention, hyperactivity, mood lability, and unpredictable outbursts. Addressing the family's challenges in raising a child with autism is central to management and may include referral to family support groups, provision of educational material, and referral for behavior management counseling. There is insufficient evidence to recommend dietary supplements or restrictions at this time.

Language and Reading Disorders

Delays and disturbances in language development are most frequently associated with intellectual disability, ASD, hearing impairment, and environmental deprivation. However, language difficulties may occur in an otherwise normal child; in such cases, they are referred to as specific language impairment, usually of unknown etiology. Some theories stress difficulties with high-level concepts and symbolic capabilities, and others stress auditory perceptual impairments as the root of specific language disorders.

Physical Examination

No specific physical signs are associated with language disorders. The physician's role is in large part to rule out other disorders with different etiologies and prognoses.

Hearing assessment is indicated for any child with delays or deviancies in language development because hearing loss is a treatable condition. Universal newborn hearing screening, now available in most states in the United States and in many other countries, allows identification and treatment of sensorineural hearing loss before it leads to delays in language, speech, and other developmental domains. The screenings use otoacoustic emissions or automated auditory brainstem responses, two inexpensive techniques that assess physiologic responses to sound without requiring voluntary responses from the child. If a newborn does not pass the screen, then definitive testing with the brainstem auditory-evoked response, an electrophysiologic measure that records brain waves as a function of sound exposure, should be performed. Universal newborn hearing screening has successfully lowered the mean age of detection of sensorineural hearing loss. However, in children with language and speech delays, repeating the audiometric assessment is important because hearing loss may be progressive or missed in the newborn period. In older infants and toddlers, conditioning techniques or conventional audiometry assess actual hearing rather than associated physiologic markers. The use of earphones allows for evaluation of each ear independently (Fig. 3-42).

Syndromes known to be associated with hearing loss include Treacher Collins syndrome, Waardenburg syndrome, and osteogenesis imperfecta. Children with abnormalities of the external ear including preauricular tags and pits, the palate, or facial structures may also have sensorineural hearing loss (Table 3-11). Repeated evaluations may be required in congenital rubella or cytomegalovirus infections because of progressive hearing loss. Several genetic causes of congenital hearing loss have been identified. Conditions associated with varying degrees of hearing loss, their disabling effects, and the interventions required for children with these conditions are listed in Table 3-12. Children with congenital hearing loss that is treated with amplification or hearing aids should be evaluated for their responses to spoken words, patterns of vocalization and sound production, visual and verbal attentiveness, social rapport, and development of communication.

Otitis media with effusion is associated with mild, variable, intermittent hearing loss. Randomized clinical trials of otherwise healthy children with prolonged middle ear effusion have compared early insertion of tympanostomy tubes with delayed or no tube insertion if the effusion clears. The results found no short-term or long-term advantages of early tympanostomy tube insertion in terms of levels of speech, language, or cognitive skills.

AUDIOGRAMS

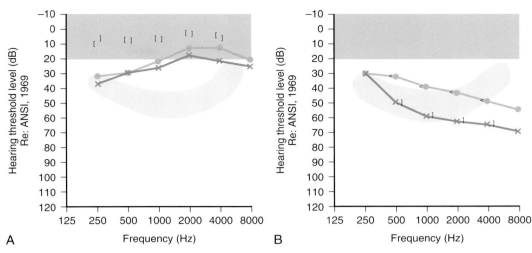

A   Frequency (Hz)   B   Frequency (Hz)

Figure 3-42 Audiograms. The purple X indicates the threshold for the left ear, and the blue circle indicates the threshold for the right ear. Brackets indicate bone conduction. **A,** This audiogram indicates mild conductive hearing loss in both ears. Notice that more energy is required for detection of sound in the low-frequency range. Bone conduction is normal. **B,** This audiogram demonstrates sensorineural hearing loss. The left ear shows a sloping pattern with mild to moderate loss in the low-frequency range and severe loss in the high-frequency range. The right ear shows mild to moderate loss throughout the frequency range.

Prognosis

Many toddlers with speech or language disorders develop adequate speech, language, and communication skills by early elementary school. No variables are consistently associated with a good prognosis; however, the prognosis for communication is clearly improved through early communication therapy. Physicians should not hesitate to refer children with speech and language delays for assessment and treatment.

Many toddlers and preschoolers with selective problems in language acquisition develop reading difficulties during the school-age years. A reading disorder (dyslexia) is a frequent finding in a child with an early history of language delay and a positive family history of language impairment or reading disability (Fig. 3-43). With increasing age, children with reading difficulties tend to improve. However, in many cases, reading remains an area of relative weakness compared with other cognitive and academic skills.

Children with reading disorders show abnormal or inefficient eye movements in the course of reading. This observation has led to visual training as a treatment strategy. However, the literature supports the notion that in most cases, a reading problem is a high-level language difficulty, not a visual or visuomotor problem.

Attention-Deficit/Hyperactivity Disorder

Attention-deficit/hyperactivity disorder (ADHD) is a syndrome characterized by persistent inattention, hyperactivity, and impulsivity compared with what is expected for a child at a particular developmental level. Judgments about the degree of deviance in these behaviors are based on the degree of interference they cause in the child's social, academic, or other functioning. The diagnosis of ADHD requires that symptoms have been long-standing, that they be present before at least 7 years of age, and that they occur in multiple settings and not just at home or school. Multiple genetic, neurologic, toxic, and psychosocial conditions are associated with the presence of ADHD. Among children born prematurely and children with intellectual disability, ADHD is more prevalent than in the general population.

Table 3-11	Conditions Associated with Sensorineural Hearing Loss

Family history of childhood hearing impairment

Congenital perinatal infection (CMV, rubella, herpes, toxoplasmosis, syphilis)

Anatomic malformations of the head or neck

Birth weight <1500 g

Hyperbilirubinemia above levels indicated for exchange transfusion

Bacterial meningitis

Severe asphyxia

Exposure to ototoxic medications

CMV, cytomegalovirus.

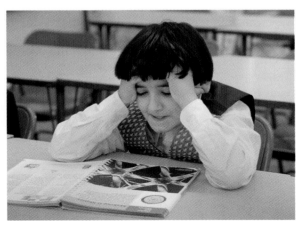

Figure 3-43 Child experiencing reading difficulties. *(Courtesy Robert Louis and the Hispanic/Latino Community of Southwestern Pennsylvania. Picture from Kaczmarek L, Chaves-Gnecco D: Special education services. In Carey WB, Crocker AC, Elias ER, et al, editors:* Developmental–behavioral pediatrics, *ed 4, Philadelphia, 2009, Elsevier, Figure 93-1.)*

Table 3-12	Disabling Effects of Hearing Loss				
Average Hearing Deficit at 500-2000 Hz (ANSI)	**Description**	**Condition**	**Sounds Heard without Amplification**	**Degree of Disability (If Not Treated in First Year of Life)**	**Probable Needs**
0-15 dB	Normal range		All speech sounds	None	None
15-25 dB	Minimal hearing loss	Serous otitis, perforation, monomeric membrane, sensorineural loss, tympanosclerosis	Vowel sounds heard clearly; may miss a few consonant sounds	Possible mild auditory dysfunction in language learning	Environmental modifications, such as preferential seating in school and face-to-face communication; auditory training, speech therapy
25-40 dB	Mild hearing loss	Serous otitis, perforation, tympanosclerosis, monomeric membrane, sensorineural loss	Hears most louder-voiced speech sounds	Possible auditory learning dysfunction, possible mild language retardation, mild speech problems, inattention	Hearing aid, auditory training, speech therapy; environmental modifications, such as preferential seating
40-65 dB	Moderate hearing loss	Middle ear anomaly, sensorineural loss	Misses most speech sounds at normal conversational level	Speech problems, language retardation, learning dysfunction, inattention	All of the above, plus consideration of special education services as required
65-90 dB	Severe hearing loss	Sensorineural or mixed loss from sensorineural loss plus middle ear disease	Hears no speech sounds of normal conversation	Severe speech problems, language retardation, learning dysfunction, inattention	All of the above, plus probable special education services as required
>90 dB	Profound hearing loss	Sensorineural or mixed loss	Hears no speech or other sounds; candidate for cochlear implantation	Severe speech problems, language retardation, learning dysfunction, inattention	All of the above, plus probable special education services as required

ANSI, American National Standards Institute; dB, decibel.
   Modified from Stewart JM, Downs MP: Medical management of the hearing-handicapped child. In Northern JL, editor: *Hearing disorders,* ed 2, Boston, 1984, Little, Brown. Reprinted by permission of Allyn & Bacon.

Although precise diagnostic criteria have changed over the past three decades, certain features have recurred in the lists of defining characteristics. Children with ADHD have difficulty sustaining attention and persisting to task completion. They become easily distracted. Frequently they fail to organize and plan before beginning a task. Because of all these features operating concurrently, these children fail to complete work assignments and eventually may avoid long and demanding tasks. Impulsivity in young children is frequently demonstrated by difficulty waiting for a turn. As children get older, impulsivity is expressed as difficulty in delaying responses, blurting out answers, interrupting others, and generally acting before thinking.

There are three different subtypes of ADHD. Most children demonstrate ADHD combined type, a variant that includes symptoms of inattention and hyperactivity–impulsivity. However, ADHD predominantly inattentive type is appropriate for children with symptoms of inattention without hyperactivity or impulsivity. An alternative diagnosis is ADHD predominantly hyperactive–impulsive type, in which inattention may be a feature but is less prominent than hyperactivity. The degree of hyperactivity varies in part with the child's age, developmental level, temperament, and style. Young school-age boys with ADHD tend to display excessive fidgetiness and activity, whereas adolescents and girls may be inattentive but not hyperactive (Fig. 3-44).

Most children with ADHD show age-appropriate attention in some highly motivating situations. For example, parents routinely report that their children with ADHD sit for computer games or captivating movies. For this reason, up to 80% of children whose behavior at home and at school meets diagnostic criteria do not show characteristics of the disorder in the physician's office. Diagnosis rests on historical information from parents and confirmatory reports from teachers. Standardized questionnaires are often used in diagnosis to quantify the degree of inattention, hyperactivity, and associated behavioral problems.

Children with ADHD are likely to have other neurobehavioral disorders such as anxiety, depression, conduct disorder, oppositional defiant disorder, and learning disabilities. In conduct disorder, as opposed to ADHD, the child violates the basic rights of others and age-appropriate social norms. In oppositional defiant disorder, the child shows severe and

Figure 3-44   Child with attention-deficit/hyperactivity disorder (ADHD), inattentive type. The girl in the picture is daydreaming while her classmates are paying attention to the teacher. *(Courtesy Robert Louis and the Hispanic/Latino Community of Southwestern Pennsylvania. Picture from Kaczmarek L, Chaves-Gnecco D: Special education services. In Carey WB, Crocker AC, Elias ER, et al, editors: Developmental–behavioral pediatrics, ed 4, Philadelphia, 2009, Elsevier, Figure 93-2.)*

persistent disobedience and hostility directed against authority figures. The evaluation of ADHD should include evaluation for these coexisting conditions.

Physical Findings

On physical examination, it is important to assess the general characteristics of the child to rule out other similar psychiatric disorders such as autism, depression, anxiety, or oppositional disorder. Physical findings in ADHD may be completely noncontributory. However, findings such as short stature or dysmorphic features may suggest an associated genetic or dysmorphic syndrome such as alcohol-related birth defects. Focal neurologic findings may suggest a static or progressive neurologic cause such as periventricular leukomalacia from prematurity. The presence of motor or vocal tics with ADHD raises the diagnostic possibility of a chronic tic disorder or Tourette syndrome.

The physical and neurologic examination of children with suspected ADHD often includes a set of specific maneuvers and tasks referred to as *neurologic soft signs* or *neuromaturational indicators*. Nonnormative performance on these specific motor and sensory tasks can be obtained in children who otherwise show no evidence of a localizing neurologic disorder or pathognomonic patterns indicative of generalized encephalopathy. The soft signs are of clinical interest because they serve as an index for cognitive or behavioral dysfunction.

Table 3-13 includes several tasks for eliciting soft signs, the typical ages of acquisition, and indications of immature or positive findings. On rapid alternating pronation–supination of the hands, developing children typically show resolution of dysdiadochokinesia by age 7 years. On the same task and on repeated finger-to-thumb apposition and alternating squeezing and relaxing of handgrip, children usually show a marked decrease in synkinesis after age 9 years.

Including these maneuvers in the physical examination is useful for unmasking a child's inattention, impulsivity, and disorganization that may otherwise go undetected in the clinical setting. Parents may be relieved when the physician observes those traits that have brought the family in for evaluation. In some cases parents have the opportunity to observe the traits that teachers find challenging in the classroom. Difficulty executing discrimination of right and left and particularly crossed commands on themselves and the examiner beyond 8 years of age may be found in children with ADHD. In addition, they may also show problems in executing four or more sequential commands from memory. However, persistence of abnormal findings on these tasks is not diagnostic of ADHD.

Prognosis

Research suggests that ADHD is a lifelong condition. The signs and symptoms of hyperactivity are likely to resolve during adolescence, but relative inattention persists into adulthood. Many individuals with ADHD do better as adolescents and adults than they did as children because they can choose educational programs or occupations that allow them to work with their strengths. They often prefer vocations that permit frequent shifts in attention and a high energy level and that do not require sustained attention to challenging tasks. Nonetheless, individuals with ADHD have poorer educational attainment, higher rates of automobile accidents, lower job attainment, and greater instability in relationships compared with siblings who do not have the disorder, presumably related to persistent inattention. The prognosis is more favorable in individuals with isolated ADHD, good cognitive skills, no learning disorders, and positive family and peer relationships.

Treatment options for ADHD fall into three categories: behavior management, educational interventions, and psychopharmacology. Combinations of these options often are more effective than a single treatment.

Visual Impairment

Visual experience assists the learning of many important concepts of space and form, important in the development of motor skills, perception, cognition, and social skills (Table 3-14). Thus in situations of congenital blindness or visual impairment, developmental patterns may be altered and delayed, demonstrating the close interrelationships that exist among developmental domains. Children with visual impairments can learn to increase the use of residual visual functioning and other sensory modalities. The physician's understanding of the impact of visual impairment is important to evaluate whether developmental progress is being achieved as expected in this population and to ensure that unexpected delays and deviancies are appropriately diagnosed and treated.

Table 3-13	Indicators Associated with Neurologic Immaturity	
Task	**Immature Response**	**Norms**
Rapid pronation–supination	Dysdiadochokinesia	Mature by age 7-8 yr
Repeated finger-to-thumb apposition	Synkinesis	Markedly decreased after age 9 yr
Alternation of squeezing and relaxation of single handgrip	Synkinesis	Markedly decreased after age 9 yr
Sensory integration—tactile recognition from visual presentation	Astereognosis	>90% accurate by age 7 yr
Identification of right and left on self	Inaccurate	>90% correct by age 7 yr
Execution of crossed commands (e.g., touch left eye with right hand)		
On self	Inaccurate	>90% correct by age 8 yr
On examiner	Inaccurate	>70% correct by age 8 yr

Table 3-14	Visually Related Behaviors
Age of Infant	**Behavior**
Term	Focuses on face, briefly tracks vertically and horizontally, turns toward diffuse light source, widens eyes to object or face at 8-12 in.
1 mo	Blinks at approaching object, tracks 60 degrees horizontally, 30 degrees vertically
2 mo	Tracks across midline, follows movement 6 ft away, smiles to a smiling face, raises head 30 degrees in prone position
3 mo	Eyes and head track 180 degrees, looks at hands, looks at objects placed in hands
4-5 mo	Reaches for object (12-in. cube) 12 in. away, notices raisins 1 ft away, smiles at familiar adult
5-6 mo	Smiles in mirror
7-8 mo	Rakes at raisin
8-9 mo	Notes visual details, pokes at holes in pegboard and at elevator buttons
9 mo	Neat pincer grasp
12-14 mo	Stacks blocks, places peg in round hole

Gross and Fine Motor Development

Apparently, much of the motivation for the infant with normal vision to raise the head 90 degrees when in the prone position is to increase the visual field. Without the feedback of interesting sights, the infant with severe visual impairment may not attain this milestone until 11 to 12 months of age. In contrast, rolling occurs in infants who are blind at close to the same age as in infants with normal vision. If sitting independently is an active goal, it can occur by 6 to 7 months of age. However, transitional movements from lying to sitting or from sitting to standing occur several months later in infants without sight than in infants able to see.

Protective reactions develop more slowly in infants with severe visual impairment, and these are expected to appear in the 10- to 12-month age range. This delay, as well as the inability to integrate visual cues in attaining balance and equilibrium, and the lack of a visual impetus to explore distant toys, may contribute to a typical delay in crawling or walking. Paired auditory–tactile cues presented to children with severe visual impairment may stimulate their interest in objects beyond their reach, thus accelerating gross motor development.

Regarding fine motor development, information gathering by index finger and manual manipulation may be more accurate in the child who is blind than in the child with normal vision. However, the youngster who is blind may experience a delay in the acquisition of precise prehension, which sometimes never develops, with raking favored as a more efficient means of exploration.

Cognitive Development

The development of cognitive skills in the child with visual impairment must of necessity depend on use of the other sensory modalities. For this reason, careful global evaluation of the child with severe visual impairment should be conducted early in infancy to ensure that the other senses are intact.

A child with normal vision develops the understanding that objects are permanent even when they cannot be seen, felt, heard, sniffed, or tasted. For the child with severe visual impairment, the opportunities for object perception are fewer, and thus the understanding of object permanence typically develops later, stimulated by encouragement of the infant to reach for sound cues. Similarly, in a child with severe visual impairment, the understanding of conservation of continuous quantity, that a cup of water contains the same volume of liquid in a tall thin container as it does in a short fat one, also develops later than in the child with normal vision. Haptic perception, the acquisition of information about objects or spaces by exploration with the hands, appears to be more important in the cognitive development of the child with severe visual impairment than in that of the child with normal vision. For this reason, tactile exploration in the child who is blind cannot be promoted at too early an age. In fact, without such encouragement, these children may be fearful and resistant to unfamiliar new feelings.

Language and Intellectual Development

Verbal imitation and receptive language skills may develop normally in healthy children who are blind. As one might expect, these children may have difficulty with words relating to visual concepts, such as *light, dark,* and *color.* They may also have problems with words referring to large things that cannot be touched (*sky* and *stars*), things that change slowly (*age* and *growth*), and the concept "I." However, some children with severe visual impairment show accurate use of all of these concepts and even make the distinction between the words *look* and *see.* In these cases the child probably uses available linguistic information to substitute for visual information.

Although standard IQ tests cannot be used to assess intellectual capabilities of children with severe visual impairment, standardized instruments have been developed to assess their cognitive development. Receptive and expressive language skills figure prominently in these assessments. In addition, interview schedules of adaptive behavior in communication and self-help skills have been developed specifically for children with visual impairment.

Social Development

Infants who are blind lack the opportunity to benefit from face-to-face contact with their caregivers, from the visual reinforcement of smiling, from the use of facial expressions to assist in the interpretation of voices or actions, and from the experience of tracking parents across the room to know that even when they cannot be heard or felt they are still there. These differences in sensory input affect their social and emotional development. Parents of infants with severe visual impairment frequently need to be coached to use touch and sound to reinforce smiling and other desired behaviors in their child.

At about the same time that children with normal vision smile at familiar faces, children who are blind smile in response to familiar touching and kinesthetic handling. Smiling in response to a familiar voice, however, may occur inconsistently up to 1 year of age. The infant who is blind demonstrates attachment by calming to the tactile exploration of the caregiver's familiar face or hands.

Blind children of about 1 year of age may have stranger awareness, although a greater hurdle will be their reaction to separation. Because these children have a limited capacity to track their caregivers, separations from them may induce panic states even among older ones. Similarly, the development of independent caregiving and play may be delayed and may require specific interventions.

Parents should be advised that, without purposeful stimulation, children who are blind may engage in nonpurposeful motor activities such as eye rubbing or rocking and that these stereotypical behaviors, referred to as *blindisms,* are difficult to extinguish. Blindisms can often be channeled to purposeful stimulation by directing the child's hands to exploration of a toy or by distracting the child with conversation or music. These efforts will serve to channel the child's activities in a more socially adaptive direction.

SUMMARY

The tasks of routine developmental surveillance supplemented by standardized screening, identification of children with variations, and referral for appropriate developmental services (especially during infancy and in the preschool years) fall largely, and often exclusively, to the primary care clinician. Although we have provided estimates regarding the expected chronology of development, these developmental milestones are guidelines rather than fixed time frames within which skill acquisition may be judged as normal or abnormal. In evaluating a child, the physician must use these guidelines, the results of screening tests, and clinical judgment, taking into account the child's own personality traits, experiences, and degree of cooperation.

Recommendations for further assessment and treatment should be made in consultation with the family.

Resources

Validated Developmental Screening Tests
http://www.developmentalscreening.org/index.htm

Ages & Stages
www.brookespublishing.com/tools/asq/index.htm
Child Development Inventories
http://www.childdevrev.com/page15/page17/cdi.html
Denver II
http://www.denverii.com/
Parents' Evaluation of Developmental Status (PEDS)
http://www.pedstest.com/default.aspx

Bibliography

Allen MC: Neurodevelopmental assessment of the young child: the state of the art, *Ment Retard Dev Disabil Res Rev* 11:274–275, 2005.

Batshaw ME, editor: *Children with disabilities*, ed 5, Baltimore, 2002, Paul H. Brookes.

Carey WB, Crocker AC, Coleman W, et al, editors: *Developmental–behavioral pediatrics*, 4th ed. Philadelphia, 2009, WB Saunders.

Committee on Children with Disabilities: Developmental surveillance and screening of infants and young children, *Pediatrics* 108:192–195, 2001.

Cooley WC, McAllister JW: Building medical homes: improvement strategies in primary care for children with special health care needs, *Pediatrics* 113:1499–1506, 2004.

Dixon SD, Stein MT: *Encounters with children: pediatric behavior and development*, ed 3, St. Louis, 2000, Mosby.

Feldman HM: Evaluation and management of language and speech disorders in preschool children, *Pediatr Rev* 26:131–142, 2005.

Glascoe FP: Early detection of developmental and behavioral problems, *Pediatr Rev* 21:272–280, 2000.

Johnson CP, Blasco PA: Infant growth and development, *Pediatr Rev* 18:224–242, 1997.

Joint Committee on Infant Hearing, American Academy of Audiology, American Academy of Pediatrics, American Speech-Language-Hearing Association, Directors of Speech and Hearing Programs in State Health and Welfare Associations: Year 2000 position statement: principles and guidelines for early hearing detection and intervention programs, *Pediatrics* 106:798–817, 2000.

Jones KL: *Smith's recognizable patterns of human malformation*, ed 6, Philadelphia, 2006, Elsevier Saunders.

Kaleida PH, Shaikh N: *Digital visual diagnosis in pediatrics teaching and review module: "Assessing infant development"* (CD-ROM). Pittsburgh, 2003, University of Pittsburgh.

Levine MD, Carey WB, Crocker AC, editors: *Developmental–behavioral pediatrics*, ed 3, Philadelphia, 1999, Saunders.

Lichtenberger EO: General measures of cognition for the preschool child, *Ment Retard Dev Disabil Res Rev* 11:197–208, 2005.

Perrin E, Stancin T: A continuing dilemma: whether and how to screen for concerns about children's behavior, *Pediatr Rev* 23:264–276, 2002.

Vargas C, Prelock PE, editors: *Caring for children with neurodevelopmental disabilities and their families: an innovative approach to interdisciplinary practice*, Mahwah, NJ, 2004, Lawrence Erlbaum.

Note: A lengthier list of tool choices is accessible in the 2006 AAP policy statement: Council on Children with Disabilities, et al: Identifying infants and young children with developmental disorders in the medical home: an algorithm for developmental surveillance and screening, *Pediatrics* 118:405–420, 2006.

ALLERGY AND IMMUNOLOGY

4

Andrew MacGinnitie | David Nash | Todd Green | David Stukus

Disorders of the immune system are diverse and range from mild to severe in their manifestations and impact on normal function. In this chapter, we review the physical findings and characteristic symptoms of children with hypersensitivity reactions and immune deficiencies, as well as diagnostic techniques and radiographic findings. Topics have been chosen on the basis of their prevalence and importance in the pediatric population and their association with characteristic physical findings.

IMMUNOLOGIC HYPERSENSITIVITY DISORDERS

Hypersensitivity disorders of the human immune system have been classified by Gell and Coombs into four groups (Table 4-1). Type I reactions occur promptly after the sensitized individual is exposed to an antigen and are mediated by specific IgE antibody. Cross-linking of IgE on the surface of mast cells and basophils leads to release of histamine and other inflammatory mediators. This mechanism is responsible for the common disorders of immediate hypersensitivity, such as allergic rhinitis and urticaria. So-called "anaphylactoid" reactions are clinically similar, but are caused by degranulation of mast cells and basophils in the absence of specific IgE. Type II reactions involve antibodies directed against antigenic components of peripheral blood or tissue cells or foreign antigens, resulting in cell destruction. Examples of this type include autoimmune hemolytic anemia and Rh and ABO hemolytic disease of the newborn. In type III reactions, antigen–antibody complexes form and are deposited in the lining of blood vessels, stimulating tissue inflammation mediated by complement or activated white blood cells. Examples of this type of reaction are serum sickness and the immune complex–mediated renal diseases. Type IV reactions involve T cell–mediated tissue inflammation and typically occur 24 to 48 hours after exposure. Examples of this type are tuberculin (purified protein derivative, PPD) reactions and contact dermatitis (see Chapter 8).

TYPE I DISORDERS

The development of type I hypersensitivity depends on hereditary predisposition, sensitization by exposure to an antigen, and subsequent reexposure to the antigen leading to an allergic reaction. Antigens that stimulate allergic reactions are known as *allergens,* and the mechanism of allergen-induced mediator release in type I hypersensitivity reactions is shown in Figure 4-1. IgE antibodies directed toward specific allergens are bound to the high-affinity IgE receptor on mast cells and basophils. When allergen causes cross-linking of IgE antibodies on the cell surface, the cell becomes activated, leading to the release of preformed mediators and the generation of the

early and late mediators of anaphylaxis. The preformed mediators include histamine, tryptase, chymase, heparin, and other proteases that drive the earliest symptoms of anaphylaxis. A serum tryptase level is currently the best biologic marker of anaphylaxis, but it is still a relatively insensitive test. Serum tryptase levels should be obtained close to the onset of anaphylaxis because levels peak in 1 hour and remain elevated for only 4 to 24 hours. The early and late mediators generated by mast cell activation include prostaglandins, leukotrienes, and cytokines. These mediators, which are generated over minutes to hours, continue to drive the clinical symptoms of the allergic reaction and initiate an inflammatory cascade that leads to the recruitment of eosinophils, basophils, and lymphocytes.

Type I reactions may occur in one or more target organs including the upper and lower respiratory tracts, cardiovascular system, skin, conjunctivae, and gastrointestinal (GI) tract. Manifestations depend on the systems involved, as shown in Figure 4-2. The most common manifestation of type I reaction is seasonal allergic rhinitis with a prevalence of at least 25%. The most serious manifestation of type I hypersensitivity is anaphylaxis, which can simultaneously involve all of the organ systems mentioned above.

Type I hypersensitivity has been diagnosed by skin testing for more than 100 years. The percutaneous skin test, also known as either the scratch or prick test, is an in vivo method to detect the presence of IgE antibody to specific allergens. The skin prick test is the safest and most specific test and correlates best with symptoms. The skin prick test is typically performed with a plastic lancet on either the forearm or upper back and involves a superficial disruption of the epidermis that is nearly painless (Fig. 4-3). The test leaves a barely visible mark, and when performed properly, the prick site should not bleed. The test is interpreted after 15 to 20 minutes by measuring the maximal diameter of both the wheal and the flare. Skin test results are compared with a negative control, which is usually saline, and a positive control, which is typically histamine. Historically, intradermal tests have been considered to be more sensitive than prick tests, but the specificity is poor and these tests should be used only when ruling out allergic disease is essential.

Allergy skin testing is contraindicated in four clinical situations: (1) when antihistamines have been used in the recent past—this will typically manifest as a negative histamine control; (2) when skin disease limits the area available for testing; (3) during either an asthma exacerbation or episode of anaphylaxis; and (4) when a patient is taking a β-blocking medicine, because these can interfere with epinephrine treatment in rare cases of test-induced anaphylaxis. When skin testing is not possible, in vitro testing is a good alternative. The in vitro tests can be accomplished with just a few milliliters of serum and also may be advantageous for some patients who have a difficult time sitting through allergy tests. In vitro

111

Table 4-1	Classification of Hypersensitivity Disorders				
Hypersensitivity Type	**Time Interval between Effector Exposure and Reaction**	**Cell or Antibody**	**Target or Antigen**	**Examples of Mediators**	**Disorder(s)**
Type I: Anaphylaxis		IgE	Pollens, foods, drugs, insect venoms		Anaphylaxis
a. Immediate	<30 min			a. Histamine	Allergic rhinitis
b. Late phase	2-12 h			b. Leukotrienes	Allergic asthma
Type II: Cytotoxic	Variable (minutes to hours)	IgG, IgM	Red blood cells, lung tissue	Complement	Immune hemolytic anemia
					Rh hemolytic disease
					Goodpasture syndrome
Type III: Immune complex mediated	4-8 h	Antigen with antibody	Vascular endothelium	Complement Anaphylatoxin	Serum sickness
					Poststreptococcal glomerulonephritis
Type IV: Delayed type	24-48 h	Lymphocytes	*Mycobacterium tuberculosis,* chemicals	Cytokines	Contact dermatitis
					Tuberculin skin test reactions

From Gell PGH, Coombs RRA: *Clinical aspects of immunology,* ed 2, Philadelphia, 1968, FA Davis.

allergy tests are more expensive and less sensitive than allergy prick tests (Table 4-2). In vitro tests are especially helpful in the evaluation of patients with possible food allergies; this is discussed further below.

SYSTEMIC ANAPHYLAXIS

Anaphylaxis results from widespread degranulation of mast cells after cross-linking of IgE on the mast cell surface. A clinically similar reaction in which mast cells degranulate without cross-linking of antigen-specific IgE is termed *anaphylactoid.* Anaphylaxis is a clinical diagnosis, and a report issued jointly by the National Institute of Allergy and Infectious Diseases and the Food Allergy and Anaphylaxis Network established criteria to define likely anaphylactic episodes (Table 4-3). Onset of anaphylaxis is typically rapid and often explosive after bee stings, drug administration, or food ingestion (Fig. 4-4). The pattern of organ system involvement can vary, based on the antigen, dose, and route of exposure, and can range from isolated urticaria to cardiovascular collapse (Fig. 4-5). Airway obstruction and hypotension are the most severe manifestations of anaphylaxis. The upper or lower airway, or both,

can be affected. Upper airway obstruction is due to laryngeal edema, whereas lower airway involvement is due to edema and bronchospasm. Hypotension is caused by vasodilation, which may be complicated by loss of intravascular volume. Vascular collapse may be aggravated by decreases in myocardial function. In addition to the airway and cardiovascular system, other organ systems are also involved in anaphylaxis. The skin is the most commonly involved organ, with urticaria being nearly universal and angioedema often present. GI involvement can manifest as vomiting, diarrhea, and abdominal pain due to gut edema.

For all reactions but isolated skin symptoms, intramuscular epinephrine is the therapy of choice. Studies have demonstrated the superiority of intramuscular injections compared with subcutaneous injections of epinephrine (Fig. 4-6). Patients at risk should carry self-injectable epinephrine and be trained in its use. There are currently four different epinephrine autoinjector devices: EpiPen, Adrenaclick, Twinject, and a generic autoinjector (Fig. 4-7). All come in two doses: either 0.15 mg or 0.3 mg. Operating technique varies somewhat among the devices, so it is important for families to become familiar with their specific device. Epinephrine is most effective when it is

IgE

FcεRI binding site

Allergens

FcεRI

Immediate release
Granule contents:
histamine, TNF-α,
proteases, heparin

Over minutes
Lipid mediators:
prostaglandins
leukotrienes

Over hours
Cytokine production;
specifically IL-4, IL-13

Figure 4-1 IgE is bound to the mast cell surface, and when cross-linked by antigen, the mast cell becomes activated. The activated mast cell releases preformed mediators and generates additional mediators over minutes to hours. FcεRI, high-affinity IgE receptor; IL-4 and IL-13, interleukin-4 and interleukin-13; TNF-α, tumor necrosis factor-α. *(From Broide DH: Molecular and cellular mechanisms of allergic disease,* J Allergy Clin Immunol *108:S65-S71, 2001.)*

Figure 4-3 Allergy prick tests. **A,** The skin prick test is typically performed with a plastic lancet on either the forearm or upper back. **B,** The test leaves a barely visible mark and should be nearly painless. **C,** The test is interpreted after 15 to 20 minutes by measuring the maximal diameter of both the wheal and the flare.

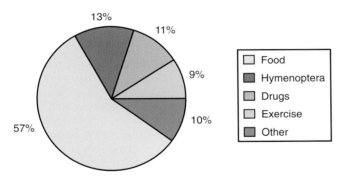

Figure 4-2 Type I hypersensitivity reactions. Note the characteristic physical findings of each affected organ system.

CAUSES OF ANAPHYLAXIS

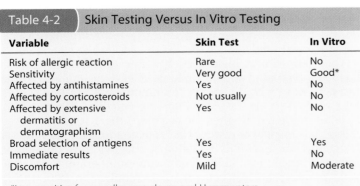

Food
Hymenoptera
Drugs
Exercise
Other

Figure 4-4 Relative frequency of causes of anaphylaxis in children. *(From Novembre E, Cianteroni A, Bernardini R, et al: Anaphylaxis in children: clinical and allergological features, Pediatrics 101:E8, 1998.)*

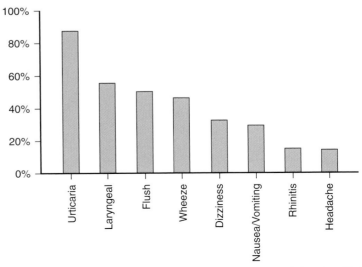

Figure 4-5 Relative frequency of symptoms associated with anaphylaxis. *(Modified from Lieberman P: Anaphylaxis: how to quickly narrow the differential diagnosis, J Respir Dis 20:221-232, 1999.)*

Table 4-2	Skin Testing Versus In Vitro Testing	
Variable	**Skin Test**	**In Vitro**
Risk of allergic reaction	Rare	No
Sensitivity	Very good	Good*
Affected by antihistamines	Yes	No
Affected by corticosteroids	Not usually	No
Affected by extensive dermatitis or dermatographism	Yes	No
Broad selection of antigens	Yes	Yes
Immediate results	Yes	No
Discomfort	Mild	Moderate

*Less sensitive for aeroallergens, drugs, and Hymenoptera.

Table 4-3	Criteria to Define Likely Anaphylactic Episodes

Anaphylaxis is highly likely when any *one* of the following three criteria are fulfilled:

1. Acute onset of an illness (minutes to several hours) with involvement of the skin, mucosal tissue, or both (e.g., generalized hives, pruritus or flushing, swollen lips/tongue/uvula), and at least one of the following:

   a. Respiratory compromise (e.g., dyspnea, wheeze/bronchospasm, stridor, reduced PEF, hypoxemia)

   b. Reduced BP or associated symptoms of end-organ dysfunction (e.g., hypotonia [collapse], syncope, incontinence)

2. Two or more of the following that occur rapidly after exposure to a likely allergen for that patient (minutes to several hours):

   a. Involvement of the skin/mucosal tissue (e.g., generalized hives, itch/flush, swollen lips/tongue/uvula)

   b. Respiratory compromise (e.g., dyspnea, wheeze/bronchospasm, stridor, reduced PEF, hypoxemia)

   c. Reduced BP or associated symptoms (e.g., hypotonia [collapse], syncope, incontinence)

   d. Persistent gastrointestinal symptoms (e.g., crampy abdominal pain, vomiting)

3. Reduced BP after exposure to known allergen for that patient (minutes to several hours):

   a. Infants and children: low systolic BP (age specific) or greater than 30% decrease in systolic BP*

   b. Adults: systolic BP less than 90 mm Hg or a greater than 30% decrease from that person's baseline

*Low systolic blood pressure for children is defined as less than 70 mm Hg from 1 month to 1 year, less than (70 mm Hg + [2 × age in yr]) from 1 to 10 years, and less than 90 mm Hg from 11 to 17 years.
BP, blood pressure; PEF, peak expiratory flow.

Figure 4-7   Anaphylaxis. The EpiPen requires three steps: (1) Remove the gray cap to activate the device; (2) press the black tip firmly against the lateral aspect of the thigh (do not touch the end of the EpiPen); and (3) hold the EpiPen in place for 10 seconds.

used within 30 to 60 minutes of the onset of anaphylaxis, and other medications should not delay prompt delivery of epinephrine, which is often lifesaving. In cases of hypotension, large-volume fluid resuscitation and intravenous epinephrine may be required. Any administration of epinephrine should be followed by a call to 911 and observation in an emergency department. Albuterol inhalation may be useful for lower airway symptoms, and steroids may prevent late-phase reactions. Antihistamines can be used for reactions confined to the skin and as an adjunct to epinephrine in more severe reactions.

Hymenoptera Sensitivity

Contrary to common opinion, life-threatening reactions to Hymenoptera are rare in childhood. The most common reactions are large local reactions or generalized urticaria. Large local reactions represent a late-phase IgE-mediated response to the sting. The swelling associated with large local reactions is contiguous with the sting, begins 12 to 24 hours after the sting, peaks in 2 to 3 days, lasts approximately 1 week, and should be treated with antihistamines and nonsteroidal anti-inflammatory drugs (NSAIDs). Patients with large local reactions have an excellent long-term prognosis, do not need allergy testing, and do not need to carry epinephrine.

Children 16 years of age or younger who have had generalized urticaria and no respiratory, cardiovascular, or GI symptoms after an insect sting also have a good long-term prognosis. The risk for systemic anaphylaxis from stinging insects in children with symptoms confined to the skin is equal to the risk in the general population. These children do not need allergy testing or desensitization with immunotherapy. At present, consensus among allergists suggests that children with a history of generalized urticaria from stinging insects carry epinephrine.

Children with a history of systemic anaphylaxis after a Hymenoptera sting should undergo allergy testing and, if the test is positive, should receive immunotherapy. Testing should take place 4 weeks or more after the reaction. When testing is done immediately after the reaction, there is an increased rate of false-negative test results. Allergen immunotherapy for Hymenoptera sensitivity is the most effective form of allergen immunotherapy available. Venom immunotherapy for wasps, yellow jackets, and hornets provides complete protection from

Figure 4-6   During anaphylaxis, intramuscular delivery of epinephrine in the lateral aspect of the thigh produces the highest serum levels of epinephrine. A, anterior deltoid; IM, intramuscular; SC, subcutaneous; T, thigh. *(From Simons FE: Epinephrine absorption in adults: intramuscular versus subcutaneous injection,* J Allergy Clin Immunol *108:871-873, 2001.)*

Figure 4-8 Hymenoptera sensitivity. The honeybee is golden brown with black markings. The honeybee has a barbed stinger and leaves the stinger and venom sac after it stings.

anaphylaxis, while on immunotherapy, in 95% to 100% of patients. Venom immunotherapy for honeybees is slightly less effective, providing complete protection to 80% of patients while on therapy. Most venom immunotherapy protocols require weekly injections for about 16 weeks and then every 1 to 3 months while on maintenance therapy. The duration of immunotherapy should be 3 to 5 years in most cases.

The Hymenoptera that have been associated with anaphylaxis come from three subfamilies: Apidae (honeybees); Vespidae (yellow jackets, wasps, and white- and yellow-faced hornets); and Formicidae (fire ants). In the United States, yellow jackets are the most common cause of Hymenoptera-induced anaphylaxis. Yellow jackets typically nest in the ground, are scavengers for food, and, consequently, are frequently encountered at picnics and around garbage cans. The yellow jacket is small with tight yellow and black bands. The honeybee is the least aggressive of the Hymenoptera family. Stings from honeybees occur most commonly in beekeepers and after accidental contact. The honeybee's stinger is barbed and is retained in the skin after stings (Fig. 4-8). If the stinger is visible, it should be quickly flicked away from the skin with a fingernail. The stinger and venom sac should not be removed by pinching between the thumb and forefinger as this process can express additional venom. Wasps and hornets are very territorial and will sting to protect their nests. The fire ant is an increasingly important cause of Hymenoptera-induced anaphylaxis. Fire ants are found in the southeastern United States, but their natural habitat appears to be expanding.

Food Allergy

Food allergy can be divided into two broad groups on the basis of the mechanism of disease: (1) type I (IgE-mediated) hypersensitivity and (2) other immunologically mediated reactions (Fig. 4-9). Other food reactions (e.g., lactose intolerance) do not have an immune basis and are referred to as *intolerant reactions.* Food allergic reactions are highly reproducible (i.e., occur with any exposure to a food), and often are triggered by ingestions of very small quantities. Anaphylaxis is the best described and understood type I hypersensitivity to food. Although contact reactions (erythema, pruritus, hives) are common if an individual touches her or his food allergen, the most severe allergic reactions occur with ingestion. Milk, egg, wheat, soy, and peanut account for more than 90% of food allergic reactions in children. The onset of type I hypersensitivity to milk and egg is almost always in the first year of life. Fortunately, these two foods rarely cause more than generalized urticaria and the sensitivity is eventually outgrown in the vast majority of patients, frequently by school age.

Most allergic reactions to foods occur with the first few ingestions of a food. In contrast to type I hypersensitivity to milk and egg, less than 25% of patients will outgrow their peanut or tree nut sensitivity. Peanuts and tree nuts cause the majority of life-threatening reactions to foods, and all patients with this hypersensitivity should carry epinephrine. In addition to peanut or tree nut allergy, other risk factors for life-threatening reactions from food-induced anaphylaxis include asthma, adolescence, and the delayed administration of epinephrine. A past history of mild reactions does not rule out the possibility of a future life-threatening episode of food-induced anaphylaxis. A substantial minority of patients with type I hypersensitivity to peanut will develop type I hypersensitivity to one or more tree nuts; and conversely, patients with hypersensitivity to a tree nut have an increased risk of developing peanut hypersensitivity. Nuts are also frequently processed together, increasing the risk of cross-contamination exposures with nuts. Many allergists therefore recommend avoiding all nuts if a patient is allergic to either peanuts or tree nuts, although recommendations are individualized and many tree nut–allergic children continue to ingest peanut butter as long as they are cautious with this and avoid peanut-containing foods that may contain tree nuts.

An increasingly common form of type I–mediated hypersensitivity to food is the oral allergy syndrome (also known as pollen food syndrome). Patients with oral allergy syndrome have underlying seasonal allergic rhinitis and develop pruritus and angioedema of the oropharynx when ingesting fresh fruits and vegetables. The reaction is due to cross-reactivity between heat-labile proteins in some fruits and vegetables and outdoor seasonal pollens. The reaction is often eliminated by heating the vegetable or fruit. The reaction does not typically extend beyond the oropharynx, and patients typically do not need to carry epinephrine, although in a minority of cases reactions can be systemic and may be severe, so taking a good history is essential before recommendations are made for avoidance and the need for epinephrine.

Type I hypersensitivity to foods can be an unrecognized trigger in up to one third of children with severe atopic dermatitis and is an uncommon trigger in children with mild atopic dermatitis. It has rarely been described in adults with atopic dermatitis. The evaluation of type I hypersensitivity to foods in children with atopic dermatitis should be reserved for patients whose disease cannot be managed with good skin care and intermittent use of low- to moderate-potency topical antiinflammatory medications. When food hypersensitivity plays a role in poorly controlled atopic dermatitis, six foods account for the vast majority of reactions: milk, egg, wheat, soy, peanut, and fish.

One of the challenges with diagnosing type I hypersensitivity to foods is the poor specificity of both the skin prick and in vitro tests. The "gold standard" for diagnosis of food allergy is a double-blind, placebo-controlled food challenge (DBPCFC). A distinction is drawn between patients who are "sensitized,"

SPECTRUM OF FOOD ALLERGY

IgE mediated ← → Non-IgE mediated

Anaphylaxis
Oral allergy syndrome

Food protein enteropathy
Milk protein enterocolitis
Lactose intolerance

Eosinophilic gastroenteritis
Atopic dermatitis

Figure 4-9 Reactions to foods can be broadly divided into two mechanistic groups: (1) type I (IgE-mediated) hypersensitivity; and (2) immune (non–IgE-mediated) reactions. Atopic dermatitis and eosinophilic gastroenteritis can be caused by either or both mechanisms.

based on skin or serum testing, and those who are clinically allergic, based on a history of reactions to ingestions. IgE-mediated reactions occur quickly and reproducibly with ingestion of the triggering food. Research using in vitro allergy tests has identified levels of specific IgE against certain foods that predict with 95% certainty a reaction during a DBPCFC. In vitro food-specific IgE levels are most useful clinically when used in association with a patient's ingestion history and (if indicated) skin test results; in a nationally representative survey study, approximately 17% of the overall population in the United States displayed serum sensitization to either cow's milk, egg, peanut, or shrimp, and this prevalence rate was even higher (28%) among children ages 1 to 5 years. Yet, on the basis of these serum levels in the same study, only approximately 2.5% of the U.S. population was predicted to be clinically allergic to one of these foods. The data concerning positive predictive levels depend on the age of the patient and are not available for all foods (Table 4-4). The in vitro allergy test may also be repeated over time to try to help with the identification of patients who may have outgrown their sensitivity. The sensitivity of both the skin prick and in vitro tests is excellent, but not 100%. If there is a strong clinical history of a type I reaction to a food, it may be necessary to perform an oral challenge in a medically supervised setting before food hypersensitivity can be fully ruled out.

Eosinophilic gastroenteritis is an especially difficult problem to evaluate because eosinophilic infiltration of the gut may be caused by either type I (IgE-mediated) hypersensitivity or other immune pathways. Patients with type I hypersensitivity causing eosinophilic gastroenteritis can be sensitive to either foods or inhaled allergens (pollens/molds) that are inadvertently swallowed. Because eosinophilic gastroenteritis can also be caused by non–IgE-mediated pathways, a negative skin prick or in vitro test does not eliminate the possibility that food allergy may be causing the disease; similarly, a positive skin test to a food does not definitely establish causation. Patch testing has been studied in patients with eosinophilic gastroenteritis to try to identify foods that are causing eosinophilic inflammation through a non–IgE-mediated pathway; at the present time, this method of testing with foods is nonstandardized and still felt to be experimental. Patients with eosinophilic inflammation of the upper GI tract tend to have problems with dysphagia, food impaction, abdominal pain, and vomiting. Patients with eosinophilic inflammation of the lower GI tract tend to have diarrhea, failure to thrive, and abdominal pain. Eosinophilic gastroenteritis appears to have an increasing incidence, and the long-term prognosis is not completely understood, although the disease often seems to follow a relapsing and remitting course.

The term *food allergy* also encompasses the food reactions elicited through non–IgE-mediated immune pathways. The classic example of a non–IgE-mediated hypersensitivity to food is seen in the milk protein enterocolitis of infancy (also known as food-induced eosinophilic proctocolitis or dietary protein proctitis). These children usually present in the first few months of life with bloody diarrhea that improves within days of removing milk proteins from the diet. Many of these children are breast-fed, and react to either cow's milk or another protein in the maternal diet. Milk protein enterocolitis is not IgE mediated, so neither allergy skin prick nor in vitro testing is helpful in the evaluation of this condition. Approximately half of children with milk protein enterocolitis will also experience symptoms with soy protein–based formulas. Almost all infants will outgrow milk protein enterocolitis by 1 to 2 years of age.

Food protein–induced enterocolitis syndrome (FPIES) is another non–IgE-mediated reaction with a more severe presentation. Infants typically present two or more hours after an ingestion of the triggering food, with profuse vomiting often to the point of dehydration, hypotension, and lethargy. Fecal leukocytes, a rise in the peripheral absolute neutrophil count, acidosis, and methemoglobinemia may also be seen, whereas skin findings are typically not present. Cow's milk and soy are the most common triggers of FPIES, although it has been described with a variety of other foods as well. Because the presentation is so different from IgE-mediated allergic reactions, it is often not recognized and infants frequently undergo multiple rule-out sepsis workups before a diagnosis is made.

Drug Reactions

Drug allergy reactions are immunologically mediated responses that result in the production of drug-specific antibodies, T cells, or both. Type I hypersensitivity to drugs can range from mild reactions involving only the skin (generalized urticaria and/or angioedema) to laryngeal edema, bronchospasm, hypotension, and cardiovascular collapse. The reactions are mediated by drug-specific IgE bound to mast cells and basophils. IgE is cross-linked by the drug, leading to mast cell and basophil activation and release of mediators that drive the clinical reaction. These reactions occur within minutes of exposure and require prior sensitization. IgE-mediated reactions occur early in the treatment course, usually after the first or second dose of a drug. A rash that develops after more than a few days of therapy is seldom due to IgE-mediated mechanisms.

Penicillin is the only drug that has been widely studied as a cause of type I hypersensitivity, and consequently, it is the only drug for which well-standardized allergy testing is available. Once penicillin enters the body, it undergoes spontaneous conversion to a reactive intermediate that then binds to nearby proteins, forming penicilloyl amides. Penicilloyl amides account for 95% of tissue-bound penicillin and are known as the major antigenic determinant. A small percentage of penicillin can be found in the body as the native drug, penicillin, or other metabolites called minor antigenic determinants (penicilloate and penilloate). Skin testing done with the major antigenic determinant, penicillin, and the minor determinants

Table 4-4	Food-Specific IgE Concentrations Predictive of Clinical Reactivity				
Allergen	**Decision Point (kU/L)**	**Sensitivity (%)**	**Specificity (%)**	**Positive Predictive Value (%)**	**Negative Predictive Value (%)**
Egg	7	61	95	98	38
Infants, ≤2 yr*	2			95	
Milk	15	57	94	95	53
Infants, ≤2 yr†	5			95	
Peanut	14	57	100	100	36
Fish	20	25	100	100	89
Soybean	30	44	94	73	82
Wheat	26	61	92	74	87
Tree nuts	~15	—	—	≈95	—

*Boyano-Martinez T, Garcia-Ara C, Diaz-Pena GM, et al: Validity of specific IgE in children with egg allergy, *Clin Exp Allergy* 31:1464-1469, 2001.
†Garcia-Ara C, Boyano-Martinez T, Diaz-Pena GM, et al: Specific IgE levels in the diagnosis of immediate hypersensitivity to cow's milk protein in infants, *J Allergy Clin Immunol* 107:185-190, 2001.
Modified from Sampson HA: Utility of food-specific IgE concentrations in predicting symptomatic food allergy, *J Allergy Clin Immunol* 107:891-896, 2001.

has a negative predictive value approaching 100%. At present, in the United States only the major determinant and the drug itself, penicillin G, are available for skin testing. Although some studies have shown that the minor determinants alone account for up to 10% to 20% of positive skin tests, a negative test to the penicilloyl amides and penicillin G has excellent negative predictive value.

The use of cephalosporins in patients with a history of penicillin allergy is controversial. Before 1980, between 10% and 20% of penicillin-allergic patients reacted to cephalosporins; but since 1980, that number has dropped to 2%. Much of the concern about cross-reactivity between these two classes of drugs is based on the presence of their common molecular structure, known as a β-lactam ring. When cephalosporins were first introduced there was occasional contamination with trace amounts of penicillin. Although clinical cross-reactivity between these two drugs has lessened over the years, there are clear reports of anaphylactic reactions after the use of cephalosporins in penicillin-allergic patients. The combination of all these factors has contributed to the persistent concern about the safety of cephalosporins in patients with penicillin allergy. Unfortunately, skin testing for cephalosporins has not been standardized and the negative predictive value of these tests is not known. There is no consensus regarding the use of cephalosporins in patients with penicillin allergy. In patients with a remote clinical history and mild reactions, it may be reasonable to treat with second- or third-generation cephalosporins without either testing or challenge dosing. Patients who have had either severe or recent reactions should be treated the most cautiously. One option is to test for penicillin, and if the test is negative then the history is not confirmed and precautions with cephalosporins are not necessary. If testing cannot be performed then the options are as follows: (1) find an alternative drug; (2) challenge dose with cephalosporin; or (3) treat by using an induction-of-tolerance protocol.

Anaphylaxis from drugs other than penicillin must be diagnosed on the basis of clinical presentation. Patients with type I hypersensitivity to drugs can still receive the drug with the induction of drug tolerance, also called *drug desensitization*. Inducing drug tolerance involves slow delivery of increasing drug doses over a period of 6 to 12 hours. The mechanism by which tolerance is induced is not well understood. Patients remain tolerant of the drug as long as they are receiving the medication, but once the drug is discontinued future treatment requires repeating the protocol to induce tolerance.

A variety of drugs can cause anaphylactoid (also called *pseudoallergic*) reactions. Anaphylactoid reactions are due to generalized mast cell mediator release not caused by cross-linking of specific IgE on mast cell surfaces. The exact mechanism of anaphylactoid reactions is not known, and no diagnostic testing is available. The two most common drug-induced causes of anaphylactoid reactions are radiocontrast media and nonsteroidal antiinflammatory drugs.

Drugs can also induce type II, III, and IV Gell and Coombs reactions. The classic Gell and Coombs type II reaction is due to IgG antibodies directed against drug bound to cell surfaces, causing either hemolytic anemia or thrombocytopenia. Serum sickness represents a Gell and Coombs type III reaction. Serum sickness usually begins 1 to 3 weeks after drug exposure and involves various symptoms including fever, malaise, arthralgias, arthritis, urticaria, and lymphadenopathy. Many patients with serum sickness will develop a characteristic serpiginous, erythematous, or purpuric eruption at the junction of the palmar or plantar and dorsolateral aspects of the hands and feet, respectively (Fig. 4-10). Patients with serum sickness may have reduced levels of complement components C3 and C4 along with the presence of circulating immune complexes. Serum sickness can be treated with antihistamines, and if the patient fails to improve systemic steroids can be used. Symptoms usually resolve within a few weeks. Future avoidance of the drug inciting the reaction is recommended.

Erythema multiforme minor (EM) and Stevens-Johnson syndrome (SJS) are drug reactions that do not conform to the Gell and Coombs classification scheme. EM can be caused by drugs or infection or be idiopathic. EM lesions typically begin as dusky, red macules or erythematous papules that evolve into target lesions after 24 to 48 hours (see Chapter 8). The diagnosis is made on the basis of the clinical appearance and the absence of significant mucosal involvement. The symptoms can persist for a few weeks, and if discomfort is significant, either antihistamines or steroids can be used. Patients with EM do not experience long-term sequelae from their disease. Patients with Stevens-Johnson syndrome (SJS) have skin symptoms similar to those of EM, but also manifest significant mucosal involvement as well as elevated temperature, and constitutional symptoms. Severe disease with extensive skin and mucous membrane involvement may produce long-term complications. Skin findings with SJS evolve from targetoid lesions to vesicles and bullae followed by sloughing of the skin. SJS and toxic epidermal necrolysis (TEN) are most likely manifestations of a single disease that exists along a

Figure 4-10   Cutaneous eruptions on the sides of the hands and feet of patients with serum sickness. **A,** A scalloped band of erythema can be seen on the side of the finger at the margin of the palmar skin. **B,** A band of purpura is seen at the margin of the plantar skin. The purpura was preceded by a band of erythema. *(From Lawley TJ, Bielory L, Gascon P, et al: Prospective clinical and immunological analysis of patients with serum sickness, N Engl J Med 311:1407-1413, 1984. Copyright © 1984 Massachusetts Medical Society. All rights reserved.)*

clinical spectrum. Patients with SJS have less than 10% of the body affected by epidermal detachment and those with TEN have more than 30% of the body affected. TEN is almost always drug induced whereas SJS may be induced by either drugs or infection with *Mycoplasma* or herpes simplex virus. When drug exposure is the inciting cause, the exposure precedes the onset of skin findings by 1 to 3 weeks. There is no universally accepted therapy, with some studies showing a benefit from high-dose intravenous immunoglobulin and other studies showing no benefit. Glucocorticoids are relatively contraindicated in this condition in children because some studies have shown a deleterious effect.

Another drug reaction that does not easily conform to a Gell and Coombs category is the syndrome known as DRESS (drug rash with eosinophilia and systemic symptoms). The mechanism of this clinical syndrome is unknown. DRESS was initially described with anticonvulsant therapies but is now known to be caused by a number of different drugs. DRESS reactions usually begin 2 to 6 weeks into drug therapy. Clinical characteristics involve a generalized rash, fever, eosinophilia (found in only 50% of cases), and multiorgan dysfunction. The liver is the most commonly involved organ, but any internal organ can be involved. Treatment involves discontinuation of the inciting drug and supportive therapy. The use of systemic glucocorticoids has not been well studied but is believed to be effective for this condition.

Allergic Rhinitis

Allergic rhinitis, characterized by inflammation, edema, and weeping of the nasal mucosa, is the most common allergic disorder and occurs in up to 25% of the population. Diagnosis is based on characteristic history, physical findings, and testing for antigen-specific IgE. Common presenting symptoms include nasal congestion and pruritus, clear rhinorrhea, and paroxysms of sneezing. Whereas older children may blow their noses frequently, younger children do not. Instead, they sniff, snort, and repetitively clear their throats. Nasal pruritus stimulates grimacing and twitching (Fig. 4-11) and picking or rubbing of the nose ("allergic salute"). Picking, repetitive sneezing, and blowing along with underlying inflammation may produce enough irritation to cause epistaxis. In the case of allergy to seasonal pollens, the symptoms may be acute, have a sudden onset, and be confined to the period during which the particular airborne pollen is detectable. Seasonal allergic rhinitis tends to be due to trees in the spring, grasses in the summer, and ragweed or other pollens in the fall.

Interestingly, seasonal allergic rhinitis is often called "hay fever," although hay is not involved and fever is not a symptom. However, the manifestations can be severe enough to induce flulike symptoms of fatigue and malaise. In contrast, symptoms may be chronic and more indolent in the case of allergy to perennial allergens including molds, house dust mites, and animal dander.

Many patients have prominent itching and watering of the eyes with nasal symptoms, and some experience pruritus of the throat or ears. Associated symptoms include (1) disturbed sleep and snoring; (2) morning dryness and irritation of the throat as a result of mouth breathing; (3) lassitude, fatigue, and irritability from sleep interruption; (4) early nighttime cough; and (5) if the maxillary, frontal, and ethmoidal sinuses are affected, a sensation of pressure over the cheeks, forehead, and bridge of the nose. The extent to which allergic rhinitis affects a patient's quality of life is often underappreciated.

Many children with long-standing allergic rhinitis can be recognized by their facial characteristics. Ocular manifestations of the allergic disposition include cobblestoning of the conjunctivae (see Fig. 4-33), the allergic shiner, and Dennie's sign. Allergic shiners, that is, bluish discolorations or dark circles beneath the eyes, are commonly observed in patients with allergic rhinitis (Fig. 4-12). This finding represents chronic venous congestion secondary to inflammation. *Dennie's sign* refers to prominent folds or creases on the lower eyelid (Fig. 4-13) running parallel to the lower lid margin. Although these lines were originally thought to indicate a predisposition to allergy, data suggest that they may be present in any condition associated with periocular pruritus and scratching or chronic nasal congestion. Frequent upward rubbing of the nose with the palm of the hand (the allergic salute; Fig. 4-14) promotes development of a transverse nasal crease across the lower third of the nose (Fig. 4-15). Chronic obstruction produced by nasal mucosal edema may result in mouth breathing and a typical open-mouthed, adenoid-type facies (Fig. 4-16).

On nasal examination, attention should be focused on the position of the nasal septum; nasal patency; mucosal appearance; and presence and character of secretions, polyps, or foreign bodies (see Chapter 23). The typical physical examination findings in allergic rhinitis include a marked decrease in nasal patency resulting from swollen inferior turbinates, which appear pale, edematous, and bluish gray (Fig. 4-17). The

Figure 4-11   Facial grimacing and twitching caused by nasal itching in a patient with allergic rhinitis. These are frequently repeated and easily noted during patient evaluation.

Figure 4-12   Allergic shiners, or dark circles beneath the eyes, in a patient with allergic rhinitis.

Figure 4-13   Dennie sign. Lines originate in the inner canthus and traverse one half to two thirds the length of the lower lid margin in an arc nearly parallel to it.

Figure 4-15   Allergic rhinitis. The nasal crease across the lower third of the nose results from chronic upward rubbing of the nose with the hand (allergic salute). *(Courtesy Meyer B. Marks, MD, Miami, Fla.)*

mucosa appears edematous, and secretions are clear and watery to mucoid in character.

Depending on the specific allergens, allergic rhinitis may be acute, recurrent, or chronic and must be distinguished from a number of nonallergic conditions. This necessitates a thorough medical and family history and careful examination. In some instances, response to a trial of medication and/or observations over time may be necessary to confirm the diagnosis. When symptoms are seasonal or regularly associated with exposure to specific allergens, the distinction is generally clear. In evaluating patients with perennial or recurrent but nonseasonal symptoms, allergy, recurrent infection, the nonallergic rhinitis with eosinophilia syndrome (NARES), and vasomotor rhinitis must be considered.

Children with frequent upper respiratory infections and/or persistent nasal congestion can present a diagnostic challenge.

In some cases the phenomenon is due to recurrent viral infections, particularly in children in their first year of day care or nursery school. In other patients, tonsillar and adenoidal hypertrophy provides favorable conditions for recurrent infections (see Chapter 23). Atopic (allergic) children may have increased risk of infection because of impaired flow of secretions due to mucosal edema. Although viral infections tend to produce clear or white discharge in contrast to bacterial infections, which typically produce a purulent yellow or green discharge, there is considerable overlap, limiting the value of this distinction.

Other forms of rhinitis that must be distinguished from allergic rhinitis are enumerated in Table 4-5. Although characterized by eosinophilia, NARES does not produce nasal pruritus, and patients lack specific IgE antibodies as measured by skin testing or in vitro serum testing. Patients with

Figure 4-14   Allergic rhinitis. The allergic salute is characteristic of children with allergic rhinitis and nasal itching and is usually noticed by parents.

Figure 4-16   Nasal obstruction. Characteristic adenoid-type facies in a patient with long-standing allergic rhinitis. Note the open mouth and gaping habitus.

Figure 4-17 Pale, edematous inferior nasal turbinate of a patient with allergic rhinitis, as seen through a fiberoptic rhinoscope. Even though this tool is not routinely used in evaluations, the physical findings are well illustrated, including watery nasal secretions.

vasomotor rhinitis do not complain of pruritus, have a clear discharge without eosinophils, and also lack specific IgE antibodies. Vasomotor rhinitis is thus considered a form of noninflammatory rhinitis, the etiology of which is unknown, although it is often triggered by nonspecific stimuli such as cold air exposure or smoke. The condition is diagnosed most frequently in adults but may affect children. Congestion or rhinorrhea may predominate in this disorder. Rhinitis medicamentosa is a condition seen in patients who have been using α-adrenergic vasoconstrictor nose drops (phenylephrine or

oxymetazoline) as decongestants for prolonged treatment periods. The disorder is characterized by rebound vasodilation that produces an erythematous, edematous mucosa in association with a profuse clear nasal discharge.

Some children with perennial allergic rhinitis have congestion so constant and severe that it produces signs of chronic nasal obstruction. This must be distinguished from other acquired and congenital causes (see Chapter 23). The history, physical findings, and results of allergy tests for specific IgE and nasal smears, along with therapeutic trials of antihistamines and intranasal corticosteroids, will all help lead to a diagnosis.

Many patients with allergic rhinitis have mild symptoms that are adequately controlled by intermittent antihistamine administration and/or environmental controls. In many of these patients the pattern of symptoms suggests the responsible allergens, and testing for specific IgE is not indicated. Those with severe symptoms only partially alleviated by antihistamines, topical antiinflammatory agents, and environmental controls and those with perennial symptoms who require daily therapy should be referred for specific IgE testing. Desensitization (allergy shots) is an effective treatment for patients who are not well controlled with medications or who prefer not to use them regularly.

Respiratory Disease

Respiratory Distress

Respiratory distress in children (tachypnea with or without grunting, flaring, retractions, and cyanosis) should be promptly evaluated and treated. The first step in approaching respiratory distress is to differentiate upper from lower airway disorders. At times, various degrees of upper and lower airway obstruction may coexist, as in laryngotracheobronchitis.

Upper airway obstruction causes difficulty moving air into the chest, whereas lower airway obstruction causes difficulty moving air out of the chest. This difference results in characteristic physical findings. In general, lower airway obstruction produces prolongation of the expiratory phase of respiration and typical expiratory wheezing, whereas upper airway obstruction prolongs the inspiratory phase. *Wheezing* is defined as musical or whistling auscultatory sounds heard more often on expiration than on inspiration, although in severe obstruction both inspiratory and expiratory wheezing are often present. Inspiratory stridor, seen with upper airway obstruction, can mimic wheezing. Both can be detected concomitantly. *Stridor* is defined as a crowing sound usually heard during the inspiratory phase of respiration. It tends to be loud when the obstruction is subglottic and quiet when obstruction is supraglottic. Mild to moderate increases in respiratory and heart rates are common in upper airway obstruction, whereas lower airway disorders such as pneumonitis and asthma often lead to markedly increased respiratory and heart rates. Retractions are often generalized (suprasternal, intracostal, and subcostal) in severe airway obstruction of any etiology.

Asthma

Asthma is the most common chronic respiratory condition affecting children. Defining characteristics of asthma, as elucidated by the National Heart, Lung, and Blood Institute (NHLBI) *Guidelines for the Diagnosis and Management of Asthma* (see Bibliography), include the following: (1) lower airway obstruction that is partially or fully reversible either spontaneously or with bronchodilator or antiinflammatory treatments, (2) the presence of lower airway inflammation, and (3) increased lower airway responsiveness (bronchial

Table 4-5	Comparison of Allergic and Nonallergic Rhinitis		
		NONALLERGIC	
	Allergic	**NARES**	**Vasomotor**
Usual onset	Childhood	Childhood	Adulthood
Family history of allergy	Usual	Coincidental	Coincidental
Collateral allergy symptoms	Common	Unusual	Unusual
Sneezing	Frequent	Occasional	Occasional
Itching	Common	Unusual	Unusual
Rhinorrhea	Profuse	Profuse	Profuse
Congestion	Moderate to marked	Moderate to marked	Moderate to marked
Physical examination			
Edema	Moderate to marked	Moderate	Moderate
Secretions	Watery	Watery	Mucoid to watery
Nasal eosinophilia	Common	Common	Occasional
Allergic evaluation			
Skin tests	Positive	Coincidental	Coincidental
IgE antibodies	Positive	Coincidental	Coincidental
Therapeutic response			
Antihistamines	Fair to good	Fair	Poor to fair
Decongestants	Fair	Fair	Poor to fair
Corticosteroids	Good	Good	Poor
Cromolyn	Fair	Unknown	Poor
Immunotherapy	Good	None	None

NARES, nonallergic rhinitis with eosinophilia syndrome.
Modified from Fagin J, Friedman R, Fireman P: Allergic rhinitis, *Pediatr Clin North Am* 28:797-806, 1981.

hyperreactivity). The last is characterized by inherent hyperreactivity of the airways to stimuli including allergens, infection, exercise, chemical agents such as methacholine, cold or dry air, emotions, and weather changes. Many cases of asthma, particularly in children, have an atopic basis. Specific allergens implicated in atopic patients are pollen, mold spores, house dust mites, and animal dander, whereas drugs, food, and insect venoms typically cause similar symptoms of wheezing and respiratory distress as part of anaphylaxis (see earlier discussion). On exposure, these allergens, via cross-linking specific IgE, produce the characteristic features of asthma: mucosal edema, increased mucus production, and smooth muscle contraction that result in airway inflammation, airway hyperreactivity, and bronchoconstriction. These responses combine to produce a state of reversible obstruction of the large and small airways that is the hallmark of asthma.

Patients with asthma should be evaluated to determine the important triggers for their disease. Affected individuals are often aware of the specific stimuli that trigger exacerbations of their asthma. Viruses are the most common precipitants of acute asthma in children, especially rhinoviruses, respiratory syncytial virus, and parainfluenza viruses. These infections usually affect the upper and lower airways, producing rhinorrhea, nasal congestion, and often fever in addition to wheezing, which tends to develop insidiously. In contrast, allergen-triggered episodes typically lack fever and have a more abrupt onset of wheezing.

Asthma is one of the leading causes of pediatric morbidity. Indeed, approximately 10% to 12% of children in the United States show signs and symptoms compatible with asthma at some time during childhood. Peak incidence of onset is before the age of 5 years (Fig. 4-18). In childhood, boys are affected more often than girls and tend to have more severe disease. Beyond puberty, the gender distribution is equal because onset in the teenage years is more common in girls, perhaps due to hormonal factors involved in menarche. Asthmatic children with respiratory allergy and eczema usually have more severe courses than those who wheeze only with upper respiratory infections.

An unexplained, worldwide increase in asthma-related morbidity and mortality rates has been noted, although these rates have apparently stabilized during the previous decade (Fig. 4-19). Indeed, deaths resulting from asthma exceed 3000 per year in the United States, although these occur mostly in adults.

Emergency department visits, hospitalizations, and intensive care unit admissions for asthma usually peak in the late

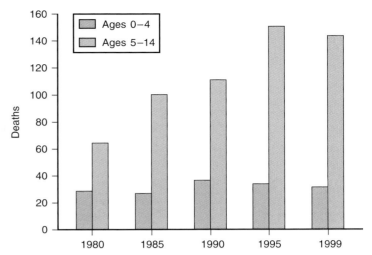

Figure 4-19 Number of pediatric asthma deaths in the United States from 1980 to 1999. *(Modified from Mannino DM, Homa DM, Akinbami LJ, et al: Surveillance for asthma—United States, 1980-1999, MMWR Surveill Summ 51:1-13, 2002.)*

autumn or early winter months and, to a lesser extent, in the spring (Fig. 4-20). These seasonal patterns may be related to environmental temperature and humidity changes, allergen exposure, or respiratory infections.

The diagnosis of asthma is frequently based on historical findings alone, indicating the importance of taking a thorough history. Updated NHLBI and American Academy of Pediatrics guidelines have stressed the importance of complementing good history taking with objective measurements of lung function. This can include in-office pulmonary function testing in children 5 years of age and older, but it is important to understand that normal results at a time when the patient is asymptomatic do not exclude asthma. Peak flow monitoring is not recommended for use in diagnosis, but can sometimes be used for monitoring. The greatest shortcomings of peak flow monitoring are that it is effort dependent, requires compliance, and does not measure small-airway function. In addition, there is a wide variability in types of peak flow meters, along with different reference ranges. When peak flow monitoring is used, patients should be given a written plan with instructions on what to do as their peak flow falls along with increase in symptoms.

As with many common diseases, asthma incidence is influenced by both genes and environment (Fig. 4-21). Family

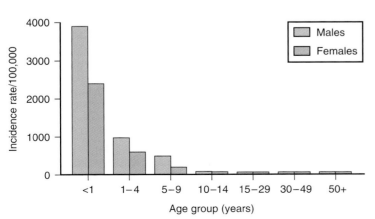

Figure 4-18 Incidence of asthma by age and gender in Rochester, Minnesota, from 1964 to 1983. Eighty percent of asthma has its onset by 5 years of age. *(Modified from Yunginger JW, Reed CE, O'Connell EJ, et al: A community-based study of the epidemiology of asthma: Incidence rates, 1964-1983, Am Rev Respir Dis 146:888-894, 1992.)*

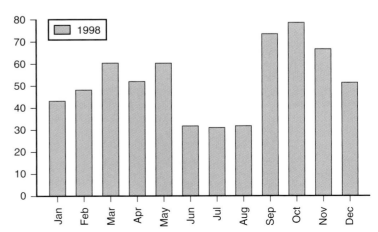

Figure 4-20 Number of asthma admissions (1998) to Children's Hospital of Pittsburgh by month of year. There is a biphasic peak in spring and fall. *(Courtesy Eliseo Villalobos, MD, and Gilbert Friday, MD, Children's Hospital of Pittsburgh, Pittsburgh, Pa.)*

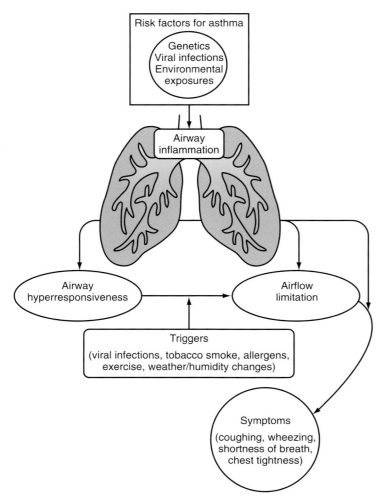

Figure 4-21   An interaction between genetic and environmental factors is involved in the pathogenesis of asthma. *(Reprinted with permission from Rachelefsky GS, Shapiro GG, Bergman D, et al, Pediatric Asthma Committee:* Pediatric asthma: promoting best practice guide for managing asthma in children, *Milwaukee, Wis, 1999, American Academy of Allergy, Asthma, & Immunology.)*

Table 4-6	When Is It Asthma?*

History of recurrent:
- Coughing
- Wheezing
- Shortness of breath or rapid breathing
- Chest tightness

Symptoms made worse by:
- Viral infection
- Tobacco smoke, wood smoke, and other irritants (e.g., strong odors or fumes)
- Exercise
- Allergens (e.g., house dust mites, pollens, cockroaches, molds, animal dander)
- Changes in weather/humidity
- Crying, laughing

Symptoms occur/worsen at night, waking the child and/or parent
Reversible airflow limitation by spirometry in children older than 4 yr of age and diurnal variation in peak flow
- Wheezing (high-pitched whistling sounds when exhaling) may or may not be present

*No single indicator is diagnostic in itself, but the presence of several increases the probability of asthma. *Objective measures are essential to establish the diagnosis of asthma.* For children younger than 4 years of age or who cannot conduct spirometry, clinical judgment and/or response to asthma treatment may be the only reliable means for diagnosing asthma.

Reprinted with permission from Rachelefsky GS, Shapiro GG, Bergman D, et al, Pediatric Asthma Committee: *Pediatric asthma: promoting best practice guide for managing asthma in children,* Milwaukee, Wis, 1999, American Academy of Allergy, Asthma, & Immunology.

history often reveals affected siblings, parents, or other relatives. An environmental survey can determine possible provocative factors, especially allergens, infections, occupational exposures, smoking, exercise, stress, climate, and medication use (NSAIDs, β-blockers). The history should emphasize the frequency, duration, and intensity of suspected episodes (Table 4-6). A description of symptoms between acute episodes aids in the determination of chronicity (night cough, exercise intolerance, fatigue, school absenteeism, social function). Individuals with asthma commonly present with recurrent episodes of wheezing that, depending on the severity, may require emergency treatment. Episodes may be infrequent and/or seasonal or may occur daily. The spectrum of presenting complaints, however, is broad, and affected individuals may complain only of mild, occasional wheezing or shortness of breath with exercise and/or colds or a persistent dry, hacking cough (particularly at night or in the morning). Breathlessness and chest tightness are also symptoms commonly reported. The frequency and severity of acute asthma episodes and the level of symptoms between episodes can be used to grade asthma severity and to guide therapy on the basis of published guidelines (Table 4-7).

The early stages of an asthma exacerbation in children are characterized by the onset of cough, chest tightness, and chest retractions or audible wheezing. The parents should be educated to critically and accurately observe their child for the warning signs and, in collaboration with the managing

physician, identify the onset of asthmatic exacerbation at home. A written asthma action plan that details use of rescue medicines such as albuterol can minimize emergency department visits for asthma.

Asthma should be considered part of the differential diagnosis in any child with recurrent or chronic lower respiratory symptoms or signs. Even though a high index of suspicion must be maintained, excessive or erroneous diagnoses may result if they are made hastily without appropriate supportive evidence; normal children or those with potentially more severe disorders may be mistakenly diagnosed with asthma and inappropriately treated. Parents must be instructed that physician assessment is essential during suspected episodes of asthma so that wheezing or other signs of lower airway obstruction and reversibility may be documented. If the diagnosis is unclear on clinical grounds, then specific laboratory studies must be performed to document asthma and rule out disorders that mimic asthma (Table 4-8). Pulmonary function tests in asthmatic children older than 5 years of age may show airway obstruction at baseline or after appropriate challenge with methacholine, exercise, or cold air and document reversibility after administration of an aerosolized bronchodilator (Fig. 4-22). For children younger than 5 years of age or for those in whom testing is unreliable, the diagnosis must be made on the basis of historical and physical findings and clinical response to bronchodilator or antiinflammatory medication. Lack of an immediate response to a bronchodilator does not eliminate asthma as a diagnostic consideration, however. In the instance of poor response to prescribed medications, appropriate inhaler technique should be addressed, as well as the importance of using a spacer device with any metered dose inhaler to ensure adequate medication delivery to the distal airways.

A thorough physical examination provides valuable information regarding the diagnosis of asthma and its severity and chronicity. The physical findings in asthma vary with the chronicity and state of activity of the disease process at the

Conjunctivitis, angioedema

Rhinitis

Anaphylactic laryngeal edema (upper airway obstruction, stridor)

Shock

Asthma (lower airway obstruction, wheezing)

Gastrointestinal edema (vomiting)

Urticaria

Intestinal edema (diarrhea)

Angioedema

Figure 4-2 Type I hypersensitivity reactions. Note the characteristic physical findings of each affected organ system.

CAUSES OF ANAPHYLAXIS

13%

11%

9%

10%

57%

- Food
- Hymenoptera
- Drugs
- Exercise
- Other

Figure 4-4 Relative frequency of causes of anaphylaxis in children. *(From Novembre E, Cianteroni A, Bernardini R, et al: Anaphylaxis in children: clinical and allergological features,* Pediatrics 101:E8, 1998.)

Figure 4-3 Allergy prick tests. **A,** The skin prick test is typically performed with a plastic lancet on either the forearm or upper back. **B,** The test leaves a barely visible mark and should be nearly painless. **C,** The test is interpreted after 15 to 20 minutes by measuring the maximal diameter of both the wheal and the flare.

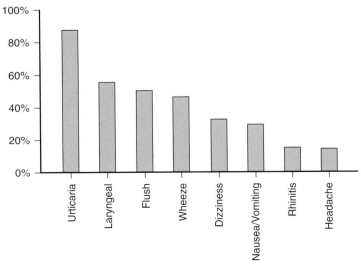

Figure 4-5 Relative frequency of symptoms associated with anaphylaxis. *(Modified from Lieberman P: Anaphylaxis: how to quickly narrow the differential diagnosis,* J Respir Dis 20:221-232, 1999.)

Table 4-2	Skin Testing Versus In Vitro Testing	
Variable	**Skin Test**	**In Vitro**
Risk of allergic reaction	Rare	No
Sensitivity	Very good	Good*
Affected by antihistamines	Yes	No
Affected by corticosteroids	Not usually	No
Affected by extensive dermatitis or dermatographism	Yes	No
Broad selection of antigens	Yes	Yes
Immediate results	Yes	No
Discomfort	Mild	Moderate

*Less sensitive for aeroallergens, drugs, and Hymenoptera.

Table 4-7	Guidelines for Defining Asthma Severity: Clinical Features before Treatment			
Asthma Severity Classification	**Symptom Severity**	**Nighttime Symptoms**	**Lung Function in Patients Who Can Use a Spirometer or Peak Flowmeter**	**Short-acting β₂-Agonist Use**
Severe persistent	• Continual symptoms • Limited physical activity • Frequent exacerbations interfere with normal activities	Frequent	• FEV₁ or PEFR ≤60% predicted • PEFR variability >30%	Used four times a day; does *not* completely relieve symptoms
Moderate persistent	• Daily symptoms • Exacerbations ≥2 times/wk; may last days; may affect activities	>1 time/wk	• FEV₁ or PEFR >60% to <80% predicted • PEFR variability >30%	Daily
Mild persistent	• Symptoms >2 times/wk but <1 time/d • Exacerbations may affect activities	>2 times/mo	• FEV₁ or PEFR >80% predicted • PEFR variability 20%-30%	>2 times/wk but <1 time/d
Mild intermittent	• Symptoms ≤2 times/wk • Asymptomatic and normal PEFR between exacerbations • Exacerbations brief (from a few hours to a few days); intensity may vary	≤2 times/mo	• FEV₁ or PEFR >80% predicted • PEFR variability <20%	≤2 times/wk

FEV₁, forced expiratory volume in 1 second; PEFR, peak expiratory flow rate.
Reprinted with permission from Rachelefsky GS, Shapiro GG, Bergman D, et al, Pediatric Asthma Committee: *Pediatric asthma: promoting best practice guide for managing asthma in children,* Milwaukee, Wis, 1999, American Academy of Allergy, Asthma, & Immunology.

time of examination. The findings of acute asthma are markedly different from those of chronic and latent or quiescent asthma. Between episodes, the examination is usually entirely normal. Prolongation of the expiratory phase is often noted. Clubbing as a sign of chronic asthma is rare and, if present in a wheezing child, suggests another chronic pulmonary disease.

During acute asthma, the following historical features should be noted: time of onset, possible triggers, present medications, comparison with previous episodes, and presence of complicating factors (e.g., vomiting, fever, chest pain). Examination should document accessory muscle use, retractions, and color. Auscultation should be done to assess air exchange, wheezing, and inspiratory-to-expiratory ratio. The ability to speak (words, phrases, or complete sentences) is a useful measure of dyspnea. Lethargy, decreased air exchange, and increased work of breathing are the most worrisome signs indicating acute deterioration.

In addition, rales are often heard, and pulse, respiratory rate, and blood pressure are frequently elevated. Pulsus paradoxus, an exaggerated decrease in systolic blood pressure during inspiration (Table 4-9), correlates highly with the degree of airway obstruction, although it is rarely measured clinically. This phenomenon may result from physical forces on the pericardium that impede venous return and reduce cardiac output during forced inspiration. Normally, the inspiratory decrease in systolic blood pressure is less than 10 mm Hg and is not discernible during routine sphygmomanometry. In acute asthma, it is usually greater than 10 mm Hg (up to 30 and 40 mm Hg) and is easily detectable.

Individuals with asthma may be distinguished by their characteristic symptoms and signs during acute episodes, which typically change as the degree of airway obstruction increases. Symptoms secondary to a viral illness usually consist of progressively increasing shortness of breath and

Table 4-8	Additional Tests That May Be Needed to Confirm the Diagnosis of Asthma in Children
Reason for Additional Tests	**Suggested Test(s)**
Child has symptoms (coughing, wheezing, breathlessness, chest tightness), but spirometry is (near) normal	• Bronchoprovocation with histamine, methacholine, or exercise (if negative, may rule out asthma)
Suspect other factors are contributing to severity of asthma symptoms	• Nasal examination • Allergy tests, gastroesophageal reflux tests, sinus radiology*
Symptoms suggest infection, large-airway lesions, heart disease, or obstruction by foreign object	• Routine chest x-ray, high-resolution CT scan*
Suspect coexisting chronic obstructive pulmonary disease or restrictive defect	• Additional pulmonary function tests; diffusing capacity test*

*Referral to a specialist is recommended for consultation or comanagement.
CT, computed tomography.
Reprinted with permission from Rachelefsky GS, Shapiro GG, Bergman D, et al, Pediatric Asthma Committee: *Pediatric asthma: promoting best practice guide for managing asthma in children,* Milwaukee, Wis, 1999, American Academy of Allergy, Asthma, & Immunology.

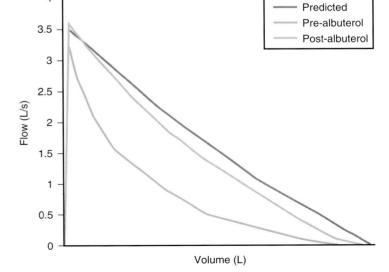

Figure 4-22 Asthma. Flow–volume loop showing predicted values, initial values, and substantial reversibility after albuterol administration. Note the downward scooping of curves, which is typical in patients with asthma with ongoing obstruction.

Table 4-9	Measurement of Pulsus Paradoxus

	BLOOD PRESSURE IN RELATION TO TIME AND RESPIRATORY PHASE (MM HG)				
	Expiration	**Inspiration**	**Expiration**	**Inspiration**	**Expiration**
Normal (no airway obstruction)	125/70	120/70	125/70	120/70	125/70
Asthma (airway obstruction)	125/70	100/70	125/70	100/70	125/70

Method
1. Pump sphygmomanometer cuff to occlude the peripheral pulse.
2. As the cuff pressure falls, listen carefully for the onset of the first Korotkoff sound.
3. Note the pressure at which the first Korotkoff sound is detected. This should be heard only during expiration. (In the above example, 125 mm Hg = normal and asthma.)
4. Continue to slowly decrease the cuff pressure until the first sound is detected during inspiration and expiration. Note this pressure. (In the above example, 120 mm Hg = normal; 100 mm Hg = asthma.)
5. When the difference between the two pressures is greater than or equal to 10, pulsus paradoxus is present.

difficulty breathing with or without rhinorrhea, low-grade fever, and vomiting. On examination, expiratory wheezing or a prolonged expiratory phase may be the only manifestation of mild asthma. However, as the obstructive process progresses, the expiratory phase becomes longer and the wheezing becomes louder and occurs on both inspiration and expiration. Eventually, airways collapse and signs of hyperinflation develop (low diaphragms, decreased lateral excursions of the chest wall with breathing, and hyperresonance to percussion). Visible sternocleidomastoid contractions; increased anteroposterior chest diameter; circumoral cyanosis; and suprasternal, intercostal, and substernal retractions occur. Subjectively, the patient experiences chest tightness and anxiety and works harder to breathe. Accessory muscle use and retractions can develop with or without marked wheezing on auscultation. To maximize air exchange, the child assumes a characteristic sitting posture, bending slightly forward. Frequent examinations are warranted, and any change in sensorium requires prompt evaluation. As respiratory muscles tire, the patient becomes lethargic and cyanotic, even with

supplemental oxygen. A decrease in wheezing with increased air entry represents response to therapy. Decreased wheezing with decreased air entry is an ominous sign. With extreme fatigue, respiratory muscles fail, retractions decrease, and respiratory failure is imminent unless appropriate therapy is promptly initiated. After initial examination, serial assessment of the degree of respiratory distress, using the parameters outlined in Table 4-10, assists determination of the response to therapy.

A particularly useful aspect of the physical examination is the respiratory rate, which increases as the degree of airway obstruction progresses. Respiratory rates of normal children are shown in Table 4-11.

The underlying pathology of asthma is lung inflammation. Histopathologic features of acute asthma include airway infiltration with inflammatory cells, increased intraluminal mucus with plugging of small airways, edema, bronchoconstriction, and smooth muscle hypertrophy. Because asthma has bronchoconstrictive and inflammatory components, the ideal therapeutic regimen should incorporate a combination of

Table 4-10	Estimation of Severity of Acute Exacerbations of Asthma in Children

	Mild	**Moderate**	**Severe**	**Life-Threatening**
Symptoms				
Breathlessness*	While walking	While at rest (infant— softer, shorter cry, difficulty feeding)	While at rest (infant—stops feeding)	
Talks in:	Sentences	Phrases	Words	
Alertness	May be agitated	Usually agitated	Usually agitated	Drowsy or confused
Signs				
Respiratory rate[†]	Increased	Increased	Significantly increased	Often normal or decreased
Accessory muscle use	Unusual	Common	Common	Paradoxic abdominal movements
Wheeze	Moderate, often only end-expiratory	Loud, throughout exhalation	Usually loud, in both inspiration and expiration	Absence of wheeze and air movement
Pulse	Normal to tachycardic	Tachycardic	Tachycardic	Bradycardic
Pulsus paradoxus[‡]	<10 mm Hg	10-20 mm Hg	20-40 mm Hg	Absence suggests respiratory muscle fatigue
Functional Assessment				
PEF (percent predicted or personal best)	>70%	40%-69%	<40%	<25%
Pa_{O_2} (room air)	Normal	>60 mm Hg	<60 mm Hg; possible cyanosis	Cyanosis
Pa_{CO_2}	<42 mm Hg	<42 mm Hg	>42 mm Hg	>42 mm Hg
Sa_{O_2} percent (room air)	>95%	90%-95%	<90%	<90%

Note: Within each category, the presence of several parameters, but not necessarily all, indicates the general classification of the exacerbation.

*Parents' or physician's impression of degree of child's breathlessness.

[†]See Table 4-11 for normal respiratory rates by age.

[‡]Pulsus paradoxus does not correlate with phase of respiration in small children.

Pa_{O_2}, arterial oxygen pressure; Pa_{CO_2}, arterial carbon dioxide pressure; PEF, peak expiratory flow; Sa_{O_2}, arterial oxygen saturation.

Adapted from National Asthma Education and Prevention Program: Expert Panel Report 3 (EPR3): Guidelines for the diagnosis and management of asthma (Publication No. 08-5846). Bethesda, Md, 2007, National Institutes of Health.

| Table 4-11 | Respiratory Rates of Normal Children, Sleeping and Awake* | | | | | |

	SLEEPING			AWAKE		
Age	No.	Mean	Range	No.	Mean	Range
6-12 mo	6	27	22-31	3	64	58-75
1-2 yr	6	19	17-23	4	35	30-40
2-4 yr	16	19	16-25	15	31	23-42
4-6 yr	23	18	14-23	22	26	19-36
6-8 yr	27	17	13-23	28	23	15-30

*In breaths per minute.
  From Waring WW: The history and physical exam. In Kendig E, Chernick V, editors: *Disorders of the respiratory tract in children*, Philadelphia, 1983, WB Saunders. As appears in National Asthma Education and Prevention Program: Expert Panel Report: Guidelines for the diagnosis and management of asthma (Publication No. 91-3642). Bethesda, Md, 1991, National Institutes of Health.

bronchodilator and antiinflammatory agents. Characteristic features of asthmatic inflammation include mast cell activation, inflammatory cell infiltration, edema, denudation and disruption of the bronchial epithelium, collagen deposition beneath the basement membrane, goblet cell hyperplasia, and smooth muscle thickening. These morphologic changes may not be completely reversible and may contribute to airway remodeling (Fig. 4-23). Education is a key component of asthma therapy, incorporating information about disease pathogenesis; avoidance of environmental triggers (including second-hand tobacco smoke exposure); benefits and risks of medications; and a written, individualized therapeutic plan for chronic and acute management that outlines the goals of asthma therapy as well as indications and correct use for prescribed medications.

The radiographic features of hyperinflation, peribronchial cuffing, and atelectasis, which are characteristic of uncomplicated acute asthma, are illustrated in Figure 4-24. Complications are generally diagnosed radiographically but may be suggested by symptoms and signs. Pneumothorax (Fig. 4-25) should be suspected in any asthmatic person who develops pleuritic chest pain associated with dyspnea, cyanosis, tachypnea, and occasionally cough. Examination reveals respiratory distress, marked hyperinflation and decreased chest wall excursion, and decreased or absent breath sounds on the affected side. With tension pneumothorax, the trachea, mediastinum, and cardiac landmarks may be shifted to the opposite side. Pneumomediastinum and subcutaneous emphysema (Fig. 4-26), usually involving the neck and supraclavicular areas, are more common than pneumothorax. When mild, they may be asymptomatic and may be detected incidentally on chest or neck radiograph. With more extensive air dissection, the patient may complain of neck and chest pain, and the subcutaneous emphysema may be visibly evident as a soft tissue swelling of the neck and chest that is *crepitant* (i.e., produces a crunching sensation) on palpation. Pneumothorax and pneumomediastinum can produce characteristic auscultatory findings including a crackling "mediastinal crunch" at the base of the heart and a systolic crunch or knock. The latter sound has been referred to as *noisy pneumothorax* and is frequently audible to the patient and physician without the aid of a stethoscope.

Other complications that may be observed on physical examination include those induced by chronic systemic steroid use, such as weight gain, "moon-type" facies, hirsutism,

PROGRESSION TO AIRWAY REMODELING

Healthy ⟷ Acute ⟷ Chronic ⟷ Remodeling (permanent changes)

Cells	Mast cells	Eosinophils, lymphocytes	Myofibroblasts
Mediators	Histamine, other inflammatory mediators	Neuromechanisms, inflammatory mediators, cytokines	Growth factors
Actions	During an acute asthma attack, mast cells release inflammatory mediators, resulting in epithelial cell edema, muscle constriction, vascular leakage, and mucus hypersecretion.	In chronic asthma, mast cells and eosinophils release inflammatory mediators. Epithelial cells are shed, resulting in exposed nerves. Epithelial cells start to lose their cilia, and increased numbers of glandular cells are observed. Changes include increased muscle mass, sub-basement membrane collagen deposition, and vascular enlargement.	Remodeling can occur leading to permanent changes. Continued loss of epithelial cells, deposition of sub-basement membrane collagen, and increased muscle mass are observed.

Figure 4-23   Asthmatic inflammation may result in permanent changes in the airways. This process is known as *remodeling*. *(Reprinted with permission from* The Allergy Report: Diseases of the Atopic Diathesis, *vol 2, Milwaukee, Wis, 2000, Task Force on Allergic Disorders, American Academy of Allergy, Asthma, & Immunology.)*

Figure 4-24   Anteroposterior chest radiograph of child with acute asthma. Note the flattened diaphragm, hyperinflation, peribronchial thickening, and right middle lobe atelectasis.

Figure 4-25   Chest radiograph showing right-sided pneumothorax in an intubated patient with acute asthma and respiratory failure. Clinical manifestations include pleuritic chest pain, dyspnea, cyanosis, tachypnea, and cough. Also, note the marked hyperinflation of the lungs, which can result in cardiac compression (narrow cardiac shadow) and compromise of cardiac venous return, as well as extensive right-sided subcutaneous emphysema. *(Courtesy Beverly Newman, MD, Pittsburgh, Pa.)*

polycythemia (red, ruddy complexion) (Fig. 4-27), and short stature (see Chapter 9). The introduction of effective antiinflammatory therapy, particularly inhaled corticosteroids, has made such sequelae rare.

In children with recent onset of wheezing, asthma must be differentiated from other disorders associated with wheezing. In infants, this differentiation includes bronchiolitis, the features of which are listed in Table 4-12 (also see Chapter 16). This differentiation may be difficult because 30% to 50% of children with recurrent bronchiolitis are later diagnosed with asthma, and asthma exacerbations are often triggered by viral infection. However, the distinction remains a clinically useful one for the following reasons: (1) the children with bronchiolitis who do not develop asthma may be inappropriately labeled as asthmatic; and (2) children younger than 2 years of age frequently do not respond to inhaled bronchodilators. In infants and young children who wheeze with viral upper respiratory infections, different patterns of illness may emerge over time.

The Tucson Children's Respiratory Study, a large, longitudinal assessment of respiratory illnesses in children, identified different patterns of wheezing illness in children. As summarized in Figure 4-28, 51.5% of children enrolled in this study never wheezed, 19.9% had transient infant wheezing (defined as wheezing during the first 3 years of life but no wheezing at 6 years of age), 13.7% had persistent wheezing (defined as wheezing during the first 3 years of life with wheezing present at 6 years of age), and 15% had late-onset wheezing (defined as no wheezing during the first 3 years of life but wheezing present at 6 years of age). Children with transient wheezing had significantly lower lung function in infancy (before any wheezing illness) than all the other groups (Table 4-13). At

Figure 4-26   Asthma with pneumomediastinum in a 16-month-old child with asthma. Note the dissection of air in the soft tissues just anterior to the vertebrae **(A)** and in the mediastinum and subcutaneous tissues of the right arm **(B).** This highlights the often subtle findings of pneumomediastinum in the chest and the more striking findings in the neck. Also note the hyperinflation **(B).** *(Courtesy Beverly Newman, MD, Pittsburgh, Pa.)*

Figure 4-27 Steroid-dependent asthma. Shown are complications of corticosteroid therapy for chronic asthma: moon-type facies **(A)** and buffalo hump **(B)**, both resulting from abnormal fat distribution.

the age of 6 years, children with early transient wheezing had significantly lower lung function than those who had never wheezed, and children with persistent wheezing had the lowest levels of lung function of all the groups.

It is hypothesized that children with early transient wheezing have congenitally smaller airways, which predispose to wheezing with viral illnesses in early life. As their airways grow in absolute size with age, these children outgrow their wheezing during viral infections. In contrast, children with persistent wheezing are born with normal airway function, which deteriorates over time, reflecting the effects of the chronic asthmatic disease process. Distinguishing transient versus persistent wheezing during infancy and early childhood remains problematic. Infant pulmonary function testing is still experimental and not widely available, there are currently no reliable genetic markers, and the use of any single biochemical

marker is controversial. However, a combination of clinical and biochemical markers may be useful in predicting persistent wheezing (Table 4-14). These include an increased serum IgE level at 9 months of age, atopic dermatitis and rhinitis (unrelated to upper respiratory infection) during the first year of life, severe lower respiratory infections requiring hospitalization, and diminished airway function as measured by spirometry at 6 years. Other factors associated with persistent wheezing include a family history of asthma and/or allergy and perinatal exposure to passive tobacco smoke. A clinical index has been developed to predict which children with recurrent wheezing are at risk for persistent asthma (Table 4-15).

Although children with pneumonia (particularly of viral origin) may wheeze, they are more likely to have rales or normal findings on auscultation, with the diagnosis suggested by tachypnea in association with retractions, nasal flaring, or expiratory grunting. Other causes of wheezing are listed in Table 4-16. Airway compression by anomalous vessels (see Chapter 5) or mass lesions are often distinguishable from bronchiolitis by virtue of the absence of signs of infection, and from asthma by failure to respond to bronchodilators. The

Table 4-12	Differentiating Features of Asthma and Bronchiolitis in Children	
	Asthma	**Bronchiolitis**
Primary etiologies	Viruses, allergens, exercise, and so on	Respiratory syncytial virus, other viruses
Age at onset	50% by 2 yr of age 80% by 5 yr of age	<24 mo
Recurrent wheezing	Yes (characteristic)	70% (≤2 episodes) 30% progress to asthma (≥3 episodes)
Onset of wheezing	Acute if allergic or exercise induced	Insidious
Concomitant symptoms of upper respiratory infection	Yes, if infectious	Yes
Family history of allergy and asthma	Frequent	Infrequent in children with ≤2 episodes
Nasal eosinophilia	With allergic rhinitis	Absent
Chest auscultation	If viral, as in bronchiolitis Nonviral: high-pitched expiratory wheezes	Fine, sibilant rales, and coarse inspiratory and expiratory wheezes
Concomitant allergic manifestations	Yes, if allergic asthma	Usually absent
IgE level	Elevated (if allergic)	Normal
Response to bronchodilator	Yes (characteristic)	Unresponsive or partially responsive

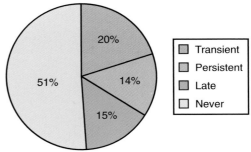

Figure 4-28 Asthma. The Tucson Children's Respiratory Study has shown that in children who wheeze, different patterns of illness may emerge over time. About half the patients in this study had evidence of wheezing before 6 years of age. In the transient group, wheezing occurred during the first 3 years of life but resolved by 6 years of age. In the persistent group, wheezing occurred during the first 3 years of life and persisted to 6 years of age. In the late group, wheezing did not occur during the first 3 years of life but was present by 6 years of age. (*Modified from Martinez FD, Wright AL, Taussig LM, et al: Asthma and wheezing in the first 6 years of life.* N Engl J Med 332:133-138, 1995.)

Table 4-13	Lung Function during Infancy and at 6 Years of Age according to Wheezing History in Patients Enrolled in the Tucson Children's Respiratory Study

	LUNG FUNCTION ($\dot{V}_{max}$FRC)		
Group	**n (%)**	**Infancy**	**6 Years of Age**
No wheezing	425 (51.5%)	Normal	Normal
Transient wheezing	164 (19.9%)	Diminished	Diminished
Persistent wheezing	113 (13.7%)	Normal	Diminished
Late-onset wheezing	124 (15%)	Normal	Normal

$\dot{V}_{max}$FRC , maximal expiratory flow at functional residual capacity, expressed as milliliters per second.
   Modified from Martinez FD, Wright AL, Taussig LM, et al: Asthma and wheezing in the first six years of life, *N Engl J Med* 332:133-138, 1995.

Table 4-15	Clinical Index to Define Asthma

Major Criteria	**Minor Criteria**
1. Physician diagnosis of parental asthma 2. Physician diagnosis of atopic dermatitis	1. Physician diagnosis of allergic rhinitis 2. Wheezing apart from colds 3. Eosinophilia (≥4%)

The loose index for prediction of asthma consists of early wheezing plus at least one of two major criteria or two of three minor criteria. The stringent index for prediction of asthma consists of early *frequent* wheezing plus at least one of two major criteria or two of three minor criteria.
   Modified from Castro-Rodriguez JA, Holberg CJ, Wright AL, et al: A clinical index to define risk of asthma in young children with recurrent wheezing, *Am J Respir Crit Care Med* 162:1403-1406, 2000.

history and presence of infiltrates help in the diagnosis of aspiration, which can mimic asthma closely, often responding to bronchodilator therapy. Radiographic studies such as barium swallow with fluoroscopy can be helpful in distinguishing among these entities (Fig. 4-29). pH probe testing may be required to identify gastroesophageal reflux (see Chapter 16), although a trial of antireflux medicines is often attempted.

In older children who have sudden onset of wheezing and respiratory distress, the differential diagnosis includes respiratory infections, left ventricular failure, aspiration, and vocal cord dysfunction. Respiratory infections such as croup may be distinguished by their characteristic histories and tendencies to involve the upper airways (see Chapter 16). Lower respiratory infections (pneumonia) generally produce fever and more localized findings of rales, a decrease in the number of and change in the quality of breath sounds, and egophony. Left ventricular failure, especially with pulmonary edema, may present with acute respiratory distress and wheezing. A history of cardiac disease, diffuse crackles or basilar rales, and a third heart sound on auscultation help distinguish this condition from asthma. Aspiration of a foreign body that lodges in a mainstem bronchus may produce wheezing (Fig. 4-30). A history of a choking episode and physical findings of unilateral wheezing and hyperresonance aid in distinguishing aspiration from asthma but do not confirm the diagnosis. Remembering that wheezing resulting from foreign body aspiration may respond at least in part to bronchodilator therapy is important. Vocal cord dysfunction is becoming more recognized in children and adolescents and is often confused with asthma by families, school nurses, as well as primary care and emergency room physicians. Symptoms include acute-onset dyspnea and often stridor, which can be mistaken for wheezing to the untrained observer, secondary to partial or complete adduction of the vocal cords during inspiration. Symptoms rarely awaken individuals from sleep and there are many triggers that are similar to asthma, including exercise, inhalational irritants, psychosocial stressors, and rhinitis. Bronchodilators are not effective and objective measurements of pulmonary function, including pulse oximetry and chest radiographs, are unremarkable during acute episodes. Some episodes of vocal cord dysfunction can become severe enough to result in syncope from hyperventilation, which often successfully resolves the acute episode as the vocal cords relax.

Table 4-14	Factors Predictive of Persistent Asthma

Family history of asthma (maternal > paternal)
- Atopy
  - ↑ IgE or positive allergy skin tests
  - Eczema
  - Rhinitis
- Allergen exposure (dust mites, animals)
- RSV bronchiolitis
- Gender (males > females)
- Environmental smoke exposure
- Severity in childhood

RSV, respiratory syncytial virus.
   Modified from Martinez FD, Wright AL, Taussig LM, et al: Asthma and wheezing in the first six years of life, *N Engl J Med* 332:133-138, 1995.

Table 4-16	Associated Symptoms and Signs in the Wheezing Child That Are Helpful in Differential Diagnosis

	DISEASES ASSOCIATED WITH WHEEZING	
Symptoms and Signs	**In Infants**	**In Older Children**
Positional changes	Anomalies of the great vessels, gastroesophageal reflux	Gastroesophageal reflux
Failure to thrive	Cystic fibrosis, tracheoesophageal fistula, bronchopulmonary dysplasia	Cystic fibrosis, chronic hypersensitivity pneumonitis, α_1-antitrypsin deficiency, bronchiectasis
Factors associated with feeding	Tracheoesophageal fistula, gastroesophageal reflux	Gastroesophageal reflux
Environmental triggers	Allergic asthma	Allergic asthma, allergic bronchopulmonary aspergillosis, acute hypersensitivity pneumonitis
Sudden onset	Allergic asthma, croup	Allergic asthma, foreign body aspiration, croup, acute hypersensitivity pneumonitis
Fever	Bronchiolitis, pneumonitis	Infectious asthma, acute hypersensitivity pneumonitis, croup
Rhinorrhea	Bronchiolitis, pneumonitis	Infectious or allergic asthma, croup
Concomitant stridor	Tracheal or bronchial stenosis, anomalies of the great vessels, croup	Foreign body aspiration, croup
Clubbing	—	Cystic fibrosis, bronchiectasis, bronchopulmonary dysplasia

Figure 4-29 Vascular ring/compression. Barium swallow (lateral chest radiograph) shows upper airway compression by a right-sided aortic arch with aberrant left subclavian and diverticulum at the left subclavian origin. Note the round indentation on the posterior wall of the esophagus and the anterior displacement and compression of the trachea, which can cause wheezing and mimic asthma. *(Courtesy Beverly Newman, MD, Pittsburgh, Pa. From Fireman P, Slavin RG: Atlas of allergies, New York, 1990, Gower.)*

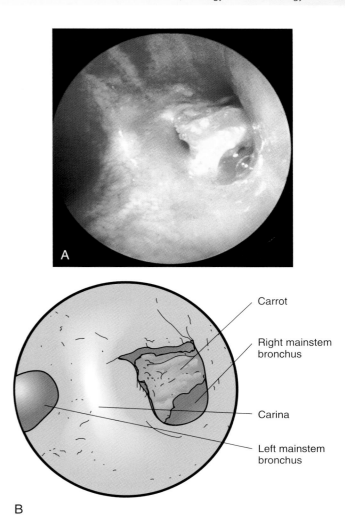

Figure 4-30 Airway foreign body. A piece of carrot is lodged in the right-stem bronchus just below the carina, as visualized during bronchoscopy. Foreign bodies such as this can cause airway obstruction that is partially responsive to bronchodilator therapy. *(Courtesy Sylvan Stool, MD, Pittsburgh, Pa. From Fireman P, Slavin RG: Atlas of allergies, New York, Gower, 1990.)*

In the older child with mild, infrequent episodes of wheezing that respond to bronchodilator therapy, asthma is readily diagnosed. However, with daily wheezing, frequent exacerbations, lack of response to bronchodilators, or poor growth, other diagnoses must be considered including chronic obstructive pulmonary disease, cystic fibrosis, α_1-antitrypsin deficiency, and immunodeficiency. Chronic obstructive pulmonary diseases, which include chronic bronchitis, emphysema, bronchiectasis, and bronchopulmonary dysplasia, are distinguished by their lack of significant reversibility with bronchodilator therapy. Cystic fibrosis may present with chronic cough, wheezing, and recurrent infections. In addition, malabsorption with bulky, foul-smelling stools; failure to thrive; and clubbing of the nail beds are common. α_1-Antitrypsin deficiency, an inherited autosomal recessive disorder, is characterized by the onset of progressive emphysema in a young adult and is one cause of neonatal hepatitis.

Hypersensitivity Pneumonitis

Although IgE-mediated allergic respiratory diseases (allergic rhinitis, asthma) are the most common manifestations of inhalant sensitivities in humans, other immunologic respiratory diseases, involving non-IgE immune mechanisms, may result from the inhalation of antigens from the susceptible individual's environment. A wide variety of inhaled biologic dusts may induce an inflammatory lung disease involving the interstitium, alveoli, and airways. The most common form of hypersensitivity pneumonitis is caused by inhalation of thermophilic actinomycetes *(Saccharopolyspora rectivirgula,* formerly *Micropolyspora faeni),* antigens present in moldy vegetable compost, and is termed *farmer's lung.* Other forms (and their causative dusts and antigens) include malt-worker's lung (moldy malt, *Aspergillus* species) and bird-breeder's lung (avian dust, avian proteins). The disorder is termed

hypersensitivity pneumonitis or *extrinsic allergic alveolitis* and appears to be mediated by a complex immune response involving both immune complexes (type III) and T cells (type IV).

Hypersensitivity pneumonitis is a syndrome with a broad spectrum of presenting symptoms and signs that have been subdivided into acute, subacute, and chronic. The clinical features depend on the following factors: (1) the nature of the inhaled dust, (2) the intensity and frequency of inhalation exposure, and (3) the immunologic responsiveness of the exposed individual. A concomitant upper respiratory infection or another pulmonary insult may be an important factor in induction. Development of sensitization to the inhaled organic dust requires several months to years, although organic dust toxic syndrome can present similarly after a single exposure to a large dose of antigen. The acute form of hypersensitivity pneumonitis is usually readily differentiated from asthma by the lack of wheezing, prominence of rales, and presence of severe systemic symptoms such as high fever and myalgia. Subacute and chronic forms generally present with insidious development of respiratory symptoms.

Allergic Bronchopulmonary Aspergillosis

Aspergillus species, in addition to being one cause of hypersensitivity pneumonitis and allergic asthma, cause a disorder termed *allergic bronchopulmonary aspergillosis* (ABPA). This entity is characterized by migrating pulmonary infiltrates and peripheral blood and sputum eosinophilia. Type I and type III hypersensitivity are thought to be involved in the pathogenesis. Affected individuals are usually atopic and have a history of asthma and/or cystic fibrosis. They often present with systemic symptoms and difficulty weaning off systemic corticosteroids. Sputum production is prominent. Physical findings include the general signs of lower airway obstruction (see the earlier section, Asthma).

Laboratory studies that assist in diagnosis include the following:

- Peripheral blood examination reveals eosinophilia (generally >1000/mm³).
- The serum IgE level is markedly elevated, often greater than 1000 ng/mL, and specific IgE to *Aspergillus fumigatus* is elevated.
- Skin testing for *A. fumigatus* is positive. Although mold-sensitive patients with asthma without ABPA may have a positive reaction, a negative reaction rules out ABPA.
- Serum precipitating antibody (IgG) to *A. fumigatus* is found in most patients, but the titer has a poor correlation with disease activity.
- Chest radiography commonly shows infiltrates in active ABPA. The upper lobes are commonly involved, and infiltrates characteristically shift rapidly from one site to the other. Remarkably, radiographic findings do not correlate well with clinical severity, and patients with extensive consolidation may be asymptomatic (Fig. 4-31).
- High-resolution CT scanning may show bronchiectasis, especially late in the course of the disease.

Ocular Allergy

Ocular allergic reactions may involve the eyelid and/or conjunctiva. The eyelids have a rich blood supply and loose connective tissue assisting edema collection from either allergic inflammation or trauma. Immediate hypersensitivity reactions that produce eyelid angioedema may be triggered by a number of stimuli including pollens, dusts, insect stings or bites, foods, or drugs. The most common cause of mild reactions is topical exposure to environmental allergens. These reactions are characterized by periorbital edema, pruritus, and erythema after exposure to an allergen (Fig. 4-32). Severe acute episodes can be distinguished from cellulitis by lack of induration, absence of tenderness and fever, and the fact that involvement is usually bilateral (see Chapter 23).

Allergic conjunctivitis may be acute or chronic and seasonal or perennial, depending on the allergens to which the individual is sensitized. Commonly implicated allergens include

Figure 4-32   Angioedema. Eyelid angioedema in a child with a venom allergy. The onset was explosive after exposure to the bee sting. *(From Fireman P, Slavin RG: Atlas of allergies, New York, 1990, Gower.)*

weed, tree, and grass pollens; molds; dust; and animal dander. In the acute seasonal form, onset may be rapid and may coincide with the appearance of pollen. This condition frequently accompanies seasonal allergic rhinitis and is commonly due to ragweed, grass, and tree pollens. Itching and excessive tearing are the most prominent symptoms. Pruritus often interferes with sleep, and vision may be impaired by excessive discharge.

Physical findings depend on the degree of chronicity. In the acute form, these findings consist of diffuse bilateral conjunctival edema and hyperemia. Photophobia, profuse tearing, and mild lid swelling are commonly associated. In the chronic form, the conjunctivae appear pale, with mild edema and hyperplasia of the papillae. This may result in a fine, granular appearance of the conjunctivae, which is termed *allergic cobblestoning* (Fig. 4-33). The clinical diagnosis may be

Figure 4-31   Chest radiograph of patient with allergic bronchopulmonary aspergillosis. These patients are frequently asymptomatic despite extensive areas of consolidation. *(Courtesy Raymond G. Slavin, MD, St. Louis, Mo.)*

Figure 4-33   Allergic cobblestoning of the conjunctiva in chronic allergic conjunctivitis. This granular appearance is due to edema and hyperplasia of the papillae.

Mucopurulent discharge

B

Figure 4-34 Atopic keratoconjunctivitis with chronic papillary conjunctivitis. Note the stringy mucopurulent discharge often seen in this disorder. *(From Fireman P, Slavin RG: Atlas of allergies, New York, 1990, Gower.)*

Figure 4-35 Vernal conjunctivitis, palpebral form. The giant papillary elevations are easily seen without magnification. *(From Fireman P, Slavin RG: Atlas of allergies, New York, 1990, Gower.)*

confirmed by finding eosinophilia on a smear of conjunctival secretions and skin testing for the suspected allergens.

The differential diagnosis of allergic conjunctivitis includes atopic keratoconjunctivitis, and vernal conjunctivitis. Atopic keratoconjunctivitis occurs in patients with atopic dermatitis and is characterized by erythema and thickening of the conjunctivae (Fig. 4-34). This may progress to scarring and vascularization of the cornea in severe cases. Ocular disease activity parallels that of cutaneous disease. It generally presents in adults.

Vernal conjunctivitis is uncommon and chronic in nature. Young, atopic boys are affected most frequently. Symptoms include severe itching, photophobia, blurring of vision, and lacrimation. Physical examination reveals white, ropy secretions containing many eosinophils. A palpebral form manifests hypertrophic nodular papillae that resemble cobblestones on the upper eyelids (Fig. 4-35). The papillae consist of dense fibrous tissue with eosinophilic infiltrates. In the bulbar form, nodules appear as gelatinous masses called *Trantas' dots*, usually found at the corneoscleral junction (Fig. 4-36). The symptoms are generally severe and frequently require referral to ophthalmology for topical steroids. This disease usually remits with maturity and is rarely seen in adults. Giant papillary conjunctivitis, which appears clinically and histologically to be a mild form of vernal conjunctivitis, is associated with the use of hard and soft contact lenses (Fig. 4-37). The stimulus is believed to be foreign material that accumulates on the surface of the contact lenses. Whether this material is antigenic and the condition an immune-mediated disease is not known.

Urticaria and Angioedema

Hypersensitivity reactions in which the skin is the major target organ are manifested clinically as diffuse erythema, urticaria, or angioedema. Type I hypersensitivity to inhalants, foods,

Gelatinous papillary elevations

B

Figure 4-36 Vernal conjunctivitis, limbal form. Note the gelatinous papillary elevations of the limbal tissue. *(From Fireman P, Slavin RG: Atlas of allergies, New York, 1990, Gower.)*

Figure 4-37 Giant papillary conjunctivitis. These hobnail-like elevations of the upper tarsal conjunctiva, evident on eversion of the upper eyelid, occur when the upper lid meets a foreign body such as a contact lens, prosthesis, or exposed suture. *(From Fireman P, Slavin RG:* Atlas of allergies, *New York, 1990, Gower.)*

Figure 4-38 Urticarial lesions. Note the well-demarcated borders, redness, elevation, and occasional confluence of the palpable lesions. *(Courtesy Michael Sherlock, MD, Bloomfield, NJ.)*

insect venoms, and drugs is the most common mechanism, but urticaria and angioedema may also accompany type II (transfusion reaction) or type III reactions (cutaneous vasculitis, serum sickness). These disorders result from increased vascular permeability. The resultant edema collects in the dermis in urticaria and primarily in the subcutaneous tissues in angioedema. Although frequently seen in combination, urticaria and angioedema may also appear individually. Urticaria is most frequently an acute disorder that resolves spontaneously. In children it is often secondary to viral illnesses, allergen exposure (food, medication, or environmental), or idiopathic in nature. When the duration of recurrences exceeds 6 weeks, the condition is arbitrarily termed *chronic urticaria*. In contrast to acute urticaria, an underlying allergic cause of chronic urticaria is often not found, even with extensive investigation. Thus this is most frequently deemed idiopathic. In approximately one third of cases an autoimmune etiology can be demonstrated, with evidence of an autoantibody to the IgE receptor on mast cells and basophils; thus individuals experience degranulation of these cells in the absence of specific IgE to an allergen.

Urticarial lesions are well circumscribed, raised, palpable wheals that blanch with applied pressure (Fig. 4-38). They are usually erythematous but may be pale or white with red halos. Typically, the lesions are intensely pruritic; however, in some instances the pruritus is mild. Angioedema is characterized by diffuse subcutaneous tissue swelling with normal or erythematous overlying skin. Angioedema may be more painful than pruritic. The face, hands, feet, and perineum are most commonly involved (Fig. 4-39).

Skin involvement may be generalized or localized to body parts exposed to a provoking stimulus. Careful history taking concerning recent exposures and medications is often rewarding, because if there is an allergic cause of acute urticaria it is most likely to be determined from the history. In cases with associated fever and respiratory and/or GI symptoms, infectious diseases resulting from viruses (including enterovirus, hepatitis B virus, and Epstein-Barr virus), group A β-hemolytic streptococcus, and helminth infestation should be considered. Generalized urticaria with or without angioedema may also be the initial manifestation of erythema multiforme or Henoch-Schönlein purpura. In general, urticaria that is not associated with pain, respiratory or GI symptoms, or residual skin changes, and in which individual lesions are red/pink and last less than 24 hours, is benign and can be managed symptomatically.

A subgroup of urticarial disorders results from hypersensitivity to physical and mechanical factors. These include cold urticaria, pressure-induced urticaria and angioedema, aquagenic and solar urticaria, and exercise-induced urticaria. The

Figure 4-39 Angioedema. **A,** Onset was sudden. **B,** Resolution was complete within 24 hours.

Figure 4-40 Positive ice cube test in a child with cold urticaria. An ice cube placed on the arm for 10 minutes results in urticaria of the exposed skin. Onset is usually immediate but may be delayed for up to 4 hours after cold exposure.

history and distribution of lesions often help in identifying the source, which can then be confirmed by challenge (Fig. 4-40).

Dermographism, translated literally as the "ability to write on the skin" (Fig. 4-41), is a form of trauma-induced pressure urticaria. It is elicited by stroking the skin with a fingernail or tongue blade. The initial white line secondary to reflex vasoconstriction is supplanted by pruritic, erythematous linear swelling, as seen in a classic wheal and flare reaction. The condition is chronic and the etiology unclear. Patients with dermographism suspected of having an atopic disorder must be skin tested with caution for specific IgE antibody, because all test results appear positive.

Hereditary Angioedema

Hereditary angioedema (HAE) is an autosomal dominant disorder characterized by the absence or abnormal function of a protein in the complement cascade known as *C1 esterase inhibitor.* Inhibitors of the complement system are part of the complement pathway and are capable of blocking activated complement components. C1 esterase inhibitor binds to activated C1 and thereby prevents further activation of the classical pathway. It also serves to regulate other blood protein

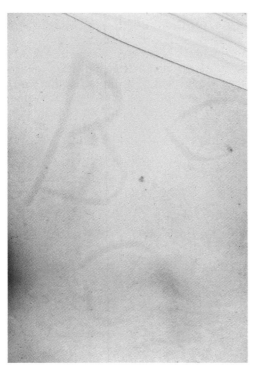

Figure 4-41 Dermographism, or "writing on the skin," is the most common type of urticaria induced by physical or mechanical factors. Firm stroking of the skin with a fingernail or tongue blade results in urticaria of the traumatized skin.

cascades including the bradykinin system. In the absence of C1 inhibitor, these cascades can proceed unchecked. This results in increased vascular permeability and the observed clinical features of angioedema. This disorder is characterized by recurrent bouts of swelling that involve any part of the body with the face, extremities, genitals, and respiratory and GI tracts most frequently involved. The swelling is generally self-limited, episodic, and commonly triggered by minor trauma. The swelling is distinguished from idiopathic angioedema (which is frequently accompanied by urticaria) by its longer duration (1 to 3 days) and the absence of urticaria. Laryngeal edema is a frightening, life-threatening complication that may result in asphyxiation. Involvement of the GI tract is characterized by severe abdominal pain, bloating, vomiting, and rarely intestinal obstruction resulting from intussusception. Other components of the complement system affected in hereditary angioedema are C2 and C4: C4 levels are consistently low in 95% of patients, and C2 levels are decreased during attacks. The diagnosis of hereditary angioedema can be confirmed by measuring the C1 esterase level and function. Until more recently, anabolic steroids were prescribed widely as treatment for HAE, with problems with efficacy, side effects, and toxicity. Fortunately, there are now two different forms of purified C1 esterase inhibitor, one kallikrein inhibitor, and one bradykinin receptor antagonist available for treatment, with options for both prophylactic and acute use, and other products are under investigation.

IMMUNOLOGIC DEFICIENCY DISORDERS

Normal Development of the Immune System

The immune system, which protects against infections, can be divided into innate and adaptive components. The innate immune system starts with mechanical barriers, such as the skin, and also includes cells that cannot generate antigen-specific receptors, such as neutrophils, eosinophils, and monocytes/macrophages. The innate immune system also includes the complement system and other soluble molecules that recognize pathogens. The innate immune system encodes a variety of receptors that recognize pathogen-associated molecular patterns (PAMPs), which are expressed by pathogens, as well as danger-associated molecular patterns (DAMPs), which are endogenous products derived from stressed or dying cells.

In contrast, the adaptive immune system is capable of generating a nearly infinite variety of antigen-recognizing receptors. The adaptive immune response is composed of B cells, which produce antibodies, and T cells, which, through T-cell receptors, recognize antigens presented by the major histocompatibility complex (MHC) on antigen-presenting cells. There is extensive bidirectional interaction between the innate and adaptive arms of the immune system. For example, activation of complement helps prime B cells for antibody production while recognition of microbes or foreign antigens by antibody can activate components of the innate immune system, including complement and natural killer cells. Immune deficiencies have been divided broadly into defects in the antibody (B-cell), cellular (T-cell), phagocytic, and complement systems, although many cellular defects also have defects in antibody responses and are therefore termed *combined deficiencies.*

Adaptive immunity depends on the maturation of two distinct lymphoid cell lines, T lymphocytes and B lymphocytes, both originating from the same stem cells in the bone marrow. T lymphocytes and B lymphocytes undergo a complex series of maturational changes that generate incredible diversity before arriving at a stage in which they are capable of

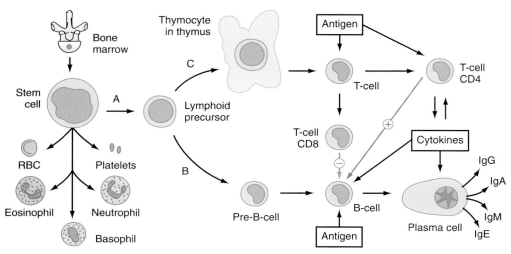

Figure 4-42 Immune development. Shown is a schematic representation of T- and B-lymphocyte ontogeny. Defects along pathway A result in combined immunodeficiencies. Pathway B is responsible for normal antibody production, whereas normal cell-mediated immunity requires the integrity of pathway C. Cytokines are soluble products of activated lymphocytes and include interleukins and interferons.

antigen-stimulated differentiation (Fig. 4-42). T lymphocytes can be divided into two main classes, CD4+ and CD8+. CD4+ T lymphocytes, via both cell-to-cell contact and production of soluble signaling molecules called *cytokines*, help orchestrate the immune response by variously activating CD8+ cells and monocytes/macrophages to kill infected cells, stimulating production of antibodies by B cells, and, in the case of T-regulatory lymphocytes, decreasing inflammation to avoid autoimmunity. CD4+ T lymphocytes have been subdivided into four major classes: Th1, Th2, Th17, and Treg. Th1 cells produce interferon-γ and are responsible for elimination of intracellular pathogens. Th2 cells are characterized by the production of interleukin (IL)-4 and IL-13. Although CD4+ Th2 cells likely evolved to fight parasitic infections, in the developed world they are more often responsible for allergic responses. Th17 cells produce IL-17 and limit infection with fungi and extracellular bacteria, and play a key role in autoimmune processes. Last, Treg cells are antiinflammatory and help limit immune-mediated destruction of tissue and development of autoimmunity, via production of IL-10 and transforming growth factor (TGF)-β.

Thymus-independent B lymphocytes produce the various classes of immunoglobulins, also known as *antibodies*. Four main subclasses of antibodies are produced: IgM, IgA, IgG, and IgE. Antibody deficiencies are the most commonly recognized primary immunodeficiencies. The ability to generate antibodies against specific antigens, as well as sufficient total antibody levels, is important for fully effective humoral immunity. Abnormalities in the maturation of T lymphocytes result in cellular immunodeficiency, and abnormalities of B lymphocytes result in humoral immunodeficiency.

Presentation of Primary Immunodeficiency

Deficiencies of the immune system can involve lymphocytes (e.g., humoral and/or cellular immunodeficiencies), phagocytes (e.g., chronic granulomatous disease), the complement system (e.g., C3 deficiency), and mucosal barriers (e.g., immotile cilia syndrome). Approximate frequencies of the different categories of immunodeficiencies are shown in Figure 4-43. Humoral (antibody) deficiencies are typically characterized by recurrent infections with extracellular encapsulated bacterial pathogens and chronic sinopulmonary infections. In contrast, cellular deficiencies are manifested by infections with opportunistic organisms such as *Candida* or *Pneumocystis jirovecii*

and an inability to clear common viral infections. They are also associated with failure to thrive in infants and poor growth in older children, wasting, and diarrhea. These patients may be susceptible to graft-versus-host disease if given nonirradiated blood transfusions and may have life-threatening infections after live virus vaccination. Some combined immunodeficiencies are associated with an increased risk of malignancy. Patients with phagocytic deficiencies present with an inability to kill certain organisms, while those with complement deficiencies are often characterized by recurrent *Neisseria* infections, although sinopulmonary infections may also be seen.

More common immunodeficiencies may present in a subtle fashion, with few life-threatening infections and normal growth. Thus the clinician is frequently confronted with the question of whether a patient should be evaluated for immunodeficiency. A set of warning signals has been widely disseminated (Fig. 4-44). In general, children with infections that are frequent, are recurrent or chronic, are caused by unusual organisms, or respond poorly to therapy should be evaluated for immunodeficiency. Moreover, growth retardation or a family history of early death from infection should raise the clinician's level of suspicion. In the screening for immunodeficiency, quantitative and functional aspects of the components of the immune system are considered (Table 4-17). Laboratory evaluation for immunodeficiency should be guided by the history and physical examination.

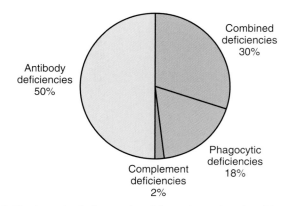

Figure 4-43 Approximate frequencies of the various categories of immunodeficiency. *(From Stiehm ER: Immunologic disorders in infants and children, ed 5, Philadelphia, 2004, Elsevier Saunders.)*

10 WARNING SIGNS OF PRIMARY IMMUNODEFICIENCY

Primary immunodeficiency (PI) causes children and young adults to have infections that come back frequently or are unusually hard to cure. In America alone, up to 1/2 million people suffer from one of the 140 known primary immunodeficiency diseases. If you or someone you know is affected by two or more of the following warning signs, speak to a physician about the possible presence of an underlying primary immunodeficiency.

1. Eight or more new ear infections within 1 year.
6. Recurrent deep skin or organ abscesses.

2. Two or more serious sinus infections within 1 year.
7. Persistent thrush in mouth or elsewhere on skin, after age 1.

3. Two or more months on antibiotics with little effect.
8. Need for intravenous antibiotics to clear infections.

4. Two or more pneumonias within 1 year.
9. Two or more deep-seated infections.

5. Failure of an infant to gain weight or grow normally.
10. A family history of primary immunodeficiency.

Figure 4-44 Ten warning signs of primary immunodeficiency disease. *(From the Jeffrey Modell Foundation.)*

Humoral (B-Lymphocyte) Immunodeficiency

Congenital Agammaglobulinemia

Congenital agammaglobulinemia is usually X-linked (Bruton's) but can rarely be autosomal recessive. Affected infants are clinically well for the first few months of life because of placentally acquired maternal IgG antibodies but subsequently develop recurrent or chronic infections with virulent bacterial pathogens such as gram-positive cocci and *Haemophilus influenzae.* The infections may localize in the upper and lower respiratory tracts, resulting in sinusitis, otitis media, and pneumonia. Sepsis, meningitis, and skin infections are also seen. Over time, recurrent lung infections can lead to bronchiectasis. This is characterized clinically by chronic cough with increased sputum production and by abnormal chest imaging (Fig. 4-45). Treatment consists of immunoglobulin (IgG) replacement, which can be given either subcutaneously or intravenously, and appropriate antibiotics. In the absence of chronic lung disease, growth is usually unimpaired, and survival to adulthood is expected.

The physical findings are those of localized infection, with specific signs depending on the particular structures infected. In addition, these children generally lack adenoidal, tonsillar,

Figure 4-45 Hypogammaglobulinemia and bronchiectasis. Bronchogram reveals bronchiectasis of the left lower lobe in an older child with hypogammaglobulinemia. Symptoms consisted of chronic cough and sputum production.

and other lymphoid tissues (Fig. 4-46). The diagnosis of agammaglobulinemia should be considered in any child who has recurrent infections with virulent bacterial pathogens and is confirmed by findings of markedly decreased levels of the immunoglobulin classes (IgG, IgA, IgM) in the serum.

Transient Hypogammaglobulinemia of Childhood

As shown in Figure 4-47, term infants are born with high levels of serum IgG because of active placental transport of maternal IgG. The serum IgG level normally declines during the first 7 months of life until endogenous IgG production matures. Delays in this maturation may lead to transient hypogammaglobulinemia. Serum IgG levels in these infants usually attain age-appropriate values by school age. Despite the low levels of serum IgG, these infants can generally synthesize specific antibodies to tetanus and other antigens. Patients with this condition typically present with ear, sinus, and lung infections. IgG replacement is generally not indicated for this condition, but some patients may benefit from prophylactic antibiotics.

IgG Subclass Deficiency and Selective IgA Deficiency

Serum IgG can be subdivided into four subclasses. Patients have been identified with low or absent levels of specific IgG subclasses and frequent infections, but whether isolated

Table 4-17	Suggested Laboratory Screening Tests for Children with Suspected Immunodeficiency	
Immune System Component	**Example of Immunodeficiency**	**Screening Tests**
B lymphocyte	X-linked agammaglobulinemia	Quantitative immunoglobulin serum levels (IgG, IgA, IgM)
		Serum antibodies to tetanus, diphtheria, *Pneumococcus*
T lymphocyte	22q11 (DiGeorge) syndrome	T-cell lymphocyte subsets
		Lymphocyte mitogen stimulation test
Phagocyte	Chronic granulomatous disease	Total neutrophil count
		Dihydrorhodamine 123 assay
Complement	C3 deficiency	CH_{50} (hemolytic complement assay)

Figure 4-46 Agammaglobulinemia. Lateral neck radiograph shows absent adenoids.

Figure 4-47 Immune development. Serum immunoglobulin levels before and after birth.

subclass deficiency represents a true immune deficiency, particularly in the absence of impaired specific antibody responses, is controversial. Many immunologists prefer to assess functional antibody response to immunization rather than to examine IgG subclasses.

Selective IgA deficiency, which affects about 1 in 600 members of the general population, is the most common humoral antibody deficiency. Patients must have a complete absence of IgA, and the diagnosis cannot be made until 4 years of age because of the slow development of IgA production in normal children. Even though these patients are deficient in both serum and mucosal secretory IgA, only a minority of affected individuals manifest frequent infections. Synthesis of IgG and IgM is generally normal. Individuals with IgA deficiency have a modestly increased incidence of autoimmune syndromes, atopy, celiac disease, and inflammatory bowel disease.

Common Variable Immunodeficiency

Common variable immunodeficiency (CVID) can occur at any age and requires decreased levels of IgG, as well as of IgM and/or IgA. In addition, specific antibody responses are significantly depressed. Although defined by decreased antibody responses, many patients with CVID also have evidence of decreased T-cell function. Therefore in addition to the expected ear, sinus, and lung infections, patients may have infections with unusual pathogens, as well as autoimmune and granulomatous complications. Several different genetic defects underlying CVID have been identified, but the cause of most cases and the reason for delayed onset, often in middle age, remain unknown.

T-Cell and Combined (B- and T-Lymphocyte) Immunodeficiency

Isolated defects of T-lymphocyte, or cell-mediated, immunity are unusual. Because T-lymphocyte function is necessary for antibody production, most cellular immunodeficiencies are also associated with humoral immunodeficiency. Patients with T-lymphocyte deficiencies experience an increased frequency

of severe infections with viral agents such as herpes simplex virus and cytomegalovirus, certain fungi, intracellular parasites, and other organisms of relatively low virulence. Figure 4-48 demonstrates severe disseminated varicella infection in a child with congenital cellular immunodeficiency.

22q11.2 (DiGeorge or Velocardiofacial) Syndrome

22q11.2 syndrome is a T-cell immunodeficiency characterized by low to absent T-cell numbers with normal or near-normal B-cell numbers and function. Because the names *DiGeorge syndrome* and *velocardiofacial syndrome* were applied to specific syndromes that are now recognized to have the same underlying genetic defect, the broad term *22q11.2 deletion syndrome* is preferred. Thymic hypoplasia, which results from abnormal development of the third and fourth branchial pouches during embryogenesis, is the proximate cause of immunodeficiency in 22q11.2 syndrome. The thymus provides the necessary microenvironment for the maturation of lymphoid precursors into functioning T lymphocytes. When the thymus is absent, maturation does not proceed, resulting in cellular immunodeficiency. Because major cardiovascular structures and the parathyroid glands are derived from the same branchial pouches, affected children frequently present with signs of congenital heart disease and hypocalcemic tetany

Figure 4-48 Cellular immunodeficiency. An adolescent with abnormal T-lymphocyte function and disseminated varicella, in whom pneumonia resulted in respiratory failure.

Figure 4-49 22q11 syndrome. Characteristic facial features: frontal **(A)** and lateral **(B)** views. Note the micrognathia; hypertelorism; low-set, malformed ears; and smooth philtrum. Also note the midline scar from repair of a cardiac defect.

or seizures within the first few days of life. Patients often evidence characteristic facies (Fig. 4-49). The 22q11.2 deletion may occur as frequently as once in 3000 to 4000 live births, and rare cases with a similar phenotype but without the 22q11.2 deletion have been described.

Most patients with 22q11 syndrome have some thymic tissue and therefore have a low level of T lymphocytes and avoid infections with low-virulence pathogens. Such patients can often have the sinopulmonary infections typical of antibody deficiency. A minority (<0.5%) of patients with 22q11 syndrome do not have a thymus and present without functional T cells. They appear similar to infants with severe combined immunodeficiency (SCID) and will die of infection unless they receive a bone marrow or thymus transplant.

Chronic Mucocutaneous Candidiasis

Chronic mucocutaneous candidiasis (CMC) is a T-lymphocyte disorder typified by superficial candidal infections of the mucous membranes, skin, and nails. It can be associated with polyendocrinopathy, a disorder linked to deficiency in the *AIRE* (autoimmune regulator) gene. CMC may be sporadic or familial. Treatment of chronic mucocutaneous candidiasis involves long-term antifungal therapy. Fluconazole given orally has resulted in dramatic clinical improvement and decreased morbidity in affected patients. HIV infection is prominent in the differential of severe or recurrent candidal infections.

Severe Combined Immunodeficiency

SCID comprises a heterogeneous group of disorders with varying etiologies (Table 4-18). The consequent defects in lymphocyte maturation ultimately result in abnormalities of humoral and cellular immunity (see Fig. 4-42). Affected infants have recurrent severe bacterial, viral, fungal, and protozoal infections. Manifestations typically appear in the first few months of life and are often associated with failure to thrive, diarrhea, and severe candidiasis (Fig. 4-50). Affected infants may be distinguished from normal babies by the frequency and severity of infections and their resistance to appropriate antimicrobial therapy. Presenting symptoms usually involve

Figure 4-50 Severe combined immunodeficiency. Widespread fungal dermatitis with *Candida albicans* over the trunk **(A)** and foot **(B)** and nails **(C).**

Table 4-18   Classification of Selected Primary Immunodeficiency Diseases

Category	Designation	T-cell Levels	B-cell Levels
Combined lymphocyte defects	X-linked severe combined immunodeficiency	Low	Normal to high
	JAK3 deficiency	Low	Normal to high
	Adenosine deaminase deficiency	Progressive decrease	Progressive decrease
	Purine nucleoside phosphorylase deficiency	Progressive decrease	Normal
	Major histocompatibility complex class II deficiency	Low CD4$^+$ T cells	Normal
	ZAP-70 kinase deficiency	Low CD8$^+$ T cells	Normal
	Recombinase-activating gene deficiency	Low	Absent
	Reticular dysgenesis	Low	Low
	Omenn syndrome	Low	Low
	X-linked hyper-IgM syndrome	Normal	Normal
	DiGeorge syndrome	Normal to low	Normal
Antibody deficiencies	X-linked agammaglobulinemia	Normal	Very low to absent
	μ Heavy chain deficiency	Normal	Absent
	Immunoglobulin deficiency including IgA deficiency and IgG subclass deficiency	Normal	Normal
	Common variable immunodeficiency	Normal	Normal or low
Other distinctive syndromes	Wiskott-Aldrich syndrome	Normal to low	Normal
	Ataxia-telangiectasia	Normal	Normal
	Bloom syndrome	Normal	Normal
	Hyper-IgE syndrome (Job syndrome)	Normal	Normal
	X-linked lymphoproliferative syndrome	Normal	Normal
	Autoimmune lymphoproliferative syndrome	Normal to high: elevated CD4$^-$CD8$^-$ T cells	High
Phagocyte disorders	Chronic granulomatous disease	Normal	Normal
	Leukocyte adhesion deficiency	Normal	Normal
	Chédiak-Higashi syndrome	Normal	Normal
Complement disorders	Individual component deficiencies	Normal	Normal

Immunoglobulin Levels	Gene Defect and Pathogenesis	Genetic Locus
Low	Defect of γ chain of interleukin (IL)-2 receptor and receptors for other cytokines, IL-4, IL-7, IL-9, IL-15	IL2RG (SCIDX1), Xq13.1
Low	JAK3 intracellular signaling kinase defect	Jak3, 19p13.1
Low	Selective lymphocyte-toxic effects of purine pathway intermediates	ADA, 20q13.11
Normal or low	Lymphocyte-toxic effects of purine pathway intermediates	PNP, 14q13
Normal or low	Mutation in factors controlling major histocompatibility complex II gene expression	CIITA, 16p13; RFX5, 1q
Normal	Thymocyte intracellular kinase defect; blocked maturation of T cells	ZAP-70, 2q12
Absent	No T-cell or B-cell receptor rearrangement; blocked lymphocyte development	RAG1, RAG2, 11p13
Low	Unknown bone marrow stem cell defect	Autosomal recessive
Low	Unknown	Autosomal recessive
Normal to high IgM; low IgA, IgG	Defect of CD40 ligand, expressed on T cells: block in B-cell isotype switch	HIGMX, Xq25-q26
Normal to low	Embryologic defect of thymic development: variable associated defects of heart, parathyroid, face	22q11.2 and other loci
Low to absent	Defect of B-cell–specific Bruton's tyrosine kinase	XLA, Xq22
Absent	Defect of cell surface μ chain expression	IGHM, 14q32.3
One or more immunoglobulin types low	Unknown defects in B-cell isotype expression; IgG subclass deficiencies associated with immunoglobulin heavy- or light-chain gene deletions	
One or more subtypes low	Unknown late-onset variable defects in B- and T-cell function and regulation	Complex
Normal (some low IgM)	Defect of WASP gene involved in cytoskeleton; sparse, small platelets; eczema	WASP, Xp11.23
Normal	DNA repair defect in ATM gene; ataxia, progressive neurodegeneration; cancer; radiation sensitivity	ATM, 11q22-q23
Normal	DNA repair defect in BLM gene, progressive neurodegeneration, cancer, radiation sensitivity	BLM, 15q26.1
High IgE	Unknown, susceptibility to cutaneous boils and lung abscess formation	Unknown
Normal	Fatal infection or immune compromise on Epstein-Barr virus encounter	XLP, Xq24-q26
High	Impaired Fas-mediated apoptosis of B and T cells; lymphadenopathy, autoimmunity	FAS, 10q24; complex
Normal	Impaired killing of ingested organisms due to defects in four genes encoding enzymes of the cytochrome oxidase system	CYBB (gp91^{phox}), Xp21.1; CYBA (p22^{phox}), 16q24.1; NCF1 (p47^{phox}), 7q11.23; NCF2 (p67^{phox}), 1q25
Normal	Defects of CD18 or other leukocyte surface proteins required for motility, adherence, and endocytosis	CD18, 21q22.3
Normal	Defect of LYST gene causing faulty lysosomal assembly, giant cytoplasmic granules	LYST, 1q42-q44
Normal	C1, C2, C4, C3 deficiencies associated with autoimmunity and pyogenic infections; C3, C5-C9, and properdin deficiencies with neisserial infections	Autosomal recessive: chromosomes 6p, 1q, etc.; X-linked: properdin

Figure 4-52 Chest radiograph of infant with severe combined immunodeficiency disease. Note the absent thymic shadow and bilateral pulmonary infiltrates.

Figure 4-51 Severe combined immunodeficiency. Absolute lymphocyte counts in normal infants and infants with severe combined immunodeficiency disease *(closed circles).* The *heavy line* indicates the mean lymphocyte counts in normal infants in relation to age. The *light dotted lines* indicate the 95% confidence limits. *(From Gossage DL, Buckley RH: Prevalence of lymphopenia in severe combined immunodeficiency, N Engl J Med 322:1422-1423, 1990. Copyright © 1990 Massachusetts Medical Society. All rights reserved.)*

and components of the T-cell receptor–associated signaling apparatus.

Partial Combined Immunodeficiencies

Wiskott-Aldrich Syndrome

Wiskott-Aldrich syndrome (WAS) is an X-linked recessive disorder characterized by eczema, thrombocytopenia, and small platelets with cutaneous petechiae, and recurrent infections that begin in infancy (Fig. 4-53). Inability to form antibody to bacterial capsular polysaccharide antigens is the most commonly reported immunologic defect, but some patients also

the respiratory tract, with pneumonia resulting from *P. jirovecii* or virulent bacterial pathogens being common. In addition to the clinical findings of infection, examination discloses hypoplastic or absent tonsils and lymph nodes. Laboratory abnormalities include peripheral blood lymphopenia (Fig. 4-51), decreased serum immunoglobulin levels, and defective lymphocyte responses to mitogens such as phytohemagglutinin. Histologic examination of tonsillar, adenoidal, and lymph node remnants reveals immature lymphoid tissue. The thymus is typically dysplastic histologically and radiographically (Fig. 4-52); normal lobulation and corticomedullary differentiation are lacking, and the number of lymphocytes is decreased.

Once the diagnosis of SCID is considered, the child must be placed in protective isolation and given appropriate supportive therapy including IgG replacement. All administered blood products must be irradiated to prevent the development of severe graft-versus-host disease, and live virus vaccines are contraindicated. These patients can be essentially cured by bone marrow transplantation. Children with SCID have been the initial recipients of gene therapy, which is curative but has led to an unexpectedly high incidence of leukemia.

Various genetic defects have been identified in patients with SCID, most of which result in a developmental block in T-cell maturation. Most common is the X-linked common γ chain that is a component of several cytokine receptors. Lack of IL-7 signaling also prevents maturation of functional T cells. Some enzyme deficiencies, such as inherited deficiency of adenosine deaminase (ADA), are also associated with SCID. This disease causes the accumulation of metabolic substrates that are toxic to T and B lymphocytes. ADA deficiency can also lead to other symptoms including skeletal changes, hearing loss, and behavioral issues due to systemic toxicity of adenosine metabolites. Other defects leading to SCID include mutations in *Jak3,* which is responsible for signaling via the common γ chain,

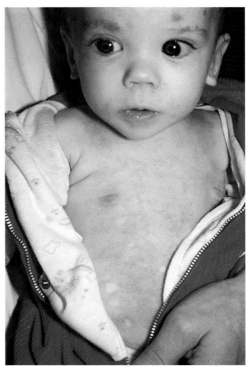

Figure 4-53 Wiskott-Aldrich syndrome. The skin eruptions on the trunk and face are eczematoid and pruritic but not always similar to atopic dermatitis in flexural distribution. *(From Fireman P, Slavin RG: Atlas of allergies, New York, 1990, Gower.)*

manifest a partial defect in T-lymphocyte responses, which seems to worsen with age. The most common cause of death is intracranial hemorrhage secondary to thrombocytopenia. As boys with Wiskott-Aldrich age they have an increased risk of malignancy, particularly lymphoma. Bone marrow transplantation is curative but has a high mortality rate in the absence of an HLA-matched sibling donor. The defective protein in WAS is termed WASP (Wiskott-Aldrich syndrome protein) and serves to link T-cell signaling at the cell surface to changes of the cytoskeleton.

Ataxia-Telangiectasia

Ataxia-telangiectasia (AT) is a complex and intriguing immunodeficiency disorder with autosomal recessive inheritance and an unusually pleiotropic presentation: telangiectasia, progressive ataxia, and variable immunodeficiency. Most patients develop ocular telangiectasia and ataxia during the first 6 years of life (see Chapter 15). The ataxia is cerebellar in nature and characteristically progressive. Neurologic involvement may be extensive, including abnormalities of speech, movement, and gait and mental retardation. The progressive, variable immunodeficiency commonly consists of humoral defects and depressed T-lymphocyte function. Recurrent sinus and pulmonary infections, which may lead to bronchiectasis, are common and may be responsible for early death. These patients have a dramatically higher incidence of neoplasia, consistent with the gene underlying AT, which limits cell division in the presence of DNA damage. Exposure to ionizing radiation, including in medical imaging, should be avoided as much as possible in patients with ataxia-telangiectasia.

Hyper-IgM Syndrome

Hyper-IgM syndrome, although defined on the basis of abnormal immunoglobulin production, is actually a combined immune deficiency. Hyper-IgM syndrome is due to an inability of B lymphocytes to class switch from the germ line–encoded IgM heavy chain constant region to other isotypes (e.g., IgA, IgM, IgE). Patients have normal to elevated IgM levels but reduced or absent levels of IgA and IgG. Specific antibody responses are also deficient. The most common form of hyper-IgM syndrome is deficiency of CD154 (CD40 ligand), which is expressed by T lymphocytes and required for B-cell class switching. In addition to sinopulmonary infections, *Pneumocystis* pneumonia and *Cryptosporidium* diarrhea are often seen, demonstrating that defects in both humoral and cellular immunity are present. Although CD154 deficiency is X-linked, defects in other, autosomal genes required for class switching lead to a similar phenotype.

Hyper-IgE Syndrome

Hyper-IgE syndrome is a disorder with both autosomal dominant and autosomal recessive inheritance and is characterized by marked elevation of serum IgE. Clinical features include recurrent staphylococcal infections, a pruritic eczematous dermatitis, and coarse facial features (Fig. 4-54). Recurrent staphylococcal skin infections including impetigo and furuncles are especially common and typically resistant to therapy. Staphylococcal pneumonia complicated by pneumatocele formation (Fig. 4-55) and lung abscesses are frequent. Other organisms of relatively low virulence, including *Candida albicans,* may cause infection. Immunologic findings include markedly elevated IgE levels (>2000 IU/mL); eosinophilia; abnormal cell-mediated immunity; and, in certain patients, abnormal polymorphonuclear leukocyte chemotaxis. The autosomal dominant, but not the autosomal recessive, form is also associated with frequent fractures of long bones and delayed eruption of secondary teeth. It should be stressed that many patients with atopic dermatitis

Figure 4-54   Hyper-IgE syndrome. Note the coarse facial features of the girl on the left, including the broad nasal bridge, fleshy nasal tip, and mild prognathism compared with her unaffected sister.

have elevated IgE levels, often markedly so, but do not have the hyper-IgE syndrome.

PHAGOCYTIC DISORDERS

Polymorphonuclear leukocytes and mononuclear cells play vital roles in the defense against acute infections. Normal neutrophil numbers, intact neutrophil chemotaxis, phagocytosis, and killing are necessary for elimination of microorganisms that invade the skin or mucous membranes. Patients with neutropenia are vulnerable to bacterial infections, as are patients with disorders of phagocyte function. The neutropenias and Chédiak-Higashi syndrome are discussed in Chapter 11.

Chronic granulomatous disease (CGD) is the most common phagocytic immunodeficiency. Neutrophil chemotaxis and phagocytosis are intact, but killing of ingested microorganisms is defective. The responsible biochemical defect results in abnormal activation of oxidative metabolism in neutrophil granules and inability to kill microorganisms. The mechanism underlying generation of the characteristic granulomas is unclear, but may involve defective inactivation of inflammatory markers. A test of neutrophil oxidative burst is used to diagnose CGD. Historically, the nitroblue tetrazolium (NBT) test has been used for diagnosis, but the NBT test has been supplanted by a flow-cytometric assay based on reduction of the dye dihydrorhodamine 123 (DHR).

Figure 4-55   Hyper-IgE syndrome. Note the clearly outlined pneumatocele in the right lung. This encapsulated lesion frequently complicates *Staphylococcus aureus* pneumonia.

Figure 4-56 Chronic granulomatous disease (CGD). The neutrophil NADPH oxidase complex is shown. Components in which mutations have been detected in patients with chronic granulomatous disease are shown in *tan*. X-linked deficiency of gp91^{phox} is the most common cause of CGD, accounting for about two thirds of cases. *(From Bonilla FA, Geha RS: Primary immunodeficiency diseases, J Allergy Clin Immunol 111:S571-S581, 2004.)*

The cytooxidase complex has four subunits (Fig. 4-56). The most common defect is X-linked, but defects in the other subunits are due to an autosomal recessive pattern of inheritance. The X-linked form is generally more severe. Clinically, most children with chronic granulomatous disease become symptomatic early in life, developing infections with catalase-positive bacteria and fungi. The skin, lungs, liver, and lymph nodes are the most common sites of infections, and five organisms account for the majority of infections: *Staphylococcus aureus, Burkholderia cepacia, Serratia marcescens, Aspergillus* species, and *Nocardia*. Liver abscesses and invasive *Aspergillus* lung infection in the absence of known immunosuppression strongly suggest CGD. Hepatosplenomegaly is a frequent physical finding and presumably represents involvement of the reticuloendothelial system. Granulomas may also develop in other organs. In the patient whose radiograph is seen in Figure 4-57, the diagnosis of chronic granulomatous disease was suggested by the finding of antral narrowing secondary to granulomatous involvement of the gastric antrum. Effective antimicrobial prophylaxis with trimethoprim-sulfamethoxazole and itraconazole, as well as cytokine therapy with interferon-γ, helps minimize infectious complications of CGD.

Leukocyte Adhesion Deficiency

Leukocyte adhesion deficiency (LAD) is rare, but most commonly results from a deficiency in CD18. This molecule is a component of β$_2$ integrins, which are required for neutrophils to exit blood vessels and enter tissue. The patients have a variety of symptoms including delayed umbilical cord separation (Fig. 4-58, *A*), a persistent and dramatic peripheral blood granulocytosis (due to the inability of neutrophils to migrate through the endothelium and into tissue), recurrent soft tissue infections, and impaired wound healing. The vast majority of infants with delayed cord separation, however, will not have LAD. Because these patients do not mobilize neutrophils in response to infection, many aspects of the normal inflammatory response are lacking including the formation of pus (Fig. 4-58, *B*). LAD deficiency should be suspected in any infant with periumbilical problems and persistent peripheral blood leukocytosis (frequently >50,000 cells/mm^3). Other rare causes of LAD have also been described.

Figure 4-58 Leukocyte adhesion deficiency. **A,** Infection involving and surrounding the umbilical cord. **B,** Histopathologic appearance of a scalp abscess. Note the presence of bacterial colonies (purple staining) and distinct lack of host cellular inflammatory response. (**A,** *Courtesy Kenneth Schuit, MD, Pittsburgh, Pa;* **B,** *courtesy Kenneth Schuit, MD, and William Robichaux, MD, Pittsburgh, Pa.)*

Figure 4-57 Chronic granulomatous disease (CGD). Barium contrast radiogram demonstrating the "string sign," a thin line of barium that represents narrowing of the gastric antrum secondary to granuloma formation. This child had persistent vomiting but none of the usual stigmata of CGD.

Figure 4-59   Characteristic facial features of NEMO deficiency. These include fine sparse hair, few teeth, conical incisors, depressed nasal bridge, and frontal bossing.

COMPLEMENT SYSTEM DISORDERS

The complement system is a complex system of serum proteins that require serial activation through the classical, alternative, or mannose-binding lectin (MBL) pathway. Complement mediates and amplifies many of the biologic functions of the immune system. These functions include (1) enhancement of phagocytosis (opsonization) and viral neutralization, (2) mediation of inflammation via chemotaxis and alteration of vascular permeability, (3) cell lysis, and (4) modulation of the immune response. Although rare, inherited deficiencies of most complement components have been reported. Clinical presentation varies, depending on the specific complement protein involved. Frequent modes of presentation for complement component deficiencies are collagen vascular diseases for defects in components C1 through C4, disseminated infections with pyogenic bacteria for C3, and disseminated neisserial infections for C5 through C8. C9 deficiency is often asymptomatic. The CH_{50} assay is a simple screening test for complement deficiency. A normal result effectively rules out complement dysfunction. Workup for complement deficiency should be undertaken in patients with severe or recurrent neisserial infection or in patients with recurrent sinopulmonary infections and normal antibody studies. A defect in C1 esterase inhibitor results in hereditary angioedema, which is discussed in an earlier section.

There is wide variation in MBL levels in the general population, with some reports showing increased rates of infection in individuals with low or absent MBL levels. However, a substantial portion of the population (5% to 8%) has low or undetectable levels and most of these patients do not have unusually frequent or severe infections.

Other Innate Defects

Several innate immune defects predisposing to infections have been identified. These include deficiency in nuclear factor (NF)-κB essential modifier (NEMO, also known as IKK-γ). This disorder is characterized by mutations that disrupt the function of NEMO, which is encoded on the X chromosome. Boys with NEMO are susceptible to a variety of infections including infection with pyogenic bacteria, mycobacteria, and viruses. They also have ectodermal dysplasia with sparse hair, few conical teeth, and frontal bossing (Fig. 4-59).

Toll-like receptors (TLRs) are among the receptors responsible for recognizing PAMPs, and signaling through TLRs helps alert the immune system to the presence of infections. Defects in TLR signaling, including the molecules MyD88 and IRAK4, which transduce signals from the membrane-associated TLRs to the interior of the cell, have been recognized in patients with recurrent pneumococcal infections. Defects in signaling via TLR-3, which recognizes double-stranded RNA, has been implicated in susceptibility to herpes simplex virus (HSV) infections.

ANATOMIC AND MUCOSAL DISORDERS

Preventing the entry of microorganisms into sterile sites and clearance of infections from these sites represent the first line of defense. Intact mucosal barriers are of crucial importance in preventing the entrance of microorganisms into the host. The respiratory and GI mucosa aid in host defense by secreting antibodies (predominantly IgA) into their lumina. Also, physical factors such as saliva flow in the oral cavity, intestinal peristalsis, and the coughing reflex are important in the "washing out" effect on potential pathogens. Anything that prevents clearance may predispose to infections in the upper airway. Hypertrophy of the adenoids can inhibit both eustachian tube function and drainage from the sinuses, predisposing to ear and sinus infections. Patients with unusual anatomy due to cleft palate or other craniofacial abnormalities (see Chapter 22) often have frequent infections despite an intact immune system.

Immotile cilia syndrome is characterized by a defect in mucociliary transport, another component of the mucosal barrier. This disorder was first described as Kartagener

Figure 4-60 Kartagener syndrome. Dextrocardia and situs inversus of the abdominal organs. Abnormal ciliary motion is thought to result in malrotation during embryogenesis.

syndrome, which consists of a triad of situs inversus (Fig. 4-60), chronic sinusitis, and bronchiectasis. These patients were also noted to be infertile because their spermatozoa were poorly motile, due to the lack of dynein arms in their tails. Studies revealed similar defects in mucosal cilia and led to recognition of the fact that the phenomenon could exist in the absence of situs inversus. The resultant ciliary dysfunction impedes mucus clearance and produces a combination of the following signs and symptoms: (1) early onset of chronic rhinorrhea, (2) chronic otitis media, (3) chronic

sinusitis with opaque sinuses on radiography, (4) chronic productive cough, (5) bronchiectasis, (6) digital clubbing, and (7) nasal polyps. The disorder should be suspected in any child with chronic or recurrent upper or lower respiratory tract infections. When situs inversus is not present, the diagnosis of immotile cilia syndrome requires confirmation by electron microscopic analysis of cilia obtained from a biopsy of the nasal or tracheobronchial mucosa (Fig. 4-61).

Bibliography

Adkinson NF, Yuninger JW, Busse WW, et al: *Middleton's allergy: principles and practice*, ed 6, St. Louis, 2003, Mosby.

American Academy of Allergy, Asthma, & Immunology: *The allergy report: diseases of the atopic diathesis*, Vol 2, Milwaukee, Wis, 2000, American Academy of Allergy, Asthma, & Immunology.

Bonilla FA, Bernstein IL, Kahn DA, et al: Practice parameter for the diagnosis and management of primary immunodeficiency, *Ann Allergy Asthma Immunol* 94:S1–S63, 2005.

Bonilla FA, Geha RS: Primary immunodeficiency diseases, *J Allergy Clin Immunol* 111:S571–S581, 2004

Borish L: Allergic rhinitis: systemic inflammation and implication for treatment, *J Allergy Clin Immunol* 112:1021–1031, 2003.

Castro-Rodriquez JA, Holberg CJ, Wright AL, et al: A clinical index to define risk of asthma in young children with recurrent wheezing, *Am J Respir Crit Care Med* 162:1403–1406, 2000.

Global Initiative for Asthma: Global strategy for asthma management and prevention. Web publication, 2005. Available at http://www.ginasthma.com

Gruchella RS: Drug allergy, *J Allergy Clin Immunol* 111:S548–S559, 2003.

International Rhinitis Management Working Group: International consensus report on the diagnosis and management of rhinitis: allergy, *Eur J Allergy Clin Immunol* 49:1–34, 1994.

Laitinen LA, Laitinen A, Haahtela T: Airway mucosal inflammation even in patients with newly diagnosed asthma, *Am Rev Respir Dis* 147:697–704, 1993.

Lawley TJ, Bielory L, Gascon P, et al: A prospective clinical and immunologic analysis of patients with serum sickness, *N Engl J Med* 311:1407–1413, 1984.

Liu AH, Jaramillo R, Sicherer SH, et al: National prevalence and risk factors for food allergy and relationship to asthma: results from the National Health and Nutrition Examination Survey 2005-2006, *J Allergy Clin Immunol* 126:798–806, 2010.

Martinez FD, Stern DA, Wright AL, et al: Differential immune responses to acute lower respiratory illness in early life and subsequent development of persistent wheezing and asthma, *J Allergy Clin Immunol* 102:915–920, 1998.

Martinez FD, Wright AL, Taussig LM, et al: Asthma and wheezing in the first six years of life, *N Engl J Med* 332:133–138, 1995.

Moffet JE, Golden DKB, Reisman RE, et al: Stinging insect hypersensitivity: a practice parameter update, *J Allergy Clin Immunol* 114:869–886, 2004.

National Asthma Education and Prevention Program: *Expert Panel Report 3 (EPR-3): guidelines for the diagnosis and management of asthma*. Bethesda, Md, 2007, National Institute of Health. Available at http://www.nhlbi.nih.gov/guidelines/asthma.

Ochs HD, Smith CIE, Puck JM, editors: *Primary immunodeficiency diseases*, New York, 1999, Oxford University Press.

Puck JM: Primary immunodeficiency diseases, *JAMA* 278:1835–1841, 1997.

Rachelefsky GS, Shapiro GG, Bergman D, et al, Pediatric Asthma Committee: *Pediatric asthma: promoting best practice guide for managing asthma in children*, Milwaukee, Wis, 1999, American Academy of Allergy, Asthma, & Immunology.

Rosenzweig SD, Holland SM: Phagocyte immunodeficiencies and their infections, *J Allergy Clin Immunol* 113:620–626, 2004.

Sampson HA, Munoz-Furlong A, Campbell RL, et al: Second symposium on the definition and management of anaphylaxis: Summary report—second National Institute of Allergy and Infectious Disease/Food Allergy and Anaphylaxis Network symposium, *J Allergy Clin Immunol* 117:391–397, 2006.

Shearer WT, Leung DYM, eds. 2008 mini-primer on allergic disease, *J Allergy Clin Immunol* 121:S363–S426, 2008.

Stiehm ER, Ochs HD, Winklestein JA, editors: *Immunologic disorders in infants and children*, ed 5, Philadelphia, 2004, Elsevier Saunders.

Figure 4-61 Immotile cilia syndrome. **A,** Electron micrograph of cilia from a patient with immotile cilia syndrome. Note the absence of dynein arms from the outer doublets. **B,** Normal cilia with dynein arms. *(From Bluestone C, Stool S: Pediatric otolaryngology, vol 1, Philadelphia, 1983, WB Saunders.)*

CARDIOLOGY

5

Lee B. Beerman | Jacqueline Kreutzer | Vivek Allada

This chapter addresses the initial approach to a patient with suspected or known heart disease by physical examination, chest x-ray, and electrocardiogram. A proper initial assessment helps to avoid the expense of unnecessary testing. However, the practice of cardiology as a pediatric subspecialty continues to evolve rapidly with expansion and enhancement of imaging technology and therapeutic options. Complex structural congenital anomalies can be precisely defined by a combination of techniques that include echocardiography, cardiac catheterization with angiography, nuclear imaging, magnetic resonance imaging (MRI), and computed tomographic (CT) angiography. Concomitant with advances in diagnostic capabilities have come remarkable advances in therapy, both surgical and by interventional catheterization. Therefore we have included considerable material on echocardiography and color flow Doppler studies, which remain the preeminent imaging modalities in pediatric cardiology. In addition, we have described the common surgical procedures used and added an updated section on the expanding array of therapeutic options in the cardiac catheterization laboratory.

The three prerequisites to a good cardiovascular examination are a proper environment, a cooperative child, and the conviction on the part of the physician that the examination is important. A heart murmur is not the only part and often is not even the most important part of the cardiac physical examination. Blood pressure determination, character of the pulse and precordial activity, observation of cyanosis, clubbing of the nail beds of the fingers or toes, and dysmorphic facial or other physical features may provide clues to the diagnosis and nature of congenital heart lesions before auscultation is even performed.

PHYSICAL DIAGNOSIS OF CONGENITAL HEART DISEASE

Cyanosis and Clubbing

Even before mild desaturation is detectable, early clubbing and cyanosis may be seen (Figs. 5-1 and 5-2). The base of the nail, especially the thumbnail, may show loss of the angle as early as 3 months of age (see Chapter 16). Elevated hemoglobin and hematocrit and loss of nail angle indicate hypoxemia and the presence of a right-to-left intracardiac shunt (Fig. 5-3). If heart disease is excluded, chronic pulmonary disease should be considered as another potential cause of clubbing.

Observation of the lips and mucous membranes for the presence of cyanosis is best done in good daylight because fluorescent lighting may produce a false cyanotic tinge. In the presence of polycythemia with hemoglobin in the 18 to 20 gm/dL range and hematocrit greater than 60%, the conjunctival vessels become engorged and plethoric (see Fig. 5-2). Conversely, when a patient is anemic, visible cyanosis can be easily missed (this is particularly important in infancy, when babies reach the physiologic nadir in hematocrit). Differential cyanosis between the upper and lower extremities is an unusual

clinical finding. If the patient has pulmonary vascular disease, reverse flow through a patent ductus arteriosus with no right-to-left intracardiac shunting, cyanosis, and clubbing may be found in the lower extremities but not in the hands (Fig. 5-4).

Blood Pressure and Pulse

Blood pressure determination in infants and children is an integral part of the cardiac physical examination. Attention to proper cuff size prevents the misdiagnosis of systolic hypertension from an undersized cuff. In general, it is better to use an oversized cuff because overestimation of systolic blood pressure can be avoided. Blood pressure can be tracked in children over time, and tables depicting normal blood pressure range for age have been published. Blood pressure determination in both arms and a lower extremity will detect coarctation of the aorta, lend support for the diagnosis of supravalvular aortic stenosis (blood pressure higher in the right arm than in the left arm, due to the Coanda effect), and help to assess the severity of aortic valve disease including aortic valve stenosis (narrow pulse pressure) and aortic regurgitation (wide pulse pressure).

Heart Murmur Evaluation

Murmurs are relatively common in the newborn period. A common innocent heart murmur (peripheral pulmonic stenosis) during this period originates from the branch pulmonary arteries because of their relatively small size compared with the main pulmonary artery; this is a result of the normal fetal flow pattern, which delivers limited flow to the right and left pulmonary arteries. Characteristically, this murmur is early systolic and loudest over both axillae and the back. The murmur of branch pulmonary artery stenosis has the same distribution as the structural lesions that cause increased pulmonary blood flow. A transient systolic murmur at the middle-low left sternal border in the normal newborn can be due to tricuspid regurgitation, and a soft systolic ejection murmur at the upper left sternal border may arise from a closing patent ductus arteriosus. A large ventricular septal defect does not produce a murmur in the newborn period because the initially high pulmonary vascular resistance results in minimal shunting across the defect. On the other hand, pathologic systolic murmurs in the newborn are caused by restrictive ventricular septal defects and lesions producing left and right ventricular outflow tract obstruction (i.e., tetralogy of Fallot and valvular aortic or pulmonary stenosis). In the newborn it can be difficult to distinguish the murmur of a small restrictive ventricular septal defect from that of a severe right ventricular outflow tract obstruction in tetralogy of Fallot or left ventricular outflow obstruction. The implications of this differential diagnosis are such that an echocardiogram is recommended for infants with this clinical presentation.

Contrary to popular belief, the presence of a continuous murmur from a patent ductus arteriosus is extremely rare in

Figure 5-1   Mild cyanosis. **A,** This child shows no obvious cyanosis of the face and lips, although the photograph in **B** demonstrates clubbing; note the loss of nail angle and curvature of the nails, especially of the thumb.

a full-term newborn. This is because the normal elevation of pulmonary artery pressure at this age minimizes the diastolic gradient between the aorta and pulmonary artery, attenuating or eliminating any diastolic component of the murmur. If a continuous murmur is heard in the newborn, patent ductus–dependent pulmonary blood flow or systemic to pulmonary

collateral vessels in association with pulmonary atresia complex should be considered.

Preschoolers and school-age children are commonly referred for evaluation of a heart murmur. Innocent murmurs of childhood fall into four major categories: systolic ejection murmurs at the base; vibratory, or Still's, murmur; venous hums; and

Figure 5-2   Moderate cyanosis. This child demonstrates moderate cyanosis of the lips **(A)** and nails **(B).** Note also the reddish discoloration of the eyes resulting from conjunctival suffusion.

Figure 5-3   Severe cyanosis. Severe cyanosis of the lips, tongue, and mucous membranes can be noted in **A,** associated with marked clubbing and cyanosis of the nails in **B**.

Figure 5-4 Differential cyanosis and clubbing resulting from reverse shunting through a patent ductus arteriosus in a patient with pulmonary vascular disease. Note the marked cyanosis and clubbing of the toes, although the finger appears to be normal. *(Courtesy J.R. Zuberbuhler, MD, Pittsburgh, Pa.)*

Table 5-1	Innocent Murmurs Mimicking Congenital Heart Disease
Innocent Heart Murmur	**Structural Congenital Heart Disease**
Systolic Ejection Murmur at the Base of the Heart	

High left sternal border	Pulmonary valve stenosis
	    Ejection click
	    Transmission to back
	Atrial septal defect
	    Parasternal lift*
	    S₂ wide split*
	    Diastolic murmur of tricuspid flow*

High right sternal border	Aortic valve stenosis
	    Ejection click*
	    Radiation to neck*

Still Murmur	

Vibratory quality
Location: left midsternal border
	Ventricular septal defect
	    Character of murmur*
	Discrete subaortic stenosis
	    Radiation to aortic area*
	Subpulmonic stenosis
	    Radiation to pulmonic area*
	    Soft P₂*

Venous Hum	

Continuous
Location: neck and under clavicles
Usually loudest when sitting,
    disappears in supine posture
	Patent ductus arteriosus
	    Location under left clavicle*
	    No change with position*
	Coronary AV malformation
	    Accentuated in diastole*

Carotid and Cranial Bruits	

Murmur over carotids and head	Aortic stenosis
	AV malformation
	    Continuous murmur would support
	    AV malformation*

*Distinguishing features.
AV, atrioventricular; P₂, pulmonic second sound; S₂, second heart sound.

carotid and cranial bruits. In most instances there are associated clinical and laboratory studies that can distinguish the innocent from the pathologic murmur. Table 5-1 summarizes the distinguishing features and differential diagnosis. Figure 5-5 illustrates the sites where murmurs resulting from various cardiovascular lesions are best heard.

Syndrome-associated Physical Findings

Dysmorphology of the face and habitus suggests certain syndromes associated with congenital heart disease (Table 5-2).

The typical features in *Down syndrome (trisomy 21)* are discussed in Chapter 1. About 40% of children with this syndrome have structural lesions such as atrioventricular septal defects (complete or partial AVSD), isolated ventricular septal defects, patent ductus arteriosus, or anomalous origin of the subclavian arteries. Although many infants with Down syndrome and congenital heart disease have chronic congestive heart failure and growth failure, there is a subset of infants with a significant septal defect who may grow and develop appropriately. This is related to abnormally high pulmonary vascular resistance not decreasing in the usual fashion in this group, leading to early pulmonary vascular disease. Because this presentation may be silent, it is important that all children with Down syndrome be thoroughly evaluated during early

Figure 5-5 Sites where murmurs resulting from various cardiovascular lesions are best heard.

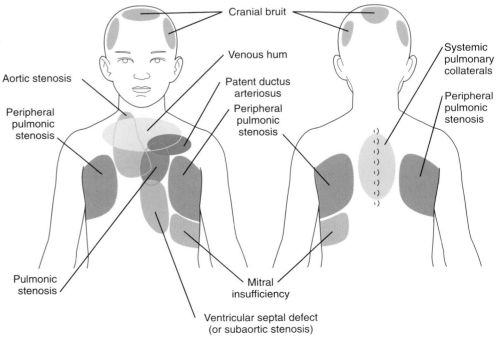

Table 5-2	Dysmorphology Syndromes and Trisomies with Associated Cardiovascular Abnormalities
Syndrome	**Common Cardiac Defect**
DiGeorge/ velocardiofacial (22q11 deletion)	Aortic arch abnormalities: interrupted arch (type B), right aortic arch Conotruncal abnormalities: truncus arteriosus, tetralogy of Fallot, pulmonary atresia with ventricular septal defect
Ellis–van Creveld	Atrial septal defect or single atrium
Fetal alcohol	Ventricular septal defect
Holt-Oram	Atrial and ventricular septal defects, arrhythmias
Marfan	Dilation of ascending aorta/aortic sinus, aortic and mitral insufficiency
Noonan	Dysplastic pulmonic valve, atrial septal defect
Turner	Coarctation of the aorta, bicuspid aortic valve
Williams	Supravalvular aortic stenosis, pulmonary artery stenosis
Trisomy	
13	Patent ductus arteriosus, septal defects, pulmonic and aortic stenosis (atresia)
18	Ventricular septal defect, polyvalvular disease, coronary abnormalities
21 (Down)	Atrioventricular septal defects, ventricular septal defect, patent ductus arteriosus, anomalous subclavian artery

infancy. The evaluation should include an echocardiogram to rule out congenital heart disease.

DiGeorge and *velocardiofacial syndromes* are related developmental disorders involving the third and fourth pharyngeal pouches. They have been shown to be caused by deletions within a critical region of chromosome 22q11 (which can be evaluated by a blood test, namely, fluorescence in situ hybridization [FISH], for 22q11 deletion). Cardiac abnormalities, particularly the conotruncal type and aortic arch anomalies, occur in 75% of patients with 22q11 deletion (see Table 5-2). Other findings include hypocalcemia, cleft palate, renal anomalies, immunologic defects, facial dysmorphisms, and variable developmental delay with educational and behavioral issues (see Chapter 4).

Ellis-van Creveld syndrome is an autosomal recessive disorder characterized by multiple gingival frenula, natal teeth, and polydactyly (Fig. 5-6). The patient with this syndrome frequently has an atrial septal defect or a common atrium.

Holt-Oram syndrome, an autosomal dominant disorder, is associated with upper limb deformities consisting of narrow shoulders, hypoplasia of the radius, and phocomelia (Fig. 5-7). Absence of both radius and thumb or proximal displacement of the thumb is the most frequent finding. Commonly

associated cardiovascular abnormalities include an atrial septal defect, ventricular septal defect, and arrhythmias (atrial and ventricular ectopy and atrioventricular block).

Marfan syndrome also has autosomal dominant inheritance; it manifests as a connective tissue disorder in which the elastic fibers are disrupted, causing cystic medial necrosis of the aorta, as well as joint laxity and subluxation of the ocular lens. Affected patients are tall, with increased limb length compared with the trunk. Their arm span exceeds their height. The cardiovascular abnormalities nearly always found in this syndrome include aneurysmal dilation of the aorta and aortic sinuses and mitral valve prolapse. Associated aortic and mitral valve regurgitation are common (Fig. 5-8) (see Chapter 1).

The most common cardiac defects in *Turner syndrome* are coarctation of the aorta and a bicuspid aortic valve. (See Chapters 1 and 9 for a detailed discussion of Turner syndrome).

Patients with *Noonan syndrome* have features characteristic of Turner syndrome but possess a defect on chromosome 12 and may be male or female. Clinically, these children have the findings of webbing of the neck, pectus excavatum, shield chest with widely spaced nipples, short stature, epicanthal folds, low-set ears, and increased carrying angle of the arms (Fig. 5-9). Common cardiovascular defects include pulmonary stenosis in association with a dysplastic pulmonary valve, atrial septal defect, and hypertrophic cardiomyopathy. On occasion, there may be dysplasia of all cardiac valves. The syndrome appears as an autosomal dominant disorder; multiple members of a family are often affected.

Patients with *Williams syndrome* characteristically have "elfin" facies: a broad maxilla, a small mandible with full mouth and large upper lip (philtrum), upturned nose, and a full forehead (Fig. 5-10). This syndrome has been associated with hypercalcemia in infants, a strikingly affable personality despite variable degrees of developmental delay, and has an identifiable genetic abnormality. Supravalvular aortic stenosis and pulmonary artery branch stenosis are the common cardiovascular abnormalities associated with this syndrome.

In addition, there are many other genetically determined diseases and inborn errors of metabolism with cardiac involvement, the most common of which are listed in Table 5-3.

Visible Clues in Acute Rheumatic Fever

Examination of the skin in a patient with acute rheumatic fever may reveal the typical rash of erythema marginatum, although this rash is not specific for rheumatic fever. It is

Figure 5-6   Ellis–van Creveld syndrome. Note the gingival frenula and natal teeth **(A)** and multiple digits (polydactyly) **(B).**

Table 5-3	Other Genetic Syndromes and Inborn Errors of Metabolism with Associated Cardiovascular Findings

Genetically Determined Diseases	Cardiac Findings
Metabolic	
Pompe disease (glycogen storage)	Cardiomyopathy (storage of glycogen in myocardium)
MPS	Storage of MPS in arteries and coronary arteries, valves with insufficiency and stenosis
	Hurler syndrome (MPS IH), Hunter syndrome (MPS II), Scheie syndrome (MPS IS), Hurler-Scheie syndrome (MPS IH/S), Morquio syndrome (MPS IV)
Hyperlipoproteinemia, familial type II	Premature atherosclerosis of arteries including coronary arteries
Neurologic	
Friedreich ataxia	Cardiomyopathy (congestive or hypertrophic)
Muscular dystrophies	Myocardial degeneration and fibrosis

Inborn Error of Metabolism (No Proven Genetic Basis)	Cardiac Findings
Progeria	Hypercholesterolemia, atherosclerotic changes in arteries including coronary arteries

MPS, mucopolysaccharidosis.

evanescent, nonpruritic, has sharp serpiginous margins, and is found on the inner aspects of the upper arms and thighs and on the trunk (Fig. 5-11). The differential diagnosis includes (1) drug rash, which is papular and pruritic; (2) erythema multiforme, which has target lesions; (3) rash of juvenile rheumatoid arthritis, which is pink, macular, and lacks wavy margins, and which may be transient; and (4) the cutaneous findings of Kawasaki disease (see Chapter 7).

Subcutaneous nodules are rare in chronic rheumatic heart disease, but if found, they are almost always associated with severe carditis. These movable, nontender, cartilage-like swellings vary in size from 2 mm to 1 cm and are persistent. They are seen over the bony prominences of the large joints and external surfaces of the elbows and knuckles of the hands, knees, and ankles. They may also be felt along the spine and over the skull. Although difficult to photograph, they are easily palpated (Fig. 5-12).

Signs of Bacterial Endocarditis

Although the clinical presentation of bacterial endocarditis varies according to the infecting organism, it should be suspected in any patient with congenital or acquired heart disease who has prolonged fever without apparent cause. The classic skin lesions include petechiae, splinter hemorrhages of the nails, conjunctival hemorrhages, and Janeway lesions (Fig. 5-13), all of which are manifestations of vasculitis. Vegetations occasionally dislodge and embolize in an end artery, which results in hemorrhagic or gangrenous lesions (Fig. 5-14). Osler's nodes, which present as small tender erythematous nodules, are found in the intradermal pads of the fingers and toes or in the thenar or hypothenar eminences (Fig. 5-15). All the aforementioned findings are often associated with a new heart murmur, splenomegaly, spiking fever, and positive blood culture. Clubbing of the fingers may occur in chronic cases.

Kawasaki Disease

This multisystem disease has surpassed acute rheumatic fever as the most common form of acquired heart disease in children. It is characterized by fever, conjunctivitis, erythema of the lips and oral mucosa, extremity changes, rash, and cervical adenopathy. Coronary artery aneurysms develop in 15% to 25% of untreated patients and may result in myocardial ischemia, infarction, or sudden death. The incidence of coronary abnormalities is markedly decreased with timely treatment (~5%). This disease is discussed in detail in Chapter 7. Coronary artery aneurysms are well demonstrated by echocardiography (Fig. 5-16), and this imaging modality plays an essential role in the diagnosis and management of Kawasaki disease.

Figure 5-7   Holt-Oram syndrome. Note the absence of the radius and thumb **(A).** The associated cardiovascular abnormality is an atrial septal defect. Radiographic examination **(B and C)** demonstrates the absence of a radius shadow; the missing thumb is apparent.

Figure 5-8   Infant with Marfan syndrome. **A,** Note the narrow elongated face, pectus excavatum, and long arms and fingers. **B,** A close-up view of the infant's hand.

LABORATORY AIDS IN THE DIAGNOSIS OF CONGENITAL HEART DISEASE

In addition to a comprehensive physical examination, the chest roentgenogram, electrocardiogram, and, most notably, echocardiography provide invaluable information concerning specific congenital heart lesions and have allowed therapeutic decisions to be made without cardiac catheterization.

Chest Roentgenography

The chest x-ray examination is useful to screen patients with suspected congenital heart disease. It is particularly useful in differentiating cardiac from pulmonary pathology such as pneumonia, pneumothorax, pneumomediastinum, or other parenchymal lung disease that may mimic congenital heart disease. The review of any chest roentgenogram requires a systematic approach.

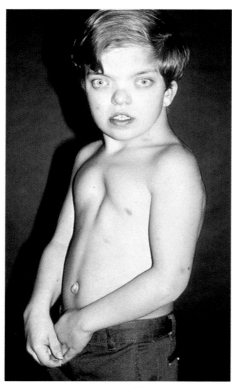

Figure 5-9   Noonan syndrome. Note the widely spaced eyes, low-set ears, webbing of the neck, shield chest, pectus, and increased carrying angle of the arms.

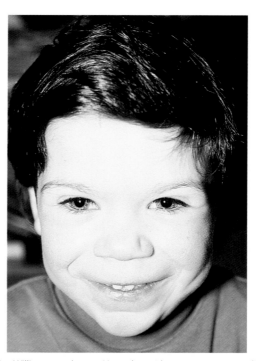

Figure 5-10   Williams syndrome. Note the wide-set eyes, upturned nose, large maxilla, prominent philtrum, and pointed chin. *(Courtesy R.A. Mathews, MD, Philadelphia, Pa.)*

Figure 5-11 Erythema marginatum rash in a child with acute rheumatic fever. Note the wavy margins in the distribution on the trunk.

Cardiac Apex and Visceral Situs

The location of the cardiac apex and visceral situs provides important diagnostic information. Discordance of the situs and cardiac apex (i.e., apex to the right with situs solitus [normal arrangement] or apex to the left with situs inversus) is often associated with structural congenital heart disease (Figs. 5-17

Figure 5-14 Acute bacterial endocarditis. Note the hemorrhagic lesions **(A)** and subungual splinter hemorrhages **(B).**

Figure 5-12 Subcutaneous nodules. Note their presence over the bony prominences of the elbow in a patient with chronic rheumatic heart disease.

and 5-18). Dextrocardia (apex to the right) or mesocardia (apex to the middle) with situs solitus is a frequent presentation of ventricular inversion or corrected transposition of the great arteries (see Fig. 5-17). Dextrocardia can also be seen with primary pulmonary problems. Scimitar syndrome is composed of dextrocardia with hypoplasia of the right lung (Fig. 5-19). In this case a major portion of the right lung (usually the right lower lobe) is "sequestered" and has its arterial supply by way of a systemic artery from the descending aorta, and the pulmonary venous return from that lung drains

Figure 5-13 Janeway lesions. Note the small (painless) nodules on the sole of a patient with bacterial endocarditis.

Figure 5-15 Osler's nodes. Note the (painful) erythematous nodular lesions resulting from infective endocarditis. *(Courtesy J.F. John, Jr., MD.)*

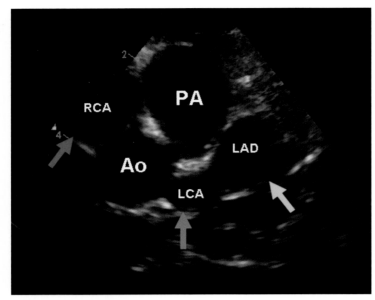

Figure 5-16 Kawasaki disease: Giant coronary artery aneurysms. Multiple giant coronary aneurysms of the right (RCA, *red arrow*), left (LCA, *green arrow*), and left anterior descending (LAD, *yellow arrow*) coronary arteries. Ao, aorta; PA, pulmonary artery.

Figure 5-18 Levocardia with situs inversus. Discordance of the apex of the heart and visceral situs is often associated with structural congenital heart defects. The hepatic portion of the inferior vena cava is absent in this patient, and there is azygos vein continuation. (Note the prominence of the shadow at the high right-sided cardiac border.) Note air in the stomach under the right hemidiaphragm.

abnormally into the inferior vena cava via a vein forming a scimitar (see Fig. 5-19). Patients with levocardia (apex to the left) with either situs inversus or situs ambiguus frequently have complex congenital heart diseases such as transposition of the great arteries, pulmonary atresia, and atrioventricular septal defects. Atrial isomerism is associated with bilateral morphologic right or left lungs and can be recognized as bilateral symmetrical right (short) or left (long) bronchi. This is best demonstrated with a magnified penetrated chest x-ray examination focusing on bronchial anatomy (Fig. 5-20). Almost all patients with this anomaly have complex congenital heart disease.

Shape and Size

Cardiac size is important, but the shape of the cardiac image may also provide a clue as to which heart chambers are enlarged and the likely structural diagnosis. In the cyanotic newborn with transposition of the great arteries, the cardiac image appears as an "egg on a string" (Fig. 5-21). If the thymic shadow does not obscure it, the mediastinal shadow shows a

A

B

Figure 5-19 Scimitar syndrome. **A,** Note the hypoplastic right lung and scimitar-shaped shadow formed by pulmonary veins draining the sequestered segment and connecting to the inferior vena cava. **B,** Note also the systemic artery coursing diagonally upward from the abdominal aorta to the sequestered lobe.

Scimitar shadow

Systemic artery

Figure 5-17 Dextrocardia (heart in the right side of the chest) associated with situs solitus. Note the prominent vascular shadow along the left-sided cardiac border that is caused by the aorta. This pattern is commonly associated with ventricular inversion (corrected transposition of the great arteries).

Figure 5-20   Atrial isomerism. Note the symmetrical bronchial anatomy. Atrial isomerism should be suspected when the heart is midline on the chest radiograph and situs ambiguus is present. The best radiographic sign of right or left atrial isomerism pertains to the symmetry of bronchial anatomy, with right atrial isomerism being related to bilateral right bronchi and left atrial isomerism to bilateral left bronchi.

Figure 5-22   Tetralogy of Fallot with pulmonic stenosis produces a "boot-shaped" heart, which results from right ventricular hypertrophy, upward tilt of the apex, and the concavity at the left upper heart border caused by a small right ventricular infundibulum and main pulmonary artery. Note also the right aortic arch.

narrow waist resulting from the posteromedial position of the main pulmonary artery. This produces the "string." Pulmonary vascular markings are usually increased, although vascularity may be normal in the immediate newborn period.

In tetralogy of Fallot with pulmonic stenosis, the heart appears "boot-shaped" because right ventricular hypertrophy causes the apex (toe of the boot) to turn upward (Fig. 5-22).

Figure 5-21   Transposition of the great arteries. Note the "egg on a string" heart shadow, which results from the position of the main pulmonary artery posterior and slightly to the left of the aorta, contributing to the narrow waist (the "string").

The concavity of the left upper cardiac border is due to the small right ventricular outflow tract and main pulmonary artery segment.

In tetralogy of Fallot with pulmonary atresia, the heart is shaped like an "egg on its side" (Fig. 5-23). The pulmonary blood flow to the lungs may be supplied by either a patent ductus arteriosus or systemic arterial collateral vessels. The pulmonary vascular markings are decreased if pulmonary blood flow is patent ductus dependent and increased if large systemic collaterals supply pulmonary blood flow.

In congenitally corrected transposition of the great arteries, the heart has a "valentine" or "heart" shape with the apex pointing downward just to the left of the midline, as shown in Figure 5-24. The fullness at the left upper border of the cardiac shadow is due to the ascending aorta arising from the left-sided morphologic right ventricle.

Although an enlarged and globular heart shadow may be associated with a cardiomyopathy, massive cardiac enlargement (so-called "wall-to-wall" heart) is typical in patients with Ebstein anomaly. In this anomaly there is a malformation of the tricuspid valve with downward displacement of the inferior and septal leaflets of the valve into the ventricle, causing severe tricuspid valve regurgitation or stenosis. As a result, the right atrium becomes markedly enlarged and, along with the "atrialized" portion of the right ventricle, contributes significantly to the cardiac image of a large box-shaped heart (Fig. 5-25).

Left-to-right shunt lesions from atrial septal defects, ventricular septal defects, or a patent ductus arteriosus demonstrate specific chamber enlargement and increased pulmonary vascular markings. A significant atrial defect shows enlargement of all right-sided cardiac chambers including the right atrium, right ventricle, and pulmonary artery (Fig. 5-26). A patent ductus arteriosus shows enlargement of all left-sided cardiac chambers including the aorta. In patients with a

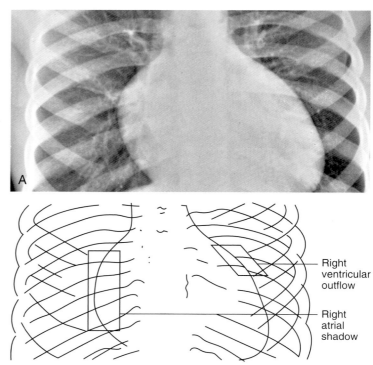

Figure 5-23 Tetralogy of Fallot with pulmonary atresia. Note the "egg on its side" appearance of the heart, due to the uplifted apex resulting from the right ventricular hypertrophy. The absence of a right ventricular outflow and the diminutive main pulmonary artery segment produce a concavity at the left upper heart border. Note also that a right aortic arch is present.

Figure 5-25 Ebstein anomaly of the tricuspid valve. Note the radiographic appearance of a "box-shaped" heart, enlarged right atrium, and prominent right ventricular outflow tract.

Figure 5-24 Corrected transposition of the great arteries. Note the characteristic "valentine-shaped" heart and the left-sided ascending aorta.

ventricular septal defect, the right atrium is the only heart chamber that is not enlarged.

Great Vessels

The radiographic appearance of the great arteries may also suggest a specific structural congenital heart defect. The main and left branch pulmonary arteries are usually enlarged in patients with pulmonary valve stenosis, due to poststenotic dilation (Fig. 5-27). The characteristic radiographic finding of congenital aortic valve stenosis is dilation of the ascending aorta, best seen as an overlapping shadow with the superior vena cava along the right upper cardiac border (Fig. 5-28).

Figure 5-26 Atrial septal defect. Note the enlarged right atrium, right ventricle, and pulmonary artery, as well as the increased pulmonary vascular markings on this radiograph.

Figure 5-27 Pulmonic valve stenosis. Note the typical radiographic abnormalities of a prominent main and left pulmonary artery.

Coarctation of the aorta not diagnosed in a timely fashion may show the distinct radiographic finding of a "reversed E" or "3" sign caused by prestenotic and poststenotic dilation of the descending aorta (Fig. 5-29). If a significant coarctation remains unrepaired for 5 to 10 years, rib notching may appear (see the section Skeletal Abnormalities, below).

The normal left aortic arch causes a shift of the tracheal air column to the right, whereas a right arch causes a similar deviation to the left (Fig. 5-30). The position of the thoracic descending aorta also helps define the side of the arch and can be determined by noting obscuring of either the left or right side of the thoracic vertebral bodies. A right aortic arch should always raise the suspicion of congenital heart disease and is found in approximately 30% of patients with tetralogy of Fallot or truncus arteriosus.

The addition of a barium swallow to the chest x-ray examination has historically been an important diagnostic tool in the assessment of patients with upper airway obstruction from vascular rings. Current practice favors the imaging techniques of MRI or CT scan, which provide clear and precise imaging of the aortic arch and great vessel anatomy and their

A

B

Figure 5-29 Coarctation of the aorta. Note that the site of the stenosis can be observed at the center of the "3" sign formed by the prestenotic and poststenotic dilation of the aorta in this characteristic radiograph in a 5-year-old child.

Figure 5-28 Aortic valve stenosis. Note the dilation of the ascending aorta, which is the only radiographic sign in children.

Figure 5-30 Right aortic arch in a child with truncus arteriosus. Note the deviation of the tracheal air column to the left.

Figure 5-31   Barium esophagram with a double aortic arch. **A,** Note the bilateral compressions on the anterior view. **B,** Note the marked retroesophageal indentation on the lateral view. **C,** Schematic of the double aortic arch. Ao, aorta; LCCA, left common carotid artery; LSCA, left subclavian artery; PA, pulmonary artery; RCCA, right common carotid artery; RSCA, right subclavian artery.

relationship to the airway and esophagus. Nevertheless, one may find vascular anomalies as findings on a barium swallow performed for the evaluation of dysphagia or upper airway respiratory symptoms: If a bilateral indentation is noted on the barium esophagram, a double aortic arch should be suspected (Fig. 5-31). A right aortic arch with distal origin of the left subclavian artery or a left aortic arch with distal origin of the right subclavian artery produces a posterior indentation on the barium esophagram, but the aberrant right subclavian artery is not associated with airway compromise. An anterior esophageal indentation is almost always caused by distal origin of the left pulmonary artery, resulting in this vessel coursing between the trachea and esophagus and causing a pulmonary artery sling (Fig. 5-32).

Pulmonary Vascularity

Left-to-right shunt lesions are associated with increased pulmonary blood flow that causes primarily arterial or a combination of arterial and venous markings on the chest radiograph. Hyperinflation seen on the chest x-ray film is a characteristic finding in infants with a large left-to-right shunt associated with pulmonary hypertension (Fig. 5-33). Patients with pulmonary venous obstruction, such as infradiaphragmatic total anomalous pulmonary venous return, show a fine reticular pattern of pulmonary venous obstruction, which may mimic respiratory distress syndrome in the neonate (Fig. 5-34). It should be cautioned that the interpretation of pulmonary vascularity can be quite difficult and should always be interpreted within the context of other clinical findings.

Oligemic lung fields indicate reduced pulmonary blood flow, as seen in most types of cyanotic congenital heart disease, the classic example being tetralogy of Fallot.

Skeletal Abnormalities

Attention should also be given to the thoracic cage including the spine and ribs. Although abnormal fusions of ribs and hemivertebrae are not pathognomonic for specific congenital heart lesions, there is a higher incidence when these findings are present. Rib notching is a distinct radiographic finding in patients older than 5 to 10 years of age with coarctation of the aorta (Fig. 5-35). Scoliosis is a common finding in teenage patients with cyanotic congenital heart disease. Pectus excavatum may cause a false impression of cardiac enlargement because of a "pancaking" effect on the heart from a narrow anteroposterior thoracic diameter. Because of its association with chest wall and spine abnormalities, mitral valve prolapse (and associated connective tissue disorders such as Marfan syndrome) should be considered in this context.

Electrocardiography and Arrhythmias

Electrocardiography

Although electrocardiography (ECG) is an invaluable diagnostic tool in the assessment of pediatric heart disease, it is impractical and unnecessary for pediatricians to have a thorough knowledge of detailed electrocardiogram interpretation. However, it is valuable to be able to recognize certain typical

PULMONARY VASCULAR SLING

Figure 5-32 Anomalous left pulmonary artery (pulmonary artery sling). **A,** Anterior view of barium-filled esophagus. **B,** Lateral view: note the anterior rounded indentation in the barium-filled esophagus and the posterior bulge into the air-filled trachea anteriorly. **C,** Diagram of vascular anatomy and relationships to trachea and esophagus. LPA, left pulmonary artery; PA, pulmonary artery; RPA, right pulmonary artery.

electrocardiographic patterns that yield important diagnostic information. For instance, most normal children have a frontal plane axis that is either normal (0 to 90 degrees) or in the mild right axis deviation range from 90 to 120 degrees. The presence of a *superior axis* (180 to 270, or 0 to –90 degrees) suggests certain specific cardiac defects. A *left axis deviation* that includes an axis in the range of 0 to –90 degrees associated with a QR pattern in leads I and AVL is frequently seen in the following situations: a cyanotic newborn with tricuspid atresia (Fig. 5-36), an atrioventricular septal defect with or without Down syndrome, Noonan syndrome, or some varieties of a single ventricle. When the frontal plane axis falls

Figure 5-33 Large left-to-right shunt from a ventricular septal defect. Posteroanterior **(A)** and lateral **(B)** radiographs from a 2-month-old infant. Note the increased pulmonary vascular markings and lung hyperinflation. The flattened hemidiaphragms are clearly seen on the lateral projection, a finding predictive of associated pulmonary hypertension.

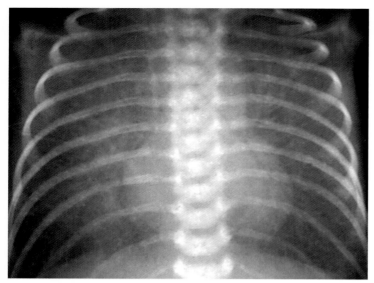

Figure 5-34   Total anomalous pulmonary venous return below the diaphragm. Note the radiographic findings of severe pulmonary venous obstruction and pulmonary edema, mimicking respiratory distress syndrome or some other primary pulmonary pathology.

Table 5-4	Pediatric Dysrhythmias	
Treatment Not Required	**Treatment Required**
Sinus arrhythmia	Supraventricular tachycardia
Wandering (ectopic) atrial pacemaker	Ventricular tachycardia
Isolated premature atrial contractions	Third-degree atrioventricular block
Isolated premature ventricular contractions	with symptoms
First-degree atrioventricular block	

seen in children is a *sinus arrhythmia*. This is a normal variant that reflects a healthy interaction between autonomic respiratory and cardiac control activity in the central nervous system. Typically the heart rate increases during inspiration and decreases during expiration and may sound wildly irregular on auscultation unless careful attention is paid to the relationship between the heart rate and respirations (Fig. 5-39). Another normal variant occurs when the atrial pacemaker transiently shifts from the sinus node to another atrial site with only minimal variation in the heart rate. This is often

between 180 and 270 degrees, it is usually referred to as a *northwest axis* and is frequently found in atrioventricular septal defects (Fig. 5-37) or other lesions that lead to severe right ventricular hypertrophy. When prominent Q waves are seen in leads I and AVL with associated ST-T wave depression in the lateral leads (V5 and V6) the clinician should suspect cardiac ischemia associated with anomalous left coronary artery from the pulmonary artery (Fig. 5-38).

Being certain about hypertrophy in the pediatric age group is difficult because of the wide range of normal values that vary with age. This is particularly true of right ventricular hypertrophy, which can be a physiologic finding in the first several years of life. On the other hand, left ventricular predominance in the newborn is almost always a pathologic finding and usually indicates one of the hypoplastic right heart syndromes, such as tricuspid atresia (left ventricular predominance is shown in Fig. 5-36) or pulmonary atresia with an intact septum.

Conduction abnormalities, such as Wolff-Parkinson-White syndrome, prolonged corrected Q–T interval, and atrioventricular block are readily apparent on the 12-lead electrocardiogram and are discussed further in the following section on arrhythmias.

Arrhythmias

Disorders of heart rate or rhythm are not nearly as common in childhood as they are in adulthood, but it is vital that pediatricians be familiar with arrhythmias that may occur in otherwise healthy children. An outline of these disorders, based on the need for treatment, is presented in Table 5-4. For the numerous rhythm disorders not listed, management must be individualized, taking into account the presence or absence of associated heart disease.

Transient arrhythmias may present in the following manner: an asymptomatic child with an irregular heartbeat noted on examination, palpitations, chest pain (a common complaint among children younger than 10 years of age when they sense a tachycardia), dizziness or presyncope, or actual syncope with or without seizure activity. More sustained arrhythmias may lead to congestive heart failure, cardiogenic shock, or even death. The most common irregularity of heart rhythm

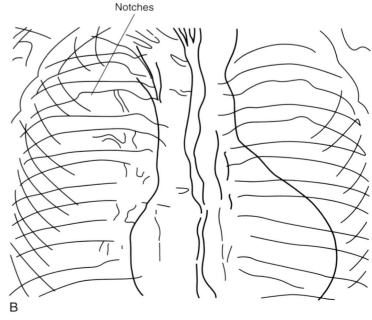

Notches

Figure 5-35   Coarctation of the aorta. Note the rib notching that can be observed in an older child.

TRICUSPID ATRESIA

Figure 5-36 Electrocardiogram of a child with tricuspid atresia. Note the left axis deviation, left atrial enlargement, and left ventricular hypertrophy. Ao, aorta; LA, left atrium; LV, left ventricle; PA, pulmonary artery; RA, right atrium; RV, right ventricle.

referred to as a *wandering atrial pacemaker* (Fig. 5-40). *Premature atrial contractions* are generally benign when they occur in the absence of underlying heart disease. They are particularly common during the newborn period, when they are often associated with aberrant conduction (Fig. 5-41) or apparent pauses (Fig. 5-42) resulting from failure of the premature atrial impulse to conduct to the ventricle. *Isolated premature ventricular beats* are not common but may be seen with an incidence of 0.3% to 2.2% and rarely require treatment as long as there is no associated heart disease. This form of ectopy is recognizable by a wide QRS, a T wave opposite in direction to the QRS in any given lead, dissociation from the P wave, and usually a full compensatory pause (Fig. 5-43). For the above-mentioned abnormalities, an appropriate initial workup includes a 12-lead electrocardiogram and rhythm strip and brief exercise in the office to see if the ectopy is suppressed or becomes more frequent as the heart rate increases. An exacerbation of the arrhythmia with this maneuver would warrant further cardiologic investigation.

By far the most common arrhythmia requiring treatment in the pediatric population is *supraventricular tachycardia* (SVT). The most frequent age of presentation is in the first 3 months of life, with secondary peaks occurring at 8 to 10 years of age and again during adolescence. This rhythm disorder is

ATRIOVENTRICULAR SEPTAL DEFECT

Figure 5-37 Electrocardiogram of a child with an atrioventricular septal defect. Note the superior (northwest) axis deviation and right ventricular hypertrophy. Ao, aorta; LA, left atrium; LV, left ventricle; PA, pulmonary artery; RA, right atrium; RV, right ventricle.

Figure 5-38   Electrocardiogram of an anomalous left coronary artery from the pulmonary artery. Note the pathologic Q waves in I, AVL, V5, and V6 leads *(arrows)*, and ST and T wave changes in the same leads.

Figure 5-39   Sinus arrhythmia. Note variable QRS cycle lengths without change in the P wave–QRS relationship.

Figure 5-40   Wandering atrial pacemaker. Note the variable morphology of the P wave, indicating origin from either the sinus node *(upward arrows)* or an ectopic atrial site *(downward arrows).*

Figure 5-41   Premature atrial contractions. Note that these premature complexes may be associated with aberrant conduction of the QRS *(open arrow)* or normal conduction *(solid arrow).*

Figure 5-42 Nonconducted premature atrial contractions. Note the premature atrial beats that are not conducted *(arrows)*, resulting in apparent pauses.

characterized by a regular, narrow QRS complex tachycardia with rates that vary with the patient's age. The overall average rate for SVT at all ages is 235 beats/minute; however, in the first 9 months the average is 270 beats/minute compared with 210 beats/minute in older children (Fig. 5-44). Discrete P waves are usually difficult to define, but if present, there is always a one-to-one relationship to the QRS. Dramatic ST segment changes that may occur during tachycardia resolve shortly after conversion to sinus rhythm.

Two important points regarding SVT include differentiating this arrhythmia from sinus tachycardia in an infant and the value of the 12-lead electrocardiogram after conversion to sinus rhythm. In a child younger than 1 year of age, during periods of severe stress such as sepsis, dehydration, or high fever, the sinus rate may reach 220 to 250 beats/minute. At this rate the P wave is lost in the T wave. Facial ice water immersion or intravenous adenosine may be invaluable in differentiating rapid sinus tachycardia from SVT: In the latter case the intervention terminates the tachycardia abruptly, whereas in the former it produces only transient slowing and the P waves become evident on the downstroke of the T wave.

Regarding the postconversion 12-lead electrocardiogram, it is important to recognize the presence of Wolff-Parkinson-White syndrome, which occurs in 25% of patients with SVT. This syndrome is characterized by a short P–R interval, a delta wave, and prolongation of the QRS complex (Fig. 5-45) and is not evident when the tachycardia is present.

A discussion of the treatment for SVT in the pediatric patient is beyond the scope of this chapter, and detailed algorithms are available in other sources. However, it should be noted that, in more recent years, radiofrequency ablation or cryoablation of the common arrhythmia substrates for SVT, accessory atrioventricular (AV) connections or dual AV nodal pathways, has become a frontline treatment for older children and adolescents. The abnormal pathway can be accurately mapped during an electrophysiology study, and application of radiofrequency energy or cryoablation at the appropriate site can result in immediate disappearance of the delta wave in a patient with Wolff-Parkinson-White syndrome (Fig. 5-46). When the arrhythmia substrate is in proximity to the AV node (AV node reentry or septal accessory pathways), cryoablation provides a larger safety margin than radiofrequency ablation

Figure 5-43 Premature ventricular contractions. Note the obvious wide QRS premature complexes with abnormal T waves, a fully compensatory pause, and absence of a preceding P wave.

Figure 5-44 Supraventricular tachycardia. Note the normal QRS complex tachycardia at a rate of 214 beats/minute without visible P waves.

Figure 5-45   Wolff-Parkinson-White syndrome. Note the characteristic findings of a short P–R interval, slurred upstroke of QRS (delta wave), and prolongation of the QRS interval.

because of the reversibility of cryoablation lesions terminated at the first sign of AV nodal injury.

Sustained *ventricular tachycardia* is distinctly uncommon in childhood, and the patient must be thoroughly investigated for underlying heart disease. This arrhythmia is most often associated with hemodynamic compromise and is characterized by a regular wide-complex tachycardia, usually with atrioventricular dissociation if P waves are visible (Fig. 5-47). This life-threatening disorder most commonly occurs in children who have had open-heart surgical repair for tetralogy of Fallot or other complex anomalies or who have a cardiomyopathy, myocarditis, congenital ion channel abnormality

(long QT, Brugada syndrome, catecholamine sensitive ventricular tachycardia) or myocardial tumor. Looking for a prolonged corrected Q–T interval (Q–T$_c$) is also important because this abnormality of repolarization may lead to recurrent syncope and sudden death secondary to ventricular tachycardia or fibrillation (Fig. 5-48). The Q–T$_c$ can be calculated using the Bazett formula: the Q–T interval divided by the square root of the preceding R–R interval. Symptomatic bradycardia is rarely encountered in the pediatric age group. One condition that needs to be recognized is congenital *third-degree atrioventricular block* (Fig. 5-49). This may occur with associated structural heart disease, but it occurs

Figure 5-46   Radiofrequency catheter ablation. Note the prompt disappearance of the delta wave *(arrow)* after radiofrequency (RF) ablation of an accessory pathway in a patient with Wolff-Parkinson-White syndrome.

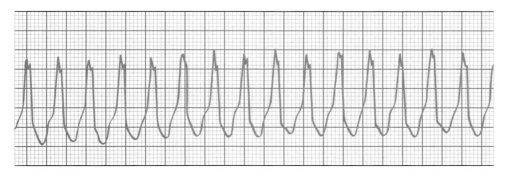

Figure 5-47   Ventricular tachycardia. Note the wide QRS complex tachycardia at a rate of 188 beats/minute.

Figure 5-48 Prolonged Q–T syndrome. Note that the corrected Q–T interval is prolonged at 0.57 second (upper limit of normal is 0.44 second). The Q–T interval must be corrected for heart rate by using the Bazett formula: measured Q–T interval (0.56 second) divided by the square root of the preceding R–R interval (0.96 second).

Figure 5-49 Complete heart block. Note that atrial activity *(arrows)* is independent of a slower ventricular rhythm.

more frequently with an otherwise normal heart. The presence of maternal connective tissue disease or anti-nuclear antibodies should always be sought as a possible cause when congenital atrioventricular block is detected in a newborn.

When a patient is evaluated for a history of syncope or new-onset seizures, it is highly recommended that the physician obtain an electrocardiogram to look for "footprints" of a possible arrhythmic cause. The possibilities include Wolff-Parkinson-White syndrome (providing a substrate for rapid supraventricular tachycardia), prolonged corrected Q–T interval (predisposing to severe ventricular arrhythmias, most often a type known as *torsades de pointes*), or atrioventricular block (leading to Stokes-Adams attacks).

Echocardiography

Echocardiography with Doppler interrogation first provided remarkable advances in the investigation of congenital heart defects in the early 1980s and is now the standard imaging modality for the diagnosis of congenital heart disease. Echocardiographic imaging and color flow Doppler allow accurate anatomic definition of even complex congenital defects, as well as providing a reliable noninvasive hemodynamic assessment of the patient. These tools complement and, in most cases, replace the need for diagnostic cardiac catheterization and angiography in the management of patients with congenital heart disease.

Accurate diagnosis of most structural congenital heart diseases, whether simple or complex, can be made by echocardiography. A systematic approach to define major intracardiac connections is a useful starting point: (1) venoatrial (systemic or pulmonary venous return to the right or left atrium), (2) atrioventricular (atria to the ventricles), and (3) ventriculoarterial (ventricles to the great vessels).

All types of septal defects can be readily visualized by echocardiography. The atrial septal defects are reliably demonstrated by the subcostal approach. The most common type

is the secundum defect (Fig. 5-50), which involves the middle portion of the atrial septum in the region of the fossa ovalis. The sinus venosus type of atrial septal defect is located in the posterosuperior portion of the atrial septum adjacent to the junction of the right atrium and superior vena cava (this vessel effectively overrides the defect) and is associated with partial anomalous pulmonary venous return of the right upper pulmonary vein (Fig. 5-51). An ostium primum defect known as a *partial form of an atrioventricular septal defect* is seen in Figure 5-52. The complete form of an atrioventricular septal defect consists of a large defect in the center of the heart, in association with a common AV valve (Fig. 5-53). During diastole, with the AV valve open, all four chambers are in direct communication; whereas during systole, the closed AV valve

Figure 5-50 Secundum atrial septal defect. Note the large defect in the fossa ovalis area *(*)* on the subcostal view *(left)*. Color Doppler *(right)* confirms a prominent left-to-right shunt (red flow). LA, left atrium; LV, left ventricle; RA, right atrium; RV, right ventricle.

Figure 5-52 Partial atrioventricular septal defect. Note the defect *(arrow)* on the apical four-chamber view *(left)* in the inferior portion of the atrial septum. A left-to-right atrial shunt is shown on the color Doppler image *(right)*.

Figure 5-51 Sinus venosus defect. Note the defect *(*)* in the posterosuperior portion of the atrial septum, with the superior vena cava (SVC) overriding the defect on the subcostal short axis view *(left)*. Color Doppler *(right)* shows left-to-right shunt across the defect. Anomalous drainage of the right upper pulmonary vein is not shown on this view. IVC, inferior vena cava; LA, left atrium; RA, right atrium.

Figure 5-53 Complete atrioventricular (AV) septal defect (four-chamber view): **A** and **B,** Diastolic frames with and without color Doppler. Note large central defect *(red asterisk)* between atria and ventricles **(A).** Red Doppler flow indicates large atrial and ventricular shunt **(B).** **C** and **D,** Systolic frames demonstrate atrial *(yellow asterisk)* and ventricular *(green asterisk)* components of the defect **(C).** Blue Doppler flow *(arrow)* indicates valve regurgitation **(D).** LA, left atrium; LV, left ventricle; RA, right atrium; RV, right ventricle.

Figure 5-54 Perimembranous ventricular septal defect. Note that the defect *(arrow)* is located in the superior portion of the septum as seen on the apical four-chamber view *(left)*. Color Doppler image *(right)* shows left-to-right ventricular shunt. LA, left atrium; LV, left ventricle; RA, right atrium; RV, right ventricle.

Figure 5-56 Muscular ventricular septal defect (small). Note that no apparent defect in the ventricular septum could be visualized by two-dimensional image *(left)* on the apical four-chamber view. However, a color Doppler image *(right)* identifies a small defect in the muscular septum near the apex by showing a left-to-right jet *(arrow)*. LA, left atrium; LV, left ventricle; RV, right ventricle.

functionally separates the defect into atrial and ventricular components. Figure 5-53, *D*, illustrates AV valve regurgitation, which is very common with this type of septal defect.

Ventricular septal defects are well defined by echocardiography and are usually seen clearly, using the apical four-chamber view. The most common defect is in the perimembranous septum located in the subaortic area and bordered by the tricuspid valve (Fig. 5-54). Moderate defects in the muscular portion of septum are easily visualized in multiple views. A short axis view of such a defect is shown in Figure 5-55. Although small defects located in the muscular septum can be difficult to image, particularly if located in the apical trabecular area, they can be readily detected by color flow Doppler interrogation (Fig. 5-56).

Typical findings in the most common cyanotic heart lesion, tetralogy of Fallot, are a dilated aortic root that overrides the ventricular septum, a large perimembranous ventricular septal defect, and right ventricular outflow obstruction (Fig. 5-57). Truncus arteriosus is a related conotruncal anomaly associated with a large ventricular defect and a common arterial trunk (truncus) arising from both the right and left ventricles, with the pulmonary arteries arising directly from this vessel just above the semilunar valve (Fig. 5-58). Transposition of the great arteries presents with severe cyanosis immediately after birth and can be recognized by the characteristic finding of parallel takeoff of the great vessels from both ventricles, with the aorta arising anteriorly from the right ventricle and the pulmonary artery originating posteriorly from the left ventricle (Fig. 5-59).

The most common cause of cardiogenic shock or congestive heart failure in the first several days of life is hypoplastic left heart syndrome, which is associated with either aortic atresia or critical aortic stenosis (Fig. 5-60). Coarctation of the aorta or an interrupted aortic arch may also present with severe

Figure 5-55 Muscular ventricular septal defect (moderate). Note the moderate-size defect *(arrow)* in the muscular septum on the parasternal short axis view *(left)*. Color Doppler image *(right)* shows left-to-right shunt *(arrow)*. LV, left ventricle; RV, right ventricle.

Figure 5-57 Tetralogy of Fallot. Aortic root (Ao) overriding a large ventricular septal defect is shown on the subcostal long axis view *(left)*. The anterior deviation of the outlet ventricular septum *(*)* resulting in narrowing of pulmonary outflow tract *(right)* is shown on the subcostal short axis view. LV, left ventricle; PA, pulmonary artery; RV, right ventricle.

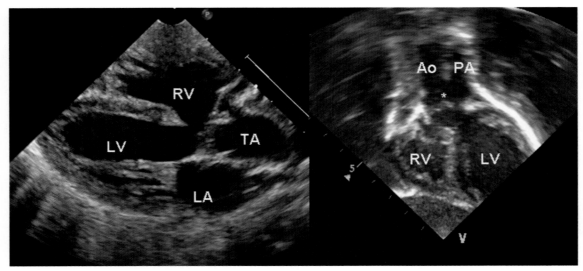

Figure 5-58 Truncus arteriosus. Parasternal long axis view *(left)* shows large truncal root (TA) overriding the ventricular septum receiving outflow from both the right ventricle (RV) and left ventricle (LV). Ascending aorta (Ao) and pulmonary artery (PA) arising directly from the proximal truncal root *(*)* are shown on the subcostal long axis view *(right)*.

heart failure in the neonate. Aortic arch anomalies are best visualized by a suprasternal approach, and the diagnosis of interrupted aortic arch or coarctation of the aorta can be readily made in most cases (Fig. 5-61).

If the pulmonary veins do not communicate directly with the left atrium, total anomalous pulmonary venous return should be suspected. Congenitally corrected transposition is the most likely diagnosis when the atrioventricular connection is discordant (right atrium to morphologic left ventricle and left atrium to morphologic right ventricle).

CARDIAC SURGICAL PROCEDURES

The remarkable progress in treating children with severe congenital heart disease, progress that has greatly accelerated during the past two decades, is due largely to dramatic achievements in the field of pediatric heart surgery. Although the first patent ductus arteriosus ligation was done in 1938, the first Blalock-Taussig shunt in 1944, and the initial repair of coarctation of the aorta in 1945, open-heart repair of complex malformations did not become relatively commonplace until the late 1960s and 1970s. Since then there have been progressive improvements in precise preoperative diagnosis, development of stunning technical skills by specialized pediatric heart surgeons, and important advances in the perioperative management of infants with critical heart disease. All of these factors have made it possible to offer successful palliative or corrective surgery for the great majority of even the most severe forms of congenital heart disease.

Although the large number of possible malformations and various operations applied to them may seem bewildering and complex, in reality only a relatively small number of types of surgical procedures are performed. Most of these procedures are associated with an eponym that designates the surgeon who developed a particular technique. The purpose of the following section is to provide schematic diagrams and brief explanations for the commonly used surgical procedures and the types of defects to which they are applied.

Figure 5-62 demonstrates the surgical approach to tetralogy of Fallot. Various types of systemic-to-pulmonary artery shunt procedures are illustrated. These palliative operations are performed in newborns and infants with complex congenital

Figure 5-59 Transposition of the great arteries. Parasternal long axial view **(A)** shows parallel arrangement of the great vessels. Apical four-chamber views confirm origination of the pulmonary artery (PA) from the left ventricle (LV) **(B)** and the aorta (Ao) from the right ventricle RV) **(C).**

Figure 5-60 Hypoplastic left heart syndrome. Markedly hypoplastic left ventricle (LV) with dilated right ventricle (RV) is shown on the apical four-chamber view *(left)*. Small ascending aorta (Ao) is demonstrated on the parasternal long axis view *(right)*. LA, left atrium; RA, right atrium.

Figure 5-61 Coarctation of the aorta. Suprasternal notch view shows discrete narrowing in the proximal portion of the descending aorta *(arrow)*. DAo, descending aorta.

heart disease associated with severe obstruction to pulmonary blood flow that is not amenable to early complete repair. These lesions generally have in common either severe subvalvular or valvular pulmonic stenosis or pulmonary atresia leading to inadequate pulmonary blood flow. In the previous era of cardiac surgery, the most common lesion in this category was tetralogy of Fallot. At present, most children with this entity now have a complete repair in infancy without a prior shunt. The original *classic Blalock-Taussig shunt* was performed by dividing the subclavian artery and creating an end-to-side anastomosis of the proximal subclavian artery stump to the ipsilateral pulmonary artery. The most common type of shunt performed in the current era is a *modified Blalock-Taussig shunt,* which uses a Gore-Tex interposition graft between the innominate or subclavian artery and pulmonary artery without dividing the distal subclavian artery. On occasion, unusual anatomy of the aorta or proximal pulmonary arteries leads to placement of a *central shunt* (a short interposition graft between the ascending aorta and main pulmonary artery). Other procedures, frequently used in the early decades of congenital heart surgery, includea *Waterston shunt* (creation of a window between the ascending aorta and right pulmonary artery) and a *Pott shunt* (creation of a window between the descending aorta and left pulmonary artery).

Figure 5-62 Palliative shunt procedures and definitive operative procedure for tetralogy of Fallot.

TETRALOGY OF FALLOT

AORTIC ATRESIA AND
HYPOPLASTIC LEFT HEART SYNDROME

Norwood procedure (first stage)

Figure 5-63   Initial palliative (Norwood) procedure for hypoplastic left heart syndrome (aortic atresia complex).

Figure 5-62 also demonstrates the technique of complete repair for tetralogy of Fallot, which includes closure of the ventricular septal defect, relief of right ventricular outflow tract obstruction with resection of subvalvular muscle, pulmonary valvotomy, and usually a transannular patch.

Figure 5-63 illustrates the initial palliation for aortic atresia and hypoplastic left heart syndrome, which is the most common cause of congestive heart failure in the first several days of life. A *Norwood procedure* is the first of a three-stage operative approach designed to provide long-term stability for a circulation supported by only one ventricle. In the first stage the aortic atresia is functionally converted to pulmonary atresia. A "neoaortic outflow" for the right ventricle is created by transecting the main pulmonary artery near its bifurcation and anastomosing the proximal root to the hypoplastic ascending aorta, making liberal use of a homograft patch to enlarge the entire aortic arch. Relieving the coarctation that is invariably part of the complex is important. A shunt is subsequently performed to provide pulmonary blood flow, and a large atrial septal defect is created to allow unimpeded flow from the left to the right atrium. A modification (Sano procedure) of this operation substitutes a conduit from the right ventricle to the

pulmonary artery for the shunt as the source for pulmonary blood flow. The second and third stages of this approach are described and shown as follows.

Figures 5-64 and 5-65 show the approach to palliation of hearts with a functional single ventricle. Any malformation that is associated with a hypoplastic right or left ventricle can be treated in this manner, with the two most common examples being tricuspid atresia with a hypoplastic right ventricle and aortic atresia with a hypoplastic left heart, status post–first-stage Norwood procedure. Figure 5-64 demonstrates the first step in separating the systemic and pulmonary circulations in the setting of a functional single ventricle. The initial procedure directs approximately one half of systemic venous return directly to the pulmonary artery by creating an anastomosis between the superior vena cava and the right pulmonary artery. In the *classic Glenn procedure*, the right pulmonary artery is divided, the superior vena cava–right atrial junction is closed, and the superior vena cava is anastomosed to the distal right pulmonary artery. This operation has been modified to a *bidirectional Glenn procedure*, which separates the superior vena cava from the right atrium and creates an end-to-side connection to the pulmonary artery,

TRICUSPID ATRESIA

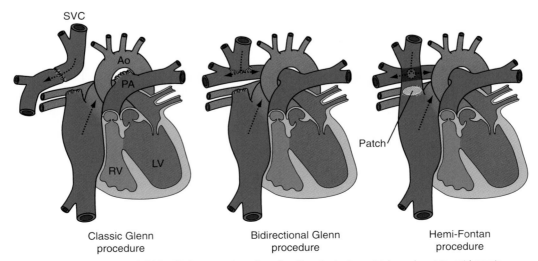

Classic Glenn
procedure

Bidirectional Glenn
procedure

Hemi-Fontan
procedure

Figure 5-64   Various initial palliative procedures for a functionally single ventricle, such as tricuspid atresia.

TRICUSPID ATRESIA

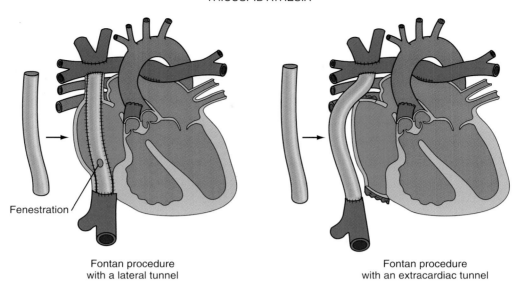

Fenestration

Fontan procedure
with a lateral tunnel

Fontan procedure
with an extracardiac tunnel

Figure 5-65   Completion of palliation for a functionally single ventricle, such as tricuspid atresia.

allowing flow to both the right and left pulmonary arteries. A variation of this latter procedure is the *hemi-Fontan*. In this operation, which produces the identical physiologic results as the bidirectional Glenn, a large superior vena cava–pulmonary artery connection is created, but the superior vena cava–right atrial connection is left intact and the orifice of the superior vena cava is closed with a patch. The *Fontan procedure* completes the process of diverting the entire systemic venous return to the pulmonary artery and is shown in Figure 5-65. This may be done by a *lateral tunnel* approach, in which a tunnel within the right atrium is created with a U-shaped graft attached to the right atrial wall. The current approach uses an *extracardiac tunnel,* which avoids incorporating right atrial tissue into the connection in the hope of preventing postoperative atrial arrhythmias related to right atrial scarring. In many Fontan operations, a small opening or *fenestration* in the tunnel is created to allow a small amount of right-to-left shunting to decompress the relatively high-pressure systemic venous conduit.

Figures 5-66 and 5-67 depict the various surgical approaches to transposition of the great arteries. The *Mustard* and *Senning procedures* were the original procedures used until the 1980s to correct the circulation in children with transposition. In both of these operations the atrial venous return is "switched" by placing a baffle that directs the superior and inferior vena caval systemic venous return posterior and to the left behind the baffle to the left ventricle, while allowing the pulmonary venous return to flow anteriorly in front of the baffle to the right ventricle. Figure 5-66 demonstrates the preoperative and postoperative flow patterns in transposition in the right and left diagrams, respectively, showing how rerouting systemic venous return allows fully oxygenated blood to go to the aorta. The only difference in the Mustard and Senning operations is the use of more native atrial tissue and less patch material in the latter operation. Because of long-term morbidity with the atrial switch procedures, including baffle obstruction and dysfunction of the systemic right ventricle, in the past 25 years all pediatric cardiology centers have been using the *arterial*

TRANSPOSITION OF THE GREAT ARTERIES

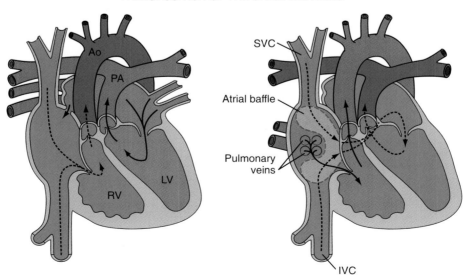

Ao

PA

SVC

Atrial baffle

Pulmonary
veins

LV

RV

IVC

Mustard or Senning procedure

Figure 5-66   Intraatrial baffle (Mustard or Senning) procedure for transposition of the great arteries.

TRANSPOSITION OF THE GREAT ARTERIES

Arterial switch
(Jatene procedure)

Figure 5-67   Arterial switch (Jatene) procedure for trans-position of the great arteries.

switch (Jatene) procedure (see Fig. 5-67) to correct the circula-tion in transposition of the great arteries. The aortic and pul-monary roots are transected and "switched" to the appropriate ventricles. The most difficult aspect of this operation is the transfer of the right and left coronary arteries from the anterior native aortic root to the posterior pulmonary root that will become the neoaorta.

The key elements of the *Rastelli procedure,* closure of a ventricular septal defect and placement of a conduit to connect the right ventricle to the pulmonary artery, are shown in Figure 5-68. This procedure is used for tetralogy of Fallot with pulmonary atresia, transposition of the great arteries with ventricular septal defect and severe pulmonic stenosis, and truncus arteriosus (pulmonary arteries arising directly from a truncal root that overrides a large ventricular septal defect, as shown in the diagram, on the left). The operation for a truncus arteriosus consists of closing the ventricular septal defect to direct all left ventricular outflow to the aorta, detachment of the pulmonary arteries from the aorta (truncus), and place-ment of a homograft conduit between the right ventricle and pulmonary arteries.

Figures 5-69, 5-70, and 5-71 show operations designed to treat aortic valve and systemic outflow tract disease. The *Ross procedure* (see Fig. 5-69) is an ingenious approach to the treat-ment of severe aortic stenosis or insufficiency when a valve replacement is required. The diseased aortic valve is removed, and the patient's own pulmonary valve is autotransplanted to the aortic position. The coronary arteries must be reimplanted into the neoaortic root, and a pulmonary homograft is used to reconstruct the right ventricular outflow tract. This opera-tion avoids the lifelong anticoagulation that would be required by a prosthetic aortic valve, but has a relatively high rate of reintervention, predominantly for dysfunction of the right ventricle-to-pulmonary artery homograft. Aortic stenosis with a small annulus is usually treated with a *Konno procedure* (see Fig. 5-70), which uses patch enlargement of the base of the ventricular septum to increase the size of the aortic annulus, allowing placement of an appropriately sized prosthetic aortic valve. This procedure may be combined with the Ross proce-dure. Figure 5-71 shows the *Konno-Rastan procedure,* in which a patch is used to enlarge the ventricular septum in order to relieve diffuse subaortic stenosis.

TRUNCUS ARTERIOSUS

Rastelli procedure

Figure 5-68   Creation of a right ventricle–to-pulmonary conduit and closure of a ventricular septal defect for truncus arteriosus (Rastelli procedure).

Figure 5-69 Replacing the diseased aortic valve with the native pulmonary valve (Ross procedure).

AORTIC VALVE DISEASE

Autograft of pulmonic valve

Pulmonary homograft

Ross procedure

Figure 5-70 Enlargement of the limited aortic annulus associated with severe aortic valve disease by patch enlargement of the ventricular septum and placement of a prosthetic valve (Konno procedure).

AORTIC STENOSIS WITH SMALL AORTIC ANNULUS

Prosthetic valve

Patch enlargement of ventricular septum

Konno procedure

Figure 5-71 Enlargement of diffuse subaortic stenosis by patch enlargement of the ventricular septum and resection of a subaortic ridge (Konno-Rastan procedure).

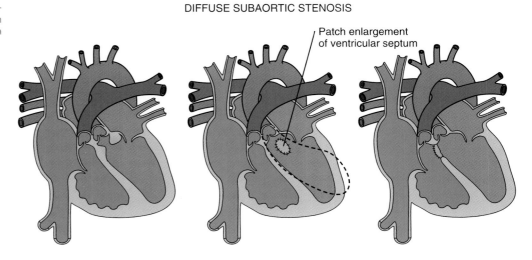

DIFFUSE SUBAORTIC STENOSIS

Patch enlargement of ventricular septum

Konno-Rastan procedure

DOUBLE INLET LEFT VENTRICLE
WITH RESTRICTIVE VENTRICULAR COMMUNICATION

Modified Blalock-Taussig shunt

Ventricular communication

MRV

MLV

Ao

PA

Damus-Stansel-Kaye procedure

Figure 5-72 Bypass of subaortic stenosis due to a restrictive ventricular communication by creation of aortopulmonary anastomosis (Damus-Stansel-Kaye procedure).

Figure 5-72 illustrates the *Damus-Stansel-Kaye procedure,* which is used to relieve aortic outflow tract obstruction in the setting of complex heart disease. A double-inlet left ventricle with a restrictive ventricular communication that results in severe "functional" subaortic stenosis is one such example. The main pulmonary artery is transected, and the distal opening is oversewn along with connection of the proximal pulmonary root to the ascending aorta, in essence creating a bypass around the small ventricular communication that leads to the aorta. A modified Blalock-Taussig shunt is created to provide pulmonary blood flow. In Figure 5-72, "MLV" refers to the dominant morphologic left ventricle, which receives both atrioventricular valves. "MRV" refers to the hypoplastic morphologic right ventricle, which receives blood only via the ventricular communication and supports the aortic valve.

INTERVENTIONAL CARDIAC CATHETERIZATION

Interventional cardiology developed as a subspecialty after William Rashkind introduced the balloon septostomy in the 1960s to alleviate cyanosis in transposition of the great arteries. In recent years the field has expanded explosively so that currently it plays a role in the treatment of almost every heart defect. Interventions can be classified according to the purpose to treat:

1. Valvular obstruction

2. Vascular stenosis

3. Creation or enlargement of defects

4. Closure of defects

5. Other

Valvular Obstruction

Pulmonary Valve Stenosis/Atresia

In general, intervention is indicated when peak-to-peak (right ventricle to pulmonary artery systolic) gradients are above 40 mm Hg as measured via cardiac catheterization. Balloon dilation has become the standard first-line treatment. In

pulmonic stenosis, balloon dilation is highly effective in the large majority of patients. However, the success rate is not as high for the so-called *dysplastic pulmonary valve* (common in Noonan syndrome), in which the valve is thick and often has associated supravalvular narrowing. For these valves, high-pressure balloons may be necessary to achieve success. Efficacy is long lasting in most cases, although about 8% of individuals do require repeat dilation for restenosis. A special group of patients are the newborns with critical pulmonary valve stenosis, for which repeat dilation within the first year of life is not uncommon. Although dilation frequently results in regurgitation of the valve, because pulmonary artery resistance is normally quite low, the physiologic consequences of the insufficiency are rarely significant. Thus the main long-term issues are observation for the rare case of restenosis.

In the newborn period intervention is necessary in those with critical pulmonary stenosis and ductal-dependent circulation, presenting with severe cyanosis. In this setting it is common to see associated variable degrees of right ventricular hypoplasia and even cavitary obliteration. The right ventricle most often remodels over time to allow a normal biventricular circulation; however, it may take several weeks or months for resolution of right-to-left shunt across the patent foramen ovale. Typically, the prostaglandins that are used to promote ductal patency before the procedure are discontinued after balloon dilation. Some patients may require ongoing prostaglandin therapy for a few days or even weeks, particularly if the severity of the right ventricular hypoplasia is marked. Transcatheter placement of a stent in the ductus arteriosus has become an attractive alternative to surgical palliation for those patients who cannot wean off prostaglandins.

Patients with membranous pulmonary atresia can undergo radiofrequency-assisted valve perforation followed by balloon valvotomy (Fig. 5-73). Although successful perforation has been reported in up to 75% to 90% of selected patients, the procedure is definitive for only 35% because they commonly require additional intervention, either transcatheter or surgical.

Aortic Valve Stenosis

Although a few centers in the world continue to perform surgical valvotomies for aortic stenosis, most prefer balloon valvotomy as the procedure of choice. In the newborn, severe

Figure 5-73 Pulmonary valve stenosis or atresia. **A,** A right ventricular angiogram in the lateral projection shows atresia of the pulmonary valve. **B,** After radiofrequency perforation of the pulmonary valve, balloon dilation is performed. **C,** After dilation there is an open pathway between the right ventricle (RV) and pulmonary artery (PA).

aortic stenosis can present as critical with ductal-dependent systemic circulation. Transcatheter balloon dilation can be performed with antegrade (femoral vein or umbilical vein to left ventricle and aorta via the foramen ovale) or retrograde (umbilical artery or femoral artery). For premature babies, the carotid artery approach is a good alternative to avoid femoral arterial damage. At present the procedure can be performed with low-profile balloons, which can be advanced via a 3-French sheath in the femoral artery, with significantly reduced incidence of iliofemoral artery thrombosis.

Natural history data for aortic stenosis have suggested that a peak-to-peak gradient across the valve of more than 50 mm Hg represents obstruction severe enough that intervention is preferable to observation and "medical management." Aortic stenosis represents a very different circumstance regarding success compared with pulmonary valve stenosis. All known forms of therapy including balloon dilation, surgical valvotomy, or replacement of the valve are palliative given that further surgery will be necessary at some point in almost all cases. Balloon dilation of the aortic valve creates small tears in the fused commissures of leaflets that result in an increase in the valve orifice size. Some degree of aortic insufficiency is commonly present after the procedure. Attempts to completely alleviate obstruction by using overly large balloons result in an unacceptable amount of regurgitation. Thus even after successful balloon dilation, patients commonly have residual obstruction and/or insufficiency. The benefit achieved after aortic valve dilation is of variable duration. In one report the intervention-free rate of survival was 50% to 60% at 10 years after dilation. The need for subsequent intervention may be due to recurrent obstruction, insufficiency, or both. In the first instance repeat valve dilation is an option.

Mitral Stenosis

Isolated congenital mitral valve stenosis is rare, occurring more commonly in association with other left-sided obstructive lesions, as in patients with Shone syndrome or other complex congenital heart disease. Congenital mitral valve stenosis has proven to be a somewhat intractable condition, with a high mortality rate. Given the palliative nature of any intervention for patients with congenital mitral stenosis, newborns that present with a severe form of this condition are typically managed as patients with hypoplastic left heart syndrome.

Mitral balloon valvotomy beyond the newborn period can be effective and may have a lasting beneficial result, especially for rheumatic mitral valve stenosis. However, for congenital mitral valve stenosis, the procedure should be considered palliative and potentially able to delay the need for mitral valve replacement in a small child.

Vascular Stenosis

Pulmonary Artery Stenosis

Peripheral pulmonary artery stenosis can be congenital or acquired after cardiac surgery and constitutes 2% to 3% of congenital heart disease. Congenital pulmonary artery stenosis can occur in isolation or be associated with other congenital heart defects (most commonly, tetralogy of Fallot with or without pulmonary atresia). As a primary lesion, it may be idiopathic or occur in the presence of syndromes, such as congenital rubella, Williams syndrome, and Alagille syndrome. Results of surgery for any of these branch pulmonary artery stenoses have been quite unsatisfactory. In addition, surgery cannot treat peripheral stenoses within the lungs. Thus balloon angioplasty has become the first-line therapy for these patients.

In general, indications for balloon dilation include an elevated right-to-left ventricular systolic pressure ratio of more than 50%, right ventricular failure, angiographic narrowing, contralateral pulmonary arterial hypertension, and abnormal perfusion by lung scintigraphy. Although there are no contraindications to this procedure by age or size, newborns with severe branch pulmonary artery stenosis should undergo balloon angioplasty only if severely symptomatic. Either discrete stenoses or long diffuse hypoplastic pulmonary arteries can be dilated, with success rates of 50% to 75%. With the use of high-pressure balloons, the success rate is on the order of 75%. Most recently the cutting balloon (Fig. 5-74) has been used for resistant lesions, significantly increasing the success rate of balloon pulmonary angioplasty. In addition, stent implantation allows a significant improvement in success rates to more than 90% (Fig. 5-75). However, not all lesions

Figure 5-74 Cutting balloon. Note the four tiny blades along the balloon surface.

Figure 5-75   Pulmonary artery angioplasty. Note the left pulmonary artery (LPA) stenosis demonstrated on the pulmonary artery angiogram **(A)**; after stent implantation the stenosis has been eliminated **(B)**.

are amenable to stent implantation. There are theoretical disadvantages to placing stents in infants, including more difficult vascular access and the need for subsequent dilations to keep up with somatic growth. Nevertheless, some lesions that have not responded to dilation alone or surgery can be managed successfully by stent implantation, regardless of the patient's age.

Aortic Coarctation

Balloon dilation of native coarctation of the aorta remains a controversial subject. In general, indications for intervention in infants and children, whether surgical or transcatheter placement, include the presence of anatomic coarctation associated with a systolic pressure gradient between the upper and lower extremities of more than 20 mm Hg or a systolic blood pressure greater than 95% for age or the presence of left ventricular dysfunction. Because of the high restenosis rate during the first month of life, intervention is indicated in this age group only in symptomatic patients with congestive heart failure, failure to thrive, or upper extremity hypertension associated with left ventricular dysfunction. Surgery is considered the management approach of choice for neonates and young infants with severe coarctation, given the unacceptably high incidence of restenosis after balloon angioplasty (at least 50%). However, there are specific clinical conditions in which

balloon dilation of a native coarctation in infants can be considered as the procedure of choice: patients with high surgical risks due to severe left ventricular dysfunction and unstable hemodynamic condition, severe pulmonary hypertension or other pulmonary diseases that would significantly increase the risk of thoracotomy, and recent intracranial hemorrhage or other major systemic disorders.

Recurrence of stenosis after balloon dilation decreases as the patient's age increases, reaching about 10% for children older than 2 years of age. The procedure is generally safe, with a mortality rate less than 1% and aneurysm formation rates of 7%.

In patients who present after adolescence and into adulthood, transcatheter stenting of the coarctation is widely gaining acceptance as appropriate first-line treatment or at least as an acceptable alternative to surgery (Fig. 5-76). The transcatheter approach is particularly appealing in the absence of any significant collateral vessels when surgical repair would have higher risk for spinal cord ischemia. Dilation with stent placement results in effective relief of the obstruction in 92% to 100% of cases.

For patients with postoperative recurrent or residual coarctation, balloon angioplasty is considered the procedure of choice, regardless of the type of previous surgical repair. Success occurs in more than 90% with a restenosis rate of

Figure 5-76   Coarctation angioplasty. Note the severe coarctation of the aorta *(*)* shown by angiography in the descending aorta (Ao) **(A)**; after balloon angioplasty and stent implantation the coarctation has been eliminated **(B)**.

less than 20%. Mortality is 0.7%, with a low incidence of aneurysm formation of less than 2%.

Systemic or Pulmonary Vein Stenosis

Symptomatic systemic venous obstruction can occur in infants and children after cardiac surgery or after placement of chronic indwelling lines. Indications for intervention include symptoms of systemic venous hypertension, superior vena cava syndrome, and chronic pleural effusions (associated with elevated central venous pressure). Balloon dilation of venous stenoses has been performed since the mid-1980s. Although the immediate success rate is more than 90% for balloon dilation alone, the restenosis rate is more than 50%, suggesting that stent implantation should be considered as first-line therapy.

Pulmonary vein stenosis is generally an intractable disease, occurring either as a congenital lesion or postoperatively. Balloon dilation and stent implantation can serve only as short-term palliation for symptomatic patients awaiting heart–lung transplantation. Hemodynamic and angiographic improvement are seen immediately in almost all patients. However, restenosis occurs in virtually all cases within a few months of intervention.

Creation or Enlargement of Defects

Balloon Atrial Septostomy

After its initial introduction by Rashkind and Miller in 1966, balloon atrial septostomy to improve atrial mixing and increase systemic oxygen saturation has become an essential intervention in the management of most patients with transposition of the great arteries and other forms of congenital heart disease with transposition-like physiology (i.e., some forms of double-outlet right ventricle). At most centers, balloon atrial septostomy is performed routinely on patients with dextrotransposition of the great arteries and intact ventricular septum, many times in the intensive care unit under echocardiographic guidance. In patients with left-sided obstructive lesions, a thick atrial septum, small left atrium, and restrictive atrial septal defect, balloon atrial septostomy is rarely successful. For these patients, other techniques of atrial septal defect creation and septoplasty (using a static balloon dilation approach) are preferred. The success rate of balloon atrial septostomy in newborns is higher than 98%, with a low complication rate.

Atrial Septoplasty/Blade Septostomy

Because balloon atrial septostomy is not feasible in newborns with an intact atrial septum or a thick septum, other techniques for septal defect creation are warranted for these patients. Blade atrial septostomy was developed by Sang Park for this purpose (Fig. 5-77). Alternative techniques currently used are a combination of Brockenbrough transseptal puncture followed by serial balloon dilations using angioplasty balloons, including the cutting balloon, and occasionally stent implantation.

Closure of Defects

Atrial Septal Defects

At present, most secundum atrial septal defects are closed via the transcatheter deployment of devices. However, some atrial defects are not amenable to device closure because of the lack of an adequate rim of tissue around the defect to anchor the device. Atrial septal defects of the sinus venosus type or ostium primum defects cannot be closed with devices. Although devices are available to close large holes (up to 38 mm in diameter), the larger devices will fit only in a large

Figure 5-77 Atrial septostomy devices. Note the Rashkind balloon *(top)* and Park blade *(bottom)* septostomy catheters (Cook Medical, Bloomington, Ind).

adult heart. Two devices are currently approved in the United States for closure of an atrial septal defect: the Amplatzer septal occluder (AGA Medical, Golden Valley, Minn) (Fig. 5-78) and the Gore Helex septal occluder (W.L. Gore & Associates, Flagstaff, Ariz). The procedure is performed under transesophageal or intracardiac echocardiographic guidance (Fig. 5-79). Several studies have documented that the efficacy of device closure compares favorably with surgery, with high closure and low complication rates. Late perforations after device closure have been reported to occur up to several years after device implantation; however, these have been rare.

Ventricular Septal Defects

Most ventricular septal defects (VSDs) cannot be closed with devices because of the significant size of the defect in relatively small hearts, as well as the proximity to intracardiac valves, particularly the tricuspid and aortic valves. An option to overcome the limitations of the technique in a small child is a combined hybrid catheterization–surgical approach. In this method the heart is exposed via a thoracotomy and the device delivery catheter advanced through the free wall of the right ventricle and across the defect. The device is then opened under echocardiographic guidance. This technique has the advantage of avoiding cardiopulmonary bypass and may be particularly useful for ventricular septal defects located in portions of the heart difficult to reach by standard open surgical technique. The CardioSEAL device (NMT Medical, Boston) (Fig. 5-80) as well as the Amplatzer muscular VSD occluder are currently approved for closure of muscular ventricular septal defects. The latter is the most widely used.

Figure 5-78 Device closure of atrial septal defect. Note the Amplatzer septal occluder device held outstretched from each disk to demonstrate its architecture. Two disks and a central waist, which occludes the defect, are shown.

A   B

Figure 5-79 Illustration of placement of Amplatzer septal occluder. Note that the delivery sheath is advanced across the defect into the left atrium, and the device is partially extruded out of the sheath with opening of the left atrial disk **(A)**; after withdrawal of the sheath the device has been deployed with the right atrial disk opened on the right side of the septum, and the device has been detached from the delivery cable **(B)**.

Figure 5-80   CardioSEAL device (NMT Medical, Boston, Mass).

Although high success rates have been reported with transcatheter closure of ventricular septal defects, in the United States the procedure is currently still reserved for defects that are difficult to close surgically or for a combined surgical–interventional catheter approach in some patients.

Patent Ductus Arteriosus

In patent ductus arteriosus (PDA), small and moderate patent ducts are typically closed in the catheterization laboratory with either embolization coils or the Amplatzer duct occluder (Fig. 5-81), whereas large symptomatic PDAs in the newborn are treated surgically. Transcatheter closure of patent ducts has been highly successful, with efficacy of more than 97% and a low complication rate.

Other Transcatheter Techniques

Closure of Collaterals

Lesions amenable to closure by embolization therapy include systemic venous anomalies (i.e., left superior vena cava to left atrium) or aortopulmonary collaterals, pulmonary sequestration, or congenital arteriovenous malformations. Coil embolization of collaterals is one of the most common procedures in children with congenital heart disease associated with aortopulmonary collateral vessels.

Percutaneous Pulmonary Valve Implantation

In January 2010 the U.S. Food and Drug Administration approved the Melody valve (Medtronic, Minneapolis, Minn) for percutaneous implantation in the pulmonary position in patients with dysfunctional right ventricle-to-pulmonary

A   B

Figure 5-81   Closure of patent ductus arteriosus. Note that the descending aorta (Ao) angiogram shows a patent ductus *(arrow)* entering the main pulmonary artery (MPA) **(A)**; a repeat angiogram after placement of an Amplatzer duct occluder demonstrates that the ductus is completely closed **(B)**.

Figure 5-82   Melody percutaneous pulmonary valve. A bovine jugular venous valve is sewn on a platinum iridium stent. Valve leaflets within the stent are shown on oblique view *(left)*.

artery conduits implanted surgically at the time of repair of certain congenital heart defects. This novel technology may delay the need for surgical conduit replacement. The valve is a bovine jugular venous valve mounted on a CP stent (NuMED, Hopkinton, NY), which is a platinum iridium stent, and is MRI compatible (Fig. 5-82). This has become an option for patients with pulmonary conduit stenosis and/or insufficiency, allowing restoration of pulmonary valve function. The valve is implanted within the existing conduit, which is expanded up to the original size. Available sizes range from 18 to 22 mm in diameter. The technique of Melody valve implantation within a stenotic right ventricle-to-pulmonary artery conduit is illustrated in Figures 5-83 through 5-85. This procedure may also benefit selected patients with tetralogy of Fallot who were initially repaired without a conduit and have developed severe pulmonary regurgitation years later.

Miscellaneous

Reopening of thrombosed vessels or surgical anastomoses can be performed by transcatheter thrombolysis with good results, although the experience in pediatrics is relatively limited. Other interventions include retrieval of foreign bodies, preservation of ductal patency by means of stents, coil embolization of coronary artery fistulae, and some novel catheter interventions such as prenatal interventions (for opening of stenotic valves or a restrictive atrial septum). Many complex hemodynamic and anatomic abnormalities are now addressed by a "hybrid approach," with the surgeon and interventional cardiologist working side by side in the catheterization laboratory, which also functions as an operating room. These innovative procedures are likely to be only a preview of what will be possible and even commonplace in the next decade as the field of interventional catheterization continues to advance and expand.

Figure 5-83   Stenotic right ventricle–to–pulmonary artery conduit. Severe conduit stenosis *(arrow)* is demonstrated in right anterior oblique view *(left)* and lateral projection *(right)* in a patient after surgical repair of congenital heart disease. Conduit was 22 mm in diameter at implantation and over time developed progressive stenosis resulting in less than half the original dimension, causing severe right ventricular hypertension.

Figure 5-84   Partially expanded Melody valve within stent. After expansion of conduit by balloon dilation and stent implantation *(arrows)*, the Melody valve is advanced into the stent and partially expanded with inner balloon. Right anterior oblique *(left)* and lateral *(right)* projections are shown.

Figure 5-85   Melody valve deployment. Valve is fully expanded by outer balloon and deployed within the stent in the conduit *(left)*. Angiogram in pulmonary artery (PA) after Melody valve implantation *(arrow)* demonstrates competent valve with no opacification of the right ventricle.

Bibliography

Beerman LB, Arora G, Park SC: Arrhythmias in the intensive care unit. In Munoz RA, Morell VO, da Cruz EM, Vetterly CG, editors: *Critical care of children with heart disease*, London, 2010, Springer-Verlag.

Bush DM: Evaluating cardiovascular presentations: what does an electrocardiogram have to offer? *Pediatr Ann* 34:858–869, 2005.

Case CL: Diagnosis and treatment of pediatric arrhythmias, *Pediatr Clin North Am* 46:347–354, 1999.

Chun TUH, Van Hare GF: Advances in the approach to treatment of supraventricular tachycardia in the pediatric population, *Curr Cardiol Rep* 6:322–326, 2004.

Du ZD, Hijazi ZM, Kleinman CS, et al: Comparison between transcatheter and surgical closure of secundum atrial septal defect in children and adults: results of a multicenter nonrandomized trial, *J Am Coll Cardiol* 39:1836–1844, 2002.

Ettedgui JA, Tersak JM: Cardiological aspects of systemic disease. In Anderson RH, Macartney FJ, Shinebourne EA, et al, editors: *Paediatric cardiology*, vol 2, ed 2, Edinburgh, 2002, Churchill Livingstone, pp 1777-1808.

Fischer DR, Baker EJ, Anderson RH: Echocardiographic manifestation of ventricular septal defects. In Anderson RH, Neches WH, Park SC, et al, editors: *Perspectives in pediatric cardiology*, vol 2, Mount Kisco, NY, 1988, Futura Publishing, pp 25-33.

Fontan F, Baudet E: Surgical repair of tricuspid atresia, *Thorax* 26:240–248, 1971.

French JW, Guntheroth WG: An explanation of asymmetric upper extremity blood pressures in supravalvular aortic stenosis: the Coanda effect, *Circulation* 42:31–36, 1970.

Glenn WW, Patino JF: Circulatory bypass of the right heart. Preliminary observations on the direct delivery of vena caval blood into the pulmonary arterial circulation: azygos vein pulmonary artery shunt, *Yale J Biol Med* 24:147, 1954.

Greenwood RD: Cardiovascular malformations associated with extracardiac anomalies and malformation syndromes, *Clin Pediatr* 23:145–151, 1984.

Hernandez-Pampaloni M, Allada V, Fishbein MC, et al: Myocardial perfusion and viability by positron emission tomography in infants and children with coronary abnormalities: correlation with echocardiography, coronary angiography, and histopathology, *J Am Coll Cardiol* 41:618–626, 2003.

Humpl T, Soderberg B, McCrindle BW, et al: Percutaneous balloon valvotomy in pulmonic atresia with intact ventricular septum: impact on patient care, *Circulation* 108:826–832, 2003.

Kirklin JW, Barratt-Boyes BG, editors: *Cardiac surgery*, vol 1, ed 2, New York, 1993, Churchill Livingstone, p 546.

Konno S, Imai Y, Iida Y, et al: A new method for prosthetic valve replacement in congenital aortic stenosis associated with hypoplasia of the aortic valve ring, *J Thoracic Cardiovasc Surg* 70:909–917, 1975.

Kreutzer J, Lock JE, Jonas RA, et al: Transcatheter fenestration dilation and/or creation in postoperative Fontan patients, *Am J Cardiol* 79:228–232, 1997.

Kreutzer J, Perry SB: Stents. In Lock JE, Keane JF, Perry SB, editors: *Diagnostic and interventional catheterization in congenital heart disease*, ed 2, Norwell, Mass, 2000, Kluwer Academic Publishers, pp 221-243.

Kugler JD, Danford DA: Management of infants, children and adolescents with paroxysmal supraventricular tachycardia, *J Pediatr* 129:324–328, 1996.

McElhinney DB, Hellenbrand WE, Zahn EM, et al: Short- and medium-term outcomes after transcatheter pulmonary valve placement in the expanded multicenter US Melody Valve Trial, *Circulation* 122:507–516, 2010.

National High Blood Pressure Education Program Working Group on High Blood Pressure in Children and Adolescents: The fourth report on the diagnosis, evaluation, and treatment of high blood pressure in children and adolescents, *Pediatrics* 114(Suppl 2):555–576, 2004.

Newburger JW, Takahashi M, Gerber MA, et al: Diagnosis, treatment, and long-term management of Kawasaki disease: a statement for health professionals from the Committee on Rheumatic Fever, Endocarditis and Kawasaki Disease, Council on Cardiovascular Disease in the Young, American Heart Association, *Circulation* 110:2747–2771, 2004.

Norwood WI Jr: Hypoplastic left heart syndrome, *Ann Thorac Surg* 52:688–695, 1991.

Park SC, Neches WH, Zuberbuhler JR, et al: Clinical use of blade atrial septostomy, *Circulation* 56:600–606, 1978.

Park SC, Zuberbuhler JR: Vascular ring and pulmonary sling. In Anderson RH, Macartney FJ, Shinebourne EA, et al, editors: *Paediatric cardiology*, vol 2, ed 2, Edinburgh, 2002, Churchill Livingstone, pp 1559-1577.

Pelech AN: Evaluation of the pediatric patient with a cardiac murmur, *Pediatr Clin North Am* 45:167–188, 1999.

Perry SB, Radtke W, Fellows KE, et al: Coil embolization to occlude aortopulmonary collateral vessels and shunts in patients with congenital heart disease, *J Am Coll Cardiol* 13:100–108, 1989.

Rashkind WJ, Miller W: Creation of an atrial septal defect without thoracotomy: palliative approach to complete transposition of the great arteries, *JAMA* 196:991–992, 1966.

Robinson B, Anisman P, Eshaghpour E: A primer on pediatric ECGs, *Contemp Pediatr* 11:69–94, 1994.

Rome JJ, Kreutzer J: Pediatric interventional catheterization: reasonable expectations and outcomes, *Pediatr Clin North Am* 51:1589–1610, 2004.

Rowan S, Adroques H, Mathur A, et al: Pediatric hypertension: a review for the primary care provider, *Clin Pediatr* 44:289–296, 2005.

Senning A: Surgical correction of transposition of the great vessels, *Surgery* 45:966–980, 1959.

Sharieff GQ, Rao SO: The pediatric ECG, *Emerg Med Clin North Am* 24:195–208, 2006.

Spicer RL: Cardiovascular disease in Down syndrome, *Pediatr Clin North Am* 31:1331–1343, 1984.

Swenson JM, Fischer DR, Miller SA, et al: Are chest radiographs and electrocardiograms still valuable in evaluating new pediatric patients with heart murmurs or chest pain? *Pediatrics* 99:1–3, 1997.

Tingelstad J: Consultation with the specialist: cardiac dysrhythmias, *Pediatr Rev* 22:91–94, 2001.

Yeager SB, Flanagan MF, Keane JF: Catheter intervention: balloon valvotomy. In Lock JE, Keane JF, Perry SB, editors: *Diagnostic and interventional catheterization in congenital heart disease*, ed 2, Norwell, Mass, 2000, Kluwer Academic Publishers, pp 151-178.

Yi MS, Kimball TR, Tsevat J, et al: Evaluation of heart murmurs in children: cost-effective and practical implications, *J Pediatr* 141:504–511, 2002.

Zuberbuhler JR: *Clinical diagnosis in pediatric cardiology*, Edinburgh, 1981, Churchill Livingstone.

CHILD ABUSE AND NEGLECT

Holly W. Davis | Mary M. Carrasco

Child abuse and neglect constitute a pediatric public health problem of enormous magnitude. Their relative contribution to morbidity and mortality in children is likewise huge. In addition to the fact that more than 900,000 children are identified as substantiated victims each year, approximately 140,000 incur serious injuries and nearly 20,000 are left with permanent physical disabilities such as cerebral palsy and blindness. The toll on emotional development is even more significant.

The incidence of reported cases of abuse and neglect has increased within much of the twentieth century, in part due to improved identification and reporting. Whereas in the past 20 years there has been a decline in substantiated cases of physical and sexual abuse, there has been no change in mortality rates. Caffey in the late 1940s and then Kempe and coworkers in the early 1960s fostered a marked increase in the recognition of the physical manifestations of abuse and of the very real needs and problems of child abuse victims. Subsequent passage of legislation in all 50 states mandating that suspected cases be reported to the proper authorities has further increased the incidence of reporting. Thus, although some of the increasing incidence is real, much is probably the result of these developments. In addition, societal standards have changed, for some of what is currently regarded as abuse was once sanctioned as discipline.

Four major forms of abuse have been delineated: physical abuse, sexual abuse, physical neglect, and emotional abuse. Not infrequently, an individual child is found to be the victim of more than one form and there is some degree of emotional abuse with all forms. For purposes of reporting under child protection laws, the abuse or neglect generally must result from the acts or omissions of a parent, guardian, custodian, or other caretaker of the child.

Of reported cases about 60% involved neglect, 19% physical abuse, 9% sexual abuse, and 5% were identified as emotionally maltreated. These figures may significantly underestimate the actual number as it is estimated that for every case reported, at least two go unreported. Clearly, some, perhaps many, reports concerning truly abused children are inaccurately determined to be unfounded, sometimes because regulations preclude this if a perpetrator cannot be clearly identified despite the fact that the child has clearly been the victim of abuse. Misleading/deceptive histories, limited investigative resources, lack of witnesses, inability or unwillingness of victims and family members to attest to the fact that abuse has occurred, and jurisdictional regulations all contribute to this phenomenon.

Fatality statistics have also been found to have limited accuracy. The National Child Abuse and Neglect Data System (NCANDS) estimates that there were about 1740 deaths in 2008. This is an increase from approximately 1500 cases in 2003 and is likely due to recent improvements in the reporting and investigation of child fatalities. This in turn probably reflects improved recognition of child abuse–related deaths as a result of the institution of child death review teams in most states. Of fatal victims, 40% to 50% are younger than 1 year of age, and 85% to 90% are 5 years of age or younger. Researchers looking at data from additional sources have determined that many, perhaps the majority, of deaths due to abuse are misclassified as due to accident, sudden infant death syndrome (SIDS), or natural or unknown causes. Reasons for misclassification include incomplete medical evaluation; delay in or inadequate death scene investigation, or no scene investigation; lack of sufficient training of coroners and pathologists regarding child abuse and the techniques and studies necessary to identify abuse at autopsy; failure to require manner of death, as well as cause, on death certificates; and poor communication among investigative agencies. Thus most authorities believe 2000 deaths per year is a more accurate figure, although this, too, may be a significant underestimate. To put this in further perspective, the number of deaths due to abuse of children younger than 5 years is greater than the number due to motor vehicle accidents and fires combined and is more than twice the number of deaths due to accidental choking or suffocation, drowning, and falls combined.

The most common causes of death due to abuse are head trauma, abdominal trauma, and suffocation. Of these, intentional suffocation is most likely to go undetected, as autopsy findings may simulate SIDS. It now appears that a large percentage of cases of SIDS are actually due to accidental suffocation as a result of sleeping prone on a soft surface, of getting the face covered in bed clothing, or of co-sleeping with one or more adults whether in bed or on a sofa or easy chair. The Back to Sleep campaign, begun by the National Institute of Child Health and Human Development, and efforts to educate parents about the risks of co-sleeping have dramatically reduced the incidence of these tragic deaths. Further review of co-sleeping deaths points to a disturbing number of cases in which the adult sleeping with the child has a history of substance misuse.

All sudden unexpected deaths in infancy warrant thorough investigation to facilitate accurate determination of cause, assess for possible foul play, and aid in future prevention. Certain historical points and physical findings may aid in distinguishing SIDS from intentional suffocation. Infants dying of SIDS are usually younger than 6 months of age, previously well (or have only mild symptoms of an upper respiratory infection), and found unresponsive in the early morning when their parents awaken. In contrast, those dying of intentional suffocation may range from weeks to 2 or 3 years of age and are more likely to be "found" sometime between mid-morning and late afternoon or evening, after a period of being with a single caretaker. In some, subtle bruises or petechiae of the face and/or neck or scant bleeding from the nose or mouth may be noted. Many of these infants have a history of a recent hospitalization for an unexplained illness or for apnea, seizure-like activity, or an apparent life-threatening event (ALTE), for which no cause could be found despite an extensive medical workup. This or a past history of multiple apparent life-threatening events and/or a history of two or more prior sibling deaths attributed to SIDS should raise strong suspicion of intentional smothering.

EPIDEMIOLOGY

Child abuse is a phenomenon found in *all* socioeconomic, cultural, racial, ethnic, and religious subsets of society. The reported incidence per capita is greatest in lower socioeconomic groups. This stems in part from the numerous chronic stresses and uncertainties of living in poverty, problems of socialization, and different attitudes regarding what constitutes appropriate discipline. It is also clear, and must be recognized by physicians and other professionals, that well-educated parents of higher socioeconomic status can be abusive; however, when they are, they are less likely to be suspected. This is in part because they "come across well" as they tend to be well dressed, well spoken, more sophisticated, and have a more confident demeanor than parents who are less well off. Also, they are often better able to fabricate a plausible history of how the injury occurred "accidentally." Furthermore, when suspected, they are less likely to be reported, and when reported, they are more likely to have the resources and legal assistance to have the case dropped or dismissed, or to be acquitted of the charges. Hence in evaluating potential abuse victims and their families, it is important *not* to rush to judgment of parents on the basis of appearance, dress, and level of sophistication, and professionals should appreciate that many parents who are poor, unsophisticated, and not well dressed are loving and caring despite their limited means and resources.

The most valuable information is gained by a nonjudgmental approach while keeping an open mind in obtaining a thorough history, making careful behavioral and interactional observations, performing meticulous examination, and ordering a well-considered laboratory and imaging evaluation before arriving at a diagnosis.

Parental Risk Factors for Child Abuse and Neglect

1. *Past history of being abused or neglected as a child.* Although this is a significant risk factor, it is important to note that not all abused children grow up to become abusive adults. Those who do not have been found to have had a strong, long-standing, and supportive relationship, from early childhood, with a nurturing and nonabusive adult who loved them unconditionally, helped them recognize their own worth, and taught them how to make good choices. This enables them to develop trusting relationships and, hence, better social support systems.

2. *Poor socialization and emotional and social isolation.* Inadequately nurtured themselves as children, these parents are poorly equipped to adequately nurture their offspring. Their own mothers may not have bonded well with them, and/or their trust may have been betrayed repeatedly by those they loved unconditionally and should have been able to count on most. They may have been shuttled back and forth between the parental home and relatives' or foster homes or placed in a series of foster homes over the course of years. As a result, they have trouble with trust and forming close attachments, and hence, are poorly equipped to develop and use support systems. They tend to have little understanding of child development and of children's emotional and other needs and, therefore, of good child-rearing practices and reasonable expectations of child behavior. E-Tables 6-1 and 6-2 present common features of many of the families of origin of abusive parents/

caretakers, as well as their child-rearing practices, which then tend to be repeated by these younger parents and by ensuing generations. E-Table 6-3 presents common character traits and historical revelations of many poorly socialized parents/caretakers and of those with character disorders.

3. *Limited ability to deal adaptively with stress and negative emotions such as fear, anger, and frustration, compounded by a tendency to lash out violently, verbally and/or physically, in response to negative feelings.* This behavior is often learned by example in their families of origin.

4. *Alcoholism/substance abuse.* When intoxicated or high, such parents may be "out of it" or may be disinhibited in approaching or dealing with their children. They also may be away for extended periods, seeking their substance of choice or the wherewithal to obtain it.

5. *Mental illness* (e-Table 6-4).

6. *Domestic violence in the parental relationship.*

7. *Being subjected to a sudden spate of major life stresses/crises such as loss of job and financial security; loss of home; loss of parent, spouse, or sibling.*

8. *Membership in certain fringe group cults or sects.*

Child Risk Factors

1. *Age younger than 3 years.*

2. *Being separated at birth from a mother at high risk for problems with attachment because of illness or prematurity, resulting in impaired bonding.*

3. *Being the product of an unplanned/unwanted pregnancy, with a mother who sought little or no prenatal care.*

4. *Being small for gestational age, born with congenital anomalies, and/or having a chronic illness (possibly due to parental grieving and guilt, compounded by the chronic stress of caring for a handicapped child).*

5. *Being perceived as difficult or different.*

6. *Having attention-deficit/hyperactivity disorder (ADHD) or being oppositional or defiant.*

7. *Foster children and adopted children.*

Two situations place children at particularly high risk for abuse. One involves a couple with an unplanned pregnancy that one parent did not want and then pushed for abortion, and which the other insisted on carrying to term. After delivery, such infants can be at significant risk when left alone in the care of the parent who opposed the pregnancy. The other involves a common pattern in which a young (often teenage) mother who has trouble with attachment and low self-esteem mistakes "attention" and sex for love and, thus, has poor judgment in her selection of boyfriends. These young women may then have a revolving door for paramours who opportunistically move in for weeks to months and then leave only to be replaced by another. These men also tend to have attachment issues and often have poor impulse control. Further, they have no vested interest in her offspring by other men and thus may have no compunction about "batting them around" when they become a source of irritation, misbehave, or have accidents while these men are "babysitting."

One common thread connecting all of these risk factors appears to be one of *unmet expectations,* due to either unrealistic parental expectations of the child or the child's inability to meet realistic expectations as the result of developmental delay, illness, temperament, hyperactivity, or inconsistent disciplining. Typically this stems from lack of parental understanding of normal child behavior and emotional development, and of their children's basic needs for nurturing. The combination can then lead the parent or caretaker to attribute *malicious intent* to an infant who will not stop crying or to a toddler who has had a toilet training accident, is stubborn, or misbehaves. Once "malicious intent" is suspected, this can incite rage in someone with a short fuse.

With this background information, the approach to diagnosis of the major forms of abuse can now be addressed more specifically.

PHYSICAL ABUSE

Physical abuse is defined as the infliction of bodily injury that causes significant or severe pain, leaves physical evidence, impairs physical functioning, or significantly jeopardizes the child's safety. Individual states have varying definitions of what constitutes abuse reportable to Child Protective Services (CPS) and law enforcement agencies, and practitioners should become familiar with the guidelines in their own states. Many of the methods used by perpetrators are listed in Table 6-1, and weapons commonly employed are detailed in Table 6-2.

Infants and toddlers are at greatest risk for physical abuse because they are unable to escape attack, and are developmentally incapable of meeting many expectations and of knowing when to "keep a low profile." Given their small size and physical immaturity, they are also the most vulnerable to severe injury. *Common triggers for abusive behavior* toward infants are *crying*, especially prolonged or inconsolable crying, and *feeding problems*. Crying may be due to hunger; pain with illness such as otitis media and esophagitis with gastroesophageal reflux; gas pain due to aerophagia either precipitated by or induced by respiratory disease or frequent feeding interruptions in avid feeders; and pain from prior inflicted trauma (rib or extremity fractures or CNS irritability from head injury). Feeding problems may stem from neurologic or oral–motor disorders, oropharyngeal deformities (such as cleft palate), or pain on swallowing due to oral lesions or reflux-induced esophagitis. With toddlers, difficulties in toilet training, *toileting accidents,* getting into things they are not supposed to touch, and stubbornness or negativism are common inciting factors. Failure to follow orders or instructions, oppositional or defiant behavior, and getting into trouble at school are notable triggers of abuse of older children.

The spectrum of severity of injuries caused by physical abuse ranges from isolated surface bruising that may be a product of overzealous discipline to fatal head and abdominal trauma that is the result of extremely violent rage reactions. Important to remember is that relatively unimpressive surface marks or injuries may be associated with far more significant underlying skeletal, abdominal, and CNS trauma (see Fig. 6-13). In addition, it is well known that physical abuse tends to be repetitive and that the severity of attacks tends to escalate over time; so does, correspondingly, the severity of injuries. Given this, early recognition, reporting, and intervention are essential in prevention of increased morbidity and mortality. Early recognition can be difficult for a number of reasons. Children with milder injuries generally are not brought to medical attention and may even be kept from those outside the immediate family until visible bruises or other surface injuries fade. Further, when care is sought, a misleading or deceptive history is almost always given. If a plausible history of accidental injury is provided (as can be the case with more sophisticated abusive parents), abuse may go unsuspected. However, when emergency department physicians make it a general practice to disrobe children and perform a complete surface examination on all those who present with mild or minor trauma, the diagnosis of otherwise unsuspected abuse rises dramatically because of identification of suspicious physical findings on other areas of the body, especially those ordinarily covered by clothing. Because presenting signs and symptoms are often nonspecific, recognition can be particularly challenging when the victim of mild to moderate inflicted trauma is a young infant and has no surface injuries or ones that are subtle and easily overlooked. Listlessness or lethargy, irritability or fussiness, vomiting (usually without diarrhea), low-grade fever, and vague complaints of trouble with breathing in infants with milder degrees of inflicted head injury can easily be interpreted as being due to early viral infection. Irritability due to pain from rib and metaphyseal fractures may be mistakenly diagnosed as due to colic or constipation (which may coexist due to stool withholding secondary to pain). Grunting respirations due to rib pain are likely to be attributed to early pulmonary disease such as bronchiolitis or pneumonitis. Relatively rapid dissipation of pain and tenderness (often within 2 to 5 days) in infants with nondisplaced fractures (due to their thick periosteal covering, which resists tearing and promotes prompt healing) can add to the diagnostic difficulty, particularly when presentation is delayed.

Hence diagnosis requires a high index of suspicion when infants, especially young infants, present with unexplained irritability and/or lethargy, with or without grunting respirations, and with vomiting without diarrhea. Unusual thoroughness in history taking and physical examination is a must. This includes asking if fussiness or irritability is or was worse with movement, on being picked up, or when held by the chest.

Table 6-1	Methods Used in Physical Abuse
Hitting—hand, fist, weapon	
Grabbing with squeeze, pinch, twist, yank, or snap	
Shaking	
Throwing	
Swinging	
Kicking	
Stomping	
Burning—scalds, contact burns	
Biting	
Hair pulling	
Holding hand over face to stifle crying	
Prolonged squeezing of chest	
Smothering/strangling	
Holding under water	

Table 6-2	Weapons Commonly Used in Physical Abuse
Hands/fists/feet	
Switch/rod/stick/TV antenna/ruler/broom	
Looped extension or cable TV cord	
Paddle	
Kitchen utensil—wooden spoon/spatula/fork	
Hairbrush/comb	
Coat hanger	
Shoe/slipper	
Rope/cord/chain/tourniquet	
Hot liquids	
Hot objects—iron/curling iron/hair dryer/space heater/cigarette/match/lighter/stove burner	

The physical examination should include a meticulous surface assessment searching for faint bruises or petechiae including a Wood's lamp examination (see the section Bruises, Welts, and Scars); careful palpation of ribs and extremities for tenderness (with particular attention to posterior ribs and long bone metaphyses); and dilated retinoscopy, all of which can be revealing. When a history of pain on motion or bony tenderness is found or when subtle surface injuries are noted, a skeletal survey is indicated, perhaps followed by a bone scan (see the sections on fractures, under Skeletal Injuries). The presence of metaphyseal and rib fractures and/or retinal hemorrhages mandates a head computed tomography (CT) scan (because of their association with subdural hematomas).

Regardless of whether or not abuse is the source of crying and irritability, when presented with an infant with these complaints, physicians should *not* be quick to jump to the diagnosis of colic, constipation, or "normal fussiness." Rather, they should institute a thorough search for a precise cause including inflicted trauma in the differential. Once the cause is found, appropriate measures should be taken and clear recommendations should be given to parents with irritable infants as to what they can do to relieve the baby's symptoms, as this may save some from future abuse.

Of note, there is a demonstrated increase in admissions for serious inflicted injury of infants around 6 to 8 weeks of age. This has been attributed to a normal increase in crying from birth to 2 to 8 weeks "unrelated to any underlying pathology." The majority of this crying does not have an identifiable cause and is observed across cultures. Given the fact that many, if not most, young infants admitted with serious inflicted trauma

have evidence of prior painful injuries, often of differing ages, it is likely that the true cause of their crying went undetected. This could be because no prior care was sought or because when sought, signs of tenderness had abated, symptoms were nonspecific, or the exact cause was not assiduously sought and was therefore missed.

The disturbing incidence of severe and fatal cases of physical abuse has led to an effort to detect identifiable risk factors that might be predictive of fatal outcome. The majority of perpetrators of such abuse who have been studied were abused themselves as children. Poverty, unemployment, a long history of family violence, drug and alcohol abuse, and adolescent parenthood were common threads. Fathers and paramours are by far the most common perpetrators, responsible for up to 58% of the cases of severe and fatal beatings, followed by babysitters in up to 21% and mothers in up to 13%. Crying and toilet training accidents were the most common triggering events. Victims frequently had histories or evidence of prior suspicious injuries, often of a series of injuries of increasing severity, before the final beating. Mothers are more likely to be the perpetrators of death by suffocation and neglect.

The diagnosis of inflicted injury is established on the basis of a constellation of factors including historical, physical, and behavioral observations. Approaching the case with an open mind, obtaining a thorough present and past medical and psychosocial history, and meticulous physical examination are crucial to ensuring accurate diagnosis of inflicted trauma as well as in preventing overdiagnosis of abuse. Important elements are detailed in Tables 6-3 and 6-4. Radiographs and

| Table 6-3 | History Guidelines for Suspected Physical Abuse |

General Guidelines	History of Present Illness	Past Medical History	Psychosocial History	Behavioral Review of Systems
Start with open-ended questions	• What brings you to see us today?	Pregnancy—planned/unplanned, wanted/unwanted	Family:	Nightmares/sleep difficulties
Follow up with specific clarifying questions	• Onset, course, specific symptoms, pertinent positives and negatives	Emotional stresses during pregnancy	Living situation—housing, who lives in household	Increased aggression
If two parent figures are present, try to take history from each separately and out of child's presence	• Who has been with the child during this time frame?	Gravidity, parity, spontaneous/induced abortions	Handling of major developmental hurdles (weaning, toilet training)	Anxiety
	• If irritability reported: Does it increase with movement or during diaper changes?	Prenatal/perinatal/neonatal course/complications	Methods of discipline	Depression
			Caretakers when parents are not home	Low self-esteem
Child should be interviewed alone, if age and condition permit (questions should be nonleading and age appropriate)	• Have bruises or other skin marks been noted?	Prior child losses	Support systems	Withdrawal from social interaction
	• If injury reported:	Well-child care—primary care provider(s), visits attended	Family stresses	Regression
	What happened?	Immunization status	Parent/parent figures:	Increased activity/anxiety
	When did it occur?	If not up to date on visits/immunizations, why?	Duration and quality of relationship	PTSD symptoms
When possible, quote questions and answers verbatim	Where did it occur?	Growth and development	History of their families of origin:	Phobias
	In what circumstances and position was the child found?	Major medical problems	Parental relationship(s)	Change in appetite
	Was the incident witnessed and if so by whom?	Hospitalizations (where)	Quality of interaction/nurturing of parent as child	Self-abuse
	What kind of forces were involved?	Surgery (where)	Methods of discipline	Decrease in academic performance/school failure
	If a fall, what precipitated it, from what height onto what surface, position on landing?	Injuries (where treated)	Levels of education/employment	Running away
		Ingestions	History of drug or alcohol abuse	Drug/EtOH use
	If child ambulating, at what speed and what led to fall?		History of psychiatric illness	Fire setting
			History of prior CPS involvement	Animal abuse
	MEDICAL REVIEW OF SYSTEMS		History of childhood physical or sexual abuse	Involvement with the law
			History of involvement with law enforcement, incarceration	
			History of domestic violence	

EtOH, ethyl alcohol; PTSD, posttraumatic stress disorder.

Table 6-4	Physical Examination for Suspected Physical Abuse

Vital signs

General appearance, demeanor

Nutritional status and growth parameters

Complete body surface examination

Palpation of each bone

Full general examination including the following:

    Head and scalp, including head circumference in infants

    Ears, nose, mouth (all mucosal surfaces), throat and dentition

    Cardiopulmonary examination

    Palpation of abdomen and serial re-examinations to assess for evolving signs of intraabdominal injury

    Palpation of regional nodes

    Genitalia including inspection of urethral, vaginal, and anal orifices

Neurologic examination

Ophthalmologic examination including conjunctivae, sclerae, pupils, anterior chamber, and dilated retinoscopy

Developmental assessment

laboratory studies (complete blood count [CBC] and differential, liver function tests [LFTs], amylase, lipase, prothrombin time/partial thromboplastin time [PT/PTT], coagulation profile) are useful, not only in identifying and confirming injuries, but also in detecting evidence of occult trauma and ruling out other differential diagnostic possibilities.

Common Historical Red Flags

In many instances one or more of the following historical red flags may provide the first clue to abuse:

1. *Despite no history of injury, injury is found.*

2. *The history is incompatible with the type or degree of injury.* For example, the distribution of lesions or type of injury does not fit the mechanism reported; the history is consistent with a minor injury (shortfall, rolled off couch), but evidence of major trauma is found; or multiple injuries of differing ages are found for which no prior care has been sought or adequate explanation provided.

3. *The history of the way in which the injury occurred is vague, or incomplete.*

4. *The history changes* each time it is told to a different health care worker, or even to the same worker who comes back with clarifying questions.

5. *The parents, when interviewed separately, give contradictory histories.*

6. *The history is not credible.* The child may be said to have done something developmentally impossible (e.g., having climbed and fallen when he or she cannot even sit, or a younger sibling caused it).

7. *No history is reported of changes in behavior in an infant or child who has older injuries of differing ages that would have caused significant pain.*

Miscellaneous Historical Red Flags

1. *A history or evidence of repeated visits* necessitated by "accidents" or injuries (often to a number of different facilities).

2. *A history or evidence of repeated fractures or old scars suggestive of prior inflicted injury.*

3. *A history of repeated ingestions.*

4. *Poor compliance with well-child care:* missed visits, immunization delay.

Behavioral/Interactional Red Flags

1. *A significant delay between the time of injury and the time of presentation often exists.*

2. *The parent may not show the degree of concern appropriate* to the severity of the child's injury.

3. *A pathologic parent–child interaction may be observed.* A parent demonstrates unusually rough/angry/impulsive behavior toward the child (yells, yanks, hits). A parent displays inappropriate expectations of child ("sit still," i.e., don't explore; "watch your brother"). A parent is often clearly unaware of the child's needs and insensitive to behavioral cues (crying with hunger, dirty diaper, wants to be held or comforted).

Few victims of physical abuse are brought in with a chief complaint of abuse. Most present with a chief complaint of an accidental injury or of an unrelated (cold, rash) or somewhat peripheral (lethargy, irritability) chief complaint. Whenever the physician's suspicion is aroused by historical or observational findings, he or she (or a designated social worker) should obtain a detailed psychosocial history, seeking more information concerning the family's current living situation, stresses, and emotional support systems. Particular attention should be paid to recent family crises including personal (ill health, job loss, separation) and environmental (pending eviction, heat or utilities discontinued) crises; degree of isolation (no family or social supports, no phone); and prior problems with family violence, mental health, alcohol, or drugs. Answers to questions about methods of discipline and parental reactions to common triggering events such as prolonged crying, toilet training accidents, and stubborn behavior can be most illuminating, as can answers to questions about how they felt when they learned of the baby's pregnancy, when they first saw the baby, and what the baby is like (see Table 6-3). Although a detailed history takes time, it can be invaluable in facilitating accurate diagnosis, individualizing care, arranging appropriate family supports, and assisting CPS and law enforcement in their investigations. This and the medical history should be obtained in a supportive, nonjudgmental manner because aggressive interrogation will only serve to alienate the parent, limiting the value of the data obtained.

During the evaluation one should bear in mind that the person who has brought the child in for care may not be the abuser, and that many parents of abused children truly want help, whether they have been directly abusive or unable to protect their child from abuse. In many cases a parent may have been unaware that abuse was occurring, had suspicions but no confirmation, suspected on some level but did not want to believe that abuse could be occurring, or was too fearful of an abusive mate to come in earlier. In some cases an abusive parent accompanies the child and the nonabusive parent in an effort to keep up a good front and to prevent disclosure. In occasional instances the nonabusive parent may actually be supportive of the abuser's "harsh discipline."

Table 6-5 presents additional historical and behavioral clues that may become apparent in the course of interviewing the parents/caretakers of an abused child.

Table 6-5	Historical and Behavioral Clues from Caretakers' Demeanor during Interview

Lack of affect in describing the baby (does not glow, even when asked about when he or she first saw the baby after delivery)

Relative lack of concern regarding severity/extent of injury

Negative comments regarding the child's (especially an infant's) behavior, appearance, or personality:

"She has a bad temper."

"She's mean."

"He's fussy, cries all the time."

"She's greedy, eats like a pig, is never satisfied."

"He likes to irritate me."

Betrayal of unrealistic expectations:

"She should know better than to cry when I have a headache."

Openly more invested in spouse/significant other.

Note: Perpetrators often disclose a watered-down version of what they did when abusing the child when asked what they think might have happened to cause the injuries found.

In approaching abused children, one must recognize that their parents are the only ones they know; that they love them and, usually, their other caretakers; and that at times, they may even feel in some way deserving of abuse. Young children rarely acknowledge that a parent or other caretaker has injured them, especially when questioned directly, often because they have been threatened or sworn to secrecy. If they can be interviewed alone (when old enough to give a history) in pleasant, nonthreatening surroundings, helpful historical information can often be obtained by means of nonleading questions and through drawings or play. In some cases in which the perpetrator is a paramour of the mother, and has not been around long, the child may be more willing to disclose, especially when he or she can honestly be reassured that they will have no further contact with him and is, therefore, safe from further assault.

It is also important to remember that siblings, especially older siblings, can often provide useful historical information. Strong consideration should be given to interviewing them as soon as possible after abuse is identified. Their histories can be quite helpful, and they may prove to be good witnesses in subsequent hearings.

PHYSICAL FINDINGS AND PATTERNS OF INJURY

Surface Marks

The most obvious manifestations of physical abuse are those visible on the surface of the skin. They include bruises, welts, scars, abrasions, lacerations, tourniquet and bite marks, and burns. Despite differing opinions on the appropriateness or inappropriateness of physical methods of discipline, there is a good rule of thumb in distinguishing the boundary between discipline and abuse: Discipline does not inflict significant pain and does *not* cause physical injury or leave marks.

All external signs of trauma found should be carefully documented in writing, on body diagrams, and in photographs (preferably with a ruler and color wheel in the frame).

Bruises, Welts, and Scars

Bruises are the most common clinical finding in cases of physical abuse, seen in up to 75% of victims, and their presence should prompt a search for other, deeper injuries. Inflicted bruises and welts may be the result of direct blows or of impacts with firm objects when pushed, shoved, thrown, or

swung into them. They frequently involve more than one plane of an extremity, the torso, and/or head, and are often found in places that are unusual sites for accidental injury (see the section Differential Diagnosis of Inflicted Injuries versus Findings Caused by Accident or Illness, later). These include the back, buttocks, upper arms, thighs, abdomen, perineum, and feet, all of which are typically covered by clothing and, thereby, hidden from public view (Figs. 6-1 and 6-2). When due to slaps or blows, these locations suggest some forethought in site selection. Among other unusual sites are the face (including the periorbital area and eyelids, cheeks, sides of the forehead, lateral aspects of the chin and mouth), ears, neck, hands, calves, and volar or ulnar (defensive posture) aspects of the forearms. Being more exposed, bruises in these areas may reflect greater impulsivity on the part of the perpetrator.

Bruises involving the head, face, mouth, neck, and ears (Fig. 6-3) are seen in a substantial percentage of physical abuse victims: approximately 50% of infants and 38% of toddlers. Subgaleal hematomas and contusions and petechiae involving the scalp may be the result of direct blows or impacts against hard surfaces. On occasion they are caused by forceful hair pulling (Fig. 6-4). Slaps of moderate force may produce diffuse bruising with petechiae (Fig. 6-5). More forceful slaps leave handprint marks, consisting of petechial outlines of the fingers of the perpetrator as maximal capillary distortion occurs at the margins of the fingers on impact (Fig. 6-6). Periorbital and eyelid bruises in the absence of evidence of an overlying forehead hematoma or abrasion, or of an accidentally incurred frontal skull fracture, are likely to be inflicted and caused by direct blows to the face (Fig. 6-7, *A* and *B*).

Surface injuries involving more than one plane of the head or face are highly suspicious for abuse. It is also important to recognize that contusions of the head, face, and ears are often associated with underlying intracranial injury, especially in infants. Such injuries are indicative of severe loss of control and intent to harm on the part of the perpetrating caregiver and have serious implications for the child's future safety unless he or she is removed from contact with the offender.

Round impressions of the thumb and forefinger may be seen on the cheeks, sides of the forehead, or sides of the chin in infants and young children who have been grasped and forcefully squeezed (see Fig. 6-1, *B*). Similar fingerprint bruises may be noted on the upper arms, trunk, abdomen, or extremities where the infant has been grasped and held tightly while being shaken or forcibly restrained (see Fig. 6-13). More elongated grab marks may also be found on the extremities (Fig. 6-8). When round bruises similar to fingerprint marks are found in a linear pattern, they may be fingertip impressions or knuckle marks from punching (see Fig. 6-2, *B* and *C*). In the latter instance, one may note partial central clearing of the rounded contusions. Fingerprints or grab marks located on the thighs, especially the medial surfaces, should prompt careful examination for signs of concurrent sexual abuse. Pinching produces apposed fingerprint marks with a shape that may be reminiscent of a butterfly or figure-of-eight. These may be seen singly or in rows, usually on clothing-covered areas (Fig. 6-9).

Attempted smothering, choking, or severe and prolonged thoracic compression may produce showers of petechiae over the shoulders, neck, and face (Fig. 6-10, *A-D*). The oral and conjunctival mucosa may be involved as well and should be carefully inspected. If a hand or other object is held forcefully over the nose and mouth of a child with erupted teeth, imprint bruises, abrasions, or lacerations left by the teeth on the labial mucosa may be noted in addition to facial petechiae (see Fig. 6-10, *E*). When strangulation is the mechanism, neck bruises are usually visible (see Fig. 6-10, *B*). These petechiae may

Figure 6-1   Inflicted bruises found in unusual locations. **A,** Multiple ecchymoses are evident over the back and upper chest of this child who presented in a poorly nourished condition. **B,** The same patient with multiple bruises involving differing planes of the face and forehead. Note the fingerprint bruise on the cheek. **C** and **D,** This child had severe contusions over the hands and feet, which were inflicted with a ruler. **E,** He also had a markedly swollen and contused ear and patches of hair loss where the perpetrator had pulled out hanks of hair. Both boys had been removed from abusive mothers and placed with maternal grandmothers who had physically abused their daughters in the past.

Figure 6-2   This toddler, the victim of repetitive beatings by her mother's boyfriend while the mother was hospitalized, had **A,** postauricular bruising, **B,** a line of fingerprint or knuckle bruises over the posterior left shoulder, and **C,** extensive bruising over the lower back in a pattern suggestive of knuckle marks, along with a large contusion over the right iliac crest. **D,** Rounded bruises over the lower abdomen and mons pubis may represent grab or punch marks. Some of her injuries were due to impacts against stairs and furniture when thrown forcefully by the perpetrator. Other injuries included a healing left radius fracture, refracture through a healing distal clavicle fracture, and evidence of old CNS trauma (see Fig. 6-26; Fig. 6-39, *B*; and Fig. 6-55).

Figure 6-3   Ear bruising. This infant was hit so forcibly on the side of his head that he has an impression bruise on his scalp in the shape of his external ear. The linear bruise over the top rim of his ear is the result of capillary distortion caused by compression between the impacting hand and the child's skull.

range from florid to faint and may be especially subtle when there has been a delay in seeking care. They can be mistaken for a rash if the examiner fails to check for blanching. Failure to detect such lesions has resulted in a number of subsequent deaths.

Bruises are often seen over the curvature of the buttocks and across the lower back after severe spankings, whether with a hand or an object such as a paddle, belt, or hairbrush (Fig. 6-11). When linear marks from fingers, belt, or brush edges are seen, these tend to be horizontally or diagonally oriented (see Fig. 6-11, *B*). However, in some cases a linear pattern of petechiae may be noted on either side of the gluteal crease (see Fig. 6-11, *C*). Despite their vertical orientation, these are also the result of forceful horizontal blows across tightly tensed glutei, as when the blows are delivered, the involved sites are closely apposed along the crease and thus are subject to maximal capillary distortion on impact.

Figure 6-4   Subgaleal hematomas. This toddler, in the care of mother's paramour, was reportedly well until about 45 minutes after being put to bed, when she "woke up screaming." On being picked up, she was noted to have a "mushy head." At the hospital, she was found to have large bilateral subgaleal hematomas, with surface bruising and petechiae over the occipitoparietal scalp. She also had semicircular bruises behind her left ear consistent with fingernail marks. Skull radiographs and a head CT scan showed no evidence of skull fracture or intracranial injury. Further examination revealed extensive bruising and lacerations of the introitus consistent with sexual assault (see Fig. 6-92 *B*). The perpetrator apparently grabbed her by her hair and by her head, leaving fingernail marks while in the process of assaulting her. Her hair was pulled so forcibly that the scalp was pulled away from the skull, leading to the extensive subgaleal bleeding, which continued to expand over the ensuing 72 hours. **A,** Thinning of the hair from hair loss and bruising of the scalp are evident, and the subgaleal hematoma over her left temporal area is so large that it is pushing her external ear out laterally. **B,** Curvilinear marks behind her left ear are fingernail impressions.

Figure 6-5   Facial slap marks. **A,** Diffuse facial bruising and petechiae seen over the side of the face and head of this 3-week-old infant were the result of repeated slaps by his father, a paranoid schizophrenic who had stopped taking his medication. He acknowledged slapping his son to make him cry, after which he would give him his bottle, the purpose being to teach him to cry when hungry. The baby also had metaphyseal chip fractures due to forced hyperextension of the knees to the point of screaming because "his muscles were tight" and "needed to be loosened up." **B,** This older infant has even more extensive petechiae and bruises that were tender on palpation.

Figure 6-6 Handprints. **A** and **B,** These children were slapped so forcefully that the outlines of their abuser's fingers are clearly evident.

Figure 6-7 **A,** Bilateral black eyes are seen in this 12-day-old baby. His father, who was well-to-do, well dressed, and sophisticated, reported that he had fallen on the stairs while holding the baby in a football hold and that in the fall, the baby hit the steps face first with father landing on top of him. Bruises involving multiple planes of the face, the absence of an associated forehead hematoma or frontal fracture, and the presence of an occipital fracture consistent with impact against a hard surface (not the father's chest) belied this story. Nevertheless, abuse was not suspected, and the baby was sent home. He returned 6 weeks later in extremis with massive intracranial injury and died. On this occasion, the father said he had found the infant choking and gasping for breath and had picked him up and shaken him to revive him. **B,** This infant's bilateral black eyes are the result of direct blows to the periorbital areas bilaterally.

Bruises involving the abdominal wall below the rib cage and above or anterior to the pelvic girdle are rarely seen with accidental injury and are relatively unusual in cases of abuse (see Fig. 6-2, *D* and Fig. 6-13). This is because of the great flexibility of the abdominal wall and its padding with adipose tissue. In fact, many children with inflicted intraabdominal injuries have little or no cutaneous evidence of trauma over the abdomen, although in some cases their absence may be due to delayed presentation. When abdominal bruises are present, they are indicative of forceful grabbing or pinching or of forceful blunt impact (such as a punch or kick). In these cases, abuse should be strongly suspected and evidence of internal injury should be sought (see the section Abdominal and Intrathoracic Injuries, later; and Fig. 6-57).

In many instances the surface marks are recognizable imprints of the edge of a weapon used to inflict the injury, because the edge causes maximal capillary deformation on impact. Those most commonly seen are looped-cord marks, caused by whipping the child with a looped electrical cord (Fig. 6-12, *A* and *B*), belt and belt-buckle marks (see Fig. 6-12, *C*, *D*, and *F*; see also Fig. 6-11, *B*), and switch marks (see Fig. 6-12, *E* and *F*); but almost any implement can be used including hairbrushes (see Fig. 6-11, *B*), shoes (see Fig. 6-12, *G* and *H*), kitchen utensils (see Fig. 6-12, *I*), and chains (see Fig. 6-12, *J*).

The size, nature, and rate of healing of bruises depend on the amount of force applied; the firmness and shape of the impacting object or surface; and the duration of impact, as well as on the degree of skin thickness, its vascularity and depth, elasticity, and adipose padding of the underlying subcutaneous tissue. Hence the initial appearance of bruises and the time it takes for them to resolve vary widely. Superficial bruises appear almost immediately and resolve more quickly than deeper contusions. The latter may not discolor the overlying skin for days and may take up to 2 weeks to resolve. Bruises of the face and perineum, where the skin is more loosely attached to underlying soft tissues and where blood vessels are less well supported, also appear early. Furthermore, the evolution of bruises in terms of color change is also variable. Although red, blue, and purple are more typical of fresh bruises, these colors can persist in some cases until resolution. Yellow, green, and brown are more characteristic of

Figure 6-8 Linear finger grab marks are seen on the outer aspect of this infant's upper arm. A thumbprint bruise was present medially. *(Courtesy Kent Hymel, MD, Inova Fairfax Hospital for Children, Falls Church, Va.)*

Figure 6-9 Pinch marks. A row of fading bruises secondary to pinching, used as a method of discipline by his mother, is seen on the lateral aspect of the thigh of this preschool-age boy. More than a year later, his sister nearly died of multiple stab wounds also inflicted by their psychotic and delusional mother (see Fig. 6-16).

older bruises but can be seen relatively early in superficial bruises. Hence it is difficult if not impossible to determine the ages of ecchymotic lesions and to be certain that bruises of differing colors are truly of different ages. However, if tenderness, swelling, and/or fresh overlying abrasions are present, one can be more confident that the lesions are new.

Some additional considerations regarding inflicted bruises warrant mention. In many cases of abuse, surface bruises and petechiae are faint or even imperceptible to the naked eye. This may be because they are early in their evolution or it may be the result of fading due to delay in seeking care. *In cases in which blows or impacts involving surface tissues also cause severe internal bleeding in the head, chest, or abdomen, bruises may be delayed in forming, may never appear, or may be subtle in their appearance.* This stems from the intense cutaneous vasoconstriction that occurs in response to shock, which severely restricts the flow of red blood cells to injured

Figure 6-10 A-D, Petechial lesions secondary to choking. **A,** Numerous petechiae are seen over this boy's face. **B,** Linear marks noted on the side of his neck correspond with the hand and finger placement demonstrated in **C** and **D**. The boy was choked to a point of near-unconsciousness by his mother's boyfriend for tracking grass onto a freshly vacuumed carpet. **E,** Central facial petechiae were present bilaterally in this infant. The perpetrator confessed to holding his hand over her mouth and nose and squeezing her cheeks with thumb and forefinger to stop her crying. *(Courtesy Kent Hymel, MD, Inova Fairfax Hospital for Children, Falls Church, Va.)*

Figure 6-11 Buttock bruises. **A,** At first glance, this toddler appeared to have a diaper rash, but on closer inspection the lesions were found to be petechiae produced by a severe spanking. **B,** The severe contusions of the buttocks and lower back seen in this child were inflicted by hand, hairbrush, and belt. **C,** A linear pattern of petechial hemorrhages is seen on either side of the gluteal cleft in this boy who was subjected to repeated rapid-fire blows across the gluteal crease.

surface capillaries, thus minimizing their extravasation. Appreciation of the potential subtlety of bruises and petechial lesions (which may provide the only clinical clue that abuse has occurred and that other injuries may be present) can enhance recognition of the importance of taking special care in performing the surface examination and checking the oral mucosa. It is also important to remember that petechiae may be mistaken for a fine macular rash if the clinician does not check to see if the lesions blanch or not. Research has demonstrated that Wood's lamp examination may increase the visibility of faint or subtle bruises and can reveal bruising that is invisible under regular light (Fig. 6-13).

When bruising is severe, deep, and extensive, underlying muscle breakdown may occur, resulting in myoglobinuria (Fig. 6-14). When severe, this may precipitate renal failure unless the risk is recognized, appropriate tests performed, and aggressive treatment measures are instituted.

Although bruises are relatively easy to see in victims with fair skin, they can be difficult to appreciate in children with darkly pigmented skin unless extra care is taken. Bruises may be further obscured when such children have dry skin with a fine surface scale, sometimes termed "ashy skin." Application of baby oil or a moisturizing cream clears the "ashy" surface, making lesions more readily visible. Small scalp lesions in children with thick dark hair can easily elude detection unless the scalp is inspected inch by inch for evidence of contusions, abrasions, and sometimes hair loss. Last, all infants with bruises and all children between 1 and 2 to 3 years of age with multiple bruises suspicious for abuse should have a skeletal survey to search for clinically occult fractures and blood work to screen for occult intraabdominal injury.

Clearly documenting the size, color, and configuration of bruises is important in potential abuse cases. This is best done with photographs that have a ruler and a standard color wheel in the frame, thereby ensuring that the lesion's true dimensions and color can be determined even if there are problems with exposure or photographic technique. Despite the difficulties in determining the ages of bruises, finding old scars that reflect prior use of a weapon in a child with acute injuries can be helpful in identifying abuse or confirming prior abuse (see Fig. 6-12, *B*).

To avoid errors in diagnosis, children who present with multiple bruises in unusual locations that do not reflect use of a weapon should be thoroughly examined to check for evidence of an underlying coagulopathy, and screening coagulation studies should be performed before arriving at a final diagnosis.

Abrasions and Superficial Lacerations

Abrasions are also seen in abuse victims, although less commonly than bruises. In some cases outline bruises of forcefully applied weapons have an overlying abraded or even lacerated surface (see Fig. 6-14). Abrasions also may result from friction on impact with a hard surface or from being dragged across a carpet or other rough surface (Fig. 6-15, *A*). Fingernails can be dug into the skin on grabbing the child or holding him or her down, or they can be used to poke at the skin, leaving small straight or arc-shaped abrasions or superficial lacerations (Fig. 6-15, *B*; and see Fig. 6-4, *B*). They can also be raked across the skin, leaving parallel linear abrasions. Simple lacerations, especially of the scalp, face, and upper extremities, although usually accidental in origin, can be the result of inflicted blows or impacts. Child abuse experts suspect that in many such cases a plausible history is provided, and the injury is classed as accidental. Here again, the practice of performing a complete surface examination on all children with minor wounds can provide clues that abuse may be the actual cause.

Slashing knife wounds and deep stab-induced lacerations are fortunately rare and are usually inflicted by caretakers with severe mental disorders (Fig. 6-16).

Strangulation, Restraint, and Tourniquet Injuries

Strangulation and restraint marks result from attempts to hang; choke; or, in some instances, tie the child to a crib, bed, or chair. Abraded or blistered circumferential ligature marks, often reflecting the surface pattern of the type of restraint used, are seen in these cases, due to friction either in forceful tightening or in the child's struggle to get free (Fig. 6-17). When extremities are involved, distal edema and often early signs of skin breakdown are seen (see Fig. 6-17, *B*). On rare occasions involving tight and prolonged tourniquet application, severe ischemia results in gangrene (see Fig. 6-17, *C*). In these unusual cases the perpetrator is likely to be psychotic, a drug addict, or both.

Bite Marks

Bite marks can be another manifestation of physical abuse. Lesions tend to be oval or semicircular. The impressions of the incisal surfaces may be variably clear, depending on the force applied and the age of the bite. Suction petechiae

Figure 6-12 Imprint marks reflecting the weapons used to inflict them. **A,** Fresh looped-cord marks and **B,** hypopigmented and hyperpigmented scars that were the result of beatings with a looped electrical cord. **C,** The characteristic pattern of parallel lines that results from blows with a belt. **D,** This contusion in the configuration of a closed horseshoe with a central linear abrasion was inflicted with a belt buckle. **E,** The red linear contusions on this child's thigh were the result of repeated blows with a switch. **F,** These acute linear contusions over the back and buttocks were inflicted with a belt and a switch. **G,** This boy was hit with a slipper with such force that imprints of the heel are evident. **H,** The heel prints of a running shoe left on this boy's arm and thigh were distinct enough to enable identification of his abuser. **I,** This girl was hit forcefully with a spatula because she was acting out while her mother was trying to prepare dinner. **J,** This boy was struck with a chain, leaving a clear imprint of the links.

may be noted centrally in some fresh lesions. In children in whom the resulting imprint is distinct, it is as identifiable as a fingerprint, and its size enables the examiner to clearly distinguish between the bite of another child and that of an adult, the latter being greater than 3 cm in diameter (Fig. 6-18, A-C). Each bite mark should be carefully photographed in its

entirety, and then photos should be taken perpendicular to the plane of the imprint of each arch, with a ruler or measuring tape in each photo. Such evidence can enable a forensic dentist to make a model of the perpetrator's dentition, which can specifically reveal his or her identity. Ultraviolet photography can disclose a clear image of bite marks weeks or

Figure 6-13 Wood lamp enhancement of visualization of bruises. **A,** Medics were called to the home of this 2-month-old baby with a report of apnea. Examination and computed tomography revealed bilateral retinal hemorrhages, subdural hematoma with edema, and loss of gray/white matter differentiation. The only external signs of trauma were three fingerprint-like bruises, two on the back and one on the lower abdomen seen here. **B,** Viewed from the opposite side under a Wood lamp, the lower abdominal bruise is seen to be even larger in extent, and a suprapubic bruise that was invisible in regular light is revealed. **C,** This 5-month-old baby presented with a history of decreased responsiveness following a crying/choking spell, after which she vomited. Subtle surface bruises were missed, and she was discharged with a diagnosis of gastroesophageal reflux. She returned a few hours later with persistent vomiting and increasing lethargy. At the second visit, multiple faint bruises were noticed over the chest, abdomen, back, buttocks, thighs, and scalp. Bruises over the chest and abdomen are barely visible in regular light. **D,** Under a Wood lamp they are seen with much greater clarity. Other injuries included an occipital fracture with diastasis of the lambdoid suture, a posterior interhemispheric subdural hematoma (see Fig. 6-44), and a metaphyseal fracture of the distal radius seen in Fig. 6-28B. *(Courtesy Eva Vogeley, MD, Children's Hospital of Pittsburgh, Pittsburgh, Pa.)*

months after all surface marks have disappeared (see Fig. 6-18, *D*). This has proved highly useful in identifying abusers of children who have a past history of being bitten but who have no acute lesions. Last, if the patient has not bathed or washed the bite wound since it was inflicted, swabbing the area with a saline-soaked, cotton-tipped applicator is indicated to obtain a sample of the perpetrator's saliva. Crime laboratory analysis of this material can positively identify the perpetrator.

Burns

Burns are generally accidental, but they are also a fairly common mode of abusive injury. Although there is no one pattern that is absolutely pathognomonic for abuse, dip burns, back and buttock burns in infants and toddlers, burns over the dorsum of the hand, and deep contact burns with a clear imprint of the hot surface are highly suspect. Here, too, inconsistency of history, the pattern of injury, and delay in seeking medical attention are valuable clues.

Immersion scalds or dip burns are among the most common forms of inflicted burns. Typical patterns include symmetrical burns of both hands or both feet in a stocking-glove distribution, with a sharp line of demarcation at the level of the water line (Fig. 6-19, *A*); circumferential burns of the feet and lower legs along with burns of the perineum and flexor surfaces of the thighs are seen in children who are held under the axillae and knees and have their legs and bottoms dipped in scalding water (see Fig. 6-19, *B* and *C*). If the child is forcibly held down in a sink or tub as it fills with scalding water, partial sparing of the palms, soles, and buttocks may be noted because these sites were pressed against the cooler sink or tub surface. Sparing of apposed skin surfaces in flexor creases may also be noted in these cases. Lower extremity/perineal burns and tub burns are typically inflicted after toileting accidents.

Figure 6-14 Severe bruising with underlying muscle damage. This toddler was covered from head to toe with severe looped cord contusions and lacerations. He had secondary myoglobinuria necessitating intensive care management to prevent renal failure.

Figure 6-15 Inflicted abrasions/lacerations. **A,** A pattern of parallel abrasions that overlie ribs and vertebral bodies is seen on the back of this infant who was dragged over a carpet. The lesions are at least one to a few days old, and surface scabs have separated from two areas. A displaced spiral fracture of the right humerus, with marked soft tissue swelling and pain on motion, was also detected. **B,** This 3-month-old had numerous small linear and arc-shaped abrasions and superficial lacerations over both legs, consistent with fingernail marks. She also had many other bruises of varying hues, an occipital skull fracture, a posterior interhemispheric subdural hematoma, multiple metaphyseal chip fractures, and an abscessed nasal septal hematoma (see Fig. 6-25).

Despite claims to the contrary, immersion burns are rarely accidental. Table 6-6 shows the time required to produce a full-thickness burn in adult skin at various water temperatures. Although the time may be slightly shorter for a child, normal children would, if they accidentally put a hand or foot into water higher than 120° F, withdraw it in a fraction of a second after the tips of their fingers or toes made contact with the water, leaving them with only superficial burns of the tips of their fingers or toes.

Table 6-6	Duration of Exposure Required to Produce Full-thickness Burn in Water at Various Temperatures
Water Temperature (° F)	**Duration of Exposure**
120	10 min
130	30 s
140	5 s
150	2 s
158	1 s

Figure 6-16 Slashing and stab wounds. This 22-month-old toddler was viciously and repeatedly attacked by her psychotic mother wielding a carving knife. She was left to die outside in the snow and, on rescue, was severely hypothermic and in shock. **A,** A superficial laceration is seen over the left eyelid. **B,** A deeper stab wound over the right flank penetrated into the subcutaneous tissue. **C,** A 3-cm wrist laceration sutured in the operating room had partially severed the median nerve. **D,** Eviscerated bowel projected through this 13-cm mid-abdominal laceration, which did not need to be extended for exploration. A through-and-through stomach laceration and a tear of the colonic mesentery were the only internal injuries found. Her throat had also been slit. Her brother had been seen a year earlier (see Fig. 6-9).

Figure 6-17 Strangulation, restraint, and tourniquet injuries. **A,** This circumferential cord burn was the result of an attempted strangulation. **B,** A deep, circumferential rope burn of the wrist with considerable edema and early skin breakdown of the hand is seen in this infant, who had been tied to the side rails of her crib. **C,** This toddler was brought in with severe skin, soft tissue, and muscle necrosis of his entire lower leg. His mother, a paranoid schizophrenic and heroin addict, reported finding a strap wrapped tightly around the leg below the knee on checking him in the morning. She did not know how it had gotten there and denied hearing his cries of pain, which surely lasted for hours.

Figure 6-18 Bite marks. **A,** In this bite mark inflicted on a toddler by a much older child with mature dentition, the configuration of the upper central incisors is clearly seen (note the diastema, or wide spacing, between them). **B,** At first glance this fading bite mark could be mistaken for a bruise; however, on close inspection, the outline of the dental arch becomes evident. The size of the arch is clearly that of an adult or adolescent. **C,** A child-size bite inflicted on an adolescent baby sitter illustrates the difference in size of the dental arch between children and adults. **D,** Viewed under ultraviolet light, bite marks that are weeks to months old can still be identified, even though the skin overlying the site has returned to normal. (*A, B, and C, Courtesy Michael N. Sobel, MD, Pittsburgh, Pa; D, courtesy Thomas J. David, MD, Atlanta, Ga.*)

Figure 6-19 Inflicted scalds. **A,** After getting his hands into something he was not allowed to touch and making a mess, this child's hands were held down in hot water, resulting in severe second-degree dip burns. Note the sharp line of demarcation just above the wrist joint and the uniform depth of the burn. **B,** This toddler was dipped in a tub of scalding water while being held under the arms and knees, as an object lesson after a toileting accident. **C,** Close-up of severe second-degree burns of the foot and lower leg of the same child. *(Courtesy Thomas Layton, MD.)*

Contact burns, sometimes termed *branding injuries,* show the imprint of the instruments used to inflict them and have a depth or degree of burn that is relatively even throughout. For example, one may see the imprint of a hot iron or of the grill of a space heater or radiator cover (Fig. 6-20, *A-D*). No child with normal sensation would remain in contact with these objects long enough to incur such a burn. Burns caused by holding a hot hair dryer next to the skin leave an imprint of the screen that covers the heating element (see Fig. 6-20, *E*), and those inflicted with a curling iron produce cigar-shaped, deep partial- or full-thickness imprints (see Fig. 6-20, *F*). Most contact burns are found in unusual locations for accidental burns or over areas such as the extensor surfaces of the upper arms or legs, the back, chest, abdomen, or buttocks that are usually covered by clothing.

Inflicted *cigarette burns* usually leave sharply circumscribed, full-thickness imprints approximately 7 to 8 mm in diameter (5 mm if a slim cigarette is used). These are surrounded by a deep, partial-thickness halo blister and then a rim of superficial erythema (Fig. 6-21, *A*). A thick, black eschar soon forms over the central, full-thickness burn. If this eschar is removed, one sees full-thickness skin loss. Subacutely, these lesions fill in with granulation tissue (see Fig. 6-21, *B*), and on completion of healing the child is left with a deep, punched-out scar (see Fig. 6-21, *C*). When a lit cigarette is held on the skin for only a fraction of a second, the resulting partial-thickness burn heals to form a uniform macular scar (see Fig. 6-21, *D*).

An unusual pattern of serrated first- and second-degree burns in parallel lines is made when the wheels of a butane lighter are heated and then pressed or run over the child's skin (Fig. 6-22).

Oral and Nasal Injuries

On occasion, child abuse results in oral bruises and lacerations. One of the most typical patterns is bruising of the mucosa of the upper lip or the maxillary gingiva associated with tearing of the frenulum (Fig. 6-23). This can be produced when the perpetrator holds a hand tightly over the child's mouth to silence screaming and can be associated with facial petechiae (see Fig. 6-10, *E*). Attempts to force a bottle or pacifier into a crying infant's mouth can also produce semicircular central gingival bruising or ulcerations. Force-feeding with a spoon may produce contusions or lacerations of the lips, floor of the mouth, and tongue. Gag marks at the corners of the mouth can be mistaken for cheilosis or for impetiginous or candidal lesions. On rare occasions, bizarre intraoral lacerations are found (Fig. 6-24). Their usual mode of presentation is a complaint of spitting or vomiting up blood.

Even more rarely, oral injuries inflicted with fingers or utensils can result in penetration of the posterior pharynx.

Figure 6-20   Contact burns or branding injuries. **A,** This child, who was acting out while his mother ironed, was punished when she held the tip of the iron against his cheek. **B,** A healing full-thickness burn in the shape of an iron was found when this boy's shirt was removed prior to his being given vaccine injections. He had been sent home after his first day in kindergarten with instructions not to return until he was caught up on his immunizations. **C,** These linear full-thickness burns were incurred when this 6-week-old infant was forced to sit on the hot grill of a space heater. The history given was that she had crawled over to the space heater, knocked it over, and then sat on it. **D,** Another infant presented with a history of irritability and a rash. The "rash" has a honeycomb configuration that matched that of a radiator cover in her home. She also had multiple fractures. **E,** These facial burns are the result of being branded with the grill of a hair dryer. The boy had been acting out while he was supposed to be getting ready for school and his mother was drying her hair. **F,** The hot wand of a curling iron leaves a cigar-shaped, partial- to full-thickness burn.

Most of these cases involve infants who may present with subcutaneous emphysema or with fever, drooling, and respiratory distress caused by a secondary retropharyngeal abscess (see Chapter 23).

In older children, punches; forceful slaps, especially with the back of a hand; or kicks can cause lip lacerations and contusions, frenulum and gingival tears (see Fig. 6-23), dental fractures, displacement injuries and avulsions, chin lacerations, and even mandibular fractures. These injuries can also stem from impact with hard surfaces when the child is violently pushed or thrown (see Chapter 20). Often these older victims present with a plausible history of accidental trauma and are not recognized as abuse victims. Sometimes the only clue that the injuries are abuse related is that the lesion is more severe than would be expected from the reported mechanism, the child is unusually reticent in providing the history, or the parent appears determined not to let the child talk.

Nasal injuries may be due to direct blows or impacts. When mild, epistaxis may be the only manifestation. More severe injuries can result in fractures of the nasal bone or cartilage, septal deviation, and septal hematoma. The abused child with a septal hematoma is especially vulnerable to developing a septal abscess due to delay in presentation, and affected infants tend to present with external nasal swelling, fever, and respiratory distress due to nasal obstruction (Fig. 6-25; and see Chapter 23).

Skeletal Injuries

Skeletal injuries are second only to bruises in terms of frequency in abused infants and children. Most fractures involve infants younger than 1 year of age. Approximately 60% of inflicted fractures are seen in children younger than 18 months, and the vast majority occur before age 3 years. This contrasts sharply with the low incidence of accidental fractures in infants and toddlers. Often, fractures are clinically occult and in many, if not most, cases no history of trauma is provided. When a history of injury is given, it is often one of a minor mechanism (fall off a couch) that does not fit with radiographic findings. Furthermore, parents of abused children tend to minimize reports of pain, discomfort, and loss of function. The high frequency of inflicted fractures in the very young and their potential for clinical subtlety necessitate that examination of suspected abuse victims include careful palpation of all bones for tenderness, crepitus, or palpable callus, and that all children younger than 2 to 3 years of age undergo skeletal survey; after that age and up to age 5 years children should be evaluated on a case-by-case basis.

Figure 6-21   Cigarette burns. **A,** This sharply circumscribed burn was inflicted through the child's sock. The burn is perfectly circular with a blistered rim and a full-thickness punched-out center to which charred fabric adheres. The configuration did not fit the history that he had accidentally stepped on a cigarette. **B,** The eschar has separated from this older burn, revealing underlying granulation tissue. **C,** Punched-out scars of healed full-thickness cigarette burns. **D,** These uniform macular scars are the result of cigarette burns in which the coal is held against the skin for only a fraction of a second. (**D,** *Courtesy Kent Hymel, MD, Inova Fairfax Hospital for Children, Falls Church, Va.*)

Figure 6-22   Cigarette lighter burns. **A,** Two pairs of lesions with the appearance of parallel serrated lines and a deep burn in the shape of a butterfly were found on examining this infant, who was brought to the emergency department for treatment of a rash. **B,** Astute deduction by a resident and social worker led to the discovery that heated cigarette lighter wheels had been used to inflict the burns. The full-thickness butterfly is the result of repeated application.

Figure 6-23 Frenulum tear. This badly beaten boy incurred a torn frenulum when his abuser tried to muffle his cries by forcibly holding his hand over the child's mouth. Note the facial bruises. *(Courtesy Robert Hickey, MD, Children's Hospital of Pittsburgh, Pittsburgh, Pa.)*

Figure 6-26 Medullary sclerosis seen in the left radius reflects the later stages of healing. The fracture line is no longer visible, and the bone has remodeled. This is the child whose surface injuries are shown in Fig. 6-2. She also had a refracture of an old clavicle fracture (see Fig. 6-39, *B*) and evidence of prior head trauma on MRI (see Fig. 6-55).

Figure 6-24 Inflicted palatal lacerations. This infant's soft palate was shredded by repeated stabs with a sharp object. He presented with a complaint of spitting up blood and no history of trauma.

Diagnosis of inflicted fractures can be especially challenging in infants because nondisplaced rib and spiral fractures, metaphyseal chip and buckle fractures, and periosteal stripping injuries have minimal swelling, even acutely, and heal with great rapidity, as is detailed later. Further, in infants a history of trauma is especially unlikely to be reported. Rather, the chief complaint may be of unexplained irritability or grunting respirations (due to rib pain) or the child may be brought in with a totally unrelated complaint such as a cold or a rash. Some present with a history of minor accidental injury (often when the infant has surface bruises), usually with a reported mechanism that does not fit the fracture pattern or severity. Furthermore, as healing is faster in the infant or young child (due to the thickness of the periosteum, which resists tearing, reducing risk of displacement, and due to its being richly invested with osteoblasts that facilitate healing), tenderness and pain on being picked up, or on motion, may abate within a few days. This is particularly true of rib and metaphyseal fractures, periosteal stripping injuries, and other nondisplaced fractures.

When presentation occurs after tenderness has disappeared but before radiographically visible signs of healing have developed, the diagnosis is likely to be missed. In these cases, when other findings raise suspicion, it is wise to obtain a second skeletal survey in 10 to 14 days. Fortunately, delay in presentation in many cases is great enough that radiographic signs of healing are noted. These include medullary sclerosis (Fig. 6-26), callus formation (Fig. 6-27; and see Figs. 6-29 and 6-31), and the presence of subperiosteal new bone (Fig. 6-27; and see Fig. 6-32). It should be noted that symmetrical thin rims of subperiosteal new bone (>2 cm in width) can be a normal finding in the long bones of infants younger than 3 to 6 months of age. Because many fractures are often not brought to medical attention and are thus not immobilized, and given

Figure 6-25 Abscessed nasal septal hematoma. This 3-month-old baby brought to the emergency department with complaints of fever and difficulty breathing was found to have **A,** a red swollen nose and **B,** erythematous bulging of the nasal septum bilaterally, obstructing her nasal passages. Note the small central lip laceration. She also had multiple bruises, fingernail abrasions (see Fig. 6-15, *B*), an occipital skull fracture, a subdural hematoma, and multiple metaphyseal chip fractures.

Figure 6-27   Multiple fractures of varying ages. This boy was seen with a chief complaint of refusing to bear weight. On examination, he was found to have marked swelling, tenderness, and crepitance over the distal left femur. **A,** Radiographic examination confirmed the presence of an acute transverse fracture and also revealed multiple additional fractures in various stages of healing. These include an old transverse fracture of the distal right femur with callus and subperiosteal new bone formation that is in the process of remodeling. Relatively new metaphyseal chip fractures are seen involving the right proximal tibia, and vigorous subperiosteal new bone formation encompasses the left tibia. **B,** On skeletal survey he was also found to have a healing fracture of the distal humerus with vigorous callus and subperiosteal new bone formation and considerable soft tissue swelling. Note that the cortices of his long bones are of normal thickness. No care had ever been sought for the older fractures. *(Courtesy Department of Radiology, Children's Hospital of Pittsburgh, Pittsburgh, Pa.)*

that abuse tends to be repetitive, reinjury at sites of prior injury is not uncommon. When this occurs, it can result in unusually "exuberant" callus formation (Fig. 6-27; and see Fig. 6-31).

In evaluating skeletal injuries, one must bear in mind the child's developmental capabilities because accidental skeletal fractures are rare in infants who are not crawling or cruising and are quite uncommon in children younger than 3 years. Likewise, being knowledgeable regarding the mechanisms of injury and the magnitude of the forces that result in different fracture patterns makes it less likely to be misled by deceptive histories.

A paradigm of child abuse is the finding of multiple, unexplained, often symmetrical fractures of varying ages involving the ribs and/or long bones of an infant or young child who has otherwise normal bones (see Fig. 6-27). Many of these fractures are clinically inapparent and therefore unsuspected. Metaphyseal fractures in infants and toddlers and rib fractures are also findings highly specific for abuse.

Metaphyseal Fractures

In infancy the cartilage of the chondro-osseous junctions adjacent to the metaphyses of long bones is poorly mineralized, making these structures the weakest points in long bones and predisposing to planar fractures through these sites when the bones are subjected to shearing forces. The periosteum overlying the epiphyseal cartilage is firmly adherent and extends close to the diaphysis to cover the subperiosteal bony collar. Thus when fractures do occur, their peripheral segments are thicker. In toddlers and older children, who have slower growth rates and a much greater amount of chondro-osseous mineralization, the same forces that produce metaphyseal fractures in infants are more likely to result in fractures through the physeal cartilage.

Metaphyseal fractures can be produced by the application of torsional or tractional forces, delivered when an extremity is grabbed and yanked. Frequently, they are caused by rapid, repetitive acceleration and deceleration as the extremities flail back and forth in the process of violent shaking. They also result from forced hyperextension of the knees. Metaphyseal fractures can be found in any long bone but are most commonly seen in the distal femur, proximal and distal tibias, and proximal humerus. They are often bilateral. They may traverse the entire metaphysis or only a portion of it. Clinically, they are not associated with any significant soft-tissue swelling, and pain and tenderness (which can be quite localized) tend to abate within 2 to 5 days.

Radiographic manifestations of metaphyseal fractures have led to the terms "metaphyseal chip" or "corner" fractures and "bucket handle" fractures. The first derives from the fact that in the anteroposterior (AP) view the central portion of the fracture is often invisible and only a chip of bone is seen on either the lateral or medial aspect of the metaphysis, or both (Fig. 6-28; and see Fig. 6-27). Chips may also be seen on lateral projections. In some cases a thin central metaphyseal lucency can be detected (see Fig. 6-28, *B*). Special oblique views are necessary to reveal the true extent of the fracture, as in this projection the separation of the metaphyseal disk becomes readily evident, resembling a bucket handle (see Fig. 6-28, *D*). Healing of metaphyseal fractures is not usually accompanied by prominent callus or extensive subperiosteal new bone formation. Reinjuries, however, can result in prominent fragmentation and sclerosis at the metaphyseal margins.

Rib Fractures

Rib fractures are also relatively unique to abused infants. Because of the plasticity and pliability of the thoracic cage in infancy, application of major forces is required to break ribs, and accidental rib fractures are rarely seen short of major motor vehicle accidents. Causative mechanisms include violent shaking while holding the child by the chest. This is done with the attacker's palms to the sides, thumbs in front, and fingers over the back. In the process of shaking, the ribs are subjected to marked AP compression forces and the posterior ribs are levered against the fulcrum of the vertebral bodies and their transverse processes. This often produces rows of multiple, often bilateral ("mirror image") posterior rib fractures, located near the costovertebral articulations (Fig. 6-29). Extreme squeezing of the chest with or without shaking can produce fractures at multiple sites along the rib arcs, as

Figure 6-28 Metaphyseal fractures. **A,** Metaphyseal chip fractures involving the medial aspects of the distal right femur and proximal tibia were found in this infant whose mother confessed to repeated episodes of shaking, after which she would throw the baby down onto a bed or couch. Note the subperiosteal new bone along the lateral aspect of the femur and medial margins of the tibia. The baby had presented with a large subgaleal hematoma and a history of having been hit on the head with a plastic nursing bottle by a toddler. Bilateral skull fractures (see Fig. 6-47), a distal right clavicle fracture (see Fig. 6-39, A), and a healing radius fracture were also found. **B,** In another child, metaphyseal chips are seen on either side of the radial metaphysis in the anteroposterior view, along with a faint central metaphyseal lucency. In the lateral projection, metaphyseal chips of both radius and ulna are evident. Subtle rims of subperiosteal new bone can be seen along the diaphyses of both bones. This is the same 5-month-old whose faint surface bruises are shown in Fig. 6-13, C and D. Her skull radiograph is presented in Fig. 6-44, B. **C,** A prominent diagonal metaphyseal fracture of the medial aspect of the proximal right tibia was found on a skeletal survey obtained of this 10-month-old infant, who presented with an unexplained supracondylar fracture (see Fig. 6-38). His proximal tibia was nontender clinically, yet no evidence of healing is seen, suggesting that the fracture is older than a few days and newer than 10 days old. Failure to detect this and rib and metacarpal fractures (see Fig. 6-40, A) on films obtained because of hand swelling and decreased movement of the right leg noted during an admission for gastroenteritis and dehydration (vomiting without diarrhea) had subjected him to this further trauma a month later (see Fig. 6-38). **D,** In the oblique projection the planar nature of metaphyseal fractures is more easily appreciated. Fracture lines traverse the entire metaphysis of each tibia, and the disk-shaped distal fragments appear offset, giving rise to the term "bucket handle fracture." (**D,** Courtesy Bruce Rosenthal, MD, Children's Hospital of Pittsburgh, Pittsburgh, Pa.)

can stomping on the chest. Direct blows with the edge of a hand or blunt instrument, kicks, and slamming or hurling resulting in chest wall impact against the edge of a table or door jamb produce fractures at the site of impact. Stomping and slamming usually produce fractures that are more severe and extensive, more likely to be displaced, and associated with intrathoracic and intraabdominal injuries (see Fig. 6-59). Most of these infants have no history of trauma and symptoms are nonspecific and include respiratory difficulty with shallow grunting respirations, and irritability especially with

movement, being picked up while held by the chest, and while being patted, burped, or rocked.

Like metaphyseal fractures, rib fractures tend not to be associated with soft tissue swelling or bruising, and tenderness often resolves in 3 to 5 days, the exception being unusually severe and displaced fractures as shown in Figure 6-59. In some cases of repetitive injury with unusually florid callus, lumps can be palpated at healing fracture sites. When fractures involve the lower rib cage, associated abdominal injury should be considered.

Figure 6-29 Rib fractures due to shaking. **A,** This 3-month-old infant has bilateral and nearly symmetrical posterior rib fractures with fairly mature callus involving the second through eighth ribs on the left and the third through sixth on the right. The latter are partially obscured by the mediastinal shadow and the right heart border. **B,** This 10-week-old, who presented with "shaking spells" and no history of trauma, has healing posterior rib fractures of the second through fifth ribs on the right and second through seventh on the left. Those of the right second and third and the left seventh appear newer than the others with less well-defined margins. He also has lateral rib fractures on the right involving the third and fourth and possibly seventh ribs. Additional fractures "appeared" during his hospital stay as healing proceeded. His CNS findings are shown in Figs. 6-51 and 6-52.

Figure 6-30 Use of bone scan to detect occult rib fractures. **A,** At 3 months of age, this infant presented with low-grade fever, nasal congestion, cough, tachypnea, and intermittent grunting respirations. Pneumonia was suspected, and a chest radiograph was obtained. On review of the films, a subtle, nearly completely remodeled fracture of the posterolateral aspect of the right third rib was detected. In addition to his tachypnea, he was noted to cry when picked up by the chest. **B,** Bone scan revealed occult posterior fractures of the second through fifth ribs on the left and the eighth and ninth ribs bilaterally, as well as the one fracture seen on the chest film. The occult fractures became visible radiographically over the ensuing 2 weeks.

Radiographically, rib fractures tend to be invisible before the appearance of callus and/or subperiosteal new bone. This is because the periosteum is only partially disrupted, and it and the arc of the rib cage keep the fracture ends apposed. These breaks can, however, be detected by bone scan at this early stage. Hence this procedure should be strongly considered when there are no visible fractures but examination reveals thoracic bruises or tenderness; when one or a few rib fractures are seen and others are suspected, or when other injuries associated with shaking—metaphyseal chip fractures, retinal hemorrhages, CNS findings—are found in the absence of visible rib fractures. Bone scans often reveal multiple fractures not visible in standard radiographs (Fig. 6-30, B).

Alternatively, one can wait and obtain a repeat skeletal survey 10 days to 2 weeks later, if assured that the infant can be protected in the interim. These follow-up films can reveal fractures invisible on the first study. An early sign of healing, seen 5 to 10 days postinjury on standard radiographs, consists of a vertical lucency at the site of the fracture surrounded by soft callus with indistinct margins (Fig. 6-31, A). Subsequently (at 14 to 21 days), callus takes on a more nodular appearance with sharper margins and is then termed *hard callus* (see Fig. 6-30, A and Fig. 6-31, B). Reinjury can result in florid callus formation (see Fig. 6-31, B). Complete remodeling and radiographic disappearance occur within a few months in the absence of reinjury.

Figure 6-31 Healing rib fractures. **A,** This infant was seen because of a history of vomiting and irritability. An abdominal film obtained to rule out intestinal obstruction showed a normal bowel gas pattern but revealed posterior rib fractures in the early stages of healing. Note the vertical lucencies surrounded by soft callus. The fractures were missed. **B,** When the infant was finally tracked down 2 months later, her chest radiograph showed in excess of 20 healing rib fractures, some posterior and others lateral and anterolateral. The exuberance of the callus in many places reflects repetitive reinjury. Some of these were palpable clinically. *(Courtesy Department of Radiology, Children's Hospital of Pittsburgh, Pittsburgh, Pa.)*

The frequent association of rib and metaphyseal fractures with head injury in infants is so great (~70%) that when these fractures are discovered, a CT scan of the head should be obtained, even when neurologic status appears normal. Not infrequently, this study will reveal evidence of prior intracranial injury that is subclinical or nonspecific in its manifestations at the time of presentation. Studies have documented the rarity of rib fractures associated with resuscitation; however, most of these studies predated the relatively new recommendation for two-handed resuscitation in infants.

Long Bone Fractures

The high incidence of long bone fractures in abused children has been attributed to the fact that the extremities serve as "convenient handles" for inflicting trauma. Formation of subperiosteal new bone is seen commonly in infants and toddlers with healing diaphyseal fractures (see Fig. 6-27, *A* and *B* and

Fig. 6-32, *A* and *B*). In infancy, it can also be seen in the absence of cortical fractures when a long bone is subjected to twisting or torsional forces short of those required to produce cortical breaks. These result in separation of the periosteum from the outer cortex and subperiosteal hemorrhage. Termed *periosteal stripping injuries,* they are relatively specific to infants, for although the epiphyseal segment of the periosteum is firmly attached, the diaphyseal portion is more loosely adherent because of sparseness of the Sharpey fibers that anchor it. As the complement of Sharpey fibers increases in early childhood, periosteal separation becomes less and less likely. Because of the attendant subperiosteal hemorrhage, the formation of subperiosteal new bone after periosteal stripping tends to be prominent and greater than 2 mm in width. This, too, becomes visible on radiographs in about 5 to 10 days in infants (10 to 14 days in toddlers). Initially, it is seen as periosteal haziness, and subsequently increasing calcification becomes evident (Fig. 6-32). These findings are easy to miss unless the physician inspects diaphyseal margins with great care. Like metaphyseal fractures, periosteal stripping injuries are clinically subtle, even acutely, because they are not associated with any significant degree of soft tissue swelling, and associated tenderness may disappear in as little as 2 to 5 days.

Although metaphyseal and periosteal stripping injuries are more common in young infants, diaphyseal or shaft fractures are not at all unusual and become even more common in older infants and toddlers who are victims of abuse. Although not specific for inflicted injury, diaphyseal fractures are highly suspect when found in infants who are not yet crawling or walking, especially when seen in the absence of a history of significant trauma; as noted, accidental fractures are also relatively uncommon in toddlers as compared with older children. Spiral, oblique, torus, transverse, and compression/distraction (or three-point bending) fractures may all be seen. An understanding of the direction and magnitude of force required to produce a given type of diaphyseal fracture and a comparison of that with the history given often enable the clinician to distinguish between accidental and inflicted injury.

Spiral fractures of the long bones (Fig. 6-33), which, in cases of abuse, are usually the result of grabbing an extremity and rapidly twisting it, are relatively low-energy injuries in comparison with other fracture types and are not uncommonly seen as a result of accidents. However, when these injuries are caused by abuse, fracture edges are more likely to be widely separated, suggesting somewhat greater force application than is true of most accidental spiral fractures. *Oblique fractures* can also be the product of torsional forces or of slowly applied bending forces. They appear to require application of significantly greater energy than with spiral fractures, especially when the fracture is complete and displaced (Fig. 6-34). When a spiral or oblique fracture of a long bone is found in a nonambulatory infant or in a mobile young child with no history of an injury that fits the fracture, abuse should be suspected.

Though more commonly accidental in origin, *torus* or *buckle fractures* can be the result of abuse, especially in very young children. When mild with only slight cortical buckling, they are the result of mild-to-moderate compression forces delivered in a direction parallel or nearly parallel to the axis of a long bone. When higher energy forces are delivered, whether accidental or inflicted, there is usually some degree of angulation; in such cases it may be more accurate to classify them as a form of compression/distraction injury. Milder fractures tend to have little associated soft tissue swelling and often only mild discomfort on motion. As degree of severity of angulation increases, so do swelling and pain. As is true of accidental fractures, they most commonly involve the distal

Figure 6-32 Periosteal stripping injuries. Wide strips of subperiosteal new bone were noted along the diaphyses of both humeri **(A)** and both femurs **(B)** of this infant. Their width was too great to be considered physiologic. She also had severe intracranial injury and multiple healing rib fractures. Dating of the periosteal stripping and rib fractures coincided with a 3- to 4-day period of nearly constant crying, "even when we picked her up," that had occurred more than 2 weeks earlier and was attributed to constipation.

radius and ulna, but volar angulation is more common in inflicted fractures, and dorsal angulation is more typical of those incurred accidentally. The usual scenario is that of a child who is thrown or forcefully pushed and lands on a out-stretched arm (Fig. 6-35; and see Chapter 21, Fig. 21-27 for the appearance of an accidental buckle fracture). Another involves grabbing by the wrist and bending it forcefully. More severe forms involving the femur or tibia can be caused by throwing or slamming a child feet first or onto the knees on a hard surface.

Figure 6-34 This partially displaced oblique fracture of the left humerus has faint evidence of early callus formation. The persistence of soft tissue swelling may be due to lack of proper immobilization and/or reinjury. *(Courtesy Robert Hickey, MD, Children's Hospital of Pittsburgh, Pittsburgh, Pa.)*

Figure 6-33 Spiral fracture. This 8-month-old presented with unexplained swelling of his right upper arm and decreased use of the extremity. He had no history of trauma. A spiral fracture courses from the distal portion to the upper third of the diaphysis. Moderate associated soft tissue swelling is also seen.

Figure 6-35 Torus or buckle fracture. This 5-year-old girl with mild cerebral palsy presented with a history of unresponsiveness lasting more than an hour, following a possible seizure, and was found to have a hyperacute subdural hematoma similar to the one shown in Fig. 6-48. Subsequent skeletal survey found a previously unrecognized and clinically silent torus fracture of the left distal radius. After an initial history reporting two falls on stairs, her mother's live-in boyfriend, who was frustrated with her slowness at toilet training, confessed to having pushed her down forcibly and to slamming her into an entertainment cabinet. When buckle fractures are displaced to this extent, they are perhaps more accurately described as compression/distraction injuries.

Figure 6-36 Transverse fractures. An acute transverse fracture of the proximal radius with associated soft tissue swelling is seen in this toddler who has another nondisplaced transverse fracture with early callus formation distally and a healing displaced transverse fracture of the mid-ulna with subperiosteal new bone formation.

Transverse and three-point bending fractures are high-energy injuries that are much more likely to be accompanied by acute soft tissue swelling and deformity. Severe pain on motion with secondary splinting and limitation of motion are the rule. *Transverse fractures* are often the result of a rapidly delivered direct blow perpendicular to the long axis of a bone, such as "karate chop" or "night stick" injury (Fig. 6-36). They can also occur when a child is thrown or swung and, in the process, hits an extremity against a hard edge such as that of a table, as a result of falls of greater than 6 feet, and when half of an extremity is held with both hands and snapped.

Violently yanking a child up from his crib while holding an extremity or grabbing an arm and yanking it upward or sideways when the child is fixed in position by the belt of a high chair or infant seat are common scenarios for *compression/distraction* or *three-point bending fractures* (Fig. 6-37), as is the snapping mechanism described earlier. Inflicted

Figure 6-37 Compression/distraction (three-point bending) fracture. **A,** A comminuted and angulated fracture of the distal femur with irregular margins is seen in this child who was brought in for refusal to bear weight, after a "fall" down wooden steps. **B,** The degree of angulation is better appreciated in the lateral view. The nature of the fracture indicates a high-energy mechanism inconsistent with the history. The father later confessed to throwing the child at a coffee table, which broke on impact. **C,** A more typical example of a completely displaced three-point bending fracture is seen in another child.

supracondylar humerus fractures of the compression/distraction type are the result of grabbing an arm and yanking it into hyperextension (Fig. 6-38; and see Fig. 6-27, *B*).

Other Fractures

Fractures of the clavicle as a result of abuse are fairly unusual. Like accidental fractures, they can be located at the junction of the outer third with the middle two thirds. When they involve the very distal portion (Fig. 6-39), they are highly suspect for abuse and are often associated with chip fractures of the acromion process and fractures of the proximal humerus and the upper ribs. Direct impact when thrown or slammed down and forceful yanking or pulling of the arm upward are common mechanisms. Medial clavicular and sternal fractures are extremely rare and reflect massive impacting forces. The same is true for fractures of the first rib and scapular body.

Fractures of the hands and feet are relatively uncommon but have a strong likelihood of being inflicted and tend to be clinically inapparent when first seen. Grabbing and yanking, twisting, or bending the hand or foot tend to produce metacarpal/metatarsal fractures, most commonly the second and third in the hand and the first in the foot. Subtle subperiosteal new bone formation and/or medullary sclerosis are common radiographic findings (Fig. 6-40, *A*). Repetitive knuckle raps with a ruler or other hard object produce radiographic changes that consist of widening and sclerosis of the distal metaphyses of the metacarpals. Forced hyperextension of the phalanges can cause buckle fractures at their bases (see Fig. 6-40, *B*).

Figure 6-39   Inflicted distal clavicle fractures. **A,** Fracture of the distal right clavicle is seen in this infant victim of shaken impact syndrome. Lack of associated soft tissue swelling and absence of callus suggest the fracture is between 3 and 10 days old. Her metaphyseal fractures are shown in Fig. 6-28*A*, and her skull fractures in Fig. 6-47. **B,** A refracture through the callus of a healing distal right clavicle fracture is seen in the toddler whose surface injuries are shown in Fig. 6-2. She had been repeatedly thrown or shoved down stairs and into furniture.

Figure 6-38   Supracondylar fracture. An inflicted supracondylar humerus fracture caused by forced hyperextension is seen in a 9-month-old infant who was brought to his local emergency department for unexplained arm swelling. Note the diagonal linear lucency over the posterior aspect of the distal humerus and the prominent soft tissue swelling. Early signs of callus formation distal to the new fracture indicate that this is a repeat injury. He had been seen a month earlier with irritability, vomiting, hand swelling, and decreased movement of his right leg. Although chest, leg, and hand films were obtained at that time, his tibial and metacarpal fractures were missed (see Fig. 6-28, *C* and Figure 6-40, *A*).

Vertebral fractures are reported infrequently, although it is thought that many may be missed. In most cases, compression of a vertebral body is found. Cervical fractures are usually the result of violent hyperflexion or hyperextension (hangman's fracture, or bilateral fractures through the pedicles of C2). More rarely, the child may be held by the head and the neck twisted or the head is used as a handle while the assailant violently swings or shakes the child, usually resulting in catastrophic cervical cord injury. Below the cervical spine, most fractures occur near the thoracolumbar junction. Axial loading (slamming the buttocks onto a hard surface) and violent hyperflexion are the major mechanisms reported. Forced hyperflexion can also result in multiple avulsion fractures of the spinous processes as they are torn from their ligamentous attachments.

Diagnostic Imaging of Skeletal Injuries

Radiographic examination of infants and children for reasons other than suspected fractures (e.g., chest and abdominal films) may provide the first clue to inflicted trauma if clinicians and radiologists follow the maxim of carefully looking at each structure on the film (see Fig. 6-30, *A* and Fig. 6-31, *A*). Too often, fractures are missed because complaints of respiratory distress or vomiting lead clinicians to focus exclusively on lungs and heart or the abdominal gas pattern. This results in missed diagnoses, especially when bony abnormalities are subtle, and return of the child to the family with major risk of even more severe subsequent injury.

When evaluating an infant or child younger than 2 or 3 years of age who is found to have multiple bruises and/or fractures, fractures of differing ages, and fractures with high (metaphyseal, rib) or moderate (vertebral body, hand, foot, and complex skull fractures) specificity for abuse, it is essential to obtain a skeletal survey because of the greater probability of finding multiple clinically occult fractures. Surveys may also yield valuable additional information in selected cases of children 3 to 5 years of age, especially if they are developmentally delayed or have other evidence of severe abuse and/or neglect. After age 5 years, careful history and physical

Figure 6-40 Hand fractures. **A,** A healing fracture of the left third metacarpal is seen in this 9-month-old infant who was brought to his local emergency department with a 2-day history of marked irritability, vomiting, and hand swelling. Subperiosteal new bone is evident along the shaft of his left middle metacarpal along with slight medullary sclerosis proximally. This, rib, and proximal tibial fractures (see Fig. 6-28, C) were missed until the films were reread when he returned a month later with an unexplained distal humerus fracture. **B,** Buckle fractures of the proximal phalanges due to forced hyperextension of the fingers are seen in this infant, who presented with redness and swelling of his hand and no history of trauma. He returned 6 weeks later in extremis with a hyperacute subdural hematoma (see Fig. 6-48).

examination should point to areas that warrant radiographic evaluation.

We cannot emphasize enough the importance of optimal imaging techniques in the identification of inflicted skeletal trauma. High-detail skeletal surveys with two views of each bone and additional oblique views of the hands and feet maximize the potential for detection but must be specifically ordered because many surveys show only one view of each bone plus two views of the head. We also advocate four views (AP, Towne's, left, and right) of the skull. These radiographs should be examined with meticulous care, comparing paired structures from left to right and comparing adjacent structures. This is most important in order to avoid missing subtle metaphyseal fractures and early collections of subperiosteal new bone. Given that some occult fractures may be invisible at the time of initial evaluation, consideration should be given to obtaining a bone scan or a repeat skeletal survey with oblique views of the ribs 2 weeks later when callus will be evident.

Although bone scans are not ideal as a primary imaging modality in detecting inflicted fractures, they can serve as a good complementary adjunct to skeletal surveys, especially in infants who have multiple bruises (highly suspicious for abuse) but no visible fractures, rib or metaphyseal fractures, retinal hemorrhages, or obvious CNS findings consistent with shaking (see Fig. 6-30), when further evidence is needed to ensure the child's protection. Scans are particularly helpful in detecting occult rib fractures and periosteal stripping injuries that are no longer tender on examination but have not yet formed radiographically visible callus or subperiosteal new bone (Fig. 6-41, A). There is some evidence that bone scans may be able to detect fractures that have already remodeled (see Fig. 6-41, B). They are not good at detecting metaphyseal injuries because the adjacent growth centers have high uptake. They are also poor at detecting skull fractures. Ultrasound, CT, or magnetic resonance imaging (MRI) examination may be useful when injuries of unossified growth centers or epiphyseal separation injuries are suspected in toddlers or older children.

Strong consideration should be given to obtaining a head CT scan, a complete blood cell count and differential with platelets, prothrombin and partial thromboplastin times, liver function tests, and amylase lipase when evaluating children, especially infants, with multiple fractures and those with injuries of moderate to high specificity for abuse because clinically inapparent CNS and intraabdominal injuries can be associated findings.

Last, we cannot give enough emphasis to the importance of considering fractures in the differential diagnosis of unexplained irritability or of grunting respirations in infants who have no pulmonary findings. Failure to identify the cause of irritability has the potential to subject previously abused babies to further, often more severe, trauma and to place infants from high-risk families who have not yet been abused at risk for future inflicted injury.

Central Nervous System Injuries

The incidence of recognized head injury in child abuse victims ranges from 7% to 19% as reported in various large case studies. Up to 80% of victims are younger than 1 year of age, and the majority of the remaining 20% are toddlers. Numbers have risen over the past decade because more infants with subtle or subclinical intracranial injuries are imaged and abnormalities are detected because of greater recognition of associated surface and/or skeletal injuries. To put inflicted head trauma in infants in perspective, findings reported in the recent literature (Billmire) reveal that approximately 65% of all head injuries (excluding uncomplicated calvarial fractures) and 95% of all serious intracranial injuries in infants younger than 1 year of age are inflicted. Further, 60% to 80% of head injury deaths in children younger than 2 years are due to abuse.

Head injuries are also the major source of morbidity and mortality due to abuse. From 20% to 25% of known victims of inflicted head trauma die, and they account for up to 80% of fatal abuse cases. Survivors are often left with sequelae, ranging from microcephaly with neurodevastation to mild cognitive deficits. In long-term follow-up studies of former victims of physical abuse (not selected for head injury), Martin found 5% were microcephalic; 31% were in less than the fifth percentile for height and/or weight; and 53% had abnormalities on neurologic examination, nearly one third of which were moderate to severe. Although only 30% of the previously abused children studied in follow-up by Elmer and Gregg had known CNS injury at the time of their initial identification, 57% had intelligence quotients (IQs) lower than 80, and 32%, known to have been abused before 13 months of age, had evidence of significant developmental delay. Given the fact that some head injuries go undetected because they are relatively mild and/or associated with nonspecific symptoms, and given that many victims of abuse are never recognized as such, it is probable that a fair percentage of infants and children with milder degrees of "idiopathic"

Figure 6-41 Usefulness of bone scans in detecting both acute and chronic occult injuries. **A,** This 14-month-old was seen for low-grade fever and refusal to walk. Initial standard radiographs were normal. The scan, obtained because of suspicion of infection, revealed increased uptake throughout the entire left tibia. Workup for infection was negative. Repeat radiographs obtained 2 weeks later revealed a healing fracture and extensive subperiosteal new bone formation. **B,** This 21-month-old toddler reportedly collapsed at home after falling from her crib. She had a right frontal hematoma, multiple abrasions, and a cigarette burn scar. On head CT, subdural blood and cerebral edema were found. An abdominal CT obtained because of elevated liver function tests revealed the bilateral adrenal hemorrhages shown in Fig. 6-58. This bone scan obtained after a negative skeletal survey shows increased tracer uptake in the left distal ulna, right proximal femur, and right clavicle and over the lateral aspects of the rib cage bilaterally. As callus over the distal right clavicle was the only positive finding on a repeat skeletal survey 2 weeks postinjury, it was postulated that the other areas of increased uptake represented healed and fully remodeled old fractures.

developmental delay, cognitive deficits, learning disabilities, attention-deficit/hyperactivity disorder, and behavioral problems are former victims of inflicted injury that went undiagnosed.

Pathophysiology and Biomechanics

An infant's head is uniquely vulnerable to injury, whether from impact or from shaking, for several reasons:

1. It is relatively large, accounting for up to 10% of body weight, as opposed to 2% in the adult. This weight adds to the momentum of acceleration and deceleration forces with shaking and accounts for the fact that infants who are dropped, thrown, or bodily ejected from motor vehicles tend to land on their heads.

2. Highly elastic, underdeveloped cervical ligaments; relatively weak neck muscles; shallow, horizontally oriented cervical facet joints; and incompletely ossified and anteriorly wedged cervical vertebrae hinder an infant's ability to protect against whiplash forces. Together they make the infant susceptible to extreme hyperflexion and hyperextension of the neck and greater head motion when subjected to acceleration/deceleration (A/D) forces.

3. The soft calvarium, which elongates with acceleration and deceleration, and the relatively large subarachnoid space place the bridging veins between the dura mater and cerebral cortex at greater risk of tearing. In addition, with impact, the pliable skull is more likely to transfer force to the underlying brain rather than fracturing and thereby absorbing some of the force along the fracture line. Even when fractures do occur on impact, greater inbending of the pliable calvarial bones still transfers much of the impacting force to the adjacent cortex.

4. Because of its higher water content, minimal myelination, and paucity of dendritic and glial connections, the brain of a young infant is far more gelatinous than that of an older child or adult. As a result, it is much more deformable when subjected to impact and/or A/D forces, and its thin unmyelinated axons are much more vulnerable to shearing injuries, especially at the gray/white matter interfaces.

5. The relatively flat calvarial base assists rotation of the brain about the brainstem when subjected to rotational acceleration.

In terms of biomechanics, the majority of head injuries in children, whether accidental or inflicted, are the result of rapidly applied dynamic blunt forces. Some are caused by direct contact forces, and some are caused by indirect inertial forces that result from A/D of the head. The distinction is somewhat arbitrary because in most cases of "contact" injury there is some degree of A/D, and most cases of "indirect" injury involve some impact or contact.

In direct contact injuries the calvarium, its overlying soft tissues, and potentially its underlying intracranial contents are subjected to focal strains or distortions. When applied forces are mild, they may result in abrasion, bruising, or laceration of the scalp, and when more moderate they tend to result in calvarial fracture. When the amount of force applied rises beyond mild to moderate, skull fractures are more likely to be diastatic or complex, and transmission of impacting forces inward to intracranial structures increases, producing focal injuries ranging from epidural hematomas to focal subdural hematomas and ultimately to cerebral contusions or parenchymal shearing.

The three main scenarios for contact injury are as follows:

1. A moving object such as a hand, fist, thrown missile, or swung baseball bat or golf club strikes a stationary head, which, on impact, is accelerated in the same direction as the applied force. If the head is resting against a surface (e.g., mattress or wall), it then incurs a second impact. In most cases the impacting force is linear, but if delivered with a spin, a rotational component is added.

2. A moving and thus accelerated head (in a fall while running, or as a result of being thrown, pushed, slammed, or swung and slammed) strikes a stationary object (e.g., floor, furniture, wall, lamp post). In such cases there is initial acceleration followed by deceleration on impact and then a bounce back.

3. A head in motion strikes another object in motion (e.g., two children running or backing up in opposite directions butt heads, child riding bicycle hits moving car), in which case there is acceleration in two different directions.

The degree of force involved in impact injury depends on the rate of acceleration (which, in a fall, depends on the child's weight and the distance of the fall), the type of surface struck, and the duration of impact. When an impacted or impacting surface is hard, greater focal calvarial deformation is likely to occur on impact and external signs of injury are typical. This is ameliorated to some extent by the fact that, when striking a firm or hard surface, the head tends to bounce back, reducing the duration of impact. When an infant's or child's head strikes a soft surface such as a pillow or mattress, it tends to

sink into it. This increases the surface area of contact and, as a consequence, focal deformation is reduced, along with the risk of surface injuries; however, duration of contact is prolonged, and thus the duration of force application.

Indirect trauma due to A/D forces results in inertial loading and, depending on velocity and direction, subjects the intracranial contents to shearing strains. When great enough (e.g., forceful to violent), these can result in tearing at interfaces between differing structures (e.g., bridging veins) or at the interface of tissues of differing density (e.g., gray and white matter). A/D forces can be translational or linear, as from anterior to posterior in the sagittal plane (whiplash), or they can have a rotational component, as when forces are applied from two different directions (auto in motion is broadsided) or when the force is delivered with spin (blow delivered to side of head with "english"). Because A/D forces are more likely to produce shearing strains, they are more apt to cause diffuse intracranial injury, as opposed to contact forces, which are more apt to result in focal trauma. However, in the case of young infant abuse victims, impact trauma may also produce shearing strains, especially when the victim is thrown.

Injuries caused by linear A/D forces, in the sagittal plane, may include shearing of the bridging veins between the dura and cerebral cortex, along with veins in their thin arachnoid sheaths, as well as contact injuries of frontal and occipital lobes incurred in striking their respective calvarial bones. They can be diffuse and severe, especially when the head is subjected to the to-and-fro motion of violent repetitive shaking. In this scenario, the brain and calvaria have a greater propensity to get "out of sync" in their motion, increasing shearing strains. This is further magnified by the greater deformability of the gelatinous infant brain. Application of rotational forces tends to cause even more severe injury because these are more likely to induce shearing of neuronal axons at the gray/white matter interfaces. This is because more peripheral brain structures rotate more rapidly and through a wider arc than deeper, more fixed structures.

To summarize, most head injuries are caused by some combination of acceleration and/or deceleration forces and contact or impact forces. In the majority of cases of accidental trauma, especially in infants or toddlers, the forces involved are mild and the resulting injuries minor. In most cases of abusive head trauma, the forces are moderate to major and the injuries are correspondingly more severe. A chronicle of advances in recognition of the differing magnitude of applied forces and severity of injury in accidental versus inflicted impact trauma can be found in the literature on fall-related head injuries. For many years it was believed that short falls (3 to 4 feet or less) could cause severe injury. This changed on publication of a series of studies of victims of falls witnessed by people other than caretakers, and of children who had fallen from beds and examining tables in hospitals. These studies demonstrated that indoor falls of less than 10 feet (3 meters), even onto hard surfaces, did not cause serious, let alone life-threatening, head injuries. Simple linear skull fractures tended to be the most severe injuries seen, and these were associated with mild focal underlying intracranial injury only in rare instances. Furthermore, in the case of outdoor falls, injuries tended to be mild unless the activity preceding the fall added angular momentum to the forces incurred because of the height of the fall (e.g., swinging on a swing, trapeze, or jungle gym). These findings led to the recognition that study populations described in earlier literature on pediatric head trauma had included many unrecognized child abuse victims, and to refutation of the conclusions of earlier investigators that short falls and other minor mechanisms of injury could result in serious, even fatal, head trauma. Research

has also found that accidental falls down stairs consist of a series of short falls and do not result in serious head injury unless the infant is in a walker or there was acceleration before the fall.

The major identified mechanisms of inflicted head trauma include violent shaking; throwing or slamming against a hard object or a soft surface; hitting with a hand, fist, or other object; and kicking. Each is associated with application of varying degrees of impact forces and acceleration and/or deceleration. It must also be noted that many victims of inflicted CNS trauma are subjected to injury on more than one occasion. In fact, 45% of infants confirmed as victims of inflicted head trauma had evidence of prior intracranial injury on initial neuroimaging (Jenny, 1999).

Evolution of Understanding of the Pathophysiology of Shaking

Our current understanding of the forces involved and of mechanisms, including the role of shaking in inflicted head trauma, derives from much questioning and research over the past several decades, during which time theories have been proposed and investigated, some verified, some disproved, and others modified.

In the late 1940s Caffey first described the association of subdural hematomas with multiple fractures in infants. Subsequently, the question of intentional injury was raised, and shaking was postulated as the probable mechanism, leading to the concept of the *shaken baby syndrome,* characterized by a constellation of findings that included subdural hematomas (Fig. 6-42), retinal hemorrhages (Fig. 6-43, *A* and *B*), and posterior rib and metaphyseal fractures (see Fig. 6-27, *A*; Fig. 6-28; and Figs. 6-29 through 6-31).

For many years thereafter, it was believed that these injuries were due solely to shaking. Indeed, studies using monkeys, conducted in the late 1960s by Ommaya, showed that violent shaking generates rapid A/D forces, with both linear and rotational components, and that either the rotational forces or the combination of forces was necessary to produce the subdural, subarachnoid, and retinal hemorrhages seen in the animals.

Subsequent advances in neuroimaging and forensic examination, together with improvements in the identification of inflicted head trauma, have expanded our knowledge of the spectrum of CNS injuries seen in abuse victims. In addition to subdural hematomas (seen particularly in the inter-hemispheric fissure along the falx, as well as over the cerebral convexities), subarachnoid hemorrhages, cerebral contusions, diffuse axonal injury with shearing at gray/white matter interfaces, and white matter tears have been reported. Epidural and subdural hematomas at the cervicomedullary junction in association with ventral cord contusions at high cervical levels have also been linked to shaking.

In 1987 the role of shaking in producing these injuries was called into question by a group of investigators (Duhaime and colleagues) who developed an infant model using a life-size doll with a rubber neck and weighted head. They concluded that shaking alone failed to generate sufficient g forces to cause the CNS injuries attributed to shaking in human infants and noted that, on close examination, many of their victims showed signs of impact injury. Thus they postulated that some form of impact was necessary, in addition to shaking, and suggested that the impact in patients with no external evidence of injury may have been on a soft surface such as a mattress. In reviewing old autopsy cases and carefully examining new victims, subsequent investigators have found that a majority of victims of abusive head trauma do indeed have evidence of associated impact injury, albeit at times subtle, and in some instances seen only in the form of

Figure 6-42   Diffuse subdural hematomas in abusive head trauma. **A,** Acute on chronic subdural hematomas are evident on this sagittal MRI view of an infant with abusive head trauma. **B,** This CT scan of another infant reveals chronic subdural hematomas along the falx and over the cerebral convexities. These are seen as a dark rim along the falx and between the bony calvaria and the brain substance. (**A,** *Courtesy Lynda Flom, MD, Department of Pediatric Radiology, Children's Hospital of Pittsburgh, Pittsburgh, Pa;* **B,** *courtesy Division of Neuroradiology, University Health Center of Pittsburgh, Pittsburgh, Pa.*)

Figure 6-43   **A,** Multiple retinal hemorrhages are seen on funduscopic examination of this infant, who was a victim of abusive head trauma including shaking. Subdural hematoma and multiple metaphyseal "shake" fractures are typical associated findings. **B,** RetCam photograph of preretinal, intraretinal, and subretinal hemorrhages, extending to the periphery. **C,** RetCam photograph of traumatic retinoschisis. (**A,** *Courtesy Stephen Ludwig, MD, Children's Hospital of Philadelphia, Philadelphia, Pa;* **B** and **C,** *courtesy Tineke Chen, MD, Children's Hospital of Pittsburgh, University of Pittsburgh Medical Center, Pittsburgh, Pa.*)

petechiae and contusions over the internal surface of the galea at surgery or on postmortem examination. However, a significant percentage (ranging from 11% to 50%, depending on the series), especially of very young infants, do not have any evidence of impact. Furthermore, on the basis of confessions, it does appear that severe CNS injury can result from violent shaking alone. The validity of the Duhaime infant model has also been questioned because its neck was stiffer than an actual infant's and, therefore, capable of less hyperflexion, and further, the forces required were derived from adult primates with mature brains. Thus some victims' injuries appear to be due solely to shaking; others result from a combination of shaking and impact trauma; and still others from impact alone.

In addition to the unique vulnerability of the young infant brain to deformation, there are two major explanations for the presence of severe injury in shaken babies who have no physical evidence of impact. One is that when the child's head strikes a soft surface, no external marker of impact may be left. The other relates to the fact that *repetitive impacts actually do occur with shaking alone,* especially when a very young infant with poor head control is violently shaken back and forth over and over again. These impacts consist of the chin hitting the chest and the occiput hitting the vertebral column at opposite ends of the arc of head motion. In the process, impacts of the frontal lobes against the frontal bone and the occipital lobes against the occipital bone occur with attendant brain deformation, on both impact and rebound. Further, in the course of violent shaking, the perpetrator's motion may not be consistently linear, the baby may turn its head to avert its gaze from the perpetrator, or the infant may lose consciousness (and therefore tone) in the process of being shaken, the head then lolling down and slightly sideways, thereby introducing rotational momentum to the A/D forces.

Most victims of suspected shaking are less than 1 year of age, frequently under 6 months, and most have no external signs of injury, although careful inspection may reveal faint finger impression bruises (see Fig. 6-13). On the basis of confessions and videotapes obtained with hidden cameras, it is now known that the infant is subjected to repetitive, violent shakes usually while being held by the trunk facing the perpetrator, less often when grasped by arms and shoulders or by hands or feet.

Metaphyseal fractures, posterior rib fractures, and retinal hemorrhages appear to be highly specific for shaking, especially when seen in combination with subdural bleeding. Retinal hemorrhages, typically numerous, diffuse, often extending out to the periphery, and located in multiple layers of the retina, are found in 70% to 90% of infants and children with inflicted head injury and in nearly 100% of those who suffer serious sequelae and death (see Fig. 6-43). Although the uniqueness of their association with shaking has been the subject of some controversy, studies of infants and children whose accidental severe head trauma was witnessed have shown that the incidence of retinal hemorrhages is vanishingly small and is largely limited to children who incurred severe crush injuries to the head; who suffered high-velocity, lateral impact rotational injuries; or who incurred injuries outdoors in falls while swinging on playground equipment or jumping on a trampoline, which involved significant angular momentum. In the rare reports of accidental in-home falls resulting in subdural hematomas with retinal hemorrhages, each case involved significant momentum from being swung, falling down stairs while on the move in a walker, or a straight fall of 8 to 10 feet onto concrete. Each child was brought promptly for care and had no associated injuries or history of injury. Subdural hemorrhages were small and resolved in 24 to 48 hours. Furthermore, in these accident scenarios the retinal hemorrhages seen were fewer in number and tended to be localized over the posterior pole. Similarly, research on children who have undergone prolonged cardiopulmonary resuscitation has revealed a very low incidence of retinal hemorrhages, and the majority of cases in which they were found involved victims of abuse or massive accidental head injury. A small minority were suffering from malignant hypertension, coagulopathy, or septic shock. Traumatic retinoschisis (Fig. 6-43, *C*) is not described with trauma-induced coagulopathy other than with abusive head trauma. Similarly, posterior and lateral rib fractures have not been found following prolonged cardiopulmonary resuscitation in either infants or animal models. Thus when cardiopulmonary resuscitation is given as an explanation for head trauma with retinal hemorrhages and rib fractures, it is false.

Clinical Picture of Inflicted Head Trauma

Modes of presentation of inflicted head trauma vary, depending on the age of the victim and severity of injury. When signs and symptoms are mild, no care may be sought, and if it is, there is often a significant delay between the time of the injury and time of presentation. When there are no external signs (which is often the case), a history of trauma is almost never reported. An unrelated chief complaint or a history of nonspecific symptoms such as vomiting, lethargy, irritability, or trouble breathing is likely to be given when neurologic abnormalities are not blatant. When injuries are more severe, complaints of unresponsiveness, shaking or stiffening spells, and apnea or choking are more likely to be reported. In patients with significant contact injuries and obvious surface bruising, a chief complaint of a bump on the head may be given with a history of a minor mechanism of injury such as rolling off a couch and falling 15 to 18 inches to a carpeted floor, or the caretaker may report having dropped the baby a short distance (usually <3 or 4 feet). In some cases another young child has been reported to have hit the baby on the head. These mechanisms do not explain intracranial injury.

In cases of more severe injury, presentation is more likely to be prompt, but delays in seeking care still occur. Often, when an infant loses consciousness as a result of shaking and/or impact, the perpetrator becomes frightened and delays seeking medical attention for fear of being caught. He or she then leaves the baby to rest for a while, hoping that the infant will revive on its own. During the ensuing interval, intracranial pressure may rise as a consequence of increasing cerebral edema and/or the mass effect of intracranial hemorrhage, compromising cerebral perfusion and resulting in varying amounts of cerebral ischemia. Associated alteration in level of consciousness and/or seizures can result in hypoventilation, apnea, or respiratory arrest, resulting in hypoxia. Hence hypoxic/ischemic injury may be added to that of the physical trauma (see Fig. 6-53). (*Note:* Studies have shown that the person alone with the child at the time worrisome symptoms are first noted is usually the perpetrator.)

Infants with milder degrees of injury may have nonspecific lethargy and/or irritability without focal neurologic signs. Some may have subtle surface bruises or petechiae evident only on close inspection, and some (but by no means all) may cry when picked up by the chest or moved because of new fractures. Funduscopic examination may reveal retinal hemorrhages. In other, more severely injured infants, physical findings may include lethargy, increased or decreased tone, rhythmic eye opening, eye deviation, extremity twitching or bicycling movements of the extremities, and sometimes posturing. Decreased ability to follow the examiner's face, decreased responsiveness to pain, and poor suck and grasp are important findings. The fontanelle is often full but may or may not be tense. On occasion, infants may present in shock resulting from massive subgaleal or intracranial hemorrhage. Diffuse retinal hemorrhages (see Fig. 6-43) are more likely to be found in these sicker babies, and dilated ophthalmoscopy should be performed in all infants seen for altered levels of consciousness. These infants should also undergo meticulous inspection of the skin and mucous membranes.

Inflicted impact injuries are seen in infants and children who have been thrown to the floor, against a wall, or into other objects or who have received direct blows to the head with a fist or other blunt object. Surface injuries are likely in these cases and may range from subtle bruising or a small patch of petechiae on the scalp to large subgaleal hematomas. Surface injuries of the face and other sites are also common (Fig. 6-44, *A*; and see Fig. 6-7, *A*). In these cases, skull fractures are frequently present. Simple linear fractures (Fig. 6-45), diastatic linear fractures with or without diastatic sutures (see Fig. 6-44, *B*), and more complex T-shaped and eggshell fractures (Fig. 6-46) have all been reported in cases of inflicted trauma. Given the greater magnitude of injury forces involved in most cases of abuse (as opposed to those in the majority of accidental injuries), diastatic and complex fractures, and bilateral fractures (Fig. 6-47) are more likely to be the result of abuse and are inconsistent with histories of minor mechanisms of injury. Conversely, when these types of skull fractures are seen and no major mechanism of injury is found, abuse should be strongly suspected. Associated intracranial injuries may include focal subdural hematomas (Fig. 6-48; and see Fig. 6-50) and focal cerebral contusions (Fig. 6-49) with adjacent edema, which, when severe, produces a midline shift and may be associated with focal shearing injury.

In cases due to shaking alone or shaking plus impact, diffuse subdural hematomas may be found over the convexities and along the falx (see Fig. 6-42). A combination of focal and interhemispheric subdurals is another common finding (Fig. 6-50), again often accompanied by varying amounts of cerebral edema. Extreme A/D forces with a rotational component produce loss of gray/white matter differentiation due to axonal shearing (Fig. 6-51, *A*), which on occasion is further highlighted by arc-shaped hemorrhages (see Fig. 6-51, *B*). Severe cerebral edema and ventricular effacement are typical in these cases. In the ensuing days the magnitude of neuronal loss can be appreciated, and the full extent of loss is seen in the ensuing months (Fig. 6-52). In cases of severe hypoxic or ischemic injury, the cortex appears hypodense in comparison with the basal ganglia, termed a *reversal sign* (Fig. 6-53), which is often seen when there is a long delay in seeking care.

On occasion, patients who have incurred milder trauma and are not seen acutely may present weeks later with one or more of the following symptoms: intermittent vomiting and irritability, rapidly increasing head circumference with split sutures and a full fontanelle, failure to thrive, and developmental delay typically affecting social more than motor development. Some of these patients are found to have *chronic subdural hematomas*.

Neuroimaging

Routine skull radiographs are best for detecting most skull fractures, and when abuse is suspected, four views (AP, Towne's, right, and left) should be obtained. CT has proved highly valuable in the acute assessment of CNS injuries, and an unenhanced head CT with brain and bone windows is indicated whenever there is any suspicion of intracranial injury, whether due to abnormal neurologic signs and symptoms, presence of metaphyseal and/or rib fractures, multiple

Figure 6-44   Abusive head trauma. **A,** Subtle bruising is seen over the right fronto-temporal area in this infant. **B,** Her skull radiograph reveals an occipital fracture with diastasis of the lambdoid suture. On CT scan, a posterior interhemispheric subdural hematoma was found. Other bruises are shown in Fig. 6-13.

bruises, or retinal hemorrhages. It clearly delineates most intracranial hemorrhages and cerebral edema, as well as the majority of subdural hematomas and many fractures. CT is especially effective in revealing interhemispheric subdural hematomas along the falx and in the parieto-occipital area,

Figure 6-45   Linear skull fracture. This linear occipital fracture was found in the infant with bilateral black eyes shown in Fig. 6-7, *A*.

Figure 6-46 Eggshell fracture. Multiple occipital fractures are seen in a child who presented with a history of a minor fall and scalp swelling. It was later acknowledged that he had been thrown against a brick wall. *(Courtesy Department of Radiology, Children's Hospital of Pittsburgh, Pittsburgh, Pa.)*

Figure 6-48 A focal subdural hematoma, caused by severe impact forces, is seen in the left frontal area of this 6-month-old infant who presented with decreased responsiveness after "rolling off a bed." The layering of the subdural blood was due to rapid collection and at surgery was found to consist of newly clotted blood and fresh hemorrhage, classified as a *hyperacute subdural hematoma*. Note also the acute subdural blood along the anterior interhemispheric fissure and the midline shift. Multiple phalangeal fractures found 6 weeks earlier, but not recognized as inflicted, are shown in Fig. 6-40, *B*.

which are seen frequently in victims of shaking (see Fig. 6-42). It is also effective in detecting cerebral edema (see Figs. 6-48 to 6-51), loss of gray/white matter differentiation due to axonal shearing (see Fig. 6-51, *A* and *B*), and subsequent cortical necrosis (see Fig. 6-52), as well as cortical hypodensity as a result of hypoxic/ischemic injury (see Fig. 6-53).

CT does have limitations, however. It may not reveal the full extent of injuries and may fail to detect thin subdural hemorrhages (especially over the convexities) and subtle cerebral contusions or hemorrhages. CT is also unable to distinguish between the layering of subdural blood as a result of rapid or hyperacute bleeds from layering of hemorrhages of

Figure 6-47 Shaken impact syndrome. **A** and **B,** These bilateral, diastatic, parieto-occipital skull fractures, shown in anteroposterior and oblique views, were the result of impacts on the arm of a couch after bouts of shaking. Her metaphyseal fractures are shown in Fig. 6-28, *A*, and her clavicle fracture is shown in Fig. 6-39, *A*.

Figure 6-50 Focal occipital and interhemispheric subdural blood are seen in this toddler who "collapsed at home after a fall from her crib." Note the effacement of the right lateral ventricle and slight anterior midline shift due to cerebral edema. Her bone scan is shown in Fig. 6-41, *B* and her abdominal CT in Fig. 6-58.

Bony discontinuity

Subgaleal hematoma

Subdural hematoma

Cortical contrast enhancement

Figure 6-49 Cerebral contusion. CT scan from a 4-week-old infant who allegedly rolled out of his crib while the side rails were up shows a large subgaleal hematoma obscuring an underlying fracture, severe cerebral swelling with a shift of the midline, and cortical contrast enhancement indicative of a cerebral contusion. *(Courtesy Division of Neuroradiology, University Health Center of Pittsburgh, Pittsburgh, Pa.)*

Figure 6-51 Diffuse axonal shearing. **A,** Loss of gray/white matter differentiation is evident on this 7-week-old infant's CT scan, along with focal subdural blood around the left occipital lobe and an interhemispheric subdural hematoma. **B,** This arc-shaped hemorrhage seen in a 2-month-old infant, who also has loss of gray/white matter differentiation, is located at the gray/white interface. This is a sign found occasionally with diffuse axonal shearing injuries. Note the frontal subdural hematoma. **C,** This CT scan of a normal 2-month-old shows normal gray/white matter differentiation.

Figure 6-52 Posttraumatic cerebral necrosis. **A,** One week after the injury, clear evidence of contraction of cortical tissues, as a result of extensive neuronal death, can be appreciated. **B,** Six months later, extensive cerebral atrophy is present. This is the same child shown in Fig. 6-51*B*.

differing ages (see Fig. 6-48). It should be noted that most acute subdurals appear bright white on CT, whereas older and chronic subdurals appear light gray or black.

MRI is up to 50% more sensitive in detecting small subdural hematomas over the convexities (Fig. 6-54, *A* and *B*). MRI can also identify subdural hemorrhages of differing ages because the imaging intensity changes as blood begins to break down (see Fig. 6-54, *C*). However, subdural hematomas of varying ages may be the result of repetitive injury or spontaneous rebleeding. MRI is far superior to CT in detecting subtle contusions and small parenchymal hemorrhages, in identifying diffuse axonal injury, and in detecting abnormalities of posterior fossa structures, the brainstem, and the cervical cord. It is good at detecting signs of prior or old injuries (Fig. 6-55) and is far superior to CT at differentiating subdural from subarachnoid fluid collections and in distinguishing

between cerebrospinal fluid and old blood. Its usefulness in child abuse cases is often greatest 5 to 7 days postinjury. For optimal results a T_1- and T_2-weighted conventional or fast spin echo MRI should be ordered with proton density or fluid attenuated inversion recovery (FLAIR) sequences.

Abdominal and Intrathoracic Injuries

Although less common than inflicted surface, skeletal, and head injuries, abdominal and intrathoracic injuries have been found in up to 2% of victims of physical abuse, with a mortality rate of up to 50%. Intraabdominal injuries predominate over intrathoracic injuries and range in severity from subclinical to catastrophic, with the majority identified as being moderate to severe. They are second only to head injury and suffocation as a cause of abuse-related deaths.

Intraabdominal Injuries

Young children are more vulnerable to internal abdominal injury with blunt trauma than adolescents or adults for three major reasons: their abdominal muscles are relatively weak, allowing impacting forces to be transmitted inward more easily; the distance between the abdominal wall and the vertebral column is relatively short; and their costal margins are more horizontally oriented, affording less protection to underlying viscera. Mid-abdominal structures that are fixed in place by pedicles or overlying ligaments (small intestines, liver, and pancreas) are particularly vulnerable. Typically, inflicted abdominal trauma is caused by blunt force injury and is the result of violent kicks or punches or of being thrown or slammed against hard objects. Penetrating injuries, fortunately, are rare (see Fig. 6-16, *D*). External findings are often minimal or absent (see Figs. 6-13 and 6-57, *A*).

As is the case with skeletal and CNS injuries, it is uncommon for caretakers to provide a history of trauma and the severity of attendant symptoms is often minimized. When a history of trauma is reported (usually when bruises are prominent), it is one of a minor mechanism that does not correspond with the type and severity of clinical findings. Presentation is often delayed but may be prompt if signs and symptoms are severe.

The major types of abdominal pathology seen are duodenal hematomas, small intestinal tears at sites of supporting

Figure 6-53 Hypoxic injury. This infant, who was found unresponsive in his crib, has a pattern of diffuse cortical hypodensity on CT scan, indicative of extensive cerebral infarction caused by hypoxia.

Figure 6-54   **A** and **B,** This 3-year-old abuse victim presented with lethargy, vomiting, hyporeflexia, and the acute onset of blindness. The CT scan reveals ventricular enlargement and cortical atrophy, which were the result of severe shaking 1 year earlier, but no hemorrhage. His MRI shows small, bilateral subdural hemorrhages that were missed on CT. **C,** This 5-month-old infant with head and facial bruises, bilateral retinal hemorrhages, and multiple rib fractures was found to have subdural hemorrhages of differing ages on MRI. The white subdural hematoma is between 0 and 14 days old, and the gray subdural hematoma is more than 14 days old. *(Courtesy Randall Alexander, MD, Moorehead School of Medicine, Atlanta, Ga.)*

ligaments, mesenteric tears, contusions or lacerations of the liver or spleen, and pancreatic and renal contusions.

Patients with duodenal hematomas present with signs and symptoms of high intestinal obstruction (e.g., vomiting and abdominal pain, sometimes manifest primarily as irritability, without abdominal distention). Plain radiographs may reveal an air–fluid level in a dilated duodenal loop (Fig. 6-56, *A*) proximal to the hematoma, and upper gastrointestinal series and ultrasound studies reveal narrowing of the lumen and thickening of the duodenal wall, respectively (see Fig. 6-56, *B*).

Because spillage of intestinal contents into the peritoneal cavity results in intense peritoneal irritation and rapid onset of infection, children with acute small intestinal tears generally have severe abdominal pain within an hour or two of injury. In most cases this is diffuse at the time of presentation and is associated with avoidance of any movement; marked abdominal distention, due to third spacing of fluid by the inflamed peritoneum (Fig. 6-57, *A*); along with diffuse, direct, and rebound tenderness, and signs of sepsis and shock. In cases in which the rent or tear is small and the child can wall

off the infection, signs and symptoms will be more localized, less marked, and similar to those of a youngster with an appendiceal abscess.

At a minimum, small tears of the mesentery, which carries the vascular supply to the large and small bowel, result in some bleeding with secondary, often localized, irritation and pain because bowel integrity tends to be preserved by collateral circulation. In the absence of prominent peritoneal signs and surface injuries, pain may be attributed to another cause. When rents are large (Fig. 6-57, *B*), however, interruption of the vascular supply to the adjacent bowel occurs, and as the involved segment gradually loses viability, it undergoes necrosis and ultimately perforates (Fig. 6-57, *C*). This process can take days, in part because of collateral circulation and in part because of evolution of the inflammatory process that thins the bowel wall before perforation ultimately occurs. During this time the child is likely to have significant abdominal pain, anorexia, vomiting, and markedly decreased activity. Parents, however, are unlikely to report these symptoms. Once perforation occurs, the clinical picture of diffuse peritonitis and sepsis, described earlier, rapidly evolves.

Abuse victims with hepatic and splenic injuries may have minimal symptomatology when these viscera are merely contused. Localized pain and peritoneal irritation are likely with small lacerations. With large lacerations, intense abdominal pain and often pain referred to the ipsilateral shoulder tend to develop within an hour because extravasated blood stimulates peritoneal and diaphragmatic irritation. In addition, signs of pallor and hypovolemia are likely to evolve with comparable rapidity. Sudden "unexplained" collapse is the rule when inflicted blows shatter one or both of these organs.

In the majority of cases of inflicted abdominal trauma, abuse is not confirmed until an abdominal CT scan is obtained, whether because of elevated liver function tests or findings on examination. In some instances the true origin of the problem is not identified until surgery is performed.

Findings from the study by Coant and colleagues (1992) indicate that the true incidence of intraabdominal injury in abuse victims may be significantly underestimated. Using transaminase levels as screening tests, the investigators found evidence of hepatic injury including three small liver lacerations in 4 of 49 patients with multiple bruises being evaluated for possible physical abuse. Although some patients had clinical evidence of head injury and some had facial or thoracic bruises, none had any external evidence of abdominal trauma or any abdominal tenderness. All were younger than 5 years

Figure 6-55   Evidence of prior intracranial injury. An MRI obtained of the child whose external injuries are shown in Fig. 6-2 shows evidence of prior shearing injury. Note the thinning of the corpus callosum posteriorly and the cyst, both of which reflect degeneration after axonal tearing and subsequent neuronal death.

Figure 6-56   Duodenal hematoma. **A,** Abdominal film reveals an air–fluid level in a dilated duodenal loop proximal to a duodenal hematoma. **B,** This upper gastrointestinal series shows narrowing of the duodenal lumen and widening of the duodenal wall at the site of a hematoma. The obstruction is partial because some barium has passed through the narrowed segment. This latency-aged boy was from a wealthy family, and although the victim told physicians that his father had punched him in the stomach 3 days before admission, the father, who was granted access to his son after discharge, made him recant his story and was acquitted. *(Courtesy Department of Radiology, Children's Hospital of Pittsburgh, Pittsburgh, Pa.)*

of age. This indicates that serum transaminase levels should be checked in suspected victims of physical abuse who are younger than 5 years of age, much as a skeletal survey is recommended for those younger than 2 years. If levels are elevated, an abdominal CT scan should be obtained. Unfortunately, in rare instances of small hepatic contusions or lacerations transaminase levels may be normal.

Renal and adrenal injuries (Fig. 6-58) are considerably less common than those involving other intraabdominal organs, probably because of their relatively protected location. Associated symptoms may be subtle and overshadowed by other injuries, unless there is extravasation of blood into the peritoneal cavity.

Thoracic Injuries

Because of the great plasticity of the thoracic cage in infants and young children, inflicted intrathoracic injuries are relatively uncommon, despite the frequency of rib fractures. They have high morbidity and mortality rates, however, because they are the result of application of massive forces to the chest such as stomping, slamming, or violent throws. When they are seen, they are usually associated with multiple, often displaced rib fractures (Fig. 6-59). Associated intrathoracic findings may include hemothorax, pleural effusion in response to smaller subpleural bleeds, pulmonary and myocardial contusions, and parenchymal lacerations. On rare occasions a pleural effusion may be seen on chest radiographs in the absence of visible rib fractures. In such cases a bone scan may reveal the true extent of the associated skeletal injuries.

The major mode of presentation of inflicted intrathoracic chest trauma is likely to be one of significant respiratory distress, with complaints of severe chest pain in victims old enough to speak. Less often, sudden collapse is reported. Typically, no history of injury is provided or one of a minor mechanism is given. Clinical findings may include dyspnea, tachypnea, grunting respirations, and anxiety, often with evident pain on movement and chest wall tenderness. When associated blood loss is significant, pallor, weak pulses, and hypotension are seen.

DIFFERENTIAL DIAGNOSIS OF INFLICTED INJURIES VERSUS FINDINGS CAUSED BY ACCIDENT OR ILLNESS

Although it is highly important to detect injuries resulting from abuse in order to protect children from future and potentially more serious trauma, it is also important to avoid diagnosing abuse erroneously because this subjects innocent families to the ordeal of a CPS investigation and sometimes results in removal of the child to foster care, causing tremendous emotional stress. Accurate diagnosis requires clear knowledge, not only of patterns of injury seen after abuse, but also of mechanisms of injury and their resulting findings, of

Figure 6-57 Mesenteric tears with secondary bowel necrosis. The mother of this 13-month-old infant (who was described as previously well) reported finding her unarousable in the morning, with bilious vomitus on her sheets. She was rushed to the hospital, where she was in profound shock. Her abdomen was markedly distended and tense and was noted to be exquisitely tender when her level of consciousness improved. **A,** A round, fading bruise is seen in this view over the right lower abdominal wall; a few even fainter bruises were seen around the umbilicus. Note the marked abdominal distention. **B,** At surgery she was found to have diffuse peritonitis, and two large rents were discovered in the jejunal mesentery. **C,** A long segment, found to be necrotic with a perforation, and adjacent bowel that appeared nonviable were resected. Inflammatory infiltrates on pathologic examination suggested that the inciting injury had occurred 5 to 7 days earlier.

the types of accidental injuries commonly seen at various ages, and of the diseases and congenital disorders that predispose to bleeding or increased bony fragility. In the vast majority of cases of significant accidental injury, the patient is brought in promptly for care by appropriately concerned parents who give a clear history of a mechanism that fits the findings. Typically there are no associated injuries unless the mechanism involves a motor vehicle accident or major fall, and there is no history or evidence of multiple prior injuries.

These families usually have been compliant with well-child care and although interviews may reveal an occasional risk factor, there is no worrisome pattern of risk factors and red flags, and parent–child interactions demonstrate warmth, caring, attentiveness, and affection. If doubt exists the services of experienced physicians with expertise in the fields of child abuse, orthopedics, pediatric surgery, and neurosurgery should be sought. In addition, valuable information and insight may be gained in conferring with the child's primary care physician.

Differential Diagnosis of Surface Bruises

Accidental Bruises

Ordinary, play-related bruises can be distinguished from those resulting from abuse by virtue of the fact that they tend to be small and nonspecific in configuration. They are typically located over the bony prominences of the shins, knees, elbows, extensor forearms, mid-chin, or mid-forehead (Fig. 6-60, *A*). Larger bruises and even those with configurations suggesting they were inflicted by an object can also be accidental or the result of an altercation with another child. In such cases, however, presentation for care is prompt, the mechanism of injury is consistent with the findings, and in most instances the incident was witnessed.

Black eyes subsequent to forehead contusions may be mistaken for inflicted bruises. If the initial injury produces a large forehead hematoma, subsequent tracking of blood through the soft tissue planes of the face is likely to occur over the ensuing 24 to 72 hours, producing ecchymotic discoloration along the sides of the nose and under the lower eyelids (Fig. 6-60, *B*). This gives the illusion of an injury resulting from direct periorbital trauma. The history, presence of residual forehead contusion or abrasion, and absence of tenderness in the infraorbital area help confirm the true origin of these findings.

Figure 6-58 Bilateral adrenal hemorrhages. This 21-month-old girl was admitted with a history of altered level of consciousness after falling from her crib. She had multiple bruises, a clavicle fracture, bilateral retinal hemorrhages, subdural hematomas with cerebral edema, and a midline shift (see Fig. 6-50). Her abdominal CT scan, performed when liver function tests were found to be elevated, reveals bilateral adrenal hemorrhages.

Figure 6-59 Intrathoracic trauma. This 4-month-old boy was brought in with severe respiratory distress and found to have paradoxic chest wall movement, caused by flail chest, and respiratory failure. **A,** His chest radiograph reveals bilateral rib fractures, with multiple fractures along many of the rib arcs, some with and some without callus. Three of the posterior fractures on the right are badly displaced. He has bilateral pleural effusions and bilateral soft tissue swelling over the chest wall, along with multiple pulmonary contusions seen as patchy infiltrates. **B,** Close-up of fresh, displaced fractures of the fifth to seventh ribs posteriorly. **C,** Close-up of left lateral rib fractures shows refracture through the callus of the ninth rib.

Bruises Caused by Subcultural Healing Practices

The influx of immigrants from Southeast Asia to the United States and Canada since the late 1970s has made it important to be aware of nonabusive healing practices that produce unusual bruising patterns. The most common of these is coin rubbing, in which the skin of the trunk and back is rubbed vigorously with the edge of a coin as a means of treating fever. This leaves a pattern of bruises resembling the branches of a fir tree (Fig. 6-61). In another practice, termed *cupping,* a candle is lit and placed under a small glass cup or the inner surface of the cup is coated with alcohol that is then burned off. The cup is then applied to the forehead or trunk. As oxygen is consumed by the flame, or as the cup cools, a vacuum is created, and the cup adheres to the skin. On removal, a round imprint is left on the skin. As the indentation resolves, a characteristic circular ecchymosis remains that encircles central petechiae (Fig. 6-62).

Purpura Due to Bleeding Disorders or Vasculitis

Purpuric lesions associated with coagulopathies and acute vasculitic disorders must also be recognized and distinguished from inflicted bruises. However, it is also important to recognize that children with disorders that predispose to easy bruising may on occasion be victims of abuse.

Thrombocytopenia

Patients with acute idiopathic thrombocytopenic purpura (ITP) and acute leukemia can have multiple purpuric lesions located anywhere on the body. Because they reflect thrombocytopenia, they are usually associated with petechiae (Fig. 6-63). Children with ITP commonly have a history of an antecedent viral illness, and those with leukemia may have a history of fatigue, anorexia, and weight loss, sometimes accompanied by bone pain. They usually have adenopathy and splenomegaly. Patients with aplastic anemia can have bruises with round, thick, indurated centers similar to those seen in children with clotting factor deficiencies, but typically their bruises are surrounded by petechiae (Fig. 6-64). These hematologic abnormalities are usually readily detected by a complete blood cell count with differential and platelet count.

Clotting Factor Deficiencies

Children with clotting factor deficiencies—the hemophilias and von Willebrand disease—tend to bruise easily, and their bruises are often much more impressive than one would ordinarily expect from the reported mechanism of injury. Those with factor VIII or IX deficiencies tend to have bruises with round, thick, indurated centers as are seen in aplastic anemia (see Fig. 6-64) but without the satellite petechiae. Although

Figure 6-60 Normal bruises. **A,** Numerous small, nonspecific bruises are present over the knees and shins of this active youngster. **B,** Black eyes occurring after a forehead contusion. This boy had fallen from the ladder of a slide 3 days before. Blood from his forehead hematoma had tracked down through the facial soft tissues, creating these shiners, which were nontender.

severe X-linked hemophilia is diagnosed prenatally in most males because of known family history or in early infancy (frequently after circumcision), those with milder forms of the disease who are uncircumcised may not be identified until they start crawling and develop prominent ecchymoses over their knees and palms, along with other evidence of easy bruising.

Von Willebrand disease, which occurs in both males and females, is characterized by partial factor VIII deficiency and platelet dysfunction and may escape detection for years. The disorder is diagnosed in some patients when they suffer unexpectedly severe bleeding postoperatively. In many girls or young women, it is identified when they develop menorrhagia during adolescence or have severe bleeding after childbirth. Suspicion of abuse may arise when an affected child presents with an unusually florid bruise subsequent to relatively mild accidental trauma. Clues to an underlying factor deficiency include (1) bruises with round, thick, indurated centers (see Fig. 6-64), (2) a clear mechanism of injury consistent with the configuration but not the severity of the bruise, and (3) a family and child who seem well adjusted and interact

appropriately. A positive family history for bleeding problems, especially after surgery or the birth of a baby, may also exist. Whenever any question exists about a possible factor deficiency, a full coagulation profile is recommended because platelet counts are normal and many patients with von Willebrand disease have normal prothrombin and partial thromboplastin times.

Vitamin K Deficiency

A fat-soluble vitamin, vitamin K is necessary for carboxylation of clotting factors II, VII, IX, and X. Because infants have relatively low levels of vitamin K at birth, it has been standard practice for more than 70 years to give them intramuscular vitamin K in the perinatal period; hence the incidence of deficiency is very low. In the absence of this supplementation infants can develop bleeding at any time during the first 12 weeks (usually within the first 2 weeks). Manifestations include rectal bleeding, hematemesis, hemoptysis, bruising, and intracranial bleeding (usually subarachnoid). With the latter retinal hemorrhages are rare and retinoschisis is not seen. In all cases prothrombin time (PT) and activated partial

Figure 6-61 Coin rubbing. **A,** Vigorous stroking of the skin of a febrile child with a coin produces a peculiar bruising pattern. **B,** Here the father of another child demonstrates the technique. (**A,** Courtesy Thomas Daley, MD, St. Joseph's Hospital, Paterson, NJ.)

Figure 6-62 Cupping. These circular bruises with central petechiae are the sequelae of the Southeast Asian practice of cupping. *(Courtesy Robert Hickey, MD, Children's Hospital of Pittsburgh, Pittsburgh, Pa.)*

Figure 6-64 A, Bruises with thick round centers can be seen in children with aplastic anemia or with clotting factor deficiencies. **B,** This view from the side shows the elevation of the indurated central portion of the ecchymosis in a patient with chronic aplastic anemia.

thromboplastin time (aPTT) are abnormal. Obtaining a PIVKA (Proteins Induced by Vitamin K Antagonism or Absence)-II level should be considered as this will be elevated.

Vasculitis

Patients with vasculitic disorders may develop diffuse purpuric lesions that can be mistaken for inflicted bruises. In the pediatric population, *Henoch-Schönlein purpura* is by far the most common of these. Knowledge of the pattern and course of evolution of its exanthem can help prevent misdiagnosis. Affected children often have a history of antecedent viral or streptococcal infection, followed by the appearance of the exanthem. In many children the initial lesions are urticarial, although pruritus is mild or absent. The purpuric lesions appear in crops, with the first distributed below the waist. Subsequent crops tend to involve the extensor forearms, cheeks, and ears. Periarticular swelling and stocking-glove angioedema, which wax and wane, are common, as is crampy or colicky abdominal pain (see Chapters 7 and 8 and Fig. 8-63).

Figure 6-63 Idiopathic thrombocytopenic purpura. This school-age child was seen with a chief complaint of a rash after a viral upper respiratory tract infection. Examination revealed diffuse petechiae, shown here over her ankle, and scattered purpuric lesions. Her hemoglobin and white blood cell count and differential were normal, but her platelet count was markedly reduced.

Ehlers-Danlos Syndrome

Children with various forms of Ehlers-Danlos syndrome tend not only to have hyperextensible skin but also to bruise easily and thus often have multiple bruises of varying ages that are usually located over their extremities. This has been mistaken in some cases for child abuse but can be distinguished by careful assessment for skin distensibility, joint hypermobility, and thin atrophic scars that are typical associated findings (see Chapter 1 and Fig. 1-41).

Trauma-related Coagulopathy

More than three fourths of children with traumatic brain injury (TBI) develop coagulopathy considered to be due to fibrinolysis and thrombosis, which may lead to disseminated intravascular coagulation (DIC). Retinoschisis (Fig. 6-43, *C*) does not occur with DIC and helps differentiate acute head trauma (AHT) from other causes of intracranial hemorrhage.

Hyperpigmentation

Mongolian Spots

Most infants of African, Mediterranean, and Asian descent have patchy areas of hyperpigmentation, termed "mongolian spots," in which the epithelial cells contain increased amounts of melanin. These are most commonly located over the sacrum and buttocks, although they may be found elsewhere on the trunk and extremities. These areas are flat, nontender, and typically a bit more blue or green than true acute ecchymotic lesions (Fig. 6-65; see also Chapter 8 and Fig. 8-87).

Postinflammatory Hyperpigmentation

After resolution of the acute phase of an inflammatory exanthem, many children with darkly pigmented skin are left with patchy hyperpigmentation at the sites affected (see Chapter 8, Fig. 8-124). These patches can be mistaken for bruises on occasion, particularly when the initial rash involved the buttocks or back. Lesions are brown to dark brown, nontender, and do not change in hue over a period of days or even weeks, as do bruises. A history of antecedent dermatitis helps in distinguishing the true nature of the problem.

Figure 6-65 Mongolian spots. This toddler, referred from a day care center because of "multiple bruises," actually had an unusual number of hyperpigmented mongolian spots.

The bites of blood-sucking insects, especially fleas and bed bugs, can induce a hypersensitivity reaction in some children, known as *papular urticaria* (see Chapter 8, Fig. 8-68). This is manifest clinically by symmetric chronic/recurrent eruptions of highly pruritic papules and wheals that tend to vesiculate centrally. Because itching is intense, scratching to the point of excoriation is typical. On resolution the child is left with target-shaped macular scars that are hyperpigmented peripherally and hypopigmented centrally (see Fig. 6-73). These may be mistaken for bruises or healed cigarette burns (see Fig. 6-21, *C* and *D*).

One particular type of postinflammatory hyperpigmentation is more often confused with bruising than others: *phytophotodermatitis*. In this disorder, plant-derived photosensitizers (psoralens) found in the juices of lemons, limes, figs, dill, parsley, parsnips, carrots, and celery are inadvertently wiped or spilled on the skin. Subsequent exposure to sunlight can then induce an exaggerated sunburn reaction. Initially, lesions are erythematous macules. In some cases, surface blistering occurs. Lesions then become hyperpigmented, and because the juice is often wiped on by the hands of a parent who was in the process of cutting one of the fruits, herbs, or vegetables when approached by the child, the patches often have bizarre or hand- or finger-shaped patterns that can be mistaken for grab or slap marks (Fig. 6-66). Again, the history of a preceding erythematous rash and the persistence of the same coloration over days or weeks can help in identifying the true source.

Patterned Tanning

Although not commonly mistaken for bruises, patterned tanning, resulting from sun exposure while wearing articles of clothing (often bathing suits) that have cut-out designs (Fig. 6-67), can be a source of confusion. The mistake is more likely when the cut-outs are round or linear, when different apparel is being worn at the time the child is seen, and when clinicians fail to recognize that children who have naturally dark skin tan with sun exposure, just as do those with fair complexions.

Differential Diagnosis of Accidental versus Inflicted Burns

All children incur accidental burns in the course of growing up, and it is important to be able to distinguish these from inflicted burns. Many are so small and minor that no medical care is sought. Children with more significant accidental burns usually present soon after the incident, and the history is consistent with the physical findings. Presentation may be delayed, however, if a minor burn being treated at home becomes secondarily infected.

Accidental Scalds

Accidental scalds typically occur when a hot liquid is spilled, producing a splash-and-droplet pattern in the case of a small spill (Fig. 6-68, *A*) or an inverted arrowhead in cases of larger spills over the chest (Fig. 6-68, *B*). The child usually presents with a history of having grabbed a cup of hot coffee, tea, or cocoa from the table while sitting on someone's lap, or of having reached up and grabbed the projecting handle of a pot on the stove. In some instances a parent or older sibling has stumbled while carrying a pan of hot liquid or food, and resulting burns commonly involve the chest, a hand, a foot, or occasionally the head. As noted earlier, presentation is prompt and parents/grandparents are appropriately concerned, and often feeling very guilty about this happening. Accidental spill scalds cannot be distinguished clinically from purposeful spills, unless there is a clear delay in seeking care for large burns.

Vesicular Reactions to Insect Bites

Some mites when biting inject a blistering agent that causes vesiculation. Such vesicles and blisters have been mistakenly attributed to sprinkling the child with scalding water. On close

Figure 6-66 Phytophotodermatitis. This boy was referred for concerns regarding possible inflicted bruises. The bizarre hand/finger marks are actually due to hyperpigmentation caused by a phototoxic reaction to psoralens. More than 2 weeks earlier, while his family was on vacation at the shore, he had been picked up by his father, who had just been cutting limes for a party. The family then went to the beach for the afternoon. Subsequently the child developed erythematous patches in the distribution seen, which then became hyperpigmented.

Figure 6-67 Patterned tan marks. **A,** This young girl, a former victim of abuse and neglect, was noted to have an odd, perfectly round patch of dark brown skin over her back seen during a visit for a mild acute injury. Despite its perfect shape, which was unlike those made with common weapons of discipline, bruising was suspected. Neither mother nor child could think of a related incident. **B,** Then, her new shirt was remembered.

inspection, however, the lesions (which are pruritic rather than painful) are found to be almost perfectly round with no evidence of splash, and the roof of each blister or vesicle is noted to have a thicker wall than that of the blisters of a second-degree burn (Fig. 6-69).

Accidental Iron Burns

Pulling an iron down from the ironing board by yanking on its cord is the classic scenario for an accidental iron burn in a young child. The iron, being heavier at one end, falls end over end, producing a configuration of two or three linear or patchy first- or second-degree burns separated by gaps (Fig. 6-70, *A*). On rare occasions the flat surface of the iron may land on the leg of a child seated on the floor, but the child's immediate reflex action to get the hot object off will result in at most a superficial pattern burn. In older children and adolescents, burns are more often acquired in the course of ironing and usually consist of small, superficial, linear burns of the hand or fingers. On occasion, impulsive behavior results in accidentally self-inflicted burns, which also tend to be superficial (see Fig. 6-70, *B*).

Accidental Curling Iron Burns

Accidental curling iron injuries occur most commonly when an older infant, toddler, or preschool-age child grabs the hot wand of a curling iron that has been left unattended by a parent or older sibling. The resulting first- and second-degree burns thus involve the palm and flexor surfaces of the fingers

Figure 6-69 Vesiculation due to mite bites. These vesicles, initially thought to be due to burns, are relatively thick walled and almost perfectly round, and they show no evidence of splash. Furthermore, the lesions were pruritic, not painful.

Figure 6-68 Accidental scalds. **A,** The splash-and-droplet pattern of an accidental scald is evident on the foot of a toddler who grabbed a hot cup of tea from the table while sitting on his grandmother's lap. **B,** This toddler grabbed a pot handle projecting out over the edge of a stove, spilling hot soup over her chest and shoulder. Cooling of the hot liquid as it flowed downward produced the inverted arrowhead pattern, the burn being wider and of greater depth proximally and narrowing and becoming more superficial distally. There is also a descending droplet and splash pattern to the left of the midline.

Figure 6-70 Accidental iron burns. **A,** These linear and patchy burns are characteristic of an accidental iron burn. In this case the patient's brother pulled the iron down by grabbing the cord while she had her back turned. **B,** This hyperactive boy decided to test the iron on his cheek while his mother went to answer the phone. Although the imprint of the iron is clear, the superficial depth of the burn is more consistent with an accidental than with an inflicted burn.

Figure 6-71 Accidental curling iron burn. First- and second-degree burns are seen over the palm and flexor surfaces of the fingers of this toddler who grabbed her mother's curling iron.

of one hand and are of varying depths (Fig. 6-71). Preadolescent and adolescent girls may incur superficial burns of the ears or nape of the neck if they are not careful when curling their hair.

Accidental Space Heater Burns

During winter months, accidental burns can be incurred as a result of brushing up against the grid of a space heater while walking or running by it or when engaging in wrestling or horseplay near it. The lesions produced tend to be superficial and tangential and usually involve the dorsum of a hand or occasionally the lateral aspect of the lower leg or forearm. Less commonly, crawling infants and toddlers engaged in exploration may grab the grid, incurring palmar burns, or may fall against it.

Blistering Distal Dactylitis

Blistering distal dactylitis, an acute infection usually caused by group A streptococci (less often by group B streptococci or *Staphylococcus aureus*), is characterized by the formation of 0.5- to 1-cm blisters on the tips and distal pads of the fingers or toes (see Chapter 8, Fig. 8-50). Because of their location, they are sometimes mistaken for fingertip burns. The fact that the vesicular fluid is cloudy, in contrast to the clear fluid of acute partial-thickness burn blisters, distinguishes these lesions from burns, and Gram stain of the fluid is positive for organisms. It should also be noted that fingertip burns are more likely to be accidental than inflicted.

Accidental Cigarette Burns

Unintentional cigarette burns usually occur when a child accidentally brushes against the lit end of an adult's cigarette.

They tend to be single superficial, tangential burns and usually involve one hand, a forearm, or the cheek.

Lesions Often Mistaken for Cigarette Burns

On occasion, impetiginous lesions have been mistaken for cigarette or cigar burns. This is often the case with bullous impetigo, after the initial central bulla has ruptured and crusted over. On careful inspection, one can detect the formation of bullous rims around the more central crusts, and other lesions can usually be found nearby (Fig. 6-72). Removal of the crust will reveal that the lesion is superficial, in contrast to the full-thickness depression seen on removal of the eschar from most inflicted cigarette or cigar burns.

On resolution of the acute inflammatory phase of insect bites or papular urticaria, children are often left with round target-shaped macular scars that are hyperpigmented peripherally and hypopigmented centrally. These have been mistaken for healed cigarette burns (Fig. 6-73). However, their usual distribution is over the lower legs above the sock line in older children, or over the arms, legs, face, neck, and scalp in crawling infants and toddlers. The fact that these are macular and not punched-out scars should enable the clinician to distinguish between these and the scars left by full-thickness cigarette burns (see Fig. 6-21, *C*). Flea bite scars also

Figure 6-72 Impetigo. This infant was initially suspected of having a cigar burn, but close inspection revealed a new peripheral bullous rim. This and the presence of another early impetiginous lesion on the cheek enabled the correct diagnosis to be made.

Figure 6-73 Postinflammatory hyperpigmentation subsequent to insect bites or papular urticaria. When this child was seen at a follow-up visit for the treatment of flea bites, he was found to have a multitude of round, hyperpigmented spots at the sites of the original bites. Their macular appearance, distribution, and target configuration distinguish them from cigarette burn scars. *(Courtesy Michael Sherlock, MD, Lutherville, Md.)*

tend to have a target pattern, probably because of the central punctum within the wheal of the acute bite. This differs from the uniform surface of most macular cigarette burn scars (see Fig. 6-21, *D*).

Accidental Tourniquet Injuries

Perhaps the most common form of accidental tourniquet injury is that caused by a hair that becomes tightly wrapped around the toe of an infant (Fig. 6-74). The constriction causes pain and irritability, which prompts the parent to seek the cause. Hence such patients are brought in promptly before

Figure 6-74 Hair tourniquet. The erythema and edema of the third and fourth toes seen here are the result of constriction by hairs that accidentally became wrapped around them. *(Courtesy Thomas J. Daley, MD, St. Joseph's Hospital, Paterson, NJ.)*

circulatory compromise occurs. If they are not and the toe is gangrenous, neglect should be suspected. We have also seen young children with mild hand edema as a result of putting colored rubber bands that are too small and tight around their wrists for bracelets.

Differentiation of Accidental and Pathologic Fractures from Inflicted Fractures

Accidental Fractures

The vast majority of accidental fractures are seen in children who are mobile and over 2 years of age. In most instances it is relatively easy to recognize a truly accidental fracture: the incident is usually witnessed, and the mechanism of injury is clearly reported and fits the findings unless it is the result of an unwitnessed fall or fall down stairs. Care is typically sought promptly, although occasional exceptions occur, especially if the patient is a stoic athlete with a mild buckle fracture of the radius, who avoids complaining in order not to miss an important game. Families are appropriately concerned and interact well with the child. Accidental fractures are usually single or isolated or involve both bones of the forearm or lower leg, and typically there are no associated injuries and no history or evidence of prior injuries. Multiple fractures are most often seen when a child is hit by a car or is a passenger in a vehicle involved in a crash.

A thorough history and knowledge of the types of fractures produced by various mechanisms of injury assist accurate diagnosis. Some of the most common fractures and their mechanisms include buckle (torus) and greenstick fractures of the radius and ulna (see Figs. 21-26 and 21-27) due to a fall forward onto an outstretched arm; mid-clavicular fractures caused by a direct blow to the clavicle or a fall sideways onto the shoulder or outstretched arm (see Fig. 21-20); supracondylar humerus fractures (see Figs. 21-18 and 21-34) due to a fall backward onto a hyperextended outstretched arm; toddler's fractures or spiral fractures of distal to mid-tibia (see Fig. 21-43) resulting from a fall with a twist while trying to extricate a caught foot, following a sudden turn while running, or on landing from a jump; and transverse diaphyseal fractures (see Fig. 21-28) following a vertical fall of greater than 6 to 10 feet (as from playground equipment) or the result of getting the thigh caught against a firm surface (e.g., having the leg slip between the mattress and outer slat of a bunk bed) and having the upper body fall in the opposite direction.

One type of accidental humerus fracture seen in an infant can easily be mistaken for an inflicted injury. This spiral fracture of the humeral shaft can occur unintentionally when someone turns an infant from the prone to supine position without completely lifting the trunk from the surface on which the baby is lying. This occurs when an infant, lying prone, has one arm extended out from the body, palm down and, while held by the opposite arm or axilla, is rolled over to the supine position. Being unable to adduct the extended arm as he is turned, the upper arm is subjected to a twisting force, which produces the spiral fracture.

Stair falls typically involve a series of short falls unless the child makes a running jump from or trips while running from the top of the stairs. Spiral, oblique, buckle, or transverse fractures can be seen depending on how the fall occurred and the position on landing.

Accidental femur fractures usually involve the midshaft. They can result from a fall while running, and then sliding into a hard object; a trip fall with a twist in which one leg folds under the body; being hit by a fast-moving object such as a car; as well as falls from heights.

Accidental rib fractures are unusual and are typically the result of severe blunt chest trauma such as being hit by a car. Those seen in infants are very rare and tend to be the result of a difficult delivery or prolonged CPR in a low-birth-weight infant; in the latter case they are typically located anterolaterally. Nonabusive metaphyseal fractures are seen equally rarely and tend to stem from a difficult breech delivery or the series of manipulations involved in corrective surgery for clubfeet.

Conditions Associated with Pathologic Fractures

Three relatively unusual conditions account for most pathologic fractures seen in the pediatric population: osteogenesis imperfecta (OI), demineralization from disuse, and bone cysts.

Osteogenesis Imperfecta

OI is a family of disorders characterized most notably by brittle bones. See Chapters 1 and 21 for a more extensive review of osteogenesis imperfecta.

Differentiating Osteogenesis Imperfecta and Abuse. Distinguishing infants and children with mild OI who incur accidental fractures from normal children with inflicted injuries is usually quite feasible. Those with OI typically are brought promptly to medical attention by appropriately concerned parents who interact warmly with their child. Unless the fracture is the result of an unwitnessed fall, they give a clear history of a mechanism of injury that fits the fracture pattern found, although the amount of force involved may be somewhat less than that usually required to cause a fracture. In general, a single fracture of the diaphysis of a long bone, or both bone diaphyseal fractures of a forearm or lower leg, are found. Furthermore, one does not see evidence of multiple fractures of differing ages for which no prior care has been sought (especially not fractures in close succession). Instead, when the child has suffered prior fractures, care for these also has been sought promptly, and parents readily report this in the history along with details of the treatment prescribed. Further, if OI has not previously been diagnosed and there is no positive family history, they may even ask if anything can be done to determine why their child is so prone to fractures.

Several other points warrant emphasis. Blue sclerae are evident in the vast majority of children with type I OI. Short stature, bowing or valgus deformities of the lower extremities, and the dental discoloration of dentinogenesis imperfecta, once teeth have erupted, are found in children with both types I and IV OI. The "classic metaphyseal lesions" and rib and skull fractures, so common in young abuse victims, are rare in infants and children with mild forms of OI. The same is true of subdural hematomas and retinal hemorrhages (see the section Differential Diagnosis of Accidental versus Inflicted Head Injuries, later), and visceral injuries have not been reported. When these findings are present, one must seriously consider the possibility of abuse of a child with OI.

The major potential source of confusion involves a young infant with type IV OI or the rare baby with type I OI whose sclerae are not noticeably blue and who has incurred one or more nondisplaced fractures in utero or during delivery that went undiagnosed in the newborn period. If this infant then has an accidental fracture in the ensuing few months, radiographs may reveal old, "unexplained" healing fractures. Even in this situation, careful clinical evaluation with close attention to timeliness of presentation with the acute fracture, consistency of reported mechanism with fracture type, and parental demeanor, combined with lack of evidence of other signs of injury and family and psychosocial history, can aid in making the correct diagnosis. Reviewing radiographs including skull films with an experienced pediatric radiologist is also useful to check for wormian bones and any signs of osteopenia. Last, it can be most helpful to confer with the child's primary care physician regarding prior experience with the family and older siblings and the family's compliance with care.

Another scenario that can be a source of concern may occur when an older child with mild OI who has a high pain threshold incurs a mild nondisplaced fracture. In such instances the child may experience pain or an aching sensation that seems "not worth complaining about," until it persists, thereby resulting in a delay in seeking care. Again, using the same principles of careful and open-minded evaluation, as described earlier, can assist correct diagnosis. Furthermore, in older children, osteopenia is more likely to be evident radiographically.

In the rare case in which a clinical diagnosis cannot be made with any degree of assurance, and where an exact diagnosis is necessary, a skin biopsy can be obtained for analysis of collagen synthesis by cultured fibroblasts. However, this procedure takes several weeks and will be negative in about 5% of cases (see later).

Three other types of OI (V through VII) that have no detectable defect of type I collagen have been described more recently. All are rare, and each has distinct clinical and/or radiographic findings that help distinguish affected from normal infants and children (see Chapter 21). These likely account for many, if not most, of the negative findings on analysis of collagen synthesis.

"Temporary Brittle Bone Disease"

"Temporary brittle bone disease" is a disorder proposed by Paterson and Miller as a transient phenomenon seen only in the first year of life, in which affected infants are unusually vulnerable to fractures with minimal trauma. On review, the few articles published on the subject not only are not peer reviewed but also have poor methodology. Cases presented are not well documented and include infants with unequivocal findings of inflicted trauma. Among these are cases in which signs of callus formation became apparent during the course of hospitalization for suspected abuse, which the authors describe as having "occurred in hospital." This is a clear misinterpretation of a well-known phenomenon seen especially in abused infants who are admitted with inflicted head trauma, as many of these babies have at least some nondisplaced fractures less than 10 days old when admitted. Initially invisible radiographically, these fractures then become apparent as healing progresses, often being seen on repeat chest films in intubated infants or on follow-up skeletal surveys. There are no scientific data, and there is no corroborative evidence to support the existence of this "disorder" or the hypotheses of transient metabolic defects proposed to explain it.

Demineralization from Disuse

Children with severe cerebral palsy, myelodysplasia, advanced neuromuscular diseases, paraplegia, or quadriplegia that essentially leaves them confined to bed or a wheelchair develop muscular atrophy and bony demineralization as the result of disuse. Cortical thinning is marked (Fig. 6-75) and makes the patient vulnerable to fractures after the application of mild forces, whether in minor falls or in the process of manipulation during physical therapy.

Bone Cysts

Benign bone cysts in pediatric patients are usually seen near the metaphyseal ends of long bones. As they enlarge, they cause cortical thinning, leaving the bone vulnerable to fracture (Fig. 6-76). Similar pathologic fractures may occur at sites of osteomyelitis or in portions of bone replaced by tumor.

Figure 6-75 Demineralization from disuse. Severe osteopenia and a femur fracture incurred during physical therapy are evident in this child who was left quadriplegic as the result of an earlier injury. Note the lack of muscle mass. *(Courtesy Department of Radiology, Children's Hospital of Pittsburgh, Pittsburgh, Pa.)*

Figure 6-77 Congenital pseudarthrosis of the clavicle. The overlapping ends of bone near the midpoint of this infant's clavicle are smooth, rounded, and well corticated, distinguishing this congenital anomaly from a fracture.

Conditions Associated with or Mimicking Fractures

Congenital Pseudarthrosis of the Clavicle

Congenital pseudarthrosis of the clavicle is a rare congenital anomaly that usually involves the right clavicle and probably results from failed maturation of an ossification center. The clavicle appears foreshortened and has a visible bulbous deformity near its mid-portion (see Fig. 21-82). Hypermobility and crepitance are felt on palpation over the bump. This is distinguishable from a fracture because the site is nontender and the patient has full range of motion of the shoulder without pain. On radiography the two ends of the clavicle at the point of deformity are seen to be smooth and rounded and covered with a well-formed bony cortex (Fig. 6-77). Pseudarthroses of the tibia, fibula, femur, or clavicle can also be seen in children with neurofibromatosis type 1 (see Chapter 15 and

Fig. 8-131, *B*). Hence neurofibromatosis type 1 should be considered whenever a pseudarthrosis is detected.

Vitamin D Deficiency and Rickets

In view of its role in regulating calcium and phosphorus metabolism, vitamin D plays a key role in normal bone development and growth. When born to a mother with normal levels of vitamin D, newborns will have received enough vitamin D via placental transfer to have adequate levels for the ensuing 3 months. Premature infants and those born to mothers with deficient levels will have lesser amounts. The two main sources of vitamin D are sunlight and foods (fortified milk or formula, eggs, and fish). Supplemental vitamins are beneficial and especially important for breast-fed infants, as breast milk has low levels. They are also indicated for infants and children with darkly pigmented skin, as the amount of melanin in their skin cells absorbs much of the UVB radiation, leaving less available to stimulate skin production of vitamin D. Heavy emphasis on sunscreen use and avoidance of sun exposure because of fear of skin cancer, and low exposure during cold winter weather add to the risk of insufficient levels of the vitamin. The prevalence of low levels has ranged from 1% to 78%, in part depending on the population studied.

The clinical findings of rickets are seen only in infants with moderate to severe deficiency. The peak season for presentation is spring, because of the very limited sun exposure during winter months. Affected patients are often from latitudes distant from the equator, tend to be breast fed, are often darkly complected, with no vitamin D supplementation or those fed primarily unfortified milk. A small percentage of children with rickets have been raised on a vegan diet, with no dairy products and no supplemental vitamins.

Because of poor mineralization, the bones of infants and young children with rickets are prone to bending. Radiographic changes include loss of the provisional zone of calcification, widening of the epiphysis, metaphyseal cupping and fraying, cortical thinning, and periosteal reaction (Fig. 6-78, *A* and *B*; see also Fig. 10-11). Clinical findings include widening of the ends of the long bones (see Fig. 6-78, *C*), especially noticeable at the wrists, ankles, and knees; costochondral beading (rachitic rosary) (see Fig. 10-10); bowing of the forearms in infants and legs in toddlers (see Fig. 10-9). One can also note delayed fontanelle closure, softening of the calvarial bones (craniotabes), and frontal/parietal bossing.

Laboratory findings are inevitably abnormal and include decreased calcium early in the course (sometimes presenting

Figure 6-76 Fracture through a unicameral bone cyst. This boy was seen because of intense pain and swelling of his upper arm after a relatively minor fall (due to slipping on wet grass while running to get out of the rain). The radiograph reveals a pathologic fracture through a unicameral bone cyst, which has caused considerable cortical thinning. *(Courtesy Department of Radiology, Children's Hospital of Pittsburgh, Pittsburgh, Pa.)*

Figure 6-78   Rickets. This 3-month-old African-American infant presented with pain and decreased movement of his right leg. Symptoms had appeared after playtime with his much older brother, who was bouncing him up and down. **A,** A skeletal survey revealed a greenstick fracture of the right femur and **B,** the fraying and cupping of the metaphyses characteristic of rickets. Reduced sunlight absorption due to his darkly pigmented skin and prenatal and postnatal factors appear to have contributed etiologically. The baby's mother had not taken vitamins for the last half of her pregnancy and did not eat dairy products. The baby was small for gestational age and had more than doubled his birth weight; hence his need for vitamin D outstripped the amount provided by his formula. **C,** In this older child who developed rickets after being placed on a vegan diet by his mother, the wrist is nearly as wide as his hand because of underlying metaphyseal widening and fraying of the radius and ulna.

as tetany), low 25-hydroxy vitamin D, and often decreased phosphate and increased alkaline phosphatase levels.

Premature infants who are born before much of the mineralization of bone that occurs during gestation is complete, and who, because of severe illness or lung disease, have prolonged nutritional problems necessitating total parenteral nutrition are particularly vulnerable to developing rickets with attendant bony fragility. Because they often require chest physiotherapy, they may incur multiple rib fractures. When these are detected on chest radiographs obtained during evaluation of a respiratory illness after discharge from the nursery, abuse is often suspected. Given a history of prematurity and prolonged hospitalization, it is wise to contact the hospital where the child was cared for and review prior films before diagnosing abuse. Careful inspection of the current films often shows residual metaphyseal and costal changes characteristic of rickets. It must be noted that infants born prematurely are at increased risk for abuse in part because of the impaired bonding and the exigency of increased care needs.

It must be noted that a number of articles have been published in which authors hypothesize that vitamin D deficiency is responsible for fractures typical of child abuse. However, the preponderance of evidence from a large amount or research shows that although vitamin D insufficiency is fairly common in young children with fractures it is no more common than in children without fractures. Not one study to date has been able to document that vitamin D is associated with an increased risk of fracture. Furthermore, children with clear clinical and radiographic findings of rickets have a low incidence of fractures, and when seen such fractures are found only in mobile infants and children. Most such fractures are accidental in origin, and present with a history that fits the fracture pattern seen.

Copper Deficiency

Copper deficiency is an exceptionally rare phenomenon that should be readily distinguishable from abuse. It occurs in nutritional and inherited forms. Prematurity; a change in early infancy to whole, powdered, or evaporated milk; severe malabsorption syndromes; and prolonged total parenteral nutrition without copper supplementation are the major predisposing factors. Clinically, affected infants have pale skin, hypopigmented hair, edema, enlarged scalp veins, and seborrhea, with or without failure to thrive or developmental delay. All have neutropenia and a hypochromic microcytic anemia that is resistant to iron therapy; radiographically, their bones are grossly abnormal. Findings include overt osteoporosis; cupped metaphyses; metaphyseal spurs; widened anterior ribs; periosteal reaction; and, at times, soft tissue calcification (see Fig. 10-12).

Menkes' kinky hair syndrome is the inherited form and results from an X-linked recessive defect in copper absorption. These children are markedly pale and have a characteristic facies with pudgy cheeks; horizontal, twisted eyebrows; and little facial expression. Their hair is dull or lusterless, sparse, and kinky with pili torti (see Fig. 8-142). Affected infants are also grossly abnormal neurologically, with hypertonia, decreased movement, lethargy, myoclonic seizures, and difficulty maintaining normothermia being major findings.

Scurvy

Children with vitamin C deficiency (now exceedingly rare) usually present after 6 months and may have been fed on evaporated or boiled milk. Clinically they tend to bruise easily because of vascular fragility; however, the diagnosis of scurvy should be readily distinguishable from abuse on the basis of radiographic findings. Although a periosteal reaction resulting

Figure 6-79 Scurvy. Note the increased density of the zones of provisional calcification and the lucency of the underlying spongiosa. The metaphyses are also widened, and early spur formation is seen medially. *(Courtesy Department of Radiology, Children's Hospital of Pittsburgh, Pittsburgh, Pa.)*

from subperiosteal hemorrhage is seen and there may be fractures through the zone of provisional calcification and through metaphyseal spurs, bony cortices are thin and the ends of the long bones show characteristic changes consisting of increased density of the zone of provisional calcification and increased lucency of the underlying spongiosa (Fig. 6-79). These infants are irritable, tend to move little because of bone pain, and often have gingival bleeding. Serum vitamin C level is low.

Hypervitaminosis A

Chronic vitamin A intoxication produces a thick, wavy periosteal reaction that most commonly involves the ulnas and metatarsals, although other long bones can be affected. Hard, tender swellings may be evident on palpation. Absence of fractures and metaphyseal abnormalities should help distinguish this from abuse. The history and findings of papilledema

or split sutures on skull radiograph resulting from concomitant pseudotumor cerebri also aid in differentiation.

Leukemia

Children with acute leukemia may develop diffuse demineralization, periosteal reactions, and osteolytic lesions. Lucent metaphyseal bands, termed *leukemic lines,* are also seen (see Fig. 11-85). The relative osteopenia and typical absence of fractures, combined with the antecedent history, often of fatigue, anorexia, and weight loss; physical findings that may include petechiae, adenopathy, visceromegaly, and sternal tenderness; and the results of hematologic tests should distinguish these findings from those of abuse.

Caffey Disease

A rare disorder of unknown etiology, Caffey disease is characterized by cortical thickening and a painful periosteal reaction (Fig. 6-80). Bones are otherwise normally mineralized, and fractures are not seen. Involvement of the mandible, seen in 75% of affected patients, results in dramatic thickening. The clavicle and ulna are also common sites, although other bones can be involved. Most patients are younger than 6 months of age, and all have fever, anorexia, and marked irritability. The skin overlying affected areas is neither warm nor discolored. There is no soft tissue swelling, and palpation reveals bony-hard thickening below the subcutaneous tissues, which are adherent to the underlying bone.

Differential Diagnosis of Accidental versus Inflicted Head Injuries

Accidental head injuries are common in childhood as a result of falls and other accidents, and the majority are minor. Presentation is usually prompt because a head injury, no matter how minor, tends to provoke considerable parental anxiety. Again, the history is usually clear, and the mechanism reported is consistent with the physical findings observed. Mild forehead and scalp contusions with or without small lacerations or abrasions are by far the most common injuries. Simple (usually nondiastatic) linear skull fractures often involving the parietal bones can result from falls of greater than 4 feet onto hard surfaces (as from a changing table or a shopping cart), but these do not tend to be associated with significant changes

Figure 6-80 Caffey disease. **A,** Intense periosteal reaction and cortical thickening are seen in the lower extremities. **B,** Mandibular involvement has resulted in dramatic thickening. These findings, associated symptoms, and absence of fractures distinguish this condition from the skeletal changes characteristic of abuse. *(Courtesy Department of Radiology, Children's Hospital of Pittsburgh, Pittsburgh, Pa.)*

in level of consciousness or with intracranial injury. More severe injuries are incurred as a result of more serious mechanisms including major falls (>10 feet and falls with angular momentum as from swings, trapezes, or trampolines), bicycle and sports accidents, and motor vehicle accidents.

In evaluating an infant or toddler who presents with a history of minor trauma but is found to have intracranial bleeding, especially one with subdural hematomas and retinal hemorrhages, it is important to rule out coagulopathy or the presence of an underlying disorder that makes the child unusually susceptible to development of subdural bleeding. A coagulopathy can be ruled in or out by obtaining a complete blood cell count with differential and platelet count, prothrombin and partial thromboplastin times, and, if necessary on the basis of family history, a von Willebrand or full coagulation profile.

In two disorders, benign extraaxial fluid collections (BEAFCs) and glutaric aciduria type 1 (GA1), subdural hematomas and retinal hemorrhages can be seen following minimal trauma. These must be considered in the evaluation and distinguished from abuse.

Disorders Simulating or Predisposing to Subdural Hemorrhage

Benign Extraaxial Fluid Collections

In BEAFCs, also known as *benign external hydrocephalus,* macrocephaly is associated with bilateral symmetrical widening of the subarachnoid space (SAS), most prominently in the frontal and frontoparietal areas and along the anterior interhemispheric fissure and the sylvian fissures. This expanded space is filled with cerebrospinal fluid. Usually the ventricles are normal in size or only slightly enlarged, and there is no evidence of increased intracranial pressure (ICP). The condition is thought to be due to transient mild impairment of cerebrospinal fluid resorption by the arachnoid villi. Widening of the SAS results in significant stretching of the bridging veins that run from the cerebral cortex to the dural venous sinuses, and it is thought that being stretched makes them more vulnerable to tearing in the face of minimal or minor trauma.

Infants with BEAFCs are usually diagnosed as a result of imaging performed as part of an evaluation for macrocephaly or enlarging head circumference. Most are neurodevelopmentally normal, although some may have mild delays and hypotonia. Many have a family history of macrocephaly that suggests autosomal dominant transmission. Usually the abnormality resolves spontaneously with normalization of findings on imaging by 2 to 5 years of age.

Approximately 10% of infants monitored with BEAFCs develop subdural hematomas in association with retinal hemorrhages, either "spontaneously" or after a minor head bump. Although some of these infants have had associated seizures and/or mild transient alterations in consciousness, most appear relatively normal neurologically even on presentation with subdurals. On MRI the subdural hemorrhages are usually small, and diffuse enlargement of the subarachnoid space (occupied by cerebrospinal fluid) is easily appreciated. Importantly, these infants tend to be brought in promptly for care when symptomatic or after falls, are accompanied by appropriately concerned parents, and have no associated injuries.

BEAFCs can be distinguished from cerebral atrophy as the sulci are not widened and because of the greater prominence of SAS widening frontally. In communicating hydrocephalus ventricular enlargement is much more prominent, and symptoms of increased ICP may be present.

Glutaric Aciduria

Glutaric aciduria type 1 (GA1) is an autosomal recessive disorder resulting in deficiency of glutaryl-CoA dehydrogenase. Affected infants appear relatively normal at birth, although approximately 40% are born with mild macrocephaly, and over ensuing months, these infants gradually cross toward the 97th percentile. Nonspecific neurologic signs consisting of irritability, jitteriness, mild hypotonia, and feeding problems are common in the first 6 months, then improve, and by a year most appear normal except for slight gross motor delays. If undiagnosed and untreated, most affected infants develop an acute encephalopathy between 12 and 18 months of age usually in association with an acute upper respiratory or gastrointestinal infection. Subsequently, they are left with severe dystonias and dyskinesias and suffer major regression in milestones.

Findings on neuroimaging, whether performed before or after the severe encephalopathic event, include marked bilateral frontotemporal atrophy along with prominent widening of the sylvian fissures and delayed myelination. Twenty to thirty percent have associated chronic subdural effusions and/or hematomas. After the encephalopathy, basal ganglia atrophy also becomes evident. As in children with BEAFCs, it is thought that the marked widening of the subarachnoid space due to cortical atrophy results in stretching of the bridging veins, making them more vulnerable to shearing with minimal trauma. When subdurals are present, retinal hemorrhages are also seen. Interestingly, the subdurals may or may not be associated with symptoms. The presence of marked cerebral atrophy in association with subdural hematomas (Fig. 6-81) helps distinguish GA1 from both inflicted head trauma and BEAFCs. No skeletal abnormalities are associated with GA1, and usually no other evident injuries exist unless irritability has provoked abuse.

Strong evidence indicates that diagnosis and institution of treatment before an encephalopathic event can prevent the encephalopathy and subsequent movement disorder. Hence neuroimaging and testing for GA1 should be strongly considered in the evaluation of infants with mild macrocephaly, especially if they are fussy, jittery, and/or hypotonic.

Subdural Hematomas and Osteogenesis Imperfecta

There have been scattered reports regarding a small number of children with OI who have presented with subdural hematomas and retinal hemorrhages. On close review the numbers are small, the histories given often incomplete, and the presence of associated injuries (i.e., femur fracture in a child with mild OI who was not yet walking, and three spiral fractures in three different long bones in another) raises suspicion of inflicted injuries. Hence, it is not clear and probably unlikely that infants with OI are more susceptible to developing subdural hematomas than normal children.

Differentiation of Accidental from Inflicted Oral Injuries

Falls and sporting and bicycle accidents are the usual sources of accidental oral injuries. These include lip and chin lacerations (see Fig. 20-55); fractured, loosened, or avulsed teeth (see Figs. 20-59 through 20-64); and gingival, lingual, palatal, or retropharyngeal lacerations, the latter resulting from falls with an object in the mouth (see Figs. 20-54, 20-56, and 23-72). These injuries, like head injuries, provoke considerable parental anxiety and result in prompt presentation for care, with a clear history and consistent mechanism of injury.

Figure 6-81   Glutaric aciduria type 1. This 3-month-old infant was brought to the emergency department with complaints of being limp and unresponsive with a recent history of pneumonia. The initial history given was that while alone with his father, he had suddenly become lethargic, his eyes had rolled back, and he had stopped breathing for a few seconds. Lethargy resolved soon after arrival. **A,** A head CT obtained because retinal hemorrhages were found revealed diffuse acute and subacute/chronic subdural hemorrhages over the convexities in the frontotemporal areas, as well as more acute collections along the posterior interhemispheric fissure and over the right frontal area. **B** and **C,** On MRI large acute on chronic subdural hemorrhages were confirmed, along with early signs of atrophy including mild flattening of the gyri, sulcal widening, and mild ventricular enlargement. This prompted testing for possible glutaric aciduria, which was positive in results obtained 1 week later. Interestingly, in the interim, the father acknowledged having shaken the baby after he didn't feed well, whereupon he went limp.

Differential Diagnosis of Accidental versus Inflicted Chest and Abdominal Injuries

Accidental chest and abdominal injuries in children are predominantly the result of major blunt force trauma and may be similar in nature to those caused by abuse. However, victims of accidental injuries have a clear history of a major mechanism of injury, such as a major motor vehicle accident, that was often witnessed. Immediate care is sought, and findings are consistent with the history.

SEXUAL ABUSE

Sexual abuse is defined as the misuse of a child for the sexual gratification of an adult. In sexual abuse the perpetrator misuses his or her power over a child, involving her or him in sexual activities that may or may not involve physical contact. The best available data indicate that in the 1980s there was a significant rise in the number of reports of sexual abuse, stemming in part from increased public and professional awareness, and in part as a consequence of a greater willingness of victims to disclose the abuse. This trend appears to have reversed since 1992, and data from 2009 indicate that there has been a 61% decrease in substantiated sexual abuse cases between 1992 and 2009. Given the fact that 20% of adult women and 5% to 10% of adult men report having been sexually abused before 18 years of age, it appears that sexual abuse still continues to be underreported, especially among males, and it is estimated that substantiated cases constitute less than one third of all cases of sexual abuse.

Extrapolating prevalence data to a pediatric practice of 1500 children, it is likely that 12 of them will be abused each year, only 8 of whom will disclose their abuse to a professional, not necessarily a pediatrician. It is of concern that only 40% of cases disclosed to professionals are then reported to authorities, despite mandatory reporting laws in all 50 states. Also worrisome is the fact that CPS will be able to substantiate only half of the cases disclosed and reported to them, for a variety of reasons, sometimes unrelated to the veracity of allegations.

Forms of sexual abuse may include visual exposure to exhibitionistic, masturbatory, or copulatory behavior; fondling, masturbation, and digital manipulation; oral/genital contact; and direct genital contact including penetration or attempted penetration of the vagina, anus, or mouth. Approximately 25% of cases reported retrospectively by women involve vaginal or orogenital penetration. Data regarding perpetrators indicate that approximately 40% are parents or stepparents, and 25% are other relatives. Strangers probably constitute no more than 10% of perpetrators. The rest are people who are known by but unrelated to the victim. By far, the majority of perpetrators are male. Adult females, who are responsible for 20% of abusive sexual contact with prepubertal males, are much less likely to be reported.

Adults who prefer children and young adolescents for physical sexual gratification are *pedophiles*. They should not be confused with homosexuals who mutually prefer same-sex partners in their own age range. Although some pedophiles may be more restrained than others, many tend to be compulsive in seeking their victims. It is also important to recognize that they often marry or cohabit with an opposite sex partner, in part as cover and in part so as to victimize their children. Most perpetrators of sexual abuse do not fit the definition of pedophile.

Of increasing concern is the fact that more and more children are disclosing that they have been exposed to pornography and have been used as subjects in pornographic photographs and videotapes, which have ever more sophisticated distribution over the Internet. Furthermore, the Internet, through use of chat rooms, has become a major vehicle for pedophiles to seek, find, and entice victims.

The issue of "sexually reactive" children is another concern, and it is important to distinguish this behavior from normal sexual play. Children who entice or coerce other children into sexual behavior, simulate intercourse, or try to insert foreign objects into themselves or other children may be evincing "sexualized behavior" because they themselves have been victims of sexual abuse. Hence they too should be evaluated in addition to their victims.

Rape, which by legal definition is "forced sexual intercourse" and may involve penetration, however slight, may occur with the use of physical force or coercion and the misuse of a power relationship. Adolescents have the highest rates of rape of any age group and, in general, tend to delay or avoid seeking care after being assaulted. Male victims are even less likely to report the assault or seek care. Not infrequently, adolescents who are raped have been using drugs or alcohol or have been given drugs surreptitiously before the event. The "date rape drug" flunitrazepam (not legally available in the United States), which is colorless and tasteless and usually administered in a drink or beverage, is reported to have increased the incidence of rape, despite the fact that *reported* rapes have been decreasing in frequency since 1992.

If the perpetrator of sexual abuse is a family member or acquaintance, the encounter is more likely to be physically nonviolent, with persuasion, bribery, or threats used to enlist the victim's cooperation. Not infrequently, these experiences are repetitive and occur over long periods of time. There is a well-described pattern of escalating levels of involvement, with initial fondling and digital manipulation progressing to actual penetration. The victim's cooperation and subsequent silence may be ensured by various means including persuasion, bribes, gifts, praise, fear of the perpetrator's power, and/ or threats of dire consequences if the child discloses the abuse. Thus the victim bears both the guilt of engaging in unwanted sexual activity and the pressure of keeping it secret. Absence of physical violence or injury *does not* imply consent, as the offender is usually in a position of power over the victim, making it difficult for the child both to refuse to engage in the activity and to disclose it. It is very common for children to disclose sexual abuse long after the abuse occurred or not at all. There is evidence that less than 40% of adults sexually

abused as children disclosed their abuse during childhood. Children abused by family members or family friends have also disclosed fears of being harmed or of having other loved ones or pets injured, or even killed, by the abuser. Episodes perpetrated by strangers are more likely to be isolated incidents and involve physical violence, adding the emotional stress of being in a potentially life-threatening situation.

Forensic requirements for a detailed history, physical examination, and multiple laboratory specimens (all carefully documented) necessitate a lengthy evaluation that, if not sensitively handled, can compound existing emotional trauma. This can be minimized if the physician approaches the patient and family with patience, gentleness, and tact. If the disclosed sexual abuse does not involve allegations requiring collection of evidence of ejaculate and/or if there is no bleeding or significant discomfort, the physical examination may be postponed; conducted in stages; or, if necessary, performed under anesthesia or conscious sedation.

Because physical findings are normal in up to 96% of cases, and, even if abnormal, are frequently nonspecific, the history is the most important aspect of the evaluation. Hence it is essential that historical information be documented meticulously, if possible verbatim, because many of these cases have the potential for legal prosecution, usually months to years later. Ideally, this history is obtained by an experienced clinician, using forensic interviewing principles. Clinicians should avoid asking leading questions, although in certain situations, after all other avenues have been exhausted, such questions may be necessary in order to elicit enough information to ensure protection of the child. When possible, the parent or persons accompanying the child should be interviewed first, apart from each other and separately from the child. During this interview one can obtain information about the youngster's emotional status and recent behavior, present and past history, family psychosocial situation, household members or other persons caring for the child, people who share or visit the home frequently who might have unwitnessed access to the child, the events that appear to have led to the disclosure or suspicion of abuse, and terms used by the child for body parts. When the chief complaint is not sexual abuse, but findings on examination point to molestation, this information should be sought in a further interview with the parent, or parents, after the examination, with the child out of the room.

In approaching the child, it is essential for the clinician to show kindness, empathy, and gentleness. Importantly, one should not convey shock or disgust or presume what the child's reactions to the abuse may have been. If the child is willing and able to give a history, it, as well as the exact phrasing of the questions asked, should be documented verbatim. In the initial portion of the interview, talking about favorite subjects such as friends, favorite toys, games, and activities can help reduce the child's anxiety and establish rapport between him or her and the clinician. Thereafter, it is best to begin with general questions, reserving more specific questions for clarification. If the child is unwilling or unable to discuss the episode or episodes, and there is a strong suspicion that sexual abuse has occurred, a return visit or referral for a session with a forensically trained clinician is recommended. In such interviews a variety of alternative techniques can be used if the child still has difficulty disclosing verbally. These include having the child try to draw what happened (Fig. 6-82), demonstrate what happened with anatomically correct dolls, or write about the incidents.

Documentation of the manner in which disclosure occurs is important. When children give spontaneous detailed descriptions of sexual experiences in language appropriate to their

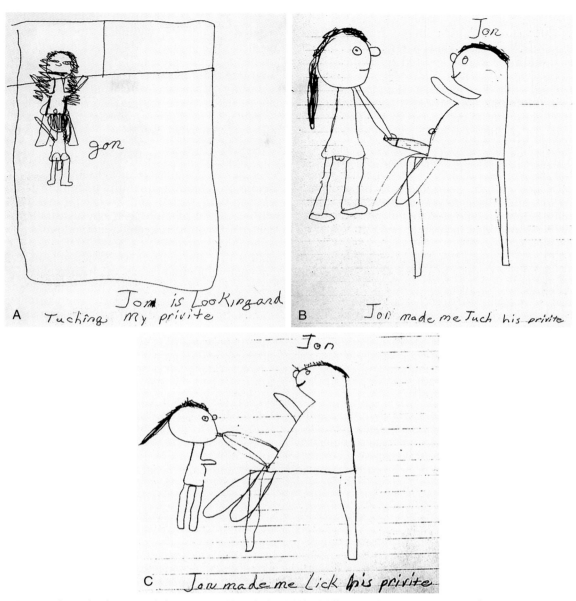

A   Tuching my privite   Jom is Looking and

B   Jon made me Tuch his privite

C   Jon made me Lick his privite

Figure 6-82   A to **C,** Drawings by a school-age sexual abuse victim. Although the child had difficulty verbalizing a description of the abuse, she was able to clearly depict the acts in her drawings.

developmental level, these are usually accurate. Asking non-directive developmentally appropriate questions to ascertain the site where the activity occurred and the number of times it happened, as well as questions related to such things as clothing worn, can be useful in documenting the child's credibility. Also important is determining the patient's understanding of the need for accuracy in relating the history and of the difference between telling the truth and telling a lie. This further aids in determining not only the child's credibility but also his or her ability to testify in court. Most areas now have access to child advocacy centers with trained forensic interviewers whose interviews can be videotaped and are conducted in a manner that is forensically defensible. If the physician sees the child first they should obtain enough history so that they can help determine what testing is appropriate and can contribute to determining appropriate placement so that the child is not continuing to be exposed to the same perpetrator.

Recognition of the problem of false accusations of sexual abuse made in the heat of child custody battles has raised questions regarding the veracity of many such claims. Findings from ongoing research suggest that if the child's disclosure is made without benefit of leading questions and is reported with feeling and often some hesitancy, and in age-appropriate terms, the report is more likely to be accurate. In contrast, children coached to make false claims tend to relate the history in a rote manner and often use adult-oriented words.

Other problems have arisen when the child has been required to repeat the history to multiple authorities—family members, physicians, CPS workers, psychologists, attorneys, and detectives. When this occurs, many victims begin to sound robotic in their reports (raising questions regarding their truthfulness) and others become so traumatized by the repetition and the impact on their family that they recant their story to avoid further painful questioning. In an effort to address this, many centers have developed a team approach in which an experienced clinician trained in forensic interviewing techniques conducts the interview while being observed by members of law enforcement and CPS and/or videotapes the interview, thereby reducing the number of interviews the child must undergo. It is important to caution distraught or unbelieving parents and family members against asking the child repeated questions about the abuse.

Before proceeding with the physical examination, one should convey to the child that the purpose is not to determine the veracity of the history but to ensure his or her continuing health. Sharing details of the examination process with the adults accompanying a young child and providing reassurance that a speculum will not be used is also helpful as many fear that the examination will be invasive. This can allay much parental anxiety, which in turn helps them to reassure the child during the process. After physical assessment, it is important to convey that there is no permanent damage related to physical function because that is another common concern for both parents and children.

Giving the child some feeling of control over the examination process in a number of small ways helps avoid further trauma and may aid in starting the child along the process of recovery. This can be accomplished with a surprisingly high proportion of children by an examiner who is comfortable with the process. Letting the child look at familiar objects such as an item of clothing through the colposcope or demonstrating to a young child, in a playful way, that the light on the colposcope is not hurtful may help. Allowing the child to choose the order in which various nonessential areas are examined can be calming, as well.

A thorough and complete physical examination is warranted for all patients suspected of having been sexually abused, with inspection of the genitalia and rectum deferred until last. Each part of the process should be explained as the examiner proceeds. If possible, and the child so chooses, a parent or supportive adult should be present. In our experience with prepubescent patients, external inspection of the genitalia suffices in the majority of cases and the insertion of a speculum is almost never indicated.

If the attempt to examine the perineum provokes anxiety that cannot be allayed and there is gross bleeding, pain, discharge, or suspicion of sexually transmitted disease, the examination and specimen collection should be performed with the patient under general anesthesia or deep conscious sedation. When the patient is too anxious to proceed and is asymptomatic with no evidence of trauma, bleeding, discomfort, or discharge, the procedure can be deferred and performed at a follow-up visit. The child *must not* be made to feel that he or she is being assaulted yet again during the examination and interview process.

Modes of Presentation

The majority of cases of sexual abuse do not involve physical violence; most patients have no signs of injury. In most instances (up to 96%), either there are no physical findings specific for sexual abuse or the examination is completely normal. Many reasons for the absence of physical findings exist even when there is a confession of vaginal penetration by the perpetrator. These include the fact that penetration may only extend to the labia, the hymen being recessed from and internal to the labia; the delay in disclosure so common in young victims; the rapid healing of injuries involving the mucosa; the elasticity of hymenal tissue; the fact that hymenal tissue is capable of regrowth and that, with the onset of puberty and increased estrogen production, the hymen regrows and becomes more elastic; the fact that the anal sphincter can distend considerably; and the possibility that perpetrators of sexual abuse may have erectile and/or ejaculatory dysfunction, as do many adult rapists.

In cases of sexual assault involving violence and resulting in major injury, a significant proportion of victims seek medical care promptly. Most acknowledge the nature of the problem at the time of presentation, and physical findings are more often positive. However, even in some of these cases a history of an accidental mechanism of injury that does not fit the physical findings is given. In these cases too there is evidence of the resolution of physical findings over time, although rarely in cases of complete transection of the hymen (Fig. 6-84, A-F).

Although there has been a significant increase in the percentage of patients who have disclosed inappropriate touching before presentation, it continues to be true that some victims of long-term sexual abuse may present with vulvovaginitis with vaginal discharge caused by a sexually transmitted pathogen or with substitute chief complaints generated by physical or emotional sequelae (Table 6-7). There are many such complaints that are somewhat age dependent, and each of which has many potential causes other than sexual abuse. Although there is a wide range of differential diagnostic possibilities in patients presenting with many of these problems, sexual abuse should be considered and addressed among the differential diagnostic considerations, and not merely after all other causes have been ruled out. When a child presents with a substitute chief complaint and/or has a history of compulsive masturbation, witnessed self-insertion of foreign objects into the vagina, and unusually sexualized behavior, the likelihood that he or she has been a victim of sexual abuse is high. In older preteen and teenage victims, signs of self-inflicted injury may be seen on occasion (see Fig. 6-83).

During the evaluation of children presenting with substitute chief complaints, it is appropriate to ask questions of parent and child separately about the possibility of inappropriate touching, and if there is any suspicion of this, a more detailed psychological assessment performed by a specially trained clinician is warranted. Even with skilled evaluation, a significant proportion of these victims do not disclose immediately. This, in our experience, seems to be particularly true of children seen for signs and symptoms of a sexually transmitted disease. However, after repeated visits with a single clinician during a stepwise evaluation for the underlying cause of their problem, many are able to develop enough trust to disclose sexual abuse or another source of their stress. A team approach may be particularly valuable in such cases.

Table 6-7	Most Common Substitute Chief Complaints in Sexual Abuse Cases*		
Any Age	**Preschool Age**	**School Age**	**Adolescence**
Abdominal pain	Excessive	Decreased school	Same as school
Anorexia	clinging	performance	age plus:
Vomiting	Sudden onset of	Truancy	Runaway
Constipation	excessive	Lying, stealing	behavior
Sleep disorders	thumb	Tics	Suicide
Dysuria	sucking	Anxiety reaction	attempts
Vaginal discharge‡	Speech disorder	Phobic and	Self-inflicted
Vaginal bleeding‡	Encopresis/	obsessional	injury
Rectal bleeding	enuresis	states	Commission
	Excessive	Depression	of sexual
	masturbation†	Conversion	offenses†
		reaction	
		Encopresis/	
		enuresis	

*Most of these complaints are also symptomatic of disorders more prevalent than sexual abuse.
†Symptoms highly suggestive of sexual abuse.
‡Symptoms somewhat suggestive of sexual abuse.

Figure 6-85   Use of Foley catheter to enhance visualization of the full extent and margins of the hymenal membrane. The catheter is inserted through the hymenal orifice, and the balloon is inflated while in the vagina and then gently pulled forward. It can then be angled to the left or right or downward to ensure a full view of all segments. *(Courtesy Earl Greenwald, MD, Harrisburg, Pa.)*

Figure 6-83   Self-inflicted injury, a finding that should raise concern about abuse and depression.

Examination Techniques

Perineal Examination

Several techniques may be used for examination of the genital and perianal areas in different age groups. In the *postpubertal age group*, a standard gynecologic examination can usually be performed with the patient in the lithotomy position (see Chapter 18). When an estrogenized hymen is redundant, a saline-moistened swab (see Fig. 6-84, *A* and *B*), or a glove-covered swab (see Fig. 6-84, *C-F*) may be inserted through the orifice and then used to spread out the membrane segment

by segment in order to better assess for the presence of contusions, tears, notches, or scars. This is not painful and is therefore possible in adolescents and peripubertal children because, once estrogenized, the hymen is not nearly as sensitive as it is before puberty. Alternatively, a Foley catheter may be inserted, the balloon inflated within the vagina, and then gently pulled forward as a means of spreading out the hymenal tissue for better visualization (Fig. 6-85). In cases of acute injury, consideration must be given to the severity and extent of the injuries before proceeding. If examination and specimen collection are likely to cause severe physical pain or emotional distress to an adolescent patient, or if internal injuries are likely, strong consideration should be given to examination under conscious sedation or even general anesthesia.

Figure 6-84   Prior sexual abuse: complete transection of the hymen. **A,** This young teen reported sexual assault several months earlier. Examination was performed by labial separation. **B,** Examination with a Calgiswab demonstrates a complete hymenal transection that would have been missed had this technique not been used. **C,** Pregnant adolescent showing what appears to be a normal redundant hymen. **D,** However, a complete transection at the 8 to 9 o'clock position was found using a large swab covered with a blue glove. **E,** Blue swab. **F,** Swab on blue glove. (**C-F,** *Courtesy Joyce Adams, MD, Rady Children's Hospital, San Diego, San Diego, Calif.)*

In the *prepubertal child* the purposes of the perineal examination are (1) to obtain full visualization of the patient's perineal and perianal anatomy; (2) to detect any evidence of acute injury, infection, distortion of anatomy, or scarring indicative of prior injury; (3) to assess the amount and appearance of hymenal tissue and to determine the size and configuration of the hymenal orifice; and (4) to collect specimens as indicated. If abnormalities of the hymen are seen, the membrane may be "floated" up by inserting saline into the vaginal area. As noted earlier, internal examination is not necessary unless there is evidence of internal extension of injury, and, in such cases, the examination, specimen collection, and repair should be done in the operating room under general anesthesia.

In examining prepubescent patients, a number of positions may be used to achieve visualization of the genital area. The one most commonly used is the *supine frog-leg position,* with the patient lying supine on the examining table. This position can also be achieved with the child semireclining on the parent's lap—the *semisupine frog-leg position.* We have also had good success with the *semisupine lithotomy position* (see Fig. 18-6, *A* and *B*). The latter is accomplished by having the parent sit on the examining table and lean back. The child sits on her lap, with the buttocks resting just above the parent's knees, and leans back. The parent then places her hands under the patient's knees, flexing them and abducting the hips. The *knee–chest position* (Fig. 6-86, *A*) provides the best exposure of perineal structures and generally a clearer picture of anatomic features and abnormalities (Fig. 6-87; see also Fig. 6-96). Most experts now tend to use the knee–chest position only in situations in which suspicious findings are found in the supine position and are to be confirmed or negated, or when the hymen has not been adequately visualized in the supine position. The child's shoulders and chest must touch the table, achieving a swayback posture. The knee–chest

position is difficult for children younger than 2 years of age, however, and some older children object to it. Nevertheless, most children can be made comfortable with the knee–chest position and helped to relax by engaging them in an ongoing conversation about an unrelated subject, having the child count as high as she can, or using a variety of visually interesting toys (e.g., kaleidoscopes, oil-based timers) held by an assistant at eye level. We also have the child practice the position while fully clothed before the examination (Fig. 6-86, *B-E*).

To assist visualization of the introitus in the supine or semisupine frog-leg or lithotomy position, the labia must be separated manually. In the *labial separation* method, the examiner places the index fingers over the lower portion of the labia majora and gently presses downward and laterally. In the *labial traction* technique, the labia majora are grasped between the thumbs and index fingers and gently pulled toward the examiner and very slightly downward. The latter usually achieves better visualization of the hymen and its orifice and the greatest hymenal opening with the child in these positions, and it is often possible to see the posterior aspect of the lower third of the vagina by this technique (see Figs. 18-2 and 18-7). It is important to bear in mind that one should be careful not to use undue force when applying labial traction so as to avoid tearing any labial adhesions present or causing undue discomfort. On occasion, these tears created during the process of examination may be mistaken for acute physical findings. It is important to examine this area carefully before applying any pressure or starting examination by labial separation or traction.

In the knee–chest position, exposure of the introitus is assisted by placing the thumbs over the edge of the gluteus muscles at the level of the introitus and lifting them upward. As the hymen drops down with gravity in the knee–chest

Figure 6-86   Knee–chest position. **A,** The sway-back position with knees widely separated assists examination and provides the best visualization of anatomic structures and abnormalities. **B-E,** After looking at enlargements of this series of photographs, the patient practices getting into position while still fully clothed. The steps are **(B)** kneel, **(C)** sit back, **(D)** stretch arms out and place arms and chest on table, and **(E)** move forward. This helps children become more comfortable with being examined from behind.

Figure 6-87 Variation in the transverse or horizontal hymenal diameter with position and technique. **A,** Supine with labial separation. **B,** Supine with labial traction. **C,** Lithotomy with more labial traction. **D,** Knee–chest position. Note that the hymenal orifice is widest with good traction and that the hymen appears wrinkled and thickened in **B** and **C**. This is due to a mild redundancy. In the knee–chest position, the hymen unfolds and drops down with gravity and is seen to be thin with smooth, sharp edges having fully stretched out.

position, its width and margins are more easily assessed. Transverse diameter of the hymenal orifice varies with position and amount of relaxation and by itself is no longer considered a useful measurement in assessing for signs of sexual abuse (see Fig. 6-87 and Fig. 6-88, *A* and *B*; and see Fig. 18-7). Rather, assessment of the appearance of the hymen and surrounding tissues is far more valuable.

Good lighting and magnification are also important. Use of a colposcope is ideal, but most practitioners do not have access to this device. Alternatively, a magnifying halogen lamp or an otoscope may be used. The latter device is most readily available, but the child must be reassured that this is being used only to get a good view with the light and that no speculum will be used as it is for ear examinations.

A complete description of the appearance of the genitalia, using anatomically correct terms, must be documented in the chart (Fig. 6-89). If at all possible, magnified photographs of the genital area should be taken, as these may obviate the need for reexamination if a second opinion is requested. Documentation should include (1) Tanner staging; (2) the presence or absence of an abnormal degree of erythema or of discharge; (3) the presence or absence and location of bruises, abrasions, or lacerations of the labia majora and perineum; (4) the appearance of the vestibule and (5) of the labia minora; (6) the presence, extent, and character of labial adhesions (thin and translucent or thickened); (7) the appearance of the posterior fourchette and presence or absence of scarring; (8)

the configuration of the hymen (annular, crescentic, redundant), and the appearance of its edges (e.g., thin and sharp, thickened or rolled, notched); and (9) the width of hymenal tissue from its attachment to its margin, especially if it is less than 1 mm wide (see Fig. 6-88, *A* and *B*), and its regularity. Also important is recording the patient's position and method used to separate the labia. Such documentation requires knowledge of basic gynecologic anatomy and terminology, which are shown in Figures 6-89 and 6-90 and given in Table 6-8 (see also the section Differential Diagnosis of Sexual Abuse, later; and the section Normal Female Genitalia in Chapter 18).

If acute external contusions or tears are seen, internal injury must be suspected. The prepubertal girl is particularly vulnerable to severe internal trauma as a result of forceful penetration of either the vagina or rectum (Fig. 6-91). This stems from the fact that the structures are relatively small and the tissues more delicate and rigid than is the case after estrogenization. Young children with relatively mild external injuries may, in fact, have major internal tears including perforation of the peritoneum and damage to pelvic vessels, mesentery, and intestine (see Figs. 18-18 to 18-20). Signs of internal injury may be subtle, but such patients will have evidence of vaginal bleeding or of a vaginal hematoma, and some may have lower abdominal tenderness or evidence of occult blood loss. Therefore when such findings are present, an exami-nation under anesthesia is indicated. In contrast, the postpubertal female

Table 6-8	Gynecologic Anatomic Terminology
Anal verge	The tissue overlying the subcutaneous external anal sphincter at the most distal portion of the anal canal, extending exteriorly to the margin of the anal skin
Anterior commissure	The union of the two labia minora anteriorly
Clitoris	A cylindrical, erectile body situated at the superior portion of the vulva, covered by a sheath of skin called the *clitoral hood* or *prepuce*
Fossa navicularis/posterior fossa	Concavity of the lower part of the vaginal vestibule situated inferiorly to the vaginal orifice and extending to the posterior fourchette (posterior commissure)
Hymen	A thin membrane located at the junction of the vestibular floor and the vaginal canal that partially covers the vaginal orifice
Labia majora	Rounded folds of skin forming the lateral boundaries of the vulva
Labia minora	Thin longitudinal folds of tissue enclosed within the labia majora; in the prepubertal child they extend from the clitoral hood to the midpoint of the lateral wall of the vestibule. After puberty they lengthen and join posteriorly (inferiorly), thereby enclosing the structures of the vestibule
Median raphe	Ridge or furrow that marks the line of union of the two halves of the perineum
Mons pubis	Rounded, fleshy prominence, created by the underlying fat pad, which overlies the symphysis pubis
Perianal folds	Wrinkles or folds of the skin of the anal verge that radiate from the anus
Perineal body	The central tendon of the perineum located between the vulva and the anus in the female and between the scrotum and anus in the male
Perineum	The pelvic floor and associated structures bounded anteriorly by the symphysis pubis, laterally by the ischial tuberosities, and posteriorly by the coccyx
Posterior fourchette	The junction of the two labia minora inferiorly (posteriorly). This is termed the *posterior commissure* in the prepubertal child, as the labia minora are not completely developed and have not extended and joined posteriorly or inferiorly as they do after puberty
Vagina	The uterovaginal canal extending from the inner aspect of the hymen to the uterine cervix
Vaginal vestibule	Anatomic cavity containing the opening of the vagina, the urethra, and ducts of the Bartholin glands; bordered by the clitoris superiorly, the labia laterally, and the posterior commissure (fourchette) inferiorly, and encompassing the fossa navicularis immediately inferior to the vaginal introitus
Vulva	The external genitalia or pudendum of the female; includes the clitoris, labia majora, labia minora, vaginal vestibule, urethral orifice, vaginal orifice, hymen, and posterior fourchette (or commissure)

Modified from the American Professional Society on the Abuse of Children.

can usually be adequately assessed by careful pelvic examination, with use of a Foley catheter or Q-tip to enhance visualization of the hymenal surface and margins (see Fig. 6-84, *A* and *B*, and Fig. 6-85). However, if, despite good emotional support, reassurance, and careful preparation, she is emotionally unable to tolerate the procedure, an examination under anesthesia is also advisable.

Perianal Examination

Rectal penetration (sodomy) is a common form of sexual abuse in both boys and girls. Care should be taken to look for evidence of abrasions, tears, fissures, and other lesions.

Immediate dilation of the sphincter to greater than 2 cm on adopting the knee–chest position has been considered suspicious for sexual abuse, when there is no visible stool in the rectum. The significance of this finding is debated. Venous congestion of the perianal area occurs within minutes of the child being placed in the knee–chest position, may also occur in the lithotomy position, and does not indicate evidence of abuse (see Fig. 6-106, *B*). The absence of physical findings is the norm and does not make the history any less credible. In most cases of sexual abuse, external inspection of the perianal area with spreading of the anal folds is sufficient; however, after specimen collection, rectal examination is necessary in

Figure 6-88 The superiority of visualization using the knee-chest position is demonstrated in a child. **A,** The hymenal rim appears narrowed to less than 1 mm in the supine position. **B,** In the knee-chest position, more hymenal tissue is observed and has a thin smooth edge. This is considered normal.

A   B

Figure 6-89 Documentation of physical findings required in sexual abuse evaluation.

Interview
Personnel involved, timing
Record exact questions
  asked and answers verbatim
  (may be used in court)
Avoid leading questions
  if possible

Physical exam
General exam
Tanner staging
Scarring/bruising

Past history
Especially of
  ano-genital symptoms
Behavioral changes

Genital exam
Magnification used
Position/technique
  Supine or semisupine
  frog-leg or lithotomy
  with labial separation
  Supine or semisupine
  frog-leg or lithotomy
  with labial traction
  Knee-chest, sway-back
Degree of relaxation

Perianal exam
Position
Degree of relaxation

Perineum/labia
Location { Lacerations
  Abrasions
  Erythema
  Bruising
  Discharge }

Hymen
Configuration
  (annular,
  crescentic,
  redundant,
  septate)
Edges
  Thin and sharp
  Thickened
  Rolled
  Projections
  Notching
  Vascularity

Vagina
Visualized
Not visualized
Ridges
Rugae
Discharge

Perianal area
Pigmentation
Erythema
Venous congestion
Anal wink/reflex
Paradoxic
  relaxation/dilatation
  (timing, measurements)
Presence of stool
Fissures
Skin tags
Lacerations
Sphincter folds
Sphincter tone

Vestibule
Erythema
Urethra

Posterior fourchette
Labial adhesions
Neovascularization
Friability

Hymenal orifice
Horizontal diameter
  (position in which
  measured)
Vertical diameter

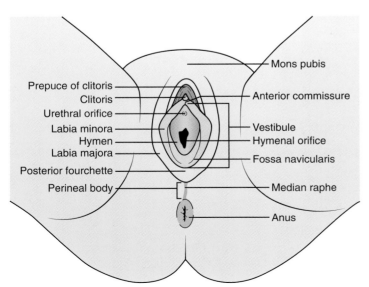

Prepuce of clitoris
Clitoris
Urethral orifice
Labia minora
Hymen
Labia majora
Posterior fourchette
Perineal body

Mons pubis
Anterior commissure
Vestibule
Hymenal orifice
Fossa navicularis
Median raphe
Anus

Figure 6-90 Normal anatomy. Location of the genital structures of the prepubescent female.

cases of acute anorectal injury in order to assess for internal rectal tears, pelvic tenderness, and sphincter tone and for bimanual palpation. When there is evidence of forceful penetration (marked bruising or lacerations) or if perineal findings suggest possible internal extension of other injuries, thereby necessitating an examination under anesthesia, the rectal examination should be deferred and performed in the operating room with the patient heavily sedated but not yet fully anesthetized. This is important because complete sphincter relaxation and anal dilation occur with full anesthesia.

Physical Findings

The changes in appearance of the female genitalia with age are described in Chapter 18. Practitioners must become familiar with the normal anatomy at different ages and with normal variations. Extensive, carefully done studies (McCann, Berenson) have documented in detail numerous normal variants, some of which have been mistaken for abnormal findings in the past (see the section Differential Diagnosis of Sexual Abuse, later). One example is apparent enlargement of the hymenal orifice. Although once thought significant, it is now known that the appearance of increased transverse diameter, in the absence of other abnormal findings, should not be used in isolation as evidence for sexual abuse. Also, for unknown reasons, obese children may have an increased anteroposterior hymenal diameter, the significance of which is unclear. Thanks to the work of McCann, Berenson, and colleagues, we now have a much better understanding of what is normal and what is abnormal.

Perineal Abnormalities

Abnormal and Suspicious Findings in Cases of Sexual Abuse

As noted earlier, findings on examination in victims of molestation or incest are totally normal in up to 96% of cases. In the remainder, abnormal or suspicious findings can be detected with careful examination. Little remaining hymenal tissue, less than 1 mm, may be suspicious for sexual abuse (see Fig. 6-91) as is deep notching of the rim through greater than 50% of hymenal width, especially when located between the 3 and 9 o'clock positions (see Fig. 6-91, A-C), which also may be seen as a result of prior sexual abuse. In addition, we have observed lichenification of the labial skin of the medial surfaces of the labia majora and marked thickening of labial adhesions due to chronic abrasive action (see Fig. 6-91, D; and see Fig. 18-26). It should be noted that acute perineal injuries often heal quickly and, at times, completely with no residual scarring. Hence patients who have incurred injuries in the past may have no abnormal findings.

Acute Traumatic Findings of Sexual Assault and Sexual Abuse

It is important to recognize that victims of sexual assault who present acutely may show evidence of physical trauma other than genital injuries. Bruises and abrasions of the head, face, neck, chest, abdomen, forearms, knees, and thighs are common (see Fig. 6-4). On occasion, even more severe nongenital injuries are encountered.

Genital and perianal examination may reveal contusions, erythema, abrasions, or lacerations (Fig. 6-92; see also Figs. 18-16 to 18-21). Perineal lesions due to sexual abuse tend to be located in the posterior portion of the introitus, as opposed to those caused by straddle injury, which are usually more anterior, are often unilateral, and rarely involve the hymen in isolation (see Fig. 6-103; and see Figs. 18-16, A and B, and 18-18).

Erythema is a common but totally nonspecific finding that may be significant within the context of a specific history. However, it is more likely to be a normal finding or one resulting from nonsexual irritation or scratching (see Chapter 18) and should not be interpreted as specific for abuse when it is the sole finding.

Figure 6-91 Abnormal findings as a result of prior sexual abuse. **A,** The hymen is almost completely absent, and the portion remaining has slightly thickened, rolled margins. A subtle bump exists at 7 o'clock, and a notch at 5 o'clock. **B,** This hymen has a posterior notch deeper than 50% of the rim, which persists in the knee–chest position (not shown here). **C,** Scarring, edema, and fresh excoriations of the perineal body extending to the anterior anal rim are seen in this child who was repetitively abused. **D,** The adhesed labia minora in another child are markedly thickened secondary to chronic frictional trauma incurred during sexual abuse. (**C,** Courtesy Pat Bruno, MD, Sunbury, Pa; **D,** courtesy John McCann, MD, University of California at Davis, Davis, Calif.)

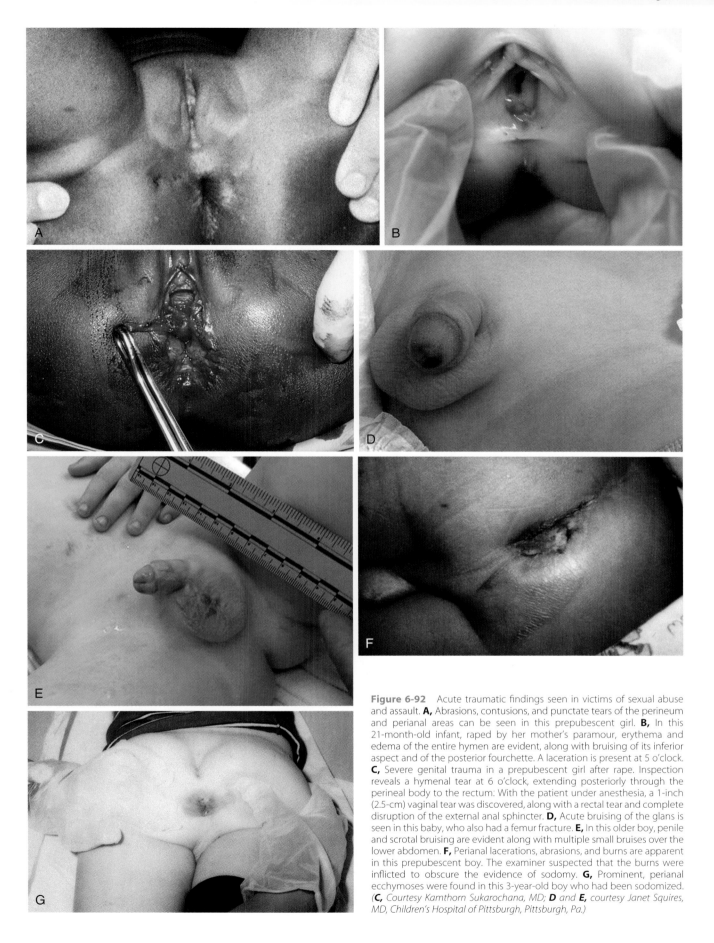

Figure 6-92 Acute traumatic findings seen in victims of sexual abuse and assault. **A,** Abrasions, contusions, and punctate tears of the perineum and perianal areas can be seen in this prepubescent girl. **B,** In this 21-month-old infant, raped by her mother's paramour, erythema and edema of the entire hymen are evident, along with bruising of its inferior aspect and of the posterior fourchette. A laceration is present at 5 o'clock. **C,** Severe genital trauma in a prepubescent girl after rape. Inspection reveals a hymenal tear at 6 o'clock, extending posteriorly through the perineal body to the rectum: With the patient under anesthesia, a 1-inch (2.5-cm) vaginal tear was discovered, along with a rectal tear and complete disruption of the external anal sphincter. **D,** Acute bruising of the glans is seen in this baby, who also had a femur fracture. **E,** In this older boy, penile and scrotal bruising are evident along with multiple small bruises over the lower abdomen. **F,** Perianal lacerations, abrasions, and burns are apparent in this prepubescent boy. The examiner suspected that the burns were inflicted to obscure the evidence of sodomy. **G,** Prominent, perianal ecchymoses were found in this 3-year-old boy who had been sodomized. (**C,** Courtesy Kamthorn Sukarochana, MD; **D** and **E,** courtesy Janet Squires, MD, Children's Hospital of Pittsburgh, Pittsburgh, Pa.)

Figure 6-93   Microscopic appearance of seminal fluid removed from a young rape victim. If a vaginal discharge is found in a patient presenting within 24 hours of sexual abuse, a wet mount may reveal sperm. A portion of the discharge should also be collected for acid phosphatase, blood grouping, and enzyme studies.

At times, evidence of seminal products in the form of a vaginal discharge may be observed if the patient is seen within 24 hours of the latest incident and has not bathed in the interim (Fig. 6-93). Seminal fluid has been reported to fluoresce under Wood's lamp, but in our tests we have found only weak fluorescence when fluid has been wet and none when dry. Urine may also fluoresce, although it is reported to fluoresce differently from semen. The BlueMaxx 500 is reported to be the most accurate forensic ultraviolet light for detecting semen on clothing. Under normal light, dried seminal products are practically invisible, but the naked eye may not be significantly inferior to use of the Wood's lamp. If a history of ejaculation is obtained and the area has not been washed, swabbing the perineum and inner thighs with saline-moistened cotton swabs *may* yield a sample of dried seminal fluid that can be identified by the crime laboratory. Swabs should be air-dried after the collection process. Clinicians should note, however, that seminal products are rarely found in the prepubertal child, in part because disclosure tends to occur long after the event.

In some cases, when labial separation or traction is performed with the victim in the supine or semisupine frog-leg or lithotomy position, findings can be obscured by redundant hymenal tissue that has folded over on itself. Hence when suspected abuse victims appear to have posterior hymenal narrowing in a supine position, an assessment in the knee–chest position is indicated. If the posterior portion of the hymen was indeed folded over when supine, it will tend to unfold because of gravity in the knee–chest position, revealing the true hymenal edge (see Fig. 6-87). Application of a few drops of saline can assist this. Examination with the child in the knee–chest position, with its superior visualization, also assists recognition of normal findings (Fig. 6-94).

Male victims may have evidence of urethral discharge and mild abrasions and contusions of the penis, scrotum, or median raphe (see Fig. 6-92, *D* and *E*).

Oral Abnormalities

Although most children forced to perform oral sex have no physical findings, forceful orogenital contact may result in perioral and intraoral injuries. These may include fissuring or tears at the corner of the mouth, as well as gingival and palatal contusions. Rarely, forceful oral penetration and thrusting can cause lacerations of posterior pharyngeal tissues, with potential complications of subcutaneous air dissection and abscess formation. Whereas oral lesions are unusual, asymptomatic gonococcal infection of the pharynx is relatively common.

Anal and Perianal Abnormalities

Patients who have been repetitively sodomized may have normal findings or may manifest paradoxical anal sphincter relaxation in response to gluteal stroking done to assess for an anal wink reflex. They also may exhibit immediate dilation of the anal sphincter to greater than 2 cm when placed in the knee–chest position. If the latter phenomenon is seen in the absence of stool in the rectal vault, the findings have been considered suspicious, although there is some debate about this. The presence of tears in the perianal area and fissures is

Figure 6-94   The superiority of visualization using the knee–chest position is demonstrated in this sexual abuse victim, whose redundant tissue made it difficult to see the true configuration of her hymen when she was supine with labial separation **(A)** or labial traction **(B)**. **C**, In the knee-chest position, narrowing and thickening of the hymenal rim can be seen more clearly. *(Courtesy Dr. John McCann, University of California at Davis.)*

also suspicious. However, fissures are not specific to sexual abuse, as they are seen frequently in children with chronic or recurrent constipation, whereas tears that extend beyond the hair follicle–bearing areas are thought to be more characteristic of abuse. Burns may be inflicted in an attempt to obscure injuries resulting from sodomy. Hence evidence of perianal burns may be suggestive of abuse, as is perianal bruising (see Fig. 6-92). Thickening and irregularity of the rectal folds may be suspicious (see Fig. 6-92); however, wedge-shaped smooth areas in the midline and skin tags are commonly seen without abuse (see Figs. 6-106, *A* and 6-107). The observation of venous congestion after the child has been in the knee–chest position for a few minutes is a normal finding.

Evidence of Sexually Transmitted Disease

The presence of sexually transmitted diseases in the prepubescent child is strongly suggestive of sexual abuse, except when other modes of transmission can be documented, or are known to be common, as in the case of genital warts in patients less than 2 years of age. In fact, some victims are identified on presenting with a vaginal or urethral discharge that is positive for a sexually transmitted pathogen. In females, this is usually manifest as vulvovaginitis with a vaginal discharge, with *Neisseria gonorrhoeae* and *Chlamydia*

trachomatis the most commonly identified pathogens (see Chapter 18 and Fig. 18-41). Although asymptomatic vulvovaginal infection is quite unusual before puberty, oral and rectal gonococcal infections are typically subclinical. Males may have overt urethritis or asymptomatic urethral infection. Girls presenting with a history of vaginal discharge should also be tested for sexually transmitted diseases.

Gonococcal vulvovaginal, urethral, oral, and rectal infections are almost always acquired through sexual contact, as are vulvovaginal *Chlamydia* infection in the child older than 2 to 3 years (see later discussion) and *Trichomonas* infection in the peripubescent child.

Development of condylomata acuminata caused by *human papillomavirus* (HPV) during infancy can be due to transmission from the mother during delivery. Because the latency period can be as long as 9 to 12 months, lesions having their onset in the first year cannot be considered as likely due to abuse. When lesions appear thereafter they are suspicious, although not diagnostic, for abuse (Fig. 6-95) as it is now thought that many of these cases are the result of nonsexual transmission from warts on the hand of a parent or caretaker of a child who still needs assistance with toileting. However, when the warts are restricted to the hymen in a prepubertal child, sexual abuse is the likely source. When human

Figure 6-95 Condylomata acuminata. **A,** Although human papillomavirus infection is not specific for abuse and is perhaps more commonly transmitted nonsexually, when condylomata are restricted to the hymen, as seen in this child, sexual abuse is the likely source. In this case the victim reported that the perpetrator had visible genital warts. **B,** Coalescent and discrete condylomata are seen in the perianal area of this 4-year-old boy with a history of being sodomized. **C,** More extensive lesions involving the mons, the introitus, the labia, and perianal area developed in another child. (**C,** *Courtesy Robin Gehris, MD, Children's Hospital of Pittsburgh, Pittsburgh, Pa.*)

papillomavirus is strongly suspected but no lesions are visible, application of a 3% to 5% solution of acetic acid for 3 to 5 minutes will impart an "aceto-white" appearance to any lesions present.

In the very young child, *genital herpes* infections may be acquired through sexual contact but are more often the result of spread from oral or hand lesions from the patient, or from a parent with a cold sore, as a result of poor attention to hand washing (see Fig. 18-38, *A*). In the latency-aged child, however, sexual contact is the more likely source. Nonspecific vaginal discharges that are culture-negative for sexually transmitted, respiratory, and enteric pathogens, especially if chronic or recurrent, are also suspect, and testing for seminal fluid should be considered.

Nonsexual transmission of gonococci, *Chlamydia, Trichomonas,* and human papillomavirus occurs primarily during vaginal delivery. Gonococcal infections tend to produce symptoms early in the neonatal period. Perinatally acquired *Trichomonas* infection causes a copious vaginal discharge in the neonate, which abates even without treatment, although the organism can persist for months. In contrast, *Chlamydia* infection acquired neonatally may persist for 18 months to 3 years. Hence finding this organism in the very young child cannot be considered diagnostic of sexual abuse. As noted earlier, because of its prolonged incubation period, the human papillomavirus acquired during delivery may not produce lesions until several months later.

Last, it must be noted that in some instances children acquire sexually transmitted diseases as the result of sexual contact with other infected children. In such cases aggressive case finding can result in identification of the index child, who is highly likely to be a victim of sexual abuse.

Specimen Collection

Laboratory studies are designed to augment the physical assessment of injury, identify sexually transmitted pathogens, and document the presence or absence of seminal fluid. Data confirm clinical experience that the yield for evidence of ejaculate on the body of a prepubertal patient presenting more than 24 hours after the abuse is extremely low. Hence studies to detect semen may be omitted if the patient seeks attention later than this. However, it is particularly important to collect articles of unlaundered clothing and bed linens that may have evidence of ejaculate on them because semen may be retrieved from these items even 12 months (or more) later. Unfortunately, this is often overlooked in the process of evidence collection in sexual abuse cases. Because the yield of positive results from vaginal cultures obtained from asymptomatic prepubertal victims is so low, the collection of specimens sometimes uncomfortable, and the cost high, many centers are advocating a more selective approach in obtaining cultures in this age group on the basis of the level of risk. However, oral and rectal cultures should be strongly considered because oral and rectal gonococcal infections are typically asymptomatic, and nucleic acid amplification tests (NAATs) are not recommended.

In the prepubescent child with vaginal discharge, all cultures, except for *Chlamydia,* may be obtained from discharge present on the perineum. It is important not to confuse smegma with discharge (Fig. 18-22). *Chlamydia* cultures necessitate swabbing the vaginal wall. Note that when NAATs are done in cases of sexual abuse a second laboratory-based confirmatory test is required. Although cultures are still recommended there is increasing evidence that the newer NAATs are both more sensitive and specific than cultures, especially in a low-incidence population (check for updated guidelines at the Centers for Disease Control and Prevention website http://

www.cdc.gov/std/treatment/2010/sexual-assault.htm#a2). This requires great care in specimen collection because the hymen, before puberty and estrogenization, is extremely sensitive, and touching it with a swab induces a significant amount of pain in most patients. Saline-moistened calcium alginate swabs on thin metal wires are the easiest to insert atraumatically. As the knee–chest position produces maximal hymenal opening, this is the optimal position for vaginal specimen collection, if the child will tolerate it.

Testing should be considered in the adolescent, regardless of time of presentation or of the presence or absence of symptoms, because sexually transmitted diseases (STDs) may be asymptomatic in postpubertal girls, and may have been acquired earlier as a result of consensual sexual activity. Cervical cultures for gonorrhea and *Chlamydia* infection in addition to cultures of the vaginal pool are indicated. The possibility of pregnancy must also be considered in all such patients, and a pregnancy test must be performed.

In obtaining rectal specimens for gonorrhea and *Chlamydia* cultures, the swab should be inserted no more than 1 to 2 cm to avoid fecal contamination, which interferes with culture results.

There has been much debate about what STD testing is appropriate and legally acceptable in cases of child sexual abuse. There are data showing that certain nucleic acid amplification tests are both more sensitive and more specific than culture for both *Chlamydia* and gonorrhea from certain sites. For the latest recommendations please check http://www.cdc.gov/std/LabGuidelines/rr5115.pdf.

Patients with evidence of trauma need urinalysis and rectal examination to check for evidence of bleeding and may require sonography or CT if physical findings are suggestive of internal extension of injury. However, if anal rape is reported or if anal inspection suggests evidence of forceful anal penetration with marked bruising or lacerations, especially in a prepubertal child who has clearly been traumatized emotionally and physically, rectal examination should be deferred until the patient is sedated before full anesthetic administration in the operating room. Loss of sphincter tone and anal dilation occur normally when a child is fully anesthetized and should not be mistaken for abnormal findings. Prepubescent girls with evidence of vaginal bleeding or a vaginal hematoma must have an internal examination performed under anesthesia to check for internal extension of injury. In such instances, specimen collection is deferred until that time.

Table 6-9 presents guidelines for specimen collection in sexual abuse cases, and Table 6-10 enumerates the additional specimens required by law enforcement authorities in rape cases. Note that, given the extremely low yield in prepubertal children presenting after 24 hours, a full rape kit is not indicated in such situations. Because the examination is for the purpose of gathering forensic evidence, in addition to assessing the patient's physical status, procedure must be meticulous. Each specimen for the crime laboratory should be packaged and labeled immediately on collection. All evidence should then be kept together and must remain under the direct supervision of the physician or nurse who was present at the time of collection until it is signed over to hospital security or law enforcement. Last, police should sign a receipt for release of evidence on accepting the specimens. Commercially available rape assessment kits greatly assist this process. Failure to adhere to these procedures breaks the chain of evidence and invalidates its use in legal proceedings. If the assault or rape has been perpetrated by a stranger (e.g., not a caretaker), the patient or parent usually must sign a consent form before collection of evidence.

Table 6-9	Documentation Required in Sexual Abuse Evaluation: Guidelines for Specimen Collection in Sexual Abuse Examination

| | **GENITAL CONTACT** | | |
Orogenital Contact	**No Evidence of Penetration**	**Evidence Consistent with Vaginal Penetration**	**Anal Contact**

1. Swabs: use two at a time*
   a. For wet mount for sperm[†]
   b. For two air-dried slides[†]
   c. For GC culture
   d. Consider *Chlamydia* culture if patient older than 3 yr
 2. Consider baseline RPR (repeat in 4-6 wk if initial test result is negative)[§]
 3. Consider HIV testing with repeat test in 3-6 mo[§]
	1. Urinalysis for occult blood
	 2. Vaginal swabs or aspirate*[‡]
	   a. For wet mount for sperm,[†] *Trichomonas,* and *Candida*
	   b. For two air-dried slides[†]
	   c. For GC and routine culture[‡]
	   d. For *Chlamydia* culture if patient older than 3 yr[‡]
	   e. For Gram stain if vaginal discharge is present[‡]
	 3. Consider baseline RPR (repeat in 4-6 wk if initial result is negative)[§]
	 4. Consider HIV testing with repeat test in 3-6 mo[§]
		1. Urinalysis for occult blood
		 2. If vaginal bleeding or hematoma seen in prepubertal child:
		   a. Consult pediatric surgeon or gynecologist for possible EUA
		   b. If EUA done, collect specimens, then:
		 3. Vaginal swabs or aspirate*[‡]
		   a. For wet mount for sperm,[†] *Trichomonas,* and *Candida*
		   b. For two air-dried slides[†]
		   c. For GC and routine cultures[‡]
		   d. For *Chlamydia* culture if patient older than 3 yr[‡]
		   e. For Gram stain if vaginal discharge present[‡]
		 4. Consider RPR (repeat in 4-6 wk if initial result is negative)[§]
		 5. Consider HIV testing with repeat test in 3-6 mo[§]
			1. If marked bruising or external tears seen:
			   a. Consult pediatric surgeon or gynecologist for possible EUA
			   b. If EUA done, collect specimens, then:
			 2. Swabs: Use two at a time and insert no more than 1 cm* (must be done before rectal examination)
			   a. For wet mount for sperm[†]
			   b. For two air-dried slides[†]
			   c. For GC and routine cultures
			   d. For *Chlamydia* culture if patient older than 3 yr
			 3. If no major bruising or tears:
			   a. Rectal examination
			   b. Stool test for blood: if positive, consult general surgeon
			 4. Consider baseline RPR (repeat in 4-6 wk if initial result is negative)[§]
			 5. Consider HIV testing with repeat test in 3-6 mo[§]

*Two of the swabs used to obtain specimens should be air-dried and placed in a sterile test tube for acid phosphatase, blood group, DNA, and enzyme studies. When specimens are obtained by vaginal aspirate, a small amount of aspirate should be applied to two swabs, which should then be processed in the same manner.
[†]Omit if seen more than 24 hours after the last incident, except in patients with vaginal discharge.
[‡]In postpubescent patients, cervical swabs must be obtained for GC and *Chlamydia* cultures and for Gram stain.
[§]These studies are indicated in cases of abuse by an unknown stranger or by a perpetrator known to be at high risk for these diseases (intravenous drug user), especially in areas where these diseases are endemic.
Note: Follow-up in 2-4 weeks is recommended, with additional specimen collection as needed.
EUA, examination under anesthesia; GC, gonococcal; RPR, rapid plasma reagin test.

Table 6-10	Additional Specimens Needed in Rape Cases (Seen within 72 Hours*)

SPECIMENS MAY BE OBTAINED BY THE PHYSICIAN OR NURSE. ALL CONTAINERS USED IN EVIDENCE COLLECTION SHOULD BE PAPER AND MUST BE LABELED WITH:

	Patient's name	Body site	Initials of collector
	Type of specimen	Date and time	
Clothing	If the patient is wearing the same clothes, they should be collected along with any debris because this may provide valuable clues regarding the assailant. The patient should disrobe while standing on a towel or sheet. Each article including the towel or sheet should then be placed in a separate paper bag. Avoid shaking the articles. Each bag is then labeled and sealed.		
Fingernail scrapings[†]	These may provide bits of skin, fiber, and debris from the assailant. Scrapings from beneath the nails or nail clippings should be obtained. Specimens from each hand should be collected over separate sheets of paper and placed in separate paper envelopes, sealed, and labeled.		
Hair samples[†]	Any loose or suspected foreign hairs should be collected, placed in an envelope, and labeled. If patient is postpubescent, comb pubic hairs onto a sheet of clean paper, fold, place in an envelope with the comb, label "combed pubic hair," and seal. Then, gently pull pubic hairs from the patient (12 hairs are needed), place on clean paper, fold, put in envelope, label "standard pubic hair," and seal. Then, comb and pull head hairs in this same manner.		
Blood sample	Five milliliters of blood should be drawn for blood grouping and enzyme typing and placed in a purple-top tube.		
Saliva sample	This enables testing of the patient's secretory status. The specimen should be obtained either by wiping the patient's oral mucosa with a gauze pad or by having the patient expectorate onto a gauze pad. The pad is then placed in an envelope, sealed, and labeled.		

Destination of Specimens

The following specimens are handled by the hospital laboratories or performed in the emergency department:

Urinalysis	Gram stains	RPR
Wet preps	Stool test for blood	Cultures

All other specimens are to be signed over to police custody for transport to the crime laboratory

Maintaining an Unbroken Chain of Evidence

Evidence should be packaged and labeled on collection. All evidence should be kept together and must remain under the direct supervision of the collecting physician or nurse until signed over to hospital security or the police. Receipt for release of evidence to law enforcement should be signed before evidence is given over to security or the police.

*The yield is very low after 24 hours and almost zero if the child is prepubertal.
[†]Omit if patient has already bathed and shampooed.
RPR, rapid plasma reagin (test).

Differential Diagnosis of Sexual Abuse

Not only is there a wide range of nonabusive causes of the physical and behavioral symptoms that serve as presenting complaints of many sexual abuse victims, but also physical findings, when present, are also variable and often nonspecific and many have a variety of other potential causes. Furthermore, as a result of McCann's pioneering work, the wide range of normal anatomic variations is being increasingly appreciated.

Normal Anatomic Variations

A wide variation in normal hymenal configuration and shape of orifice exists (Fig. 6-96; see also Figs. 18-3 and 18-7), as well as some amount of variation in diameter that must be appreciated by the examining physician (see Fig. 18-3). Several normal anatomic variants are now recognized as well. *Septal remnants* (Fig. 6-97), seen as tags near the midline on either

the anterior or posterior portion of the hymenal membrane (see Chapter 18), and even anterolateral *hymenal flaps* (Fig. 6-98) are normal findings, as are periurethral bands. These and *intravaginal ridges* (Fig. 6-99) were once erroneously thought to be the result of scarring. Thin *labial adhesions* are a common finding in normal children as well (Fig. 6-100; and see Fig. 18-12).

Vulvar Erythema and Inflammation

Erythema of the vaginal vestibule is common in asymptomatic, nonabused, prepubescent girls. It can also be seen in abuse victims and in children with irritant and other forms of vulvovaginitis (see Figs. 18-24, 18-25, 18-31, 18-38, and Table 18-4). *Vulvovaginitis* has a wide variety of causes, many of which are noninfectious, including chemical irritation, poor perineal hygiene or aeration, nonabusive frictional trauma, contact dermatitis, or itching and scratching due to pinworms

Figure 6-96   Variations in normal hymenal configuration. **A,** A redundant hymen. **B,** A crescentic hymen with thin smooth edges. **C,** A somewhat redundant hymen with an annular orifice. **D,** A septate hymen resulting from failure of lysis of the embryonic hymenal septum.

Figure 6-97 Septal remnant. This skin tag at the 6 o'clock position is a remnant of the vaginal septum present earlier in fetal development and constitutes a normal finding seen in about 5% of girls.

Figure 6-98 Hymenal flap. This child has a redundant hymen with an everted anterolateral flap, another normal variant.

or other sources of irritation. These conditions may be associated with nonspecific erythema, maceration, or superficial abrasions/excoriations (see Figs. 18-22, 18-24, and 18-25). Many infectious cases are caused by respiratory or gastrointestinal pathogens (the former transmitted from nose or throat by the child's hands, the latter often due to perineal contact with infected stool) or are seen concurrently with urinary tract infections (see Chapter 18). Thus vulvovaginitis resulting from sexually transmitted disease probably constitutes a minority of vulvovaginal complaints in prepubescent children. To avoid misdiagnosis of abuse, it is wise to defer diagnosis until definitive culture results are obtained.

Urethral Prolapse

The clinical findings of *urethral prolapse* (Fig. 6-101) have been mistakenly attributed to sexual abuse because the purplish-red prolapsed mucosal tissue that protrudes between the labia minora bleeds easily and often overlies the vaginal orifice, simulating edematous, traumatized, redundant hymenal folds. The condition is often first discovered when blood or a serosanguineous discharge is found on the diaper or underwear, because associated dysuria is unusual and urination is not impeded. With magnification, the urethral orifice can be seen at the center of the mass, which is soft and markedly tender to touch. After application of topical anesthetic,

Figure 6-99 Intravaginal ridges. The bands of tissue along the vaginal walls that appear here to extend medially and downward from the 11 and 2 o'clock positions are normal features of the vaginal walls; in the past they were erroneously thought to be the result of scarring. *(Courtesy John McCann, MD, University of California at Davis, Davis, Calif.)*

Figure 6-100 Labial adhesions. The labia minora are fused in the midline as a consequence of prior inflammation. They are separated by a thin lucent line, and the epithelium of the labia is normal.

Figure 6-101 Urethral prolapse. This child was referred for evaluation for possible sexual abuse when blood was noted on her underwear, and "traumatized tissue" was seen on examination. On close inspection, this was found to be edematous, friable prolapsed urethral mucosa.

the prolapse can be lifted, revealing the hymen underneath. The condition is unusual and tends to occur only in children younger than 12 years of age; two thirds of affected girls are African American. The cause is unknown, although many affected girls have a history of constipation.

Lichen Sclerosus

Lichen sclerosus et atrophicus has often been mistakenly attributed to sexual abuse. The involved perineal skin is paper-thin and tends to be hypopigmented. During periods of acute inflammation, hypopigmentation may be partially obscured by erythema and areas of superficial ulceration that bleed easily (Fig. 6-102; and see Fig. 18-29 and accompanying text). Its cause remains unknown.

Accidental Trauma

As noted earlier, trauma inflicted in the course of attempted or actual sexual penetration generally results in contusions and tears of the posterior portion of the hymen and introitus. In contrast, *straddle injuries* produce lesions of the anterior and anterolateral portions because these are tissues most likely to be crushed between the pubic ramus and the object on which the child falls. Findings include contusions, abrasions, and superficial lacerations, the latter being frequently found at the junction of the labia majora and minora (Fig. 6-103; and see Fig. 18-16).

Vaginal Foreign Bodies

The presence of foreign objects within the vaginal canal sometimes precipitates an inflammatory response with production of a copious brown, sometimes blood-tinged, discharge with a foul odor. The discharge and its odor generally prompt presentation. Foreign bodies may or may not suggest abuse. Whereas finding firm objects within the vagina and witnessing a child stroking herself with crayons or similar objects and then inserting them are suspicious for prior sexual abuse, the not uncommon finding of a small wad of toilet tissue lodged within the vagina is more likely an inadvertent consequence of vigorous wiping (Fig. 6-104).

Midline Defects

Perineal midline fusion defects are an unusual phenomenon in which a small portion of the median raphe adjacent to the anus fails to fuse in utero. The anomaly, seen only in female infants, is present at birth and may be located anteriorly or posteriorly to the anus. When the unfused edges of the median raphe are spread apart they reveal an underlying pink or reddish mucosal-like surface (Fig. 6-105). The defect often goes unnoticed until days or weeks after delivery during a diaper change, bathing, or a well-child care visit. When first detected by a parent or physician unfamiliar with the problem,

A

B

Figure 6-102 Lichen sclerosus et atrophicus. **A,** Multiple small points of bleeding dot the atrophic mucosa in this child. **B,** In another girl, acute inflammation has largely subsided, leaving an hourglass pattern of hypopigmentation extending from the mons to below the anal folds. (**B,** *Courtesy Robin Gehris, MD, Children's Hospital of Pittsburgh, Pittsburgh, Pa.*)

Figure 6-103 Accidental trauma caused by a straddle injury. **A,** This child with a straddle injury was brought in immediately for care because of slight bleeding. Superficial abrasions and contusions extend from the anterior portion of the labia minora to the posterior fourchette. Note that the lesions are largely unilateral. **B,** Another child complained of dysuria and was noted to have a small amount of blood on her underwear after a straddle injury. The superficial laceration between the hymen and labia minora was barely visible in regular light but was brought out by viewing it through a green filter.

findings may be mistaken for a laceration due to sexual abuse. Medical recognition of the true nature of the abnormality is enhanced by knowledge of its existence, and by the fact that the edges of the outer layer of tissue and of the underlying "mucosal" surface are smooth and intact. Other features that help distinguish midline defects from abuse-related injury are the absence of associated introital and anal abnormalities and of bleeding.

Normal Anal and Perianal Variants

Anal fissures and *perianal skin tags* (Fig. 6-106) are common sequelae of constipation. The fissures caused by the passage of hard or large-caliber stools are superficial and usually do not extend beyond the perianal skin bearing hair follicles, whereas tears produced by sodomy usually exceed this limit.

Infantile perianal pyramidal protrusion consists of a single benign papule with a pyramidal shape located in the midline of the perineal raphe, usually just anterior to the anus (occasionally just posterior). It is smooth, soft, pink, and totally asymptomatic (Fig. 6-107). The protrusion is either present at birth or noted shortly thereafter, and there is no association

with antecedent fissures or fistulas. The "lesion" usually resolves spontaneously over weeks to months. Exact etiology is as yet unclear, although an association with lichen sclerosus et atrophicus has been noted.

Spontaneous anal sphincter relaxation occurring 30 seconds to 3 or 4 minutes after adopting the knee–chest position is normal. Immediate sphincter dilation when there is stool present in the rectal vault is also considered normal, as is anal dilation in the fully anesthetized child. However, reproducible immediate sphincter dilation to greater than 2 cm on adopting the knee–chest position is considered to be suspicious for repetitive prior anal penetration. Perianal erythema, hyperpigmentation, and venous engorgement are other common findings seen in normal children.

PASSIVE ABUSE OR NEGLECT

Passive abuse or neglect is by far the most commonly reported type of child abuse, accounting for more than 50% of cases each year. In its mildest form, this may consist of a pattern of lack of vigilance and safeguarding of young children, who are

Figure 6-104 Vaginal foreign body. **A,** A white object is noted within the vagina on perineal inspection. **B,** This was better visualized by labial traction. Toilet paper had become enlodged in the process of wiping after toileting.

Figure 6-105   Perineal midline fusion defect. This toddler was referred for concern of sexual abuse when this defect was noticed by her new foster mother during a diaper change. The unfused edges of the median raphe are spread apart to reveal an underlying mucosal-like surface. Both are smooth and intact with no evidence of inflammation or bleeding. Note that she has another congenital anomaly, an anteriorly displaced anus. A normal redundant hymen is also seen. *(Courtesy Carol Byers, CRNP, Children's Hospital of Pittsburgh, Pittsburgh, Pa.)*

from caring for a doll. Once the demands are evident, they may become disenchanted and lose interest. Disinterest may be manifested by bottle propping; talking on the phone during feedings; leaving the baby in a crib much of the time; leaving the baby home alone; or frequently dropping the baby off with relatives, friends, acquaintances, or neighbors (often with dubious child care skills) so that they can go out when they want. A challenging subset of adolescent mothers are those who are pseudo-independent with "attitude." Despite limited knowledge and experience, these girls are convinced they know all they need to know about caring for their baby and are resistant to and often suspicious of suggestions, advice, and offers of help.

Economic situation and lack of education also play a role. *Poverty* with its stresses and pressures, its association with

thereby at greater risk for accidents and ingestions. This may include leaving them unattended for long periods, placing them in a hazardous environment, or leaving an older child in charge who is too young and/or unprepared to take on responsibility for the care of younger siblings. In its most severe form, the patient presents with severe growth failure and developmental delay as a result of inadequate provision of calories and minimal or ineffective nurturing.

Typically, in severe cases, the patient has been fed irregularly, offered insufficient volumes of formula and food, given little interactional attention, and received minimal basic care. In some cases it appears that an infant may have picked up on maternal anxiety and/or depression and developed secondary anorexia and autonomic disturbances of intestinal motility. Some affected infants actually begin to resist contact and become difficult to feed. In addition, as malnutrition worsens, babies tend to become listless and irritable, making care more difficult and less rewarding. Furthermore, secondary malabsorption worsens nutrient utilization.

Risk factors are similar to those seen in cases of active physical abuse, with a few additions. More of these infants were *unplanned* and *unwanted*. Often *little or no prenatal care* was sought. In numerous cases there is a history of the father having abandoned the mother after learning of the pregnancy. Mothers of these babies are more likely to be frankly depressed or cognitively limited and to have had difficulty caring for the children they already have. In some cases the mother appears to have been coping reasonably well with the children she'd already had, but this last baby has proved one too many. The incidence of maternal *drug abuse* as a predisposing factor has increased substantially over the past few decades.

Infants born to a *teenage mother* have twice the risk of suffering neglect as those born to older women, often because of the deprivation of nurturing, love, attention, and affection they suffered themselves as infants and children. As a consequence, these young women are emotionally needy yet have difficulty with attachment and bonding, not only to their infants but also to friends and family who might be of support. Further, they have neither the emotional wherewithal nor the experience necessary to nurture their offspring. Some fantasize that the unconditional love of a child will meet their unmet needs for love. Often emotionally immature and self-focused, the teenage mothers may have little concept of what is involved in caring for a child, thinking it not much different

Figure 6-106   **A,** Perianal skin tag. This is a common finding, particularly in children with a history of constipation and prior problems with anal fissures. **B,** Venous congestion noted in the perianal area. This can occur after a few minutes in either the knee–chest or lithotomy positions and is a normal finding.

Figure 6-107 Infantile perianal pyramidal protrusion. This smooth, soft, pink papule, located in the midline just anterior to the anus, has a pyramidal shape. It was noted by the mother shortly after birth and was totally asymptomatic.

poor housing conditions (nonfunctioning appliances, poor sanitary conditions, and general disrepair); lack of utilities because of unpaid bills; or homelessness is another common thread. This is further complicated by social isolation, lack of transportation, and mental health problems that can interfere with a mother's ability to mobilize herself to sign up for food stamps and the Women, Infants, and Children program (Food and Nutrition Service, U.S. Department of Agriculture) to which she is entitled.

Limitations in knowledge and understanding of the importance of nutrition and children's needs are also common and, when combined with ill-informed dietary beliefs (juice is as good as formula because the Women, Infants, and Children program gives it out) or fears (regarding obesity, cholesterol or animal products [vegans], and milk/food allergy), contribute to inappropriate feeding practices.

Major *infant risk factors* are prematurity; being born small for gestational age; being the last of a large sibship or the latest of three or four born in rapid succession; being passive and undemanding; or being perceived as difficult.

Psychosocial Failure to Thrive

On presentation, the mother of an infant with *psychosocial failure to thrive* often appears relatively unconcerned about her baby's state of nutrition, even when this has reached the point of emaciation. When asked about it, she may report not having noticed it or may state that all her babies are small. Typically, she has brought the child for treatment of a minor unrelated problem, such as a cold, rash, vomiting, or constipation. Some present with a history of colic, crying "all the time," or a feeding problem. In many cases there are glaring inconsistencies in the feeding history (e.g., "he takes 6 ounces every 4 hours," yet "he takes 16 ounces in 24 hours"). Many mothers readily acknowledge that they often do not hold the baby for feedings but instead prop the bottle on a towel or against the side of the crib. When observed, even when they do hold the infant during a feeding, they often do not make

good eye contact and tend to put him or her down immediately afterward. A high percentage of these infants have received little or no professional well-child care and are behind on their immunizations.

On examination, the infant or child with psychosocial failure to thrive is usually found to be significantly undergrown. Weight may be below the third percentile, or there may be evidence of plateauing of weight gain. In long-standing cases, height and head circumference are abnormally low as well. Comparison with birth parameters and measurements made at prior visits (if any) reveal that the child has "fallen off the growth curve" (Fig. 6-108). In the more severe case the child presents with decreased subcutaneous tissue (most notably over the buttocks, thighs, and upper arms); a pinched face; and sunken prominent eyes. In some there are frank physical findings of multiple vitamin deficiencies, which include a nonspecific or seborrhea-like dermatitis that can progress to skin breakdown, cheilosis, glossitis and stomatitis, and erythema and thinning of the skin over the palms and soles (Fig. 6-109, *A-E*).

Affected infants tend to look serious, smile infrequently, appear apathetic and withdrawn when left alone, and often lie on their backs with their arms up beside their heads. They show more interest in inanimate objects than in people, and although they appear vigilant toward people at a distance, they

Figure 6-108 Growth chart of a child with psychosocial failure to thrive. This boy's growth was normal until he was 15 months of age, when his mother became addicted to crack. His weight gain slowed between 15 and 19 months, after which he showed a precipitous weight loss and slowing of height growth. He showed rapid catch-up growth within a week of removal from the home. (*Courtesy Robin Gehris, MD, Children's Hospital of Pittsburgh, Pittsburgh, Pa.*)

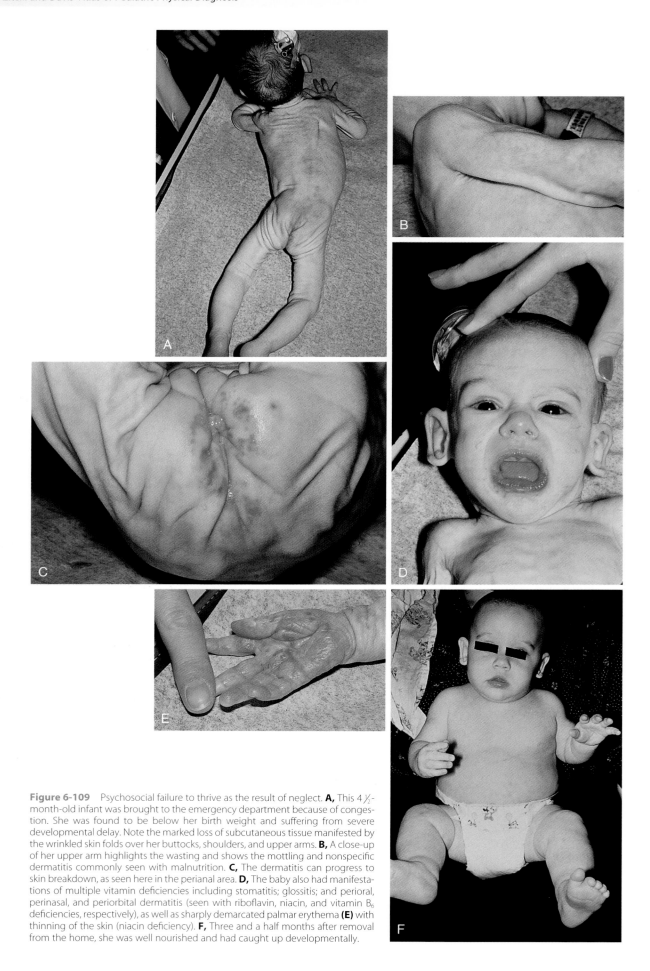

Figure 6-109   Psychosocial failure to thrive as the result of neglect. **A,** This 4½-month-old infant was brought to the emergency department because of congestion. She was found to be below her birth weight and suffering from severe developmental delay. Note the marked loss of subcutaneous tissue manifested by the wrinkled skin folds over her buttocks, shoulders, and upper arms. **B,** A close-up of her upper arm highlights the wasting and shows the mottling and nonspecific dermatitis commonly seen with malnutrition. **C,** The dermatitis can progress to skin breakdown, as seen here in the perianal area. **D,** The baby also had manifestations of multiple vitamin deficiencies including stomatitis; glossitis; and perioral, perinasal, and periorbital dermatitis (seen with riboflavin, niacin, and vitamin B$_6$ deficiencies, respectively), as well as sharply demarcated palmar erythema **(E)** with thinning of the skin (niacin deficiency). **F,** Three and a half months after removal from the home, she was well nourished and had caught up developmentally.

Figure 6-110 Neglect. **A,** Another infant with severe failure to thrive has a badly neglected case of irritant diaper dermatitis. **B** and **C,** Severely neglected baby-bottle caries were among the findings noted on evaluation of a toddler with failure to thrive. She was examined after her marasmic baby brother was referred by Women, Infants, and Children personnel. Their mother was suffering from immobilizing depression. In **B,** one can see that the upper teeth are markedly discolored by decay and have eroded down to the gingiva. In **C,** note the abscesses over the upper left gingiva.

tend to become upset when someone approaches and avoid making eye contact. They often object to being touched, held, or cuddled. When health care personnel persist in trying to get them to interact, they find they must work hard to get the baby to calm down and sit in their lap; when put back in the crib, the child cries only briefly, if at all. Vocalization is sparse, and development is delayed and uneven, with social milestones being farther behind than motor development. We have seen some who have had abnormal tone, scissoring, and posturing suggestive of a neurologic problem, which promptly abated within a few days of hospitalization.

Poor hygiene, dirty clothes, badly neglected diaper rashes, and severe baby-bottle caries are common additional findings suggestive of neglect (Fig. 6-110, *A-C*).

The easiest, least traumatic way to confirm the diagnosis of psychosocial failure to thrive is to remove the infant from its home and observe its growth in a nurturing environment. Infants and children with milder cases will gain weight promptly, whereas marasmic infants may take 1 to 2 weeks before resuming growth (see Fig. 6-109, *F*).

Although pure psychosocial failure to thrive is the most common form of growth failure in infancy, accounting for between 33% and 50% of cases, up to 25% of cases are of purely organic origin; in another 25%, growth failure is due to a combination of organic and psychosocial factors. In the latter instances, affected infants often have suffered prenatal or perinatal insults that have resulted in growth retardation and/or physical conditions that make them difficult to feed and care for.

Organic Causes of Failure to Thrive

Of cases of *organic failure to thrive,* CNS, gastrointestinal, cardiac, genetic, pulmonary, renal, and endocrine disorders account for organically based growth failure, in descending order of frequency. The majority of such disorders can be recognized during physical examination because of the obvious

abnormalities seen. The remainder tend to be revealed by history or can be readily diagnosed on the basis of a few simple screening laboratory tests.

Neurologic Disorders

Severe cerebral palsy, neuromuscular disorders, encephalopathies, and neurodegenerative diseases are the major CNS problems associated with failure to thrive. Poor suck; problems coordinating sucking and swallowing; and lethargy, irritability, and altered level of consciousness are the more common factors that impede adequate intake in these infants. Some also have excess losses because of vomiting. Neurologic dysfunction may also impair an infant's ability to provide interactive feedback to the mother.

Gastrointestinal Disorders

A variety of gastrointestinal problems cause growth failure, and numerous mechanisms are responsible. Oral malformations including cleft lip and palate, severe micrognathia, and macroglossia interfere with sucking and swallowing. Many of these conditions are also associated with chronic or recurrent ear and nasopharyngeal infections. Esophageal and gastric disorders can interfere with growth by causing pain on swallowing, resulting in decreased intake, or by causing repetitive vomiting (abnormal losses), with or without aspiration. These include gastroesophageal reflux (GER), esophageal stricture, stenosis, or atresia; external esophageal compression by abnormal vessels, an enlarged heart, or mass lesions; chalasia; and achalasia. Among these, GER predominates, and it must be remembered that this disorder has varied manifestations. Although vomiting and repetitive spitting are common modes of presentation, they are not uniformly present. Other symptoms include crying after every few swallows during feedings (with or without writhing or arching) and/or feeding refusal due to esophagitis. In some cases snoring, coughing, wheezing, and even apnea are prominent and tend to worsen during sleep or while recumbent (see Chapters 10 and 23).

With the exception of pyloric stenosis, which can cause failure to thrive due to repeated vomiting when diagnosis is delayed, malabsorption is the major mechanism of growth failure in patients with small or large intestinal disorders and pancreatic disease. These infants may also experience pain associated with eating caused by gas, hyperperistalsis, or inflammation, each of which may also cause anorexia. Further, they typically have a history of excessive stool losses, and stool examination may suggest the underlying cause. Carbohydrate malabsorption is characterized by large, watery stools, which are positive for reducing substances, have a low pH, and are accompanied by considerable gas. Fat malabsorption results in large, bulky, greasy stools, and protein malabsorption in foul-smelling stools. Infants with blind-loop syndromes resulting from webs, bands, or stenoses have large, watery stools as a result of bacterial overgrowth in the gut lumen proximal to the site of partial obstruction. Short-gut syndrome subsequent to surgical resection and parasitic infections with *Giardia* or *Strongyloides* organisms are other causes of malabsorption.

Impaired bile acid metabolism results in fat malabsorption in infants with severe liver disease. Associated anorexia, malaise, and fatigue further impede intake in these children, and vomiting contributes to caloric losses. It must also be remembered that malnutrition itself causes malabsorption.

Infants and toddlers with symptomatic *celiac disease* or gluten-sensitive enteropathy may present between 6 months and 2 years of age with failure to thrive. In the "textbook case" the child has diarrhea with foul-smelling stools, vomiting, abdominal distention, anorexia, and pallor, and has an irritable, unhappy demeanor. A wide range of symptomatology exists, however. Some patients may only have vomiting and growth retardation, others only short stature, and a majority of affected children are probably asymptomatic. The disorder and its symptoms stem from a genetic susceptibility to intolerance to the gliadin fraction of gluten, which then sets off a T cell–mediated immunologic response. This results in chronic inflammation of the mucosa of the small intestine, impairing its absorption and digestive functions. Because gluten is found in wheat, rye, barley and, to a lesser extent, oats, symptoms cannot develop until the infant or child has been exposed to cereals, breads, or crackers containing these grains for some period of time.

Cardiac Disease

Severe cardiac disorders including those characterized by chronic congestive heart failure, large shunts, or pulmonary hypertension appear to result in growth failure primarily as a result of dyspnea with feeding and secondarily decreased intake. Slow feeding and a history of diaphoresis with feeding and during sleep are commonly noted. The role of hypoxia and malabsorption (resulting from impaired intestinal lymphatic drainage in children with congestive heart failure) remains unclear. Many of these patients also have recurrent pulmonary infections, and in some, intrauterine growth retardation, congenital infections, and genetic disorders play a role.

Genetic Disorders

The genetic disorders associated with impaired growth include chromosomal disorders, storage diseases, skeletal disorders and dysplasias, inborn errors of metabolism, idiopathic hypercalcemia, and heritable CNS defects. Nearly all are characterized by obvious physical stigmata.

Pulmonary Disease

Of the pulmonary disorders associated with failure to thrive, bronchopulmonary dysplasia and persistent viral infections are the two main sources. Dyspnea with feeding and secondarily decreased intake appear to be the major underlying mechanisms, often compounded by recurrent infection. *Cystic fibrosis* can be put in this category, but it is malabsorption due to pancreatic enzyme deficiency more than pulmonary dysfunction that appears to affect the growth of these patients.

Renal Disease

Renal diseases that involve the interstitium and tubular structures are the major nephric sources of growth failure. These include dysplasia, multicystic or polycystic kidney disease, severe hydronephrosis with azotemia, chronic obstructive uropathy, renal tubular acidosis, nephrogenic diabetes insipidus, chronic or recurrent urinary tract infections with severe reflux or other anatomic abnormalities, and chronic renal failure. Inability to concentrate the urine, abnormalities of urinary sediment, and abnormal serum chemistry values are found on screening tests in these patients. Inadequate intake stemming from anorexia and protein restriction, malabsorption, abnormal vitamin D absorption and secondary hyperparathyroidism with renal osteodystrophy, decreased somatomedin levels, and abnormal peripheral use and degradation of insulin may contribute to growth failure in these children.

Endocrine Disease

Among the endocrine disorders, *diabetes mellitus* and pituitary, thyroid, and adrenal disorders can all be associated with growth impairment. Urinary losses of glucose, dehydration, and excessive protein catabolism result in weight loss in children with diabetes mellitus. A history of polyuria, polydipsia, or polyphagia and tests for serum and urine glucose readily enable diagnosis. The growth curves of children with *isolated growth hormone deficiency* and *panhypopituitarism* level off between 9 and 12 months of age, with height affected more than weight. Such patients appear well nourished for height but often have an elfin physiognomy. *Congenital hypothyroidism* is characterized by an open posterior fontanelle, umbilical hernia, macroglossia, mottled skin, prolonged physiologic jaundice, and severe constipation. Although height is short and bone age markedly delayed, weight is normal or increased for height. Characteristic physical stigmata assist diagnosis. *Congenital hyperthyroidism* results in failure to thrive because of poor feeding and frequent loose stools. Affected infants are irritable and hyperactive and have tachypnea, tachycardia, and diaphoresis. The presence of goiter makes this condition obvious. Patients with *adrenocortical insufficiency* grow poorly because of anorexia, vomiting, and diarrhea, which also predisposes them to dehydration. Basic serum chemistry tests reveal hyponatremia and hyperkalemia.

Other Organic Factors

In late infancy and early childhood, severe tonsillar and adenoidal hypertrophy with secondary sleep apnea assumes significance as a cause of impaired growth. Difficulty swallowing, whether mechanical (due to mass effect) or secondary due to tonsillopharyngeal pain; immune stress from chronic or recurrent adenotonsillar and middle ear infection; and the effect of sleep interruptions on nocturnal growth hormone secretion are contributing factors.

Nursing or baby bottle syndrome secondary to being put to bed with a bottle of milk or juice at night and poor dental hygienic practices (little or no brushing) tends to develop in late infancy or during the second year. When severe, numerous deep caries, enamel erosion, and abscesses make sucking and chewing painful, and the chronic infection adds immune stress, which also can contribute to inadequate intake and secondary growth impairment. This age group is also the most likely to be given large quantities of juice throughout the day, damping their hunger for more nutritious foods and milk.

Of all the organic causes of or contributors to failure to thrive, gastroesophageal reflux, whether with decreased feeding due to esophagitis or increased losses from vomiting, or both, and chronic nonspecific diarrhea are the major contributors. The latter may stem from diet (high juice, sorbitol intake), recurrent infection with its combination of immune stress and cycles of antibiotic administration, or malabsorption due to malnutrition, among other factors.

Whether of psychosocial, organic, or combined origin, growth failure in infancy and early childhood is the result of insufficient provision, retention, and/or absorption of nutrients—protein, fat, carbohydrates (and often micronutrients and vitamins)—to meet the needs for protein and energy required for normal growth and development of the child. This insufficiency can result from failure of the mother to offer adequate amounts of breast milk, formula, and, later, foods and milk or from inappropriate feeding (psychosocial); inadequate intake by the infant (anorexia, feeding refusal, feeding/swallowing difficulty); inability to retain adequate nutrition (vomiting/malabsorption); growth inefficiency (chronic infection, cardiopulmonary disease, hypothyroidism); or unusually high caloric needs (malignancy, chronic illness, hyperthyroidism).

Once undernutrition reaches a significant level (generally when weight, height, and head circumference growth are all impaired), the infant tends to become caught up in a vicious cycle: with malnutrition impairing immune function, which increases frequency/chronicity/severity of infection, which causes anorexia with decreased intake and decreased nutrient absorption while adding to caloric needs, thereby further exacerbating the malnutrition. In addition to this cycle there is another involving maternal–child interaction: the malnourished infant, regardless of cause, tends to become progressively more irritable and listless; less engaging and engageable; and, therefore, less rewarding to care for. Hence a combination of physical and psychosocial factors comes into play in all cases of severe failure to thrive.

Evaluation and Management of Failure to Thrive

Given the vicious cycles described earlier; given the prevalence of undernutrition, variably estimated at between 2% and 10% in the United States; given the high percentage of cases in which psychosocial factors are the primary cause or a prime contributor in an infant with organic disease; and given the stresses of caring for infants with severe organic disorders, it is essential in evaluating the infant with poor growth to obtain a thorough psychosocial and family history, as well as a detailed medical history (Table 6-11). The latter should include information regarding duration of the problem, mode of onset, and pattern of growth. Asking the parents how easy or difficult it is to take care of this child is also helpful. A complete review of systems (gastrointestinal,

Table 6-11	Findings in Failure to Thrive in Infancy			
Cause	**Approximate Percentage of All Cases**	**History**	**System-specific Physical Findings**	**System-specific Laboratory Studies**
Psychosocial	Up to 50% or more	Vague, inconsistent feeding history, history of bottle propping	None, may have soft neurologic signs	None
Central nervous system	13%	Poor feeding, gross developmental delay, vomiting	Grossly abnormal neurologic findings	Frequent gross abnormalities on EEG and CT scan or grossly abnormal tests of neuromuscular function
Gastrointestinal	10%	Chronic vomiting and/or diarrhea, abnormal stools, crying with feedings, nocturnal cough/snoring	Often negative, may have abdominal distention	Abnormal barium, pH probe, or endoscopic study; abnormal stool findings (pH, reducing substances, fat stain, Wright stain)
Cardiac	9%	Slow feeding, dyspnea and diaphoresis with feeding, restlessness and diaphoresis during sleep	Often cyanotic or have signs of congestive heart failure	Abnormal echocardiogram, ECG, catheterization findings
Genetic	8%	May have positive family history or a history of developmental delay	Often have facies typical of a syndrome, skeletal abnormalities, neurologic abnormalities, or visceromegaly	May have typical radiographic findings, chromosomal abnormalities, abnormal metabolic screens
Pulmonary	3.5%	Chronic or recurrent dyspnea with feedings, tachypnea	Grossly abnormal chest examination findings	Abnormal chest radiographs
Renal	3.5%	May be negative or may have history of polyuria	Often negative, may have flank masses	Abnormal urinalysis, frequently elevated BUN and creatinine, signs of renal osteodystrophy on radiographs
Endocrine	3.5%	With hypothyroidism, constipation and decreased activity level; with diabetes, polyuria, polydipsia	With hypothyroidism, no wasting but mottling, umbilical hernia, often open posterior fontanelle. With diabetes, often without specific abnormality, but may have signs of dehydration, ketotic breath, and hyperpnea. With hypopituitarism and isolated growth hormone deficiency, growth normal until 9 mo or later, then plateaus, but normal weight for height; delayed tooth eruption	Decreased T_4, increased TSH; glucosuria and hyperglycemia; abnormal pituitary function study results

BUN, blood urea nitrogen; CT, computed tomography; ECG, electrocardiogram; EEG, electroencephalogram; T_4, thyroxine; TSH, thyroid-stimulating hormone.

cardiorespiratory, neurologic, genitourinary, and endocrine), emphasizing intake and output, is often helpful. A thorough, specific, and concrete feeding and dietary history is essential, including the following:

1. Specific items offered and amounts taken at each feeding, with calorie counts

2. Times fed—regular or erratic, of sufficient frequency?

3. Feeding situation—place in home, fed by whom, held for feeding or bottle-propped

4. Feeding atmosphere—noise level, calm or chaotic, discord

5. Feeding method:
   - Breast—time at each breast, sufficient to empty?
     - Child's positioning
     - Milk production
     - Adequacy of mother's diet
   - Bottle—type of formula
     - How mixed?
     - How much fed, how often?
     - Total volume per 24 hours

6. Infant's demeanor/behavior during feedings:
   - Disinterest/anorexia
   - Refusal

7. Mother's dietary beliefs/concerns/fears

8. Home facilities for food storage/preparation

It is also highly important to observe the maternal–child interaction, especially during feedings, to assess the behavior and demeanor of each and their degree of mutuality, cueing, and attentiveness to cues. A thorough general physical examination will reveal gross abnormalities in patients with underlying CNS, cardiopulmonary, or genetic problems.

A few basic screening tests (complete blood count and differential; urinalysis and culture; stool pH, reducing substance, and fat stain; and urea nitrogen, electrolytes, and creatinine) can serve to rule out most other organic causes of failure to thrive. If onset of poor growth follows introduction of wheat into the diet, a celiac panel should be obtained. Table 6-11 summarizes the most common causes of infantile growth failure and their major findings on evaluation.

The earlier that growth impairment/undernutrition is recognized, evaluated as to cause(s), and treatment instituted, the better, because the more long-standing the problem, the more difficult it is to treat, and the greater the risk of long-term sequelae, especially in cases of neglect and primary psychosocial failure to thrive. The latter include developmental delay and cognitive deficits secondary to impaired brain growth and inadequate stimulation that may not be fully reversible with therapy and early intervention. There is evidence that even if good nutrition is reestablished and catch-up growth is achieved, failure to improve emotional nurturing perpetuates developmental delays. An increased incidence of behavior problems and of affective and motivational disorders has also been found later in childhood in children who had psychosocial failure to thrive as infants and toddlers.

Effective treatment depends on helping the mother (in a supportive and nonthreatening manner) understand the nature of the problem, her child's nutritional needs, and the need for increased caloric density to accomplish catch-up growth (1.5 to 2 times normal requirements), thereby enlisting her as part of the treatment team and the process. This must be supplemented by education regarding her baby's emotional and developmental needs and the importance of warm, consistent nurturing. The process may also necessitate helping her to get and accept help with feeding support, early intervention

services, housing, and mental health issues. This is often best accomplished by a specialized multidisciplinary team.

EMOTIONAL ABUSE

It must be emphasized that emotional abuse accompanies *all* of the other forms of abuse described previously. It can also occur in isolation and can range from inattentiveness to frank rejection, scapegoating, or even terrorizing. Because isolated emotional abuse is difficult to document, leaving no visible stigmata, it accounts for the smallest proportion of reported cases. Victims may present with chronic severe anxiety, hyperactivity, depression, agitation, or frank psychotic reactions. Many victims are socially withdrawn, have trouble relating to peers, and generally perform poorly in school. Low self-esteem is the rule. If emotional abuse is suspected, psychological testing and psychiatric examination may prove helpful in confirming its existence and directing treatment.

REPORTING

Each state has regulations requiring health care providers, hospitals, and professionals involved in child care to report suspected cases of abuse and neglect to CPS agencies. Although these regulations are similar, they vary from state to state, and clinicians should become familiar with the regulations in their respective states. The suspected abuse or neglect must result from the acts or omissions of a parent, stepparent, or other person in a caretaking role. For abuse to be reported, *reasonable* grounds for suspicion are required, not clinical certainty. There is no penalty for reporting in good faith after careful evaluation, but there can be severe penalties for failure to report.

Many states require physicians and hospitals to notify police regarding cases involving severe abuse (potentially lifethreatening or threatening a vital sense organ or limb), as well as sexual abuse. This can be done by the clinician evaluating the patient or by CPS, but, unfortunately, the latter often do not notify police promptly. Cases of stranger rape, physical assault, or abuse perpetrated by a person in a noncaretaking role must be reported to law enforcement and not CPS because such situations usually do not involve caretakers. CPS should be notified, however, if it is suspected that parental negligence was also contributory.

Pediatricians may be unaware of the definition of statutory rape, which varies by state. In these cases a child may "consent" to intercourse but may, by legal definition, not be considered old enough to give consent. These laws usually specify the age difference between the sexual partners. Particularly when dealing with adolescents, who may hesitate to disclose either consensual activity or sexual assault for fear of mandatory reporting to the police and having to testify, one must consider what, in the clinician's best judgment, is in the best interest of the patient, given the information at hand. In rare instances the child may be at further risk if the physician reports the abuse (e.g., believable threats of suicide by the patient). In those instances one must document reasons for failure to report the event to the authorities and try to ensure follow-up with the patient.

CONCLUSION

Although treatment and follow-up are beyond the scope of an atlas of physical diagnosis, a few additional points bear emphasis. Use of a team approach including physicians, nurses, and social workers or psychologists greatly assists evaluation of victims of abuse and their families, and it reduces the burden on any one health care worker. Reporting requirements necessitate only reasonable grounds for suspicion and place the onus of full investigation on state agencies. Unfortunately, close follow-up, although highly important, is often neglected, especially when patients get caught up in large bureaucratic systems. Having improved our performance on identification and documentation of cases, we must increasingly apply ourselves to assisting better long-term follow-up to ensure that victims not only are safe from harm but also have access to medical, educational, and mental health services to help them cope with, and when possible, overcome physical and emotional sequelae, thereby improving outcomes.

Bibliography

Ablin DS, Greenspan A, Reinhart M, et al: Differentiation of child abuse from osteogenesis imperfecta, *Am J Radiol* 154:1035-1046, 1990.

Ablin S, Sane SM: Nonaccidental injury: Confusion with temporary brittle bone disease and mild osteogenesis imperfecta, *Pediatr Radiol* 27:111-113, 1997.

Adams JA, Kaplan RA, Starling SP, et al: Guidelines for medical care of children who may have been sexually abused, *J Pediatr Adolesc Gynecol* 20:163-172, 2007.

Alexander R, Crabbe L, Sato Y, et al: Serial abuse in children who are shaken, *Am J Dis Child* 144:58-60, 1990a.

Alexander R, Sato Y, Smith W, et al: Incidence of impact trauma with cranial injuries ascribed to shaking, *Am J Dis Child* 144:724-726, 1990b.

Alexander RC, Schor DP, Smith WL: Magnetic resonance imaging of intracranial injuries for child abuse, *J Pediatr* 109:975-979, 1986.

American Academy of Pediatrics, Committee on Child Abuse and Neglect: Distinguishing sudden infant death syndrome from child abuse fatalities, *Pediatrics* 107:437-441, 2001.

Amodio J, Spektor V, Pramanik B, et al: Spontaneous development of bilateral subdural hematomas in an infant with benign infantile hydrocephalus: color Doppler assessment of vessels traversing extra-axial spaces, *Pediatr Radiol* 35:1113-1117, 2005.

Bauer CH, editor: Failure to thrive, *Pediatr Ann* 7:737-795, 1978.

Bays J, Jenny C: Genital and anal conditions confused with child sexual abuse trauma, *Am J Dis Child* 144:1319-1322, 1990.

Berenson AB, Heger AH, Hayes JM, et al: Appearance of the hymen in prepubertal girls, *Pediatrics* 89:387-394, 1992.

Case ME, Graham MA, Corey Handy T, et al: National Association of Medical Examiners Ad Hoc Committee on Shaken Baby Syndrome: Position paper on fatal abusive head injuries in infants and young children, *Am J Forens Med Pathol* 22:112-122, 2001.

Centers for Disease Control and Prevention: CDC Sexual assault and STD guidelines, 2010: Sexual assault or abuse of children. Available from http://www.cdc.gov/std/treatment/2010/sexual-assault.htm#a2

Chadwick DL: The diagnosis of inflicted injury in infants and young children, *Pediatr Ann* 21:477-483, 1992.

Chadwick DL, Berkowitz CD, Kerns DL, et al: *Color atlas of child sexual abuse*, Chicago, 1989, Year Book.

Chadwick DL, Chin S, Salerno C, et al: Deaths from falls in children: how far is fatal? *J Trauma* 31:1353-1355, 1991.

Christian CW, Lavelle JM, DeJong AR, et al: Forensic evidence findings in prepubertal victims of sexual assault, *Pediatrics* 106:100-104, 2000.

Coant PN, Kornberg AE, Brody AS, et al: Markers for occult liver injury in cases of physical abuse in children, *Pediatrics* 89:274-278, 1992.

Dubowitz H, Bross DC: The pediatrician's documentation of child maltreatment, *Am J Dis Child* 146:596-599, 1992.

Duhaime AC, Gennarelli TA, Thibault LE, et al: The shaken baby syndrome: a clinical, pathological and biomechanical study, *J Neurosurg* 66:409-415, 1987.

Ewing-Cobbs L, Prasad M, Kramer L, et al: Acute neuroradiologic findings in young children with inflicted or noninflicted traumatic brain injury, *Childs Nerv Syst* 16:25-34, 2000.

Finkelhor D: Current information on the scope and nature of child sexual abuse, *Future Child* 4:31-53, 1994.

Finkelhor D: Improving research, policy, and practice to understand child sexual abuse, *JAMA* 280:1864-1865, 1998.

Gilliand MGF, Folberg R: Shaken babies—some have no impact injuries, *J Forens Sci* 41:114-116, 1996.

Girardet RG, Lahoti S, Howard LA, et al: The epidemiology of sexually transmitted infections in suspected child victims of sexual assault, *Pediatrics* 124:79-86, 2009.

Green FC, editor: Incest and sexual abuse, *Pediatr Ann* 8:1-103, 1979.

Hadley MN, Sonntag VKH, Rekate HL, et al: The infant whiplash-shake injury syndrome: a clinical and pathological study, *Neurosurgery* 24:536-540, 1989.

Heger A, Emans SJ, Muram D: *Evaluation of the sexually abused child*, ed 2, New York, 2000, Oxford University Press.

Helfer RE: The neglect of our children, *Pediatr Clin North Am* 37:923-942, 1990.

Helfer RE, Kempe HC, editors: *The battered child*, ed 5, Chicago, 1997, University of Chicago Press.

Herman-Giddens ME, Brown G, Verbiest S, et al: Underascertainment of child abuse mortality in the United States, *JAMA* 282:463-467, 1999.

Hodge D, Ludwig S: Child homicide: Emergency department recognition, *Pediatr Emerg Care* 1:3-6, 1985.

Hoffman GF, Athanossopoulos S, Burlina AB, et al: Clinical course, early diagnosis, treatment and prevention of disease in glutaryl-CoA dehydrogenase deficiency, *Neuropediatrics* 27:115-123, 1996.

Homer MD, Ludwig S: Categorization of etiology of failure to thrive, *Am J Dis Child* 135:848-851, 1981.

Hymel KP, Hall CA: Diagnosing pediatric head injury, *Pediatr Ann* 34:358-370, 2005.

Hymel KP, Jenny C: Abusive spiral fractures of the humerus: a videotaped exception, *Arch Pediatr Adolesc Med* 150:226-227, 1996.

Jenny C, Hymel KP, Ritzen A, et al: Analysis of missed cases of abusive head trauma, *JAMA* 281:621-627, 1999.

Jenny C, Committee on Child Abuse and Neglect: Evaluating infants and young children with multiple fractures, *Pediatrics* 118:1299-1303, 2006.

Johnson CF: Inflicted injury versus accidental injury, *Pediatr Clin North Am* 37:791-814, 1990.

Kellogg ND, Committee on Child Abuse and Neglect: Clinical report—the evaluation of sexual behaviors in children, *Pediatrics* 124:992-998, 2009.

Kessler DB, Dawson P, editors: *Failure to thrive and pediatric undernutrition, a transdisciplinary approach*, Baltimore, 1999, Paul H. Brookes.

Kleinman P: *Diagnostic imaging of child abuse*, ed 2, St. Louis, 1998, Mosby.

Kleinman PK, Blackbourne BD, Marks SC, et al: Radiologic contributions to the investigation and prosecution of cases of fatal infant abuse, *N Engl J Med* 320:507-511, 1989.

Krugman RD: Recognition of sexual abuse in children, *Pediatr Rev* 8:25, 1986.

Lavy U, Bauer CH: Pathophysiology of failure to thrive and gastrointestinal disorders, *Pediatr Ann* 7:10-33, 1978.

Levin AV, Magnusson MR, Rafto SE, et al: Shaken baby syndrome diagnosed by magnetic resonance imaging, *Pediatr Emerg Care* 5:181-186, 1989.

McCann J, Voris J, Simon M, et al: Perianal findings in prepubertal children selected for non-abuse: a descriptive study, *Child Abuse Negl* 13:179-193, 1989.

McCann J, Wells R, Simon M, et al: Genital findings in prepubertal girls selected for non-abuse: a descriptive study, *Pediatrics* 86:428-439, 1990.

McCann JJ, Kerns DL: *The anatomy of child and adolescent sexual abuse: a CD-ROM atlas/reference*, St. Louis, 1999, InterCorp.

Morris AAM, Hoffmann GF, Naughton ER, et al: Glutaric aciduria and suspected child abuse, *Arch Dis Child* 80:404-405, 1999.

Ophthalmology Child Abuse Working Party, Royal College of Ophthalmologists: Child abuse and the eye, *Eye* 13:3-10, 1999.

Paradise JE: The medical evaluation of the sexually abused child, *Pediatr Clin North Am* 37:839-862, 1990.

Piatt JH Jr: A pitfall in the diagnosis of child abuse, external hydrocephalus, subdural hematomas and retinal hemorrhages, *Neurosurg Focus* 7:4, 1999. Available at http://www.aans.org/education/journal/neurosurgical/oct99/7-4-4.asp

Pierce MC, Bertocci GE, Janosky JE, et al: Femur fractures resulting from stair falls among children: an injury plausibility model, *Pediatrics* 115:1712-1722, 2005.

Pierce MC, Bertocci GE, Vogeley E, et al: Evaluating long bone fractures in children: a biomechanical approach with illustrative cases, *Child Abuse Negl* 28:505-524, 2004.

Reece RM: Unusual manifestations of child abuse, *Pediatr Clin North Am* 37:905-922, 1990.

Reece RM, Ludwig S, editors: *Child abuse: medical diagnosis and management*, ed 2, Philadelphia, 2001, Lippincott Williams & Wilkins.

Reece RM, Sege R: Childhood head injuries, accidental or inflicted? *Arch Pediatr Adolesc Med* 154:11-22, 2000.

Reiber GD: Fatal falls in childhood: How far must children fall to sustain fatal head injury? Report of cases and review of the literature, *Am J Forens Med Pathol* 14:201-207, 1993.

Rosenberg NM, Marino D: Frequency of suspected abuse/neglect in burn patients, *Pediatr Emerg Care* 5:219-221, 1989.

Rosenn DW, Loeb LS, Jura MB: Differentiation of organic from nonorganic failure to thrive syndrome in infancy, *Pediatrics* 66:698-704, 1980.

Schwartz ID: Failure to thrive: an old nemesis in the new millennium, *Pediatr Rev* 21:257-264, 2000.

Sills RH: Failure to thrive, *Am J Dis Child* 132:967-969, 1978.

Starling SP, Holden JR, Jenny C: Abusive head trauma: the relationship of perpetrators to their victims, *Pediatrics* 95:259-262, 1995.

Stephenson T, Bialas Y: Estimation of the age of bruising, *Arch Dis Child* 74:53-55, 1996.

Sugar NF, Taylor JA, Feldman KW: Bruises in infants and toddlers: those who don't cruise rarely bruise, *Arch Pediatr Adolesc Med* 153:399-403, 1999.

West MH, Billings JD, Frair J: Ultraviolet photography: bite marks on human skin and suggested technique for exposure and development of reflective ultraviolet photography, *J Forensic Sci* 32:1204-1213, 1987.

Woodlong BA, Kossosis PD: Sexual misuse, *Pediatr Clin North Am* 28:481-499, 1981.

RHEUMATOLOGY

Kathryn Torok | Paul Rosen

The rheumatic diseases of childhood are a heterogeneous group of disorders usually manifested by signs and symptoms of inflammation. Although significant progress has been made in the understanding of the pathophysiology of these disorders, their etiologies remain largely unknown. Despite available laboratory markers, the cornerstones of diagnosis remain the history and physical examination. Knowledge of the natural history of these disorders is also helpful for diagnosis and management.

The majority of the common rheumatic diseases that occur during childhood are classified as inflammatory arthritis or enthesitis syndromes, connective tissue disorders, and vasculitides, although overlap does occur. Noninflammatory disorders that cause musculoskeletal pain include joint hypermobility syndromes and pain amplification syndromes. This chapter illustrates the more distinctive clinical features of these unique disorders.

MUSCULOSKELETAL HISTORY

A meticulous rheumatologic history is the foundation of accurate diagnosis (Table 7-1). The exact location that the patient complains about should be given careful attention. Muscle, bone, and tendon or ligament insertion pain (enthesitis) may be interpreted as joint pain unless the clinician asks specifically for the parent or child to describe the symptoms. Often it is helpful for the clinician to ask the child to point with one finger to the site of maximal discomfort.

The patient's age and gender serve as initial guides to a possible etiology. The clinician must then try to discern whether musculoskeletal symptoms are inflammatory or mechanical. Pain that involves swelling, morning stiffness, warmth, redness, and improvement with movement is indicative of inflammation. Pain that is worse at the end of the day, worse with activity, and lacking persistent swelling is more mechanical in nature.

A history of prior illnesses, medications, immunizations, trauma, and bites, and the acuteness of symptoms, can be a clue to diagnosis. Joint pain (arthralgia) is a common symptom of childhood. However, the symptoms associated with inflammatory joint pain (arthritis) are uncommon in the pediatric population. In children with arthritis, the duration and pattern of the symptoms can be telling. Acute migratory arthritis affecting large and small joints is seen in acute rheumatic fever (ARF). Arthritis resolving within a few weeks is consistent with a reactive arthritis (i.e., *Streptococcus*, Epstein-Barr virus, parvovirus B19). An additive arthritis persisting for more than 6 weeks is consistent with a chronic form of arthritis (i.e., juvenile idiopathic arthritis [JIA]). The chronic arthritides cause indolent and persistent joint changes. Joint stiffness, or gel phenomenon, can be seen not only in the morning, but also after a child has napped or been immobile in a vehicle. As the day progresses, the child with chronic arthritis may become more limber and may even appear normal.

Differences in the quality and duration of arthritis exist among the various rheumatoid diseases. The arthritis in patients with systemic lupus erythematosus (SLE) may feature less swelling with more intense pain, whereas the arthritis of children with JIA is characterized by more stiffness and swelling and less pain. The joint pain of the patient with SLE may be intermittent in nature. The joint stiffness of JIA is usually a daily occurrence without treatment. The joints of ARF can also be distinguished from those of JIA by the presence of exquisite pain that is out of proportion to physical findings. A rapid response to nonsteroidal antiinflammatory drugs further supports a clinical impression of ARF.

A careful family history can be helpful. Children with an extensive family history of autoimmune diseases in their first-degree relatives are at slightly greater risk for developing a rheumatologic condition. Because these diseases are complex genetic traits, there is often little direct genetic linkage. Some diseases such as psoriasis, SLE, acute rheumatic fever, and autoimmune thyroiditis have a stronger genetic penetrance than other rheumatic diseases. Other conditions have little or no penetrance. A child with first-degree relatives with adult rheumatoid arthritis is not at increased risk for developing juvenile idiopathic arthritis.

PHYSICAL EXAMINATION OF THE MUSCULOSKELETAL SYSTEM

The only way to confirm the diagnosis of JIA is to demonstrate arthritis by physical examination of the joints. The elucidation of joint inflammation by examination may be the only indication of a rheumatic disease. Because most joints are near the surface of the body, the examiner has an excellent opportunity to obtain significant information about many diseases. A rheumatologic diagnosis requires a thorough joint examination and meticulous general physical examination with special attention to the skin, mucous membranes, nail beds, and muscles.

The physical examination begins with observation of the child and parents walking from the waiting area to the examination room. The physician notes the general appearance of the patient and interactions among family members. Nutritional status and an incremental graph of height and weight must be carefully documented. Certain skin and mucous membrane changes provide valuable information (Table 7-2). Muscle strength must be evaluated first by attempting to elicit a Gowers sign (Fig. 7-1) and then by testing resistance capacity of individual muscle groups and grading them on a standard scale (Table 7-3).

The hallmark of a good physical examination of the musculoskeletal system is a careful examination of the joints, consisting of inspection, palpation, and measurement of each joint's range of motion. The examiner should develop a standard order for examining joints and follow the same pattern so that no joints are missed. Large effusions are easily felt and often ballotable; synovial hypertrophy may be more subtle and has a doughy, spongy, boggy feel. Synovial outpouchings are common in children with arthritis and can resemble ganglion cysts, especially in the wrists and ankles. A ganglion cyst does

Table 7-1	Distinguishing Features of the Rheumatologic History

1. Musculoskeletal pain
2. Joint swelling
3. Morning stiffness that improves with activity
4. Constitutional symptoms (e.g., recurrent fevers, fatigue, weight loss, growth disturbance)
5. Ocular symptoms (e.g., eye redness, visual change)
6. Cardiopulmonary symptoms (e.g., dyspnea, chest pain, hemoptysis)
7. Gastrointestinal symptoms (e.g., dysphagia, abdominal pain, melena)
8. Neurologic symptoms (e.g., vascular headache, weakness, seizure, altered mental status)
9. Cutaneous and mucous membrane symptoms (e.g., photosensitive rash; Raynaud phenomenon; oral, nasal, or genital ulcerations; xerostomia; and keratoconjunctivitis sicca)
10. Psychosocial history (e.g., family dysfunction, fibromyalgia, depression, chronic pain)
11. Family history (e.g., psoriasis, rheumatic fever, systemic lupus erythematosus)

not cause pain. In children with arthritis the findings may be subtle and often appreciated only because of pain or decreased range of motion.

Temporomandibular Joint

The temporomandibular joint (TMJ) permits three types of motion: (1) opening and closing of the jaw, (2) anterior and posterior motion, and (3) lateral or side-to-side motion; each type should be carefully measured. Careful observation of the TMJ may reveal micrognathia, a clue to the diagnosis of JIA (Fig. 7-2).

Table 7-2	Mucocutaneous Signs of the Rheumatic Diseases

1. Malar rash
2. Discoid rash—rare in childhood; often heals with atrophy and scarring
3. Periungual erythema
4. Telangiectasias
5. Fingertip ulcers
6. Alopecia and fracturing of frontal hair
7. Heliotrope-violaceous eyelid edema
8. Gottron papules—scaly, symmetrical, erythematous papules over MCP and PIP joints
9. Skin thickening, contractures, calcinosis
10. Palpable purpura
11. Livedo reticularis—lacy, fishnet appearance of skin
12. Evanescent salmon-pink rash
13. Erythema nodosum—panniculitis with septal inflammation
14. Rheumatoid extensor nodules
15. Psoriasis
16. Onycholysis (lifting up of the distal portion of the nail), nail pits
17. Balanitis circinata—small, shallow, painless ulcers of the glans penis and urethral meatus
18. Keratoderma blennorrhagicum—clear vesicles on erythematous bases that progress to macules, papules, and keratotic nodules

MCP, metacarpophalangeal; PIP, proximal interphalangeal.

Table 7-3	Standard Muscle Strength Grading

Muscle Grade	Description
5	Complete range of motion against gravity with full resistance
4	Complete range of motion against gravity with some resistance
3	Complete range of motion against gravity
2	Complete range of motion with gravity eliminated
1	Evidence of slight contractility; no joint motion
0	No evidence of contractility

Cervical Spine

In children the neck can be extended so that the head can touch the back and flexed so that the chin touches the chest; 90-degree rotation and 45-degree lateral bending in each direction is also normal (Fig. 7-3).

Cricoarytenoid Joint

The cricoarytenoid joint is rarely involved in JIA but can present a life-threatening complication if edema and scarring interfere with respiration. An early symptom is hoarseness because arytenoid movement is important to phonation.

Acromioclavicular Joint

The acromioclavicular joint is formed by the lateral end of the clavicle and the medial margin of the acromial process of the scapula; it allows for "shrugging" of the shoulders.

Sternoclavicular Joint

The two sternoclavicular (SC) joints are the only points of articulation between the shoulder girdle and trunk; they move with any motion of the shoulders. The SC joints can be involved in the spondyloarthropathies, in which they become ankylosed (fused).

Shoulder

The shoulder is usually involved only in severe polyarticular JIA. It is an extremely complicated joint, but range of active motion can be conveniently tested by having the child perform three simple maneuvers (Fig. 7-4). These maneuvers require 180 degrees of abduction, 45 degrees of adduction, 90 degrees of flexion, and 45 degrees of external rotation of the glenohumeral joint and related articulations.

Elbow

The examiner must distinguish swelling in the olecranon bursa from involvement of the true elbow joint. The elbow is frequently affected in all forms of JIA and is the most common upper extremity joint affected in spondyloarthropathy. Range of motion of the elbow is easily tested (Figs. 7-5 and 7-6).

Wrist and Hand

Children do not require much extension to perform most activities of daily living and thus can lose strength and mobility in the wrist, which may go unnoticed. The wrist is frequently affected in childhood arthritis, and thus a careful range of motion examination is essential. Normal is 70 degrees

Figure 7-1 Gowers sign. The child begins in a prone position and is asked to stand. The child is unable to rise without rolling over and progressively pushing to the knees and using hands to push up to a standing position.

Figure 7-2 Micrognathia. Note the underdevelopment of the jaw and retracted chin. This occurs in patients with juvenile idiopathic arthritis.

of extension, 80 degrees of flexion (Fig. 7-7), 20 degrees radially, and 30 degrees to the ulnar side.

Metacarpophalangeal (MCP) joints extend 30 degrees and flex 90 degrees. Normal range of motion for the proximal interphalangeal (PIP) joints is illustrated in Figure 7-8.

Hip

The normal hip examination consists of 45 degrees of abduction and 20 degrees of adduction (Fig. 7-9) with the knee bent 20 degrees. The hip can extend 30 degrees, externally rotate to 45 degrees, and internally rotate to 35 degrees. An increase in lumbar lordosis may be the first sign of decreased hip flexion. Normally, hip flexion reaches to about 135 degrees (Fig. 7-10).

Knee

The knee is the joint most commonly involved in childhood arthritis. Swelling of the knee may be diffuse or localized to the suprapatellar bursa, which communicates with the true knee joint, or to the gastrocnemius-semimembranosus bursa (Baker cyst) (Fig. 7-11), which may dissect down the leg. The patella must be carefully evaluated for "roughening of the undersurface" indicative of chondromalacia patellae, which is not uncommon in teenage girls. Normal knee range of motion is illustrated in Figure 7-12.

Figure 7-3   A child's neck normally can be extended so that the head touches the back **(A)**, flexed so that the chin touches the chest **(B)**, rotated 90 degrees **(C)**, and tilted laterally 45 degrees **(D)**.

Figure 7-4   Testing range of motion of the shoulder. **A,** Place hand behind head and touch opposite shoulder (external rotation and abduction). **B,** Place back of hand behind the back and touch opposite scapula. **C,** Place hand on opposite shoulder. (Movements in **B** and **C** test internal rotation and adduction.)

Figure 7-5   Supination and pronation of the elbow. The elbow should be held flexed at 90 degrees and against the body. **A,** The fist is held in a neutral vertical position and then **B,** rotated 90 degrees in pronation and **C,** 90 degrees in supination.

Figure 7-6   **A,** The elbow should extend from 0 degrees with the arm held down and **B,** flex to 150 degrees.

Figure 7-7 The wrist should extend to 70 degrees **(A)** from a neutral position **(B)** and flex to 80 degrees **(C)**.

Figure 7-8 The metacarpophalangeal joints can extend 30 degrees **(A)** and flex 90 degrees **(B)**. Note the normal range of motion for the proximal interphalangeal joints **(C)**.

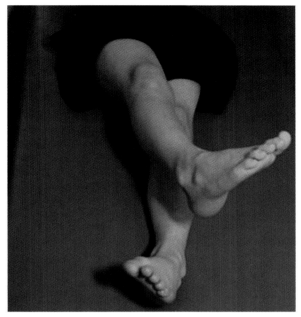

Figure 7-9 The normal hip can be adducted 20 degrees.

Figure 7-10 The normal hip can be flexed 135 degrees.

Figure 7-11 Arthrogram demonstrates communication of Baker's cyst with synovial cavity of the knee joint.

Figure 7-12 Normal knee range of motion extends from 10 degrees of hyperextension *(left knee)* to 130 degrees of flexion *(right knee).*

Foot and Ankle

The foot and ankle can offer valuable clues to the diagnosis of arthritis in childhood. Evidence of Achilles tendinitis or plantar fasciitis can suggest a spondyloarthropathy. First metatarsophalangeal (MTP) joint involvement is also a strong clue to the diagnosis of a spondyloarthropathy. Normal ranges of motion of the true ankle joint and subtalar joint are illustrated in Figure 7-13, and decreased range of motion is common in oligoarticular JIA.

Careful flexion and extension of all interphalangeal joints of the feet must be evaluated, especially the first MTP joint

(80 degrees of extension to 35 degrees of flexion). The MTP joints should be squeezed enough to wrinkle the skin.

Leg Length

Leg length discrepancy (Fig. 7-14) is common in JIA because of hyperemia of an affected joint and subsequent overgrowth. Compensatory scoliosis may also develop.

Thoracic Spine/Lumbar Spine/Sacroiliac Joints

The entire spine including all spinous processes should be carefully palpated to elicit tenderness. Flexion, extension, and lateral motion of the spine should be measured, using S1 as the focal point. Thirty degrees of extension and 50 degrees of lateral motion are normal. Careful examination of the sacroiliac joints (Fig. 7-15) may give an important clue to the diagnosis of a spondyloarthropathy in an adolescent. Chest expansion, occiput-to-wall, and finger-to-floor measurements (Fig. 7-16) are useful in monitoring patients with inflammatory back disease. To detect limitation of forward flexion of the lumbar spine, the Schober test is quite useful. The patient is asked to stand erect, and the skin overlying the spinous process of the fifth lumbar vertebra (usually at the level of the "dimples of Venus") and another point 10 cm above in the midline are marked. The patient is asked to maximally bend the spine forward without bending the knees. If the lumbar spine is mobile, the distance between the two points increases by 5 cm or more; that is, the distance between the two points becomes equal to or greater than 15 cm. An increase of 4 cm or less indicates decreased mobility of the lumbar spine.

JUVENILE IDIOPATHIC ARTHRITIS

Juvenile idiopathic arthritis (JIA) is the most common rheumatic disease in children. JIA is a broad term that is used to describe chronic arthritis in children. The group of diseases placed under the JIA rubric combines diverse entities, generally divided into seven categories: (1) oligoarthritis (persistent or extended), (2) polyarthritis (rheumatoid factor negative), (3) polyarthritis (rheumatoid factor positive), (4) enthesitis-related arthritis (ERA), (5) psoriatic arthritis, (6) systemic arthritis, and (7) undifferentiated arthritis. The JIA onset type is based on the disease presentation during the first 6 months of illness. The presenting subtype of JIA may differ from the child's ultimate disease course. Of note, no laboratory tests, such as a positive anti-nuclear antibody or rheumatoid factor, are required to make a diagnosis of JIA.

The incidence of JIA is approximately 10 cases per 100,000 population per year. The prevalence of JIA is approximately 100 per 100,000 population. JIA in the United States is estimated to affect more than 300,000 children.

Figure 7-13 The ankle normally can flex to 20 degrees **(A)** and extend to 45 degrees **(B)**. Inversion occurs to 30 degrees **(C)**, and eversion occurs to 20 degrees **(D)**.

Figure 7-14 Leg length is measured from the anterosuperior iliac spine to the medial malleolus.

Figure 7-15   Clinical tests for sacroiliitis. **A,** Application of direct pressure by thumbs over the sacroiliac joints to elicit tenderness. **B,** With knee flexed and hip flexed, abducted, and externally rotated, downward pressure is applied on the flexed knee and the contralateral anterosuperior iliac spine. **C,** Compression of the pelvis with patient lying on side. **D,** Patient lying supine, with flexed knee pushed maximally toward the opposite shoulder. **E,** Anterosuperior iliac spines forced laterally apart.

The first clear description of these entities was presented by George Still in 1897. He postulated multiple etiologies for childhood arthritis, and this concept is still supported today. All forms of JIA feature inflammation of the synovial tissue as one of the cardinal features. Synovium is usually hypertrophied, and joint effusions may occur. On physical examination (Fig. 7-17), joint swelling, loss of normal anatomical landmarks, tenderness, decreased joint mobility (Fig. 7-18), warmth, erythema, and joint deformity may be noted. It is typical for the child with JIA to have more joint stiffness than pain. Symptoms often develop gradually over a period of weeks or months before evaluation. Morning stiffness is often reported. The duration of morning stiffness correlates well with the degree of inflammation in children with JIA. Immobility and weather changes may exacerbate symptoms, although they have no impact on the underlying inflammatory component of the disease. Although arthralgia alone can be the initial presentation of JIA, the diagnosis cannot be confirmed without the presence of arthritis on physical examination.

Despite objective signs of arthritis, the patient with JIA may not experience pain. When inflammation persists for a long enough period of time, destruction of the articular surface and bony structures may occur (Fig. 7-19). Because of the poor regenerative properties of articular cartilage, these deformities are usually permanent. Fortunately, most cases of JIA are not associated with permanent joint deformity.

Oligoarthritis (Persistent or Extended)

Oligoarthritis is defined as arthritis in one to four joints. The large joints (knees, ankles, and elbows) are often asymmetrically involved. Systemic symptoms do not dominate the clinical picture. Persistent disease affects no more than four joints throughout the disease. Extended disease affects more than four joints after the first 6 months.

Polyarthritis (Rheumatoid Factor Negative)

Polyarthritis accounts for approximately 30% of all children with JIA. To make the diagnosis, five or more joints must be involved in the absence of prominent systemic signs and symptoms. Rheumatoid factor–negative polyarthritis can occur at age 1 year, with a peak incidence at age 2 years.

The onset of polyarthritis may be insidious or acute. Children with seronegative disease generally have a better prognosis, but a subset can progress to joint destruction and flexion contractures. Any synovial joint may be involved in the inflammatory process including the knees, wrists, elbows, ankles, small joints of the feet, and proximal interphalangeal (PIP) and MCP joints. The lumbosacral spine is usually spared.

Polyarthritis (Rheumatoid Factor Positive)

The seropositive group is believed to be nearly identical to the adult entity of rheumatoid arthritis (RA). Although onset of rheumatoid factor–positive polyarthritis can occur as early as 8 years of age, it usually occurs in the early teens and girls predominate. Whereas 80% of all adult patients are

Figure 7-16   With feet together, the child bends forward. The measurement from floor to fingertip is recorded and compared with subsequent examination.

Figure 7-17   Juvenile idiopathic arthritis (JIA). **A,** Erythema of the knee in a patient with systemic-onset JIA (Still disease). **B,** Swelling and inflammation of the small joints of the hands in a patient with polyarticular JIA. Note the inability to fully extend the fingers. **C,** Swelling of the right thumb interphalangeal joint. **D,** Right knee swelling in a patient with pauciarticular JIA.

seropositive, only 5% of children with JIA are positive for rheumatoid factor. The seropositive subgroup tends to progress to destructive synovitis and a prolonged chronic course.

Seropositive disease provides some additional clues to diagnosis. The subcutaneous nodules that occur in seropositive disease are firm, nontender nodules on the skin surface with a predilection for pressure points or extensor areas. The most common location is the elbow, but the nodules also occur on the heels, hands, knees, ears, scapula, sacrum, and buttocks. Other features of seropositive disease may include cutaneous vasculitis, Felty syndrome (leukopenia and splenomegaly), and Sjögren syndrome (keratoconjunctivitis sicca and xerostomia with or without parotid swelling).

Psoriatic Arthritis

Psoriatic arthritis is diagnosed in a child with arthritis and psoriasis. Criteria are also met when a child with arthritis has two of the three findings: dactylitis ("sausage digit"), nail

Figure 7-18   Oligoarticular juvenile idiopathic arthritis. **A,** A 2-year-old girl with arthritis of the left knee. Note that the left lower extremity is bent at the knee as she bears weight on the extended right lower extremity. **B,** A closer look at the knees reveals left knee swelling. **C,** The left knee can be extended only to 35 degrees (secondary to a flexion contracture).

Figure 7-19   Juvenile idiopathic arthritis. Demineralization of the left femur and tibia with soft tissue swelling and hypertrophy of the epiphyses secondary to hyperemia.

pitting (or onycholysis), or psoriasis in a first-degree relative. Whereas the forms of arthritis previously discussed have weak genetic penetrance, psoriasis and its related disorders are often found through a given family's pedigree. A patient may often present to their physician with just dactylitis of one or multiple toes. In such a situation, in addition to a detailed joint examination, a detailed skin and nail examination should be performed (Fig. 7-20). Special attention should be paid to the scalp, the umbilicus, posterior ears, gluteal cleft, and shins.

Enthesitis-related Arthritis

Arthritis with enthesitis features inflammation of the tendon and tendon insertion site (i.e., Achilles). The other features that distinguish this disease group include sacroiliitis, HLA-B27 positivity, male predominance, and acute uveitis (presenting with eye pain and redness). This group also has a strong family predominance with first-degree relatives with ankylosing spondylitis, inflammatory bowel disease, and Reiter syndrome. A male patient older than 6 years presenting with arthritis should raise suspicion for ERA. Younger patients present with peripheral arthritis. Axial arthritis affecting the spine often does not present until the late teen years or second decade.

Systemic Arthritis

Systemic arthritis (Still disease) accounts for approximately 10% of all children with JIA. Fever, rash, irritability, arthritis, and visceral involvement dominate the clinical presentation. The patient's temperature usually rises to greater than 39° C, and this often occurs twice daily in a double quotidian pattern. Chills are associated with fever, but rigors rarely occur.

Although the late afternoon is a typical time for a temperature rise, many other patterns may occur. Other manifestations of systemic arthritis, such as rash and joint symptoms, may wax and wane during febrile periods. A helpful clinical feature during the febrile phase is one subnormal temperature during every 24-hour period, which suggests JIA.

The rash of JIA is macular, 2 to 6 mm in diameter, evanescent, and salmon or red in color, with slightly irregular margins (Fig. 7-21). An area of central clearing often exists. The rash usually occurs on the trunk and proximal extremities, but it may also be distal in distribution, with palms and soles affected. Although the rash generally does not produce discomfort, some older patients report pruritus. Superficial mild trauma to the skin, exposure to warmth, and emotional upset may precipitate the rash (Koebner phenomenon). Arthritis may not occur invariably at the onset of systemic arthritis, and thus the diagnosis may not be readily apparent. When fever of unknown origin is the sole initial presentation of systemic arthritis, it must remain a diagnosis of exclusion until the clinician observes inflammatory arthritis during the physical examination. Arthralgia and myalgia can be prominent early, as can hepatosplenomegaly and lymphadenopathy. Serositis, pleuritis, pericarditis, hyperbilirubinemia, liver enzyme elevation, leukocytosis, and anemia are supporting clinical features. About 50% of patients with systemic arthritis progress to having chronic inflammatory arthritis, which often is destructive (Fig. 7-22).

Extraarticular Manifestations

Patients with JIA are at risk of developing iridocyclitis (or uveitis). Although photophobia, eye pain, and erythema can occur, uveitis is often asymptomatic. For that reason, children

Figure 7-20 Psoriatic arthritis. **A,** Erythematous plaques with silver scale. **B,** Dactylitis (sausage toe) of the bilateral third and fifth toes. **C,** Diffuse nail pitting.

Figure 7-21   Systemic-onset juvenile idiopathic arthritis. **A** and **B,** The rash is erythematous, macular, and often evanescent. It can be more prominent during periods of fever. Featured on trunk and extremities.

Figure 7-22   Systemic-onset juvenile idiopathic arthritis (JIA). The femoral head from a 13-year-old girl with a hip replacement shows significant bony erosion. Patients with systemic and polyarticular JIA are more likely to suffer joint destruction than are patients with oligoarticular juvenile idiopathic arthritis.

Figure 7-23   Iridocyclitis. An irregular pupil in a patient with oligoarticular juvenile idiopathic arthritis. Note synechiae projecting posteriorly toward the lens.

with oligoarticular and polyarticular JIA must receive slit-lamp examinations frequently.

The first clinical sign of uveitis is cellular exudate in the anterior chamber. If the uveitis is left untreated, synechiae (adhesions) between the iris and lens may develop, leading to an irregular and poorly functioning pupil (Fig. 7-23). Further along in the clinical course, band keratopathy (calcium deposits in the cornea) (Fig. 7-24) may occur, as well as cataracts or glaucoma. For these reasons, strict adherence to the recommendations for eye examination outlined in Table 7-4 is necessary to help prevent visual loss in these children. Ophthalmologic complications do not parallel the activity of the arthritis.

Linear growth retardation may occur in the child with active JIA, especially with systemic or polyarticular disease. The degree of growth retardation and the ultimate prognosis for reaching adult height are related to the severity and duration of inflammation and the use of corticosteroids. Treatment with steroid-sparing agents such as nonsteroidal antiinflammatory drugs (NSAIDs), disease-modifying agents (i.e., methotrexate), and biologic agents (i.e., etanercept, adalimumab, and infliximab) is currently preferred compared with the heavy steroid usage of the past. Oligoarticular arthritis can present with bizarre growth abnormalities, usually confined to leg length discrepancy or an enlarged hand or foot related to refractory ankle or wrist involvement. During early illness,

Figure 7-24   Band keratopathy. Note the calcium deposits in the Bowman layer in this patient with juvenile idiopathic arthritis.

Type	ANA	Age at Onset (yr)	Duration of Disease (yr)	Risk Category	Eye Examination Frequency (mo)
Oligoarthritis or polyarthritis	+	≤6	≤4	High	3
	+	≤6	>4	Moderate	6
	+	≤6	>7	Low	12
	+	>6	≤4	Moderate	6
	+	>6	>4	Low	12
	–	≤6	≤4	Moderate	6
	–	≤6	>4	Low	12
	–	>6	NA	Low	12
Systemic disease (fever, rash)	NA	NA	NA	Low	12

Table 7-4 Recommended Frequency of Ophthalmologic Examinations in Juvenile Idiopathic Arthritis

Recommendations for follow-up continue through childhood and adolescence.
ANA, antinuclear antibodies; NA, not applicable.
From Cassidy J, Kivlin J, Lindsley C, et al: Ophthalmologic examinations in children with juvenile rheumatoid arthritis, *Pediatrics* 117:1843-1845, 2006.

Figure 7-25 Macrophage activation syndrome (MAS). Bone marrow aspirate shows activated macrophages with foamy cytoplasm engulfing surrounding erythrocytes and neutrophils. *(Courtesy Alexi Grom, MD, Cincinnati, Ohio.)*

bony development may be advanced; later in the course of the illness the opposite may be true. Premature epiphyseal fusion may occur.

Cardiac involvement occurs in more than one third of patients with systemic arthritis. Pericarditis, myocarditis, and endocarditis occur, with pericarditis being the most common. Chest pain, a friction rub, tachycardia, dyspnea, and supportive chest radiograph, electrocardiogram, and echocardiographic findings may occur. These episodes may last for weeks to months and are usually associated with a generalized flare of disease. Various other extraarticular manifestations including hepatosplenomegaly and lymphadenopathy are particularly common in systemic arthritis.

Patients with systemic arthritis are at risk for developing a potentially fatal disorder called *macrophage activation syndrome* (MAS). Patients present with a toxic appearance, fever, hepatosplenomegaly, lymphadenopathy, and mucosal bleeding. If not recognized early, MAS can progress to hepatic failure, encephalopathy, and disseminated intravascular coagulation. Laboratory testing that supports a diagnosis of MAS includes evidence of hepatitis and coagulopathy. In addition, the white blood cell count, hemoglobin, and platelet counts are depressed with a normal or low sedimentation rate (Table 7-5). Diagnosis is confirmed by bone marrow aspiration demonstrating activated macrophages engulfing surrounding cells (Fig. 7-25).

Differential Diagnosis

Because JIA is a clinical diagnosis, strict clinical criteria have been established to make the diagnosis. Most authors suggest the presence of objective joint findings (arthritis) for a minimum of 6 consecutive weeks coupled with the exclusion of other causes of arthritis in children (Table 7-6).

Table 7-5 Characteristics of Macrophage Activation Syndrome in Patients with Systemic-onset Juvenile Idiopathic Arthritis

Acutely ill with bruising, purpura, mucosal bleeding

Hepatosplenomegaly

Lymphadenopathy

Decrease in white blood cell count, hemoglobin, and platelet count

Decrease in erythrocyte sedimentation rate

Elevation of alanine aminotransferase, aspartate aminotransferase, prothrombin time, partial thromboplastin time, fibrin split-products, ferritin, and triglycerides

Decrease in fibrinogen, clotting factors

Tissue biopsy (i.e., bone marrow, liver) may demonstrate active phagocytosis by macrophages

Modified from Cassidy JT, Petty RE: *Textbook of pediatric rheumatology,* ed 5, Philadelphia, 2005, WB Saunders.

Table 7-6 Differential Diagnosis of Juvenile Idiopathic Arthritis

Systemic Onset

Systemic lupus erythematosus

Kawasaki syndrome

Acute rheumatic fever

Henoch-Schönlein purpura

Polyarteritis nodosa

Dermatomyositis

Systemic sclerosis

Inflammatory bowel disease

Malignancy (leukemia, neuroblastoma)

Lyme disease

Viral syndrome

Familial Mediterranean fever

Polyarticular Onset

Systemic lupus erythematosus

Psoriatic arthritis

Hypermobility syndrome

Enthesitis syndrome

Reactive arthritis

Oligoarticular Onset

Septic joint (monoarthritis)

Reiter syndrome

Juvenile ankylosing spondylitis

Pigmented villonodular synovitis

Psoriatic arthritis

Lyme disease

Figure 7-26   Lyme disease. The lesion of erythema migrans may be a large erythematous macule with central clearing, occurring singly or multiply.

Because of its destructive nature, pyogenic arthritis (e.g., staphylococci, streptococci, *Haemophilus influenzae*) must be ruled out in any child with active joint disease, especially monoarthritis. The intensely red and tender joint should raise suspicion of a bacterial pathogen. This combined with systemic symptoms of infection (fever, chills, malaise, rigors) should prompt the clinician to perform an arthrocentesis early in the course of the illness.

Lyme arthritis can mimic oligoarticular JIA. This spirochetal form of arthritis is tick-borne and usually affects the knee, elbow, or wrist in a monoarthritic pattern with spontaneous exacerbations and remissions. Malaise, fever, myalgia, lymphadenopathy, headache, meningismus, and weakness also may occur in the first phase of the illness. The distinctive rash, known as *erythema migrans* (Fig. 7-26), begins as an erythematous macule or papule. After this clears, the borders of the lesion expand to form an erythematous circular lesion that can be as large as 30 cm in diameter. These lesions can initially occur singly but can progress to multiple lesions over the legs, arms, and trunk. Other manifestations of Lyme disease include neurologic complications such as seventh nerve palsy, meningitis, radiculoneuritis, and the cardiac manifestations of heart block and myopericarditis. Bilateral Bell's palsy or seventh nerve paralysis even more strongly suggests the diagnosis of Lyme disease.

Other infections cause a reactive arthritis that dissipates in less than 6 weeks. *Salmonella, Shigella, Yersinia,* and *Campylobacter* organisms should also be considered. A multitude of viruses cause arthritis. These include rubella; hepatitis B; adenovirus; and herpesviruses including Epstein-Barr virus, cytomegalovirus, varicella zoster, and herpes simplex. Parvoviruses, mumps, and enteroviruses including echovirus and coxsackievirus are associated with acute polyarthritis and occasionally have been recovered from joints. Other viruses result in reactive arthritis and may not infect the joint directly.

Poststreptococcal phenomena include acute rheumatic fever (ARF) and poststreptococcal reactive arthritis. In ARF, Jones criteria are met. The child must be monitored for cardiac sequelae such as valvulitis and congestive heart failure. In poststreptococcal reactive arthritis, Jones criteria are not met. Arthritis will resolve but arthralgia can last for 6 months. The joint pain may be axial and affect the spine. In both cases, children are given prophylactic antibiotics to try and prevent future streptococcal infections.

Malignancies such as neuroblastoma and leukemia may present with musculoskeletal pain. More careful evaluation generally reveals bone pain. Sickle cell disease, particularly in the form of dactylitis, can have prominent digital involvement. Hemophilia, tuberculosis, and gonorrhea infection must be considered in the patient with arthritis. Differential diagnoses of JIA are proposed in Table 7-6.

SYSTEMIC LUPUS ERYTHEMATOSUS

Systemic lupus erythematosus (SLE) is a multisystem autoimmune disease with a myriad of clinical presentations. SLE may present in an insidious fashion and hence escape early diagnosis, or it may present acutely and progress rapidly, leading to the patient's demise. Frequently, children will present with nonspecific constitutional symptoms, such as fever, diffuse alopecia, weight loss, fatigue, and evidence of diffuse body inflammation with lymphadenopathy and hepatosplenomegaly. All organ systems have the potential to become involved, but the most common are skin, musculoskeletal, and renal systems in pediatric SLE (pSLE). As with other collagen vascular diseases, the etiology of SLE is unknown. Because of the large number of serologic markers known to occur in SLE, it is considered by many to be the prototype of autoimmune diseases. To increase diagnostic accuracy, the American College of Rheumatology (ACR) revised its classification criteria of lupus (Table 7-7). This classification, which combines clinical and serologic markers, is highly sensitive and specific for the diagnosis of this disease, reaching almost 100% sensitivity and specificity when 4 of the 11 criteria are present; however, the criteria are not meant for the clinical application of diagnosis and should be used as a study guide rather than applied to the clinical arena.

The word *lupus,* which means wolf, alludes to the erosive nature of the rash of SLE ("wolf bite") (Fig. 7-27). This feature of the disease was critical to the diagnosis of SLE until the discovery of the lupus erythematosus (LE) cell in 1948. The LE cell represents a healthy neutrophil that has phagocytosed the nuclear debris of a nonliving cell that has been coated with antibody. The antibody is directed against deoxyribonucleoprotein (DNP), which is made up of both DNA and histones. The presence of this serologic marker for lupus greatly expanded the recognized clinical entity of SLE. Although the

Table 7-7	Criteria for the Classification of Systemic Lupus Erythematosus*

Malar (butterfly) rash

Discoid-lupus rash

Photosensitivity

Oral or nasal mucocutaneous ulcerations

Nonerosive arthritis

Nephritis[†]
   Proteinuria > 0.5 g/d
   Cellular casts

Encephalopathy[†]
   Seizures
   Psychosis

Pleuritis or pericarditis

Cytopenia

Positive immunoserology[†]
   Antibodies to double-stranded DNA
   Antibodies to Smith antigen
   Positive anti-phospholipid antibodies based on:
      IgG or IgM anti-cardiolipin antibodies or
      Lupus anticoagulant or
      Biologic false-positive test for syphilis

Positive anti-nuclear antibody test

*Four of 11 criteria provide a sensitivity of 96% and a specificity of 96%.
[†]Any one item satisfies this criterion.
Modified from Hochberg MC: Updating the American College of Rheumatology revised criteria for the classification of systemic lupus erythematosus, *Arthritis Rheum* 40:1725, 1997.

Figure 7-27 Systemic lupus erythematosus. **A,** Malar rash of systemic lupus erythematosus. Erythema, erosion, and atrophy are present. Note sparing of nasolabial folds. This patient also has a rash involving the forehead and chin. **B,** Lateral view shows ear involvement.

LE preparation has proved to be of historical interest, time has shown that it is a nonspecific immunologic phenomenon and has no specificity with respect to the diagnosis of SLE; hence, although it was included in the ACR 1982 criteria, it was not included in the ACR 1997 criteria.

SLE accounts for 10% of patients with rheumatic diseases and for less than 5% of children seen in pediatric rheumatology practices. The incidence is estimated at 0.5 per 100,000 children per year. From prevalence data, it has been inferred that there are between 5000 and 10,000 children with SLE in the United States. The disease is rare in children younger than the age of 5 years. Before menarche, the boy-to-girl ratio is equal. After menarche, the ratio of affected girls to boys approaches 8 : 1. African Americans and Asians are more commonly affected than the white population.

The incidence of other connective tissue diseases is higher among family members of patients with SLE. Hematologic malignancies and immunodeficiencies are also reported in increased frequency among the relatives of patients with SLE. These well-described phenomena may reflect a genetic alteration of immunity or, as some researchers suggest, the effects of a transmissible agent. The high incidence of the disease in girls supports the role of hormonal factors as contributing or modulating agents in the pathogenesis of SLE. Other investigators suggest the influence of viruses, sunlight, and emotional stress on those developing lupus.

Although immunologic markers contribute to making the diagnosis of SLE, a high index of suspicion is necessary to obtain these studies. The early symptoms are often nonspecific and sometimes go unrecognized as harbingers of serious disease. Fever, fatigue, malaise, anorexia, and weight loss may be the only symptoms. In the adolescent population these symptoms may be all the more difficult to interpret. Conversely, this multisystem disease may present with a plethora of physical findings and the presentation may be so dramatic that the diagnosis is readily apparent. The most common organ manifestations at disease presentation in pSLE are musculoskeletal, cutaneous, renal, and hematologic.

Cutaneous manifestations of SLE occur at some time during the course of the disease in 80% of affected individuals. There are a variety of cutaneous findings including a malar rash, photosensitive rash, palmar erythema (Fig. 7-28), annular erythema, vasculitic skin lesions with nodules or ulcerations, Raynaud phenomenon and associated ulceration, alopecia, and discoid lupus. Isolated discoid lupus is rarely seen in children, but when it occurs is usually without systemic manifestations. The same holds true for subacute cutaneous lupus, which is uncommon, presenting as a serpiginous-like

photosensitive erythematous rash associated with positive SS-A (anti-Ro) antibody. The most frequent skin manifestations of SLE are malar rash and photosensitive rash. The classic malar or butterfly rash is a maculopapular rash distributed over the cheeks (malar eminences) and extending over the bridge of the nose, while sparing the nasolabial folds (see Fig. 7-27). The malar rash is photosensitive in 30% of the patients. In general, sun exposure may not only exacerbate the skin disease but also cause a systemic flare of disease, theoretically through large exposure of the immune system to intracellular proteins through massive apoptosis of damaged skin cells. Therefore, appropriate sun protection and avoidance is strongly encouraged. An annular photosensitive rash is frequently associated with the "Sjögren syndrome antibodies" anti-Ro (SS-A) and anti-La (SS-B). The typical morphology of the rash of lupus is defined as reddish purple and raised with a whitish scale (Fig. 7-29). When the scale is removed, the underlying skin often shows "carpet tack–like" fingers on the unexposed side of the scale itself. Carpet tacking is caused by the contouring of the scale into the skin follicles. These finger-like projections on a scale strongly suggest the diagnosis of lupus. Vasculitic rashes are more violaceous and may be associated with nodules, ulceration, and palpable purpura (Fig. 7-30). These lesions are commonly found in an acral distribution, and typically result in postinflammatory hyperpigmentation. Discoid lupus, although uncommon (5% to 10% of patients with pSLE), leaves the most damage with follicular plugging and scarring. Mucosal erosions and ulcers of the oral cavity and nasal mucosa are part of lupus as well, with the most well-recognized manifestation being the "silent"

Figure 7-28 Systemic lupus erythematosus. Palmar erythema.

Figure 7-31 Systemic lupus erythematosus. "Silent" ulceration of the hard palate.

Figure 7-29 Systemic lupus erythematosus. **A,** Note the localized erythematous rash in a nonmalar distribution. **B,** The rash of SLE often has a slight white scale.

large violaceous ulceration of the hard palate (Fig. 7-31). Alopecia occurs in 20% of patients and may present as broken hair shafts or patchy, red, scaling areas on the scalp, which may eventually scar and cause permanent hair loss (Fig. 7-32). Other reported mucocutaneous findings are livedo reticularis (lacy, fishnet appearance of the skin), urticaria, atrophy, and telangiectasia. The presence of livedo reticularis may be the clinician's only clue to an associated hypercoagulable state

manifested by anti-phospholipid antibodies. This tendency can be diagnosed by obtaining a lupus anticoagulant panel, a functional assay that includes a partial thromboplastin time (PTT), anti-cardiolipin antibodies, and anti–β_2-glycoprotein antibodies. Although anti-phospholipid antibody syndrome (APS) can occur as an entity alone, it is commonly associated with SLE. APS is defined as a hypercoagulable state characterized by both positive laboratory findings of anti-phospholipid antibodies and clinical findings of a variety of venous and arterial thromboses and recurrent fetal loss.

The heart is often significantly involved in patients with lupus. Although the pericardium is involved most commonly, the myocardium and the endocardium may also be of clinical importance. Pericarditis with associated pericardial effusion can be painless and may present only as cardiomegaly on a

Figure 7-30 Systemic lupus erythematosus. Purpuric, ulcerative, and necrotic skin lesions of cutaneous vasculitis.

Figure 7-32 Systemic lupus erythematosus. Scarring alopecia.

Figure 7-33 Systemic lupus erythematosus. Large pericardial effusion with associated cardiac tamponade physiology in teenage female. Pleural effusions are also present.

chest radiograph (Fig. 7-33) or as pericardial effusion on an echocardiogram. However, chest pain may be noted, especially on deep inspiration and when lying down. Auscultation of a friction rub signifies pericarditis. Although pericarditis is usually mild, it can progress to life-threatening cardiac tamponade. If the myocardium is affected, life-threatening complications including dysrhythmias, heart failure, and infarction can result. *Libman-Sacks endocarditis* is the term given to the verrucous projections of fibrinoid necrosis in the endocardium. These lesions rarely cause clinical symptoms, although the presence of a murmur raises suspicion of endocardial disease. The mitral valve is most commonly involved, although aortic and tricuspid valves may be similarly affected. The presence of Libman-Sacks endocarditis should also alert the clinician to the possibility of an underlying anti-phospholipid antibody syndrome. The major cardiac morbidity associated with SLE, which is gaining more recognition in the adolescent pediatric SLE population, is premature atherosclerosis. Several factors contribute to the risk of atherosclerosis, including chronic inflammatory processes, altered endothelial function, lipid abnormalities, nephritis, and proteinuria. Monitoring and controlling classic Framingham risk factors in addition to factors attributable to lupus are critical for long-term morbidity.

Pulmonary manifestations of lupus are particularly difficult to diagnose noninvasively. Migrating pneumonitis, particularly involving the lung bases, suggests "lupus lung"; however, distinguishing these entities from infection may be impossible without invasive procedures. Typically, patients have atelectasis, pleural effusions, interstitial pneumonitis, or hemorrhage (Fig. 7-34). These sequelae may present as cyanosis, dyspnea, or almost any other form of respiratory distress. Pulmonary arterial hypertension is another manifestation, more commonly seen in those with positive U1 ribonucleoprotein (U1-RNP) antibodies or those patients with SLE with features that overlap with systemic sclerosis. An uncommon but well-described pulmonary manifestation of SLE is "shrinking lung" syndrome. This is manifested by diaphragmatic involvement and progressively smaller lung volumes recorded by pulmonary function testing.

Arthritis is seen in approximately 80% of patients with pSLE and is usually present at the time of diagnosis. Unlike the destructive arthritis of juvenile idiopathic arthritis (JIA), lupus arthritis is more transient and episodic and rarely results in joint contracture. Jaccoud arthropathy, which is a nonde-forming, easily reversible, soft tissue arthritis that can mimic the boutonnière (flexion of PIP joints and hyperextension of

distal interphalangeal [DIP] joints) and swan-neck (hyperextension of PIP joints and flexion of DIP joints) deformities associated with JIA, is strongly associated with the diagnosis of SLE. The fact that arthralgia is more predominant than arthritis has been noted consistently, with the degree of pain out of proportion to the degree of effusion observed at the joint. Any joint may be involved, but the fingers are particularly susceptible and usually affected in a symmetrical polyarticular manner. Myalgia and weakness also occur as features of lupus but do not dominate the clinical picture as they do in dermatomyositis. A true myositis with weakness is seen in less than 10% of patients with SLE. Musculoskeletal manifestations associated with long-term high-dose corticosteroid therapy in SLE are avascular necrosis (AVN), particularly of the hip and knee joints, osteoporosis, and vertebral fractures.

CNS signs and symptoms of lupus are a great challenge to physicians. A wide range of neurologic and psychiatric manifestations of the disease have been described. Further complicating the spectrum of CNS lupus is the difficulty in distinguishing the disease itself from side effects of therapy such as corticosteroid psychosis, emotional response to disease, and a non-CNS etiology of CNS pathology such as hypertensive encephalopathy and posterior reversible encephalopathy syndrome (PRESS). Chorea is a neurologic manifestation of lupus that must be distinguished from the chorea of rheumatic fever. Altered mental status and focal neurologic defects occurring in lupus also suggest the possibility of cerebral vascular accident and again alert the clinician to the diagnosis of the anti-phospholipid antibody syndrome. Approximately one quarter of all patients with lupus have some form of CNS disease. If headaches are included in CNS SLE manifestations, then up to 75% of pSLE would be considered to have neurologic involvement. A "true" lupus headache is described as refractory to standard analgesics, requiring narcotic analgesia. Of concern are the more severe, unremitting headaches that may be caused by pseudotumor cerebri, CNS vasculitis, or central vein thrombosis (CVT). The latter is associated with the presence of lupus anticoagulant and is captured on magnetic resonance venogram (MRV). Other CNS and peripheral nervous system findings include mononeuritis, multiplex (inflammatory lesions of multiple nerves located in anatomically unrelated parts of the body), transverse myelitis, ataxia, peripheral neuropathy, seizures, psychosis, and intellectual impairment or "lupus fog." As a direct extension of the brain, the retina may also show evidence of disease (i.e., retinal vasculitis). The best known ocular manifestation is the

Figure 7-34 Systemic lupus erythematosus. Atelectasis, pleural effusions, and pulmonary infiltrates in a teenage girl.

Figure 7-35 Systemic lupus erythematosus. **A,** A white exudate (cotton-wool spot) between the disk and macula. **B,** Papilledema with flame hemorrhages.

cotton-wool spot, an exudative, whitish lesion of the retina. Hemorrhage and papilledema are also seen (Fig. 7-35). The CNS effects of lupus are responsible for much morbidity and mortality. The majority of patients will have neurologic symptoms within the first year of onset of disease. Investigation of CNS involvement in SLE typically involves imaging with CT and magnetic resonance imaging (MRI) (Fig. 7-36) as well as analysis of cerebrospinal fluid (CSF) cell count, protein, and opening pressures. Lumbar puncture may show nonspecific findings of elevated white blood cell count (WBC) and protein, but in the absence of infection. The lumbar puncture is typically done to rule out non-SLE causes of CNS disease, especially infection. CSF anti–ribosomal P protein and anti-neuronal antibodies were found in some reports to support active SLE CNS disease, but this remains controversial as some patients without CNS disease have these antibodies.

At least as important as CNS disease in determining ultimate prognosis in pediatric SLE is the degree of renal involvement. Approximately 75% of all children with SLE have some degree of clinically apparent renal disease. This is more prevalent than in adult SLE and is more severe. This often manifests itself in the first 2 years of illness but can also appear many years after the initial diagnosis. The type of pathology largely relates to the nature of immune complex deposition at various sites in the kidney (i.e., size and electrical charge of the immune complexes). At a histologic level, renal involvement is classified according to the World Health Organization classification of lupus nephritis (Table 7-8). A pathologic diagnosis must be made in children with rapidly progressive renal problems or change in their renal disease to assist with both the diagnosis and evaluation of the severity of nephritis (i.e., focal vs. diffuse) and the degree of acute and chronic changes to help direct systemic therapy. The most common (and severe) subtype is diffuse proliferative glomerulonephritis (class IV) with the presence of subendothelial deposits on electron microscopy and a "full house" appearance on immunofluorescence (usually signifying C3 and IgG deposition). Other than the glomeruli, the tubules, interstitium, and blood vessels can be involved. In addition to the biopsy, renal serologic and urinalysis parameters, including serum albumin and total protein, microscopic urinalysis for red blood cell (RBC) casts, and 24-hour protein to quantify protein loss are essential to initial diagnosis and monitoring renal disease. Monitoring complement (C3 and C4) and double-stranded DNA (dsDNA) titers is also helpful in diagnosing and predicting lupus renal flares, as they often mirror renal disease activity. Hypertension and peripheral edema are present in approximately one third of pediatric patients with lupus nephritis, and typically are associated with class III and class IV glomerulonephritis. Control of hypertension is as important as any other therapeutic maneuver in delaying the progression to renal failure and other systemic insults, such as posterior reversible encephalopathy syndrome (PRESS) (Fig. 7-36, C and D). Advances in treatment for SLE nephritis with relatively aggressive immunosuppressive regimens have dramatically improved the renal outcome of children with nephritis in the last few decades, with a recent 5-year survival rate for class IV lupus nephritis of 93%.

Hematologic abnormalities are one of the most common initial manifestations of SLE. They are found in three quarters of patients and include leukopenia, anemia, and thrombocytopenia. The "classic" anemia in lupus, or anemia of chronic disease, is normocytic and normochromic, but over time evolves into a microcytic and hypochromic anemia with iron deficiency. The Coombs test is positive in one third of patients, but less than 10% have overt hemolysis. Increase in anemia is frequently seen at times when the patient is experiencing a lupus flare. Thrombocytopenia in lupus is typically mild but can be more severe and refractory to common therapy with intravenous immunoglobulin (IVIG) and corticosteroids. The presence of both anemia and thrombocytopenia, known as Evans syndrome, is not uncommon in SLE. Lymphopenia is much more common than granulocytopenia in SLE, with typical values of the absolute lymphocyte count (ALC) ranging between 1000 and 1500.

Wide arrays of gastrointestinal manifestations are found in association with lupus, but are not the leading sources of morbidity. They include hepatosplenomegaly, hepatitis, splenomegaly, serositis, enteritis (direct inflammation of bowel wall), pancreatitis, malabsorption, diarrhea, and abdominal pain.

Perhaps more than in any other rheumatic disease, the clinical diagnosis of lupus can be supported serologically. Anti-nuclear antibodies (ANAs) represent a group of antibodies found in serum and are directed against antigens within the cellular nuclei of patients with lupus. ANAs are usually reported as a titer and a pattern. The patterns are either peripheral, homogeneous, speckled, or nucleolar (Fig. 7-37). These patterns are typically associated with antibodies to certain extractable nuclear antigens, such as anti–SS-A, anti–SS-B, Smith, RNP, dsDNA, histone antibody, and Scl-70.

Other antibodies found in patients with SLE are listed in Table 7-9. Anti-dsDNA antibodies are detected in 50% to 60% of patients with lupus and are specific for the diagnosis of SLE. As previously mentioned, dsDNA antibody levels correlate with disease activity, especially renal and CNS disease.

Figure 7-36 Systemic lupus erythematosus (SLE). **A,** Axial and **B,** coronal images of brain with scattered cortical and subcortical foci with T_2 prolongation mostly in the posterior white matter (parietal and occipital lobes), but also in some areas anteriorly (frontal lobe). Another abnormality is in the left precentral gyrus (motor area). These abnormalities were found in a teenage male with chorea and newly diagnosed SLE. **C,** Axial and **D,** coronal T_2 images consistent with posterior reversible encephalopathy syndrome in the same patient 3 months later, associated with a hypertensive crisis.

Ribonucleoprotein (RNP), although better known for its presence in high titers in mixed connective tissue disease, is also seen in low titers in 30% to 40% of patients with lupus. Other SLE antibodies include anti–SS-A and anti–SS-B, also known as anti-Ro and anti-La, respectively, which are associated with Sjögren's symptoms of dry eyes, dry mouth, and marked

Table 7-8	World Health Organization Classification of Lupus Nephritis

Class	Characteristic
I	Normal
II	Mesangial
IIA	Minimal alteration
IIB	Mesangial glomerulitis
III	Focal and segmental proliferative glomerulonephritis
IV	Diffuse proliferative glomerulonephritis
V	Membranous glomerulonephritis
VI	Glomerular sclerosis

Modified from Cassidy JT, Petty RE: *Textbook of pediatric rheumatology,* Philadelphia, 2005, WB Saunders.

cutaneous photosensitivity. Last, the clinician may find antibodies to Smith antigen (Sm), a nonhistone antigen that is most specific for the diagnosis of lupus, but is present only in 30% of patients. Anti-phospholipid antibodies are present in approximately 50% of patients with SLE, with anti-cardiolipin antibody being the most common. The lupus anticoagulant (LAC) panel is abnormal in approximately 20% of patients with pSLE. These antibodies are associated with increased risk for thrombosis, miscarriages, chorea, migraine headaches, and livedo reticularis.

In summary, SLE is a chronic disease with a variable course and with periods of varying activity. Although the mortality and morbidity remain high, marked improvement in prognosis has occurred in recent years.

Neonatal lupus occurs in infants whose mothers have a connective tissue disease. SS-A and SS-B antibodies of the IgG class are passed via the placenta to the fetus, leading to positive serologies for the infant and systemic manifestations of neonatal lupus including the presence of erythematous annular rash (Fig. 7-38), thrombocytopenia, Coombs-positive hemolytic anemia, liver function abnormalities, and congenital heart block (CHB). The majority of infants with CHB and

Figure 7-37 Anti-nuclear antibody patterns in systemic lupus erythematosus (SLE). **A,** Peripheral, nonspecific. **B,** Homogeneous; correlates with anti-dsDNA active renal disease. **C,** Speckled; seen with SLE, mixed connective tissue disease (MCTD), and Sjögren syndrome. To further delineate a diagnosis, anti-ribonucleoprotein (RNP) is present in MCTD, and Smith (Sm) antibody is present in SLE (RNP and Sm are "coarse speckled"). Extractable nuclear antigens SS-A and SS-B are associated with Sjögren syndrome (SS-A and SS-B are "fine speckled"). **D,** Nucleolar; suggests scleroderma associated with Scl-70 antibody.

neonatal lupus have entirely asymptomatic mothers, although a percentage of these women develop Sjögren syndrome rather than SLE. Fortunately, most manifestations of neonatal lupus are transient, lasting only a few months until the disappearance of passively transferred maternal antibody; however, the congenital heart block is permanent because remodeling of the heart conduction tissue occurs from antibody interference in utero during development. Two percent of infants born to mothers with anti-Ro antibodies have CHB, and the addition of anti-La antibodies increases it to 5%. Heart block is treated with pacemakers.

Several medications induce a lupus-like syndrome, called "drug-induced lupus," and their withdrawal leads to resolution of symptoms, usually within 6 months. Many patients taking certain drugs such as minocycline, hydralazine, procainamide, isoniazid (INH), chlorpromazine, or certain anticonvulsants develop a positive result for ANA without developing a lupus syndrome, and this is not an absolute reason to discontinue the medication. Oral contraceptives have also been shown in some studies to be associated with a lupus-like syndrome.

Figure 7-38 Neonatal lupus erythematosus. Shown is a newborn on its first day of life: **A,** typical annular rash and **B,** tissue infarction of the right ear pinna. Infant and mother were positive for anti-nuclear antibody (ANA) and anti-Ro (SS-A) and anti-La (SS-B) (Sjögren syndrome antibodies). The infant also had thrombocytopenia, hypocomplementemia, and increased transaminases.

SCLERODERMA

The term *scleroderma* literally means "*skleros*," sclerosing or hardening, of the "*derma*," skin. "Scleroderma" encompasses both forms of the disease: systemic sclerosis (SSc), characterized by skin, vascular, and visceral organ fibrosis, which more commonly affects adults, and localized scleroderma (LS), characterized by fibrosis of skin and underlying tissue without vascular or internal organ involvement, which more commonly affects children. Both are quite rare in children, with the estimated annual incidence of LS being 1 to 3 per 100,000 children and that of SSc being 1 per million. The mean age of onset for both forms of pediatric scleroderma is between 7.3 and 8.8 years of age, although less than 5% of all patients with SSc have pediatric onset, and the majority of patients with LS have childhood onset. The female-to-male ratio of pediatric SSc is 4:1 and for pediatric LS it is 2:1. There is no clear evidence of racial predilection for either form of pediatric scleroderma.

Systemic Sclerosis

Systemic sclerosis (SSc) is a rare but life-threatening condition. There are three main subtypes: diffuse cutaneous SSc (dcSSc), characterized by widespread and rapidly progressive skin thickening (proximal to elbows and knees) and early visceral disease (lung, heart, and kidney); limited cutaneous SSc (lcSSc), characterized by restricted and nonprogressive skin thickening (distal extremities) and late visceral disease (pulmonary arterial hypertension, malabsorption); and overlap SSc, which can be dcSSc or lcSSc with features of another

Table 7-9	Antibodies Found in Patients with Systemic Lupus Erythematosus
Antibody	**Patients (%)**
Native DNA (double-stranded)	50-60
DNP (DNA and histone protein)	Up to 70 (usually high titer)
RNP (RNA and nonhistone protein)	30-40
Histones	
All patients with SLE	60
Patients with drug-induced lupus	95
Anti–SS-A (anti-Ro)	30-40
Anti–SS-B (anti-La)	15
Smith	30

DNP, deoxyribonucleoprotein; RNP, ribonucleoprotein; SLE, systemic lupus erythematosus.
Modified from Tan EM: Antinuclear antibodies in diagnosis and management, *Hosp Pract* 18:74-79, 1983.

Figure 7-39 Systemic sclerosis. Patients with calcinosis cutis, Raynaud phenomenon, esophageal dysfunction, sclerodactyly, and telangiectasia (CREST) syndrome. **A,** Raynaud phenomenon (note cyanosis and pallor of the fingertips). **B,** Sclerodactyly. **C,** Telangiectasia.

connective tissue disease such as dermatomyositis or SLE. Patients with CREST (calcinosis cutis, Raynaud phenomenon, esophageal dysfunction, sclerodactyly, and telangiectasia) syndrome are considered to have lcSSc (Fig. 7-39). Scleroder- matous skin findings or organ fibrosis can be secondary to another process, such as graft-versus-host disease, or induced by a chemical agent, such as bleomycin (Table 7-10). The autoantibody profile is also helpful in defining subsets of SSc and predicting their organ involvement (Table 7-11). The fre- quency of these autoantibodies in pediatric SSc also reflects the frequency of clinical subsets. In general, overlap SSc is much more common in pediatric SSc (30% vs. 7% in adult SSc), as reflected by the increased frequency of PM-Scl and U1-RNP antibodies, and is related to the higher percentage of myositis and arthritis observed in pediatric SSc. Another direct clinical correlation is the paucity of severe renal disease in pediatric SSc compared with adult SSc, which is reflected by the low RNA polymerase III antibody in childhood SSc (see Table 7-11).

Common features at the onset of pediatric SSc are Raynaud phenomenon (RP) (70%) and skin changes of hands (60%) including edema, sclerodactyly, and induration proximal to MCP joints. In the largest cohort study of pediatric SSc patients (total, 153), 53% presented with both skin induration of hands and RP, and 10% of those presenting with RP also had digital infarcts. Raynaud phenomenon (see Fig. 7-39, *A*) is a vasospastic response leading to a triphasic color change of the hands (first white because of vasoconstriction, then blue secondary to cyanosis, and finally red because of reper- fusion with subsequent swelling and pain) associated with a sensation of numbness and tingling. Healthy individuals can also experience the color changes of Raynaud without being at risk for developing an underlying connective tissue disease. In SSc, RP is more pronounced and can lead to tissue damage due to a more fixed vasospasm. This occurs because there is an underlying vasculopathy that causes endothelial damage, resulting in more narrow and stiff arterioles. These

vasculopathic changes are identifiable in the nail fold capillary beds of these patients by capillary microscopy, demonstrating dilation, tortuosity, hemorrhage, drop-off, and later arboriza- tion of the capillaries (Fig. 7-40). Poor perfusion of the fingers eventually leads to digital tip pitting, ulceration (Fig. 7-41), and, in more severe cases, autoamputation. Features that help the clinician differentiate primary Raynaud phenomenon from that secondary to a connective tissue disease are the following: lack of nail fold capillary changes, digital tip pitting and/or ulceration, and a negative ANA. These features combined have a negative predicative value of 90% of developing a con- nective tissue disease. Cutaneous manifestations frequently bring children to medical attention, but because of the insidi- ous and subtle onset of skin changes, there is often a delay in diagnosis, with a mean time of 1.9 years between first sign of disease and diagnosis. Early in the clinical course, the skin is edematous with particular predilection for the distal extrem- ities; rarely, more proximal limb, face, and trunk involvement is present. The induration phase, for which scleroderma is named, is characterized by loss of the natural pliability of the skin and the presence of a palpable skin thickness. The skin takes on a shiny, tense appearance, with distal tapering of the fingers (Fig. 7-42). The visual impression that movement might be impaired is supported by the lack of flexibility in the hands (Fig. 7-43). The typical scleroderma facies of tight skin and skin atrophy produces the appearance of a fixed stare, pinched nose, thin pursed lips, small mouth, prominent teeth, and characteristic grimace (Fig. 7-44). Subcutaneous calcium deposits (calcinosis cutis) may occur at pressure points, typi- cally found on the extensor surfaces of hand joints in SSc, and may occasionally extrude through the skin in a fashion similar to dermatomyositis (see Fig. 7-62 in the section Juvenile Der- matomyositis). These lesions may be painful and may ulcer- ate. However, they are more typically associated with chronic disease and will not be present at the time of disease onset and diagnosis. Telangiectasias are also a manifestation of SSc, most typically found in the lcSSc variant (previously known

Table 7-10	Classification of Scleroderma and Related Disorders

Primary

Systemic sclerosis

    Diffuse cutaneous scleroderma

    Limited cutaneous scleroderma (CREST syndrome)

    Overlap

Localized scleroderma

    Plaque morphea (circumscribed superficial*)

    Generalized morphea

    Deep morphea

        Subcutaneous morphea (circumscribed deep*)

        Eosinophilic fasciitis

    Linear scleroderma

        Extremity/trunk

        Scalp/face: *en coup de sabre*

    Pansclerotic

    Mixed morphea (any combination of two or more of the above subtypes*)

Diseases with Sclerodermatous Manifestations

Graft-versus-host disease

Drug or chemical induced

    Vinyl chloride

    Bleomycin

    Pentazocine

    Tryptophan

    Silicone

    Toxic oil syndrome

Phenylketonuria

Progeria

Werner syndrome

Scleredema

Porphyria cutanea tarda

Diabetic cheiroarthropathy[†]

*According to Padua preliminary classification criteria, 2004.
  [†]Arthropathy of the hand.
  CREST, calcinosis cutis, Raynaud phenomenon, esophageal dysfunction, sclerodactyly, and telangiectasia.

Table 7-11	Clinical and Laboratory Characteristics of Patients with Systemic Sclerosis According to Serum Autoantibody Type

Autoantibody	Pattern	Clinical Association	Children (%)	Adults (%)
RNA Pol III	Speckled nucleolar	dc, severe skin, renal	4*	32
Topo (Scl-70)	Speckled nucleolar	dc, ILD	20	21
Centromere	Centromere	lc, intrinsic PAH	16*	4
Th/Tho	Nucleolar	lc, ILD, intrinsic PAH	3	3
U3-RNP	Nucleolar	dc = lc, myopathy, cardiomyopathy, PAH	5	2
U1-RNP	Speckled	Overlap, myositis, ILD	16*	4
PM-Scl	Nucleolar	Overlap, myositis	14*	5
>1 antibody			8*	2
Positive for ANA, but none of the above			20*	11
Negative for ANA			3	2

*Significantly different between groups.
  ANA, anti-nuclear antibody; dc, diffuse cutaneous; ILD, interstitial lung disease; lc, limited cutaneous; PAH, pulmonary arterial hypertension; PM-Scl, polymyositis-scleroderma; Pol, polymerase; RNP, ribonucleoprotein; Scl, scleroderma; Scl-70, anti-topoisomerase.
  Modified from Scalapino K, Arkachaisri T, Lucas M, et al: Childhood onset systemic sclerosis: classification, clinical and serologic features, and survival in comparison with adult onset disease, *J Rheumatol* 33:1004-1013, 2006.

as CREST syndrome), with a "matted" appearance and commonly distributed on the face and upper extremities (see Fig. 7-39, *C*).

Other organ manifestations in SSc (in order of decreasing frequency) include gastrointestinal, pulmonary, musculo-skeletal, cardiac, renal, and neurologic. Gastrointestinal (GI) symptoms occur in approximately half of the children. More detailed investigation often indicates the presence of abnormalities in a larger percentage. Esophageal dysmotility associated with gastroesophageal reflux often leads to dysphagia and symptoms of esophagitis. Distal dysphagia, especially with solids, with a sensation of "food getting stuck" mid-chest is typical and represents dysfunction of the distal smooth muscle of the esophagus. In some affected individuals, aspiration or cough may occur and esophageal strictures can develop if the process of reflux is chronic. If the small bowel is involved, cramps, diarrhea, and constipation may result from peristaltic dysfunction. Episodes of pseudo-obstruction with postprandial abdominal distention, pain, and nausea can occur because of a functional ileus. Bacterial overgrowth, steatorrhea, weight loss, volvulus, and even perforation can occur. Colonic disease occurs in the form of wide-mouth diverticula and a loss of the normal colonic architecture. Another complication of GI involvement with SSc is acute GI bleeding associated with gastric antral venular ectasia (GAVE) requiring photocoagulation. This condition is uncommon in children and is associated with early dcSSc, RNA polymerase III–positive patients.

Pulmonary involvement in pediatric SSc is described in the literature as ranging from 30% to 70% and includes interstitial lung disease (ILD) (Fig. 7-45), pulmonary arterial hypertension (PAH) (either primary or intrinsic from vasculopathy or secondary from ILD), and abnormal pulmonary function test (PFT) results (decreased forced vital capacity [FVC] and diffusing capacity of the lung for carbon monoxide [DL_{CO}]). ILD typically presents as slowly progressive dyspnea with exertion over years and is associated with decreased FVC and a reticular–nodular (ground glass) pattern on chest CT examination. PAH, on the other hand, presents as a rapid progression of dyspnea on exertion over months with decreased DL_{CO} on PFTs, and an abnormal echocardiogram with estimated

Figure 7-40 Systemic sclerosis. Nail fold capillary changes (original magnification, ×10), enlarged capillary loops, and capillary dropout.

Figure 7-41 Systemic sclerosis. Digital pitting ulcers (**A,** early disease; **B,** late disease) represent one of the three minor diagnostic criteria for scleroderma.

Figure 7-42 Systemic sclerosis. Sclerodactyly and tapering of digits. Note the thickened cuticle tissue.

pulmonary artery (PA) or RV systolic pressure greater than 40 mm Hg, verified by right heart catheterization, with mean PA pressure greater than 25 mm Hg. Musculoskeletal involvement is more common in pediatric SSc, with inflammatory arthritis (joint effusions) in addition to the typical "dry synovitis" of scleroderma, which is reflected by the fibrosis of tendons traversing the joints, limiting their range of motion (ROM). Early in the disease process, especially among those with dcSSc, tenosynovitis/bursitis causes palpable tendon friction rubs when the joint is extended or flexed (patients claim

Figure 7-44 Systemic sclerosis. Facial features show that the skin appears tight and drawn, without evidence of wrinkles. *(Courtesy J. Jeffrey Malatack, MD, Philadelphia.)*

Figure 7-43 Systemic sclerosis. Lack of flexibility in the hands is another characteristic of scleroderma.

Figure 7-45 Systemic sclerosis. Bilateral pulmonary fibrosis.

Figure 7-46   Localized scleroderma. **A** and **B,** Active-phase lesions have an inflammatory border or "lilac ring." (**B,** *Courtesy Elena Pope, Hospital for Sick Children, Toronto, ON, Canada.*)

it feels like a creaking door). When the patient has myopathy, typically there is a symmetrical proximal weakness, especially of the shoulder girdle and humeral muscles, with pronounced atrophy at times. Myositis is also reflected by elevated muscle enzymes and changes on MRI similar to that of juvenile dermatomyositis (JDM). The muscle biopsy differs from that of JDM by having more fibrosis and by the presence of thickened capillaries. Myositis in SSc increases the risk of cardiac involvement from 10% to 20%. Cardiac involvement includes heart block, arrhythmia, congestive heart failure, electrocardiographic changes, and pericardial effusion. These abnormalities appear to be a result of myocardial fibrosis, vascular insufficiency, and inflammation. Cardiac involvement is the leading cause of death in pediatric SSc, whereas morbidity and mortality in adults with scleroderma are usually related to hypertension and renal failure. Before the advent of angiotensin-converting enzyme inhibitors, adult SSc patients with scleroderma renal crisis (SRC) had a 1-year survival rate of 20%; it is now 80%. SRC is most frequently seen early in the disease course of RNA polymerase III–positive patients with dcSSc and is characterized by accelerated hypertension and its sequelae, in addition to a clinical profile including thrombocytopenic purpura.

Despite all the potential organ involvement of pediatric SSc, in general the frequency of severe organ involvement is less than in adult SSc and it is associated with a more favorable prognosis, with 5-, 10-, and 15-year survival rates in children (89%, 85%, and 80%, respectively) compared with adults (75%, 55%, and 35%, respectively). Treatment of SSc is dependent on organ involvement but includes general measures such as GI protection with antacid medication, promotility agents, vasodilators for Raynaud (may help with PAH), NSAIDs, and physical therapy for arthritis or tendinitis. Corticosteroids for myositis, arthritis, and other inflammatory clinical features must be used with caution as they can prompt SRC.

Localized Scleroderma

Localized scleroderma, also known as "morphea," has a different pattern of skin involvement than systemic sclerosis (SSc) and encompasses several subtypes, including plaque morphea, generalized morphea, bullous morphea, linear scleroderma, deep morphea, and pansclerotic morphea. Traditional classification of these subtypes is based on the Mayo criteria, but more recently a few modifications have been

made (see Table 7-10). This group of disorders is characterized by fibrosis that is confined mainly to the skin and subcutaneous tissue; however, deeper forms also involve the fascia, muscle, tendon, and joint capsule. As in SSc, there is an earlier, more active phase of disease followed later by a fibrotic phase. Early active lesions are characterized by a violaceous inflammatory border or "lilac ring" (Fig. 7-46) and skin induration throughout the lesion, including the border. The lesions also expand and new lesions accumulate when the disease is in an active state. Over time disease damage accumulates and is represented by an increase in skin thickness, especially at the center of the lesion, sometimes leaving an ivory-colored sclerotic center (Fig. 7-47). Dermal and subcutaneous atrophy result from previous inflammation and subsequent collagen deposition. Clinically, when the dermis is atrophic there is a lack of hair growth at the site of the lesion, visible veins, and a slight "cliff drop" appearance to the skin (Fig. 7-48). Subcutaneous atrophy is identified as a flattening of the skin in mild cases to a more "scooped out" concavity appearance of the adipose tissue in more severe lesions, to such a point that one can see the muscles moving underneath the skin (Fig. 7-49). Postinflammatory hyper- and hypopigmentation also are a result of previous inflammation and are the most notable features that bring the lesion to the attention of a medical provider (Fig. 7-50). Often families will miss the early, active phase and consider the erythema/violaceous color more of a bruise or injury; it is the "bruise that does not go away"

Figure 7-47   Localized scleroderma. Pale and thickened sclerotic center of lesion on the wrist.

Figure 7-48 Localized scleroderma (LS). Dermal atrophy of LS, demonstrated by "cliff drop" lesions and visible veins in a teenage female with generalized morphea.

Figure 7-49 Localized scleroderma. **A,** Subcutaneous atrophy, moderate atrophy (divot or "scoop out" lesion) in a toddler. **B,** More severe subcutaneous atrophy of the right buttock, leaving the buttocks asymmetric.

Figure 7-50 Localized scleroderma. "Salt-and-pepper" appearance of a plaque in a patient with localized scleroderma. Note the hyperpigmentation within the hypopigmented lesion.

(postinflammatory hyperpigmentation) that is brought to medical attention. At times these patients see hematologists first for a possible bleeding disorder.

Linear scleroderma occurs on the extremities, trunk, or head, and is the most common subtype that occurs in children (50% to 60%), typically as a single, linear unilateral band (Fig. 7-51). Legs are the most commonly involved sites, followed by arms, frontal head, and trunk. When the limbs are involved, sclerosis of the muscle, tendon, and joint capsule may result in contracture across the joints and limb dysfunction with decreased ROM, leg length discrepancy, and antalgic gait. Involvement of the epiphyseal growth plate can alter growth, leading to permanent shortening or atrophy of the limb (Fig. 7-52). Linear lesions involving the scalp and

Figure 7-51 Localized scleroderma. Linear scleroderma affecting the right lower extremity, the most common site.

Figure 7-52 Localized scleroderma. **A** and **B,** Linear form of scleroderma affecting the right lower extremity of two children. **C,** Linear scleroderma affecting the entire left side of the body. Note the extensive atrophy.

Figure 7-53 Localized scleroderma. Linear scleroderma of the scalp and face: *en coup de sabre*. **A,** Teenage female with single lesion. **B** and **C,** Two views of a young girl with two linear lesions of the face and scalp with associated scalp ulceration and crust.

forehead are termed *en coup de sabre* (ECDS) because the linear depression resembles a saber wound scar (Fig. 7-53). The linear lesions of the face may progress to hemifacial atrophy, termed *Parry-Romberg syndrome* (PRS), in which hemiatrophy of the mandible, maxilla, tongue, and subcutaneous and muscle tissue may be apparent (Fig. 7-54). Certain extracutaneous manifestations are more common in patients with ECDS/PRS, including headache, uveitis, seizures, and transient ischemic attacks.

Plaque morphea is the most common presentation of LS in adults (60%) and accounts for approximately one quarter of LS in children. It is characterized by one or a few oval or rounded areas of induration, ranging from 1 to 30 cm in diameter. They typically arise on the trunk or proximal extremities (Fig. 7-55). Generalized plaque morphea is defined as three or more plaque lesions that are greater than 3 cm wide each. Typically the plaques become confluent and affect several anatomic areas; the trunk is the most common (Fig. 7-56).

Deep or subcutaneous morphea may have only subtle cutaneous changes, such as slight erythema and thinning of the dermis, but a great deal of inflammatory infiltrate in deep subcutaneous tissue and fascia, causing a great depression in the adipose tissue ("scooped out" appearance) and thickened,

Figure 7-54 Localized scleroderma. **A** and **B,** Frontal and side views of Parry-Romberg syndrome affecting the right side of the face.

Figure 7-55 Localized scleroderma. Large plaque morphea lesion of chest/abdomen in a young male.

Figure 7-56 Localized scleroderma. Generalized morphea in **A,** an African-American female (unaffected skin is lighter) and **B,** a white female.

bound-down skin (see Fig. 7-49). Many consider eosinophilic fasciitis a type of deep morphea; however, it often behaves as a mixture of deep morphea and linear scleroderma, resulting in deep infiltration and joint contractures. Pansclerotic morphea of childhood is a rare subset of LS, affecting only 1% to 2% of children with LS, and it is typically disabling. It affects the extremities first and sometimes migrates to the trunk, sparing only the face and distal areas of the fingers and toes (Fig. 7-57). There is a rapidly progressive fibrosis of the deep dermis, subcutis, fascia, and muscles, with occasional

Figure 7-57 Localized scleroderma. Pansclerotic morphea. Note that the distal toes are spared. Diffuse joint contractures are the result of progressive fibrosis.

bone involvement, which leads to significant contracture of joints, muscle atrophy, cutaneous ulcerations, and sometimes restrictive pattern respiratory insufficiency if the trunk is involved. Another rare subtype is bullous morphea; however, many experts agree that the bullous lesions are secondary to aggressive linear or deep LS disease. A final subtype that is now viewed as its own category is mixed morphea, which is seen in approximately 15% of the pediatric LS population. The most common presentation of mixed morphea is a combination of linear and generalized morphea occurring in the same patient.

Patients with LS sometimes present with extracutaneous manifestations. These manifestations occur in approximately one fifth of the patients throughout the course of disease, are more frequent in patients with linear scleroderma, and consist essentially of orthopedic complications (rate of occurrence for the entire group, 19%; for those with linear scleroderma of the extremities, 50%), neurologic or ocular findings (entire group, 5%; linear scleroderma of the head, up to 40%), and other autoimmune conditions such as thyroiditis (all subtypes, 2%). Intensive physical and occupational therapy in conjunction with systemic immunosuppressive therapy is recommended for those with linear scleroderma of the extremities to help avoid joint contractures and leg length discrepancy. Routine screening of all patients with LS by ophthalmology is recommended, but especially for those with linear scleroderma of the head, as "silent" uveitis occurs and has clinical outcomes similar to those of JIA.

No laboratory test exists to diagnose linear scleroderma. Although a "localized" disease, several autoantibodies have been associated with the disease. ANA positivity was found in 42% of a large pediatric LS cohort. Anti-histone antibodies (AHAs) have been detected in 47% of patients with LS, with a higher prevalence in the generalized morphea (GM) group. Single-stranded DNA (ssDNA) antibodies have been reported in 50% of patients with linear scleroderma, and were associated with more extensive GM. Rheumatoid factor is present in one third of patients, particularly those who have GM, and correlates with disease severity (as determined by the number of lesions). General markers of inflammation, including sedimentation rate and serum immunoglobulin levels, may be useful markers of disease activity in select patients with localized scleroderma; however, the majority of patients present with active LS lesions without elevation of these markers.

MIXED CONNECTIVE TISSUE DISEASE

A syndrome characterized by features of rheumatoid arthritis, scleroderma, SLE, and dermatomyositis and associated with high-titer anti-RNP antibodies was first described in 1972 and termed *mixed connective tissue disease* (MCTD). Clinical characteristics of MCTD in children are summarized in Table 7-12. The most common presentation encountered in our experience is the combination of Raynaud phenomenon, swollen hands with mild sclerodactyly, polyarthritis, mild myositis, and gastroesophageal reflux disease (GERD).

Cardiopulmonary disease and esophageal dysmotility are common in MCTD; nephritis occurs but is less common and is usually less severe than in SLE. Regarding pulmonary disease, both interstitial lung disease and pulmonary arterial hypertension can occur and should be screened for by chest x-ray, echocardiography (for PAH), and pulmonary function tests including a DL_{CO} test. Further evaluation is warranted with a high-resolution CT scan of the chest if interstitial lung disease is suspected and with right heart cardiac catheterization if PAH is suspected. Anti–U1-RNP antibodies are strongly associated with the diagnosis of MCTD. High-titer positive

Table 7-12	Clinical Characteristics of Children with Mixed Connective Tissue Disease

Characteristic	Patients (%)
Arthritis	93
Raynaud phenomenon	85
Thickened skin of scleroderma	49
Rash of SLE	33
Rash of DM	33
Fever	56
Abnormal esophageal motility	41
Cardiac	30
Pericarditis	27
Myositis	61
CNS disease	23
Pulmonary	43
Renal	26

DM, dermatomyositis; SLE, systemic lupus erythematosus.
   Modified from Cassidy JT, Petty RE: *Textbook of pediatric rheumatology,* Philadelphia, 2001, WB Saunders.

anti-nuclear antibody (ANA) is common. Rheumatoid factor (RF) may also be present.

The outcome and course of children with MCTD is variable. Sick children with MCTD often experience cardiopulmonary or renal complications.

SJÖGREN SYNDROME

A syndrome commonly associated with systemic lupus erythematosus in children is Sjögren syndrome, characterized by keratoconjunctivitis and xerostomia due to decreased tear production and saliva production. An additional recognizable feature is photosensitivity with an erythematous rash appearing at sun-exposed areas. Serologically, this syndrome typically features a positive result for anti-nuclear antibody, with specific extractable nuclear antigen antibodies to Ro (SS-A) and La (SS-B). Diagnosis is supported by objective evidence of decreased tear flow, using Schirmer test. Lip biopsy demonstrating a periductal lymphocytic infiltrate confirms the diagnosis. Adults with Sjögren syndrome are at a higher risk to develop lymphoma.

JUVENILE DERMATOMYOSITIS

Juvenile dermatomyositis (JDM) is a rare but distinctive disease that accounts for approximately 5% of all rheumatic disease in childhood. Although its exact etiology remains unknown, evidence supports the involvement of both the innate and adaptive (humoral and cell-mediated) immune system contributing to a vasculopathy, primarily affecting the skeletal muscle and skin. This results in the classic clinical skin findings and nonsuppurative myositis observed in JDM. Dermatomyositis affecting the adult generally carries a worse prognosis than that encountered in the pediatric age group. There is no association with malignancy in patients with JDM, although it appears to be a paraneoplastic syndrome in certain adult populations. Nevertheless, childhood dermatomyositis has a higher incidence of vasculopathy with intimal proliferation of small blood vessels, thrombosis, and sometimes infarctions, which may lead to tissue damage, such as permanent ulcerations of the skin (Fig. 7-58). Despite the potential severity of JDM, the majority of children who are treated by immunosuppression have a good outcome with favorable prospects for normal school and work performance.

Figure 7-58 Juvenile dermatomyositis. **A,** A 3-year-old girl with a vasculitic facial rash. Note the heliotrope hue and ulcerations. **B,** Ulcerations of the right ear and lateral to the eye (common sites). **C,** Ulcerations lateral to the left eye. Note the deep red/violaceous hue of the rash. **D,** Deep ulceration of the axilla, with ischemic tissue.

Figure 7-59 Juvenile dermatomyositis (JDM). **A,** Gottron papules: Erythematous, atrophic skin changes overlying the metacarpophalangeal and proximal interphalangeal joints. **B** and **C,** Typical rash of JDM, as seen on **B,** the knees and **C,** the elbow.

Although the age range for JDM is broad, presentation of the disease is usually between ages 4 and 10 years, with onset of disease at less than 5 years of age in 25% of the patients. Girls predominate by a 2 : 1 ratio. No racial bias exists, nor is there any evidence of a familial predisposition.

Clinically, patients usually have fatigue and symmetrical, progressive, proximal muscle weakness, particularly affecting the limb-girdle musculature (shoulders and hips), anterior neck flexors, and trunk muscles. Although painless weakness is the hallmark of the disease, myalgia can exist with tender, indurated, and edematous-appearing muscles. The first complaints often concern an inability to climb stairs and disturbances of gait. Although shoulders and arms are often involved, this may not be detected as easily in a child. A positive Gowers sign on physical examination (see Fig. 7-1) reflects proximal muscle weakness. Dysphasia, dysphonia, and dyspnea may occur if the respective muscles for these functions are affected. Other musculoskeletal manifestations include arthralgia and arthritis, affecting more than half of patients, typically early in the disease course; these are responsive to typical JDM immunosuppression. However, there are a minority of patients who develop long-term flexion contractures secondary to muscle tightening.

Cutaneous manifestations of JDM include the pathognomonic rashes, that is, Gottron's papules and heliotrope eyelid rash, which are found in more than three quarters of patients with JDM and can confirm the diagnosis. Gottron's papules are found symmetrically on the extensor surfaces of the knuckles (MCP, PIP, and DIP joints), elbows, and knees. They are characterized as flat-topped, erythematous or violaceous papules sometimes with associated scale (Fig. 7-59). The heliotrope rash, which is violaceous and telangiectatic, over the upper eyelids often is associated with edema of the eyelids and face, and may be confluent with a malar type of erythematous rash distributed over the cheeks and nose (Fig. 7-60). The JDM malar rash is different from that of SLE by being more diffuse, ill-defined, and typically not sparing the nasolabial folds. However, it is similar regarding the degree of photosensitivity. The cutaneous vasculopathy of JDM is most visible at the nail fold capillaries, with capillary loop dilation, hemorrhage, drop-out, and telangiectasias (Fig. 7-61). Adjacent periungual erythema, with thickened cuticle hypertrophy and periungual infarcts, further reflects vasculopathy.

Figure 7-60 Juvenile dermatomyositis. The facial rash shows heliotrope discoloration and violaceous suffusion with edema of the eyelids. Note the faint malar blush in patient **A** and diffuse light erythematous rash of the face, including the forehead and not sparing nasolabial folds, in patient **B**.

Figure 7-61   Juvenile dermatomyositis. Nail bed telangiectasia. Erythema can be seen around the nail edge. The pinpoint telangiectasia may require a magnifying lens to identify.

Other areas that commonly ulcerate because of vasculopathy are the corners of the eye (see Fig. 7-58), in the axilla, and over the elbows. Calcinosis (nodular calcium deposits) of the skin, subcutaneous tissue, and muscle is another characteristic cutaneous complication of JDM. It is more common in those with long-standing, untreated, severe disease (Fig. 7-62). Pressure points and severely affected soft tissue are particularly susceptible. These calcium deposits can be inflammatory, causing pain and eruption through the surface of the skin, and

can contribute to joint contractures. Last, lipodystrophy is another cutaneous finding that is representative of disease damage from long-standing and/or uncontrolled JDM (see Fig. 7-62, C and D). Lipodystrophy results from the slow, progressive loss of subcutaneous tissue, typically symmetrically distributed in the upper body, and is associated with glucose and lipid metabolism abnormalities.

JDM can exist with skin involvement only, and skin involvement can predate muscle involvement by months to years. Because of the pathognomonic features of the rash, the diagnosis of JDM can often be suspected before overt symptoms occur. Constitutional symptoms such as anorexia, malaise, weight loss, fever, and irritability (in young children) may be present. The illness may progress at variable rates in different patients; however, the majority of patients have a more insidious rather than acute course.

Unfortunately, long delays in diagnosis can occur, particularly in the insidious group. Other, more uncommon findings include mouth ulcers, retinitis, hepatosplenomegaly, pancreatitis, vasculopathy of the gastrointestinal tract leading to ulceration, bleeding, or perforation (Fig. 7-63), respiratory muscle weakness with a restrictive pattern on lung function studies, decreased lung diffusion capacity associated with interstitial lung disease, aspiration pneumonitis from pharyngeal muscle weakness, myocarditis, and pericarditis. To screen for some of these abnormalities, clinicians will often perform certain examinations on recently diagnosed patients, including a swallow study with an upper GI and small-bowel follow-through radiographic studies, chest radiograph, electrocardiogram and echocardiogram, and pulmonary function tests with a DL_{CO} test.

Elevated muscle enzymes may be the first clue to the diagnosis of inflammatory muscle disease. Creatine kinase, aspartate transaminase, alanine aminotransferase, aldolase, and lactate dehydrogenase should be checked serially because they can be useful in monitoring disease activity. Not all of the aforementioned muscle enzymes may be elevated in the setting of floridly active myositis. Serum neopterin, reflective of macrophage activation, is another marker of disease activity in dermatomyositis. An elevated serum von Willebrand factor

Figure 7-62   Juvenile dermatomyositis (JDM). Six-year-old male with chronic JDM and poor compliance. **A,** Calcinosis surrounding the right knee after years of untreated disease. **B,** Calcium deposits, right knee, after 2 months of intensive therapy. **C,** Sacral calcium deposits (untreated for years); note lipodystrophy of the buttocks from chronic unopposed disease activity. **D,** Sacral calcinosis after 2 months of immunosuppressive therapy. **E,** Radiologic evidence of soft tissue calcification in the same patient.

Figure 7-63 Juvenile dermatomyositis. Computed tomographic scan of the abdomen demonstrates bowel wall thickening and edema in the transverse colon. The patient's bowel eventually perforated because of active vasculitis.

antigen level is thought to be a measure of endothelial cell damage due to vasculitis.

Magnetic resonance imaging, specifically T_2-weighted imaging with fat suppression, is quite sensitive in detecting even subclinical myositis (Fig. 7-64). In the setting of a child with muscle weakness, Gottron's papules, elevated muscle enzymes, and abnormal muscle MRI, most clinicians choose to make the diagnosis of JDM and initiate therapy without a muscle biopsy or electromyography (EMG), which were previously performed as a standard for diagnosis but are more invasive and painful and are used less commonly today (usually in patients who do not have the typical rash).

Corticosteroids in conjunction with methotrexate and hydroxychloroquine are the mainstay of therapy. The initial clinical efficacy of treatment, with reduced rash and gain of muscle strength within days to weeks of treatment, is

attributable mostly to the corticosteroid effect. Severe disease with vasculitis/vasculopathy of the lungs, skin, and gastrointestinal or nervous system will typically require the addition of IVIG and/or cyclophosphamide. Early and aggressive therapy is often the key to halt disease and prevent further disease damage, such as muscle atrophy, calcinosis, and skin ulcerations.

SYSTEMIC VASCULITIDES

The vasculitides are a broad group of disorders with a common pathology characterized by blood vessel inflammation. The type of inflammation, organ system affected, and size of the vessels affected vary with each disease entity. A classification of the systemic vasculitides based on the size of the blood vessels involved is noted in Table 7-13. Further classification is made on the basis of the presence or absence of antineutrophil cytoplasmic antibodies (ANCAs) and granulomas.

Nonspecific generalized findings are present in the initial inflammatory state, such as fever, fatigue, weight loss, elevated acute-phase reactants, and failure to thrive. For many of the vasculitides, it is not until later in the disease process, after vessel damage has accumulated from chronic inflammation, that the diagnosis become more evident, reflecting vascular compromise. For example, involvement of the large vessels of the extremities leads to claudication, bruits over the site of involvement, and skin ulcerations distally on physical examination, whereas arterial insufficiency of the visceral vessels causes hypertension (renal arteries), abdominal pain and melena (mesenteric arteries), chest pain (coronary arteries), or neurologic deficits (mononeuritis multiplex). Fortunately, the two more common forms of vasculitis in children,

Figure 7-64 Juvenile dermatomyositis. Magnetic resonance imaging of the thigh (T_2-weighted image with fat suppression) illustrates marked diffuse muscle edema and inflammation. Note the patchy white area in muscle similar in appearance to fluid in the bladder.

Table 7-13	Classification of Vasculitis by Vessel Size

Large-Vessel Vasculitis
Giant cell arteritis (seen in adults only)
Takayasu arteritis
Medium-Vessel Vasculitis
Kawasaki syndrome
Polyarteritis nodosa (PAN)
Primary granulomatous central nervous system vasculitis
Small-Vessel Vasculitis (ANCA Associated)
Microscopic polyangiitis
Wegener granulomatosis
Churg-Strauss syndrome
Drug-induced
Small-Vessel Vasculitis (Immune Complex Associated)
Henoch-Schönlein purpura
Essential cryoglobulinemic vasculitis
Hypocomplementemic urticarial vasculitis
Vasculitis with lupus, rheumatoid arthritis, or Sjögren syndrome
Behçet syndrome
Goodpasture syndrome
Serum sickness
Drug-associated
Infection-associated
Small-Vessel Vasculitis (Paraneoplastic)
Lymphoproliferative
Myeloproliferative
Carcinoma
Small-Vessel Vasculitis (Inflammatory Bowel Disease)

From Jennette JC, Falk RJ: Small-vessel vasculitis, *N Engl J Med* 337:1512, 1997.

Figure 7-65   Henoch-Schönlein purpura. **A** and **B,** Rash characteristically involves the lower extremities, with purpuric coalescent lesions.

Kawasaki disease (KD) and Henoch-Schönlein purpura (HSP), typically do not result in chronic arterial insufficiency and have a more recognizable acute inflammatory state that typically resolves in a period of weeks to months. These conditions are discussed at length in the following sections, and the others are briefly described.

Henoch-Schönlein Purpura

Henoch-Schönlein purpura (HSP) is a small-vessel leukocytoclastic vasculitis mediated by IgA immune complex deposition with clinical manifestations of nonthrombocytopenic palpable purpura, arthritis, bowel angina, and renal abnormalities. Although HSP is associated with serious potential complications of the gastrointestinal tract and kidneys, the majority of cases are mild and self-resolve within weeks. Ninety percent of cases occur in children younger than 10 years of age, with the median age being 5 years. Children younger than 2 years of age generally develop milder disease with less frequent gastrointestinal and renal involvement. This syndrome may or may not occur after an identifiable trigger such as viral illness, bacterial infection, insect bite, dietary allergen, immunization, or medication usage. Seasonal peaks occur in fall and winter, suggesting an infectious trigger, but a definite etiology remains elusive. A familial predilection does not appear to exist, and all races have been affected. The clinical picture of HSP is that of a previously well child who acutely develops a distinctive skin rash, arthritis, and abdominal pain. The skin rash allows for definitive diagnosis, and hence it is said to occur in all patients with HSP. Fifty percent of patients present with rash, which usually involves the buttocks and lower extremities (waist-down distribution) (Fig. 7-65). The lesions begin as petechiae or red macules that coalesce and become confluent with nearby lesions to form purpuric plaques and patches that are nonblanching. Typically, various stages of eruption are simultaneously present. Some patients have lesions that mimic urticaria. Pruritus can be a feature of the rash, and about 25% have subcutaneous edema. The edema is nonpitting, painless, evanescent, and most commonly affects the hands (Fig. 7-66, B) and feet. The child younger than 2 years of age is most likely to have edema as a feature of this illness. The younger child is also more likely to display facial involvement (see Fig. 7-66, A and C). Infants tend to have the rash on face, ears, sacrum and buttocks, whereas older children tend to have the rash on the buttocks and lower legs because gravity causes the IgA immune complexes to deposit and incite inflammation in dependent areas. A similar-appearing purpuric skin manifestation associated with edema in infants is acute

hemorrhagic edema of infancy (AHEI) (Fig. 7-67). Although the appearance of the rash is quite concerning, the child appears well, typically does not have any internal organ involvement, and the condition self-resolves within weeks. Skin biopsy of AHEI would support a leukocytoclastic vasculitis, mainly of the venules, but without IgA deposition as seen in HSP.

HSP does have internal organ vasculitis, most notably intestinal and renal. Approximately 85% of patients display some gastrointestinal symptoms. Simple colicky abdominal pain can be the only symptom, but its severity can raise physician concerns about more threatening abdominal complications.

Figure 7-66   Infant with Henoch-Schönlein purpura (HSP). **A,** The rash may occur on the face along with edema. **B,** Rash and edema may be present in the extremities. **C,** Ulceration and vesicles are an unusual manifestation of HSP.

Figure 7-67   Acute hemorrhagic edema of infancy. **A,** A 15-month-old male with classic annular, medallion-like, and targetoid-shaped purpuric lesions on the leg, and **B,** the face (including auricles).

Massive gastrointestinal hemorrhage, intussusception (typically ilio-ileal), and perforation are potential serious complications; however, they occur in less than 5% of patients. More common manifestations are melanotic stools, vomiting, ileus, and hematemesis. Pancreatitis, cholecystitis, and protein-losing enteropathy have also been described. In rare circumstances abdominal pain precedes the rash, making it difficult to distinguish appendicitis and other acute abdominal conditions from HSP.

The periarticular swelling that occurs presents as arthritis or arthralgia and is a part of HSP in three quarters of reported cases. Knees and ankles are the most common sites of involvement. Warmth and erythema are not usually associated with the pain and swelling that occur. The joints are not affected permanently, and this feature of HSP generally resolves in several days. As with the gastrointestinal symptoms, arthritis can precede the rash. For this reason, HSP should be considered in the child with acute onset of arthritis.

Renal involvement is detected in about one half of patients with HSP and typically occurs early in the disease, during the first days or weeks. The degree of renal pathology generally affects the patient's ultimate prognosis. Renal manifestations can range from mild hematuria or proteinuria to end-stage renal disease (less than 1% of patients). Patients usually declare themselves within several months, but cases of renal failure and hypertension have occurred years after the initial illness. Overall, about 1% to 5% of patients with HSP develop some degree of chronic renal disease. Berger disease (IgA glomerulonephritis) is believed by many to be HSP without the rash and hence an alternative manifestation of the same pathologic process.

Other features of HSP include low-grade fever, malaise, scrotal swelling with pain, periorbital and scalp edema, headache, cerebral vasculitis, CNS bleeding, seizures, nosebleeds, parotitis, hydrops of the gallbladder, and cardiopulmonary disease. There are no specific diagnostic laboratory abnormities, although tissue specimen staining for IgA is helpful. Clotting functions are generally normal, and platelet counts are normal or elevated. The presence of IgA complexes in the glomeruli, skin, and serum of affected individuals may be a clue to diagnosis. Skin biopsy documents leukocytoclastic vasculitis with IgA deposits in dermal capillaries and postcapillary venules. Elevated serum IgA and IgM levels are found in about one half of patients with HSP. Because there are no diagnostic laboratory examinations for this syndrome, the history and physical examination provide clues to the successful recognition of HSP.

The course of the illness varies with age. The majority of patients self-resolve their initial illness in 4 weeks; however, approximately 40% have at least one recurrence, especially those with nephritis. Recurrences are generally less severe, have a shorter duration, and are limited to cutaneous and mild abdominal symptomatology. Recurrences typically occur during the first 4 to 6 months from onset of disease. If corticosteroids (CSs) are used to treat manifestations of HSP (which is controversial), a rapid taper has been demonstrated to trigger a flare of symptoms. Therefore it is advisable, if treating HSP with CSs, that a slow taper be conducted. In general, treatment of HSP is supportive, with the focus on maintaining adequate hydration, pain relief, and bowel rest.

Kawasaki Disease

Kawasaki disease (KD), classified as a medium-vessel vasculitis with specific mucocutaneous features affecting younger children (90% are less than 5 years old), is notorious for its effects on the coronary arteries. Although the etiology of KD has eluded investigators, the clinical features and natural history of this distinctive vasculitis are well described. The need to rapidly recognize the presentation of this disease is heightened by its potentially devastating cardiac sequelae. The early recognition of KD favorably affects morbidity and mortality.

KD, first described in 1967 in Japan by Tomisaku Kawasaki, consists of a unique constellation of clinical findings initially called *mucocutaneous lymph node syndrome*. This multisystem disease was independently described by Melish in 1976 in Hawaii. Since that time the disease has been recognized in all racial groups worldwide. Individuals of Asian ancestry are most commonly affected, and Japanese and Korean children have a particularly high incidence. The risk to African-American children is greater than the risk to white children. Boys are more commonly affected than girls by a ratio of approximately 1.5 : 1. The peak age of patients with KD in the United States is 18 months to 2 years, with 80% of cases occurring in children younger than 4 years. Middle and upper socioeconomic classes are overrepresented. A variety of etiologies have been suggested as the cause of KD, but all have fallen short of complete acceptance.

The clinical features of typical KD are remarkably consistent (Table 7-14). However, incomplete or atypical KD adds uncertainty to the clinician's approach to diagnosis. It is notable that 10% of children who develop coronary artery aneurysms never meet the full criteria for KD. The diagnosis must be considered when a child has fever for more than 4 days and has two other clinical criteria. Children younger than 1 year of age are at highest risk of developing KD without fulfilling criteria and, unfortunately, are the group with the highest risk of developing coronary artery aneurysms,

Table 7-14	Kawasaki Syndrome: Diagnostic Criteria

1. Fever for 5 or more days
2. Conjunctivitis (bilateral, bulbar, nonsuppurative)
3. Lymphadenopathy
4. Rash (polymorphous, no vesicles or crusts)
5. Change(s)* in the mucous membranes of the oropharynx, such as:

    Injected pharynx

    Injected lips

    Dry, fissured lips

    "Strawberry" tongue
6. Change(s)* of the peripheral extremities, such as:

    Hand or foot edema (acute)

    Hand or foot erythema (acute)

    Fingertip desquamation (convalescent)

*One is sufficient to establish criterion.

Diagnosis requires five of six criteria, or four criteria plus coronary artery aneurysms shown on echocardiography.

It has been suggested that in the presence of classic features, the diagnosis of KS can be made (and treatment initiated) before the fifth day of fever.

Modified from Centers for Disease Control: Multiple outbreaks of Kawasaki syndrome—United States, *MMWR* 34:33, 1985.

Figure 7-69   Kawasaki disease. Nonexudative, nonulcerative, bulbar conjunctivitis. Note sparing of the limbus.

magnifying the gravity of the situation. The importance of appropriate clinical suspicion in the *forme fruste* of the disease cannot be overemphasized.

The course of the illness is triphasic: acute (lasting 7 to 14 days), subacute (days 10 to 25), and convalescent (days 21 to 60) (Fig. 7-68). The acute phase is characterized by fever, irritability, nonexudative conjunctivitis, oropharyngeal erythema, rash, lymphadenopathy, and distal extremity edema and erythema. The onset of fever is sudden, often spiking as high as 40° C. It is remitting in character, with a mean duration of 12 days in the untreated individual. Some patients may continue to be febrile for 30 days or more without therapy. The fever has been shown to reflect elevation of proinflammatory cytokines, such as interleukin (IL)-1 and tumor necrosis factor (TNF), which are thought to mediate the underlying vascular inflammation. Fever generally precedes other clinical signs and symptoms by 1 to 2 days. The conjunctivitis appears early in the progression of the illness. The conjunctivitis is

nonexudative and nonulcerative with bulbar predominance, and it usually persists for 1 to 2 weeks in the untreated patient. Limbic sparing is a common feature (Fig. 7-69). Additional eye findings include a transient anterior uveitis in most patients during the first 2 weeks of illness. Uveitis is demonstrated by slit-lamp ophthalmologic examination. Because these findings are not seen in the differential diagnosis of KD, their presence may be a helpful diagnostic tool. Oral findings include red, cracked, fissured lips; "strawberry tongue"; and diffuse mouth erythema (Fig. 7-70). These findings may last for several weeks as well. The classic "strawberry tongue" finding results from sloughing of the filiform papillae and denuding of the inflamed glossal tissue. Other findings, such as discrete oral ulcers or vesicles and tonsillar exudate, would support more of an infectious etiology opposed to KD. The rash of KD may manifest itself in many forms: scarlatiniform, morbilliform (Fig. 7-71), macular and papular erythema, multiforme-like with target lesions, urticarial plaques, or even pustular. It can be pruritic, but the presence of vesicles, erythroderma, petechiae, or purpura suggests another diagnosis. A predilection for involvement of intertriginous areas, particularly the perineum, has been noted (Fig. 7-72). Peeling of the perineum generally occurs several days before desquamation

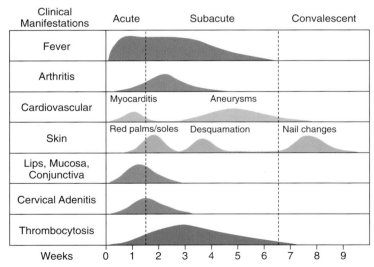

Figure 7-68   Kawasaki disease. The syndrome can be divided into three clinical phases: acute, subacute, and convalescent. The temporal characteristics described here are typical of the disease course. *(Adapted from Kawasaki T: Acute febrile mucocutaneous syndrome with lymphoid involvement and specific desquamation of the fingers and toes in children, Arerugi 16:178-222, 1967.)*

Figure 7-70   Kawasaki disease. **A,** Erythematous, cracked lips. **B,** "Strawberry tongue."

Figure 7-73   Kawasaki disease. Swollen, erythematous hands. Note the fusiform appearance.

Figure 7-71   Kawasaki disease. Morbilliform rash is one possible manifestation.

of the fingers and toes. A particularly striking feature of the acute phase of the syndrome is erythema and edema of the hands (Fig. 7-73) and feet, often associated with a refusal to walk. The characteristic desquamation of fingers and toes, beginning at the nail–fingertip junction, occurs between 10 and 21 days during the subacute phase (Fig. 7-74). The toes are involved later and to a lesser degree than the fingers. In the syndrome's most dramatic form, the entire distal extremity can peel. Months after the acute phase of illness, transverse grooves called *Beau lines* are noted in the fingernails (Fig. 7-75). Although the initial syndrome was named mucocutaneous lymph node syndrome, the presence of a 1.5-cm or greater cervical lymph node is the least consistent feature, occurring in about 50% to 75% of children. The other five features are each found in the majority of patients. The "lymphadenopathic" presentation of KD strongly mimics pyogenic lymphadenitis.

Although many of the aforementioned features are considered central to the diagnosis of KD, it is often the associated features of the disease that add credence to the diagnosis. Both an "early" and a "late" form of arthritis and arthralgia occur in one third of children with KD. The arthritis is

Figure 7-74   Kawasaki disease. Fingertip and toe tip peeling in the subacute phase.

Figure 7-75   Kawasaki disease. Beau lines of fingernails in the convalescent phase.

Figure 7-72   Kawasaki disease. **A,** Perineal rash with peeling. **B,** Neck rash with peeling. Note that peeling of an intertriginous rash occurs before extremity peeling.

Figure 7-76 Kawasaki disease. Inflammation of the urethral meatus (often associated with sterile pyuria).

typically characterized by a small-joint polyarthritis during the first weeks of illness and later a large-joint pauciarthritis. It does not persist beyond a few months and is nonerosive. Urethritis and inflammation of the urethral meatus occur and generally are accompanied by sterile pyuria (Fig. 7-76). Diarrhea, vomiting, abdominal pain, and hepatitis are frequent gastrointestinal features seen early in the illness. Other gastrointestinal manifestations include pancreatitis and transient gallbladder dilation. During the acute phase of KD, cardiac features include tachycardia, dysrhythmias, pericarditis, pericardial effusion, myocarditis, mitral or aortic insufficiency, and congestive heart failure. CNS findings such as lethargy, meningismus, aseptic meningitis, facial nerve palsy, sensorineural hearing loss, and paralysis of the extremities have been described but are uncommon. Analysis of CSF demonstrates inflammation with mononuclear pleocytosis but typically without elevation of CSF protein. Other laboratory abnormalities reflecting systemic inflammation include elevation of acute-phase markers such as the erythrocyte sedimentation rate (ESR) and C-reactive protein (CRP), leukocytosis with a left shift in the WBC count, normocytic normochromic anemia, and thrombocytosis. Because of the dynamic nature of this syndrome, meticulous and frequent physical examinations are essential.

As the syndrome progresses toward the subacute phase, thrombocytosis is considerable with platelet counts reaching 1 million. Coronary artery aneurysms (Fig. 7-77) also develop in the subacute phase and, in combination with thrombocytosis, place the patient at risk for myocardial infarction. Coronary artery aneurysms are the hallmark of KD sequelae, and since the 1980s it has been recognized that early treatment of KD (within the first 10 days of illness) with intravenous immunoglobulin (IVIG) reduces the incidence of coronary artery aneurysms by more than 70%. Approximately 20% of untreated patients develop coronary artery aneurysms. Although many regress spontaneously, approximately 1% of affected individuals die of related complications. Of these deaths, 85% occur during the first 10 to 40 days of illness.

The natural history of these aneurysms includes thromboembolism and vessel occlusion and leads to myocardial infarction in a small group of patients. Others develop coronary artery stenosis or persistent asymptomatic aneurysms of various sizes. Giant aneurysms (8 mm or more in diameter) are most likely to result in stenosis, thrombosis, and myocardial infarction. In general, smaller aneurysms (<8 mm) tend to regress over time and many may fully resolve as indicated by echocardiography; however, although their structure may appear normal their function (vascular reactivity) is not preserved, due to fibrointimal proliferation, fibrosis, and calcinosis, which occur while the vessels are healing. Particularly worrisome indicators for the development of aneurysms include male gender, age less than 1 year, fever lasting more than 2 weeks, recurrent fever after defervescence, recurrence of rash, exaggerated leukocytosis and elevated sedimentation rate, and cardiac rhythm disturbances other than first-degree heart block. Arterial aneurysms have also been found to occur in axillary, iliac, renal, hepatic, cerebral, and brachial and femoral arteries. Some experts believe in these cases with more widespread aneurysms that "infantile polyarteritis nodosa" is a more suitable diagnosis.

The late convalescent phase is a period of relatively low risk for the development of aneurysms, although the long-term impact of coronary artery vasculitis on vessel function and on the incidence and severity of atherosclerotic heart disease remains a concern.

Differential diagnosis includes scarlet fever (both streptococcal and staphylococcal), staphylococcal scalded skin syndrome, toxic shock syndrome, leptospirosis, disseminated yersiniosis, Rocky Mountain spotted fever, rubeola, adenoviral and enteroviral infection, drug reactions, reactive arthritis, JIA, PAN, and SLE. Cultures, serologic tests, patient age, and clinical course of disease help in distinguishing these other disorders (Table 7-15).

Polyarteritis Nodosa

Polyarteritis nodosa (PAN), the prototype medium-sized vessel vasculitis, is a systemic necrotizing vasculitis with segmental aneurysm formation leading to the classic "beading" of vessels pattern demonstrated in vascular imaging studies. Worldwide, PAN is associated with hepatitis B and C infections; however, pediatric PAN is quite rare, especially in North America. The average age of children affected is 9 years, with a slight predominance in boys. There is an association with

Figure 7-77 Kawasaki disease. Coronary artery aneurysms. The autopsy specimen of this infant heart shows a dilated right coronary artery filled with thrombus (dissected in cross-section). The inferior portion of the heart demonstrates a dilated left coronary artery. *(Courtesy David Witte, MD, Cincinnati, Ohio.)*

Table 7-15	Differential Diagnosis of Kawasaki Syndrome	
Agent	**Disease**	**Distinguishing Characteristics**
Bacteria	Streptococcal	Positive culture and serology, palatal petechiae, no anterior uveitis
	Staphylococcal scalded skin syndrome	Positive culture, bullous lesions, Nikolsky sign, earlier desquamation, no anterior uveitis
	Toxic shock syndrome*	Primarily females, older age predilection, toxin detection, positive culture
Rickettsia	Rocky Mountain spotted fever*	Petechial rash, positive serology, regional geography, no anterior uveitis
Spirochetes	Leptospirosis*	Positive culture and serology, muscle pain and tenderness, rigid abdominal muscles
Toxins	Acrodynia (mercury poisoning)	Photophobia, no conjunctivitis, slow onset, diaphoresis, severe pain in hands and feet, pruritus
Autoimmune/ allergic	Stevens-Johnson syndrome	History of drug or infection exposure, no predominant lymph node, corneal ulcers, blisters, more severe mucous membrane involvement
	Systemic-onset JIA	Nondesquamating evanescent rash, hepatosplenomegaly, generalized adenopathy, vasculopathy
	Polyarteritis nodosa	Vasculitic skin findings of palpable purpura, livedo reticularis, and dusky nodules
	Reiter syndrome	HLA-B27 positive, not toxic appearing
Viral infection	Epstein-Barr virus*	Positive serology, splenomegaly, atypical lymphocytes
	Rubella	Minimal enanthem, distal extremities not affected, not toxic appearing
	Rubeola	Cough, catarrh more prominent, lips not cracked, fewer oral changes, distal extremities generally not affected
	Roseola	As fever ends rash begins, shorter course
	Enterovirus*	Seasonal, epidemic, not toxic appearing

*May fulfill diagnostic criteria for Kawasaki syndrome.
JIA, juvenile idiopathic arthritis.
Modified from Lohr JA, Rheuban KS: Kawasaki syndrome, *Infect Dis Clin North Am* 1:559-574, 1987.

Figure 7-78 Cutaneous polyarteritis nodosa (PAN). Cutaneous PAN of the lower extremities in a teenage female; biopsy supportive of diagnosis.

irreversible vessel damage has occurred, causing clinical findings on examination of bruits, decreased or absent acral pulses, and blood pressure differences exceeding 10 mm Hg between arms. Laboratory findings support systemic inflammation with highly elevated ESR and CRP, leukocytosis, and moderate anemia. Diagnosis is made by angiography or magnetic resonance angiography demonstrating segmental involvement (Fig. 7-79).

Anti-neutrophil Cytoplasmic Antibody–associated Vasculitides

Wegener's granulomatosis (WG), microscopic polyangiitis (MPA), and Churg-Strauss syndrome (CSS) are small-vessel vasculitides associated with the presence of ANCA. WG is a necrotic, granulomatous disease affecting mainly the upper and lower airways and the kidneys, although other organ manifestations are found. Most children with WG present with upper respiratory symptoms such as sinusitis, otitis media,

the periodic fever syndrome familial Mediterranean fever (FMF). Systemic PAN can affect any organ system and can be quite devastating. Typical skin findings, which suggest a larger size vessel involvement, include palpable purpura, livedo reticularis, tender nodules and necrotic lesions. Other findings suggestive of the disease include hypertension, abdominal pain, myalgia, arthritis, neuropathy, weight loss, and fever. Although suspected clinically, the diagnosis requires tissue biopsy or radiologic documentation of segmental aneurysms. Cutaneous PAN is limited to the skin and musculoskeletal system and is often noted in the setting of poststreptococcal infection. The lower extremities are most commonly affected, with arthritis of knees and ankles and associated skin changes in this distribution (Fig. 7-78). Although this condition is much milder than the systemic form, chronic immunosuppressive agents are often required because of persistence of disease and relapse.

Takayasu Arteritis

Takayasu arteritis (TA), also known as the *pulseless disease*, is the prototype large-sized vessel vasculitis, affecting the aorta and its branches, and is associated with great morbidity and mortality. TA typically affects young females, especially of Asian descent. The symptoms are nonspecific, such as fever, fatigue, and weight loss, and therefore the delay in diagnosis from symptom onset is 19 months. By this time

Figure 7-79 Takayasu arteritis. Magnetic resonance angiogram of the chest, demonstrating a markedly abnormal ascending and descending aorta and its branches with gross dilation and strictures. Note the completely occluded right subclavian artery.

Figure 7-80 Wegener granulomatosis. Pansinusitis with mucosal thickening throughout and bilateral mastoid effusion in teenage female with WG.

epistaxis, or hearing loss (Fig. 7-80). Lower respiratory symptoms include cough, wheeze, hemoptysis, and dyspnea. Because the majority of these symptoms occur commonly with typical childhood viral infections, WG should be suspected if the respiratory disease is recurrent or resistant to typical therapy. Chest radiographs demonstrate nodular pulmonary infiltrates in one third of those with WG, and therefore may be helpful when considering the diagnosis. Renal disease is typically asymptomatic and not discovered until evaluated by urinalysis, 24-hour urine collections, and biopsy. Arthritis, vasculitic skin lesions, symptomatic uveitis, episcleritis, and gastrointestinal involvement are also common in WG. Longer term sequelae of WG include the classic "saddle nose" deformity and subglottic tracheal stenosis due to granulomatous destruction of the cartilage. Confirmation of a WG diagnosis relies on biopsy results (sinus, lung, or renal) (Fig. 7-81). The presence of serum cytoplasmic ANCA directed toward proteinase-3 antigen is supportive. Microscopic polyangiitis (MPA) is a nongranulomatous renal–pulmonary disease typically defined by focal segmental glomerulonephritis,

Figure 7-81 Wegener granulomatosis. Multiple pulmonary nodules in a teenage female demonstrated by a high-resolution computed tomographic scan of the chest. Pulmonary nodules may serve as source of tissue to biopsy for definitive diagnosis.

pulmonary hemorrhage, and positive peripheral ANCA with reactivity to myeloperoxidase (MPO) antigen. Typically, systemic and other organ features seen in WG are not as prominent in MPA. Churg-Strauss syndrome (CSS) is the third ANCA-associated small-vessel vasculitis with well-recognized features that distinguish it from WG and MPA. These features include a long-standing history of asthma (typically poorly controlled), peripheral eosinophilia, frequent cardiac and peripheral nerve (mononeuritis multiplex) involvement, and mild renal disease without progression. This ANCA-associated vasculitis is the most uncommon in children, given that decades of preceding asthma contribute to its pathophysiology.

Other Vasculitides

Primary angiitis of the central nervous system (PACNS), previously called *granulomatous angiitis,* is basically a diagnosis of exclusion. It is an isolated vasculitis of the CNS without systemic signs or markers of inflammation. If cerebral angiography demonstrates abnormal "beading" (alternating ectasia and stenosis) of the cerebral vessels, then the diagnosis PACNS is supported. Rarely is a tissue diagnosis confirmed in children. Symptoms of PACNS vary and include transient ischemic attack, stroke, seizures, vision loss, and neurocognitive impairment.

Behçet Disease

Behçet disease (BD) is a rare systemic vasculitis of both the arterioles and veins associated with thrombosis. It is extremely uncommon in children, and the majority of affected patients live in Japan and the Mediterranean area along the historic Silk Road route. The presence of the HLA-B51 allele is associated with susceptibility to the disease.

BD may affect virtually any organ in the body. It classically presents as a triad of findings: recurrent oral and genital ulcers and uveitis (Fig. 7-82). The well-recognized feature of Behçet disease in childhood is recurrent aphthous stomatitis. Ulcers occur on the lips, buccal mucosa, tongue, and tonsils and may involve the larynx. In general, these ulcers tend to be larger than typical viral aphthous ulcers and leave scar tissue. Genital ulcers occur frequently; the penis and scrotum are affected in the male patient, and the vulva and vagina are affected in the female patient. Ocular involvement is important to recognize because visual loss and other complications may result if untreated. Eye lesions occur in 30% to 60% of children with BD, including anterior and posterior uveitis, retinal vasculitis, retinal vein occlusion, retinal detachment, and papilledema.

All organ systems may be affected in patients with BD. The skin, joints, CNS, and blood vessels are important and frequent targets of the disease. Erythema nodosum is the most frequent skin finding followed by pseudofolliculitis and nodular acneiform lesions. Recurrent arthralgia and peripheral arthritis may be seen; the number of joints affected may vary from a single joint to multiple joints. Arthritis may be symmetrical or asymmetrical and most commonly affects the knees. CNS manifestations include headaches, meningoencephalitis, pyramidal tract and brainstem lesions, seizures, and memory loss. Vascular lesions include thrombosis of deep and superficial veins, arterial occlusion, aneurysms, and varices. Organ involvement occurs, albeit less frequently, in the heart, lungs, gastrointestinal tract, and genitourinary tract. Symptoms may be vague and nonspecific; thus the clinician must maintain a high index of suspicion that even minor symptoms could be clues to the diagnosis. The aphthous and gastrointestinal ulcers of BD can be confused with inflammatory bowel disease.

Figure 7-82 Behçet disease. **A,** Painful uveitis. **B,** Ulceration throughout oral mucosa. **C,** Genital ulceration. **D,** Pathergy test.

The diagnosis of Behçet disease is made on clinical grounds in the absence of other clinical explanations. A positive pathergy test is supportive in light of other clinical features. This phenomenon occurs when a sterile needle prick into the skin produces a sterile erythematous papule greater than 2 mm in diameter by 24 to 48 hours (see Fig. 7-82, *D*). The pathergy test is sensitive but not specific and may be seen in patients with other disorders such as Sweet syndrome. Inflammatory markers, such as the erythrocyte sedimentation rate (ESR) and C-reactive protein (CRP), tend to be elevated in patients with BD. Treatment is directed at the relief of symptoms, and close monitoring of eye involvement is imperative.

RELAPSING POLYCHONDRITIS

Relapsing polychondritis is considered a perivasculitic syndrome, which is identified by its widespread recurrent inflammation of the cartilage. The ear is the most common site affected, followed by the nasal bridge, trachea (leading to stenosis), bronchi, and cartilage of the joints. Relapsing polychondritis is also associated with uveitis, deafness, vestibular involvement, and aortic insufficiency. The most common presentation in children is a recurrent "cellulitis" of the outer ear, sometimes with spreading of erythema beyond the ear toward the face and scalp.

SARCOIDOSIS

Sarcoidosis is a multisystem autoimmune disease that can cause arthritis, lymphadenopathy, lung disease, uveitis, rash, and CNS disease. The most common initial manifestation of sarcoidosis is lymphadenopathy. Sarcoidosis is sometimes detected incidentally as hilar lymphadenopathy on chest radiograph. Laboratory features may include hypercalcemia and elevation of serum angiotensin-converting enzyme (ACE). Noncaseating granulomas are demonstrated on biopsy specimens, supporting the diagnosis of sarcoidosis.

PERIODIC FEVER SYNDROMES

The periodic fever syndromes are a group of disorders characterized by febrile attacks that occur in a predictable, periodic fashion. The fevers may reach a peak of 106 degrees and last several days before subsiding. Often the pattern is a few weeks without symptoms before the next episode of fever begins. The parents can often predict the start of the next attack on the basis of the child's pattern of fever. During the febrile illness, the child may also suffer abdominal pain, rash, arthralgia, arthritis, loss of appetite, pleuritis, and peritonitis. Markers of inflammation such as white blood cell count, platelet count, erythrocyte sedimentation rate, and C-reactive protein will be elevated during the attacks. The various phenotypes of the periodic fever syndromes depend on the genetic mutations involved. Thus far, the identified syndromes include familial Mediterranean fever (FMF), hyperimmunoglobulinemia D syndrome (HIDS), PFAPA (periodic fever, aphthous stomatitis, pharyngitis, and cervical adenitis) syndrome, TRAPS (tumor necrosis factor receptor–associated periodic syndrome), and the cryopyrin-associated periodic syndromes (CAPS). CAPS include Muckle-Wells syndrome, familial cold autoinflammatory syndrome, and neonatal-onset multisystem inflammatory disease (NOMID) (Table 7-16).

Familial Mediterranean fever is an autosomal recessive disorder affecting people of eastern Mediterranean descent. The

Table 7-16	Common Features of Hereditary Periodic Fever Syndromes					
	FMF	**HIDS**	**TRAPS**	**FCAS**	**MWS**	**NOMID**
Inheritance	Recessive	Recessive	Dominant	Dominant	Dominant	Dominant
Common ethnicities	Jewish, Armenian, Arabic, Turkish, Italian	Dutch, French	Irish, Scottish	European	Northern European	None
Chromosome	16p13	12q24	12p13	1q44	1q44	1q44
Gene	*MEFV*	*MVK*	*TNFRSF1A*	*CIAS1*	*CIAS1*	*CIAS1*
Protein	Pyrin	Mevalonate kinase	55-kDa TNF receptor	Cryopyrin	Cryopyrin	Cryopyrin
Symptom duration	1-3 d	3-7 d	>1 wk	<1 d	1-2 d	Continuous
Cutaneous findings	Erysipeloid-like erythema	Skin rash and eruptions	Migratory erysipelas-like rash	Cold-induced urticaria	Urticarial rash	Urticarial rash
Eye findings	Rare	Rare	Conjunctivitis; periorbital edema	Conjunctivitis	Conjunctivitis; episcleritis; optic disc edema	Conjunctivitis; uveitis, papilledema, visual loss
Musculoskeletal findings	Monoarthritis, sacroiliitis	Arthralgia, nonerosive polyarthritis	Arthralgia; myalgia	Arthralgia, myalgia	Arthralgia, myalgia, large joint oligoarthritis	Arthritis; epiphyseal overgrowth
Abdominal symptoms	Sterile peritonitis	Pain, emesis, diarrhea	Peritonitis, diarrhea, constipation	Nausea	Pain	Hepatosplenomegaly
Amyloidosis	Significant risk	Uncommon	Significant risk	Uncommon	Significant risk	Uncommon
Treatment	Colchicine	NSAIDs and steroids	Anti-TNF biologics	Anti–IL-1	Anti–IL-1	Anti–IL-1

FCAS, familial cold autoinflammatory syndrome; FMF, familial Mediterranean fever; HIDS, hyperimmunoglobulinemia D syndrome; IL-1, interleukin-1; MWS, Muckle-Wells syndrome; NOMID, neonatal-onset multisystem inflammatory disease; NSAIDs, nonsteroidal antiinflammatory drugs; TNF, tumor necrosis factor; TRAPS, tumor necrosis factor receptor–associated periodic syndromes.

Modified from Samuels J, Ozen S: Familial Mediterranean fever and the other autoinflammatory syndromes: evaluation of the patient with recurrent fever, *Curr Opin Rheumatol* 18:108-117, 2006.

defect is in the *MEFV* gene on the short arm of chromosome 16, and several mutations have been identified. Attacks are characterized by fever, abdominal pain, pleuropericardial pain, arthritis, myalgia, and erysipelas-like erythema. Episodes occur at intervals of days to months. Laboratory findings are nonspecific. Colchicine is the recommended treatment. Lack of treatment can be associated with the development of amyloidosis.

Hyper-IgD syndrome (HIDS) is an autosomal recessive disorder resulting from a mutation in the MVK gene on chromosome 12, which encodes mevalonate kinase. Patients are usually of Dutch, French, or other European descent. Symptoms may start in the first year of life and can include periodic fever, vomiting, diarrhea, arthritis, lymphadenopathy, splenomegaly, and maculopapular rash. Other cutaneous findings in HIDS may include urticaria, erythematous nodules, morbilliform rash, annular erythema, purpura, and petechiae. The serum IgD level may be elevated or normal during an acute attack. Elevation of IgG is not specific to HIDS as it has been found in FMF and TRAPS.

PFAPA syndrome is characterized by periodic high fevers, pharyngitis, lymphadenopathy, and splenomegaly. Typical attacks last 4 to 5 days with a symptom-free period of 4 to 7 weeks. All patients with the syndrome have periodic fever and at least one of the following: aphthous stomatitis, pharyngitis, or splenomegaly. Growth and development are normal in this syndrome. Corticosteroids or cimetidine have been beneficial in patients with PFAPA syndrome. Adenotonsillectomy has also been reported in the otolaryngology literature to be curative of the condition.

TRAPS includes the dominantly inherited periodic fever syndromes such as familial Hibernian fever. The affected gene is *TNFRSF1A*, which encodes a tumor necrosis factor receptor. Originally described in Irish and Scottish kindreds, the disease has been found in other ethnic groups including those of Middle Eastern descent. Clinical manifestations include periodic attacks of fever, abdominal pain, and myalgias. Other features include episodic erythematous patches, conjunctivitis, and unilateral periorbital edema. Unlike FMF and HIDS,

the febrile attacks in TRAPS can last for weeks. Effective treatments have included corticosteroids and TNF antagonists. Risk of amyloidosis is higher for those with mutations in cysteine residues.

Muckle-Wells syndrome (MWS), familial cold autoinflammatory syndrome (FCAS), and neonatal-onset multisystem inflammatory disease (NOMID; also known as chronic infantile neurologic cutaneous articular syndrome [CINCA]) are dominantly inherited syndromes linked to mutations in the *CIAS1* gene. The cryopyrinopathies feature FCAS as the mild form and NOMID as the most severe form of the spectrum. The cryopyrinopathies are characterized by fevers and urticarial rash. The fevers may be more regular than the typical periodicity seen with other periodic fever syndromes. Symptoms of FCAS are precipitated by exposure to cold. NOMID (or CINCA) symptoms begin in infancy and symptoms may be more severe including mental retardation, facial dysmorphism, chronic aseptic meningitis, sensorineural hearing loss, papilledema, and premature ossification and joint bony overgrowth.

In summary, the periodic fever syndromes are a heterogeneous group of disorders characterized by episodic fevers and other systemic sequelae. Because of the combination of fever and abdominal pain, an acute attack can masquerade as acute appendicitis. Cyclic neutropenia must also be ruled out when considering periodic fever. The syndromes may be difficult to distinguish clinically but can sometimes be diagnosed by genetic testing. Aggressive treatment with medications is warranted when there are disturbances of growth, development, or function.

IDIOPATHIC MUSCULOSKELETAL PAIN SYNDROMES (REFLEX NEUROVASCULAR DYSTROPHY)

The idiopathic musculoskeletal pain syndromes are characterized by intense chronic pain in the context of an essentially healthy physical examination. The nomenclature can be confusing, and it includes syndromes such as fibromyalgia, reflex sympathetic dystrophy, reflex neurovascular dystrophy, complex regional pain syndrome, myofascial pain, causalgia, pain amplification, neuropathic pain, pain-associated disability syndrome (PADS), and reflex neurovascular dystrophy (RND).

Children with chronic pain present with a mean age of onset of 12 years. The female-to-male ratio is 4:1. In the history, a triggering event may sometimes be identified. For example, the pain may begin after a minor sprain, fall, or sports injury. In other cases, the pain begins after the onset of a stressful event in the child's life such as a divorce or a death in the family. Children can present with marked pain and disability. Limp, dependence on crutches or a wheelchair, or bracing of a limb have all been observed. The pain can be described as intense, burning, sharp, and numbing, and the severity is often a 10 on a 1-to-10 scale. The pain may be exacerbated by bizarre triggers, such as the wind blowing on the skin, putting on a sock, or a light touch. Pain-relieving medications offer no relief.

A complete psychosocial history must be obtained in a child with a suspected idiopathic musculoskeletal pain syndrome. In some families, there is a model for pain. Adult family members may have fibromyalgia, chronic back pain, migraines, or other forms of chronic pain or disability. Patients are often described as high achievers, perfectionists, and having a desire to please. Many are straight-A students, successful athletes, or talented musicians. In witnessing the interaction between the parent and the patient, the examiner may note *enmeshment*, in which a child is directly asked a question and the parent acts as the spokesperson.

Children with localized idiopathic musculoskeletal pain may report changes in color, temperature, or perspiration in an affected part of the body (Fig. 7-83). The body part, such as a hand or a foot, may be guarded and braced by the child. The pain usually follows a nonanatomic distribution. On physical examination, a light touch by the examiner may elicit a wince-and-withdraw reaction. The *allodynia* has a variable border, such that successive examinations will feature different areas of pain distribution.

In generalized idiopathic musculoskeletal pain, patients often present with the triad of disorganized sleep, lack of exercise, and widespread body pain. Fatigue is a common symptom. Teenage patients often enter a cycle of sleeping irregularly with daytime napping, reducing aerobic exercise, and developing muscle and joint pain. On physical examination there may or may not be tender points as in adult patients with fibromyalgia.

Adults with fibromyalgia also feature sleep disorder, fatigue, and muscle and joint pain. However, adults with fibromyalgia tend to have a poorer prognosis than children with a pain syndrome. Adults may be treated with multiple medications, whereas it is preferable that children undergo physical therapy and cognitive behavioral therapy. Only one third of adult patients with fibromyalgia show improvement 10 years after diagnosis. The majority of children improve without medication.

Patients who present with idiopathic musculoskeletal pain syndromes often undergo extensive medical testing. Repeated phlebotomy, radiographs, nuclear scintigraphy, magnetic resonance imaging, endoscopy, and surgical biopsy have been performed in these patients to try to identify the etiology of the pain. Testing is normal or noncontributory.

Treatment begins by making the diagnosis on clinical grounds and ceasing medical testing. The patient's pain should be acknowledged without judgment. Therapy involves intensive desensitization physical therapy, aerobic exercise, normalization of sleep pattern, and psychological counseling. Comorbidities may include other chronic pain syndromes such as irritable bowel syndrome, chronic headaches, noncardiogenic chest pain, and dysmenorrhea. Screening for anxiety, depression, eating disorders, and family dysfunction should be performed. When a child presents with chronic idiopathic musculoskeletal pain, the syndrome often envelops the entire family. Delay in diagnosis can increase the family's frustration and anxiety. With physical therapy, psychology, and sometimes family therapy, the child can be returned to normal function.

ACKNOWLEDGMENTS

We extend our deepest thanks to the original author of this chapter—Dr. Aldo V. Londino. Dr. Londino, until the time of his passing in 2000, was the sole pediatric rheumatologist in western Pennsylvania and was widely recognized for his superb teaching and clinical skills. We are also grateful for the contributions of the previous authors, Drs. Andrew H. Urbach and Sara C. McIntire; as well as photograph contributors: Bernard Cohen, John Zitelli, A'Delbert Bowen, Basil Zitelli, J. Carlton Gartner Jr., J. Jeffrey Malatack, Joseph McGuire, Holly Davis, Virginia Steen, Joseph Warnicki, Albert Biglan, Cora Lennox, Sang Park, Chester Oddis, Alexi Grom, David Witte, and Susan Gelnett.

Figure 7-83   Reflex neurovascular dystrophy (RND). RND of the left leg with swelling, coolness to touch, and mild distal cyanosis.

Bibliography

Benseler SM, Silverman ED: Systemic lupus erythematosus, *Rheum Dis Clin N Am* 33:471-498, 2007.

Cassidy JT, Petty RE: *Textbook of pediatric rheumatology*, ed 5, Philadelphia, 2005, WB Saunders.

Compeyrot-Lacassagne S, Feldman BM: Inflammatory myopathies in children, *Rheum Dis Clin N Am* 33:525-554, 2007.

Dedeoglu F, Sundel RP: Vasculitis in children, *Rheum Dis Clin N Am* 33:555-584, 2007.

Hsieh Y, Wu M, Wang J, et al: Clinical features of atypical Kawasaki disease, *J Microbiol Immunol Infect* 35:57-60, 2002.

Laxer RM, Zulian F: Localized scleroderma, *Curr Opin Rheumatol* 18(6):606, 2006.

Lee BH, Scharff L, Sethna NF, et al: Physical and cognitive–behavioral treatment for complex regional pain syndromes, *J Pediatr* 141:135-140, 2002.

Lee W, Yang M, Lee K, et al: PFAPA syndrome (periodic fever, aphthous stomatitis, pharyngitis, adenitis), *Clin Rheumatol* 18:207-213, 1999.

Narchi H: Risk of long term renal impairment and duration of follow up recommended for Henoch-Schönlein purpura with normal or minimal urinary findings: a systematic review, *Arch Dis Child* 90:916-920, 2005.

Newburger JW, Takahashi M, Gerber MA, et al; Committee on Rheumatic Fever, Endocarditis, and Kawasaki Disease, Council on Cardiovascular Disease in the Young, American Heart Association: Diagnosis, treatment, and long-term management of Kawasaki disease: a statement for health professionals from the Committee on Rheumatic Fever, Endocarditis, and Kawasaki Disease, Council on Cardiovascular Disease in the Young, American Heart Association, *Pediatrics* 114:1708-1733, 2004.

Oen K, Malleson PN, Cabral DA, et al: Disease course and outcome of juvenile rheumatoid arthritis in a multicenter cohort, *J Rheumatol* 29:9, 2002.

Peterson LS, Nelson AM, Su WP, et al: The epidemiology of morphea (localized scleroderma) in Olmsted County 1960-1993, *J Rheumatol* 24:73-80, 1997.

Peterson LS, Nelson AM, Su WP: Classification of morphea (localized scleroderma), *Mayo Clin Proc* 70:1068-1076, 1995.

Petty RE, Southwood TR, Manners P, et al: International League of Associations for Rheumatology classification of juvenile idiopathic arthritis: second revision, Edmonton, 2001, *J Rheumatol* 31:390-392, 2004.

Reed AM, Mason T: Recent advances in juvenile dermatomyositis, *Curr Rheum Reports* 7:94-98, 2005.

Samuels J, Ozen S: Familial Mediterranean fever and the other autoinflammatory syndromes: evaluation of the patient with recurrent fever, *Curr Opin Rheumatol* 18:108-117, 2006.

Saulsbury FT: Henoch-Schönlein purpura: report of 100 patients and review of the literature, *Medicine* 78:395-409, 1999.

Scalapino K, Arkachaisri T, Lucas M, et al: Childhood onset systemic sclerosis: classification, clinical and serologic features, and survival in comparison with adult onset disease, *J Rheumatol* 33:1004-1013, 2006.

Schneider R, Passo MH: Juvenile rheumatoid arthritis, *Rheum Dis Clin N Am* 28:503-530, 2002.

Sherry DD: An overview of amplified musculoskeletal pain syndromes, *J Rheumatol Suppl* 58:44-48, 2000.

Zulian F: Scleroderma in children, *Pediatr Clin North Am* 52:521-545, vii, 2005.

Zulian F, Athreya BH, Laxer R, et al: Juvenile localized scleroderma: clinical and epidemiological features in 750 children: an international study, *Rheumatology (Oxford)* 45:614-620, 2006.

DERMATOLOGY

Bernard A. Cohen | Holly W. Davis | Robin P. Gehris

Most of us think of our skin as a simple, durable covering for our skeleton, muscles, and internal organs. However, the skin is a complex organ, consisting of many parts and appendages (Fig. 8-1). The outermost layer, the stratum corneum, is an effective barrier to irritants, toxins, and organisms, as well as a membrane that holds in body fluids. The remainder of the epidermis manufactures this protective layer. Melanocytes within the epidermis help protect us from the harmful effects of ultraviolet light, and Langerhans cells are one of the body's first lines of immunologic defense.

The dermis, consisting largely of fibroblasts and collagen, is a tough, leathery, mechanical barrier against cuts, bites, and bruises. Its collagenous matrix also provides structural support for a number of cutaneous appendages. Hair, which grows from follicles deep within the dermis, is important for cosmesis and protection from sunlight and particulate matter. Sebaceous glands are outgrowths of the hair follicles. Oil produced by these glands helps to lubricate the skin and contributes to the protective epidermal barrier. The nails are specialized organs of manipulation that also protect the sensitive digits. Thermoregulation of the skin is accomplished by eccrine sweat glands and changes in cutaneous blood flow, which is regulated by glomus cells. The skin also contains specialized receptors for heat, pain, touch, and pressure. Sensory input from these structures helps to protect the skin surface against environmental trauma. Beneath the dermis, in the subcutaneous tissue, fat acts as stored energy and as a soft, protective cushion.

Defects or alterations in any component of the skin may result in serious systemic disease or death. Each and every part of the skin can be affected by congenital, inflammatory, infectious, and degenerative disorders and tumors. For example, an altered stratum corneum is seen in ichthyosis; melanocytes are selectively destroyed in vitiligo; the epidermis proliferates in psoriasis; excess collagen is produced in the connective tissue nevus of tuberous sclerosis; hair is preferentially infested by certain fungi; and so on. In addition, the skin is affected by many systemic diseases and thus may provide visible markers for internal disorders. A skin examination may demonstrate lesions of vasculitis, explaining a child's hematuria. The white macules of tuberous sclerosis may give insight into the cause of seizures.

EXAMINATION AND ASSESSMENT OF THE SKIN

The skin is the largest, most accessible, and most easily examined organ of the body and is the organ of most frequent concern to patients. Therefore, physicians should be able to recognize basic skin diseases and dermatologic clues to systemic disease.

Optimal examination of the skin is performed in a well-lit room. The physician should inspect the entire skin surface including hair, nails, scalp, and mucous membranes. This may be particularly problematic with infants and teenagers because it may be necessary to examine the skin in small segments to prevent cooling or embarrassment. Although no special equipment is required, a hand lens and side lighting aid in the assessment of skin texture and small, discrete lesions. A Wood's lamp can improve precision in distinguishing hypopigmented from depigmented patches of skin.

Despite the myriad conditions affecting the skin, a systematic approach to the evaluation of a rash or exanthem assists and simplifies the process of developing a manageable differential diagnosis. After assessing the patient's general health, the practitioner should obtain a detailed history of the skin symptoms including the date of onset, inciting factors, evolution of lesions, and presence or absence of pruritus and/or fever, as well as any other systemic symptoms. Recent immunizations, infections, drugs, and allergies may be directly related to new rashes. The family history may suggest a hereditary or contagious process, and the clinician may need to examine other members of the family. Review of nursery records and photographs helps to document the presence of congenital lesions. Attention should then turn to the distribution and pattern of the rash. The term *distribution* refers to the location of the skin findings, whereas the term *pattern* defines a specific anatomic or physiologic arrangement (e.g., the distribution of a rash may include the extremities, face, or trunk, and the pattern could be flexural or intertriginous). Identification of a pattern can assist in the development of a differential diagnosis even before the detailed morphology of the skin lesions is studied. Other common patterns include photodistributed (involving sun-exposed sites), acral (involving primarily the distal extremities), and dermatomal configurations (Fig. 8-2).

Next, the clinician should consider the local *organization* of the lesions, defining the relationship of primary and secondary lesions to one another in a given location. Are the lesions scattered or clustered? Are they linear, grouped, serpiginous, confluent, or discrete?

Last, the practitioner should identify the *morphology* of the cutaneous lesions. *Primary lesions* (macules, papules, pustules, wheals, plaques, vesicles, bullae, nodules, and tumors) arise de novo in the skin. *Secondary lesions* (erosions, ulcers, crusts, excoriations, fissures, lichenification, atrophy, and scars) evolve from primary lesions or result from the patient's manipulation (e.g., scratching, picking, or popping) of primary lesions. Delineation of the primary and secondary lesions allows the clinician to develop a differential diagnosis on the basis of the *anatomic level* of the skin lesions (Table 8-1). Disorders restricted to the epidermis may be associated with macular color changes, such as in

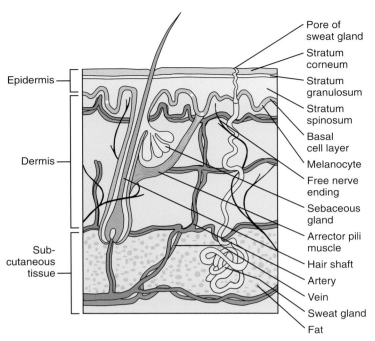

Figure 8-1　Schematic diagram of normal skin anatomy.

Labels on figure:
- Epidermis
- Dermis
- Subcutaneous tissue
- Pore of sweat gland
- Stratum corneum
- Stratum granulosum
- Stratum spinosum
- Basal cell layer
- Melanocyte
- Free nerve ending
- Sebaceous gland
- Arrector pili muscle
- Hair shaft
- Artery
- Vein
- Sweat gland
- Fat

vascular telangiectasias, freckles, and vitiligo. In *epidermal disorders,* surface markings are commonly altered by scales, vesicles, pustules, crusts, and erosions. Bullous impetigo, atopic dermatitis, and ichthyosis are primarily epidermal disorders. When the dermis is also involved, lesions usually display distinct borders because of dermal inflammation and edema. Disorders with both epidermal and dermal changes include psoriasis, lichen planus, and erythema multiforme. Inflammatory disorders or tumors restricted to the dermis do not usually alter the surface markings. Lesional borders are distinct, and color changes and edema may be present. Examples of *dermal disorders* include granuloma annulare, intradermal nevi, urticaria, and hemangiomas. The diagnosis of *subcutaneous disorders* is made by careful palpation. The surface markings are normal, and the color of the skin may be normal or red. There is altered skin firmness, and tenderness may be present. Subcutaneous lesions include lipomas,

Table 8-1	Anatomic Depth of Lesions	
Cutaneous Structure	**Physical Findings**	**Specific Skin Disorders**
Epidermis	Altered surface markings Scale, vesicle, crust Color changes (black, brown, white)	Impetigo Café-au-lait spot Atopic dermatitis Vitiligo Freckle
Epidermis and dermis	Altered surface markings Scale, vesicle, crust Distinct borders Color changes (black, brown, white, and/or red) Edema	Psoriasis Atopic dermatitis Contact dermatitis Cutaneous lupus erythematosus
Dermis	Normal surface markings Color changes Altered dermal firmness	Urticaria Granuloma annulare Hemangioma Blue nevus
Subcutaneous tissue	Normal surface markings Normal or red skin color Altered skin firmness	Hematoma Cold panniculitis Erythema nodosum

From Cohen BA: *Pediatric dermatology,* ed 2, London, 1999, Mosby.

deep hemangiomas, hematomas, subcutaneous fat necrosis, and erythema nodosum.

Because an outline of specific pediatric dermatoses defies any one scheme of organization, this text follows a clinically practical format. First, this chapter covers common papulosquamous and vesiculopustular eruptions, which account for a majority of rashes seen in children. This is followed by sections covering reactive erythemas, insect bites and infestations, tumors and infiltrations of the skin, neonatal dermatology, vascular lesions, congenital and acquired nevi, and disorders of pigmentation. The chapter concludes with a discussion of disorders of the hair and nails and complications of topical therapy.

PAPULOSQUAMOUS DISORDERS

Papulosquamous eruptions share the morphologic features of papules and scales. However, the clinician must understand that the papulosquamous disorders, which are quite diverse, are produced by a variety of different mechanisms. In psoriasis, increased turnover of keratinocytes by the basal cell layer results in a markedly thickened epidermis and stratum corneum (scaly surface layer). In dermatitic processes such as atopic dermatitis, contact dermatitis, seborrheic dermatitis, pityriasis rosea, and fungal infections, inflammation results in increased production and abnormal maturation of epidermal cells, with subsequent scale production. Increased adherence of cells in the stratum corneum may result in the retention hyperkeratosis characteristic of ichthyosis vulgaris, which is frequently found in association with atopic dermatitis.

Psoriasis

Psoriasis is a common disorder characterized by red, well-demarcated plaques covered with dry, thick, silvery scales. These tend to be located on the extensor surfaces of the extremities, the scalp, and the buttocks. In some patients, the distribution consists of large lesions over the pressure points of the knees and elbows (Fig. 8-3, *A-D*). Thickening and fissuring of the skin of the palms may also be seen (Fig. 8-3, *E*). In some children, numerous droplike (guttate) lesions are found scattered over the body (Fig. 8-4), often after a bout of group A β-hemolytic streptococcal infection (which may have been recognized or have been subclinical). In infants, psoriasis may present as a persistent diaper dermatitis (see Fig. 8-45). Lesions of psoriasis are often induced at sites of local injury such as scratches, surgical scars, or sunburn, a response termed the *Koebner phenomenon* (Fig. 8-5). Nail changes include reddish-brown psoriatic plaques in the nail bed (oil drop changes), surface pitting, and distal hyperkeratosis (see Fig. 8-148).

The factors that initiate the rapid turnover in epidermal cells that produce the psoriatic plaques are unknown, although an inherited predisposition is suspected and upper respiratory tract and streptococcal infections may precipitate lesions in children, especially in cases of guttate psoriasis. Although the increased epidermal growth causes a thickening of the skin in the psoriatic plaque, there are also areas between the epidermal ridges where the skin is thin and the scale is close to the subepidermal vessels. Thus when the scale is removed, small bleeding points are often seen. This is called the *Auspitz sign,* and it is the hallmark of psoriasis (Fig. 8-6).

Except in cases of guttate psoriasis, which can be limited to one episode, the course of psoriasis can be chronic and unpredictable, marked by remissions and exacerbations. Thirty-seven percent of adults with psoriasis first develop lesions in childhood.

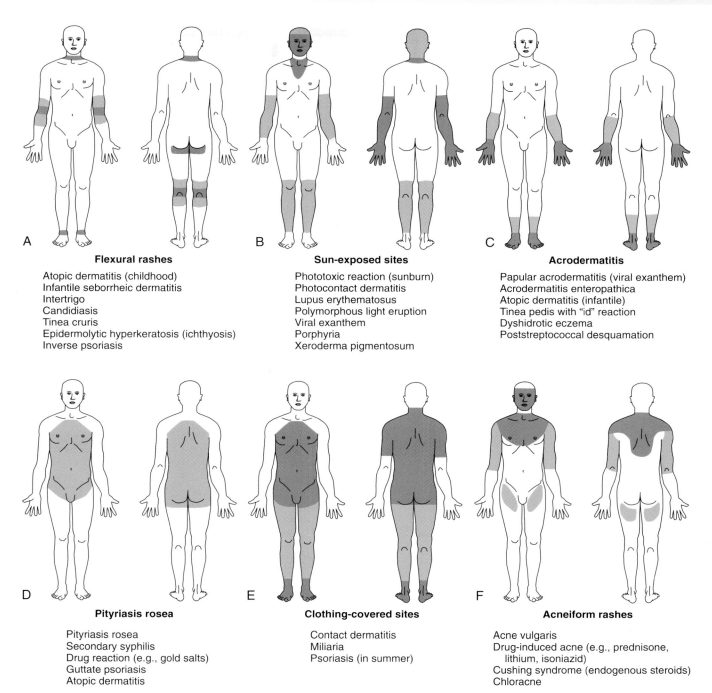

Flexural rashes

Atopic dermatitis (childhood)
Infantile seborrheic dermatitis
Intertrigo
Candidiasis
Tinea cruris
Epidermolytic hyperkeratosis (ichthyosis)
Inverse psoriasis

Sun-exposed sites

Phototoxic reaction (sunburn)
Photocontact dermatitis
Lupus erythematosus
Polymorphous light eruption
Viral exanthem
Porphyria
Xeroderma pigmentosum

Acrodermatitis

Papular acrodermatitis (viral exanthem)
Acrodermatitis enteropathica
Atopic dermatitis (infantile)
Tinea pedis with "id" reaction
Dyshidrotic eczema
Poststreptococcal desquamation

Pityriasis rosea

Pityriasis rosea
Secondary syphilis
Drug reaction (e.g., gold salts)
Guttate psoriasis
Atopic dermatitis

Clothing-covered sites

Contact dermatitis
Miliaria
Psoriasis (in summer)

Acneiform rashes

Acne vulgaris
Drug-induced acne (e.g., prednisone,
  lithium, isoniazid)
Cushing syndrome (endogenous steroids)
Chloracne

Figure 8-2   Pattern diagnosis. **A,** Flexural rashes. **B,** Sun-exposed sites. **C,** Acrodermatitis. **D,** Pityriasis rosea. **E,** Clothing-covered sites. **F,** Acneiform rashes.

The Ichthyoses

Ichthyosis refers to a group of genodermatoses characterized by dry, scaly skin. Various types have been identified according to clinical course; histopathology; biochemical markers; and, in some cases, specific genetic mutations.

Ichthyosis Vulgaris

Ichthyosis vulgaris occurs secondary to a mutation in filaggrin and is transmitted as an autosomal dominant trait and affects about 0.5% of the population. Although the rash is not present at birth, by 3 months of age thick, fishlike scales may be apparent on the shins and extensor surfaces of the arms (Fig. 8-7). On occasion, scales become more generalized, involving the trunk, but the flexures are usually spared. Lesions tend to flare during the winter (because of the drying effect of central heating) and improve during the summer, particularly with

increasing age. Biopsy of involved skin shows retention hyperkeratosis and a thinned granular layer in the epidermis. Liberal use of topical emollients usually keeps pruritus and scaling under control.

X-linked Ichthyosis

X-linked ichthyosis occurs in 1 in 6000 males as a result of a mutation in the enzyme steroid sulfatase, although findings are occasionally present in hemizygous female carriers. Affected newborns usually present between 3 and 12 months of age with generalized "dirty" brown scales, particularly on the lateral neck, abdomen, back, and anterior legs and feet (Fig. 8-8). The central face and flexures are spared. Skin biopsy demonstrates an increased granular layer and stratum corneum, and biochemical studies demonstrate decreased or absent steroid sulfatase in the serum and skin. Children with

Figure 8-3   Psoriasis. **A,** Typical erythematous plaques are topped by a silver scale. **B,** Thick tenacious scale on a red base extends from the forehead to the scalp of this 10-year-old girl. **C,** Large plaques are located over the shins and right knee. **D,** In this child lesions are prominent over the pressure point of the knee and the distal fingers. **E,** The skin of the palms is markedly thickened, with silvery fissuring of the palmar creases.

Figure 8-6 Auspitz sign. Removal of the thick scale from a psoriatic plaque produces small points of bleeding from tortuous capillaries.

Figure 8-4 Guttate psoriasis. Small droplike plaques with typical scales quickly developed in a generalized distribution in this child following streptococcal pharyngitis. *(From Cohen BA:* Atlas of pediatric dermatology, *London, 1993, Mosby-Wolfe.)*

X-linked ichthyosis are at increased risk of undescended testes as well (even independent of this risk) as testicular cancer. Decreased or absent steroid sulfatase activity during fetal life may result in decreased placental estrogen and a delay in onset of labor.

Lamellar Ichthyosis

Lamellar ichthyosis is a rare autosomal dominant disorder occurring in fewer than 1 in 250,000 births as a result of a mutation in keratinocyte transglutaminase-1. Infants are usually born with a collodion membrane (see Fig. 8-93). During the first month of life, thick, brownish gray, sheetlike scales with raised edges appear. Scaling is prominent over the face, trunk, and extremities (Fig. 8-9). In contrast to ichthyosis vulgaris, the flexural areas are involved (Fig. 8-9, *B*). Eversion and fissuring of the eyelid margins (ectropion) and lips (eclabium) are common complications (Fig. 8-9, *C*). The palms and soles show thick keratoderma with fissuring. Some improvement of the scaling occurs with age, and topical keratolytics such as lactic acid and salicylic acid may provide some benefit. Severe cases may respond to the administration of systemic retinoids such as acitretinoin or isotretinoin.

Epidermolytic Hyperkeratosis

Epidermolytic hyperkeratosis is a rare autosomal dominant form of ichthyosis characterized by the development of generalized, thick, warty scales and intermittent blistering with severe involvement of the flexures (Fig. 8-10). In newborns, blisters and erosions may be widespread and must be differentiated from epidermolysis bullosa or herpes simplex. Histologically, massive hyperkeratosis is associated with ballooning of squamous cells and formation of microvesicles. Epidermal turnover is also markedly increased. The mainstay of treatment includes use of keratolytics, lubricants, and antibiotics for secondary infection, which is common and usually caused by *Staphylococcus aureus*. Oral retinoids may also significantly decrease scaling.

The Dermatitides

Depending on duration of involvement, the dermatitides are characterized clinically by acute changes (including redness, edema, and vesiculation) and/or chronic changes (such as scaling, lichenification, and increased or decreased pigmentation) in the skin. Microscopically, these disorders are characterized by infiltration of the dermis with inflammatory cells, variable thickening of the epidermis, and scaling.

Atopic Dermatitis (Eczema)

Atopic dermatitis, or eczema, is one of the most common and stressful of all chronic skin disorders in children. This entity is divided into three phases on the basis of the age of the patient, each having a different distribution.

Figure 8-5 Koebner phenomenon in psoriasis. Lesions are often induced in areas of local trauma such as these scratches.

Figure 8-7 Ichthyosis vulgaris. The typical fish scale appearance is seen in this close-up of a fair-skinned patient's shin.

Figure 8-8   X-linked ichthyosis. "Dirty" brown scales persist on the flanks, elbows, and shoulders despite the use of topical lubricants.

Figure 8-10   Epidermolytic hyperkeratosis is characterized by thick, warty scales and intermittent blistering. The flexural creases are particular sites of involvement.

The *infantile phase* of atopic dermatitis begins between birth and 6 months of age and lasts about 2 or 3 years. Characteristically, the rash is manifest by red, itchy papules and plaques that ooze and crust. Lesions are distributed over the cheeks, forehead, scalp, trunk, and extensor surfaces of the extremities, and patches are often symmetrical (Fig. 8-11).

The *childhood phase* of atopic dermatitis occurs between ages 4 and 10 years. The dermatitis is typically dry, papular, and intensely pruritic. Circumscribed scaly patches are distributed on the wrists, ankles, and antecubital and popliteal fossae (Fig. 8-12); these patches frequently become secondarily infected, both as a result of the nonintact skin barrier as well as secondary to discrete immunologic differences in children with atopic dermatitis, namely a deficiency in two innate antiviral and antibacterial arms of the skin's immune system: β-defensins and cathelicidins. Cracking, dryness, and scaling of the palmar and plantar surfaces of the hands and feet are also common (Fig. 8-13). Remission may occur at any time, or the disorder may evolve into a more chronic type of adult dermatitis. Of children with atopic dermatitis, 75% improve between the ages of 10 and 14; the remaining children may go on to develop chronic dermatitis.

The *adult phase* of atopic dermatitis begins around age 12 and continues indefinitely. Major areas of involvement include the flexural areas of the arms, neck, and legs (Fig. 8-14). Eruptions are sometimes seen on the dorsal surfaces of the hands and feet and between the fingers and toes. Lichenification may be marked (Fig. 8-15).

Other associated findings include xerosis (dryness); ichthyosis vulgaris (see Fig. 8-7); *keratosis pilaris*, keratin plugging of hair follicles and formation of perifollicular scales over

Figure 8-9   Lamellar ichthyosis. **A,** Note the thick, brownish-black scales covering the entire skin surface. **B,** Flexural involvement helps differentiate lamellar ichthyosis from ichthyosis vulgaris. **C,** Ectropion (note the eversion of the lower lids) is a unique finding in this form of the disorder.

Figure 8-11 Infantile atopic dermatitis or eczema. **A,** This infant has an acute, weeping dermatitis on the cheeks and forehead. **B** and **C,** Involvement of the trunk and the extremities, with erythema, scaling, and crusting, is evident. Usually the diaper area is the only portion of the skin surface that is spared. (***B** and **C,** From Fireman P, Slavin RG: Atlas of allergies, New York, 1991, Gower.)*

Figure 8-12 Childhood atopic dermatitis with lesions on the arms **(A)** and the legs **(B).** In childhood, eczema involves the flexural surfaces of the upper and lower extremities. The neck, ankles, wrists, and posterior thighs also may be severely affected. (***A,** From Fireman P, Slavin RG: Atlas of allergies, New York, 1991, Gower; **B,** courtesy Michael Sherlock, MD, Lutherville, Md.)*

Figure 8-13   Involvement of the hands and feet in eczema. **A,** A 10-year-old atopic child has lichenification of the skin over the dorsum of his fingers and "buff" nails from chronic rubbing. **B,** This infant has numerous red excoriated lesions over the soles of his feet.

the extensor surfaces of the extremities and sometimes the trunk and abdomen (Fig. 8-16; and see also Fig. 8-25, *D*); hyperlinearity of the palms; Dennie-Morgan lines (double skin creases under the lower eyelid [see Chapter 4]); and hyperpigmentation and hypopigmentation, which may be marked and at times may be the predominant findings. As a result of their altered immunity in the skin, more than 90% of patients with atopic dermatitis are colonized with *Staphylococcus aureus* at the time of a flare; for the same cellular reason these patients are also unusually susceptible to cutaneous viral infections including warts, herpes simplex, and molluscum contagiosum. Patients with eczema should be warned to avoid people with cold sores because they are at great risk for developing generalized eczema herpeticum (see Fig. 12-13). Parents of children with eczema who themselves have recurrent herpes simplex lesions should be taught hygienic techniques that reduce the risk of transmitting the virus, even when asymptomatic, as shedding can still occur to their children.

In the rash of *pityriasis alba,* which is common in patients with atopic dermatitis, inflammatory changes are minimal. Poorly defined, hypopigmented, round or oval scaly patches measuring 2 to 4 cm in diameter are noted most commonly on the face and extremities (Fig. 8-17), although they may involve the trunk as well. These patches fail to enhance with

Wood's lamp examination, which distinguishes them from vitiligo. Lesions are more prominent in children with dark skin and are more noticeable during spring and summer because they do not tan like surrounding skin. Surface scaling is more evident when the skin is dry (especially in winter). The etiology is unknown. Because the disorder is usually asymptomatic and spontaneously resolves in several months to a few years, treatment is usually unnecessary, although moisturizers may help reduce surface scaling.

The cause of atopic dermatitis remains elusive. An immunologic etiology is suggested by the chronic elevation of IgE seen in a majority of patients. Some investigators propose an aberrant cutaneous response to histamine and other mediators of inflammation as a primary mechanism. However, laboratory findings vary from patient to patient and in the same patient at different times in the course of the disease. Atopic dermatitis does seem to occur in families and in association with other atopic conditions in the atopic triad, including asthma, allergic rhinitis, and food allergies, suggesting some degree of genetic predisposition. Pathophysiologically, a number of external factors including dry skin, soaps, wool fabrics, foods, infectious agents, and environmental antigens may act individually or in concert to produce pruritus, which is almost universal in atopic individuals. The resultant scratching leads to the acute and chronic changes typical of atopic dermatitis.

The differential diagnosis of atopic dermatitis includes seborrheic dermatitis, contact dermatitis, pityriasis rosea, psoriasis, fungal infections, Langerhans cell histiocytosis, and acrodermatitis enteropathica. It can be distinguished from seborrheic dermatitis on the basis of the distribution of lesions

Figure 8-14   Adult atopic dermatitis. Erythematous excoriated plaques with indistinct borders are seen in the antecubital areas. Note the dried blood from recent excoriation.

Figure 8-15   *Lichenification* refers to marked thickening of the skin seen in areas of atopic dermatitis that have been subject to chronic scratching. In addition, this patient demonstrates significant postinflammatory hyperpigmentation.

Figure 8-16 Keratosis pilaris. **A,** Diffuse fine follicular papules and sandpaper scaling are seen on the extensor surface of the arm of this adolescent. **B,** In this 5-year-old boy, characteristic white follicular papules are more widely spaced and more prominently seen on the extensor surface of his thighs and upper arms. His mother had similar lesions. *(From Cohen BA, Lehman CU, editors: DermAtlas, Baltimore, 2000-2011, Johns Hopkins University. http://dermatlas.med.jhmi.edu/derm.)*

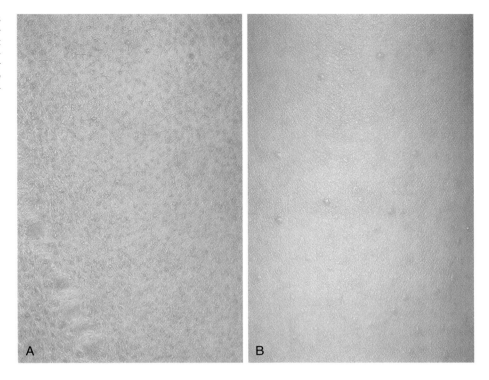

and associated pruritus; atopic dermatitis spares moist, intertriginous areas such as the axillae and perineum, where seborrheic dermatitis is prominent. Exposure history and distribution help differentiate it from contact dermatitis, as does the discreteness of lesions and their distribution in pityriasis rosea. The thick, silvery scale and Koebner phenomenon help distinguish psoriasis, and central clearing with an active border of red papules, vesicles, and/or pustules helps differentiate tinea corporis. The rash of histiocytosis is crusted, atrophic, and may be more generalized. It is associated with petechiae and is often accompanied by chronically draining ears, hepatosplenomegaly, and lymphadenopathy (see Fig. 8-85 and Chapter 11). The acral and periorificial distribution of lesions and gastrointestinal symptoms help in distinguishing eczema from acrodermatitis enteropathica.

The mainstays of atopic dermatitis treatment are elimination or avoidance of predisposing factors; hydration and

Figure 8-17 Pityriasis alba. In some atopic individuals, subtle inflammation may result in the development of poorly demarcated, hypopigmented patches that are covered by a fine superficial scale.

lubrication of the skin; the use of antipruritic agents to relieve itching, break the itch–scratch cycle, and normalize sleep patterns; and the use of topical steroids to further relieve itching and decrease inflammation. Pimecrolimus cream and tacrolimus ointment are two agents in the class of nonsteroidal topical immunomodulators that may also dramatically interrupt the itch–scratch cycle. They have been approved as second-line therapy for the management of atopic dermatitis in children older than 2 years of age. Use of these agents should be accompanied by an explanation of the boxed warning regarding the theoretical risk of lymphoma and skin cancer. However, these tumors have been seen only with prolonged systemic use at very high doses.

All children with atopic dermatitis should be monitored closely for secondary bacterial infection, which must be treated promptly with topical or systemic antibiotics to prevent progression to cellulitis. The use of a hyperdiluted bleach (1 to 2 ounces in a 30-gallon tub of water) bath several times per week is a cost-effective way of preventing infection in patients with atopic dermatitis. Herpes simplex can also occur as a secondary infection over atopic dermatitis and can rapidly disseminate in patients with active atopic dermatitis, resulting in the severe disorder known as *eczema herpeticum* (see Fig. 12-13). Hence, patients' families should be warned to have their children avoid contact with people with cold sores, and if parents have recurrent herpes labialis, they should be instructed in strict hand-washing precautions. Further, patients should be treated with antiviral agents at the first sign of infection with herpes simplex.

Dyshidrotic eczema and *nummular eczema* are clinical patterns of atopic dermatitis, and *juvenile palmo–plantar dermatosis* and *lip-licking* and *thumb-sucking eczema* represent irritant dermatitides that may be associated with atopic dermatitis.

Dyshidrotic Eczema

Dyshidrosis is a severely pruritic, chronic, recurrent, vesicular eruption affecting the palms, soles, and lateral aspects of the fingers and toes. Characteristically, the vesicles are symmetrical, multilocular, and 1 to 3 mm in diameter. These lesions

Figure 8-18 Dyshidrosis. Chronic cracking, oozing, and scaling develop after the initial tiny pruritic vesicles have been scratched.

Figure 8-20 Juvenile plantar dermatosis. This variant of atopic dermatitis is usually localized to the plantar surfaces of the toes and feet. Note the glistening erythema, scaling, and fissuring. In some patients the palms may be affected as well.

rupture, leaving scales and crust on an erythematous base (Fig. 8-18). Pathologically, this eruption demonstrates spongiotic vesicles and normal eccrine sweat glands. The cause is unknown; however, frequent exposure to water, wet or sweat-soaked shoes, or chemicals (on the hands) may trigger or exacerbate the condition. Hyperhidrosis, or excessive sweating of the palms and soles, may also play a role. Treatment is similar to that for acute atopic dermatitis.

Nummular Eczema

Nummular eczema is an acute papulovesicular eruption named for its coin-shaped configuration and probably also represents another clinical pattern found in atopic individuals. Lesions are intensely pruritic, well-circumscribed, round to oval, red, scaly patches studded with 1- to 3-mm vesicles (Fig. 8-19, *A*). They are usually located on the extensor thighs or abdomen of children who also may have atopic dermatitis. Vigorous scratching causes excoriation and crusting (Fig. 8-19, *B*). Lack of central clearing helps distinguish these lesions from tinea corporis (see Fig. 8-35). Although the rash is often resistant to therapy, it may respond to the treatment for acute dermatitis outlined previously.

Juvenile Plantar–Palmar Dermatosis

Juvenile plantar–palmar dermatosis ("sweaty sock syndrome") is common in toddlers and school-age children. Chronic, red scaly patches with cracking and fissuring typically begin on the anterior plantar surfaces of the feet and big toes (Fig. 8-20). The palms may be involved as well, although less severely. Although the cause is unknown, the condition is triggered by excessive sweating and/or repeated wetting of the skin inside the child's shoes (especially those made of synthetic materials that do not breathe), followed by drying of the skin at night. Some children experience flares in the summer, whereas in others the flares occur in winter. Consequently, the mainstay of treatment consists of emollients for prevention and occasional application of topical steroids when intense inflammation is present during flares.

Lip-licking and Thumb-sucking Eczema

The repeated wetting and drying from persistent lip licking (especially in winter) or thumb sucking can produce eczematoid changes of the perioral skin (Fig. 8-21) or the skin of the involved thumb (Fig. 8-22). Lip-licking eczema can be the result of a habit or can be a manifestation of anxiety, and

Figure 8-19 Nummular eczema. **A,** Round- to oval-shaped lesions studded with tiny vesicles are typically located over the extensor thighs or abdomen. They do not show central clearing. **B,** Vigorous scratching results in excoriation with weeping and crusting. (**A,** *Courtesy Michael Sherlock, MD, Lutherville, Md.*)

Figure 8-21 Lip-licking eczema. The perioral skin is inflamed, scaly, and thickened as a result of repetitive licking of the lips. *(Courtesy Douglas W. Kress, MD, University of Pittsburgh Medical Center.)*

sources of stress should be explored on history taking. Once the process begins, it can become a vicious cycle as the child licks with increasing frequency to moisten the dry skin.

Seborrhea

Seborrheic dermatitis is characterized by a red scaling eruption that occurs predominantly on hair-bearing and intertriginous areas such as the scalp; eyebrows; eyelashes; perinasal, presternal, and postauricular areas and the neck; axillae; and groin. Lesions often involve the intertriginous areas of the arms, legs, neck, and trunk, and occasionally become generalized (Fig. 8-23, *A-D*). In affected infants, scalp lesions consist of a thick, tenacious, scaly dermatitis that is often salmon colored and is commonly known as *cradle cap* (Fig. 8-24, *A* and *B*). In adolescents the dermatitis may manifest as dandruff or flaking of the eyebrows, postauricular areas, or flexural areas.

Although the pathogenesis of seborrheic dermatitis is unknown, *Pityrosporum* and *Candida* species have been implicated as causative agents. A role for neurologic dysfunction is suggested by the increased incidence and severity in neurologically impaired individuals.

The dermatitis of seborrhea is usually nonpruritic and mild in nature. Most cases respond to topical steroids, and many clear spontaneously, although residual postinflammatory hypopigmentation may persist for weeks or months thereafter (see Fig. 8-125). Some practitioners find that use of a topical antifungal cream or wash, as well as a low-potency topical steroid, hastens resolution. Antiseborrheic shampoos may also be helpful for patients with scalp involvement. In infants and

Figure 8-22 Thumb-sucking eczema. Repeated wetting and drying from persistent thumb sucking result in eczematoid changes with cracking, fissuring, and lichenification. *(Courtesy Michael Sherlock, MD, Lutherville, Md.)*

young children, atopic dermatitis can have a greasy, scaly appearance and may be confused with seborrhea. However, infantile atopic dermatitis produces intense pruritus and invariably spares moist sites such as the diaper area and axillae. The two are often present simultaneously in the same patient. The differential diagnosis of seborrhea includes Langerhans cell histiocytosis (in which the rash is generalized, in part petechial, and usually associated with chronic draining ears and hepatosplenomegaly) and tinea corporis (in which lesions usually are more circumscribed, with an active border and central clearing). Scalp lesions may be difficult to differentiate from psoriasis.

Hyper-IgE (Job) Syndrome

Job syndrome is a rare genetic disorder with prominent cutaneous manifestations. It has been linked to a mutation on chromosome 4q and is usually inherited as an autosomal dominant trait with variable severity of expression. Affected patients have abnormalities of the immune response involving T lymphocytes, neutrophils, cytokines, and interleukins. They also have variably but significantly elevated levels of serum IgE and circulating eosinophils.

Dermatologic features include a pruritic dermatitic rash that shares features with both atopic dermatitis and seborrhea, and which tends to develop shortly after birth (earlier than seborrhea and atopic dermatitis). It rapidly becomes superinfected with *S. aureus*, which results in the formation of weeping, crusting, and folliculitic lesions, as well as cutaneous abscesses (Fig. 8-25, *A-D*). In contrast to furuncles in patients with a normal immune response, the abscesses in children with Job syndrome cause little pain and show few signs of inflammation. Development of mucocutaneous candidiasis is also common. Other clinical manifestations include recurrent/chronic infections such as bronchitis, pneumonia (with pneumatoceles), sinusitis, otitis, gingivitis, dental abscesses, septic arthritis, and osteomyelitis. Decreased bone density is the source of multiple fractures, which cause remarkably little pain. With age and growth, facial features tend to coarsen (see Fig. 4-54, *E*) and scoliosis is common.

Treatment is aimed at controlling infections and ameliorating symptoms. The major differential diagnostic consideration is Langerhans histiocytosis (see Fig. 8-85).

Pityriasis Rosea

Pityriasis rosea is a benign, self-limited disorder that can occur at any age but is more common in adolescents and young adults. A prodrome of malaise, headache, and mild constitutional symptoms occasionally precedes the rash. The typical eruption begins with the appearance of a "herald patch" (Fig. 8-26, *A*), which is a large, isolated, oval lesion, usually pink in color and slightly scaly; it may occur anywhere on the body. On occasion, it clears centrally, simulating tinea corporis. From 5 to 10 days later, other smaller lesions appear on the body, frequently concentrated over the trunk but also seen on the proximal extremities, especially the thighs (see Fig. 8-26, *B-G*). On occasion, lesions predominate on the face, groin, and/or distal extremities including the palms and soles, a phenomenon known as *inverse pityriasis*, which is more common in African-American patients. Pityriasis lesions begin as small, round papules that enlarge to oval plaques up to 1 to 2 cm in size, with a scaly surface. They are usually somewhat raised but can be macular, and they can be erythematous, hyperpigmented, or hypopigmented. The long axes of the ovals tend to run parallel to the lines of the cleavage of the skin, creating a "Christmas tree" pattern over the thorax (Fig. 8-26, *C* and *D*). The rash reaches its peak in several weeks, and then slowly fades over 4 to 8 weeks. The average total duration is 2 to 3 months. Oral erythromycin or

Figure 8-23   Seborrhea. This slightly greasy, red, scaling eruption typically involves the hair-bearing areas of the face, axilla **(A),** and diaper area **(B). C,** The intertriginous folds of the neck are another common site of involvement. **D,** Postauricular lesions are common and often become secondarily infected as in this case, which grew group A β-streptococci. **(D,** *Courtesy Michael Sherlock, MD, Lutherville, Md.)*

Figure 8-24   Seborrhea of the scalp. **A,** Note the oily appearance and salmon-pink hue. Numerous scales, some adherent to the scalp and many interlaced through the baby's hair, are present. **B,** In this infant the scales have formed a thick crust, and erythema is less evident.

Figure 8-25 Job syndrome. This infant with markedly elevated IgE experienced early onset of a pruritic dermatitis that shared clinical features with both seborrhea and atopic dermatitis. **A,** Note the erythema and scaliness, the evidence of excoriation from scratching, and the perinasal crusting due to *Staphylococcus aureus* infection. **B,** In this view, in addition to the erythema, scaling, and thickening of the skin, there are weeping areas around the ear and crusts and scabs over the scalp. Note also the purulent ear drainage. **C,** He also had crusted palmar lesions. **D,** The skin over his abdomen had the classic features of keratosis pilaris.

doxycycline and small doses of ultraviolet light may hasten the disappearance of the eruption. Although the cause is unknown, the peak incidence in late winter and the low recurrence rate favor an infectious etiology.

Other eruptions that can resemble pityriasis rosea include guttate psoriasis, benign parapsoriasis, viral exanthems, measles-like (morbilliform) drug eruptions, and secondary syphilis (see Fig. 18-36). Secondary syphilis should specifically be considered when a patient presents with a rash resembling pityriasis rosea and the palms and soles are involved. As noted earlier, the appearance of the herald patch may simulate tinea corporis, but a potassium hydroxide (KOH) preparation is negative.

Contact Dermatitis

Contact dermatitis refers to a group of conditions in which a dermatitic or inflammatory reaction in the skin is triggered by direct contact with environmental agents. In the most common form, *irritant contact dermatitis,* changes in the skin are induced by caustic agents such as acids and alkalis, hydrocarbons, and other primary irritants. Anyone exposed to these agents in a high enough concentration for a long enough period will ultimately develop a contact dermatitis. The rash is usually acute, with well-demarcated erythema, crusting, and/or blister formation.

In contrast, allergic contact dermatitis is a T-lymphocyte–mediated immune reaction to an antigen coming into contact with the skin. Although patients typically present with acute onset of erythema, vesiculation, and pruritus, in some cases they delay seeking care until after the rash has become chronic with scaling, lichenification, and pigmentary changes. Often, the allergen is obvious, as is the case with poison ivy or nickel jewelry. However, in other cases, careful questioning may be required to detect the inciting agent.

The initial reaction occurs after a 7- to 14-day period of sensitization in susceptible individuals. Once sensitization has occurred, reexposure to the allergen provokes a more rapid reaction, sometimes within hours. This is a classic example of type IV (delayed) hypersensitivity (see Chapter 4).

Rhus Dermatitis (Poison Ivy)

The most common type of allergic contact dermatitis in the United States is poison ivy, or rhus dermatitis. This typically presents as linear streaks of erythematous papules and vesicles (Fig. 8-27, *A*); however, with heavy exposure, the rash may appear in relatively large patches (Fig. 8-27, *B* and *C*). When lesions involve the skin of the face or genitalia, impressive swelling can occur (Fig. 8-27, *D*).

Direct contact with the sap of poison ivy, poison oak, or poison sumac from leaves, stems, or roots (whether the plant is alive or dead) produces the dermatitis (Fig. 8-28). Contact with clothing that has brushed against the plant, with logs or railroad ties on which the vine has been growing, or with smoke from a fire in which the plant is being burned are other means of exposure. Areas of skin exposed to the highest concentration of plant oil develop changes first. Other sites that

Figure 8-26   Pityriasis rosea. **A,** The large herald patch on this boy's back shows evidence of central clearing, mimicking tinea corporis. **B,** Numerous oval lesions with their long axes oriented along lines of skin cleavage are seen over the trunk of this adolescent. **C** and **D,** This feature creates the appearance of a fir tree distribution on the back. **E-G,** Lesions can be raised, macular, or scaly and can be erythematous or hyper- or hypopigmented. (**A** and **C,** *Courtesy Douglas W. Kress, MD, University of Pittsburgh Medical Center; **E** and **F,** courtesy Michael Sherlock, MD, Lutherville, Md.*)

received lower doses then vesiculate in succession, giving the illusion of spreading. This is not the case, however, as within about 20 minutes of initial contact, the rhus oil becomes tissue-fixed to the epithelial cells and cannot be spread farther. Thorough washing within minutes of exposure can prevent fixation, and hence, the eruption. On occasion the oil can oxidize, leaving a black discoloration superimposed on the

contact dermatitis; this is known as "black dot" or "urushiol" dermatitis.

Other Common Causes of Contact Dermatitis

Other common offending agents are nickel (Fig. 8-29), rubber (Fig. 8-30), glues and/or dyes in shoes or diapers (Fig. 8-31), ethylenediamine in topical lotions, neomycin, and topical

Figure 8-27 Poison ivy, or rhus dermatitis. **A,** Linear streaks of pruritic vesicles are typical of contact dermatitis caused by exposure to a plant. **B** and **C,** With heavier exposure, however, the eruption can develop in relatively large patches. Also note the microvesicular appearance of the facial lesion in the child shown in **C. D,** Reactions involving the face and genitalia can provoke impressive swelling.

anesthetics (Fig. 8-32). Paraphenylenediamine dye used in amateur henna tattoos is an increasingly common cause of contact dermatitis among adolescents, and the pattern reflects the image of the original tattoo (Fig. 8-33).

Photocontact Dermatitis and Phototoxic Reactions

Photocontact or photoallergic dermatitis is a true cell-mediated delayed hypersensitivity reaction and necessitates a 7- to 10-day period of sensitization, after which sun exposure may precipitate development of a dermatitis. When caused by systemically administered drugs, it characteristically erupts in a symmetrical distribution on the face, the V of the neck, and the arms and legs distal to the end of shirt sleeves and shorts. Potentially causative agents include the tetracyclines, isotretinoin, sulfonylureas, thiazides, nonsteroidal anti-inflammatory drugs, fluoroquinolones, and griseofulvin. Topical photosensitizers (sunscreens with PABA esters or oxybenzone; fragrances in soaps, creams, lotions, or cosmetics;

Figure 8-28   A, Poison ivy. The plant has characteristic shiny leaves in groups of three. It may resemble a vine, a low shrub, or a bush. **B,** Poison oak. This also has leaves in groups of three, although the edges tend to be more scalloped than those of poison ivy. (**B,** Courtesy Mary Jelks, MD.)

Figure 8-29   Nickel contact dermatitis. The location and distribution of the rash are often helpful in determining the cause of a contact dermatitis. In this case wrist lesions were triggered by the nickel in her bracelet clasp.

Figure 8-30   Rubber contact dermatitis. This child had become sensitized to the elasticized waist bands of his underpants.

Figure 8-31   Contact dermatitis of the foot due to glues/dyes in shoes. **A,** This adolescent became sensitized to the glue under the insoles of his shoes. Note the sparing of the instep. **B,** Another child had a similar problem with the toe reinforcers in his shoes. Note that the web spaces are spared. (**A,** *Courtesy Michael Sherlock, MD, Lutherville, Md;* **B,** *courtesy Douglas W. Kress, MD, University of Pittsburgh Medical Center.*)

Figure 8-32   Contact dermatitis due to topical anesthetics. This adolescent became sensitized to the topical anesthetic Lanacaine in a moisturizing cream that she applied to her hands daily. Note the line of demarcation at the wrist.

Figure 8-33   Contact dermatitis due to henna dye. This young teenager developed vesicular lesions in the precise pattern of a henna tattoo she had had applied 2 weeks earlier.

Figure 8-34 Photocontact dermatitis. This boy developed contact dermatitis after sun exposure while outside for a day of swimming. The offending agent was found to be in his soap. *(Courtesy Michael Sherlock, MD, Lutherville, Md.)*

coal tar; furocoumarins; and halogenated salicylanilides in germicidal soaps) produce localized patches of dermatitis when used on sun-exposed sites (Fig. 8-34).

Phototoxins, when applied to the skin, are the source of a nonimmunologic exaggerated sunburn reaction in which the initial erythema progresses to hyperpigmentation. Of these, phytophotodermatitis is the most common. In this form, plant-derived photosensitizers, psoralens, found in the juice of lemons, limes, figs, dill, parsley, parsnips, carrots, and celery, are responsible for the reaction. Typically a child is touched by a parent who has been cutting the fruit, herbs, or vegetables, thereby getting the juice on the child's skin. Subsequent exposure to sunlight then results in the appearance of erythematous macules, with or without accompanying bullae, which then go on to become hyperpigmented. These patches often have bizarre or hand/finger-shaped patterns that can mimic child abuse (see Fig. 6-66).

"Id" Reaction

On occasion, the local reaction of a contact dermatitis is so severe that the patient develops a widespread secondary eczematous dermatitis. When the dermatitis appears at sites that have not been in contact with the offending agent, the reaction is referred to as autoeczematization or an "id" reaction. Id reactions can also occur in patients with tinea, especially coincident with the start of oral therapy.

Basic Principles of Management

Although localized patches of contact dermatitis are best treated topically, widespread reactions require a 2-week tapering course of systemic corticosteroids beginning at 0.5 to 1 mg/kg/day. Patients may experience rebound of the rash if treated with a shorter course. Response usually occurs within 48 hours. Oral steroids may also be indicated in localized reactions involving the eyelids, extensive areas of the face, genitals, and/or hands, where swelling and pruritus may become incapacitating.

Prevention requires identification of the offending agent and then its avoidance. Children with rhus dermatitis should be shown pictures of the causative plants and taught where they are commonly found. Patients sensitive to nickel must ensure that jewelry, particularly earring posts, are made of 24-karat gold, stainless steel, or sterling silver. However, in some patients painting watchband buckles with clear nail polish every several weeks can obviate the difficult task of trying to find watchbands with pure gold or silver buckles.

Fungal Infections

Two types of fungal organisms produce clinical cutaneous disease: dermatophytes and yeasts. Dermatophytes include the tinea or ringworm fungi, and yeasts include *Candida* species, which are associated with diaper dermatitis and *Pityrosporum* species, which cause tinea versicolor. Both *Candida* and *Pityrosporum* have been implicated as partially causative in seborrhea.

Tinea Corporis

Tinea corporis is a superficial fungal infection of the nonhairy or glabrous skin. It has been labeled "ringworm" because of its characteristic configuration consisting of pruritic, annular lesions with central clearing and an active border made up of microvesicles that rupture and then scale (Fig. 8-35, *A-C*). Lesions, which may be single or multiple, typically begin as pruritic red papules or pustules that rupture and evolve to form papulosquamous lesions, which are also pruritic. These then spread out from the periphery as new vesicles form at their outer margins, and at the same time begin to clear centrally (see Fig. 8-35, *D* and *E*). Over a period of several weeks, the patches may expand up to 5 cm in diameter. Tinea corporis can be found in any age group and is usually acquired through direct human contact (*Trichophyton tonsurans*) or from an infected pet, such as a kitten.

Clinically, tinea may be differentiated from atopic dermatitis by the propensity for autoinoculation from the primary patch to other sites on the patient's skin, by the spread to close contacts, and by the central clearing noted in many lesions. Moreover, the rash of atopic dermatitis tends to be symmetrical, chronic, and recurrent in a flexural distribution. Unlike tinea, patches of nummular eczema are self-limited and do not clear centrally. The herald patch of pityriasis rosea is often mistaken for tinea. However, it is KOH negative, and the subsequent development of the generalized rash with its characteristic truncal distribution is distinctive (see Fig. 8-26). The clinical pattern, findings, and chronic nature of psoriasis and seborrhea help differentiate them from tinea. Although granuloma annulare produces a characteristic ringed eruption, on palpation the lesions are firm and usually asymptomatic. They tend not to show epidermal changes other than occasional slight scaling (see Fig. 8-86).

The diagnosis of tinea corporis is confirmed by KOH examination of skin scrapings. The first step is to obtain material by scraping the loose scales at the margin of a lesion (Fig. 8-36, *A*). These should be mounted onto the center of a glass slide, with one or two drops of 20% KOH solution added. Next, a glass coverslip is applied and gently pressed down with the eraser end of a pencil to crush the scales (Fig. 8-36, *B*). The clinician then heats the slide, taking care not to boil the KOH solution, and again the coverslip is pressed down. When viewing the slide under the microscope, the clinician sets the condenser and light source at low levels to maximize contrast, with the objective at ×10. On focusing up and down, true hyphae are seen as long, branching, often septate rods of uniform width that cross the borders of epidermal cells

Figure 8-35 Tinea corporis. The characteristic annular lesions show many variations in appearance. **A,** This lesion has a raised, active border and shows partial central clearing. **B,** In another case the inflammatory response is intense, and only a little central clearing is seen. **C,** The lesion shown here involving the palm and flexor surfaces of the fingers is macular and scaly and has a sharply circumscribed proximal border. **D,** The evolution of lesions from papules and pustules into larger papulosquamous patches is seen on this girl's leg. **E,** In another child, small papules, plaques that have not cleared centrally, and larger lesions with varying degrees of central clearing are seen. (**B,** Courtesy Douglas W. Kress, MD, University of Pittsburgh Medical Center; **D,** courtesy Michael Sherlock, MD, Lutherville, Md.)

Figure 8-36 Potassium hydroxide (KOH) preparation. **A,** Small scales should be scraped from the edge of the lesion onto a microscope slide. **B,** To more easily visualize the fungus, the scales should be crushed, making a thin layer of cells.

Figure 8-37   Positive KOH preparation of skin scrapings. Fungal hyphae are seen as long septate branching rods at the margins and center of the scales.

(Fig. 8-37). Cotton fibers, cell borders, or other artifacts may be falsely interpreted as positive findings.

Tinea infections on glabrous skin readily respond to topical antifungal creams such as miconazole, clotrimazole, econazole, naftifine, ketoconazole, and ciclopirox. When lesions are multiple and widespread, oral therapy with griseofulvin is indicated. Itraconazole, terbinafine, and fluconazole are good alternatives for systemic antifungal therapy. Like griseofulvin, they are effective against most ringworm organisms, but unlike griseofulvin, these medications are concentrated in skin, hair, and nails for weeks to months after they are discontinued. Tinea infections should never be treated with the topical products that combine an azole antifungal with a medium or high-potency topical steroid. Paradoxically, these agents increase the likelihood that the fungal infection will spread deeper within the skin and be more resistant to topical therapy, a process called tinea incognito or Majocchi granuloma. At this stage oral therapy often becomes necessary to clear the infection.

Tinea Pedis

Commonly referred to as *athlete's foot,* tinea pedis is a fungal infection of the feet with a predilection for the web spaces between the toes. Tinea pedis is quite common in adolescence, somewhat less so in prepubertal children. The infecting organisms are acquired from contaminated shower, bathroom, locker room, and gym floors, and their growth is fostered by the warm, moist environment of shoes.

In some cases, scaling and fissuring predominate; in others, vesiculopustular lesions and maceration are found, especially in the web spaces between the third, fourth, and fifth toes. The infection begins between and along the sides of the toes, where it may remain (Fig. 8-38, *A*). However, lesions can extend over the dorsum of the foot (see Fig. 8-38, *B*) and may involve the plantar surface as well, particularly the instep and ball of the foot. Patients complain of a combination of burning and itching, which is frequently intense.

This diagnosis often can be made on clinical grounds and is confirmed by KOH preparation of skin scrapings. The mainstays of treatment are topical antifungal creams or powders, as well as measures designed to reduce foot moisture. The latter include careful drying of the feet after bathing, wearing cotton rather than synthetic socks, and wearing shoes that do not promote sweating or, better still, sandals. In patients with severe inflammatory lesions, oral antifungal agents may be required. Onychomycosis (see Fig. 8-144) responds well only to oral agents and requires treatment for 4 months,

Figure 8-38   Tinea pedis. **A,** Cracking and scaling are seen in the web space. **B,** In this patient the lesions began in the web spaces but then extended onto the dorsum of the foot. Note the active border. (**B,** *Courtesy Douglas W. Kress, MD, University of Pittsburgh Medical Center.*)

occasionally longer (see Disorders Affecting the Nails, later). Secondary bacterial infection (particularly with gram-negative organisms) may be a problem.

Tinea pedis is distinguished from contact dermatitis of the feet by virtue of the fact that the latter spares the interdigital web spaces (see Fig. 8-31). Dyshidrosis can have a similar distribution, but the KOH preparation is negative (see Fig. 8-18).

Tinea Versicolor

Tinea versicolor is a common dermatosis characterized by multiple small, oval, scaly patches measuring 1 to 3 cm in diameter, usually located in a guttate or raindrop pattern on the upper chest, back, and proximal portions of the upper extremities of adolescents and young adults (Fig. 8-39, *A* and *B*). However, all ages may be affected, including infants. Facial involvement occurs occasionally. The eruption is caused by a dimorphous form of *Pityrosporum.* Warm, moist climates, pregnancy, immunodeficiency, and genetic factors predispose people to the development of infection.

Figure 8-39   Tinea versicolor. **A** and **B,** Multiple oval patches are seen in a guttate or raindrop pattern over the upper chest and back of two patients. **C,** In areas not exposed to sunlight, lesions are darker than surrounding skin, whereas in **A** and **B** sun-exposed lesions fail to tan, remaining lighter than surrounding skin. *(Courtesy Michael Sherlock, MD, Lutherville, Md.)*

The rash is usually asymptomatic, although some patients complain of mild pruritus. Typically, patients go to the physician because they are bothered by the cosmetic appearance of the lesions. Lesions may be light tan, reddish, or lightly discolored, giving rise to the term *versicolor*. They are darker than surrounding skin in non–sun-exposed areas (Fig. 8-39, *C*) and lighter in areas that have tanned on exposure to sunlight (see Fig. 8-39, *A* and *B*).

The diagnosis of tinea versicolor can generally be made on the basis of the clinical appearance of lesions and their distribution. It can be confirmed by examining the lesions under a Wood's lamp, which reveals a characteristic tan to salmon-pink glow but no enhancement of the discoloration as in vitiligo. Although pathogenesis of the color change under a Wood's lamp is not fully understood, the fungus is known to produce a substance that interferes with tyrosinase activity and subsequent melanin synthesis. A KOH preparation of the surface scale demonstrates short hyphal and yeast forms that resemble spaghetti and meatballs (Fig. 8-40).

The differential diagnosis of tinea versicolor includes postinflammatory hypopigmentation and vitiligo. The history and distribution help to distinguish tinea versicolor from postinflammatory hypopigmentation; the presence of fine superficial scaling and some residual pigmentation (even in hypopigmented areas) that does not enhance with Wood's lamp examination helps rule out vitiligo.

Topical antiyeast agents such as selenium sulfide produce rapid clearing of the superficial lesions. Localized eruptions may be treated with topical antifungal creams such as miconazole, clotrimazole, or econazole, and recalcitrant cases respond to oral fluconazole or itraconazole. Patients must be counseled about the high risk of recurrence, which often necessitates ongoing prophylactic selenium sulfide washes for several days each month. They should also be reminded that pigmentary changes may take months to clear, even after eradication of the fungus.

Diaper Dermatitis

Because the diaper area is warm, often moist, and frequently contaminated by feces laden with organisms, diaper dermatitis is one of the most common skin disorders of infancy and early childhood.

Figure 8-40   Positive KOH preparation for tinea versicolor. The combination of hyphal and yeast forms of the fungus simulates the appearance of spaghetti and meatballs.

Figure 8-41 Irritant or ammoniacal diaper dermatitis. Note the erythema and scaling involving the convex surfaces and sparing of the intertriginous creases.

Figure 8-43 KOH preparation of skin scrapings from an infant with candidal diaper dermatitis demonstrating pseudohyphae and spores.

Irritant Diaper Dermatitis

The diaper area is a prime target for irritant dermatitis because it is bathed in urine and stool and occluded by plastic diaper covers. Failure to change diapers frequently is a major predisposing factor because it provides time for fecal bacteria to form ammonia by splitting the urea in urine. Harsh soaps, irritant chemicals, and detergents can contribute to the process. Moderate to severe diarrhea is another predisposing condition. The erythema; scaling; and, at times, maceration characteristic of irritant diaper dermatitis are usually confined to the convex surfaces of the perineum, lower abdomen, buttocks, and proximal thighs, sparing intertriginous areas (Fig. 8-41). When neglected, this may progress, with further skin breakdown and ulceration. Frequent diaper changes; gentle, thorough cleansing of the area; and application of lubricants and barrier pastes usually result in clearing of the dermatitis. A short course of low-potency steroids may hasten resolution, but this must be discontinued after a week or so and then followed by prevention with thick, unfragranced zinc oxide pastes as a barrier.

Persistent diaper dermatitis that does not resolve with conservative therapy may be due to other disorders such as contact dermatitis to the dyes present in the diaper (this has become increasingly common), candidiasis, seborrheic dermatitis, and psoriasis. These should be suspected particularly when intertriginous areas are involved.

Candidal Diaper Dermatitis

Candidal diaper dermatitis appears as a bright red eruption, with sharp borders and pinpoint satellite papules and pustules (Fig. 8-42, *A* and *B*). Examination of pustule contents by KOH preparation reveals the typical budding yeasts and pseudohyphae of *Candida* organisms (Fig. 8-43). Candidal diaper dermatitis is occasionally associated with oral thrush, and it is a common sequela of oral or parenteral antibiotic therapy. One should suspect a secondary invasion by *Candida albicans* whenever intertriginous areas are involved or when a diaper rash fails to respond to symptomatic treatment. Most cases respond well to topical antifungal therapy, but the occasional resistant case may require a brief course of oral medication.

Figure 8-42 Candidal diaper dermatitis. **A** and **B,** The eruption is bright red with numerous pinpoint satellite papules and pustules. Intertriginous areas are prominently involved.

Figure 8-44   Staphylococcal diaper dermatitis. Numerous thin-walled pustules are surrounded by erythematous halos, as well as multiple areas in which pustules have ruptured, leaving a collarette of scale around a denuded erythematous base.

Figure 8-46   Tinea diaper dermatitis. Note the prominent scaling and the elevated active border.

Staphylococcal Diaper Dermatitis

Irritant diaper dermatitis is frequently complicated by secondary staphylococcal infection, or pustules may appear as primary lesions, especially in the first few weeks of life. The presence of thin-walled pustules on an erythematous base (larger than those seen with candidiasis) alert the clinician to the diagnosis. Typically, these rupture rapidly and dry, producing a collarette of scaling around the denuded red base (Fig. 8-44). A Gram stain of pustule contents demonstrates neutrophils and clusters of gram-positive cocci. Bacterial cultures are confirmatory but are rarely necessary. Early diagnosis and treatment with oral and topical antibiotics result in rapid resolution.

Seborrheic Diaper Dermatitis

Seborrheic diaper dermatitis is characterized by salmon-colored lesions with a yellowish scale. The rash is particularly prominent in the intertriginous areas (see Fig. 8-23, B). Although concurrent infection with *Candida* or *Pityrosporum* is likely, satellite lesions are usually not seen. Typically, seborrheic dermatitis of the scalp, face, and postauricular areas is seen in association with this form of diaper dermatitis.

Psoriatic Diaper Dermatitis

Psoriasis occasionally begins as an erythematous, scaling eruption in the diaper area (Fig. 8-45, A and B), which is clinically indistinguishable from seborrheic diaper dermatitis. Perhaps because the diaper area tends to be moist, the thick silvery scale typical of psoriatic lesions at other sites is not seen. Although lesions may develop subsequently on the trunk and extremities, the rash may persist for months in the diaper area alone. Failure of a seborrheic-like diaper rash to respond to empiric therapy over several weeks or months should raise psoriasis as a diagnostic possibility. Skin biopsy is the only way to confirm the diagnosis.

Tinea Diaper Dermatitis

Although less common than the other dermatitides in the differential diagnosis of diaper dermatitis, tinea must be kept in mind when examining a scaly perineal rash. Its characteristic features are those of a recalcitrant scaly eruption with an elevated or "active" scaly border (Fig. 8-46), from which scales can be scraped and tinea demonstrated on KOH preparation. It responds well to topical antifungals alone and should not be treated with topical steroids.

Figure 8-45   Psoriatic diaper dermatitis. **A,** This child had a persistent diaper rash that did not respond to routine therapy. Note that scaling is not as intense as in psoriatic lesions seen elsewhere on the body. **B,** Another infant with inverse psoriasis involving the inguinal creases had also failed to improve despite multiple courses of topical antifungal treatment.

Figure 8-47 Lichen planus. These flat-topped violaceous papules of varying sizes and shapes overlying the anterior shin are typical. Note the linear lesions that formed after scratching, examples of the Koebner phenomenon.

Lichenoid Eruptions

Lichen Planus

Lichen planus is the prototypic lichenoid inflammatory eruption in that it displays flat-topped pruritic polygonal violaceous papules and plaques, which have a fine lacy pattern (Wickham striae) over their outer surfaces. They are often noted first over the dorsal surfaces of the extremities and can display koebnerization at sites of prior trauma (Fig. 8-47). The disorder may involve the nails (leading to dystrophy) as well as the oral mucosa, where lesions appear as lacy white plaques. Topical steroids are the mainstay of initial treatment. After resolution of primary lesions, a prolonged period of postinflammatory hyperpigmentation can be expected (see Fig. 8-124).

Lichen Striatus

Lichen striatus is one of the more common and distinctive lichenoid papulosquamous eruptions. Lesions consisting of flat-topped papules appear fairly abruptly, usually in a linear or sometimes swirled distribution along the lines of Blaschko. Although they may involve any portion of the skin, they are more typically located on the extremities, neck, or upper back. They may be slightly erythematous or hypopigmented, and their surfaces are covered with fine scale (Fig. 8-48, *A* and *B*). When lesions form on a digit, lichen striatus can lead to temporary linear nail dystrophy. The cause of this otherwise asymptomatic disorder, which has its peak incidence in school-age children, is unknown. Spontaneous resolution within 1 to 3 years is the norm.

VESICULOPUSTULAR DISORDERS

Vesiculopustular eruptions range from benign, self-limited conditions to life-threatening diseases. Early diagnosis, especially in the young child, is mandatory. Systematic evaluation of the clinical findings and a few rapid diagnostic techniques allow these various disorders to be readily differentiated from one another.

Viral Infections

Viral infections including herpes simplex and varicella-zoster produce characteristic vesiculopustular exanthems, which are discussed in Chapter 12. However, the technique of confirming the suspicion of a herpetic lesion by preparing a Tzanck test is discussed here.

The Tzanck smear is obtained by removing the roof of a vesicle with a scalpel or scissors and scraping the cells at its base. This is then spread onto a glass slide with the scalpel blade, air dried, and stained with Giemsa or Wright stain. The diagnostic finding in viral blisters is the multinucleated giant cell (Fig. 8-49). This is a syncytium of epidermal cells with multiple, overlapping nuclei; hence it is much larger than other inflammatory cells. Unfortunately, a positive Tzanck test cannot be used to differentiate one blistering viral exanthem from another, and a viral culture, or the more rapid direct fluorescent antibody test, should be done when the clinical situation mandates precise identification.

Bacterial Infections

Several common cutaneous bacterial infections present with vesiculopustular reactions as well. In impetigo, the eruption tends to be discrete and localized, whereas in staphylococcal scalded skin syndrome (SSSS) it tends to be associated with a diffuse erythroderma. A Gram stain of material aspirated from bullae or removed from the base of an impetiginous lesion is positive for organisms. However, in patients with SSSS, the organism must be sought from noncutaneous

Figure 8-48 Lichen striatus. **A,** In this school-age child, mildly erythematous scaly flat-topped papules are seen in a linear distribution on the lower leg. **B,** Another child with darker skin has lesions that are hypopigmented on the posterior thigh. (**A,** *From Cohen BA:* Atlas of pediatric dermatology, *London, 1993, Mosby-Wolfe;* **B,** *from Cohen BA:* Pediatric dermatology, *ed 2, London, 1999, Mosby.*)

Figure 8-49   Tzanck preparation. Note the multinucleated giant cell characteristic of viral infection with herpes simplex and varicella-zoster.

colonized locations (nasopharynx, conjunctivae, sinuses) because the diffuse cutaneous blistering is due to elaboration of the toxin epidermolysin by the infecting organism and not to the organism's direct action within individual lesions (see Chapter 12 and Fig. 12-18).

Blistering Distal Dactylitis

Blistering distal dactylitis is a superficial bacterial infection involving the tips of the pads of fingers or toes. Lesions consist of tense blisters 0.5 to 1 cm in diameter that are filled with thin purulent fluid and surrounded by a narrow erythematous rim. With evolution, they may coalesce and extend proximally along the lateral aspect of the nail fold. On rupture, a thick crust forms (Fig. 8-50). Group A β-streptococci are the usual causative organisms and are detected by Gram stain and culture of vesicular fluid. On occasion, group B streptococci and *S. aureus* are isolated. The disorder can be distinguished from a paronychia by the distal location of initial lesions; from a herpetic whitlow by the larger size of the initial vesicles and Gram stain of the purulent fluid; and from burns by the purulence of the vesicular fluid and Gram stain revealing white blood cells and bacteria.

Erythema Multiforme

Erythema multiforme (EM) is a distinctive, acute hypersensitivity syndrome that, in both children and adults, is most frequently triggered by recurrent herpes simplex virus (HSV) infection. EM should not be confused with either *Stevens-Johnson syndrome* (SJS) or *toxic epidermal necrolysis* (TEN),

Figure 8-50   Blistering distal dactylitis. A tense blister filled with purulent fluid first developed at the tip of the thumb pad of this child. Subsequently, the lesion ruptured and crusted and newer lesions formed more proximally along the nail fold and at the tip of the index finger. *(From Cohen BA:* Pediatric dermatology, *ed 2, London, 1999, Mosby.)*

which are severe, potentially life-threatening eruptions characterized by variably widespread cutaneous blistering and sloughing, and by involvement of multiple mucous membranes.

The classic eruption of EM is symmetrical and may occur on any part of the body. However, the dorsum of the hands and feet and the extensor surfaces of the arms and legs are affected most commonly. Involvement of the palms and soles also is typical. The initial lesions are dusky red macules or erythematous wheals that evolve into iris- or target-shaped lesions, the hallmark of EM (Fig. 8-51, *A*). In many instances the initial crop of lesions simulates diffuse urticaria, although EM lesions are typically much less pruritic, if at all, and ultimately they become painful and persistent, in contrast to true urticarial lesions, which remain pruritic and tend to migrate over a 24-hour period. The target configuration is due to formation of a central depression that may be blue, violaceous, or white, whereas the elevated periphery tends to remain erythematous. In some cases, vesicles or bullae develop centrally, and in others the peripheral rings may vesiculate or become bullous (Fig. 8-51, *B* and *C*). The eruption continues in crops that last from 1 to 3 weeks. In most patients the disease is self-limited, and systemic manifestations are relatively mild, consisting of low-grade fever, malaise, and myalgia. Mucous membranes tend to be spared, although, on occasion, the oral mucosa may be mildly involved. The major differential diagnosis is urticaria, which does not demonstrate three discrete zones of color change to form a target, as do lesions of true erythema multiforme.

Stevens-Johnson Syndrome and Toxic Epidermal Necrolysis

SJS and TEN are rare, potentially life-threatening disorders characterized by widespread epidermal and mucous membrane necrosis and sloughing. In both SJS and TEN the plane of cleavage of bullae is beneath the basement membrane zone, resulting in full-thickness sloughing. Operationally, they can be distinguished by virtue of the fact that SJS tends to involve from 10% to 30% of the body surface area, whereas in TEN anywhere from one third to 100% is affected, although there is some overlap. Although the etiology is often unclear, hypersensitivity reactions to medications, antecedent viral infections, connective tissue disorders, and malignancy have all been implicated.

Clinically, a prodrome of fever, malaise, and sore throat usually precedes the appearance of diffuse erythroderma, which is then superseded in 24 to 48 hours by necrosis and cleavage, resulting in the formation of thick-walled vesicles and bullae that often are hemorrhagic (Fig. 8-52, *A-C* and Fig. 8-53). Nikolsky sign is evident soon thereafter, and as bullae and vesicles slough, they leave deep bloody erosions, which then crust over. Mucous membrane involvement, particularly of the oral, conjunctival, and urethral mucous membranes, is routine and often severe. It consists of the formation of fragile, thin-walled bullae that rupture early, leaving ulcerations of variable depth that are rapidly covered by a gray, yellow, or white membrane (Fig. 8-52, *D*). On healing, mucosal adhesions and scarring may be noted. Conjunctival involvement can progress to involve the cornea, resulting in corneal scarring, and necessitates early and aggressive ophthalmologic treatment for possible prevention. Lid scarring may result in ectropion. Constitutional symptoms are prominent in both disorders and include high fever, cough, sore throat, vomiting, diarrhea, chest pain, and arthralgias. Fluid and electrolyte imbalances, caused by losses from ruptured bullae, and secondary infection are major risks and are proportionately greater in cases of TEN, given its more extensive body surface area involvement. Intensive supportive care is required to

Figure 8-51 Erythema multiforme. **A,** The characteristic target-shaped lesions are symmetrically distributed. **B,** These lesions are dusky centrally and their peripheral rims are beginning to vesiculate. **C,** In this case, the peripheral rims have become frankly bullous. (**C,** Courtesy Michael Sherlock, MD, Lutherville, Md.)

prevent complications from these fluid losses and from secondary bacterial infection, which is an ever-present danger. Recovery may take a month or more.

Although large, well-controlled trials are lacking, administration of intravenous immunoglobulin (IVIG) early in the course of disease has been found to mitigate progression in some cases. Systemic steroids, on the other hand, are usually contraindicated, as they have been associated with an increased risk of morbidity from secondary infection.

Differential diagnostic considerations include staphylococcal scalded skin syndrome (SSSS) and erythema multiforme. In SSSS the plane of cleavage is high in the epidermis. Hence bullae are thin walled (see Fig. 12-18), and although mucous membranes are erythematous, they do not slough. Furthermore, Gram stain and culture of exudates from the nose and conjunctivae are positive for *S. aureus*. In EM initial lesions appear as dusky-red macules or erythematous wheals, which then evolve into bullous, target-shaped lesions, which do not tend to slough, and mucous membrane involvement, if present at all, is mild.

Miliaria

Miliaria Crystallina

Miliaria crystallina is a condition in which obstruction of the eccrine sweat ducts located high in the outer layer of the epidermis results in the formation of multiple 2- to 3-mm sweat retention vesicles. Being thin walled, these vesicles are readily ruptured (Fig. 8-54). In infants, lesions form over the head, neck, and upper trunk. In older children, they more commonly occur in areas of desquamating sunburn.

Miliaria Rubra

Sweat duct obstruction deeper in the epidermal or dermal layers produces an erythematous papulopustular eruption known as *miliaria rubra*, or prickly heat (Fig. 8-55). This rash is common in infants and children, especially over the face, upper trunk, and intertriginous area of the neck, as a result of tight-fitting clothing or use of occlusive lubricants, particularly during hot, humid weather. Wearing lightweight, loose-fitting clothing, eliminating greasy topical agents, and using corn starch assists clearing of the rash.

Infantile Acropustulosis

Infantile acropustulosis, a remitting and exacerbating disorder of unknown etiology, begins as pinpoint erythematous papules, which evolve to form papulopustules or vesiculopustules (Fig. 8-56) that are highly pruritic. They appear in crops over the hands and feet, at times extending onto the wrists and ankles. After 10 to 21 days they resolve, only to recur within a few weeks. Ultimately, the disorder resolves by 2 to 3 years of age. Differential diagnostic considerations include scabies, dyshidrosis, erythema toxicum, and transient neonatal pustular melanosis. High-potency topical steroids applied sparingly up to twice a day and high doses of antihistamine may help relieve itching.

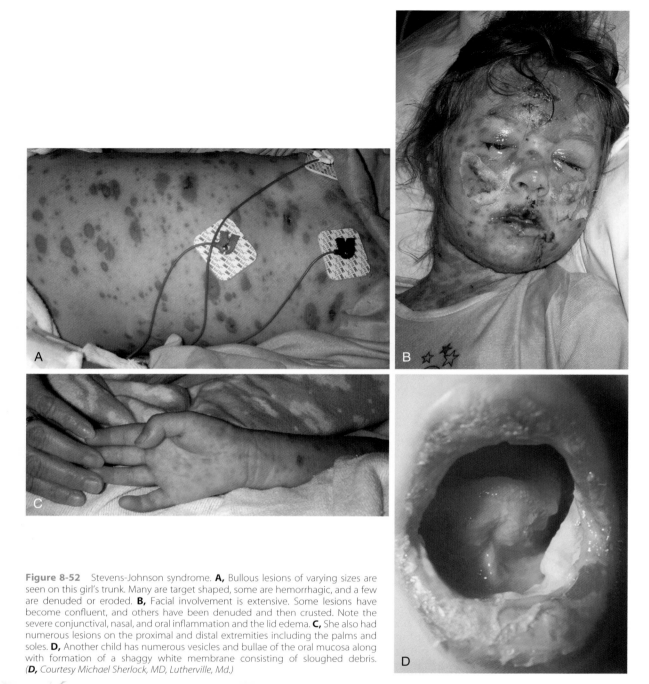

Figure 8-52   Stevens-Johnson syndrome. **A,** Bullous lesions of varying sizes are seen on this girl's trunk. Many are target shaped, some are hemorrhagic, and a few are denuded or eroded. **B,** Facial involvement is extensive. Some lesions have become confluent, and others have been denuded and then crusted. Note the severe conjunctival, nasal, and oral inflammation and the lid edema. **C,** She also had numerous lesions on the proximal and distal extremities including the palms and soles. **D,** Another child has numerous vesicles and bullae of the oral mucosa along with formation of a shaggy white membrane consisting of sloughed debris. (**D,** Courtesy Michael Sherlock, MD, Lutherville, Md.)

Figure 8-53   Toxic epidermal necrolysis. Three weeks after starting phenytoin for new-onset seizures, this 10-year-old experienced sudden onset of fever and malaise in association with diffuse erythroderma, conjunctivitis, and oral mucositis. Soon thereafter, thick-walled bullae formed, then rapidly sloughed, leaving deep bloody erosions. Note the extensive amount of surface area involved. (Courtesy http://www.dermatlas.org.)

Figure 8-54   Miliaria crystallina. Found primarily over the head, neck, and upper trunk, these tiny thin-walled sweat retention vesicles rupture readily and then quickly desquamate.

Figure 8-55 Miliaria rubra. Numerous tiny papulopustular lesions dot the skin of this infant's face, neck, and upper trunk.

Vesiculation following Insect Bites

Inflammatory reactions to insect bites, although often beginning as edematous papules, may evolve into pruritic vesicles and bullae on erythematous bases (Fig. 8-57). This is particularly true of the bites of grass and sand mites, and of fleas in sensitized individuals who react intensely. The eruption is frequently misdiagnosed as chickenpox or bullous impetigo. Severe pruritus, the lack of systemic complaints, localization to exposed areas (especially the lower legs), and seasonal occurrence point to the correct diagnosis. Furthermore, the vesicles have thicker walls than those of bullous impetigo, and they do not rapidly umbilicate and crust as is true of varicella lesions. Tzanck tests and Gram stains are also negative in bullous insect bite reactions (see Bites and Stings, later). Bedbugs can present in a similar fashion but can be widespread and occur even under clothing.

REACTIVE ERYTHEMAS

The term *reactive erythema* refers to a group of disorders characterized by erythematous patches, plaques, and nodules that vary in size, shape, and distribution. Unlike other specific dermatoses, they represent cutaneous reaction patterns triggered by a variety of endogenous and environmental agents.

Figure 8-56 Infantile acropustulosis. Intensely pruritic papulopustular lesions are seen over the foot and ankle of this infant. He had had multiple episodes and had been treated repeatedly for scabies. *(Courtesy Sylvia Suarez, MD, Centerville, Va.)*

Figure 8-57 Vesicular reaction to insect bites. This boy's lower legs are studded with numerous thick-walled vesicles and bullae that have formed in response to mite bites.

In children, the most common reactive erythemas include erythema nodosum, urticaria, vasculitis, and drug eruptions.

Erythema Nodosum

Erythema nodosum is characterized by symmetrical, red, tender nodules, 1 to 5 cm in diameter, which are usually located over the pretibial surfaces (Fig. 8-58, *A* and *B*). Most likely, it represents a hypersensitivity reaction to streptococcal infection, sarcoidosis, tuberculosis, or other bacterial or fungal infections. Noninfectious disorders such as ulcerative colitis and regional ileitis have also been implicated. In adolescent girls, oral contraceptives are the most common cause, and a number of other medications may trigger this reaction.

Erythema nodosum is most often seen in children older than 10 years. The lesions begin as red, tender, slightly elevated nodules. These enlarge to form indurated subcutaneous plaques, and the overlying skin takes on a brownish-red or purplish-red hue within a few days. The disorder usually lasts between 2 and 6 weeks, although recurrences are common. Although any site may be involved, the shins are most commonly affected.

Differential diagnosis includes cellulitis, insect bites, thrombophlebitis, ecchymoses, and vasculitis. The fact that lesions are symmetrical, recurrent, and persistent helps exclude cellulitis and ecchymoses. Their usual pretibial and extensor location helps differentiate the lesions from thrombophlebitis. Insect bite reactions typically are pruritic, and other exposed sites such as the arms, head, and neck may be involved. The deep-seated nature of the nodules in erythema nodosum should allow differentiation from the smaller, more superficial palpable lesions of cutaneous small-vessel vasculitis. However, they can mimic the cutaneous lesions seen in polyarteritis nodosum, a medium-vessel vasculitis.

Treatment is directed toward the underlying cause. Nonsteroidal antiinflammatory agents may be effective in reducing pain, and bed rest is beneficial.

Figure 8-58   Erythema nodosum. **A,** Note the typical red, raised, tender nodules overlying the pretibial surfaces of the legs. **B,** This 18-month-old boy developed tender, indurated, erythematous patches over his chest and abdomen after an upper respiratory infection. (**B,** *Courtesy Cohen BA:* Pediatric dermatology, *ed 2, London, 1999, Mosby.*)

Urticaria

Urticaria, commonly known as *hives,* is characterized by the sudden appearance of transient, well-demarcated wheals that are usually intensely pruritic, especially when arising as part of an acute IgE-mediated hypersensitivity reaction (Fig. 8-59, *A*). Individual lesions usually last 1 to 2 hours but may persist for up to 24 hours. They may have an edematous white center and macular red halo (Fig. 8-59, *B*) or the reverse—a red center with an edematous white halo. Size can vary from a few millimeters to giant lesions greater than 20 cm in diameter

(Fig. 8-59, *C*). Central clearing with peripheral extension may lead to the formation of annular, polycyclic, and arcuate plaques, simulating erythema multiforme and erythema marginatum (see Fig. 8-59, *D*). The reaction may involve the mucous membranes and can spread to the subcutaneous tissue, producing woody edema known as *angioedema.*

Urticaria can be caused by a variety of immunologic mechanisms including IgE antibody response, complement activation, and abnormal levels of or sensitivity to vasoactive amines. Most commonly, acute urticaria (lasting less than

Figure 8-59   Urticaria. **A,** Typical erythematous raised wheals are seen. **B,** The wheals on this child's face have red rims and lighter centers. **C,** This patient with cold-induced urticaria has a giant whitish wheal with an erythematous halo. **D,** Gyrate urticarial plaques have evolved from individual plaques that became confluent. (**A** *and* **C,** *Courtesy Douglas W. Kress, MD, University of Pittsburgh Medical Center.*)

6 weeks) is idiopathic, postviral, or is caused by a hypersensitivity reaction to food, drugs, insect bites, contact allergens, inhaled substances, or acute infections (especially β-streptococcal infections and viral infections including mononucleosis). Chronic urticaria (lasting more than 6 weeks) can be a sign of an underlying disorder such as occult infection (of the urinary tract, sinuses, or dentition); hepatitis B; or connective tissue disease (see Chapters 4 and 7). Urticarial lesions that remain fixed in the same location for more than 24 hours and/or heal with prolonged bruising are particularly likely to be manifestations of urticarial vasculitis.

In otherwise healthy patients who have no evidence on thorough history and physical examination to suggest occult infection or an underlying disorder and whose laboratory studies are normal, extensive testing is not warranted. Empiric treatment with oral antihistamines provides symptomatic relief and may help break the itch–scratch cycle.

Serum Sickness–like Reaction

Serum sickness–like reaction, a relatively common acute clinical picture, involves a constellation of urticarial lesions, periarticular swelling, and extremity angioedema in conjunction with acute upper respiratory infection or following use of medications such as sulfonamides, cefaclor, minocycline, or the "-cillins." The urticaria is typically either nonpruritic or only mildly pruritic, and lesions evolve into target shapes or gyrate plaques simulating erythema multiforme, although they do not vesiculate (Fig. 8-60, *A* and *B*). With this eruption, painful migratory periarticular swelling is seen, especially involving the wrists and ankles, and often associated with bluish discoloration of the overlying skin. Migratory stocking-glove angioedema, which is also painful, is common; on occasion, facial edema is seen as well (Fig. 8-60, *C*). After resolution of the respiratory infection or discontinuation of the offending agent, symptoms wax and wane over 1 to 3 weeks. This appears to be a T-lymphocyte–mediated reaction, and classic changes of vasculitis are not seen.

Drug Eruptions

Morbilliform Drug Eruption

Many different types of drug eruption are seen in children. Morbilliform rashes or exanthems account for 75% to 80% of all cutaneous drug reactions. The rash is reminiscent of measles or other viral exanthems (see Chapter 12). Erythematous macules and papules, which may range from fine to blotchy, usually begin to erupt on the face and trunk within 5 to 14 days after starting a medication. They then spread to the extremities over one to several days (Fig. 8-61, *A-C*). The rash, which may be pruritic, is occasionally restricted to the extremities, or it may appear acrally (distally) at first and then spread centrally. Lesions may become confluent and generally resolve over 1 to 2 weeks with the development of faint purpura, fine desquamation, and residual postinflammatory erythema. In cases of severe morbilliform drug eruption with facial swelling, fever, and/or malaise, the clinician should check hepatic function to rule out the more life-threatening disorder, DRESS (drug rash with eosinophilia and systemic symptoms), which can lead to hepatic failure if not identified and treated promptly. DRESS is more common with certain medications such as sulfa drugs, minocycline, and the anticonvulsants.

Fixed Drug Eruption

Fixed drug eruptions occur repeatedly at the same cutaneous site after reexposure to an offending drug. Postinflammatory hyperpigmentation is usually marked and may be the only manifestation of the rash during remissions. Morphologically and histologically, the target-shaped and bullous lesions of fixed drug reactions may be indistinguishable from erythema multiforme and may represent a localized form of EM (Fig. 8-62).

Henoch-Schönlein Purpura

Henoch-Schönlein purpura (HSP) is an inflammatory disorder with multiple predisposing conditions. It is characterized by a diffuse vasculitis involving the small postcapillary venules in the skin; gastrointestinal tract; kidneys; joints; and, rarely, the lungs and CNS. Although the exact etiology is unclear, the common history of antecedent upper respiratory or gastrointestinal infection suggests a hypersensitivity phenomenon resulting in a localized or widespread vascular insult. Other factors, including drugs, food, immunizations, and chemical toxins, have been implicated as well. Histologically, immune complex deposition in capillaries and postcapillary venules is associated with a leukocytoclastic vasculitis in the skin and other involved organs.

After a prodrome of headache, anorexia, and, occasionally, low-grade fever lasting one to a few days, patients may develop

Figure 8-60 Serum sickness–like reaction to cefaclor. **A** and **B,** Extensive urticarial, target-shaped, and gyrate lesions are seen over the back, arms, and trunk. **C,** Facial edema involving the forehead was prominent in this child.

Figure 8-61   Morbilliform drug eruption. **A** and **B,** This diffuse exanthem developed on the seventh day of treatment with amoxicillin for streptococcal pharyngitis. **C,** The palms and soles were also affected.

one or more of the following in any order: rash, abdominal pain, arthritis, and occasionally hematochezia. Cutaneous lesions consist of erythematous macules, urticarial papules, and purpuric papules and plaques that tend to appear in crops (Fig. 8-63, A-C), each resolving over 5 to 7 days, although the total duration of this waxing and waning eruption may last anywhere from 1 to 8 weeks (average, 2 to 3 weeks). Of affected children, 15% to 40% have one or more recurrences, usually within 6 weeks of resolution of the first episode.

Although in most children the initial crop consists of purpuric lesions distributed symmetrically below the waist (over the buttocks, lower abdomen, and lower extremities), in some this may be preceded by an acral or generalized urticarial eruption that is minimally pruritic and waxes and wanes over one to several days before the appearance of purpura. Subsequent crops of purpura usually involve the extensor surfaces of the arms, cheeks (Fig. 8-63, D), and tips of the ears. The rash may also involve the trunk and genitalia. In unusually severe cases, skin necrosis may occur, heralded by the appearance of bullae.

Joint involvement consists of painful, tender periarticular swelling, especially involving the wrists, ankles, and knees.

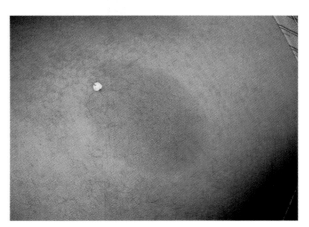

Figure 8-62   Fixed drug eruption. This hyperpigmented patch with an erythematous border developed on the flank of an adolescent taking tetracycline.

The overlying skin tends to appear ecchymotic. Stocking-glove edema of the hands and feet is also common (Fig. 8-63, E). In young children, nonpruritic angioedema of the face, scalp, sacral area, and/or genital area (Fig. 8-63, F) may be prominent. These phenomena wax and wane, as does the exanthem.

Gastrointestinal symptoms can precede, coincide with, or follow the appearance of cutaneous lesions. Segmental edema of the intestinal tract can cause crampy to colicky abdominal pain and may even serve as the lead point for an intussusception. Mucosal hemorrhage can be the source of gastrointestinal bleeding that can range from occult loss to massive hematochezia or hematemesis (see Chapter 17).

Up to 25% of patients develop nephritis between 1 and 8 weeks after the onset of symptoms (peak, 1 to 3 weeks). This is more common in older children, and it is usually mild and self-limited. It is first detected by finding evidence of hematuria and proteinuria on urinalysis. On occasion, nephritis is severe and progressive (see Chapter 13). Long-term studies suggest that the risk of subtle renal disease may be higher than initially suspected, and the routine determination of blood pressure at regular pediatric visits is a good screening tool. Moreover, children with chronic HSP with recurrences lasting more than 4 to 6 months may be at higher risk for chronic renal disease. CNS involvement is extremely rare, and its presence is usually heralded by severe headache, altered level of consciousness, and/or seizures subsequent to meningeal hemorrhage.

Treatment of HSP is generally supportive, although gastrointestinal, renal, and CNS vasculitis may respond to systemic corticosteroids.

The cutaneous lesions of HSP must be differentiated from acute bacterial, viral, and rickettsial infections (see Chapter 12). Negative blood cultures and classic findings on cutaneous examination and skin biopsy define HSP. Purpuric rashes associated with thrombocytopenia are more likely to be associated with petechiae and can be ruled out by a normal platelet count. Last, vasculitic rashes may also be seen in collagen vascular disorders such as lupus erythematosus, mixed connective tissue disease, and dermatomyositis (see Chapter 7). These disorders can usually be excluded by the

Figure 8-63 Henoch-Schönlein purpura. **A,** Palpable purpuric macules, papules, and plaques are seen over the legs and ankles of this toddler. **B** and **C,** These smaller purpuric papules are more typical and are seen initially over the buttocks, thighs, and ankles. **D,** Later crops may involve the extensor surfaces of the upper extremities, trunk, and face. **E** and **F,** Edema of the extremities, genitals, face, and scalp may be impressive.

absence of other findings. An etiology, likely related to HSP but occurring in infants, is called acute hemorrhagic edema of infancy and is characterized by purpura en cockade, annular lesions of purpura on the distal extremities, as well as swelling of those distal extremities. Unlike HSP, acute hemorrhagic edema of infancy has an extremely benign course with only a few reports of renal involvement to be found in the literature.

BITES AND STINGS

Insect and spider bites may be associated with a number of cutaneous and systemic reactions. Lesions are found on exposed areas of skin, particularly the lower legs, arms, head, and neck. During the warm summer months they may also appear on the trunk. Protected areas (including the buttocks, groin, and axillae) are invariably spared. When bites involve the face, they can cause marked pruritic swelling that, although erythematous, is nontender and minimally indurated, if at all; rather, it tends to be soft or mushy on palpation (Fig. 8-64).

Insect Bites

Insect bites, most commonly caused by mosquitoes, fleas, mites, and fleas, tend to produce mild acute local reactions including erythema, edema, and urticarial papules that are typically pruritic (Fig. 8-65, *A*). A tiny central crust or hemorrhagic punctum may be apparent on close inspection. On occasion, patients develop more intense hemorrhagic reactions (see Fig. 8-65, *B*).

Although mosquito and mite bites occur only during the warm months of spring, summer, and fall, flea bites can occur year round, typically in households with pets or in apartments

Figure 8-64   Facial swelling caused by a mosquito bite. The area was pruritic, nontender, and nonindurated. (*Courtesy Michael Sherlock, MD, Lutherville, Md.*)

or homes recently vacated by previous tenants or owners whose pets had fleas. Young children who only visit on occasion with friends or relatives who have pets are also susceptible. Bites are usually found on the lower legs above the sock line but can be more diffusely distributed on crawling infants and toddlers. Like those of bedbugs, flea bites often appear in clusters of three (a clinical finding termed "breakfast, lunch, and dinner"). This stems from the fact that although fleas can jump, they cannot fly. Hence they tend to produce a localized series of bites in the same vicinity before jumping on to a new area. Excoriation caused by scratching makes them prone to secondary impetiginization. It should also be noted that not all members of a household may be sensitive to flea bites, and therefore some may "appear" to be spared. This can be a source of confusion to people who assume that if fleas are the source, everyone should be affected.

Figure 8-65   Insect bites. **A,** Multiple erythematous papules with central puncta were thought to be the result of either flea or bedbug bites. **B,** Another child had an intense hemorrhagic reaction to flea bites. (**A,** *Courtesy Sylvia Suarez, MD, Centerville, Va.*)

On occasion, the bites of grass or sand mites can produce frank blistering because the venom they inject contains a blistering agent that affects sensitive individuals (see Fig. 8-57).

Biting flies include sandflies, blackflies, horseflies, and gnats. The bite itself causes immediate pain and is usually followed by the development of a painful papule that sometimes vesiculates centrally.

Spider Bites

Spider bites tend to provoke more intense inflammatory reactions than those of most insects. Commonly, this consists of an area of erythema and induration that frequently becomes ecchymotic and is simultaneously painful and pruritic (Fig. 8-66). Less often, the lesions may vesiculate or even progress to develop central necrosis with eschar formation. The latter is particularly typical of the bite of the brown recluse spider.

Hymenoptera Stings

Bee, wasp, hornet, and yellow jacket stings typically produce a mild local reaction consisting of pain, erythema, and edema appearing within 2 hours after the sting (Fig. 8-67, A). The honey bee leaves its stinger behind, embedded in the skin. Because this may continue to release venom for up to 1 hour, it should be removed as soon as possible, using a horizontal scraping motion with a knife or fingernail. Grasping the stinger between forceps or two fingernails can inject more venom. Evidence indicates that topical application of a paste of papain (meat tenderizer) mixed with water may reduce the severity of local reactions, if applied within minutes of the sting.

Hymenoptera stings commonly produce a late-onset increase in swelling that is more diffuse than the initial reaction and tends to peak in 48 to 72 hours. This is the result of a delayed hypersensitivity reaction, and it is described by patients as being both pruritic and painful (Fig. 8-67, B). Treatment is symptomatic.

In approximately 0.5% to 0.8% of the population (including many patients with underlying mastocytosis [see Fig.

Figure 8-66 Spider bites. A marked inflammatory response consisting of a central wheal with a wide erythematous halo is seen in this child, who complained of both pain and pruritus.

8-83]), hymenoptera stings cause severe, acute, anaphylactic reactions within 15 minutes of the sting (see Chapter 4). This necessitates education regarding avoidance of the offending insects and immediate availability of an insect sting kit (EpiPen or EpiPen Jr).

Papular Urticaria

Papular urticaria, a phenomenon seen primarily in young children, is characterized by symmetrical chronic/recurrent eruptions of highly pruritic papules and wheals that tend to vesiculate centrally. Acute lesions are round, about 3 to 10 mm in diameter, and often have a central punctum. They tend to be arranged in linear or triangular clusters on exposed body

Figure 8-67 Hymenoptera stings. **A,** This child had an acute reaction with pain, redness, and mild swelling that developed within 2 hours of the sting. **B,** In this example of a delayed hypersensitivity response to a bee sting, marked swelling of the hand and fingers developed over 24 hours after a sting between the fingers.

Figure 8-68   Papular urticaria. This severe, excoriated, papular reaction developed in response to recurrent flea bites. *(Courtesy Michael Sherlock, MD, Lutherville, Md.)*

surfaces such as the arms; legs; back; face; and in toddlers, the scalp. As itching is intense, the child scratches to the point of excoriation, incurring risk of secondary infection and scarring. During resolution, lesions tend to form a central crust with a surrounding collarette of scale, and ultimately (after 4 to 6 weeks) the child is left with target-shaped macules that are hyperpigmented peripherally and hypopigmented centrally. Often lesions in varying stages of evolution and healing are seen within a small geographic area (Fig. 8-68).

The disorder is the result of a hypersensitivity response induced by bites of blood-sucking insects, especially dog and cat fleas and bedbugs, and sometimes mosquitoes. Flea bites can be acquired by living in a home with pets that have fleas, in a house or apartment recently vacated by pet owners, or by visiting at regular intervals the home of a relative, family friend, or babysitter with pets. Bedbugs may be brought into the home in luggage by a family member on return from travel involving a stay in a hotel room or house that was infested. Because fleas live indoors and bedbugs bite year round, there is no seasonal predilection when they are the source.

Typically only one family member, usually one of the youngest children, is affected. This is because some individuals never develop hypersensitivity to the bites; others have varying thresholds of sensitization; and older individuals, sensitized in the past, have become tolerant.

Because a full-scale reaction tends to require a fairly long period of sensitization, during which the child has repeated exposure to the offending insect, few children become sensitized before their first birthdays. During this period of induction of sensitization, the child reacts minimally when bitten. Once sensitized, children go through a period of variable duration (months to years) in which they experience both immediate and delayed hypersensitivity reactions to bites. Ultimately, they develop tolerance (i.e., become desensitized) and no longer react. During peak sensitivity, many experience a phenomenon known as *reactivation*, in which new bites incite a delayed hypersensitivity reaction at old sites.

Identification of the offending vector and elimination of its presence can shorten the cycling. Other treatment measures include use of moisturizers, high-potency topical steroids, and oral antihistamines for acute lesions. Good hand and nail hygiene reduces the risk of secondary infection. Wearing protective clothing, avoiding going outdoors after dusk, and judicious use of insect repellent are helpful when mosquitoes are causative.

Treatment Principles for Insect Bites

General principles of therapy for insect bites consist of insect control, use of insect repellents, and application of topical corticosteroids supplemented by oral antihistamines for symptomatic relief. Parenteral administration of epinephrine, antihistamines, and corticosteroids combined with intensive supportive care may be lifesaving in anaphylactic reactions.

INFESTATIONS

Scabies

Scabies is a highly contagious infestation caused by the mite *Acarus scabiei*, which burrows under the skin. It is contracted by direct contact with other infested humans or fomites. The characteristic eruption appears 4 to 6 weeks after initial contact, and it is thought to represent a hypersensitivity reaction to the mites. Intensely pruritic papules, vesicles, pustules, and linear burrows appear in the finger and toe webs (Fig. 8-69, *A*), the axillae, over the flexor surfaces of the wrists and elbows, around the nipples and waist, and over the groin and buttocks. The burrow, which is produced by the female mite, is the pathognomonic sign of scabies. It consists of a small, scaly, linear papule with pinpoint vesicles at the ends (Fig. 8-69, *B*). In infants and toddlers the distribution differs, with the head; neck; trunk; palms; soles, dorsa, and lateral and instep portions of the feet; and lateral aspect of the wrists being more prominently involved (Fig. 8-70, *A-E*). This age group is also more prone to developing an intense and persistent nodular reaction to the mite (see Fig. 8-70, *F*).

In many patients, excoriation, secondary infection, or even development of a widespread secondary eczematous eruption (as a result of intense scratching) alters the appearance of or masks the primary lesions, making diagnosis more difficult. Therefore, scabies must be considered in any individual who has no history of atopic dermatitis but has severe pruritus and recent onset of an eczematous rash. The distribution of scabies in intertriginous areas and over the palms and dorsa and soles of the feet helps to differentiate it from other insect bite reactions.

Although scabies can often be diagnosed clinically, an unequivocal diagnosis can be made with a skin scraping that shows a mite, mite eggs, or feces. The most important factor in obtaining a successful scraping is choice of site. Burrows and papules are most likely to be identified on the wrists, finger webs, feet, or elbows or in an infant by scraping one of the nodules present on the trunk, palms, or soles. A fresh burrow can be identified as a 5- to 10-mm raised mound with a small dark spot resembling a fleck of pepper at one end. This spot is the mite, and it can be lifted out of the burrow with a needle or the point of a scalpel blade. If a scalpel is used to scrape the burrow, it is worthwhile to place a drop of mineral oil onto the skin to ensure adherence of the scrapings to the blade. The scrapings are placed on a slide, another drop of mineral oil is added, and a coverslip is applied.

Scabies mites are eight-legged arachnids easily visible under the scanning power of the microscope (Fig. 8-71, *A*). Care must be taken to focus through thick areas of skin scrapings so as not to miss camouflaged mites. The presence of eggs (smooth ovals, approximately one quarter to one half the

Figure 8-69 Scabies. **A,** Multiple pruritic papules, some excoriated and a few with central black dots, are seen on the wrist and dorsum of the hand. **B,** A pathognomonic scabies burrow is present in the finger web space of another child.

Figure 8-70 Infantile scabies. Widespread, pruritic papules, pustules, and vesicles are seen over the trunk and axilla **(A)**; the soles and dorsal, lateral, and instep portions of the feet **(B** and **C)**, where burrows are also evident; the palm of the hand **(D)**; and the lateral aspect of the wrist **(E)**. **F,** Infants are also more likely to develop an intense nodular reaction to the mite.

Figure 8-71 **A,** Microscopic appearance of an adult scabies mite obtained by scraping off the black dot at the end of a burrow. Note the small oval egg within the body. **B,** In a second specimen, no mite is seen but multiple eggs and mite feces are evident.

size of an adult mite) or feces (reddish-brown or black pellets, often seen in clusters) is also diagnostic (Fig. 8-71, *B*).

Eradication of scabies necessitates topical application of 5% permethrin (Elimite) cream to the patient, all household members, and close contacts (even if asymptomatic). In addition, thorough cleansing of all dirty clothing, towels, bedding, and car seat covers is essential. Two courses of treatment, 1 week apart, are necessary—the first to kill live mites, and the second to eliminate mites that had not hatched at the time of first application. Symptomatic therapy with oral antipruritic agents and topical steroids may be required long after the mites have been killed (i.e., until the secondary reaction has subsided). Although not yet approved in the United States for scabies, a single dose of oral ivermectin may be effective in recalcitrant cases.

Lice

Three varieties of lice produce clinical disease in humans, and all can involve the scalp hair in children. Crab lice *(Phthirus pubis)* are transmitted primarily by sexual contact. They are short and broad, with claws spaced far apart to grasp the sparse hairs on the trunk, pubic area, and eyelashes (Fig. 8-72, *A*). They are typically found inhabiting the pubic hair and occasionally axillary hair and other body hair in adolescents and adults. Their bites produce bluish, pruritic papules that are distributed over the lower abdomen and upper thighs. Pruritus is intense, and a secondary eczematous rash may develop, particularly in the pubic area, as a result of scratching. Young children lacking pubic and axillary hair may develop scalp or eyelash infestations after close contact with infested adults. Body lice *(Pediculus humanus corporis)* generally live in bedding or clothing, and their eggs may be found in the seams of trousers or underwear. Bites produce urticarial papules, seen primarily over the waist, neck, shoulders, and axillae, which are usually obliterated by excoriations and secondary bacterial infection.

Head lice *(Pediculus humanus capitis)* represent the most common cause of infestation in children. The lice are acquired by close physical contact; by sharing hats, combs, brushes, or scarves with an infested person; or by rubbing against upholstered furniture recently used by such a person. Head lice are long and thin, with claws spaced close together to grasp the more densely distributed scalp hairs (see Fig. 8-72, *B*). Pruritus is the principal symptom, and the resultant scratching produces excoriations of the scalp and nape of the neck that are vulnerable to secondary infection. Occipital adenopathy is common.

Nits are seen as oval, white, 0.5-mm dots glued onto the hair shafts about 1 to 3 cm from the scalp (Fig. 8-73, *A*), particularly above and behind the ears. These are firmly attached to the hair and do not move along the hair shafts, as do the hair casts for which they are frequently mistaken. Although nits may be seen along the entire length of the hair, they are deposited by the lice only near the scalp. Those far from the root indicate a span of perhaps months between infestation and examination. Nits are difficult to remove and may adhere as nonviable shells. Patients adequately treated for lice still have nonviable shells attached to the hair. Removal is assisted by use of a weak vinegar rinse (which is left on under a shower cap or towel for 15 to 20 minutes), followed by combing with a fine-toothed comb. Alternatively, the hair can be cut close to the scalp. This is important because the persistence of dead nits is a common cause of misunderstanding by school health care workers, who insist on re-treating the children or sending them home from school. Active disease is present only if a viable organism or new nits attached close to the scalp are identified.

Diagnosis of pediculosis must be considered in patients with unexplained scalp pruritus. A careful search for the organism may permit a specific diagnosis. Lice are six-legged insects visible to the unaided eye; they are commonly found on the scalp, eyelashes, and pubic areas. They are best identified close to the skin or scalp, where they can be seen moving around and where their eggs are more numerous and more obvious. Diagnosis can be made either by identifying a louse or by plucking hairs and confirming the presence of nits by microscopic examination (Fig. 8-73, *B*).

Figure 8-72 Microscopic appearance of lice. **A,** The crab louse has a short, broad body, with claws spaced far apart. **B,** The head louse has a long, thin body, with claws spaced close together.

Figure 8-73 Head lice. **A,** Nits appear as tiny white dots that adhere to the hair shafts. They are typically found 1 to 3 cm from the scalp above and behind the ears. **B,** Microscopic appearance of the nit of a head louse attached to a scalp hair. Microscopic examination distinguishes nits from hair casts and other artifacts. (**A,** *Courtesy Michael Sherlock, MD, Lutherville, Md.*)

Eradication of lice requires application of a pediculicide to infested hair-bearing areas of all household members and cleaning measures similar to those specified for ridding the house of scabies. Special attention should also be given to hats, scarves, and coat collars. Resistance to available pediculicides has been documented worldwide, and some cases may require multiple treatments or use of new agents. A permethrin 1% to 5% cream rinse is an appropriate first-line treatment, but if cure is not achieved and resistance is suspected, malathion lotion is a highly effective second-line option. However, it is important to instruct patients to avoid smoking near the patient because malathion is flammable. Four percent benzoyl alcohol lotion has been approved and a number of new products are in the pipeline. Lindane, an agent used in the past, is contraindicated for use in infants, children, and the elderly because of the potential for systemic absorption and neurotoxicity.

ACNE

Acne vulgaris, a disorder of the pilosebaceous apparatus, is the most common skin problem of adolescence. Lesions may appear on the face as early as infancy, although they usually begin to develop in the second decade of life during the onset of puberty. Other areas with prominent sebaceous follicles including the upper chest and back may be involved as well.

The exact pathogenesis of acne is unknown. However, abnormalities in follicular keratinization are thought to produce the earliest acne lesion, the microcomedone. In time, microcomedones may grow into clinically apparent open comedones (blackheads) (Fig. 8-74, *A*) and closed comedones (see Fig. 8-74, *B*). The entire process is driven by androgens, which stimulate sebaceous gland differentiation and growth and the production of sebum. The proliferation of *Propionibacterium acnes* in noninflammatory comedones and the rupture of comedone contents into the surrounding dermis may trigger the development of inflammatory papules, pustules, and cysts (Fig. 8-74, *C*). Cystic acne is typified by nodules and cysts scattered over the face, chest, and back (see Fig. 8-74, *D*). This form frequently leads to scarring.

Although therapy must be individualized, patients with mild to moderate comedonal and/or inflammatory acne respond well to a combination of topical retinoic acid, benzoyl peroxide, and antibiotics. Moderate to severe papulopustular acne warrants the use of oral antibiotics in combination with topical agents. Oral 13-*cis*-retinoic acid, or isotretinoin, should be reserved for patients with acne that has been recalcitrant to the previously described regimen or acne that is severe, scarring, or cystic.

TUMORS AND INFILTRATIONS

Persistent lumps and bumps in the skin often raise fears of skin cancer. Fortunately, primary skin cancer is extremely rare in childhood, and most tumors and infiltrated lesions are benign. Hemangiomas and nevi, which can be regarded as tumors, are discussed in subsequent sections of this chapter.

Figure 8-74 A, Comedonal acne with open comedones, or blackheads, seen over the cheek. **B,** Comedonal acne with closed comedones, or whiteheads, on the forehead, accentuated by side lighting. **C,** Papulopustular acne with inflamed papules and pustules over the cheeks, which responded well to antibiotics. **D,** Cystic acne shows deep cysts with marked erythema that can cause severe scarring.

Warts

Warts are benign tumors produced by human papillomavirus (HPV) infection of the skin and mucous membranes. In children they occur most commonly on the fingers, hands, and feet. The incubation period for warts varies from 1 to 6 months, and the majority of lesions disappear spontaneously over a period of 5 years. Local trauma promotes inoculation of the papillomavirus. Thus periungual lesions are common in children who bite their nails or pick at hangnails.

Investigators have identified more than 80 HPVs capable of producing warts, and many of these organisms produce characteristic lesions in specific locations. For instance, the discrete, round, skin-colored papillomatous (roughened) papules typical of *verruca vulgaris* (common warts) are produced by HPV types 2 and 4 (Fig. 8-75). The subtle, minimally hyperpigmented, flat warts *(verruca plana)* caused by HPV type 3 are frequently spread by picking and scratching and thus may become widespread on the face, arms, and legs (Fig. 8-76).

Plantar warts (Fig. 8-77) are associated with HPV type 1. Although not proven, the spread of these warts probably occurs through contact with contaminated, desquamated skin on shower floors, pool decks, and bathroom floors. Being much larger below the skin surface than is apparent from their external appearance, they occasionally cause pain when the patient walks. Although lesions can be confused with corns, calluses, or scars, they can be distinguished by their interruption of the normal skin lines (dermatoglyphics). Characteristic black dots in the warts are thrombosed superficial capillaries.

Warts can also be found on the trunk, oral and nasal mucosae, and conjunctivae. Anogenital lesions *(condylomata acuminata)* are usually associated with HPV types 6 and 11, and the possibility of sexual abuse must be considered in children older than 3 years (with no known exposure to warts) who present with lesions at this site (see Fig. 6-94).

Although warts are self-limited in most children, the presence of persistent and/or widespread lesions suggests the possibility of congenital or acquired immunodeficiency. Warts can become a serious management problem in immunosuppressed oncology and transplant patients, as well as those with HIV/AIDS.

Molluscum Contagiosum

Molluscum, a contagious disease caused by a pox virus, is characterized by sharply circumscribed dome-shaped papules with waxy surfaces. Lesions can occur singly or multiply and can be pruritic. Although usually umbilicated centrally, some have protruding white centers (Fig. 8-78, *A* and *B*). Lesions initially appear as pinpoint papules, and then rapidly enlarge to up to 5 mm. They are found most commonly on the trunk and face, and in the axillae and genital area. Spread occurs as a result of scratching, and thus molluscum lesions are often arranged in a linear configuration (Fig. 8-78, *B*). Frequently,

Figure 8-75 Verruca vulgaris. Dry, rough, and crusty, these common warts usually involve the hands. The periungual distribution in this girl was due in part to her habit of picking at her cuticles.

Figure 8-76 Flat warts, or verruca plana. These tiny, light brown warts are spread by scratching.

Figure 8-77   Plantar warts. Two painful lesions are seen over the ball of the foot. Note how they interrupt the normal skin lines.

Figure 8-79   Milia. These small, whitish-yellow papules are found close to the skin surface and are particularly common around the eyes and midface.

a curdlike core can be expressed from the center; microscopic examination of this material reveals typical molluscum bodies. Because most lesions are asymptomatic and many undergo spontaneous remission within 2 to 3 years, treatment may not be necessary. However, in patients with symptomatic lesions who desire removal or in those with coexisting skin disease such as poorly controlled eczema in whom molluscum can quickly become widespread, curetting after application of topical anesthetic is curative for individual lesions and carries minimal risk of scarring. Painful destructive measures such as freezing with liquid nitrogen, electrocautery, and CO_2 laser are associated with a significant risk of scarring and recurrence and should therefore be avoided in young children. Studies looking at the efficacy of a topical imiquimod cream for the treatment of molluscum showed that the immune response modifier was no more effective than placebo.

Milia

Milia are tiny (1- to 2-mm), whitish-yellow papules that develop spontaneously on the face in neonates (Fig. 8-79). They are firm and, unlike pustules, are not easily denuded by pressure. Milia consist of small epithelial-lined cysts arising from hair follicles. They are persistent, although they may resolve spontaneously after months to years. In newborns, they usually arise without any apparent cause, although in older infants and children they are often seen after skin injury, such as that caused by blistering eruptions or abrasions. They are a characteristic feature of the dystrophic form of epidermolysis bullosa (see Fig. 8-96).

Keloids

Keloids are firm, rubbery nodules or plaques that result from the proliferation of fibroblasts and deposition of collagen after injury to the skin (Fig. 8-80). They can be pruritic or tender, especially during the active growing phase, and they may extend well beyond the margins of the original wound. This latter trait distinguishes keloids from hypertrophic scars, which remain confined to the wound margins and flatten partially within 6 months of the injury. In predisposed individuals, keloids often occur after minimal injury such as abrasions, minor lacerations, acne papules, insect bites, and ear piercing. They are most commonly seen in African Americans and are more likely to develop on the ear lobes, upper trunk, and deltoid areas. Fortunately, they are not seen on the

Figure 8-78   Molluscum contagiosum. **A,** In this case centrally umbilicated dome-shaped lesions are seen. **B,** Lesions have spread on the face of this boy as a result of scratching. Note that some of these lesions have protruding white centers.

Figure 8-80 Keloids. An abnormal reparative reaction to skin injury, keloids are characterized by proliferation of fibroblasts and collagen that extends beyond the margins of the original wound.

midface. Keloids may soften or regress with topical or intralesional steroid injections alone or in combination with surgical excision. However, recurrences are common.

Neurofibromas

Neurofibromas are solitary or multiple growths of neural tissue, presenting as soft, skin-colored or pink dermal and/or subcutaneous nodules (Fig. 8-81). The central portion of an early lesion is particularly soft, and fingertip pressure creates the illusion of pressing in a buttonhole. Neurofibromatosis type 1, or von Recklinghausen disease, is a syndrome characterized by the presence of multiple neurofibromas, café-au-lait spots, axillary and inguinal freckling, Lisch nodules, and various systemic findings. When considering this diagnosis, the clinician must remember that the neurofibromas usually appear after puberty, whereas in prepubertal children, café-au-lait spots are the most important cutaneous marker of von Recklinghausen disease (see Fig. 8-131, *A* and *B*; and see Chapter 15). Solitary neurofibromas without other stigmata of neurofibromatosis occasionally develop in normal individuals.

Figure 8-81 Neurofibromatosis. A soft pink neurofibroma is seen arising within a café-au-lait spot. Usually neurofibromas arise at sites that are normally pigmented.

Mastocytosis

Cutaneous mastocytosis refers to a group of disorders characterized by dermal infiltrations of mast cells.

Mastocytoma

Isolated mastocytomas may be seen in infants. They usually appear as skin-colored or light reddish-brown, slightly indurated plaques, 1 to 2 cm in size (Fig. 8-82, *A*). Development of a wheal-and-flare reaction after firm stroking of the lesion, known as a *positive Darier sign,* confirms the diagnosis (Fig. 8-82, *B*). This is a response to the vascular effects of histamine released from infiltrating mast cells. On occasion, enough histamine may be released from a large mastocytoma to cause localized blistering or systemic symptoms of flushing, wheezing, or diarrhea. Mastocytomas can be located anywhere on the body and usually resolve spontaneously by puberty.

Urticaria Pigmentosa

Urticaria pigmentosa is another form of cutaneous mastocytosis that presents with numerous small, reddish-brown papules or plaques, most commonly on the trunk (Fig. 8-83, *A-C*). These may be present at birth or may appear later in childhood. They are often mistaken for café-au-lait spots but, unlike them, typically react to stroking with a wheal-and-flare reaction (Fig. 8-83, *B* and *C*). Urticaria pigmentosa in children is usually limited to the skin and often resolves by adolescence. However, the bone marrow, gastrointestinal tract, and other organs may be involved. Rare systemic findings in children with urticaria pigmentosa include chronic diarrhea, gastric ulcers, flushing reactions, headaches, and failure to thrive. In infancy there is a tendency for lesions to blister, and widespread erosions may rarely result in dehydration and sepsis. Unlike mastocytosis in adults, pediatric mastocytosis has never been associated with mast cell leukemia.

Patients with isolated mastocytomas and urticaria pigmentosa should be counseled to avoid certain medications and iodinated contrast media, which are known to cause sudden mast cell release of histamine, as these can be life-threatening. Affected children should carry an EpiPen Jr because they can have a severe, even anaphylactic reaction to bee stings.

Juvenile Xanthogranuloma

Infiltration of the skin by other types of cells can also occur. An example is juvenile xanthogranuloma (JXG), in which local infiltration and proliferation of histiocytes form an isolated plaque or nodule or groups of small nodules (Fig. 8-84, *A* and *B*). These asymptomatic red or yellowish-brown lesions grow rapidly in infants and young children but resolve spontaneously later in childhood. They are not associated with abnormalities of circulating lipids. In cases with multiple lesions (Fig. 8-84, *C*) there may be associated ocular involvement. This disorder is the most common cause of nontraumatic hyphema in children. Hence ophthalmologic evaluation is important in patients with multiple or diffuse micronodular xanthogranulomas.

Langerhans Cell Histiocytosis

Langerhans cell histiocytosis (formerly known as *Letterer-Siwe disease, Hand-Schüller-Christian disease,* and *eosinophilic granuloma*) is a potentially more serious disorder of proliferating histiocytes in the skin that may be associated with systemic disease. Lesions may be localized to the skin or may become more widespread with visceral involvement. Marrow failure, pulmonary disease, hepatic infiltration, and gastrointestinal lesions may result in life-threatening complications.

Figure 8-82 Mastocytoma. **A,** This solitary reddish-brown plaque on an infant's buttock contained numerous mast cells on histopathologic examination. **B,** Positive Darier sign. After firm stroking with a tongue blade, a wheal-and-flare reaction appeared with an overlying bulla as a result of histamine release. This is diagnostic for mastocytoma.

Figure 8-83 Urticaria pigmentosa. **A,** Numerous reddish-brown lesions are seen on the scalp and forehead of this toddler. **B,** Marked hyperpigmentation developed in the truncal lesions of this child. Note the wheal-and-flare reaction over the right inferior scapula. **C,** Another infant also has a wheal-and-flare reaction over the left upper abdomen after accidental rubbing.

Figure 8-84 Juvenile xanthogranuloma. **A,** This 1-cm, yellowish nodule located on the back of a 3-month-old infant is the result of infiltration and proliferation of histiocytes. **B,** Numerous satellite papules developed around the primary lesion that appeared abruptly on the chin of this 3-month-old. **C,** Another infant has multiple micronodular juvenile xanthogranulomas, a finding that should prompt ophthalmologic referral to rule out an associated hyphema. (**B,** *From Cohen BA:* Pediatric dermatology, *ed 2, London, 1999, Mosby.*)

Figure 8-85 Langerhans cell histiocytosis. **A,** The exanthem in this 3-week-old infant began in the diaper area and rapidly generalized. Lesions were erythematous and scaly with interspersed petechiae. Associated findings included hepatosplenomegaly, diffuse adenopathy, and diarrhea with poor weight gain. **B,** In this close-up of an older child, raised infiltrative lesions with scaly surfaces, some of which have become petechial, can be seen over the neck and scalp. Chronic draining otitis is another associated finding seen in some cases. *(From Cohen BA:* Pediatric dermatology, *ed 2, London, 1999, Mosby.)*

Cutaneous lesions may be subtle and few in number or diffuse with widespread scaly papules, nodules, or infiltrative plaques (Fig. 8-85, *A* and *B*). These lesions can be distinguished from seborrheic dermatitis, which they can resemble, by the presence of petechiae, bloody crusting, and firmly indurated nodules. Diagnosis is suggested by associated systemic manifestations such as hepatosplenomegaly, lymphadenopathy, and chronically draining ears (see Chapter 11). It is confirmed by skin biopsy, which shows characteristic Langerhans granules within the cytoplasm of infiltrating mononuclear cells.

Granuloma Annulare

When fully evolved, granuloma annulare is an annular eruption histologically characterized by dermal infiltration of lymphocytes around altered collagen. The lesion begins as a nodule or papule that gradually extends peripherally to form a ring. The initial papule and subsequent ring are raised and indurated, and in some cases the ring is broken into segments. The overlying epidermis is usually intact and the same color as the adjacent skin (Fig. 8-86, *A-C*). However, it may be slightly erythematous or even hyperpigmented. Most lesions are asymptomatic, although a few are mildly pruritic. In the latter instance, superficial excoriation caused by scratching may be noted. Lesions are most commonly found on the extensor surfaces of the lower legs, feet, fingers, and hands (often overlying a joint), but other areas may be involved. They resolve spontaneously within a few months to several years, and no treatment is required. Their origin is unclear.

Granuloma annulare is most commonly confused with tinea corporis, or ringworm (see Fig. 8-35). However, the thickened indurated character of the ring and the lack of

Figure 8-86   Granuloma annulare. **A,** Three raised, indurated rings with intact overlying skin and an early papular lesion on the ring finger are seen on a child's hand. **B,** In this infant an incomplete ring of dermal nodules overlies the lateral malleolus. **C,** In an older child this lesion on the dorsum of the foot is less raised.

dermatitic changes such as scales, crusts, vesicles, or pustules enable clinical distinction.

NEONATAL DERMATOLOGY

The skin of a newborn differs from that of an adult in several ways: it is thinner, less hairy, has fewer sweat and sebaceous gland secretions, and has weaker intercellular attachments. During the neonatal period, common rashes or skin abnormalities may develop, and they need to be differentiated from more serious cutaneous disorders. Transient phenomena include erythema toxicum neonatorum and transient neonatal pustular melanosis. More serious diseases to be considered include systemic Langerhans cell histiocytosis and staphylococcal scalded skin syndrome.

Mongolian Spots (Dermal Melanocytosis)

Mongolian spots are flat, slate-gray to bluish-black, poorly circumscribed macules. They are located most commonly over the lumbosacral area and buttocks (Fig. 8-87), although they can appear anywhere on the body. The spots range in size from 1 to 10 cm and may be single or multiple (see Fig. 6-65). Ninety percent of African-American infants, up to 80% of Asian infants and those of other darkly pigmented ethnic groups, and about 10% of white newborns have these macules, which contain accumulations of melanocytes deep within the dermis. No risk of malignancy is known, and Mongolian spots usually fade without therapy by age 7 years. Special variants of Mongolian spots, including nevus of Ota (involving the face, particularly the periocular area) and nevus of Ito (involving the shoulder), may persist indefinitely. Rarely, when

present along with vascular malformations, they can be part of a syndrome called phakomatosis pigmentovascularis, which can have associated internal abnormalities.

Erythema Toxicum Neonatorum

Erythema toxicum neonatorum is a benign, self-limited, asymptomatic disorder of unknown etiology. It occurs in up to 50% of full-term infants and has no racial or sexual predisposition. Lesions usually begin 24 to 48 hours after birth but may appear up to the tenth day of life. The disorder has been described as "flea-bite" dermatosis of the newborn, owing to the intense erythema with a central papule or pustule that

Figure 8-87   Mongolian spot. A typical slate-gray lesion is located over the lumbosacral area of this African-American infant.

Figure 8-88   Erythema toxicum neonatorum. Numerous yellow papules and pustules are surrounded by large, intensely erythematous rings on the trunk of this infant.

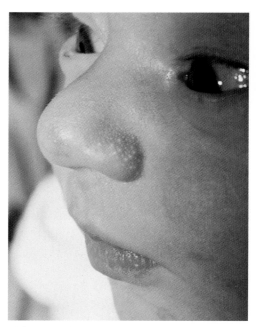

Figure 8-90   Sebaceous gland hyperplasia. Note the yellowish-white papules on the nose of this infant.

resembles a flea bite (Fig. 8-88). The central papule or pustule is typically 2 to 3 mm in diameter and is surrounded by a much larger area of erythema. There may be a few to several hundred lesions on the back, face, chest, and extremities. The palms and soles are usually spared. A smear of material from a central pustule reveals numerous eosinophils, and concomitant circulating eosinophilia is present in up to 20% of patients. The eruption fades spontaneously within 5 to 7 days. No treatment is necessary.

Differential diagnosis includes transient neonatal pustular melanosis, staphylococcal folliculitis, milia neonatorum, miliaria rubra, and herpes simplex (see also Chapter 12). Infections often can be excluded clinically or with a Gram stain, Tzanck smear, and cultures, when necessary.

Transient Neonatal Pustular Melanosis

Transient neonatal pustular melanosis (TNPM) is a self-limited dermatosis of unknown etiology that presents at birth with 1- to 2-mm vesiculopustules or ruptured pustules that disappear in 24 to 48 hours, leaving pigmented macules with a collarette of scale (Fig. 8-89, *A* and *B*). Lesions may appear anywhere on the body but are most often seen on the neck, forehead, lower back, and legs. Wright stain of a pustular smear shows numerous neutrophils; Gram stain and culture are negative for bacteria. The hyperpigmentation fades in 3 weeks to 3 months. TNPM is a benign disorder and requires no therapy. Differential diagnosis is similar to that of erythema toxicum neonatorum.

Sebaceous Gland Hyperplasia and Neonatal Cephalic Pustulosis (Formerly Neonatal Acne)

Neonatal sebaceous gland hyperplasia is a common entity consisting of multiple 1- to 2-cm yellowish-white papules usually located over the nose and cheeks of full-term infants (Fig. 8-90) and represents a normal physiologic response to maternal androgenic stimulation of sebaceous gland growth. Lesions resolve spontaneously by 4 to 6 months.

Neonates can also develop findings that resemble acne within the first few weeks of life. On close examination, however, instead of true comedones, lesions are seen to consist

Figure 8-89   Transient neonatal pustular melanosis. **A,** A myriad of tiny pustules dot the forehead and scalp of this neonate. **B,** When the pustules rupture, a pigmented macule surrounded by a collarette of scale remains.

Figure 8-91   Cephalic pustulosis (formerly neonatal acne). Erythematous papules and pustules are present over the nose and cheeks.

Figure 8-93   Collodion baby. **A** and **B,** A shiny transparent membrane covered this baby at birth; she later developed lamellar ichthyosis. Note the ectropion and eclabium (eversion and fissuring of the eyelid margins and lips). *(From Cohen BA: Pediatric dermatology, ed 2, London, 1999, Mosby.)*

of papules and papulopustules over the face, neck, and trunk (Fig. 8-91). It, too, is thought to be a result of hormonal stimulation of sebaceous glands, which creates a hospitable environment for overgrowth of yeast (*Malassezia* sp.). Formerly called neonatal acne, it is now termed *neonatal cephalic pustulosis*. The condition is benign and self-limited and is best treated by observation or with topical antifungal agents.

Cutis Marmorata

Cutis marmorata is characterized by a transient, netlike, reddish-blue mottling of the skin caused by variable vascular constriction and dilation (Fig. 8-92). It is a normal response to chilling, and on rewarming, normal skin color returns. The discoloration occurs symmetrically over the trunk and extremities in infants. In neonates the condition usually abates by 6 months, but it may persist longer in fair-skinned individuals. When cutis marmorata is fixed, asymmetrical, and does not fade with warming, the clinician should consider the diagnosis, cutis marmorata telangiectatica congenita, which is a type of a vascular malformation present at birth that can be accompanied by atrophy and other systemic findings when it is extensive.

Collodion Baby

In several variants of ichthyosis, particularly lamellar ichthyosis, the infant is born encased in a thick, parchment-like scale known as a *collodion membrane* (Fig. 8-93). This dries and is shed in large sheets within 7 to 14 days. Significant secondary fluid, electrolyte, and heat losses can occur. Although scaling may resolve completely in some infants, most go on to develop cutaneous findings typical of the underlying ichthyosis (see Figs. 8-8 and 8-9).

Epidermolysis Bullosa

Epidermolysis bullosa (EB) is a group of inherited mechanobullous disorders characterized by the development of blisters after the skin is subjected to mild friction or trauma. The three general types are EB simplex, junctional EB, and dystrophic EB. These types are classified according to the level at which blister formation occurs. Modes of inheritance vary with subtypes in each group, and blistering, with few exceptions, occurs in the newborn period.

Epidermolysis Bullosa Simplex (Epidermolytic Epidermolysis Bullosa)

In EB simplex, which is usually transmitted as an autosomal dominant trait, blister formation takes place superficially within or just above the basal cell layer of the epidermis. On

Figure 8-92   Cutis marmorata. Note the reticulated bluish-purple mottling of the skin of this infant's thigh.

Figure 8-94   Epidermolysis bullosa (EB) simplex (formerly epidermolytic EB). Blisters form easily in pressure-bearing areas, particularly the hands and feet. Scarring does not occur.

presentation, blistering can be mild or severe and widespread (Fig. 8-94). The most common form presents in later infancy, childhood, or adolescence with blisters confined to pressure-bearing areas, especially on the hands and feet, and particularly after intense physical activity. Although there is no scarring, secondary infection can occur, and atrophy may develop in some cases.

Junctional Epidermolysis Bullosa

Junctional EB, inherited as an autosomal recessive trait, usually presents at birth with bullae and erosions in a generalized distribution. Blisters form at the junction of the epidermis and dermis (Fig. 8-95). The most severe form is usually fatal during the first year of life, due to malnutrition, fluid losses, recurrent cutaneous infection, and sepsis. A milder variant resembles generalized epidermolytic EB. An uncommon subtype of this form of EB is associated with pyloric atresia and has a high mortality in the neonatal period.

Dystrophic Epidermolysis Bullosa

The dystrophic forms of EB are divided into dominant and recessive types. The plane of cleavage is deep within the upper portion of the dermis. In both, scarring occurs as the blisters heal and milia are common (Fig. 8-96, A). The dominant form usually results in more localized lesions (e.g., feet only) than the recessive form; patients with the latter show retardation

in growth and development, severe oral blisters, loss of nails, and sometimes syndactyly as the skin of the digits fuses during healing from the deeper blisters (Fig. 8-96, B).

Skin biopsies, especially for observation by electron microscopy, are helpful in distinguishing among the three general types of EB in neonates, and they are also helpful in determining prognosis. A more rapid and less costly screening study known as immunofluorescence antigenic mapping of a skin biopsy specimen can identify the location of the split in the skin. Sequencing of the suspected genes cannot be done for many of the EB variants. Although treatment has generally been symptomatic and supportive, more definitive options such as bone marrow transplantation and gene repair therapies are being evaluated. Prenatal diagnosis is now possible for many variants, and genetic counseling is advisable.

Incontinentia Pigmenti

Incontinentia pigmenti (IP) is an X-linked dominant disorder that affects the skin and may also involve the CNS, eyes, teeth, and skeletal system. It is seen predominantly in females and thus is thought to be fatal to males in utero. The exception is a male with an XXY genotype. Clinically, the disorder may present in any of four overlapping phases, and distribution along the lines of Blaschko is typical of disorders demonstrating X-linked genetic mosaicism. In the first phase, inflammatory vesicles or bullae appear on the trunk and extremities, usually within the first 2 weeks of life (Fig. 8-97, A). New blisters then develop over the ensuing 3 months. At this stage a skin biopsy shows characteristic inflammation with intraepidermal eosinophils and necrotic keratinocytes. Before the blistering phase ends, the second phase, marked by development of irregular, warty papules, supervenes (Fig. 8-97, B and C). These lesions resolve spontaneously within several months. A characteristic swirling or streaking pattern (referred to as a blaschkoid distribution) of brown to bluish-gray pigmentation on the trunk or extremities marks the third phase (Fig. 8-97, D and E). Interestingly, these pigmented whorls are sometimes located at sites other than those involved in the first two phases. The blaschkoid pigmentation, which also likely represents a form of pigmentary mosaicism (see Disorders of Pigmentation, later), fades in later infancy or early childhood in most patients, leaving subtle, streaky, hypopigmented scars that may be the only residual cutaneous findings seen in affected mothers (Fig. 8-97, F), who should be carefully examined for other markers of IP. Gene markers should also be sent for affected mothers and babies.

Figure 8-95   Junctional epidermolysis bullosa. Widespread involvement was seen in this infant at birth. **A,** Note the erosions and the large, intact blister over the thumb and dorsum of the hand. **B,** Large, denuded areas are evident over the back and flank.

Figure 8-96 Dystrophic (formerly dermolytic) epidermolysis bullosa (EB). **A,** Blisters, erosions, and hundreds of milia are seen on the foot and ankle of this newborn. **B,** In another child with the recessive form of dystrophic EB, severe scarring encased the fingers, resulting in syndactyly.

Figure 8-97 Incontinentia pigmenti. **A,** Linearly distributed vesicles on an erythematous base are seen on the legs of this neonate. **B** and **C,** Subsequently, lesions evolve into warty papules, which can have thick overlying crusts. **D,** Splotchy hyperpigmented patches replaced the warty lesions by 8 months of age. **E,** In many cases the hyperpigmentation appears in swirls and streaks. **F,** These hypopigmented reticulated lesions on the leg of an affected child's mother represent old scars in areas of prior hyperpigmentation. (**A** and **C,** From Cohen BA: Pediatric dermatology, ed 2, London, 1999, Mosby.)

A number of other systemic manifestations affecting various body systems are seen in patients with IP. The literature shows that up to 30% have CNS abnormalities such as seizures, mental retardation, and spasticity. However, this probably represents an exaggeration of the true incidence of CNS abnormalities, as there may be a selection bias toward describing these patients once they have presented to a neurologist. Ophthalmic complications including strabismus, cataracts, blindness, and microphthalmia are seen in 35%. Pegged teeth and delayed dentition are seen in 65%. Cardiac and skeletal malformations have also been reported.

Differential diagnosis of IP in the blistering stage includes herpes simplex, bullous impetigo, and EB. Warts or epidermal nevi may mimic the warty phase. The swirled pigmentation of the third phase is characteristic of IP but must be distinguished from congenital blaschkoid hyperpigmentation, which is not associated with an inflammatory phase. Although no specific therapy is usually required, early intervention for eye lesions may help to preserve vision, and systemic therapy for neonatal seizures may be lifesaving. Genetic counseling is critical.

HEMANGIOMAS AND VASCULAR MALFORMATIONS

Hemangiomas are benign vascular tumors or neoplasms that are dynamic, having the capacity for rapid growth as a result of endothelial cell proliferation. There are several subtypes including infantile hemangiomas, rapidly involuting congenital hemangiomas (RICH lesions), noninvoluting congenital hemangiomas (NICH lesions), kaposiform hemangioendotheliomas, tufted angiomas, and pyogenic granulomas. In contrast, vascular malformations (discussed later) are stable lesions that are present at birth and grow with the child.

Infantile Hemangiomas

Infantile hemangiomas constitute the most common vascular tumors of infancy and are seen in approximately 10% of infants by 1 year of age. They are seen more commonly in white infants, females, premature infants, and babies born to mothers with placental abnormalities. This latter phenomenon, combined with the fact that infantile hemangiomas and the placenta express similar tissue markers (such as the glucose transporter GLUT-1), has raised the question of whether hemangiomas may have their origin in embolized placental tissue.

Although not usually present at birth, infantile hemangiomas tend to appear within several days to weeks of delivery. The initial manifestation may be slight reddening or bluish discoloration of the overlying skin. Thereafter, in the majority of cases, rapid vascular overgrowth occurs, resulting in formation of a bright red nodule or plaque with definite elevation above the surrounding skin surface (Fig. 8-98). These lesions can then grow for up to 15 months, although most peak in size by 3 to 6 months. Thereafter, they stabilize or plateau and then gradually involute at a rate of approximately 10% a year. Hence their chances of resolution are as follows: 30% by 3 years, 50% by 5, and 70% by age 7. The onset of involution is signaled by a "graying out" of the surface (Fig. 8-99). The natural history of involution of a lesion is shown in Figure 8-100.

Although hemangiomas do involute, and families can be reassured that they will ultimately regress considerably, it is important to inform them that residual skin changes are likely. This is because in 40% of cases the skin overlying a resolved lesion shows mild redundancy with telangiectasias, and some

Figure 8-98 Superficial or strawberry hemangiomas. Multiple soft, red, raised lesions dot the back and arms of this otherwise healthy 1-month-old with benign hemangiomatosis. Note that a number of the lesions exceed 2 cm in diameter and are plaquelike.

lesions leave behind a cosmetically noticeable residue of fibrofatty tissue (Fig. 8-101).

Clinically, hemangiomas have been described or categorized as superficial, deep, or mixed lesions, depending on the level of greatest bulk (epidermal, dermal, or subcutaneous). Superficial lesions, sometimes referred to in layman's terms as "strawberry hemangiomas," form bright red rounded tumors and/or plaques that are well demarcated and clearly elevated above the surrounding skin surface. They are soft, compressible, and usually range in size from a few millimeters to 5 cm, although some can be much larger. In deep hemangiomas, the bulk of which is located deeper in the dermis or in subcutaneous fat, the overlying skin tends to have a subtle bluish hue. Further, their borders are indistinct, and they have a doughy consistency on palpation (Fig. 8-102). When placed in a dependent position, deep hemangiomas enlarge as they fill with an increased amount of blood—a finding that helps differentiate them from lymphangiomas. Most hemangiomas, however, are mixed, having both superficial and deeper components (Fig. 8-103). More than half of all hemangiomas are found on the head and neck, about 25% on the trunk, and the rest on the extremities.

Although most infants have only a single lesion, a small proportion have multiple hemangiomas, ranging from a few, to several, to 100 or more. Those with numerous lesions (in the 100s) are said to have hemangiomatosis. When these are

Figure 8-99 Involuting hemangioma. The onset of involution is signaled by a "graying out" of the surface of the lesion.

Figure 8-100 Natural history of a hemangioma. After growing for approximately 6 months, hemangiomas tend to plateau in size and then gradually involute. Note the appearance at 5 months **(A)**, at 2 years **(B)**, and almost total resolution at 5 years **(C)**.

limited to the skin, the condition is termed *benign* (see Fig. 8-98). In some, however, cutaneous lesions are associated with internal or visceral lesions. This appears most commonly in infants with numerous small (<2 cm), widely dispersed cutaneous hemangiomas (Fig. 8-104). Internal lesions can involve the liver, gastrointestinal tract, CNS, and lungs, as well as other organs. Large hepatic hemangiomas often have arteriovenous shunts that precipitate high-output congestive heart failure and affected infants tend to present between 6 and 12 weeks of age with tachypnea, dyspnea, and sweating with feedings and hepatomegaly. Gastrointestinal (GI) lesions are often manifest by gastrointestinal bleeding and CNS neoplasms by mass effects. Thus, in young infants presenting with a large number of small, widely dispersed hemangiomas, a

screening hepatic ultrasound examination and close observation for GI and CNS signs and symptoms may be advisable. It must be noted, however, that on occasion a patient with only a few or even no cutaneous hemangiomas may present with signs of an internal lesion as well (see later).

In addition to the increased risk of visceral involvement in infants with hemangiomatosis, certain sites and patterns of cutaneous hemangiomas may serve as signals for underlying lesions. Most hemangiomas are focal round or oval lesions of variable size. When there are multiple round or oval lesions they are described as multifocal. Last, when hemangiomas are large and follow certain embryologic segmental patterns, they are referred to as *segmental hemangiomas*. The presence of segmental hemangiomas over the lower face (lower lip, chin, preauricular area, and neck) in the "beard" distribution has a significant association with airway involvement (Fig. 8-105), and midline lumbosacral hemangiomas may be markers of underlying spinal dysraphism (see Chapter 15). Along these lines, an important syndrome initially described by Frieden and colleagues is *PHACES syndrome*. PHACES is an acronym for posterior fossa malformations, hemangiomas (usually a plaque-like segmental hemangioma of the face), arterial anomalies (including abnormal carotid arteries), cardiac defects, eye anomalies, and sternal clefting. The segmental

Figure 8-101 After involution of some large hemangiomas, the patient is left with a fibrofatty residue at the site.

Figure 8-102 Deep hemangioma. Most of the vessels that make up this large, partially compressible lesion lie deep beneath the skin surface but still impart a bluish hue to the overlying skin. Note the indistinctness of the margins.

Figure 8-103 Mixed hemangioma. The hemangioma on this child's nasal bridge has both superficial and deep components.

Figure 8-105 Hemangiomas involving the "beard" distribution of the lower face signal the possibility of underlying airway hemangiomas.

hemangioma associated with PHACES syndrome may be present at birth and may initially mimic a port-wine stain. However, unlike port-wine stains, they are often ulcerated at the time of presentation and begin to proliferate rapidly, becoming raised and plaque-like (Fig. 8-106).

In the past it was believed that large hemangiomas, whether cutaneous or visceral, could sequester platelets, resulting in coagulopathy, a phenomenon termed *Kasabach-Merritt syndrome*, characterized by sudden enlargement of a vascular tumor accompanied by thrombocytopenia. It is now clear, however, that this potentially life-threatening condition occurs exclusively with one of two rare vascular tumors: the kaposiform hemangioendothelioma and the tufted angioma (Fig. 8-107), two distinct pathologic entities that express more lymphatic markers than hemangiomas. Both of these lesions appear more purpuric than infantile hemangiomas and need to be treated in conjunction with an oncologist because their behavior can be aggressive.

There are certain complications seen in infants with cutaneous hemangiomas that are site specific and require close monitoring because they can be associated with significant morbidity if left untreated. Periorbital and lid lesions can cause significant narrowing of the palpebral aperture, thereby occluding the visual axis. They can also compress the cornea. This constitutes an ophthalmologic emergency because, without prompt and aggressive therapy, permanent visual axis deprivation, amblyopia, strabismus, and astigmatism can result. As noted earlier, it is important to recognize that infants with hemangiomas distributed over the lower face may have similar lesions of the airway. With growth, these can cause narrowing, resulting in stridor and respiratory distress within the first few months, at times necessitating tracheotomy.

Figure 8-104 Hemangiomatosis. This infant presented with signs of congestive heart failure due to arteriovenous shunting within a large hepatic hemangioma. Note the large number of lesions and that all are less than 2 cm in diameter, rounded, and widely dispersed.

Hemangiomas involving the lips, nose, or ears have a high potential for permanent disfigurement.

Steroids, interferon, or surgical intervention may be indicated for lesions involving the airway or the eye.

Lesions located in areas that are prone to friction and/or maceration, such as the diaper area, intertriginous folds, and perioral region, are especially at risk of developing painful ulcerations (Fig. 8-108). This can result in bleeding, secondary infection, and ultimately scarring. Hence close attention should be paid to skin care to prevent breakdown. If ulceration does occur, treatment with wet compresses and antibacterial ointment often suffices, with pulsed-dye laser therapy serving as an effective second-line treatment.

Considering that the majority of infantile hemangiomas cause no discomfort and, with the exceptions described earlier, pose no undue risk, and given their natural history of involution, conservative management (e.g., watchful waiting) is generally the best approach. When function, form, or cosmesis becomes threatened by either the current or impending growth of an infantile hemangioma, there are several medical treatment options; none of these, the authors note, are approved by the U.S. Food and Drug Administration (FDA) for the treatment of hemangiomas, but each is supported by solid clinical and empiric data. Traditionally, high-dose oral steroids were often administered as a first-morning dose until the hemangioma responded with a slowing or halting of its rapid growth phase. At that point the oral steroid dose was then tapered gradually and eventually discontinued when the infant's hypothalamic–pituitary–adrenal (HPA) axis demonstrated the ability to produce a normal first-morning cortisol response. This taper could take months, during which time the child's immunizations might need to be delayed because of possible lack of response. Other negative sequelae included an increased risk of infection, hypertension, gastroesophageal reflux, irritability, and the development of a cushingoid appearance while receiving the high-dose steroids. The use of intralesional steroids for select amenable locations such as the lip could sometimes circumvent these systemic side effects. If an aggressive infantile hemangioma did not respond to systemic steroids, then interferon was a second- or third-line option, but because it carried with it a possibility for spastic diplegia, a potentially devastating side effect, it has fallen out of favor. For hemangiomas that developed recalcitrant or painful surface ulcerations, pulsed-dye laser therapy was and still remains a viable option to aid in healing the superficial defect, but it must be stressed that this type of laser penetrates only about 1 mm into the skin, and thus does not typically cause involution of the entire lesion; it only causes coagulation and healing of the most superficial vessels.

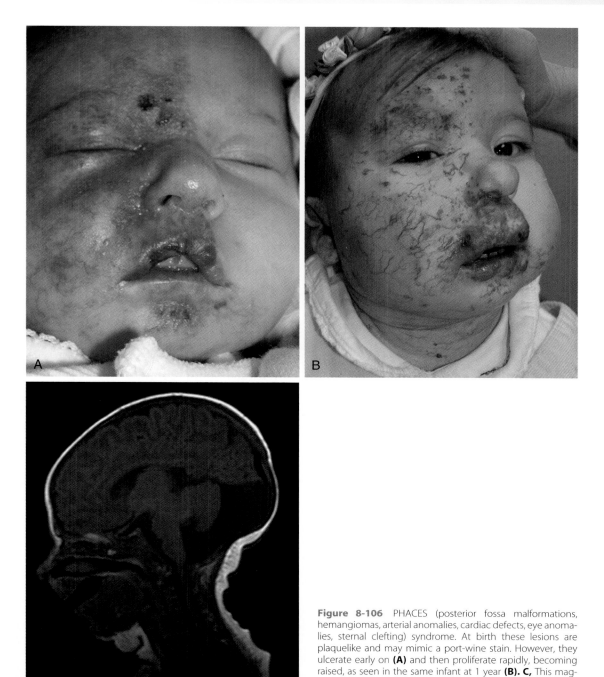

Figure 8-106 PHACES (posterior fossa malformations, hemangiomas, arterial anomalies, cardiac defects, eye anomalies, sternal clefting) syndrome. At birth these lesions are plaquelike and may mimic a port-wine stain. However, they ulcerate early on **(A)** and then proliferate rapidly, becoming raised, as seen in the same infant at 1 year **(B). C,** This magnetic resonance imaging (MRI) scan reveals a Dandy-Walker malformation in an infant with PHACES syndrome.

Figure 8-107 Tufted angioma. This lesion involving the right leg first appeared as a bruiselike plaque, which continued to grow well beyond infancy.

Figure 8-108 Ulcerated hemangioma. Hemangiomas located in friction- or maceration-prone areas are at risk for ulceration. When ulcerated, they cause significant pain and are vulnerable to infection and, ultimately, scarring, unless treated aggressively.

More recently, a new use for an age-old cardiac medication, propranolol, has begun to change the face of hemangioma therapy. Although caution must be emphasized, the authors have used oral propranolol safely and effectively in more than 150 infants with hemangiomas of infancy. Unlike oral steroids, which at best can slow or halt the growth of an infantile hemangioma, oral propranolol has proven to have the ability to both halt the growth as well as often trigger active involution of the lesion. Caution is of paramount importance, however, as propranolol can cause hypotension, hypoglycemia, and bradycardia, which are rare after the neonatal period Although there have been rare reports of unresponsiveness or lethargy as a result of hypoglycemia, there are no reports of deaths in children treated with propranolol over the last 40 years. Whereas some groups start propranolol on an outpatient basis, the authors have each chosen to initiate propranolol in a controlled inpatient hospital setting, where vital signs and glucose can be monitored closely, before discharging the infant several days later on a dose that was well tolerated in-hospital. The topical version of propranolol, which has been used for years as an ophthalmic preparation, may after further study prove useful to topically treat thin or early infantile hemangiomas.

More recently, two other types of hemangiomas, distinguished by their presence at the time of birth and therefore termed *congenital*, have been described. The noninvoluting congenital hemangioma (NICH) may grow slightly after birth but then does not regress like most hemangiomas. It has a telangiectatic surface with a rim of pallor (Fig. 8-109). The rapidly involuting congenital hemangioma (RICH) also peaks in size at the time of birth, but this subtype recedes briskly, often before 1 year of life, leaving behind a characteristic atrophied plaque (Fig. 8-110). Both NICH and RICH lesions demonstrate tissue markers different from those of infantile

Figure 8-109   Noninvoluting congenital hemangioma (NICH) lesion. These lesions are present at birth and have a telangiectatic surface surrounded by a rim of pallor. *(Courtesy http://www.dermatlas.org.)*

hemangiomas and seem to have higher vascular flow, which may explain their differing clinical courses.

Pyogenic Granuloma

Pyogenic granulomas are common benign vascular tumors that resemble small hemangiomas. They are thought to stem from vascular overgrowth of granulation tissue following minor trauma, or in reaction to a foreign body such as a thorn, splinter, or piece of glass. They are seen in children and young adults, and lesions are usually located on the face or an extremity, although on occasion, the trunk and mucous membranes may be involved. They consist of solitary bright red,

Figure 8-110   Rapidly involuting congenital hemangioma (RICH) lesion. Also present at birth, these lesions grow no larger but instead involute rapidly and have often resolved by 1 year of age. **A,** This infant has a large RICH lesion on his back, which is in the process of involuting. After involution these lesions leave behind an atrophic plaque. **B,** In this child evidence of mild residual atrophy is seen. **C,** Another child was left with marked subcutaneous atrophy at the site. *(**A,** Courtesy http://www.dermatlas.org.)*

Figure 8-111 Pyogenic granuloma. **A,** A bright red, raised, hemorrhagic papule developed on an infant's cheek. **B,** Another rapidly growing friable lesion is present between this child's fingers.

soft nodules that are often pedunculated and average 5 to 6 mm in diameter. Their surface is friable and bleeds easily (Fig. 8-111, *A* and *B*). Pyogenic granulomas are commonly confused with hemangiomas, but their onset well after the newborn period and their morphology, distribution, and course allow for distinction between these two types of benign vascular tumors. Treatment consists of shave excision followed by electrodesiccation of the "feeder" blood vessels at the base. They occasionally recur, in which case repeat surgery is recommended. It is important when the clinician surgically removes what he or she feels to be a pyogenic granuloma, particularly lesions greater than 5 mm in diameter, to have that tissue examined by a pathologist, such as a dermatopathologist, who is well versed in skin lesions, as Spitz nevus and (extremely rarely) amelanotic melanoma can present as a pyogenic granuloma-like lesion and can occur in children.

Vascular Malformations

Vascular malformations are not neoplasms, but rather develop as a result of errors in morphogenesis of capillaries, veins, arteries, or lymphatic vessels (or any combination thereof). Capillary and lymphatic lesions are present at birth and, in contrast to hemangiomas, which grow rapidly and then involute, vascular malformations are stable lesions that grow only in proportion to the child, and do not recede over time. Although they do not proliferate like hemangiomas of infancy and other neoplasms of infancy, they may become more prominent with increasing age. Arterial, venous, and arteriovenous malformations are usually present at birth but may become apparent in later childhood or adolescence. Capillary and venous malformations are macular and easily compressible. In this section we focus mainly on capillary and capillary/venous malformations because they are the most common vascular malformations seen in infancy. They include *salmon patches,* present in more than 70% of newborns, and *port-wine stains*.

Nevus Simplex (Salmon Patch or "Stork Bite")

The nevus simplex, which is commonly referred to as a *salmon patch* or *"stork bite,"* is a capillary malformation that is seen in the majority of infants and hence is considered a normal variant. Some experts believe that these may represent persistent fetal vessels as opposed to a true malformation, which may partly explain why they tend to fade slightly over time. Lesions are located at the nape of the neck and on the glabella, forehead, upper eyelids, and/or lower back (Fig. 8-112). They become more apparent clinically when the baby cries or

strains and tend to fade or become less noticeable over the first year of life.

Persistent Capillary Vascular Malformation (Port-wine Stain)

Port-wine birthmarks represent a persistent capillary vascular malformation and are usually recognized as purple-red macules in the newborn. Mature capillaries may infiltrate the superficial and/or deeper dermis and subcutaneous tissues. Unlike infantile hemangiomas, these neither enlarge nor involute over time. Left untreated, however, underlying skin and soft tissue can become hypertrophied and most develop angiomatous blebs by adolescence or adulthood. Most commonly they are located on the head and neck (Fig. 8-113) and, when present in the distribution of the ophthalmic branch of the trigeminal nerve (even more so when present bilaterally), can be associated with *Sturge-Weber syndrome,* a constellation of port-wine stain, vascular malformations of the ipsilateral leptomeninges and cerebral cortex, and glaucoma. Seizures and mental retardation are possible complications (see Chapter 15 and Figs. 15-19 through 15-22). An important differential diagnostic consideration is PHACES syndrome, in which the initial lesion may resemble a facial port-wine stain before entering its phase of rapid growth (see Fig. 8-106).

A port-wine stain located over the midline occipital scalp, especially when accompanied by a hair tuft or whorl, may overlie a CNS malformation such as an atretic encephalocele (see Fig. 15-34), just as a midline lumbosacral port-wine stain may be associated with an underlying spinal dysraphism, such as a tethered cord or lipoma (see Chapter 15). Extensive port-wine stains located on the trunk or extremities may be

Figure 8-112 Stork bite, or salmon patch. A typical light red splotchy area is seen at the nape of the neck.

Figure 8-113 Port-wine stain. This infant has a characteristic purplish-red lesion covering nearly half of his face.

Figure 8-115 Giant nevomelanocytic nevus. This lesion covers the lower back and buttocks, is uniformly pigmented, and has smaller satellite nevi.

associated with soft tissue and bony overgrowth and deeper venous anomalies such as in *Klippel-Trénaunay syndrome* and *Trénaunay-Weber syndrome* (see Fig. 15-23).

NEVI

Nevomelanocytic nevus is a term used to describe a group of congenital and acquired pigmented lesions, located in the dermis, which contain nevus cells derived from the neural crest. These cells, like melanocytes in the epidermis, have the ability to synthesize melanin. The term *nevus* also refers to a group of congenital skin lesions composed of mature or nearly mature cutaneous elements organized in an abnormal fashion. Also known as *hamartomas,* the latter may be composed of almost any epidermal or dermal structures.

Nevomelanocytic Nevi

Congenital Melanocytic Nevi

Congenital forms of nevomelanocytic nevi (CMN) consist of pigmented plaques often associated with dense hair growth. At birth, lesions may be tan or light pink, with only soft vellus hairs (Fig. 8-114, *A*). During infancy and childhood, the nevus darkens, the hair becomes more prominent, and small dark

macules or nodules may appear in a pebbly array within the larger plaque (Fig. 8-114, *B*). CMN are classified by size, specifically their greatest diameter: small being less than 1.5 cm; medium, 1.5 to 20 cm; and large, greater than 20 cm. A large CMN present in a segmental distribution is termed a *giant CMN* (Fig. 8-115).

All CMN have the potential for malignant transformation, which may be heralded by the development of new, darker, and/or bleeding nodules within the original lesion or by sudden rapid growth of the nevus. The likelihood of malignant transformation is less than 1% for small- to medium-sized CMN and perhaps 2% to 5% for giant lesions. Some evidence suggests that the greatest risk of malignancy for giant CMN may occur during the first decade of life.

Although no uniformly accepted guidelines exist for the management of small- to medium-size nevi, a reasonable

Figure 8-114 Congenital nevomelanocytic nevi. **A,** Two small nevi with differing degrees of hyperpigmentation are seen on the thigh of an infant. **B,** During adolescence this nevus developed prominent hair and dark pigmented macules and papules within its borders.

approach is to have a yearly follow-up with a dermatologist or primary care provider who is comfortable monitoring patients with pigmented lesions. Excision is recommended if a nevus begins to appear atypical and may be considered if any are located in areas that are difficult to monitor such as the scalp, groin, or interdigital spaces. Because of their higher risk, early full-thickness excision (in infancy, if possible), followed by grafting, may be considered for patients with giant CMN. However, some exceptionally large nevi may not be amenable to surgical management. In these cases impeccably close observation (facilitated by comparative photographs) is recommended, at 6- to 12-month intervals. Careful palpation of the entire lesion is necessary at each visit, as melanomas may arise deep within a large CMN and often are first detectable as a new, palpable nodule, well before any surface change occurs. Laser treatment for small, medium, or large/giant CMN has not gained wide acceptance, as the currently available lasers ablate only the superficial components of nevi, leaving behind the deeper nevus cells that could undergo malignant change. CMN must be differentiated from other congenital pigmented spots such as urticaria pigmentosa, lentigines, café-au-lait spots, and Mongolian spots, none of which carry any significant risk of malignancy. The *nevus spilus,* which consists of a light brown macule with darker brown freckling throughout, is considered a variant of congenital nevus superimposed on a café-au-lait macule with an extremely low (but not zero) risk of progression to melanoma (Fig. 8-116).

Acquired Nevomelanocytic Nevi

Acquired nevomelanocytic nevi begin to develop in early childhood as small, pigmented macules 1 to 2 mm in diameter, which are flat on palpation. At this stage the nevus cells are limited to the epidermal–dermal junction and are called *junctional nevi* (Fig. 8-117, *A*). They then enlarge slowly and become papular or even pedunculated. In such elevated nevi, the nevus cells have proliferated into the dermis to become either intradermal or *compound nevi* (Fig. 8-117, *B*). During puberty, these lesions may darken noticeably and increase in size. However, normal nevomelanocytic nevi rarely exceed 1 cm in diameter. They tend to be located on sun-exposed areas and are seen less frequently on the soles, palms, legs, genitalia, and mucous membranes. In general, these nevi change slowly over months to years and warrant only observation.

Sudden enlargement of a nevus with redness and tenderness may occur because of infection of a hair follicle within

Figure 8-116 Nevus spilus. These lesions consist of light brown macules, with darker brown speckles scattered uniformly over their surfaces.

the nevus or because of rupture of a follicular cyst with a secondary foreign body reaction. This may alarm the patient, prompting dermatologic evaluation. Another, slower change causing concern in patients is the appearance of a hypopigmented or depigmented ring associated with mild local pruritus around a benign nevus. This is called a *halo nevus* (Fig. 8-118), and the phenomenon is caused by a cytotoxic T-lymphocyte reaction against both the nevus cells and their innocent melanocytic bystanders. As a result, the nevus tends to disappear partially or completely, and the halo eventually repigments.

Nevi and Melanomas

Melanomas in childhood may occur de novo or develop within a giant congenital nevus. Unfortunately, increased exposure to sunlight and artificial ultraviolet light (e.g., tanning salons), particularly in adolescent girls, has contributed to a marked increase in melanoma arising in acquired nevi in children since the late 1990s, with an annual increase of 3% to 7%. Another cause of melanoma in the pediatric age group is transplacental transfer of maternal melanoma. Thus neonates

Figure 8-117 Acquired nevomelanocytic nevi. **A,** Junctional nevi. These brown macules are flat on palpation. **B,** This typical compound nevus is raised, with a regular border and uniform pigmentation.

Figure 8-118   Halo nevi. Large hypopigmented halos surround three relatively small nevi on the back of this boy.

Figure 8-120   Blue nevus. This blue nodule was made up of deep nevus cells; it was firm on palpation.

born to mothers with a history of melanoma should be examined and monitored carefully. Conversely, mothers of infants born with melanoma should be examined thoroughly for signs of the malignancy, and all first-degree relatives should be checked yearly for signs of melanoma.

As long as the clinical appearance of a nevus is typical, excision is unnecessary. However, a number of changes in pigmented lesions may portend the development of melanoma (Fig. 8-119). These include the following:

1. A change in size, shape, or outline, with scalloped, irregular borders

2. A change in the surface characteristics such as development of a small, dark, elevated papule or nodule within an otherwise flat plaque; or flaking, scaling, ulceration, or bleeding

3. A change in color to a different shade of black or brown or to a mixture of red, white, or blue

4. Development of burning, itching, or tenderness, which may be an indication of the body's immune reaction to malignancy

Fortunately, melanomas are still rare in children. However, their incidence is increasing (at about 3% annually), and curative treatment is contingent on early diagnosis and prompt excision. Hence it is important for clinicians to have a keen awareness of diagnostic features and of worrisome changes in benign nevi that should prompt referral for possible excision. Excised specimens should be analyzed by a pathologist specialized in dermatologic pathology and in melanomas, because many of the changes of dysplasia are subtle; experience is required to recognize the grade.

The differential diagnosis of childhood melanoma includes congenital and acquired nevocytic nevi; the *blue nevus*, a small, firm, blue papule consisting of deep nevus cells (Fig. 8-120); traumatic hemorrhage, especially under the nails or in mucous membranes; vascular lesions such as pyogenic granuloma or angiokeratoma; and the *Spitz nevus*, a red and rapidly growing nevus composed of spindle and epithelial cells that can be confused clinically and histologically with melanoma (Fig. 8-121).

Hamartomatous Nevi

Hamartomatous nevi are derived from embryonic ectoderm and can be composed of epidermal structures, hair follicles *(nevus pilosus)*, apocrine and eccrine glands *(apocrine and eccrine nevi)*, fibroblasts *(connective tissue nevi)*, blood vessels (salmon patch [see Fig. 8-112]), and multiple components *(nevus sebaceus)*.

Epidermal nevi are quite common in pediatric patients. They are composed of epidermal structures only and must be distinguished from nevus sebaceus (see later). The lesion may be present at birth or may develop during childhood and appears as a slightly hyperpigmented papillomatous or verrucous growth (Fig. 8-122, *A-C*). Development of and increases in verrucous changes are particularly common at puberty. Lesions may be small and localized, linear, dermatomal, or generalized. The number of differing clinical presentations is

Figure 8-119   Melanoma. This lesion shows the irregularity of outline, color, and thickness typical of a melanoma.

Figure 8-121   Spitz nevus. This raised red nevus grows rapidly.

Figure 8-122   Epidermal nevi. **A-C,** These raised lesions vary in color depending on the child's skin tone, ranging from lightly pigmented to markedly hyperpigmented. Note the characteristic whorled array of verrucous papules, best seen in **B.** All three of these children had localized lesions and were otherwise healthy. More extensive nevi may be associated with systemic abnormalities (epidermal nevus syndrome [see Chapter 15]).

reflected in the variety of descriptive synonyms: *nevus verrucosus* for localized disease, *nevus unius lateris* for linear or unilateral involvement, and *ichthyosis hystrix* for bilateral involvement with irregular geometric patterns. Important associations with extensive epidermal nevi are seizures, mental retardation, and ocular and skeletal defects (see Chapter 15 and Fig. 15-26). Extensive lesions have also been associated with hypophosphatemic vitamin D–resistant rickets.

Nevus sebaceus of Jadassohn is characterized by a hairless, well-circumscribed, skin-colored or yellowish waxy plaque located most commonly on the scalp, face, or neck (Fig. 8-123; and see Fig. 15-25). The lesion is usually solitary and may be linear or round. It is present at birth, although at puberty the plaque may become more verrucous, raised, and nodular (see Fig. 15-25). Histologically, epidermal proliferation is seen along with abortive hair follicles, sebaceous glands, and apocrine structures. Although it has been taught in the past that 10% to 15% of these nevi develop into secondary malignant neoplasms, more recent studies suggest that this is extremely rare in children and uncommon even in adults. Many neoplasms arising from nevus sebaceus lesions, previously thought to be basal cell carcinomas, were actually benign follicular

Figure 8-123   Nevus sebaceus of Jadassohn. **A,** This yellowish, hairless plaque was present on the temporal scalp at birth. **B,** In an adolescent boy the lesion has developed secondary warty growths, stimulated by pubertal androgens. (**A,** *Courtesy http://www.dermatlas.org.*)

Figure 8-124   Postinflammatory hyperpigmentation **(A)** arose in a child with chronic atopic dermatitis, which provoked persistent scratching. **B,** This patient with discoid lupus provides another example of the phenomenon.

growths known as trichoblastomas. As a consequence, routine excision of nevus sebaceus in childhood is not medically necessary and can be deferred to adolescence or adulthood.

DISORDERS OF PIGMENTATION

Childhood disorders of pigmentation are usually of cosmetic importance only, although some pigmented lesions are markers of multisystem disease.

Postinflammatory Pigmentary Changes

Postinflammatory hyperpigmentation (Fig. 8-124, *A* and *B*) and hypopigmentation (Fig. 8-125) are the most common forms of disordered pigmentation. The phenomenon develops following inflammatory disorders of the skin such as dermatitis, acne, infection, or injury and usually resolves spontaneously over a few months. Histologically, melanocytes appear normal, but the dispersion of pigment to other cells is disturbed. Postinflammatory hypopigmentation also must be distinguished from vitiligo (see Fig. 8-127), in which there is usually a complete absence of pigment without associated scaling or history of inflammation. Tinea versicolor may present with hypopigmented patches in sun-exposed areas (or hyperpigmented lesions in clothing-covered sites), which are covered with a fine scale. KOH examination confirms the correct diagnosis by demonstrating typical "spaghetti and meatballs" organisms (see Figs. 8-39 and 8-40).

Figure 8-125   Postinflammatory hypopigmentation is evident in this infant after treatment with topical agents for seborrheic diaper dermatitis.

Pigmentary Mosaicism

The term *pigmentary mosaicism* refers to a group of conditions in which affected children have genetic mosaicism (i.e., they are born with at least two genetically different cell lines, resulting in the existence of keratinocytes of two different pigment tones). When these different populations of skin cells migrate during development, they create a whorled, fountain-like pattern of alternating hypo- and hyperpigmentation (Fig. 8-126, *A-C*). This pattern is referred to as a blaschkoid distribution because it occurs along the "lines of Blaschko," which are lines of embryologic ectodermal development. They may be evident at birth and, if not, appear in infancy or early childhood. The bands are macular and are found most commonly over the trunk and respect the midline, but they can also be seen on the extremities, where they tend to be more linear. In contrast to the hyperpigmented macules of incontinentia pigmenti, those of pure pigmentary mosaicism have no antecedent vesicular or verrucous lesions and are not associated with atrophy.

Pigmentary mosaicism can stem from a postzygotic mutation or an error in cell division early on in the course of embryogenesis, or may be the result of random X chromosome inactivation in X-linked conditions. The phenomenon has been reported in association with a number of different types of chromosomal mosaicism including trisomies 13, 18, and 20, among others. Affected individuals may have associated abnormalities of the CNS, the musculoskeletal system, and/or the eye. Although the risk of associated anomalies has probably been overestimated because of reporting bias, children with more extensive cutaneous lesions are probably at greater risk for extracutaneous involvement and should receive careful medical examination and targeted studies.

Vitiligo

In vitiligo, an acquired condition, there is partial to complete loss of pigmentation. Lesions consist of well-demarcated hypopigmented and depigmented macules and patches that are usually seen in a characteristic distribution around the eyes, mouth, genitals, elbows, hands, and feet (Fig. 8-127), although they may appear elsewhere, as in a koebnerized distribution in areas of prior friction or trauma. They enhance dramatically under a Wood's lamp. Spontaneous but slow repigmentation may occur from the edges of a lesion and around hair follicles (which retain melanocytes), resulting in a speckled appearance. Histologically, melanocytes are absent

Figure 8-126   Pigmentary mosaicism. **A** and **B,** Swirling bands of alternating lighter and darker hues are seen on this adolescent's trunk, demonstrating a widespread blaschkoid distribution. Note that they vary in width and stop at the midline, and that the streaks on the upper arm are more linear and parallel to its long axis. The patient also had a seizure disorder and significant cognitive deficits. **C,** More extensive involvement is seen over the back of another child. (**C,** *Courtesy http://www.dermatlas.org.*)

in areas of vitiligo, and evidence suggests that they have been destroyed by an autoimmune mechanism. In a small proportion of patients with vitiligo, other autoimmune conditions, such as thyroiditis, diabetes, or pernicious anemia, can be detected concomitantly.

Ash-leaf Spots

Congenital, well-demarcated, hypopigmented macules, termed *ash-leaf spots* because of their usual lanceolate shape, are often a valuable early marker of tuberous sclerosis. They appear at birth or shortly thereafter as 1- to 3-cm macular lesions on the trunk. Because they are hypopigmented, rather

than totally depigmented, they are not as easily appreciated or as bright white as the lesions of vitiligo, and their usual truncal distribution is different (see Chapter 15, Fig. 15-13).

The identification of ash-leaf macules may be enhanced (although not as dramatically as is seen in vitiligo) by the use of a Wood's lamp, and this method of examination should be part of the assessment of any child, particularly one with a fair complexion, who develops idiopathic seizures in infancy. The visible purple light emitted is absorbed by normal melanin in the skin. Thus in a darkened room, areas of hypopigmentation or depigmentation appear brighter violet, whereas normally melanized skin reflects little visible light and appears dull purple or black. In addition to tuberous sclerosis, Wood's

Figure 8-127   Vitiligo. Completely depigmented patches are seen on the legs. On occasion, macules of repigmentation arise from epidermal appendages within the white patches. A characteristic distribution helps to distinguish vitiligo from other causes of hypopigmentation.

lamp examination may also be helpful in delineating the full extent of pigmentary changes in vitiligo and in postinflammatory hypopigmentation.

It is important to recognize that up to 0.5% of otherwise normal newborns will have an isolated hypopigmented macule, which, in the absence of other signs of tuberous sclerosis, is termed a *nevus depigmentosus* and represents a localized form of pigmentary mosaicism (Fig. 8-128). Nevus depigmentosus is somewhat of a misnomer, as the lesions are not truly depigmented; they are hypopigmented.

Albinism

The term *albinism* refers to a heterogeneous group of inherited disorders characterized by congenital hypopigmentation of the skin, eyes, and hair. It occurs in an X-linked ocular form (in which the skin appears clinically normal) and an autosomal recessive oculocutaneous form. In oculocutaneous albinism (OCA), both sexes and all races are affected equally. This form of the disorder is subdivided into a number of variants on the

basis of clinical findings and biochemical markers. In the past, tyrosinase-negative and tyrosinase-positive subtypes were identified on the basis of the ability of plucked hairs to produce pigment when incubated in tyrosine. Now, DNA markers allow for identification of specific mutations. In classic tyrosinase-negative OCA, children are born without any trace of pigment. Affected individuals have snow-white hair, pinkish-white skin, and translucent or blue irises. Nystagmus is common, as is moderate to severe strabismus and poor visual acuity (see Chapter 19). Although children with tyrosinase-positive OCA may be clinically indistinguishable from their tyrosinase-negative counterparts at birth, they usually develop variable amounts of pigment with increasing age. Eye color may vary from gray to light brown, and hair may change to blond or light brown. Most African-American patients acquire as much pigment as light-skinned white individuals.

Because they lack the protection of melanin, patients with OCA are at high risk for early development of basal cell and squamous cell skin cancers. Hence they should be instructed in the use of sunscreens and avoidance of excessive sun exposure.

Piebaldism

Piebaldism (partial albinism) is an autosomal dominant disorder characterized by a white forelock and a circumscribed congenital leukoderma. The typical lesions include a triangular patch of depigmentation and white hair on the frontal scalp. The apex of this patch points toward the nasal bridge (Fig. 8-129, *A*). Patients may also have hypopigmented or depigmented macules on the face, neck, ventral trunk, flanks, or extremities (Fig. 8-129, *B*). Within areas of decreased pigmentation, scattered patches of normal pigmentation or hyperpigmentation may appear. The lesions are stable throughout life, although some variability in pigmentation may occur with sun exposure. Special variants of piebaldism include Waardenburg syndrome, in which leukoderma is associated with lateral displacement of the inner canthi and inferior lacrimal ducts, a flattened nasal bridge, and sensorineural deafness; and Wolf-Hirschhorn syndrome, an autosomal recessive disorder associated with neurologic deficits.

Acanthosis Nigricans

Acanthosis nigricans is characterized by hyperpigmentation and hyperkeratosis in intertriginous areas and over bony prominences. Skin lines are accentuated, and the skin surface of involved areas may have a velvety, leathery, or warty appearance (Fig. 8-130, *A-C*). Four main forms of the disorder exist. The benign/idiopathic form is the most common and is obesity related. Onset is usually at puberty but can occur in childhood in concert with development of obesity. Interestingly, the prominence of lesions tends to lessen when the patients lose weight. An inherited form, transmitted as an autosomal dominant trait, usually presents in infancy or early childhood but becomes more prominent during adolescence. This form is also unassociated with other underlying disorders. In endocrine-associated acanthosis nigricans, the condition may antedate or appear in association with insulin resistance with or without polycystic ovary disease. More rarely, it is seen in patients with pituitary tumors. Malignancy-related acanthosis nigricans is extremely rare in childhood.

Other Pigmentary Disorders

Café-au-lait spots are tan macules that usually occur in otherwise healthy individuals but that can be an indication of neurofibromatosis type 1 (von Recklinghausen disease; see

Figure 8-128   Nevus depigmentosus is a localized form of pigmentary mosaicism, seen here on the nape of the neck of an otherwise healthy child.

Figure 8-129   Piebaldism. **A,** A white forelock overlies a depigmented patch of scalp and forehead. **B,** The infant also has a hypopigmented patch on his arm in which smaller areas of hyperpigmentation are seen.

Chapter 15) or McCune-Albright syndrome. In the latter, they are associated with polyostotic fibrous dysplasia of the long bones and endocrinopathy (see Chapter 9). Café-au-lait macules that are small and have smooth borders are more likely to be associated with neurofibromatosis type 1 (Fig. 8-131, *A-C*), whereas those that are large and segmental with jagged borders are more likely to be seen in association with McCune-Albright syndrome (Fig. 8-131, *D*). Children who have café-au-lait spots in the absence of a syndrome usually have fewer than four lesions that are relatively small in size.

Swirled hyperpigmentation may be a marker of the later stages of incontinentia pigmenti (see Fig. 8-97, *D* and *E*) or of pigmentary mosaicism (see Fig. 8-126). Diffuse hyperpigmentation may be seen in Addison disease and in hemochromatosis. Peutz-Jeghers syndrome is manifest by lentigo-like pigmentation of the lips (see Fig. 17-66), oral mucosa, hands, and fingers in association with benign small intestinal polyps in children (see Chapter 10 and Fig. 17-67).

DISORDERS OF THE HAIR AND NAILS

Diseases that involve the hair and nails make up an integral part of pediatric dermatology. Hair and nails are composed of keratin produced by epidermal hair follicles and the nail matrix, respectively. Some diseases are specific to these structures, whereas others affect the skin as well. In many cases, important diagnostic clues to skin diseases and systemic disorders can be found in related abnormalities of the hair and nails.

The Alopecias

The most common diseases of the hair result in some degree of hair loss, or alopecia. Evaluation begins by determining whether scarring is present. Nonscarring alopecia can be due to growth defects causing the hair to be lost at the roots (effluvium) or by defects of the hair shaft that result in breakage.

Figure 8-130   Acanthosis nigricans. **A** and **B,** Hyperpigmentation and leathery thickening of the skin are seen on the neck and in the axilla of an obese adolescent with the benign/idiopathic form of the disorder. **C,** She also had velvety hyperpigmentation and prominence of skin lines over the knuckles of her hands and other bony prominences. *(From Cohen BA: Pediatric dermatology, ed 2, London, 1999, Mosby.)*

Figure 8-131   Café-au-lait macules. **A** and **B,** Small café-au-lait spots are seen in two infants with neurofibromatosis type 1 (NF1), one fairly pigmented and one with darker pigmentation to demonstrate the differences in color of lesions with differing skin tones. Note that the lesions have smooth borders, which are typical of this disorder. The infant in **B** also has pseudarthrosis of the tibia and fibula, with foreshortening of the left lower leg (see Chapter 15). **C,** This older boy has both café-au-lait spots and axillary freckling (Crowe sign). The presence of six or more café-au-lait macules and axillary freckling is diagnostic for NF1. **D,** Another infant with McCune-Albright syndrome has a large café-au-lait macule located in a segmental distribution over his back. Note the jagged margins of the lesion. The child also had precocious puberty. (**C,** *Courtesy http://www.dermatlas.org.*)

Alopecia Caused by Systemic Insult: Telogen and Anagen Effluvium

Normal hair cycles through a growth phase lasting 3 years or more (anagen phase) and a resting phase of 3 months (telogen phase), after which the hair is shed, and the cycle then begins again. Telogen effluvium is one form of partial, temporary alopecia, which may occur 3 months after an emotional or physical stress such as a severe illness, major surgery, or high fever. It rarely causes more than 50% hair loss. In these patients the initial systemic insult induces more than the usual 20% of hairs to enter the telogen phase, and 3 months later these hairs are shed simultaneously, producing marked thinning of scalp hair until new anagen hairs regrow (Fig. 8-132). Anagen effluvium is the sudden loss of growing hairs (80% of normal scalp hairs) caused by abnormal interruption of the anagen phase. In these cases the hair shafts taper and lose

Figure 8-132   Telogen effluvium. This toddler experienced sudden partial hair loss approximately 3 months after being hospitalized for pneumococcal sepsis. *(Courtesy Alejandro Hoberman, MD, Children's Hospital of Pittsburgh.)*

adhesion to the follicle. This type of hair loss is most common after systemic chemotherapy.

Alopecia Areata

Alopecia areata is a form of localized anagen effluvium usually presenting with round or oval patches of alopecia that may be located anywhere on the scalp, eyebrows, lashes, or body.

On occasion, hair loss is diffuse or generalized. The injury causing cessation of growth is thought to be of immunologic origin. Clues to diagnosis include absence of inflammation and scaling in the involved areas of scalp and the presence of short (3 to 6 mm), easily epilated hairs at the margins of the patch (Fig. 8-133, *A* and *B*). Under magnification these hair stubs resemble exclamation points because the hair shaft narrows just before its point of entry into the follicle. Another finding in many patients with alopecia areata is Scotch-plaid pitting of the nails, consisting of rows of pits crossing in a transverse and longitudinal fashion (see Fig. 8-147). The clinical course of alopecia areata is difficult to predict. The disorder may resolve spontaneously; it may persist, with the appearance of new patches while the old patches regrow; or it may progress to total scalp *(alopecia totalis)* or even generalized whole-body alopecia *(alopecia universalis)*, either of which can be permanent (Fig. 8-133, *C*). In severe cases it is helpful to perform a thorough search to exclude coexistent autoimmune disease such as autoimmune thyroiditis because systemically treating the comorbid condition can improve the response of alopecia to topical treatment.

Trichorrhexis Nodosa

Alopecia caused by hair shaft breakage is due to a structural defect of the hair, and it is easily diagnosed by microscopic examination. The most common structural defect is acquired trichorrhexis nodosa. This defect presents at any age as brittle, short hairs that are perceived by the patient as nongrowing. On gentle pulling, many hairs are easily broken. Microscopically, the distal ends of the hairs are frayed, resembling a broom (Fig. 8-134). Other hairs may have nodules, resembling two brooms stuck together. The fragility is the result of damage to the outer cortex of the hair shaft, resulting in a loss of structural support. Without this support, the weaker fibrous medulla frays like an electrical cord with broken insulation. This disorder is most common in African Americans, often

Figure 8-133   Alopecia areata. **A,** Patches of complete hair loss with otherwise normal scalp are typical of this disorder. **B,** In this close-up, small broken hairs that pull out easily are seen at the margins. **C,** In this boy the process has progressed to alopecia totalis. Note that even his eyebrows are involved. *(C, Courtesy Michael Sherlock, MD, Lutherville, Md.)*

Figure 8-134   Trichorrhexis nodosa consists of a brittle hair shaft defect usually caused by overmanipulation of the hair or application of harsh chemicals. The frayed brown appearance is typical.

Figure 8-136   Traction alopecia. The hair thinning and loss are due to excessive traction on the hairs as a result of tight braiding.

arising from the trauma of combing tightly curled hairs. It is also seen after repeated or severe chemical damage to the cortex from hair straighteners, bleaches, and permanents. Because hair growth is normal, the disorder is self-limited and normal hairs regrow when the source of the damage is identified and eliminated.

Other common causes of hair loss associated with shaft abnormalities include friction alopecia, traction alopecia, and trichotillomania. All are caused by external trauma and breakage of an otherwise normal hair shaft.

Friction Alopecia

Friction alopecia (Fig. 8-135) is common on the posterior scalp of infants, where the head rubs on the pillow or bed clothes. Although worrisome to parents, this disorder is self-limited. It has become considerably more common since implementation of the Back to Sleep campaign to prevent sudden infant death syndrome (SIDS). It can be prevented or its severity reduced by ensuring that an infant spends plenty of time on his or her tummy when awake and able to be supervised. When unusually severe or long-standing, friction alopecia should raise the question of neglect, suggesting that the infant is being left to lie in his or her crib for extended periods of time.

Traction Alopecia

Traction alopecia (Fig. 8-136) is common in young girls whose hairstyles, such as ponytails, pigtails, braids, or cornrows, maintain a tight pull on the hair shafts. This traction causes shaft fractures and follicular damage. If prolonged, permanent scarring alopecia can result. On rare occasions, excess traction applied in the process of braiding can result in subgaleal bleeding and hematoma formation. This phenomenon can also be seen in child abuse victims who have been subjected to forceful hair pulling (see Fig. 6-4).

Trichotillomania

Trichotillomania is a fairly common disorder seen in older children and adolescents that mimics many other types of alopecia. It should be distinguished from self-limited hair pulling in preschoolers. This form of localized nonscarring hair loss presents with bizarre patterns, often in broad, linear bands on the vertex or sides of the scalp where the hair is easily twisted and pulled out (Fig. 8-137). Trichotillomania is seen more commonly on the side opposite the child's dominant hand as the other hand is free to manipulate the hair while the child is engaged in other tasks. Rarely, the entire scalp, eyebrows, and eyelashes are involved. The most important clue to the correct diagnosis is the finding of short, broken-off hairs along the scalp, with stubs of different lengths in adjacent areas. This is the result of repetitive pulling and/or twisting of the hair, which fractures the longer shafts. Once broken, the hairs are too short to be rebroken until they grow longer. The scalp appears otherwise normal.

Trichotillomania is sometimes confused with alopecia areata because there are patches of hair loss with short hairs, and there may be involvement of the eyebrows and eyelashes. However, in trichotillomania, patches of hair loss are never completely bald, and the hair shafts are normal anagen hairs that are usually difficult to remove from the scalp. In addition, there are no associated nail abnormalities.

Parents and children usually vigorously deny that the alopecia could be caused by the child, and thus diagnosis rests on a high index of suspicion and recognition of the clinical findings. Although trichotillomania may occur in children with severe psychiatric disease, most cases are associated with situational stress (e.g., school phobia, marital or social problems). Trichotillomania should be distinguished from *habitual*

Figure 8-135   Friction alopecia. Hair loss over the occiput resulted from rubbing of the head on sheets and pillows while lying supine.

Figure 8-137 Trichitillosis, or trichotillomania. **A,** This linear patch of short broken hairs along the midline is typical of hair pulling. **B,** Another child has a unilateral geometric patch of hair loss, again with short broken hairs. Note that the scalp is normal in both cases.

hair pulling, twisting, or twirling seen in preschool children. This typically occurs at bedtime and naptime. Most of these young children shed the habit by the early school years.

Scarring Alopecia

Scarring alopecia in children is considerably less common than nonscarring alopecia and may be caused by a number of disorders, both congenital and acquired. Morphea (localized scleroderma) and lupus may involve the scalp with indurated, hairless plaques. Scarring alopecia may also result from severe infection (e.g., inflammatory tinea capitis) or trauma such as oil burns from hot-comb straightening of the hair. A scalp biopsy is often helpful in determining the cause of scarring alopecia.

Aplasia Cutis Congenita

Aplasia cutis congenita is a congenital condition characterized by absence of or failure of formation of a localized area of scalp or skin. In most cases there is a single lesion located over the vertex of the scalp. More rarely, lesions may be multiple or may involve the trunk or extremities. They may be associated with limb defects and other congenital and genetic anomalies. In the majority only the dermis and epidermis are absent; however, some lesions extend to involve subcutaneous tissue, and, in rare cases, a calvarial defect may underlie a scalp lesion.

At birth, the lesion may consist of a sharply circumscribed open and weeping ulceration, or it may be covered by a thin, often hemorrhagic membrane or crust (Fig. 8-138, *A*; and see Fig. 1-27, *E*). Evaluation should include radiologic studies to assess the depth of the lesion and a search for associated anomalies. When a hair collar sign is present surrounding the lesion (see Fig. 8-138, *D*), one should rule out an underlying neural tube defect with a magnetic resonance imaging (MRI) scan. Conservative treatment designed to protect the area from infection and injury includes application of saline compresses, topical antibiotics, and sterile dressings. Depending on the size of the lesion, healing takes place over several weeks to months, leaving a smooth atrophic and hairless scar (Fig. 8-138, *B* and *C*). The disorder is easily distinguished from ulcerations due to perinatal monitor electrode insertion or blood sampling, by virtue of history. The differential diagnosis includes congenital nevus sebaceus lesions, which are raised and have an uneven, yellow, waxy surface (see Fig. 8-123),

and epidermal nevi, which are typically hyperpigmented and have a raised warty surface.

Tinea Capitis (Fungal Infections of the Hair and Scalp)

Fungal infection of the hair weakens the shaft, causing breakage. This typically results in the development of multiple patches of partial alopecia, commonly referred to as *ringworm*. *Trichophyton tonsurans* is the organism responsible for more than 95% of cases in the United States, and for unknown reasons, infection with this strain is endemic among African-American school children, although there is some evidence of spread by inadequately disinfected barber tools. *Microsporum canis* (the dog and cat ringworm) accounts for a small percentage of cases.

Clinical presentations of tinea capitis vary. In some patients mild erythema and scaling of the scalp occur in association with partial alopecia (Fig. 8-139, *A*). In other cases there is widespread breakage at the scalp, creating a "salt-and-pepper" appearance, with the short residual hairs appearing as black dots on the surface of the scalp (Fig. 8-139, *B*). On occasion, scalp lesions are annular, simulating tinea corporis. In yet other children, sensitization to the infecting organism results in more erythema, edema, and pustule formation. As the latter rupture, the area weeps and golden crusts form, simulating impetigo (Fig. 8-139, *C*). Some cases are characterized by patches of heaped-up scale in association with small pustules (Fig. 8-139, *D*). Less commonly, intense inflammation causes formation of raised, tender, boggy plaques or masses studded with pustules that simulate abscesses, termed *kerions* (Fig. 8-139, *E*). Unless treated promptly and aggressively with oral antifungal agents and, in cases characterized by severe inflammation, steroids, the latter may produce scarring and permanent hair loss. Incision and drainage of kerions is not indicated because loculations are small and septae thick. Importantly, when pustules or weeping and crusting lesions involve the scalp or hair line, the infection is far more likely to be of fungal than bacterial origin. Patients with tinea capitis often have associated occipital, postauricular, and posterior cervical adenopathy (see Fig. 12-46).

Fungal infection of the scalp is readily confirmed by a KOH examination of infected hairs (Fig. 8-140). Residual broken hairs or black dots at the surface of the scalp should be scraped for KOH preparation and/or fungal culture. In the past, when

Figure 8-138   Aplasia cutis congenita. **A,** This 2-day-old has a sharply circumscribed, punched-out ulceration over the vertex with a hemorrhagic crust. **B,** After 3 weeks of topical mupirocin therapy, the lesion has nearly healed. **C,** The typical atrophic hairless scar of a healed lesion is seen. **D,** Healed aplasia cutis congenita with the "hair collar" sign.

Microsporum audouinii was the most common causative organism and was easily identified by its fluorescence, the Wood's lamp was a useful adjunct in diagnosis. Today, however, *T. tonsurans,* the most common causative organism in the United States, does not fluoresce. Only *M. canis,* which causes 5% of cases, fluoresces bright bluish-green, still justifying its use.

Because topical antifungal agents do not penetrate deeply enough to be effective in the treatment of tinea capitis, oral antifungal agents are necessary and must be administered for at least 6 weeks to 4 months to eradicate the infection. Unfortunately, risk of recurrence is high. In the past, griseofulvin and ketoconazole were the only oral agents approved in the United States for the treatment of tinea capitis; more recently, terbinafine granules (6 weeks of therapy) have gained FDA approval for its treatment. Studies show that itraconazole and fluconazole are also effective and require shorter (6-week) courses of therapy. However, reports of severe adverse side effects of ketoconazole have sharply curtailed its use, and studies of this agent have also raised concerns about its efficacy. Concurrent use of selenium sulfide shampoo (2.5%) during a course of oral therapy reduces spore formation and shedding and thus may help minimize the risk of spread to family members, playmates, and classmates until oral treatment is complete. Other measures useful in reducing passage of organisms to others include no communal use of brushes, combs, or hair grease jars; no sharing of hats, coats, scarves, towels, or linens; and careful washing or cleaning of combs and brushes and of potentially contaminated linen, clothing, and upholstery.

Congenital and Genetic Disorders

Some structural defects of the hair shaft are congenital in origin or associated with heritable syndromes.

Monilethrix and Pili Torti

Monilethrix is a developmental hair defect that produces brittle, beaded hair. The condition is autosomal dominant, and clinical manifestations usually appear in infants 2 to 3 months after birth, when fetal or neonatal vellus hairs are replaced by abnormal beaded hairs (Fig. 8-141, *A*). The scalp is most severely affected, although hair on any part of the body can be involved. The disease is permanent, although the clinical appearance of the hair may improve as the child grows older. Microscopically, regular, periodic narrowing of the hair shafts is seen (Fig. 8-141, *B*). Breakage occurs in constricted areas close to the scalp. Care must be taken not to confuse monilethrix with *pili torti,* another structural defect in which the hair shaft is twisted on its own axis. Pili torti may be localized or generalized and also appears with the first terminal hair growth of infancy. It may be associated with Menkes kinky hair syndrome (Fig. 8-142), an inherited defect of copper absorption, which also affects the central nervous, cardiovascular, and skeletal systems.

Figure 8-139   Tinea capitis can present in many guises. **A,** In this child, mild erythema and scaling of the scalp are associated with spotty alopecia. **B,** Infiltration of hair shafts by an endothrix fungus has resulted in widespread breakage at the scalp, producing a "salt-and-pepper" appearance. **C,** Superficial papules and pustules have ruptured, producing weeping and crusting lesions simulating impetigo. **D,** This variant of tinea is characterized by thick, heaped-up scale. **E,** Kerion. A boggy mass has formed as a result of an intense inflammatory response. This child, seen relatively late in the course, had nearly total alopecia over the involved area. Note that the lesion is studded with pustules.

Disorders Affecting the Nails

Patients may seek the advice of a physician for nail disorders because of pain or cosmetic concerns. For the physician, knowledge of nail disorders can also be helpful in detecting clues to systemic disease.

Figure 8-140   Microscopic appearance of hair shafts infected with fungi. Note the tight packing of fungal arthrospores that cause hair shaft fragility and breakage (KOH mount for endothrix).

Paronychia

Paronychia is a common childhood disorder. It presents as a red, swollen, tender nail fold, usually on the side or at the base of the nail. The acute form, with sudden swelling and marked tenderness, is caused by bacterial invasion by staphylococci or streptococci after trauma to the cuticle (often from chewing), or it can develop in a child with a dermatitis that has damaged the stratum corneum barrier (see Fig. 12-32). Chronic paronychia may involve one or several nails. An associated history of chronic dermatitis or frequent exposure to water usually is present. In contrast to the acute form, tenderness is mild, although sometimes a small amount of pus can be extruded. Some degree of associated nail dystrophy often exists (Fig. 8-143). The causative organisms are *Candida* species, usually *C. albicans*. This form resolves with the use of topical antimycotics and avoidance of water.

Onychomycosis and Nail Dystrophy

Onychomycosis, or fungal infection of the nail plate (Fig. 8-144), is not as common in children before puberty as it is in adults. Thus nail dystrophy should not be treated as a fungal infection unless proven by microscopic examination or fungal culture. Dystrophic nails are seen frequently as a complication of trauma (Fig. 8-145) or of an underlying dermatosis such as psoriasis, atopic dermatitis, or lichen planus.

Figure 8-141   Monilethrix. **A,** Short, broken hairs give the appearance of diffuse alopecia. **B,** Microscopically, periodic narrowing of this hair shaft is evident. Hairs are brittle and break off at constricted points near the scalp.

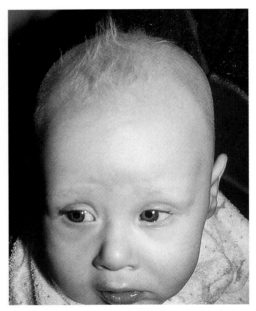

Figure 8-142   Menkes kinky hair syndrome with generalized pili torti. This infant demonstrates the characteristic features of the disorder: fair skin; blue eyes; and the fair, sparse brittle hair of diffuse pili torti. He experienced developmental regression and had a seizure disorder. *(From Cohen BA: Pediatric dermatology, ed 2, London, 1999, Mosby.)*

Figure 8-143   Chronic paronychia with nail dystrophy caused by candidal infection.

Figure 8-145   Traumatic nail dystrophy. This teenager developed median nail dystrophy as a result of chronically picking at his nails.

Figure 8-144   Onychomycosis caused by a chronic dermatophyte infection of the nail plate in a 4-year-old boy. This is relatively rare in prepubertal children.

Figure 8-146 Traumatic subungual hemorrhage. Discoloration because of traumatic hemorrhage under the toenail is common in children and athletic adults. When seen at the base of a toenail, it is commonly a result of jamming the toe into the end of the shoe while running or stopping (turf toe).

Trauma

Acute trauma to the nail bed may cause subungual hemorrhage, resulting in a brownish-black discoloration. This is particularly likely following crush injuries. Usually the diagnosis is simple, unless trauma is subtle. When a large, painful hematoma is produced, this should be evacuated by electrocautery to relieve pain and reduce risk of infection. Bluish-black pigmentation at the base of the great toenail, caused by jamming the toe into the end of the shoe at a sudden stop, is called *turf toe* and results in mild subungual hemorrhage (Fig. 8-146). This must be distinguished from melanoma. Concern for melanoma should heighten if pigmentation of the cuticle or proximal nail fold accompanies hyperpigmentation of the nail; this is called *Hutchinson sign*. When present, this should prompt immediate referral for a biopsy of the nail matrix to exclude melanoma. Hemorrhage, on the other hand, can be identified by the presence of purplish-brown pigment in the distal nail and normal proximal outgrowth of the nail. Chronic repetitive trauma due to the habit of picking at one nail with another, and to long-standing rubbing of ill-fitting shoes, is a common source of nail dystrophy (see Fig. 8-145).

Nail Findings in Other Dermatologic Disorders

As noted earlier, nail disorders may provide clues to other dermatologic or pediatric syndromes. For example, alopecia areata is associated with a characteristic Scotch-plaid pitting of the nails (Fig. 8-147). Similarly, psoriasis affects the nails in a number of ways that may help to distinguish it from other scaling disorders. Involvement of the nail matrix results in the

Figure 8-148 Psoriatic nails. Psoriasis affecting the nails results in onycholysis and pitting.

formation of scattered pits that are larger, deeper, and less numerous than those found in alopecia areata. Psoriasis of the nail bed, especially under the distal nail, causes separation of the nail from the underlying skin (onycholysis) and oil-drop discoloration with heaped-up scaling (Fig. 8-148). Onycholysis alone, without pits or discoloration, may be caused by trauma, infection, nail polish hardeners, or phototoxic reactions to drugs such as tetracycline or doxycycline.

COMPLICATIONS OF TOPICAL SKIN THERAPY

An important rule in medicine is as follows: "do no harm." To follow that rule, the physician must recognize the potential for adverse side effects of the therapies prescribed.

Topical Steroids

The most commonly used topical medications are steroids. These may be classified as low, medium, or high potency, according to their biologic activity. In general, fluorinated steroids are more potent than nonfluorinated steroids, and those in ointment bases are more active than those in cream or lotion bases. High-potency steroids should be used only for short periods of time to avoid major side effects. These side effects include skin atrophy (Fig. 8-149), telangiectases, and

Figure 8-147 Broad, shallow, Scotch-plaid pitting of the nails associated with alopecia areata.

Figure 8-149 Steroid-induced skin atrophy. Topical steroids may cause marked atrophy and fragility of the skin, especially if used under occlusion regularly for more than 1 month.

Figure 8-150   Steroid-induced striae distensae. Prolonged use of potent fluorinated steroids may cause permanent striae distensae.

Figure 8-151   Steroid-induced subcutaneous atrophy. Injection of steroids into fat instead of muscle often produces subcutaneous atrophy. Whereas in some cases this may resolve in 6 to 12 months, in others it can be permanent.

increased skin fragility; acneiform eruptions; permanent skin striae (Fig. 8-150); and masking or delayed recognition of infections and infestations such as tinea corporis and scabies.

Use of fluorinated steroids should be avoided on the face, eyelids, genitals, or intertriginous areas such as the axillae and thighs because absorption is greater and side effects are more common in these areas. Good general rules of safety are to use the weakest agent that is likely to clear the dermatitis and to avoid using topical steroids stronger than class 5 (the most potent) in high-risk locations. If topical medication is applied to large areas, if the treated area is occluded, or if therapy is continued for a long period, adrenal suppression may result. Accidental injection of steroids into fat on attempted intramuscular injection may cause permanent subcutaneous atrophy (Fig. 8-151).

Secondary local bacterial, viral, and fungal infections may progress with unusual rapidity in children receiving topical corticosteroids. Hence patients should be instructed to look for early signs of secondary bacterial infection and return promptly if they develop. The risk of systemic viral and bacterial infections is similarly increased in patients undergoing a prolonged regimen of widespread topical or high-dose oral steroids. All patients taking high-dose steroids and who have no past history of varicella should be alerted to return immediately for zoster immune globulin if they discover that they have been exposed to chickenpox.

Other Agents

Other complications from topical medications, such as contact dermatitis, can be easily prevented. Allergic contact dermatitis is frequently seen as a reaction to both prescribed and over-the-counter drugs. The most common allergens are neomycin, "-caine" topical anesthetics or antipruritics, bacitracin, and ethylenediamine (a preservative in many topical preparations).

When possible, products containing these agents should be avoided. Anaphylaxis can occur even in response to topical medications, especially if applied to broken skin. Hence obtaining a history of drug allergies is important before prescribing topical agents.

Fortunately, most complications of therapy can be avoided if the physician has clear knowledge of the disease, its treatment, and the pharmacologic agents being prescribed.

Bibliography

Cohen BA: *Atlas of pediatric dermatology*, London, 1993, Mosby-Wolfe.
Cohen BA: *Pediatric dermatology*, ed 2, London, 1999, Mosby.
Cohen BA, Lehman CU, editors: *DermAtlas*, Baltimore, 2000–2011, Johns Hopkins University. http://dermatlas.med.jhmi.edu/derm/
Frieden IJ, Haggstrom AN, Drolet BA, et al: Infantile hemangiomas: Current knowledge, future directions. Proceedings of a research workshop on infantile hemangiomas, *Pediatr Dermatol* 22:383–406, 2005.
Harper J, Oranje A, Prose N: *Textbook of pediatric dermatology*, London, 2000, Blackwell Science.
Hernandez RG, Cohen BA: Insect bites–induced hypersensitivity and the SCRATCH principles: A new approach to papular urticaria, *Pediatrics* 118:e189–e196, 2006.
Paller AS, Mancini AJ, editors: *Hurwitz clinical pediatric dermatology: a textbook of skin disorders of childhood and adolescence*, ed 3, Philadelphia, 2006, Elsevier Saunders.
Ruiz-Maldonado R, Parish LC, Beare JM: *Textbook of pediatric dermatology*, Philadelphia, 1989, Grune & Stratton.
Schachner LA, Hansen RC: *Pediatric dermatology*, ed 3, New York, 2003, Churchill Livingstone.
Weinberg S, Leider M, Shapiro L: *Color atlas of pediatric dermatology*, ed 2, London, 1990, McGraw-Hill.
Weston WL: *Practical pediatric dermatology*, ed 2, Boston, 1985, Little, Brown.

ENDOCRINOLOGY

9

Wassim Chemaitilly | Oscar Escobar | Selma F. Witchel

Clinical presentations of endocrine disease can vary widely. Alterations in hormone balance result in distinct phenotypes affecting linear growth, timing of puberty, and body composition. The steady stream of discoveries of new genes, novel mutations, and alterations in gene expression has provided and will continue to elucidate the functional genomics of the clinical presentation of insufficient or excessive hormone secretion as well as altered hormone receptor activity. Despite the explosion of new information, the clinical presentations of children with endocrine disorders remain constant. The recognition of physical signs associated with these states assists in the diagnosis and treatment of imbalances of the neuroendocrine axis. The following text highlights the physical signs associated with normal endocrine function, as well as those due to hyposecretion and hypersecretion.

NORMAL GROWTH

Growth is influenced by many factors including overall health, heredity, gender, and environmental factors such as nutrition. Growth is rapid during the first year of life and then slows between 1 and 2 years of age (Table 9-1). After 2 years of age, linear growth continues to decline slowly, averaging a growth rate of approximately 2.0 inches (5 cm) per year until it reaches a nadir just before the initiation of the pubertal growth spurt. This nadir has been referred to as the "prepubertal dip" or the "prepubertal deceleration." The "pubertal growth spurt" occurs during puberty. There are noticeable differences in the growth pattern of girls and boys during puberty. Girls generally start puberty at a younger chronologic age than boys and their pubertal growth spurt happens at an earlier pubertal stage. The pubertal growth spurt is also shorter in duration and displays a lower peak growth velocity in girls compared with boys. This sexual dimorphism is responsible for the differences in adult mature height between males and females. The average mature height of males is 13 cm greater than that of females.

Because stature varies among healthy children, incremental growth rate is one of the most important elements used to assess health in a child. Subnormal growth velocity can indicate endocrine and nonendocrine disorders. The most critical tool to evaluate normal and pathologic growth is the growth chart. In May of 2000, the Centers for Disease Control and Prevention (CDC) released updated growth charts based on a broad population sample combining many different growth studies (Fig. 9-1, *A-D*). These charts are readily available (http://www.cdc.gov/growthcharts). The charts not only define the 3rd and 97th percentiles for height and weight, but also characterize standards for head circumference and body mass index (BMI) defined as weight (kg)/height^2 (m). In contrast to adults for whom specific BMI values are used to define overweight and obesity, age- and gender-specific BMI values are used to classify children as over- or underweight. Health care professionals can use established percentile cutoff points to identify underweight and overweight children (Table 9-2).

Although it can be normal for a child to change percentiles between birth and 18 months of age, after this age children usually follow their growth curves fairly closely. When a child crosses percentiles in a relatively short period of time, he or she should be carefully evaluated through a detailed investigation regarding the etiology of the abnormal growth pattern. Between 4 years and adolescence, a growth rate below 4 to 5 cm per year for girls and boys is abnormal and should be assessed. Adolescence is the only time during which the rapid growth of the infant is recapitulated. For girls, a sharp increase in growth velocity is the harbinger of puberty.

Short stature with normal body proportions and decreased growth velocity can be due to endocrine as well as nonendocrine disorders. Endocrine causes of short stature include growth hormone (GH) deficiency, GH resistance (GH receptor mutations or defects in insulin-like growth factor I [IGF-I] action), and hypothyroidism. Exogenous pharmacologic steroid therapy often leads to growth deceleration. Nonendocrine causes include chronic illness (e.g., renal tubular acidosis, celiac disease, or inflammatory bowel disease), genetic disorders, and undernutrition. One common cause of short stature in children is familial or genetic short stature. The genetic growth potential of a child is heavily influenced by the growth achieved by both parents and their relatives. The heritability of height has been estimated to be 0.7 to 0.8, rising to as much as 0.9 between identical twins. Common endocrine and nonendocrine causes of short stature are listed in Tables 9-3 and 9-4.

Calculation of the target height provides an estimate of a child's genetic potential. The target height, also referred to as mid-parental height (MPH), is the midpoint between the heights of parents, correcting for the 13-cm difference between male and female adult mature heights. For boys, the MPH is the midpoint between the father's height and the corrected mother's height (i.e., mother's height plus 13 cm). This can be easily calculated by adding 6.5 cm (2.5 inches) to the mean of the parents' heights. For girls, the MPH is the midpoint between the mother's height and the corrected father's height (i.e., father's height minus 13 cm). This can be easily calculated by subtracting 6.5 cm (2.5 inches) from the mean of the parents' heights. Ideally, this calculation should be based on measured parental heights, given that reported heights are frequently overestimated. The standard deviation of the target has been calculated as 5 cm in boys and 4.5 cm in girls. Therefore, the target height range is MPH ± 10 cm in boys and MPH ± 9 cm in girls. This information should be obtained during the initial evaluation, especially for children with concerns of tall or short stature. As an example, calculation of the MPH of a boy whose father's height is 179 cm and mother's

Table 9-1	Normal Growth Rates in Children	
	GROWTH RATE (PER YEAR)	
Age	**Inches**	**Centimeters**
Birth to 1 yr	7–10	18–25
1 to 2 yr	4–5	10–13
2 yr to puberty	2–2.5	5–6
Pubertal growth spurt: girls	2.5–4.5	6–11
Pubertal growth spurt: boys	3–5	7–13

Table 9-3	Selected Nonendocrine Causes of Short Stature

Familial short stature (genetic)

Constitutional delay of growth and development

Malnutrition
    Inadequate caloric intake
    Pharmacologic, such as medications for ADHD
    Anorexia nervosa

Pharmacologic steroid treatment

Idiopathic short stature

Intrauterine growth retardation

Systemic disease
    Pulmonary
        Cystic fibrosis
        Asthma
    Cardiac and circulatory
        Congenital heart disease (cyanotic)
        Acquired heart disease
    Renal
        Renal insufficiency
        Pyelonephritis (chronic)
        Renal tubular acidosis
        Nephropathic cystinosis
    Gastrointestinal and hepatic
        Malabsorption
        Celiac disease
        Inflammatory bowel disease
        Hepatic insufficiency
    Neurologic
        Mental retardation with growth delay
    Musculoskeletal and connective tissue
        Storage diseases
        Hypotonia
        Skeletal dysplasias
    Immunologic
        Immune deficiencies
        HIV
    Mucopolysaccharidosis

Syndromes associated with short stature
    Chromosomal abnormalities
        Trisomy 21
        Trisomy 13
        Trisomy 18
        Turner syndrome
        Noonan syndrome
        Prader-Willi syndrome
        Progeria
        Russell-Silver syndrome
        Cockayne syndrome
        Seckel syndrome
        CHARGE syndrome
        18q deletion

Disproportionate short stature
    Achondroplasia
    Hypochondroplasia
    Spina bifida

Radiation to spine

ADHD, attention-deficit/hyperactivity disorder; CHARGE, coloboma of the eye, heart defects, atresia of the nasal choanae, retardation of growth and/or development, genital and/or urinary abnormalities, and ear abnormalities and deafness.

height is 160 cm, would be as follows: 179 + 160 divided by 2 plus 6.5 cm. This is 176 cm. The target height range would be 166 to 186 cm.

Radiographic determination of epiphyseal maturation, or bone age, is often helpful in evaluating children with short stature. By convention, a radiograph of the left hand is compared with established standard radiographs to determine the bone age or skeletal age. Before 24 months of life, epiphyseal development is better estimated by radiographic examination of the hemiskeleton. Children who have familial or genetically determined short stature generally have a bone age equivalent to their chronologic age. The term "constitutional delay of growth" refers to children who have later onset of puberty. Typically, the bone age of children with constitutional delay is delayed, being more consistent with the children's height age rather than chronologic age.

Children with constitutional delay typically have a period of decreased linear growth within the first 3 years of life. In this variation of normal growth and pubertal development, the rate of linear growth velocity and weight gain slow temporarily, often resulting in downward crossing of growth percentiles. By 2 or 3 years of age, linear growth resumes at a normal rate. Subsequently, children may grow either along the lower growth percentiles or beneath the curve but parallel to it for the remainder of their prepubertal years (Fig. 9-2). A family history of "late bloomers" or delayed puberty is common.

Genetic syndromes (such as Turner, Noonan, and Down syndromes) are examples of chromosomal abnormalities associated with short stature. Congenital disorders of bone mineralization and bone growth, such as the chondrodystrophies, represent an important cause of disproportionate short stature. When evaluating a child with a suspected chondrodystrophy, body proportions should be measured. A simple method of determining proportions consists of measuring the lower segment (symphysis pubis to floor) and subtracting this value from the total height to determine the upper segment and then calculating the upper segment–to–lower segment ratio. This ratio, along with the arm span–to–height ratio, is used to document whether the spine or limbs are more severely shortened. Arm span is usually equal to standing height. However, in children with achondroplasia, the long bones are disproportionately shortened. Sitting height (another way of calculating the length of the upper segment), determined with a special sitting stadiometer, is generally normal whereas the standing height is short. During adolescence, hypogonadism is often associated with increased limb length. For the child with short

Table 9-2	Body Mass Index Cutoff Points

Category	BMI for Age (Range)
Underweight	<5th percentile
Normal	5th percentile to <85th percentile
At risk for overweight	85th percentile to <95th percentile
Overweight	≥95th percentile

BMI, body mass index.

stature and subnormal linear growth velocity, the evaluation should be comprehensive with consideration of endocrine and nonendocrine disorders.

Pubertal Development

Puberty is the process through which reproductive competence is achieved and is initiated by reactivation of the hypothalamic–pituitary–gonadal axis (gonadarche). In humans and several nonhuman primates, adrenal pubertal maturation, indicated by increased adrenal dehydroepiandrosterone sulfate

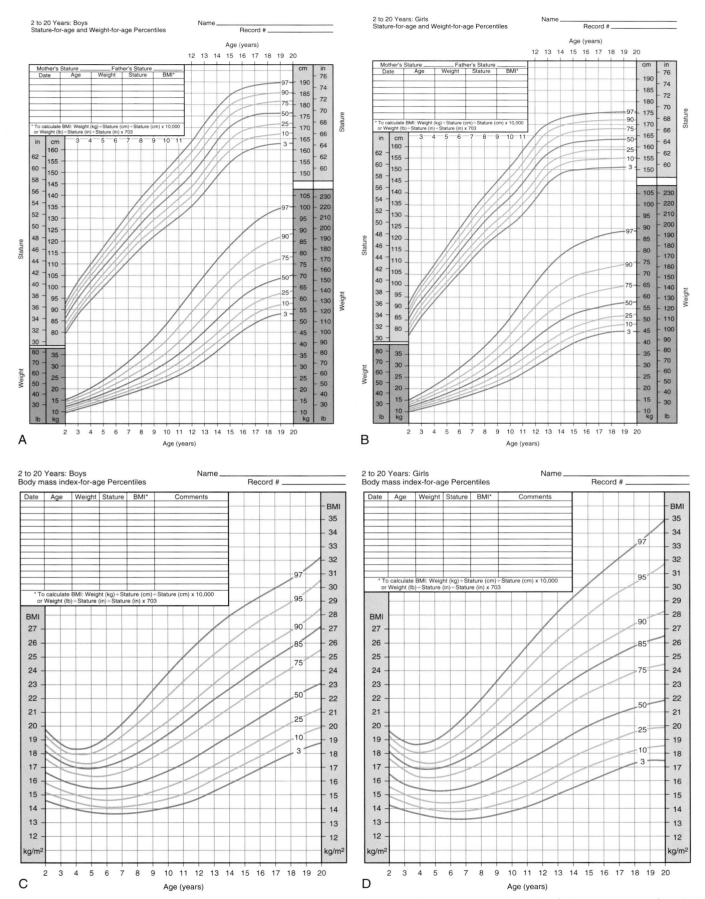

Figure 9-1   A-D, Growth charts from the Centers for Disease Control. **A,** Stature-for-age and weight-for-age percentiles (3rd to 97th) for boys 2 to 20 years of age. **B,** Stature-for-age and weight-for-age percentiles for girls 2 to 20 years of age. **C,** Body mass index-for-age percentiles for boys 2 to 20 years of age. **D,** Body mass index-for-age percentiles for girls 2 to 20 years of age. *(Developed by the National Center for Health Statistics in collaboration with the National Center for Chronic Disease Prevention and Health Promotion [2000]. Available online at http://www.cdc.gov/growthcharts.)*

Table 9-4	Endocrine Causes of Impaired Growth and Short Stature

Pituitary development
  Growth hormone deficiency
  Septo-optic dysplasia
  Mutations in HESX1, SOX2, SOX3, GLI2, LHX3, LHX4, PROP1, and POU1F1
    genes
Craniopharyngioma
Transection of pituitary stalk due to trauma
Radiation damage to hypothalamus/pituitary
GH gene mutation
Laron dwarfism (GH receptor mutation)
IGF-I deficiency
  IGF-I gene mutation
  IGF-I receptor gene mutation
  STAT5 mutation
Thyroid hormone
  Congenital hypothyroidism
  Acquired hypothyroidism
  Thyroid hormone resistance
  Consumptive hypothyroidism

Cortisol hypersecretion
  Cushing syndrome
  Cushing disease
Diabetes insipidus
  Congenital ADH deficiency
  Nephrogenic diabetes insipidus
  Wolfram syndrome
  Acquired
    Postoperative
    Neoplasms
    Infiltrative (Langerhans cell histiocytosis)
Defects in aldosterone synthase (CYP11B2)
Bone and mineral metabolism
  Vitamin D deficiency rickets
  Hypophosphatemic rickets
  Pseudohypoparathyroidism
  Pseudopseudohypoparathyroidism (hereditary Albright osteodystrophy)
Poorly controlled diabetes mellitus (Mauriac syndrome)

ADH, antidiuretic hormone; GH, growth hormone; IGF-I, insulin-like growth factor type I.

Figure 9-2 Growth curve of a child with constitutional growth delay. Note the typical pattern of growth deceleration followed by a normal growth rate.

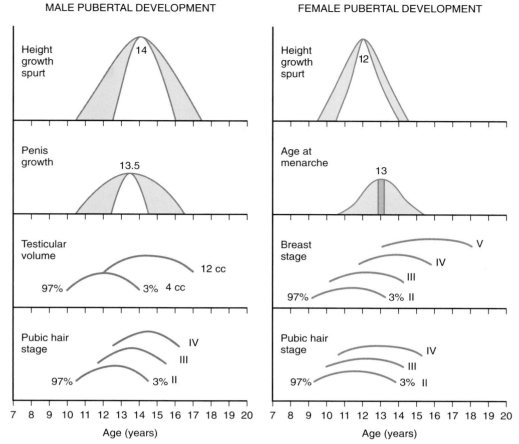

MALE PUBERTAL DEVELOPMENT   FEMALE PUBERTAL DEVELOPMENT

Figure 9-3 Schematic representation of the onset of male and female puberty. *(Modified from Johnson TR, Moore WM, Jeffries JE: Children are different: development physiology, ed 2, Columbus, Ohio, 1978, Ross Laboratories, Division of Abbott Laboratories, pp. 26-29. Used with permission of Ross Products Division, Abbott Laboratories, Inc., Columbus, Ohio 43215.)*

(DHEAS) secretion, occurs in close temporal proximity to gonadarche. Clinical studies have demonstrated that gonadarche and adrenarche are regulated through different molecular mechanisms.

The pattern of timing of pubertal events for boys and girls is generally predictable (Fig. 9-3). For both boys and girls, mean ages for the onset of puberty vary among different ethnic groups and represent the combined influences of genetic and environmental factors. In boys, puberty, first evidenced by testicular enlargement, usually begins between 9 and 14 years of age. In girls, puberty, evidenced by breast development, usually begins between 8 and 12 years of age. Among white girls, the mean age of onset of breast development and pubic hair growth occurs at approximately 10½ years of age, with menarche occurring at approximately 12½ years of age. African-American females tend to enter puberty at an earlier age. For girls, increased BMI may be associated with premature adrenarche and earlier pubertal onset. Large-scale population studies have identified a secular trend for slightly earlier (by 2.5 to 4 months) ages at menarche, suggesting changes in the timing of the onset of puberty. Boys with rapid weight gain during childhood tend to have a later onset of puberty. The physiologic basis for this intriguing discordant effect of obesity on pubertal timing in boys versus girls is unexplained. These shifts, however, have generally not altered clinical practice guidelines regarding evaluation of "off-time" puberty.

Tanner Staging

To describe the onset and progression of pubertal changes (Fig. 9-4), boys and girls are rated on five-point scales. Boys are rated for both genital development and pubic hair growth, and girls are rated for breast development and pubic hair growth. In general, for healthy children, Tanner stages of puberty for genital development and pubic hair growth are congruent. Differences in pubertal staging may be useful to formulate the differential diagnosis for children with "off-time" puberty. Attention should be paid to the Tanner staging of genital and pubic hair development especially for the child with "off-time" puberty. Inconsistent staging assists with the initial differential diagnosis.

The stages for male *genital* development are as follows (Fig. 9-4, *A*):

Stage I (Preadolescent)—The testes, scrotal sac, and penis have a size and proportion similar to those seen in early childhood

Stage II—There is enlargement of the scrotum and testes and a change in the texture of the scrotal skin. The scrotal skin may also be reddened.

Stage III—Further growth of the penis has occurred, initially in length with some increase in circumference. There is also increased growth of the testes and scrotum.

Stage IV—The penis is significantly enlarged in length and circumference, with further development of the glans penis. The testes and scrotum continue to enlarge, and there is distinct darkening of the scrotal skin.

Stage V—The genitalia are adult in size and shape.

The stages in male *pubic hair* development are as follows (Fig. 9-4, *B*):

Stage I (Preadolescent)—Vellus hair appears over the pubes with a degree of development similar to that over the abdominal wall. There is no androgen-sensitive pubic hair.

Stage II—There is sparse development of long pigmented downy hair, which is only slightly curled or straight. The hair is seen chiefly at the base of the penis.

Stage III—The pubic hair is considerably darker, coarser, and curlier. The distribution of hair has now spread over the junction of the pubes.

Stage IV—The hair distribution is now adult in type but still is considerably less than that seen in adults. There is no spread to the medial surface of the thighs.

Stage V—Hair distribution is adult in quantity and type and is described as an inverse triangle. There can be spread to the medial surface of the thighs.

The stages in female *breast* development are as follows (Fig. 9-4, *C*):

Stage I (Preadolescent)—Only the papilla is elevated above the level of the chest wall.

Stage II (Breast budding)—Elevation of the breasts and papillae may occur as small mounds along with some increased diameter of the areolae.

Stage III—The breasts and areolae continue to enlarge, although they show no separation of contour.

Stage IV—The areolae and papillae elevate above the level of the breasts and form secondary mounds with further development of the overall breast tissue.

Stage V—Mature female breasts have developed. The papillae may extend slightly above the contour of the breast as the result of recession of the areolae.

Pubic hair growth in females is staged as follows (Fig. 9-4, *B*):

Stage I (Preadolescent)—Vellus hair develops over the pubes. There is no sexual hair.

Stage II—Sparse, long, pigmented, downy hair, which is straight or only slightly curled, appears mainly along the labia.

Stage III—Considerably darker, coarser, and curlier sexual hair appears. The hair has now spread sparsely over the junction of the pubes.

Stage IV—The hair distribution is adult in type but decreased in total quantity. There is no spread to the medial surface of the thighs.

Stage V—Hair is adult in quantity and type and appears in an inverse triangle of the classically feminine type. There is spread to the medial surface of the thighs, but not above the base of the inverse triangle.

THE HYPOTHALAMUS AND THE PITUITARY GLAND

The hypothalamus is derived from neuroectodermal tissue of the diencephalon and surrounds the inferior aspect of the third ventricle. Its basilar portion consists of the median eminence and pituitary stalk, which provide the common route for hypothalamic factors to reach the pituitary gland. Various regions in the hypothalamus secrete small peptide hormones that use this pathway to regulate pituitary hormone secretion. The neurohypophysis, consisting of unmyelinated axons and axon terminals, extends from the median eminence to the posterior pituitary gland.

The pituitary gland develops as a fusion of cells of different embryonic origins. There is an upgrowth of ectodermal cells from the roof of the primitive pharynx (known as Rathke pouch), and a downgrowth of neural tissue cells from the hypothalamus. These two distinct areas form the anterior lobe (the adenohypophysis) and the posterior lobe (the neurohypophysis), respectively.

Both congenital and acquired abnormalities of pituitary function occur. Structural abnormalities of the central nervous system (CNS), such as septo-optic dysplasia (Fig. 9-5, *A* and *B*) and holoprosencephaly (Fig. 9-5, *C*), can interfere with

I
Preadolescent

II
Enlargement, change in texture

III
Growth in length and circumference

IV
Further development of glans penis, darkening of scrotal skin

V
Adult genitalia

A

Figure 9-4   **A-C,** Schematic drawings of male and female Tanner stages show male genital development **(A)**, pubic hair development **(B)**, and breast development **(C)**. *(Modified from Johnson TR, Moore WM, Jefferies JE: Children are different: development physiology, ed 2, Columbus, Ohio, 1978, Ross Laboratories, Division of Abbot Laboratories, pp. 26-29. Used with permission of Ross Products Division, Abbott Laboratories, Inc., Columbus, Ohio 43215.)*

pituitary function. Craniopharyngiomas and CNS tumors can be associated with acquired hypopituitarism (Fig. 9-6). Additional causes of acquired hypopituitarism include radiation therapy to treat CNS tumors, granulomatous infiltration, and traumatic interruption of the pituitary stalk.

I
Preadolescent
no sexual hair

II
Sparse, pigmented,
long, straight,
mainly along labia
and at
base of penis

III
Darker, coarser,
curlier

IV
Adult, but decreased
distribution

V
Adult in
quantity
and type
with spread
to medial thighs

I
Preadolescent

Areola
Papilla

II
Breast budding

III
Continued enlargement

IV
Areola and papilla
form secondary mound

V
Mature female breast

B

C

Figure 9-4, cont'd

Anterior Pituitary

The anterior pituitary, with its diverse cell types and hormonal secretory patterns, controls many important biologic processes. It contains cells that secrete three types of hormones: (1) corticotrophin-related peptide hormones, (2) glycoprotein hormones, and (3) somatomammotropins. These compounds have great biologic potency with tight regulation of hormone secretion governed by positive and negative feedback signals. Anterior pituitary hormone deficiencies cause subsequent hypofunction in the output of secondary endocrine glands, with substantial consequences for growth and development.

Figure 9-5   A-C, Congenital abnormalities of the CNS commonly associated with hypothalamic–pituitary dysfunction. **A,** Pale optic discs noted on funduscopic examination indicative of optic nerve hypoplasia, which can be associated with septo-optic dysplasia. **B,** Magnetic resonance image showing optic nerve hypoplasia. **C,** Holoprosencephaly. (**A,** Courtesy D. Hiles, MD, Pittsburgh, Pa.)

Children with midline defects have a higher incidence of hypopituitarism when compared with normal children. The child seen in Figure 9-7 has a single central incisor, an example of a midline abnormality associated with GH deficiency. Thus, specific alterations in physical appearance should alert physicians to a possible abnormality in anterior pituitary development potentially associated with secondary hormone deficiencies (e.g., thyroid-stimulating hormone [TSH] deficiency affecting thyroid function). The molecular etiologies for autosomal recessive, autosomal dominant, and X-linked disorders affecting anterior pituitary development and function have been elucidated.

Growth Hormone

GH influences linear growth and modulates several complex metabolic processes. GH secretion is regulated by the relative balance between the levels of GH-releasing hormone (GHRH) and somatostatin (Fig. 9-8). Both GHRH and somatostatin are secreted by the hypothalamus. The GH receptor is a single transmembrane protein. After the binding of GH to its receptor, a second GH receptor dimerizes with the first receptor to initiate the signal transduction process. GH generates direct effects via the GH receptor signal transduction pathway and secondary effects by promoting an increase in IGF-I and insulin-like growth factor-binding protein-3 (IGF-BP3).

In children with hypopituitarism due to growth hormone deficiency, GH treatment markedly improves growth velocity. GH stimulates an increase in lean body mass, as well as a marked increase in the size of the heart, pancreas, liver, and kidneys. It has positive effects on carbohydrate, fat, and protein metabolism and causes a decrease in body fat. GH inhibits carbohydrate uptake by muscle. This diabetogenic effect of GH action is a known complication of GH hypersecretion. Typically, children with GH deficiency have normal birth weights and normal growth patterns during the first year of life, after which time their growth velocities decelerate. As seen in Figure 9-9, GH-deficient children have a characteristic "kewpie" doll appearance. They are often described as being "cherubic" because of their short stature, excess subcutaneous fat, retarded body proportion changes, and high-pitched voices. Infants with hypopituitarism may present in the early neonatal period with hypoglycemia or prolonged jaundice. On physical examination, male infants with hypopituitarism may have small penises due to concomitant luteinizing hormone (LH) deficiency.

Figure 9-6   Craniopharyngioma. Heterogeneous, densely enhancing suprasellar mass extending from the pituitary fossa into the hypothalamus and third ventricle.

Figure 9-7   Central maxillary incisor. The presence of a single central maxillary incisor should alert the clinician to investigate the possibility of growth hormone (GH) deficiency. (Courtesy P. Lee, MD, Hershey, Pa.)

Figure 9-8 Feedback regulation of growth hormone (GH) at the level of the hypothalamus, pituitary, and target organs. GHRF, growth hormone-releasing factor.

The pulsatile nature of GH secretion necessitates provocative stimulation tests to diagnose GH deficiency. Thus, measurements of random GH concentrations are not helpful in the evaluation of short stature. IGF-I concentrations may be low in children with GH deficiency. Because IGF-I concentrations also reflect nutritional status, IGF-I concentrations may be low in children with inadequate caloric intake.

Excessive GH secretion is uncommon in children. If GH excess begins during childhood, gigantism with increased growth velocity ensues. After closure of the epiphyses, soft tissue growth of the hands and feet and coarsening of facial features are typically the first clinical manifestations of acromegaly. Random GH, IGF-I, and IGF-BP3 concentrations are usually elevated in gigantism/acromegaly.

Adrenocorticotropic Hormone

The corticotropin-related peptide hormones consist of adrenocorticotropic hormone (ACTH), α-melanocyte-stimulating hormone (α-MSH), and γ- and β-lipotropins (γ-LPH, β-LPH). These hormones are derived from a common precursor molecule, pro-opiomelanocortin. Within the subunit structure of β-LPH are the important neuroendocrine molecules α-, β-, and γ-endorphin and enkephalin. After posttranslational processing from this large precursor molecule, the secretion of ACTH is regulated by the level of corticotropin-releasing hormone (CRH), which is secreted by the hypothalamus. Cortisol secreted from the adrenal gland also influences ACTH secretion by negative feedback (Fig. 9-10). Prolonged pharmacologic glucocorticoid therapy suppresses the hypothalamic–pituitary–adrenal axis, with the potential for adrenal insufficiency as well as a significant impact on growth and development.

Gonadotropins

The glycoprotein hormones include follicle-stimulating hormone (FSH) and luteinizing hormone (LH). Each of these hormones is composed of two dissimilar peptide subunits. The α chain is identical for both hormones. However, the β chain is unique and confers specificity to each hormone. These hormones also contain significant amounts of carbohydrate and sialic acid residues along with their basic amino acid structures.

Secretion of LH and FSH is regulated by the pulsatile gonadotropin-releasing hormone (GnRH) secretion. Neurons

Figure 9-9 Growth hormone deficiency. The normal 3½-year old boy *(right)* is in the 50th percentile for height. The short 3-year-old girl *(left)* has GH deficiency.

Figure 9-10 Feedback regulation of adrenocorticotropic hormone (ACTH) at the level of the hypothalamus, pituitary, and adrenal glands. CRF, corticotropin-releasing factor.

in the hypothalamus secrete GnRH in pulses that vary in amplitude and frequency during childhood and puberty. Various neurotransmitters are involved in controlling GnRH-secreting neurons and thus modulate the GnRH pulses. Kisspeptin, which acts via its receptor GPR54 (also known as KISS1-R), has been identified as a major stimulus for GnRH and LH release. Translational studies have identified several other genes that are involved in controlling the onset of puberty. In addition to kisspeptin and its receptor, other genes include neurokinin B, its cognate receptor (*TACR3*), *PROK2*, and its receptor (*PROKR2*).

After active secretion in late gestation and in the early neonatal period, the GnRH pulse generator becomes quiescent until the onset of puberty, which is characterized by the resumption of increased GnRH secretion. Increased nocturnal LH secretion marks the reactivation of the GnRH pulse generator and the onset of puberty. In primary gonadal failure, the deficiency of sex steroids interferes with negative feedback inhibition, resulting in elevated gonadotropin secretion during infancy, puberty, and adulthood.

The primary actions of FSH and LH affect gonadal function. LH binds to the LH receptor on Leydig cells to stimulate testosterone synthesis and secretion. In the testes, FSH supports Sertoli cell development and spermatogenesis (Fig. 9-11). The ovary is characterized by a two-cell model for steroidogenesis. LH stimulates ovarian theca cells to synthesize androstenedione, which serves as the precursor for estradiol synthesis. Subsequently, in the ovarian granulosa cells, FSH increases expression of aromatase, the enzyme that converts androgens to estrogens. The negative feedback effect of sex steroids on LH and FSH production is dramatically emphasized in postmenopausal women and in individuals with gonadal failure, in whom marked elevations of these hormones occur. Inhibin B is produced by the gonads and inhibits FSH release.

Gonadotropin secretion, especially in females, is influenced by metabolic state and by the degree of adiposity. Very athletic and lean girls experience delayed puberty with low gonadotropin levels; girls with eating disorders of the restrictive type experience amenorrhea with suppressed gonadotropins. Pubertal development may be slow among boys who restrict food intake to maintain a low weight for wrestling. Leptin, a hormone produced by the adipose tissue, exerts a significant effect on the hypothalamus and is a major link between energy balance and gonadotropin secretion.

Thyroid-stimulating Hormone

Thyroid-stimulating hormone (TSH) is the third glycoprotein hormone; its α subunit is identical to the α subunits of LH and FSH. Its specificity lies in its β subunit. TSH stimulates many aspects of thyroid function. Its major role is to promote the synthesis and secretion of thyroid hormone. Mediated by the TSH receptor, TSH increases the size of the thyroid cells, vascularity of the gland, iodide uptake, thyroglobulin synthesis, and thyroid hormone secretion. The rate of TSH secretion appears to be determined by the level of circulating thyroid hormone and by the hypothalamic hormone, thyrotropin-releasing hormone (TRH), as seen in Figure 9-12. Negative feedback of TSH secretion by circulating thyroid hormone occurs mainly at the pituitary level.

Prolactin

Prolactin (PRL) acts directly on its target organs and does not require an intermediary secondary endocrine gland. The major known function of PRL in humans is the initiation and maintenance of lactation. In contrast to other anterior pituitary hormones, PRL is regulated by tonic inhibition by dopamine secreted by the hypothalamus. Congenital or acquired interruption of the hypothalamic–pituitary stalk may

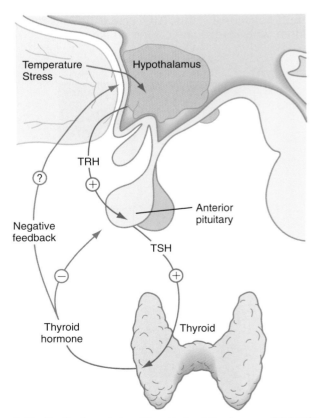

Figure 9-11 Feedback regulation of luteinizing hormone (LH) and follicle-stimulating hormone (FSH) at the level of the hypothalamus, pituitary, and gonads. GnRH, gonadotropin-releasing hormone.

Figure 9-12 Feedback regulation of thyroid-stimulating hormone (TSH) at the level of the hypothalamus, pituitary, and thyroid gland. TRH, thyrotropin-releasing hormone.

be accompanied by elevated prolactin concentrations reflecting decreased inhibition due to impaired hypothalamic–pituitary communication. Galactorrhea may be a clinical manifestation of hyperprolactinemia. Hyperprolactinemia can be observed with pituitary adenomas or secondary to medications such as neuroleptics, antipsychotics, estrogens, and antihypertensive medications. When hyperprolactinemia is secondary to medications, the prolactin concentrations are generally less than 75 ng/mL.

Posterior Pituitary

Vasopressin and oxytocin are two evolutionarily related peptides, each composed of nine amino acids. These hormones are synthesized in the hypothalamus and stored in the posterior pituitary gland. Expression of vasopressin and oxytocin genes occurs in the hypothalamic paraventricular and supraoptic nuclei. On magnetic resonance T_1-weighted images, the posterior pituitary has a characteristic high signal intensity. The presence of this high signal intensity adjacent to the median eminence with absence of the normal pituitary bright spot within the sella on T_1-weighted images is evidence of an ectopic posterior pituitary. An ectopic posterior pituitary is often associated with anterior pituitary hormone deficiencies, but typically these patients do not have diabetes insipidus (Fig. 9-13).

Vasopressin, also known as arginine vasopressin (AVP) or antidiuretic hormone (ADH), is a hormone important in water balance. It is synthesized and carried via axonal transport to the posterior pituitary, its primary site of storage. It is then released into the systemic circulation. AVP acts primarily on the kidneys at V2 receptors to aid in the reabsorption of water by affecting water permeability in the collecting duct of the kidney. At high concentrations, it also causes constriction of the arterioles through its action at V1 receptors, thereby leading to an increase in blood pressure. V3 receptors in the pituitary contribute to ACTH release by potentiating the action of CRH. Osmoreceptors in the hypothalamus detect an increase in osmotic pressure in the blood, leading to increased AVP secretion and increased thirst. The combination of increased AVP secretion leading to increased renal reabsorption of free water and increased oral fluid intake will decrease osmolality. Other factors that increase AVP secretion include pain, trauma, nausea, and vomiting.

Head trauma, brain tumors, encephalitis, pneumonia, and some drugs are associated with overproduction of AVP. This can lead to inappropriate water retention and hyponatremia, known as the syndrome of inappropriate ADH secretion (SIADH). The symptoms of SIADH include headache, apathy, nausea, vomiting, and impaired consciousness. Underproduction of AVP results in central diabetes insipidus (DI). DI can result from pituitary tumors; head trauma; infiltrative disease processes such as Langerhans cell histiocytosis, sarcoidosis, hemochromatosis, and autoimmune hypophysitis; or from any surgery that damages the pituitary gland and hypothalamus. Familial central DI, inherited in both recessive and dominant patterns, is rare and has its onset in infancy. Wolfram syndrome is an autosomal dominant form of central DI often associated with diabetes mellitus, optic atrophy, and deafness (DIDMOAD).

Nephrogenic DI is characterized by failure of the kidney tubules to respond to ADH. Genetic causes of nephrogenic DI include X-linked forms due to mutations in the V2 receptor gene and autosomal forms due to mutations in the aquaporin-2 gene. Acquired nephrogenic DI can be caused by drugs such as lithium. Psychogenic water drinking, hypercalcemia, hypokalemia, sickle cell anemia, and polycystic kidney disease can also impair renal concentrating ability.

Oxytocin secretion occurs in response to nervous stimulation of the hypothalamus. This hormone causes contraction of the smooth muscle of the uterus and also of the myoepithelial cells lining the duct of the mammary gland. Although some oxytocin is found in males, its function is unclear.

THE THYROID GLAND

The thyroid gland is situated in the neck or, in rare cases, at the base of the tongue or in the mediastinum. The gland originates in the floor of the primitive pharynx, near the base of the tongue, approximately 24 days after fertilization, forming initially the thyroid diverticulum. During the elongation of the embryo, the developing thyroid gland moves down anteriorly to the hyoid bone and laryngeal cartilages along a narrow tube, the thyroglossal duct. When reaching its final position anterior to the trachea, the thyroid divides into right and left portions called the thyroid lobes connected by a thin layer of thyroid tissue, the isthmus, which lies ventrally to the second and third tracheal rings. The thyroglossal duct degenerates and disappears. On occasion, the lower portion of the thyroglossal duct fills up with thyroid tissue forming the pyramidal lobe. On occasion, the atrophy of the thyroglossal duct is not complete, leading to the presence of fluid-filled thyroglossal duct cysts, which appear clinically as tense, painless, and movable swellings at any point along the course of the thyroglossal duct. The thyroid gland synthesizes thyroxine (T_4) and triiodothyronine (T_3); this process is dependent on the availability of iodine. Most circulating T_4 and T_3 is transported by thyroid-binding globulin (TBG), albumin, and transthyretin. The free hormone is the active moiety. T_4 and T_3 are metabolized by inner ring deiodination to reverse T_3 and diiodothyronine (T_2), respectively.

Inherited disorders affecting TBG concentration or acquired alterations in availability of binding sites may confound interpretation of thyroid hormone function studies. The gene encoding TBG is mapped to the X chromosome. Both X-linked dominant and X-linked recessive inheritance have been reported for TBG excess and TBG deficiency; such patients are typically euthyroid.

Both overactivity and underactivity of the thyroid gland may be associated with a goiter. However, the clinical features typical of hyperthyroidism and hypothyroidism are dramatically different. The medical history and examination of the thyroid gland provide important information when evaluating a suspected abnormality in thyroid function.

Figure 9-13 Ectopic pituitary. Note the absent normal posterior pituitary bright spot *(arrow)* within the sella on magnetic resonance imaging. Instead, the bright spot is located in the median eminence.

Figure 9-14 Examination of the thyroid gland. The thyroid gland is best palpated with the examiner behind the patient.

As seen in Figure 9-14, the thyroid gland usually is best palpated with the examiner behind the patient. After identification of the cricothyroid cartilage, the second and third fingers are moved laterally along the trachea just medial to the sternocleidomastoid muscles. Two distinct lobes are palpable; the right lobe is usually greater in size than the left lobe. When a goiter is present, these lobes may be quite easily identified (Fig. 9-15). The texture of the gland varies with hyperthyroidism and hypothyroidism, the former usually being soft and fleshy, and the latter usually firm or bosselated. Nodules can also be palpated and may be indicative of an adenoma or carcinoma. Because the thyroid is directly supported by the trachea, having the patient swallow will elevate and depress a palpable gland along with the trachea during the swallowing motion.

Thyroid nodules are uncommon in children. A solitary thyroid nodule should raise concerns of thyroid neoplasia. Although 70% to 80% of solitary thyroid nodules prove to be benign or cystic lesions, thyroid cancer accounts for 1% to 1.5% of all childhood cancers. Clinical features suggestive of malignancy include neck irradiation, family history of medullary carcinoma, rapid growth of the nodule, fixation to adjacent structures, and enlarged lymph nodes.

Hyperthyroidism

Hyperthyroidism refers to excessive thyroid hormone secretion by the thyroid gland. Features of hyperthyroidism include accelerated basal metabolism, tachycardia, weight loss, increased frequency of bowel movements, heat intolerance, nervousness, widened pulse pressure, and tremor. The skin is warm and moist; hair is fine and friable. Separation of the distal margin of the nail bed, Plummer nails, may be noted. Restlessness, inability to sit still, emotional lability, short attention span, excessive sweating, and fatigue may be found.

Hyperthyroidism can be due to autoimmune thyroid disease including Graves disease or the hyperthyroid phase of Hashimoto thyroiditis, commonly called hashitoxicosis. Graves disease is a condition in which a stimulating antibody directed against the TSH receptor (thyroid receptor antibody [TRAb] or thyroid-stimulating immunoglobulin [TSI]) increases the endogenous production of thyroid hormone. The transient hyperthyroidism seen in Hashimoto thyroiditis is related to the release of preformed thyroid hormone from a thyroid gland being disrupted by lymphocytic infiltration. Other, less common causes of hyperthyroidism in children include autonomously functioning adenomas, toxic multinodular goiters, activating mutations of the TSH receptor, selective pituitary T_3 resistance, and exogenous intake of thyroid hormones. Although rare, thyroid cancer can occur within an autonomously functioning "hot nodule." Exophthalmos, a characteristic finding of Graves disease, usually is less dramatic in children than adults, but proptosis and lid lag can be appreciated (Fig. 9-16). The hyperthyroid gland can become quite large, as much as three to four times its normal size, and is warm when palpated. A bruit may be heard over the gland. Thyroxine and triiodothyronine concentrations are elevated and TSH concentrations are suppressed.

Hypothyroidism

Hypothyroidism, often associated with a goiter, can be congenital or acquired. Hypothyroidism can be classified as primary when the defect lies in the thyroid gland itself, central when it is due to pituitary dysfunction (referred to

Figure 9-15 Goiter. Note the enlarged thyroid gland in a patient with Hashimoto thyroiditis, easily visualized with neck extension. *(Courtesy M. Parker, MD, Charlotte, N.C.)*

Figure 9-16 Graves disease. Mild thyromegaly and proptosis or exophthalmos are characteristic findings in patients with Graves disease.

Figure 9-17 A child with cretinism. Note the coarse facial features, broad nasal bridge, thick lips, and umbilical hernia. *(Courtesy T.P. Foley, Jr., MD, Pittsburgh, Pa.)*

Figure 9-19 Examination of the neonatal thyroid gland. Examination is performed by elevating the infant's trunk while allowing the head to fall back gently as shown.

as secondary hypothyroidism), or hypothalamic dysfunction (referred to as tertiary hypothyroidism). Iodine deficiency is one of the most common causes of primary acquired hypothyroidism in the world. The incidence of congenital hypothyroidism is 1 in 4000.

Children with untreated congenital hypothyroidism (cretinism) develop a broad nasal bridge, coarse facial features, mental retardation, short stature, a characteristic puffy appearance of their hands, protuberant tongue, and delayed skeletal maturation (Fig. 9-17). Because treatment by 3 to 4 weeks of age ameliorates these features, newborn screening programs have been implemented to identify hypothyroid infants. Despite the success of screening, thyroid function tests should still be obtained if signs and/or symptoms of congenital hypothyroidism are detected, even in the face of normal screening results. Radionuclide scanning using either technetium or iodine-123 (^{123}I) can be useful in identifying an ectopic thyroid gland or thyroid agenesis (Fig. 9-18). Absence of radioisotope uptake is consistent with thyroid agenesis.

A goiter in an infant with congenital hypothyroidism (CH) suggests an enzymatic defect in thyroid hormone biosynthesis, referred to as dyshormonogenesis. To demonstrate a goiter in a newborn, the examiner's hand is best placed gently under the back and shoulder blades of the infant, and the infant's trunk is raised from the bed (Fig. 9-19). As the head falls backward, the neck is elevated and a goiter, if present, will

be evident. Thyroid ultrasound may be useful to confirm the presence of thyroid tissue.

Acquired hypothyroidism, most frequently due to Hashimoto/chronic lymphocytic thyroiditis, may present in childhood. Typical features include dry skin, constipation, hair loss, fatigue, cold intolerance, apathy, depressed or delayed relaxation phase of deep tendon reflexes, and weakness. A sharp deceleration in growth may also be seen in children with acquired hypothyroidism, as seen in the growth curve shown in Figure 9-20. Family history is often positive for autoimmune thyroid disease. The diagnosis is confirmed by measurement of a high TSH level and low thyroxine level. Anti-thyroid antibodies (directed against thyroperoxidase and thyroglobulin) are often detected. After institution of thyroid hormone replacement therapy, growth velocity returns to normal (see Fig. 9-20). Acquired hypothalamic or pituitary disorders can cause hypothyroidism due to TRH and/or TSH deficiencies.

Thyroid hormone resistance is a rare cause of either congenital or acquired hypothyroidism. This occurs when there is either resistance to thyroid hormone or resistance to thyroid-stimulating hormone (TSH). Resistance to thyroid hormone is due to mutations in the thyroid hormone receptor β1 (TRb1) gene and can be generalized (affecting all target tissues) or limited to the pituitary. Patients with TSH resistance have been found to have inactivating mutations of the TSH receptor (TSHR) gene. Clinical manifestations such as mental retardation and delayed bone maturation have been seen in individuals with generalized thyroid hormone resistance. Patients with partial TSH resistance are usually clinically euthyroid as they are able to compensate by increasing thyroid hormone levels. Those with complete TSH resistance may have profound hypothyroidism detectable on neonatal screening for CH.

THE PARATHYROID GLANDS

The parathyroid glands are four glands located adjacent to the thyroid gland in the neck. They are responsible for the synthesis and secretion of parathyroid hormone (PTH), a hormone important in regulating extracellular calcium concentration through its effects on three principal target organs: bone, intestinal mucosa, and kidney (Fig. 9-21). An increase in extracellular calcium inhibits secretion of PTH, whereas a decrease in extracellular calcium stimulates its release. In addition to calcium, there are other regulators of PTH secretion. Hypermagnesemia inhibits PTH secretion. Conversely, in states of hypomagnesemia, PTH is stimulated.

To monitor extracellular calcium concentration and, thereby, regulate the secretion of PTH, parathyroid cells rely on a G

4   5
RT   ANT   LT   RT   ANT   LT
                            w/o marker
← Sternal notch

5 min statics
PT supine

Figure 9-18 Ectopic thyroid gland. Technetium (^{99m}Tc) scan of an 8-day-old infant with congenital hypothyroidism. A lingual thyroid gland is identified with no functioning thyroid tissue in the anatomic thyroid bed. *(Courtesy S.F. Witchel, MD, Pittsburgh, Pa.)*

Figure 9-20 Growth curve of a child with acquired hypothyroidism. Note the sharp deceleration in growth before the onset of symptoms. After thyroid hormone replacement, significant catch-up growth occurs. The inserted photographs illustrate the child before onset of acquired hypothyroidism **(A)**, the change in body habitus associated with acquired hypothyroidism **(B)**, and resolution after thyroid replacement at the indicated times **(C)**.

protein–coupled receptor, the calcium-sensing receptor (CaSR). Mutations in the CaSR gene, mapped to chromosome 3q13.3-21, have been implicated in disorders of calcium homeostasis. These disorders are associated with an altered "set point" for serum calcium concentrations. Activating mutations in the CaSR gene have been found in families with autosomal dominant hypercalciuric hypocalcemia. Heterozygous loss-of-function mutations are associated with familial hypocalciuric hypercalcemia. Homozygosity for CaSR loss-of-function mutations is associated with severe neonatal hyperparathyroidism, which can be life-threatening.

In the intestine, PTH does not appear to have a significant direct effect on calcium or phosphate absorption, but acts indirectly by promoting the synthesis of the hormonally active form of vitamin D, calcitriol [1,25-dihydroxyvitamin D_3; $1,25(OH)_2D_3$], in the kidney, the action of which is to enhance intestinal calcium absorption. In the kidney, PTH has direct effects on the reabsorption of calcium, phosphate, and bicarbonate, predominantly in the distal convoluted tubule. PTH also inhibits reabsorption of phosphate in the renal proximal tubule.

CAUSES OF HYPERCALCEMIA

Hyperparathyroidism

Hypercalcemia (Fig. 9-22) due to hyperparathyroidism may be sporadic or inherited as a common manifestation of the multiple endocrine neoplasia (MEN) syndrome type 1. Other features of MEN 1 include islet cell tumors, Zollinger-Ellison syndrome, and pituitary tumors. Collagenomas and angiofibromas are cutaneous features associated with MEN 1. Although typically a disease of adults, affected children can be identified through biochemical screening before the onset of clinical symptoms. Inherited as an autosomal dominant trait, MEN 1 is associated with mutations in the menin gene (*MEN1*).

Williams-Beuren Syndrome

Children with Williams-Beuren syndrome have distinctive "elfin" facies characterized by dolichocephaly, flat nasal bridge, epicanthal folds, long philtrum, and wide mouth. Despite cognitive impairment, affected individuals tend to be very social and empathic. Cardiac anomalies, typically supravalvular aortic stenosis, occur in approximately 30%. Hypercalcemia can occur during infancy, but generally resolves by 4 years of age, if not earlier. Hypercalciuria may occur as well. Other endocrine manifestations can include impaired glucose tolerance, subclinical hypothyroidism, and early menarche. This disorder is associated with a microdeletion involving the elastin gene (*ELN*) at chromosome 7q11.13.

Other Causes of Hypercalcemia

Less than 1% of children with malignancies develop hypercalcemia. Mechanisms responsible for the hypercalcemia include direct tumor invasion and tumor secretion of humoral factors such as parathyroid hormone–related peptide (PTHrP). Hypercalcemia may occur with granulomatous disease or other inflammatory diseases. Prolonged immobilization can be associated with increased bone resorption and hypercalcemia. Other disorders associated with hypercalcemia include excessive vitamin D or vitamin A intake and Jansen metaphyseal chondrodysplasia.

CAUSES OF HYPOCALCEMIA

Hypoparathyroidism

Hypoparathyroidism may be congenital, surgical, autoimmune, familial, or idiopathic. Regardless of the etiology, the hallmarks of hypoparathyroidism are the same. Typical features include hypocalcemia (Fig. 9-23), hyperphosphatemia (phosphaturic effect of PTH is lost), and an inappropriately low or undetectable PTH level.

Figure 9-21 Calcium and phosphorus homeostasis. **A,** Calcium homeostasis. Intestinal calcium absorption occurs mostly in the duodenum and jejunum and is regulated by a magnesium-dependent ATPase. The primary regulatory site for calcium reabsorption in the kidneys is the distal tubule. Calcitriol [1,25(OH)₂D₃] increases circulating calcium by stimulating intestinal and renal absorption and enhancing bone resorption. Parathyroid hormone (PTH) increases circulating calcium by stimulating renal absorption and bone resorption. PTH also stimulates intestinal absorption indirectly by increasing the synthesis of calcitriol. **B,** Phosphorus homeostasis. Intestinal phosphorus absorption occurs mostly in the duodenum and jejunum; most of its renal reabsorption occurs in the proximal tubule. Calcitriol [1,25(OH)₂D₃] increases circulating calcium by stimulating intestinal absorption and bone resorption. Despite its effect on bone resorption, PTH overall decreases serum phosphorus as it also suppresses renal reabsorption.

The DiGeorge syndrome is a heterogeneous developmental field defect characterized by dysmorphic features, cardiac defects, immune deficiency, thymic aplasia/hypoplasia, and hypoparathyroidism. A microdeletion at chromosome 22q11.2 is the most common etiology of this syndrome. Genetic testing can confirm the microdeletion. Approximately 10% to 20% who have hypocalcemia and DiGeorge syndrome present with hypocalcemia between 0 and 3 months of age. Up to 10% of infants will present with seizures secondary to hypocalcemia. The degree of hypoparathyroidism can vary over time.

Acquired hypoparathyroidism can be due to autoimmune disease, infiltration, or trauma. Hypoparathyroidism may be one of the first manifestations of the autosomal recessive autoimmune polyglandular syndrome type 1 (APS-1) or autoimmune polyendocrinopathy–candidiasis–ectodermal dysplasia (APECED) syndrome. Other manifestations of this disorder include mucocutaneous candidiasis, autoimmune adrenal insufficiency, alopecia, pernicious anemia, chronic active hepatitis, and gonadal failure. This disorder has been associated with mutations in the autoimmune regulator gene *(AIRE)* located at chromosome 21q22.3. Infiltration of the parathyroid glands associated with metal overload (hemochromatosis, chronic transfusion therapy), malignancy, or granulomatous disease can lead to hypoparathyroidism. Mutations in mitochondrial DNA can also be associated with hypoparathyroidism.

Pseudohypoparathyroidism

Patients with Albright hereditary osteodystrophy (AHO), also known as pseudohypoparathyroidism type 1a, have a distinct phenotype with a round facies, short stature, obesity, skin hyperpigmentation, subcutaneous calcifications, and a short thick neck (Fig. 9-24, *A*). Shortening of the metacarpals and metatarsals is common, especially for the fourth digit (Fig. 9-24, *B* and *C*). AHO results from loss-of-function mutations in Gₛ-alpha subunit (GNAS1) gene, which maps to chromosome 20q13.3. AHO should be suspected in a short child with hypocalcemia and a history of similarly affected family members. Affected patients have hypocalcemia, hyperphosphatemia, and extremely elevated PTH values. Because *GNAS1* is an imprinted gene, the phenotype depends on the parental origin of the affected allele. When the maternal allele carries the mutation, the child typically has the phenotype of AHO and hypoparathyroidism. When the paternal allele carries the mutation, the child usually manifests only AHO (pseudopseudohypoparathyroidism). Resistance to other hormones utilizing *GNAS1*, such as TSH, gonadotropins, and ADH, may be observed.

Vitamin D–deficient Rickets

Vitamin D deficiency may result from inadequate sunlight exposure, inadequate nutrition, and/or malabsorption. The term *vitamin D* refers to vitamin D₂ (ergocalciferol), which originates in plants, and vitamin D₃ (cholecalciferol), which originates in the body. Drugs that activate the catabolism of vitamin D, such as phenytoin and phenobarbital, can also worsen vitamin D deficiency in individuals with baseline marginal vitamin D stores. Vitamin D deficiency should be suspected in children with poor linear growth; delayed walking secondary to muscle weakness; and bone pain, hypotonia,

Hypercalcemia

```
                    ┌─────────────────────┐
                    │      History        │
                    │      Newborn        │
                    │ Maternal hypocalcemia│
                    │   Immobilization    │
                    │     Malignancy      │
                    │  Williams syndrome  │
                    └─────────────────────┘
```

Normal or increased parathyroid hormone → Urinary fractional calcium excretion → <0.01 → Familial hypocalciuric hypercalcemia / Neonatal severe primary hyperparathyroidism; >0.01 → Primary hyperparathyroidism / Bartter syndrome

Decreased parathyroid hormone → Parathyroid hormone–related peptide → Increased → Malignancy / HIV; Normal/Low → 25(OH)–D → Increased → Vitamin D intoxication

Figure 9-22 Hypercalcemia. Initial approach to the child with hypercalcemia.

Hypocalcemia

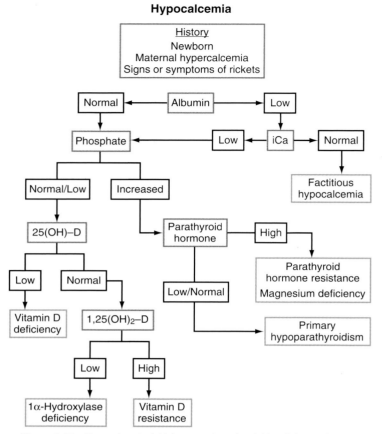

Figure 9-23 Hypocalcemia. Initial approach to the child with hypocalcemia.

and anorexia. Clinical manifestations of rickets in ambulatory infants and children include genu varum or genu valgum (bowed legs and "knock knees," respectively) and metaphyseal flaring (widening) (Fig. 9-25, *A*); prominence of the costochondral junctions (rachitic rosary) (Fig. 9-25, *B*); indentation of the lower anterior thoracic wall (Harrison groove); frontal bossing; and, occasionally, craniotabes. Darkly pigmented and exclusively breastfed infants and children who have limited exposure to sunlight are particularly prone to developing vitamin D deficiency.

Vitamin D deficiency may also be the consequence of intestinal malabsorptive disorders such as celiac disease, biliary obstruction, gastric resection, cystic fibrosis, or pancreatic insufficiency. In the majority of infants and children with rickets, total calcium levels are usually borderline-normal or low; phosphate levels are low. Alkaline phosphatase activity

and PTH concentrations are increased. Determination of 25-hydroxyvitamin D concentrations provides the best index regarding vitamin D nutritional status.

To become biologically active, vitamin D undergoes two hydroxylation steps. The first step, 25-hydroxylation, occurs in the liver to generate 25-hydroxyvitamin D. The second step, 1α-hydroxylation, takes place in the kidney to generate 1,25-dihydroxyvitamin D. The biologic actions of vitamin D are mediated by the vitamin D receptor, which is a member of the steroid/thyroid hormone nuclear receptor family.

Elucidation of the pathways involved in vitamin D metabolism has identified the molecular basis for rickets unresponsive to pharmacologic vitamin D treatment. Vitamin D–dependent rickets type 1 is an autosomal recessive disorder associated with mutations in the 1α-hydroxylase gene *(CYP27B1)*. Vitamin D–dependent rickets type 2A is associated with loss-of-function mutations in the vitamin D receptor gene *(VDR);* this form may be associated with alopecia. Additional features include growth retardation, alopecia, and extremely elevated calcitriol and PTH concentrations. Laboratory data seen in rickets are listed in Table 9-5.

CAUSES OF HYPOPHOSPHATEMIA

Phosphate, an abundant anion, plays major roles in bone mineralization, energy metabolism, cell signaling, and acid–base homeostasis. Phosphate concentrations are modulated by PTH, vitamin D, and phosphatonin concentrations. In general, approximately 85% to 90% of filtered phosphate is reabsorbed by the kidney.

Hypophosphatemic rickets is characterized by severe hypophosphatemia, postnatal growth retardation with short stature, genu varum, and dental anomalies. Muscle, bone, and joint pain may occur. The X-linked form of hypophosphatemic rickets is associated with genetic variants in the phosphate-regulating gene with homologies to endopeptidases on the X-chromosome gene *(PHEX)*. Autosomal recessive forms are associated with mutations in the fibroblast growth factor-23 *(FGF23)*, dentin matrix acidic phosphoprotein *(DMP1)*, and *SLC34A3* genes. FGF23 is a phosphatonin; mutations that prevent cleavage of FGF23 to inactive forms are associated with decreased renal 1α-hydroxylase activity and increased phosphate excretion.

Hypophosphatasia is an autosomal recessive metabolic bone disorder of varying severity due to loss-of-function mutations in the *TNSALP* gene. Decreased TNSALP activity leads to defective mineralization of skeletal osteoid. In addition to the radiographic findings of rickets, affected subjects have low alkaline phosphatase activity and increased urinary phosphoethanolamine excretion.

Table 9-5	Laboratory Findings in Rickets					
Type	**Calcium**	**Phosphate**	**Alkaline Phosphatase**	**25-Hydroxyvitamin D₃**	**1,25-Dihydroxyvitamin D**	**PTH**
Vitamin D deficiency						
Mild	N, ↓	N, ↓	↑	↓	N	N
Moderate	N, ↓	↓	↑↑	↓	↓, N, ↑	↑
Severe	↓	↓	↑↑	↓↓	↓	↑↑
X-linked hypophosphatemic rickets	N	↓↓	↑	N	N, ↓	N
Pseudovitamin D–deficiency rickets	↓↓	↓↓	↑↑↑	N	↓↓↓	↑↑↑

N, normal; PTH, parathyroid hormone.
From Sperling MA, editor: *Pediatric endocrinology*, ed 2, Philadelphia, 2002, WB Saunders.

Figure 9-24 Albright hereditary osteodystrophy (AHO; also known as pseudohypoparathyroidism). **A,** AHO is characterized by a round facies, short stature, and obesity, as seen in these three sisters with AHO. **B,** A short fourth metacarpal may be easily appreciated in this photograph. **C,** Radiograph of the hand illustrates the short fourth metacarpal seen in AHO. (**A** and **B,** Courtesy J. Parks, MD, Atlanta, Ga; **C,** courtesy J. Medina, Pittsburgh, Pa.)

Figure 9-25 Clinical manifestations of rickets. **A,** Genu varum ("knock knees"), metaphyseal flaring. **B,** Rachitic rosary. (Courtesy T. Thacher, MD.)

THE ADRENAL GLANDS

The adrenal gland consists of the inner adrenal medulla and the outer adrenal cortex. Cells destined to develop into the adrenal medulla have an ectodermal origin, whereas adrenal cortical cells have a mesodermal origin. At approximately 7 to 8 weeks of gestation, sympathetic cells derived from the neural crest invade the adrenal primordium; these cells will differentiate as the adrenal medulla, which is responsible for the production of epinephrine and norepinephrine.

During fetal life, the adrenal cortex consists of the fetal adrenal cortical zone, which involutes during the first year of life, and the outer definitive zone. Within the fetal zone, adrenal hormone biosynthesis is initiated early in gestation to provide DHEAS, which serves as the substrate for placental estrogen synthesis. At birth, the fetal adrenal is roughly twice the size of adult adrenals.

Postnatally, the definitive adrenal cortex develops into the adult adrenal cortex, comprising three distinct zones. The zona glomerulosa synthesizes mineralocorticoids (principally aldosterone). Mineralocorticoids influence electrolyte balance, intravascular volume, and blood pressure. The zona fasciculata synthesizes glucocorticoids (principally cortisol). The multiple biologic actions of glucocorticoids include effects on carbohydrate metabolism, immune function, and cell differentiation. The innermost zone, the zona reticularis, synthesizes the so-called adrenal androgens (principally DHEAS, DHEA, and androstenedione). The adrenal androgens do not bind to the androgen receptor, but are readily converted to more potent androgens by extraadrenal enzymes. Cholesterol is the precursor for all adrenal steroids. Most cholesterol used for steroid hormone biosynthesis is derived from dietary sources.

ACTH and cortisol secretion manifest a diurnal rhythm with the highest concentrations occurring during the early morning. This rhythm is generally established between 6 and 12 months of age. ACTH stimulates cortisol secretion, which then inhibits ACTH secretion by the anterior pituitary by negative feedback inhibition.

Adrenal Cortex

Cushing Syndrome

Cushing syndrome, the phenotype resulting from excessive glucocorticoids, can be due to either excessive endogenous or exogenous steroid exposure. Rounded facies, plethora, central obesity, impaired linear growth, fatigue, and hypertension are characteristic features of Cushing syndrome (Fig. 9-26).

Figure 9-26   Cushing syndrome. These photographs show how dramatic the changes associated with Cushing syndrome are and how rapidly they occur. **A,** Patient before the onset of Cushing syndrome. **B,** Patient 4 months after photograph in **A** was taken. Note the centripetal obesity of the trunk compared with the extremities after the onset of Cushing syndrome. **C,** Moon facies, clearly demonstrated, should raise the diagnostic index of Cushing syndrome. **D,** Buffalo hump. Excessive adipose tissue over the lower cervical and upper thoracic spine is characteristic of Cushing syndrome.

Impaired linear growth velocity is a frequent finding. Children with Cushing syndrome can be irritable. Muscle weakness and muscle wasting occur, resulting in comparatively thin extremities (Fig. 9-26, *B*). A buffalo hump (Fig. 9-26, *D*) can occur. The skin is often thin, friable, and easily bruised. Loss of bone mineral density and osteopenia/osteoporosis can occur with chronic glucocorticoid exposure. Delayed bone maturation may be noted. Some children manifest signs of excessive androgen secretion. Amenorrhea may occur among adolescent girls. Central nervous system effects can include mood swings, psychosis, and idiopathic intracranial hypertension.

Treatment with pharmacologic doses of glucocorticoids is the most common cause of Cushing syndrome in children. Endogenous Cushing syndrome may be caused by adrenal tumors, pituitary adenomas (Cushing disease), primary pigmented micronodular adrenal hyperplasia (PPNAD), or ectopic ACTH production. Cushing disease is rare in infants. PPNAD can occur sporadically, as a familial disorder, or as a feature of the Carney complex. The Carney complex is a heterogeneous disorder; its features include PPNAD, myxomas, testicular Sertoli cell and Leydig cell tumors, and thyroid tumors. One theme emerging from studies of PPNAD is that genetic variants are associated with abnormal cyclic AMP signaling, cortisol excess, and adrenal tumors. The differential findings in the specific etiology of Cushing syndrome are listed in Figure 9-27.

Measurement of simultaneous cortisol and ACTH concentrations may be helpful to document elevated cortisol concentrations. Elevated 24-hour urinary free cortisol excretion and salivary cortisol measurements are two additional tests used to confirm excessive glucocorticoid secretion. Measurement of midnight salivary cortisol concentrations may be helpful because individuals with Cushing syndrome typically manifest loss of normal cortisol diurnal variation. Some obese individuals have elevated cortisol secretion rates; correction for body surface area generally normalizes the results. Overnight, low-dose, and high-dose dexamethasone suppression tests may help confirm the diagnosis and discriminate among the potential etiologies. Most obese individuals show suppression of the morning cortisol concentration after an overnight dexamethasone stimulation test (1.25 mg of dexamethasone/m^2).

Once endogenous excessive glucocorticoid secretion is confirmed, additional studies are needed to identify the specific etiology. Computed tomography (CT) scans are recommended for the evaluation of adrenal tumors. When Cushing disease is suspected, pituitary magnetic resonance imaging is the study of choice. Because pituitary adenomas may be small, bilateral inferior petrosal sinus sampling may be necessary to localize the adenoma before surgery. Although rare among children, ectopic ACTH-secreting tumors can occur and may be occult.

Adrenal Insufficiency

Patients with primary adrenal insufficiency (Addison disease) typically present with weight loss, anorexia, wasting of subcutaneous tissue, and hyperpigmentation (Fig. 9-28, *A*). Primary adrenal insufficiency is characterized by glucocorticoid and mineralocorticoid deficiencies. There is little change seen in the overall growth rate. Frequently, the hyperpigmentation is striking and appears as bronzing of the skin, more obvious in flexor creases, in scars, and over the areolae of the nipples (Fig. 9-28, *B-D*). This is due to simultaneous secretion of ACTH and melanocyte-stimulating hormone (MSH). Vitiligo may occur as well. Frequently, patients may be weak and confused. If untreated, patients with Addison disease progressively weaken and vascular collapse ensues. The decreased circulating plasma volume is reflected by the thinned, narrow heart shadow seen on a chest radiograph (Fig. 9-28, *E*). Hyponatremia, hyperkalemia, and elevated plasma renin activity are usually found. Hypoglycemia and eosinophilia may occur.

Autoimmune destruction of the adrenal gland has now replaced tuberculosis as the most common cause of the disease. Two autoimmune polyendocrine syndromes have been characterized. The type 1 form is characterized by chronic mucocutaneous candidiasis, hypoparathyroidism, and adrenal insufficiency; it is associated with mutations in the *AIRE* gene. The type 2 form (Schmidt syndrome) is characterized by diabetes, hypothyroidism, and adrenal insufficiency.

Other causes of primary adrenal insufficiency include adrenoleukodystrophy, Wolman disease, hereditary unresponsiveness to ACTH, Allgrove syndrome, and congenital adrenal

	Normal	Adrenal tumor	Pituitary hypersecretion
Plasma cortisol diurnal rhythm	10–25 μg% rhythmic	High; no rhythm	High; no rhythm
Plasma ACTH	Normal	Low	High

Figure 9-27 The differential diagnosis of Cushing syndrome as interpreted from the dexamethasone suppression test. ACTH, adrenocorticotropic hormone. *(Modified from Williams RH: Textbook of endocrinology, ed 6. Philadelphia, 1981, WB Saunders, p. 272.)*

Figure 9-28   Addison disease. **A,** This patient shows the thin habitus and ill appearance characteristic of Addison disease. **B,** Hyperpigmentation of external genitalia. **C,** Hyperpigmentation of palms of hands. **D,** Hyperpigmentation of areolae. **E,** Microcardia is characteristically seen on chest radiograph. (*A-D, Courtesy M. New, MD, New York; E, courtesy J. Medina, Pittsburgh, Pa.*)

hypoplasia. Adrenoleukodystrophy is an X-linked peroxisomal degenerative disorder that affects the CNS and adrenal glands; plasma very long–chain fatty acid concentrations are elevated due to inhibition of normal metabolism in the peroxisome. Mutations in the peroxisome biogenesis factor-1 gene *(PEX1)* are associated with autosomal recessive forms of adrenoleukodystrophy such as Zellweger syndrome, infantile Refsum disease, and neonatal adrenoleukodystrophy.

The infantile form of Wolman disease typically presents with diarrhea, massive hepatosplenomegaly, failure to thrive, and calcification of adrenal glands; this autosomal recessive disorder is associated with mutations in the lysosomal acid lipase gene *(LIPA)* located at chromosome 10q24-q25. Loss-of-function mutations of the ACTH receptor gene *(MC2R)* present in infancy with failure to thrive, hyperpigmentation, and hypoglycemia. Mineralocorticoid secretion is normal, whereas ACTH concentrations are elevated because of ACTH unresponsiveness. Congenital adrenal hypoplasia is an

X-linked recessive disorder due to loss-of-function mutation of the DAX1 gene and can be associated with hypogonadotropic hypogonadism. Congenital adrenal hypoplasia may also occur as a contiguous gene defect in association with Duchenne muscular dystrophy and glycerol kinase deficiency. The autosomal recessive triple A syndrome is characterized by achalasia, absent lacrimation, and cortisol deficiency and is associated with mutations in the ALADIN gene. Acute adrenal insufficiency due to massive adrenal hemorrhage can occur with meningitis or traumatic births.

The clinical manifestations of secondary adrenal insufficiency are less fully expressed in individuals who have either isolated ACTH deficiencies or hypothalamic alterations in corticotropin-releasing factor (CRF) kinetics. This is because aldosterone secretion is preserved because it is primarily regulated by the renin–angiotensin system rather than ACTH. This is well demonstrated in the girl with isolated ACTH deficiency seen before and after treatment (Fig. 9-29). Although she has

Figure 9-29 Isolated adrenocorticotropic hormone (ACTH) deficiency. **A,** Young girl with isolated ACTH deficiency shows wasting and pallor rather than excessive bronzing. **B,** The same girl after therapy.

the clinical wasting associated with Addison disease, her skin is pale as opposed to bronze.

Congenital Adrenal Hyperplasia

The congenital adrenal hyperplasias (CAHs) are a group of autosomal recessive disorders characterized by impaired glucocorticoid biosynthesis. The specific symptoms and laboratory findings reflect the specific defect in steroidogenesis.

The most common form of CAH is 21-hydroxylase deficiency due to loss-of-function mutations in the 21-hydroxylase gene *(CYP21A2)* (Fig. 9-30). In this disorder, decreased glucocorticoid biosynthesis results in increased ACTH and adrenal androgen biosynthesis. The phenotype varies depending on the severity of the genetic mutation. Classic CAH occurs in approximately 1 of 16,000 births and is characterized by very elevated 17-hydroxyprogesterone (17-OHP) and androstenedione concentrations. In the most severe forms, mineralocorticoid biosynthesis is also inadequate, leading to chronic salt loss, hyponatremia, hyperkalemia, and elevated plasma renin activity.

Figure 9-30 Steroid biosynthesis pathway. Pathways for the synthesis of mineralocorticoids (aldosterone), glucocorticoids (cortisol), and androgens (testosterone) are shown. Deficiency in 21-hydroxylase activity *(CYP21A2)* prevents the conversion of 17-hydroxyprogesterone to 11-deoxycortisol, resulting in an elevation of 17-hydroxyprogesterone and shunting of precursors into the pathway for androgen biosynthesis. Androstenedione is secreted by the adrenal cortex and converted to testosterone or estradiol in the periphery. Testosterone may be converted by 5α-reductase *(SRD5A2)* to dihydrotestosterone (DHT). DOC, deoxycorticosterone. *(Courtesy K. LynShue and S. Witchel, Pittsburgh, Pa.)*

The excessive prenatal androgen biosynthesis is associated with masculinization of the external genitalia of affected female infants. Whereas affected females typically have ambiguous symmetrical external genitalia with nonpalpable gonads at birth, male infants have normal male external genitalia. Ovarian and uterine development are normal in virilized female infants. Hyperkalemia, hyponatremia, failure to thrive, and hypoglycemia, ultimately culminating in shock, ensue within 10 to 14 days of birth in the untreated infant as consequences of the severe mineralocorticoid and glucocorticoid deficiencies. Newborn screening for 17-OHP levels has been enormously beneficial; nevertheless, false negative screening can occur.

Those with simple virilizing 21-hydroxylase deficiency do not produce adequate amounts of cortisol but are able to make sufficient amounts of aldosterone to maintain normal electrolytes. Similar to classic CAH, females may have ambiguous genitalia, whereas affected males usually present later when signs of androgen excess develop prematurely. Children with simple virilizing CAH often present with premature pubarche, rapid growth, and advanced skeletal maturation. Affected females may have premature pubic hair and progressive clitoromegaly. Affected males often present with pubic hair, phallic enlargement, prepubertal testes, tall stature, and advanced skeletal maturation.

Patients with nonclassic 21-hydroxylase deficiency (NCAH) produce normal amounts of cortisol and aldosterone at the expense of elevated androgen production. Affected adolescent girls usually present with hirsutism, oligomenorrhea, and acne. Clinical features of adolescent girls with NCAH can be similar to the clinical features associated with polycystic ovary syndrome (PCOS). In some instances, ACTH stimulation testing may be necessary to distinguish between NCAH and PCOS. Males with NCAH generally are asymptomatic and are identified through family studies after diagnosis of NCAH in a female relative.

Less common forms of virilizing congenital adrenal hyperplasia are due to mutations in the 3β-hydroxysteroid dehydrogenase type 2 gene (HSD3B2) and 11β-hydroxylase gene (CYP11B1). Loss-of-function mutations in the 17α-hydroxylase/17,20-lyase (CYP17) gene prevents synthesis of glucocorticoids and sex steroids. Affected females show normal female external genital development and delayed puberty, whereas affected males are undervirilized at birth; elevated mineralocorticoid concentrations can be associated with hypertension. Congenital lipoid adrenal hyperplasia is characterized by inadequate virilization of affected male features, adrenal insufficiency presenting in the late neonatal period, and lipoid hyperplasia of the adrenal glands. This form of congenital adrenal hyperplasia is due to mutations in the steroidogenic acute regulatory protein (StAR) gene.

Adrenal Medulla

Pheochromocytoma

Pheochromocytomas and paragangliomas are rare catecholamine-secreting tumors derived from neural crest chromaffin cells. When located within the adrenal medulla, the tumors are pheochromocytomas. Extraadrenal tumors arising from both sympathetic and parasympathetic paraganglia are paragangliomas. Clinical manifestations result from excessive catecholamine secretion from the tumor. These catecholamines include norepinephrine, epinephrine, and rarely dopamine. Symptoms may include headache, diaphoresis, palpitations, tremor, nausea, weakness, anxiety, and weight loss. Patients may present with hypertension, which may be episodic. Altered mental status, orthostatic hypotension, syncope, or cardiac arrhythmias may occur.

Pheochromocytoma may occur in certain familial syndromes, including multiple endocrine neoplasia (MEN) 2A and 2B, neurofibromatosis type 1, and von Hippel-Lindau (VHL) syndrome. MEN 2A, also known as Sipple syndrome, and MEN 2B show autosomal dominant inheritance and occur secondary to mutations in the RET proto-oncogene. Because medullary carcinoma of the thyroid is common in MEN 2, genetic screening to identify high-risk individuals is beneficial. In those suspected of having a pheochromocytoma, fractionated plasma metanephrines and a 24-hour urinary collection for epinephrine, norepinephrine, dopamine, and their metabolites (homovanillic acid, normetanephrine, and metanephrine) can be measured.

SEXUAL DIFFERENTIATION

The process of sexual differentiation begins early in gestation and depends on the regulated expression of specific genes and interactions of specific gene products. In the usual situation, the undifferentiated gonad and related structures develop into internal and external genitalia according to chromosomal sex (Fig. 9-31). The SRY gene, located on the short arm of the Y chromosome, plays a major role in testicular differentiation by promoting differentiation of Sertoli cells. As anticipated, mutations in the SRY gene are associated with male-to-female sex reversal. Through investigation of patients with aberrant sexual differentiation, other genes involved in this process have been identified. Campomelic dwarfism and 46,XY sex reversal are associated with mutations in the SOX9 gene. Denys-Drash syndrome, due to mutations in the WT1 gene, is characterized by Wilms tumor, nephropathy, and 46,XY sex reversal.

The child with ambiguous genitalia must be evaluated promptly. In speaking with the parents, the child should be referred to as "the baby" and not as he, she, or it. An interdisciplinary approach including a pediatric endocrinologist, pediatric urologist/pediatric surgeon, and psychologist/social worker with expertise in this area can be helpful.

The physical examination of the child directs selection of the appropriate laboratory studies to confirm a specific diagnosis. Diagnoses for disorders of sex development (DSD) can be classified as XY DSD, XX DSD, and sex chromosome DSD. The external genitalia should be carefully examined to determine whether gonads are palpable. The magnitude of virilization and position of the urethral meatus should be noted. Asymmetrical external genitalia are often associated with 45,X/46,XY sex chromosome DSD (formerly known as mixed gonadal dysgenesis) (Fig. 9-32). Symmetrical external genitalia with nonpalpable gonads suggest a virilized XX fetus with CAH (see the section Congenital Adrenal Hyperplasia, earlier); the diagnosis of 21-hydroxylase deficiency is confirmed by elevated 17-hydroxyprogesterone measurement. Other disorders associated with virilization of female fetuses include congenital adrenal hyperplasia due to 11β-hydroxylase or 3β-hydroxysteroid dehydrogenase deficiency. Placental aromatase deficiency due to mutations in the aromatase gene (CYP19) is associated with virilization of female fetuses and maternal virilization during pregnancy.

Symmetrical genital development with palpable gonads suggests incomplete male sexual differentiation. Diagnostic entities include Leydig cell hypoplasia due to LH receptor mutations, inborn errors of testosterone biosynthesis due to mutations in steroidogenic enzyme genes, or androgen insensitivity. Enzyme deficiencies associated with incomplete virilization of a male fetus include 3β-hydroxysteroid dehydrogenase, 17α-hydroxylase/17-20 lyase, 5α-reductase, 17-hydroyxsteroid dehydrogenase, and congenital lipoid adrenal hyperplasia secondary to mutations in the HSD3B2, CYP17, SRD5A2, HSD17B3, and StAR genes, respectively.

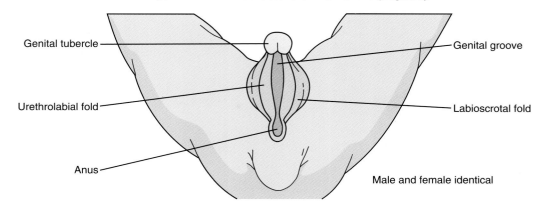

Sexual appearance of fetus at second to third month of pregnancy

Genital tubercle

Genital groove

Urethrolabial fold

Labioscrotal fold

Anus

Male and female identical

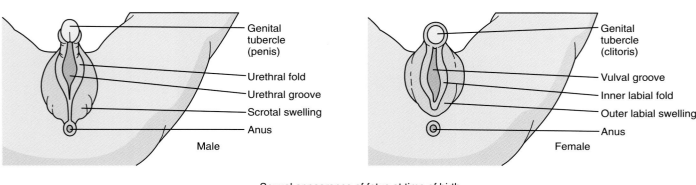

Sexual appearance of fetus at third to fourth month of pregnancy

Genital tubercle (penis)

Urethral fold

Urethral groove

Scrotal swelling

Anus

Male

Genital tubercle (clitoris)

Vulval groove

Inner labial fold

Outer labial swelling

Anus

Female

Sexual appearance of fetus at time of birth

Penis

Urethral raphe (joining line of urethral fold)

Scrotal raphe (joining line of scrotal swelling)

Scrotum

Anus

Male

Clitoris

Urethral opening

Labia minora

Labia majora

Vaginal opening

Anus

Female

Figure 9-31 Normal sexual differentiation. Schematic drawing demonstrating differentiation of normal male and female genitalia during embryogenesis.

Smith-Lemli-Opitz syndrome, an autosomal recessive disorder characterized by multiple malformations including urogenital anomalies, mental retardation, cleft palate, and developmental delay, is due to mutations in the 7-dehydrocholesterol reductase *(DHCR7)* gene. Genital ambiguity associated with craniosynostosis, midface hypoplasia, radiohumeral synostosis, and glucocorticoid deficiency may be secondary to mutations in the cytochrome P450 oxidoreductase gene *(POR)*; the skeletal dysplasia is also known as the Antley-Bixler syndrome. The phenotype associated with ovotesticular disorder can range from slightly virilized female to almost fully virilized male; this disorder is defined by the presence of ovarian tissues with follicles and testicular tissue with seminiferous cords.

Determinations of LH, FSH, 17-hydroxyprogesterone, testosterone, and dihydrotestosterone in the neonatal period are helpful because the hypothalamic–pituitary–gonadal axis is active. In complete androgen insensitivity due to loss-of-function mutations in the androgen receptor gene, external genital development appears to be female. Labial or inguinal gonads may be palpable, and uterine structures are absent.

Persistent müllerian duct syndrome is characterized by persistence of müllerian structures in an otherwise normal 46,XY male infant. Affected infants may present with cryptorchidism or transverse testicular ectopia. This disorder can be due to mutations in the anti-müllerian hormone gene *(AMH)* or the gene for its receptor *(AMHRII)*.

Some children born with anatomic variants, such as agenesis of the phallus, penoscrotal transposition, and exstrophy of the bladder (Fig. 9-33), may have neither a detectable endocrine nor biochemical defect but likely represent developmental anomalies.

Cryptorchidism

During embryogenesis, the testes migrate from their original location near the kidney through the abdomen and descend into the scrotum. Cryptorchidism, or failure of the testes to descend into the scrotum, occurs in approximately 3% of infant males. Treatment of cryptorchidism is usually delayed until 6 to 12 months of age to allow the testicle to descend spontaneously. If there is failure of descent, an orchiopexy is

Figure 9-32   Ambiguous genitalia. These cases include a true hermaphrodite **(A)** and congenital virilizing adrenal hyperplasia **(B-E)**. *(B-D, Courtesy D. Becker, MD, Pittsburgh, Pa.)*

performed. A cryptorchid testicle may be intrinsically abnormal and is more likely to undergo malignant transformation. Although surgical intervention may not completely alter the risk of malignancy, placing the testicle in its proper location allows for earlier detection of a suspicious mass.

PRECOCIOUS PUBERTY

A diagnosis of precocious or early development may be made if sexual maturation begins before age 8 years for girls, as evidenced by breast development, and before age 9 years for boys, as evidenced by testicular enlargement. The medical history should focus on the temporal sequence of the pubertal changes. Clinical features of androgen and estrogen effects should be noted during the physical examination. Gonadotropin-dependent precocious puberty, also known as central precocious puberty, is marked by a premature activation of the hypothalamic–pituitary–gonadal (HPG) axis. In girls, the causes of isosexual precocity (development along lines of the same sex), are related to alterations in gonadal or CNS function. Gonadotropin-dependent precocious puberty follows an early onset of pulsatile LH and FSH secretion and the subsequent response of the ovary. Hypothalamic hamartomas are composed of structurally abnormal nervous system tissue and may be associated with GnRH-dependent precocious puberty. Gelastic seizures can be associated with hypothalamic hamartomas and precocious puberty. Intracranial neoplasms are more commonly associated with precocious puberty in boys as compared with girls.

In GnRH-independent forms of precocious puberty, there is an increased production of gonadal steroids. This leads to physical changes of puberty, in the absence of activation of the HPG axis. McCune-Albright syndrome, characterized by irregular café-au-lait spots (Fig. 9-34, *A*), polyostotic fibrous dysplasia (Fig. 9-34, *B*), and sexual precocity, is one example of a GnRH-independent cause of precocious puberty. McCune-Albright syndrome is due to a somatic activating mutation of the gene encoding the α subunit of G protein receptor, which is located at chromosome 20q13.2. Other endocrine manifestations include gigantism, hyperprolactinemia, hyperthyroidism, and hyperparathyroidism.

Gonadal or adrenal neoplasms secreting sex steroids, such as Leydig cell tumors in boys, are rare causes of precocious puberty. In boys, human chorionic gonadotropin (hCG)–secreting tumors can also be a cause of isosexual precocity. Familial male-limited precocious puberty or testotoxicosis is characterized by premature testicular testosterone production, testicular enlargement, and precocious puberty. It is due to constitutively active mutations of the LH receptor gene. Long-standing and severe primary hypothyroidism in girls may be associated with isosexual precocity, given the partial structural homology between thyrotropin (TSH) and gonadotropins.

Premature Thelarche

Premature thelarche is a transient and self-limiting condition defined by the early onset of isolated breast development. Typically, premature thelarche develops during the first or

Figure 9-35   Premature thelarche. Isolated bilateral breast enlargement in a toddler with premature thelarche.

Figure 9-33   Agenesis of the phallus. Rare developmental anomaly with a normal male karyotype. *(Courtesy D. Becker, MD, Pittsburgh, Pa.)*

second year of life without any other signs of puberty. The breast tissue may appear unilaterally or bilaterally and may regress or persist (Fig. 9-35). Other features of pubertal development, including growth acceleration and pubic hair development, are absent. Hence, premature thelarche is a diagnosis of exclusion and cannot be made in the presence or progression of other pubertal signs. The ingestion of exogenous estrogens, such as oral contraceptives, should always be suspected in cases of breast enlargement. Premature thelarche must be differentiated from other forms of progressive precocious

puberty. Breast enlargement secondary to maternal hormones may occur in either sex in the immediate neonatal period. The etiology of premature thelarche is unclear; in some instances, activating mutations of the *GNAS1* gene encoding the α subunit of the G_s protein have been described in the absence of other elements of McCune-Albright syndrome.

Premature Pubarche

The development of pubic hair before 8 years of age in girls and 9.5 years of age in boys is considered to be premature (Fig. 9-36). Associated findings may include axillary hair, adult-type body odor, and acne. Diagnostic considerations include premature adrenarche due to premature adrenal pubertal maturation or late-onset congenital adrenal hyperplasia (CAH).

Figure 9-34   McCune-Albright syndrome. **A,** Irregular café-au-lait pigmentation over right anterior chest, shoulder, and right arm. **B,** Polyostotic fibrous dysplasia. Multiple areas of fibrous dysplasia, most commonly found in long bones and pelvis. (**A,** *Courtesy the National Institutes of Health, Bethesda, Md.)*

Figure 9-36   Premature adrenarche. Pubic hair development in a prepubertal girl with premature adrenarche.

Androgen-secreting adrenal or gonadal tumors are extremely rare. Although advanced skeletal maturation is more common in CAH, ACTH stimulation tests are often necessary to distinguish late-onset CAH from premature adrenarche. To diagnose late-onset CAH, the ACTH-stimulated 17-hydroxyprogesterone value is typically greater than 1500 ng/dL. In children with premature adrenarche, adrenal steroid hormone concentrations may be elevated for chronologic age but are normal for the degree of pubic hair development. For some girls, premature adrenarche heralds subsequent development of polycystic ovary syndrome in adolescence. Polycystic ovary syndrome is characterized by oligorrhea/amenorrhea, chronic anovulation, and hyperandrogenism.

DELAYED PUBERTY

Delayed puberty is defined in girls by the absence of breast development past the age of 12 years and in boys by the lack of testicular enlargement past the age of 13 years. A common cause of delayed puberty, especially in boys, is constitutional delay, which refers to a normal variant of the timing of puberty. Disorders of puberty can be classified as central (hypothalamic or pituitary) or as gonadal in origin. Kallmann syndrome refers to hypothalamic hypogonadism associated with anosmia due to impaired migration of GnRH and olfactory neurons; this form is often due to mutations in the *KAL1* gene located on the X chromosome. Hypothalamic hypogonadism with normal sense of smell is considered as idiopathic hypogonadotropic hypogonadism; autosomal recessive inheritance has been described.

Acquired gonadotropin deficiency can be due to trauma, neoplasms, infiltrative disorders, hyperprolactinemia, or chronic illness. Anorexia nervosa, cystic fibrosis, and sickle cell anemia may be associated with delayed puberty. Turner syndrome and Klinefelter syndrome are chromosomal disorders associated with gonadal failure. Trauma, chemotherapy, and radiation therapy are additional causes of pituitary and/or gonadal failure. Other disorders associated with delayed puberty include Prader-Willi, Noonan, CHARGE (*c*oloboma of the eye, *h*eart defects, *a*tresia of the nasal choanae, *r*etardation of growth and/or development, *g*enital and/or urinary abnormalities, and *e*ar abnormalities and deafness), and Bardet-Biedl syndromes.

Androgen insensitivity occurs secondary to mutations in the androgen receptor gene, which is located at Xq11-q12. Androgen action is essential for retention of wolffian duct derivatives, development of the prostate, and differentiation of male external genitalia. Common clinical presenting features of complete androgen insensitivity include inguinal or labial masses in an otherwise normal-appearing female infant or primary amenorrhea in an adolescent girl. In all instances, the karyotype is 46,XY.

Patients with 17-hydroxylase deficiency have mutations in the 17α-hydroxylase/17,20-lyase gene *(CYP17)* that encodes the P450c17 enzyme. This enzyme is essential for the production of cortisol and sex steroids (see Fig. 9-30). In classic 17-hydroxylase deficiency, patients with both XX and XY karyotypes are phenotypic females and both present with lack of secondary sexual development.

Mutations have been identified in association with syndromes involving dysgenesis of the müllerian or wolffian ducts, gonads, kidneys, and adrenal glands. The Wilms tumor-suppressor gene *(WT1)* is essential for both gonadal and renal formation. The SF-1 (steroidogenic factor-1) and DAX1 (duplicated in adrenal hypoplasia congenital on the X chromosome) proteins are essential for gonadal and adrenal differentiation. *SOX9* and *SRY* are two genes important in testicular differentiation. Individuals with partial or mixed gonadal dysgenesis usually present with asymmetrical genital ambiguity. Older children often present with infantile sexual characteristics, and girls may present with primary amenorrhea.

TURNER SYNDROME

Turner syndrome, due to structural or numeric aberrations of the X chromosomes, should be suspected in any short female. Typically, girls with Turner syndrome have short stature and delayed puberty due to gonadal failure. Some of the clinical presentations of Turner syndrome are shown in the pictures of young women reported in the original article by Turner (Fig. 9-37, *A* and *B*). The wide carrying angle (cubitus valgus), shieldlike chest, and webbed neck may be easily appreciated.

Figure 9-37   Turner syndrome. **A,** Turner used this photograph in 1938 to describe the syndrome that bears his name. This girl exhibits characteristic features of Turner syndrome including a webbed neck, broad chest, marked cubitus valgus, and low-set ears. **B,** Note the clinical heterogeneity within the syndrome.

Table 9-6	Common Clinical Findings in Turner Syndrome

Skeletal Growth Disturbances	*Renal Anomalies*
Short stature	Collecting system anomalies
Short neck	Horseshoe kidney
Abnormal upper-to-lower segment ratio	*Miscellaneous Defects*
Cubitus valgus	Strabismus
Short fourth metacarpals	Ptosis
Madelung deformity	Multiple pigmented nevi
Scoliosis	Selective impairment in nonverbal skills
Genu valgum	Visual–spatial organization skills
Characteristic facies—micrognathia, high-arched palate	Neurosensory hearing loss
Lymphatic Obstruction	Middle ear effusions/chronic otitis media
Webbed neck	Decreased bone mineral density
Low posterior hairline	*Associated Disorders*
Rotated ears	Hypothyroidism
Edema of hands, feet	Alopecia
Nail dysplasia	Vitiligo
Characteristic dermatographics	Celiac disease
Ovarian Function	Crohn disease
Delayed puberty	Carbohydrate intolerance
Gonadal failure	
Infertility	
Gonadoblastoma	
Cardiovascular Anomalies	
Bicuspid aortic valve	
Coarctation of the aorta	
Partial anomalous pulmonary venous connection	
Aortic dissection	
Hypertension	

Adapted from Davenport ML: Approach to the patient with Turner syndrome, *J Clin Endocrinol Metab* 95:1487-1495, 2010.

Figure 9-38 Turner syndrome growth curve. Normal female growth percentiles from the National Center for Health Statistics *(dotted lines)* and Turner syndrome growth curves *(solid lines)* are indicated. Pretreatment *(open circles)* and posttreatment *(solid circles)* heights of girls with Turner syndrome who received growth hormone treatment are illustrated. Girls with Turner syndrome were monitored for a total of 8.8 ± 1.4 years in the group receiving GH alone, to a mean age of 18.0 ± 2.2 years. *(Courtesy of Rosenfeld RG, Attie KM, Frane J, et al: Growth hormone therapy of Turner's syndrome: beneficial effect on adult height,* J Pediatr *132:319-324, 1998. Permission for use given by Elsevier Limited, Kidlington, Oxford, UK.)*

A more comprehensive list of physical findings in patients with Turner syndrome is listed in Table 9-6 and at the Turner Syndrome Society website (available online at http://www.turnersyndrome.org). It is important to evaluate for cardiac and renal anomalies. Turner syndrome can be associated with left-sided cardiovascular malformations of varying severity including aortic valve stenosis, aortic coarctation, aortic dilation, and rupture. At the time of diagnosis, all girls should be evaluated by a cardiologist with expertise in congenital heart disease. Imaging studies, echocardiography, and magnetic resonance imaging should be performed. The clinical features, especially among girls with mosaic forms of Turner syndrome, can be quite variable. Peripheral blood karyotype is often diagnostic in a clinical picture suggestive of Turner syndrome. In some instances, the karyotype of fibroblasts from a skin biopsy may be helpful to confirm a suspected diagnosis. GH treatment appears to significantly augment ultimate adult growth in Turner syndrome. A growth chart for untreated girls with this syndrome is shown in Figure 9-38.

KLINEFELTER SYNDROME

Boys with Klinefelter syndrome have a 47,XXY karyotype. With puberty, the testes are noted to be small and firm. Gynecomastia and neurobehavioral difficulties are common. Clinical features include eunuchoid body proportions with tall stature and long limbs, sparse facial hair, and small penis (see Chapter 1, Fig. 1-29). Laboratory evaluation shows elevated gonadotropin concentrations, low testosterone concentrations, and decreased sperm count. For a list of other syndromes associated with endocrine dysfunction, see Table 9-7.

DIABETES MELLITUS

Diabetes mellitus represents one of the most common chronic diseases seen by the pediatric endocrinologist. There are several forms of diabetes mellitus including type 1 diabetes (insulin-dependent diabetes mellitus, IDDM), type 2 diabetes (non–insulin-dependent diabetes mellitus, NIDDM), cystic fibrosis–related diabetes (CFRDM), drug-induced diabetes (secondary to steroids, immunosuppressive agents), monogenic forms of diabetes (maturity-onset diabetes of the young, MODY), neonatal diabetes, and ketosis-prone type 2 diabetes ("Flatbush diabetes").

Type 1A diabetes (T1DM) refers to autoimmune insulin deficiency diabetes, which is typically characterized by relatively acute onset associated with polydipsia, polyuria, nocturia, weight loss, glycosuria, and hyperglycemia. The incidence of type 2 diabetes (T2DM) has increased among American youth, especially among native American, Hispanic, and African-American youth. Individuals with T2DM manifest insulin resistance, obesity, hypertension, and dyslipidemia in addition to hyperglycemia. A cutaneous feature of insulin resistance includes acanthosis nigricans. The increased survival of children with cystic fibrosis has led to recognition of the high frequency of CFRDM.

Neonatal diabetes presents shortly after birth and can be classified into two categories: transient or permanent. Typically, infants with neonatal diabetes have low birth weights and failure to thrive. Specific genetic variants at chromosome

Table 9-7	Syndromes Associated with Endocrine Dysfunction	
Syndrome	**Clinical Features**	**Genetic Locus**
APS-1	Mucocutaneous candidiasis, hypoparathyroidism, adrenal insufficiency, ovarian failure	*AIRE* at chromosome 21q22.3
APS-2	Hypothyroidism, diabetes mellitus	
Beckwith-Wiedemann	Fetal overgrowth, hemihypertrophy, omphalocele, hepatomegaly, neonatal hypoglycemia	Duplication or deletion at chromosome 11p15.5
Denys-Drash	Ambiguous genitalia, Wilms tumor, renal failure, diffuse mesangial sclerosis, glomerulopathy, focal segmental glomerulosclerosis	*WT1* at chromosome 11p13
DiGeorge	Hypocalcemia, velocardiofacial syndrome, thymic aplasia, congenital heart disease	*TBX1* at chromosome 22q11.2
Down	Short stature, autoimmune thyroid disease, diabetes mellitus, hypogonadotropic hypogonadism	Trisomy chromosome 21
Kallmann	Hypogonadotropic hypogonadism	*KAL1, FGFR1, PROK2, PROKR2, CHD7, FGF8, KISS1, KISS1R, NKB, TACR3*
Klinefelter	Testicular failure, tall stature, hypergonadotropic hypogonadism	XXY karyotype
McCune-Albright	Precocious puberty, fibrous dysplasia, café-au-lait macules	*GNAS1* at chromosome 20q13.2
MEN 1	Hyperparathyroidism, acromegaly, hypoglycemia (Zollinger-Ellison syndrome), collagenomas	*MEN1* at chromosome 11q13
MEN 2A	Medullary thyroid carcinoma, pheochromocytoma, Hirschsprung disease	*RET* at chromosome 10q11.2
MEN 2B	Medullary thyroid carcinoma, pheochromocytoma, Hirschsprung disease, thick lips, neuromas of lips and tongue	*RET* at chromosome 10q11.2
Noonan	Short stature, triangular facies, ptosis, hypertelorism, congenital heart disease, von Willebrand	*PTPN11* at chromosome 12q24.1
Prader-Willi	Short stature, hypotonia, obesity, hypogonadotropic hypogonadism	15q12, 15q11-q13
Russell-Silver	Short stature, triangular facies, blue sclera, hypospadias	*H19* at chromosome 11p15.5; uniparental disomy at chromosome 7p11.2
Smith-Lemli-Opitz	Short stature, failure to thrive, cleft palate, congenital heart disease, hypospadias, renal anomalies	*DHCR7* at chromosome 11q12-q13
Turner	Ovarian failure, delayed puberty, streak gonads, short stature	Monosomy or isodisomy of X chromosome
von Hippel-Lindau	Retinal angiomata, pheochromocytoma, hemangioblastoma, renal cell carcinoma	*VHL* at chromosome 3p26-p25
Williams-Beuren	Short stature, supravalvular aortic stenosis, valvular aortic stenosis, developmental delay, friendly personality	Chromosome 7q11.23

APS-1, autoimmune polyglandular syndrome type 1; APS-2, autoimmune polyglandular syndrome type 2; MEN, multiple endocrine neoplasia.

6q24 have been associated with transient neonatal diabetes. Permanent neonatal diabetes can be associated with specific mutations in potassium inwardly-rectifying channel subfamily K member 11 *(KCNJ11);* glucokinase; insulin promoter factor-1 *(IPF-1);* ATP-binding cassette, subfamily C, member 8 *(ABCC8);* and insulin genes.

Before the institution of aggressive insulin therapy, children with diabetes mellitus and short stature were seen frequently in endocrine clinics and represented instances of Mauriac syndrome. This syndrome is characterized by poorly controlled diabetes, short stature, hepatomegaly, and sexual infantilism. Fortunately, it is now rare to see a child with Mauriac syndrome. In the well-controlled patient with type 1, or insulin-dependent, diabetes mellitus, the growth rate should be indistinguishable from that of a normal child. The inability to flatten the palms of the hands because of limited joint mobility and waxy thickened skin in the areas of the proximal and distal interphalangeal joints is one physical finding seen in diabetic patients. This finding is associated with poor diabetic control (Fig. 9-39). The development of specific skin lesions, such as necrobiosis lipoidica diabeticorum (Fig. 9-40) may occasionally be seen in a child with type 1 diabetes.

HYPOGLYCEMIA

Signs and symptoms of hypoglycemia reflect activation of the autonomic nervous system, epinephrine release, and central nervous system glucopenia. These signs and symptoms include lethargy, somnolence, confusion, irritability, hunger, and seizures. At the time of hypoglycemia, a "critical blood sample" should be obtained before glucose administration. Analytes to be obtained include laboratory glucose, insulin, C-peptide, bicarbonate, cortisol, growth hormone, β-hydroxybutyrate,

free fatty acids, lactate, pyruvate, ammonia, and carnitine profile. Urine for ketones and organic acids should be obtained as well.

The serum concentration of glucose, the major energy substrate, is regulated by a series of mechanisms that create a balance between substrate production and substrate use. Insulin is the mediator of substrate use. An abnormal increase in insulin leads to hypoglycemia. Substrate production, on the other hand, uses redundant but very important mechanisms that include dietary intake, followed by two sequential processes, glycogenolysis and gluconeogenesis, both of which require the use of energy provided in large part by fatty acid oxidation in the mitochondria. These processes are finely regulated and modulated by hormones that counterregulate the action of insulin, namely catecholamines, glucagon, cortisol, and growth hormone. A defect in any of these

Figure 9-39 Diabetic sclerodactyly. This patient shows an inability to flatten the palms and fingers as he presses both hands together. *(Courtesy A. Rosenbloom, MD, Gainesville, Fla.)*

Figure 9-40 Necrobiosis lipoidica diabeticorum. Characterized by the presence of yellow waxy skin lesions that exhibit reddened components. Small areas of ulceration may also be seen. *(Courtesy B. Cohen, MD, Pittsburgh, Pa.)*

Figure 9-41 Fasting hypoglycemia. Diagnostic evaluation for fasting hypoglycemia in the presence or absence of ketosis. CPT, carnitine palmitoyltransferase; GH, growth hormone; GSD, glycogen storage disease; HMG-CoA, 3-hydroxy-3-methylglutaryl-coenzyme A; LCHAD, long-chain 3-hydroxyacyl-coenzyme A dehydrogenase; MCAD, medium-chain acyl-coenzyme A dehydrogenase; SCAD, short-chain acyl-coenyzme A dehydrogenase.

substrate-enhancing processes or in the hormones that regulate them may, therefore, cause hypoglycemia.

The differential diagnosis of hypoglycemia is broad (Tables 9-8, 9-9, and 9-10). A useful classification divides hypoglycemic states into those in which ketones are absent or low and those in which ketones are present and usually elevated (Fig. 9-41). In general, nonketotic hypoglycemia should raise suspicion for a hyperinsulinemic state because insulin blocks hepatic glucose production, lipolysis, and ketogenesis. With one major exception, the presence of ketosis at the time of hypoglycemia suggests a disorder of decreased substrate production (Table 9-9). The exception is disorders of fat metabolism (see Table 9-9), in which fatty acids cannot be oxidized and ketones cannot be produced even during times of adequate endogenous insulin suppression. Hypoglycemia may occur during a period of fasting or catabolic stress (see Table 9-9) or may be iatrogenic or drug-induced such as surreptitious insulin administration (Table 9-10). Prompt diagnosis and treatment of hypoglycemia, especially recurrent or persistent hypoglycemia, is important due to the risk for subsequent neurologic impairment.

Hyperinsulinism is an important cause of hypoglycemia in infants and children. During gestation, infants of a diabetic mother may be exposed to elevated ambient glucose concentrations and compensate by increased insulin secretion. After birth, these infants may experience transient hypoglycemia due to excessive endogenous insulin secretion. Infants with intrauterine growth restriction may also develop transient hyperinsulinism. Hyperinsulinism is suspected in the neonatal period when severe hypoglycemia is refractory to treatment with intravenous administration of dextrose providing glucose infusion rates greater than 10 to 15 mg/kg/minute. Hyperinsulinism may be caused by activating mutations of enzymes, such as glucokinase and glutamate dehydrogenase, by inactivating (gain-of-function) mutations of the K-ATP channel regulating insulin secretion (*ABDD8* and *KCNJ11* genes), by exogenous administration of glucose-lowering medications such as insulin or sulfonylureas, or by an insulin-secreting

adenoma. Syndromes such as Beckwith-Wiedemann syndrome (Fig. 9-42) may also be associated with hypoglycemia in addition to macrosomia, macroglossia, omphalocele, hemihypertrophy, and embryonal tumors. In these cases, hypoglycemia has been attributed to hyperinsulinism. After Nissen fundoplication, some children develop postoperative dumping syndrome, which can be associated with postprandial reactive hypoglycemia due to excessively rapid transit of food from the stomach to the small bowel (see Table 9-8).

Table 9-9	Fasting Hypoglycemia

Increased Substrate Use

Hyperinsulinism—endogenous
    Insulinoma
    Mutations in SUR, KIR, GLUD, GCK
    Autoimmune hypoglycemia
    Infants of diabetic mothers
    Beckwith-Wiedemann syndrome
    Leprechaunism

Decreased Substrate Production

Inborn errors of carbohydrate metabolism
    Defects of gluconeogenesis
    Glycogen storage diseases

Inborn errors of protein metabolism
    Maple syrup urine disease
    Methylmalonic aciduria

Inborn errors of fat metabolism
    Systemic carnitine deficiency
    Carnitine acetyltransferase deficiency
    Hydroxymethylglutaryl-CoA lyase deficiency
    Acyl-CoA dehydrogenase deficiency

Counterregulatory hormone deficiency
    Cortisol
    Thyroid
    Glucagon
    Growth hormone
    Catecholamines

Ketotic hypoglycemia

Hepatic and renal disease

Extrapancreatic neoplasms

Reye syndrome

GCK, glucokinase; GLUD, glutamate dehydrogenase; KIR, potassium inwardly-rectifying channel; SUR, sulfonylurea receptor.

Table 9-8	Postprandial Hypoglycemia

Postgastric surgery

Diabetes mellitus

Galactosemia

Hereditary fructose intolerance

Reactive or functional hypoglycemia

Table 9-10	Drug-induced Hypoglycemia

Insulin
Oral hypoglycemic agents
Ethanol
Salicylates
Propranolol
Miscellaneous other drugs
Ackee fruit

Ketotic hypoglycemia (see Fig. 9-41) can be a manifestation of a disorder affecting substrate production (see Table 9-9). Not infrequently, young children present with ketotic hypoglycemia without an obvious cause. This has been referred to as idiopathic ketotic hypoglycemia of infancy and childhood, which usually presents between the ages of 18 months and 5 years with resolution of symptoms by age 8 to 9 years. In these cases, when a fasting challenge test is performed, the child becomes hypoglycemic within 16 hours of fasting and develops ketosis; measurement of insulin and counterregulatory hormones at the time of hypoglycemia shows appropriate physiologic responses. Relatively deficient substrate stores have been blamed for the occurrence of this condition. Hypopituitarism, glycogen storage diseases, and disorders of gluconeogenesis are additional causes of ketotic hypoglycemia. Hepatomegaly is often found in children with glycogen storage diseases.

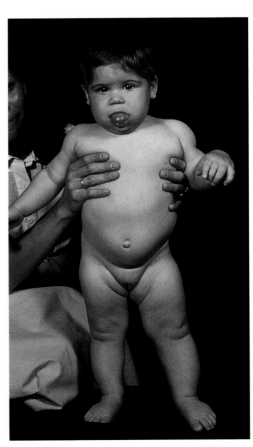

Figure 9-42 Beckwith-Wiedemann syndrome. Note hemihypertrophy on the left side, along with prominence of the tongue. *(Courtesy D. Becker, MD, Pittsburgh, Pa.)*

Table 9-11	Causes of Secondary Obesity

Endocrine Disorders
Cushing syndrome (exogenous or endogenous)
Hypothyroidism
Pseudohypoparathyroidism
Growth hormone deficiency
Type 2 diabetes mellitus
Monogenic Disorders Associated with Obesity
Leptin deficiency
Leptin receptor mutation
Pro-opiomelanocortin *(POMC)* mutation
Melanocortin receptor-4 *(MC4R)* mutation
Melanocortin receptor-3 *(MC3R)* mutation
Prohormone convertase-1 mutation
SIM-1 mutation
Obesity Associated with Mental Retardation Syndromes
Prader-Willi syndrome
Bardet-Biedel syndrome
Cohen syndrome
Alström syndrome
Carpenter syndrome
TrkB mutation
BDNF deficiency
Börjeson-Forssman-Lehmann syndrome
Central Nervous System Disorders
Hypothalamic tumor
Trauma
Inflammation
Rapid-onset obesity with hypothalamic dysfunction, hypoventilation, and autonomic dysregulation (ROHHAD) syndrome
Miscellaneous
Drug induced (e.g., risperidone, tricyclic antidepressants, steroids)
Binge-eating disorder
Bulimia nervosa

Modified from Schneider MB, Brill SR: Obesity in children and adolescents, *Pediatr Rev* 26:155-162, 2005.
    BDNF, brain-derived neurotrophic factor.

OBESITY AND ASSOCIATED ENDOCRINOPATHIES

Obesity, defined by excessive corpulence and body fat accumulation, has far-reaching long-term health consequences and is increasing at rapid rates in children. Clinicians are faced with the challenge presented by identifying children "at risk" for becoming overweight, and the diagnosis relies on the measurement of various parameters including the body mass index (see Table 9-2). Although the majority of childhood obesity cases are thought to be "exogenous" (i.e., exclusively related to excessive caloric intake), genetic syndromes, hypothalamic tumors, and endocrinopathies may also present with overweight or weight gain as the initial symptom. Causes of secondary obesity are listed in Table 9-11.

Body weight and fat mass accumulation are controlled by complex neuroendocrine circuits that regulate appetite and energy expenditure. Peripheral signals reflective of body weight and nutritional status (such as leptin secreted by adipose tissue, ghrelin produced by the stomach, or glucagon-like peptide-1 [GLP-1] secreted at the duodenum) affect appetite by regulating the release of appetite-controlling substances in the hypothalamus (orexigenic factors such as neuropeptide Y vs. anorexigenic factors such as pro-opiomelanocortin and

Table 9-12	Complications of Obesity	

Respiratory	*Endocrinologic*
Sleep apnea	Insulin resistance
Snoring	Impaired glucose tolerance
Pickwickian syndrome	Type 2 diabetes mellitus
Asthma	Polycystic ovarian syndrome
Musculoskeletal	Menstrual irregularity
Blount disease	Metabolic syndrome
Slipped capital femoral epiphysis	Hyperleptinemia
Gastrointestinal	Gynecomastia (in males)
Gallbladder disease	Premature adrenarche
Nonalcoholic fatty liver disease	*Psychological*
Cardiovascular	Depression
Dyslipidemias	Poor self-esteem
Hypertension	Eating disorders
	Social isolation

Schneider MB, Brill SR: Obesity in children and adolescents, *Pediatr Rev* 26:155-162, 2005.

melanocortin-4 receptor [MC4R]). In turn, hypothalamic neurotransmitters can regulate energy expenditure through their control of the balance between the sympathetic nervous system (aims at energy expenditure) versus the vagal system (aims at storage) with consequences on fat accumulation and body weight. The recognition of the factors involved in these control loops has changed how obesity is perceived and highlighted the contribution of inherited factors. For instance, MC4R mutations may cause up to 3% of familial and early-onset obesity cases. The recognition of theses factors has also

opened the way for novel and promising pharmacologic strategies, which can be illustrated by the recent use of GLP-1 analogues in the treatment of type 2 diabetes.

Patients who are obese are at risk for developing systemic complications as listed in Table 9-12. The combination of obesity, insulin resistance, dyslipidemia, and hypertension has been termed the "metabolic syndrome" or "syndrome X." Individuals with this syndrome are at increased risk for developing type 2 diabetes and cardiovascular disease. Adolescent girls with hyperandrogenism, irregular menses, and chronic anovulation may also have metabolic syndrome and polycystic ovary syndrome. An early sign of insulin resistance is acanthosis nigricans (Fig. 9-43), a skin finding characterized by hyperpigmented, velvety plaques most commonly seen around the neck, in the axillae, or over joints.

ROHHAD (rapid-onset obesity with hypothalamic dysfunction, hypoventilation, and autonomic dysregulation) is a recently characterized condition manifested by a series of disorders that appear in a sequential manner after apparent normality in the first 2 to 4 years of life. The earliest manifestations are related to hypothalamic dysfunction (HD) appearing at a mean age of 3 years. ROHHAD most commonly presents as rapid-onset obesity followed by alterations in water balance (hypernatremia or polydipsia) and other endocrine problems such as growth hormone deficiency, adrenal insufficiency, hypogonadotropic hypogonadism, and so on. Autonomic dysregulation (ophthalmologic manifestations, thermal dysregulation, gastrointestinal dysmotility, altered perception of pain, altered sweating, bradycardia, etc.), behavioral abnormalities (depression, flat affect, psychosis, emotional lability, etc.), and respiratory manifestations (alveolar hypoventilation, cardiorespiratory arrest, reduced carbon dioxide ventilatory response, obstructive sleep apnea, etc.), appear thereafter at mean ages of 3.6, 4.8, and 6.2 years, respectively. A genetic cause has

Figure 9-43 Acanthosis nigricans. **A** and **B,** Note the thickened skin and velvety appearance around the neck **(A)** and in the axilla **(B)** of this patient with polycystic ovary syndrome and insulin resistance. **C,** Acanthosis nigricans affecting the fingers of this patient with insulin resistance.

not been identified, but it is now clear that this is a separate entity from congenital central hypoventilation syndrome (CCHS) manifested early in the newborn period with alveolar hypoventilation and typically associated with mutations in the *PHOX2B* gene. ROHHAD should be suspected in children with obesity starting after 2 years of age in whom symptoms of autonomic dysregulation are identified. Early referral for comprehensive respiratory and endocrinologic testing and management will improve care and quality of life.

SUMMARY

As seen in the illustrations, endocrine dysfunction results in dramatic alterations in a child's phenotype. These alterations should be readily recognized and thus direct the diagnostic approach. Careful attention to the appearance of children requiring evaluation by a physician should allow early diagnosis of endocrine disorders, resulting in prompt therapeutic intervention and in restoration of the child's appearance and overall state of well-being.

Bibliography

Abrams P, Levitt Katz LE: Metabolic effects of obesity causing disease in childhood, *Curr Opin Endocrinol Diabetes Obes* 18:23–27, 2010.

Bondy CA: Turner Syndrome Study Group: Care of girls and women with Turner syndrome: A guideline of the Turner Syndrome Study Group, *J Clin Endocrinol Metab* 92:10–25, 2007.

Brown EM: Clinical lessons from the calcium-sensing receptor, *Nat Clin Pract Endocrinol Metab* 3:122–133, 2007.

Chemaitilly W, Sklar CA: Endocrine complications in long-term survivors of childhood cancers, *Endocr Relat Cancer* 17:R141–R159, 2010.

Davenport ML: Approach to the patient with Turner syndrome, *J Clin Endocrinol Metab* 95:1487–1495, 2010.

Helgeson VS, Honcharuk E, Becker D, et al: A focus on blood glucose monitoring: Relation to glycemic control and determinants of frequency, *Pediatr Diabetes* 12:25–30, 2011.

Ize-Ludlow D, Gray JA, Sperling MA, et al: Rapid-onset obesity with hypothalamic dysfunction, hypoventilation, and autonomic dysregulation presenting in childhood, *Pediatrics* 120:e179–e188, 2007.

Kappy MS, Allen DB, Geffner ME, editors: *Pediatric practice endocrinology*, New York, 2010, McGraw-Hill Medical.

Krakow D, Rimoin DL: The skeletal dysplasias, *Genet Med* 12:327–341, 2010.

Lambert SM, Vilain EJ, Kolon TF: A practical approach to ambiguous genitalia in the newborn period, *Urol Clin North Am* 37:195–205, 2010.

Lee PA, Houk CP, Ahmed SF, et al; International Consensus Conference on Intersex: International Consensus Conference on Intersex, organized by the Lawson Wilkins Pediatric Endocrine Society and the European Society for Paediatric Endocrinology: Consensus statement on management of intersex disorders, *Pediatrics* 118:e488–e500, 2006.

Lietman SA, Germain-Lee EL, Levine MA: Hypercalcemia in children and adolescents, *Curr Opin Pediatr* 22:508–515, 2010.

Lifshitz F, editor: *Pediatric endocrinology: A clinical guide*, ed 5, New York, 2007, Informa Healthcare.

Partsch CJ, Heger S, Sippell WG: Management and outcome of central precocious puberty, *Clin Endocrinol* 56:129–148, 2002.

Pescovitz OH, Eugster EA: *Pediatric endocrinology: Mechanisms, manifestations, and management*, Philadelphia, 2004, Lippincott Williams & Wilkins.

Rastogi MV, LaFranchi SH: Congenital hypothyroidism, *Orphanet J Rare Dis* 5:17, 2010.

Raymond J, LaFranchi SH: Fetal and neonatal thyroid function: Review and summary of significant new findings, *Curr Opin Endocrinol Diabetes Obes* 17:1–7, 2010.

Rivkees SA: Pediatric Graves' disease: Controversies in management, *Horm Res Paediatr* 74:305–311, 2010.

Rosenfeld RG, Attie KM, Frane J, et al: Growth hormone therapy of Turner's syndrome: Beneficial effect on adult height, *J Pediatr* 132:319–324, 1998.

Schneider MB, Brill SR: Obesity in children and adolescents, *Pediatr Rev* 26:155–162, 2005.

Semple RK, Topaloglu AK: The recent genetics of hypogonadotropic hypogonadism: Novel insight and new questions, *Clin Endocrinol* 72:427–435, 2010.

Speiser PW, Azziz R, Baskin LS, et al: Endocrine Society: Congenital adrenal hyperplasia due to steroid 21-hydroxylase deficiency: An Endocrine Society clinical practice guideline, *J Clin Endocrinol Metab* 95:4133–4160, 2010.

Sperling MA, editor: *Pediatric endocrinology*, ed 3, Philadelphia, 2008, Saunders Elsevier.

Sykiotis GP, Plummer L, Hughes VA, et al: Oligogenic basis of isolated gonadotropin-releasing hormone deficiency, *Proc Natl Acad Sci USA* 107:15140–15144, 2010.

Walvoord EC: The timing of puberty: Is it changing? Does it matter? *J Adolesc Health* 47:433–439, 2010.

Witchel SF, Azziz R: Nonclassic congenital adrenal hyperplasia, *Int J Pediatr Endocrinol* 2010:625105, 2010.

NUTRITION AND GASTROENTEROLOGY

Jeffrey A. Rudolph

Nutritional and gastrointestinal symptoms are two of the most common themes encountered in general pediatric medicine. From a global perspective, undernutrition and diarrheal disease continue to cause untold morbidity and mortality. In the developed world, nutritional assessment is at the forefront in both well-child care and the management of chronic illness. Gastrointestinal complaints are commonplace in both acute illness as well as the presenting manifestations of primary chronic gastrointestinal diseases. Because a major function of the gastrointestinal system is to provide fluid, vitamins/minerals, and the energy requirements to sustain viability and growth, the interplay between gastroenterology and nutrition is readily apparent. However, for the purposes of this chapter, nutrition and gastroenterology are divided into two sections, with a focus on the entities commonly seen by pediatric primary care physicians.

NUTRITION

Normal Infant Nutrition and Growth

The first year of life is marked by unprecedented growth when compared with any other period of life. Within the first 6 months birth weight generally doubles and by 1 year triples, with length close to doubling. As such, the normal caloric and protein requirements for growth are accordingly higher (Table 10-1). The fuel for this growth is human breast milk or formulas that have been derived to simulate the major components of breast milk. Beyond convenience and cost, there has been a growing consensus and acceptance that breast milk offers advantages that formulas to date cannot emulate (Table 10-2). Although generally considered nutritionally replete, breast milk lacks substantial amounts of vitamin D and fluoride, requiring supplementation from a multivitamin. Low amounts of vitamin K stores at birth and in breast milk have led to a standard practice of intramuscular vitamin K injection at birth. Breast milk also contains a lower amount of iron, albeit in a bioavailable form, requiring additional supplementation via a multivitamin or solid food as an infant uses the iron stores obtained in utero and reaches a physiologic nadir in the second half of the first year of life. Standard infant formulas do contain sufficient iron, vitamin K, and vitamin D and when diluted in fluoridated water are nutritionally replete. There has been a virtual explosion of the varieties of formulas available for infant feeding. Many of the "niche" formulas are designed for specific gastrointestinal illnesses and therefore are not necessary for standard infant feeding. Table 10-3 categorizes the elements of the most common variants of infant formulas used today. Although whole cow's milk and other forms of mammalian milk have features similar to human breast milk, they include a higher protein

concentration and thus higher renal solute load; the American Academy of Pediatrics recommends that their use be delayed until an infant is 12 months of age.

Normal Childhood/Adolescent Nutrition and Growth

As an infant reaches 12 months of age, the caloric requirements necessary for growth continue to diminish as the rate of growth decreases (see Table 10-1). Solid foods, typically introduced around the fourth month of life, take on the role as a major source of calories and nutrients and formula is typically replaced by whole cow's milk. Psychological and behavioral aspects of feeding from both the toddler's and caregiver's perspective take on new roles and are a common topic of discussion during health care visits. Variations of feeding patterns that do not affect growth but may lead to gastrointestinal symptoms are often recognized during this time period. Careful nutritional assessment, including dietary monitoring and simple anthropometric monitoring, continues to be essential as a marker of general health to recognize tendencies in undernutrition, overnutrition, and the recognition of both acute and chronic disease. Monitoring of nutrition continues to be important throughout childhood and adolescence as dietary habits are established, to promote overall healthy choices that remain well beyond childhood and into adult life.

Basic Monitoring of Growth and Nutrition

Growth assessment has been and continues to be commonplace in pediatric practice as both a surrogate for nutritional adequacy and general health status. Growth charts are the means by which to monitor simple anthropometric data to achieve this goal. Nationally standardized growth charts, in use since 1977, were updated in 2000 (see Chapter 9, Fig. 9-1), using data from the National Health and Nutrition Examination Survey III (NHANES III) as well as previous versions of the survey and other primary sources to obtain a percentage-based distribution of growth over a large cross-sectional population. The updated version continues to use weight for age, length/height for age, and occipital–frontal circumference for age, and has added normative data for body mass index for age after 2 years of age. The inclusion of body mass index [weight (kg)/height (m)^2] is in response to the growing epidemic of overnutrition as a measure of obesity. Other reasons for the updated changes include additional data that were previously lacking in the infant age range. As a distribution based on percentages, it should always be recognized that by definition, there will always be a population that is over the greatest isopleth (>97th percentile) and under the lowest

Table 10-1	Nutritional Requirements	
Age	**Calories (kcal/kg/d)**	**Protein (g/kg/d)**
0-6 mo	100-120	2.5-3.0
6-12 mo	90-100	2.0-2.5
1-7 yr	75-90	1.5-2.0
7-12 yr	60-75	1.5-2.0
12+ yr	30-60	1.0-1.5

isopleth (<3rd percentile). Despite this, the characteristics of growth of a child over time can be an invaluable comparative measure of what would be considered normal growth to actual growth. Growth charts have been developed for specialized populations such as infants with trisomy 21 and premature infants. Care must be taken when using these growth charts, as the numbers of patients in the sample section are less than in the standard growth charts.

Other measurements, such as triceps skinfold thickness (Fig. 10-1) and midarm circumference (Fig. 10-2), when done by a well-trained, experienced examiner can be useful when growth charts are insufficient. Examples of this would include infants with end-stage liver disease and marked ascites or vascular malformations/hypertrophy of an organ or append-age, which falsely elevates true body weight. For the great majority of infants and children, growth charts are usually sufficient to assess overall growth.

Figure 10-1   Triceps skinfold. Grasp a vertical pinch of skin and subcutaneous fat. The caliper jaw is placed over the skinfold at the midpoint mark while maintaining grasp of skinfold. Make reading to nearest 1 mm without excessive pressure. Average three readings for the final result.

Malnutrition States

Malnutrition results from an imbalance between the intake and/or absorption of calories and the consumption of calories required for growth. Obesity is the result of overnutrition and has grown to epidemic proportions in the United States and other developed nations. Obesity, in the context of both over-nutrition and hormonal imbalance, is discussed in Chapter 9. Undernutrition results from inadequate intake, absorption, or digestion of nutrients, or insufficient intake for increased metabolic needs. Careful plotting of height, weight, and body mass index as a function of time on a standard growth chart greatly aids in the diagnosis of malnutrition. The Waterlow criteria assess undernutrition by plotting weight for height, as a measure of current nutritional status, and height for age, which reflects the chronicity of the malnutrition.

A traditional classification of extreme protein energy mal-nutrition includes marasmus, kwashiorkor, and marasmic kwashiorkor. Marasmus, defined as predominantly caloric/energy deficiency, is characterized by marked emaciation; loss of subcutaneous fat and muscle; brittle, sparse hair; and poor nail growth (Fig. 10-3). Diarrhea is common as intestinal cell turnover is blunted due to lack of energy (Fig. 10-4). Secondary effects of marasmus, such as hypothermia and bradycardia, occur late in the clinical course. Marasmus is usually seen within the first year of life at the time of weaning, during famine, or at any time when there is a consistent and extreme deprivation of calories. It is the consequence of poor caloric, protein, vitamin, and mineral intake. Kwashiorkor, on the other hand, results from a diet rich in calories but lacking

Table 10-2	Advantages of Breast-feeding
Convenience/economic benefits
No sterilization required
Maternal–infant bonding
Immunologic
Less frequent hospitalizations
Innate immunity: IgA, lysozymes, epidermal growth factor, complement, nucleotides, oligosaccharides, others
Prevention of atopy
Possible protection from autoimmune diseases
Association with small but significant increase in cognitive development
Optimal absorption of nutrients
Lactoferrin: Iron
Vitamin B_{12}–binding protein
Health in later life
Decreased obesity
Decreased hypertension
Maternal health benefits

Table 10-3	Considerations in Choosing a Formula	
Carbohydrate Source		***Fat Source***
Lactose		LCT:MCT ratio
Sucrose		***Additives***
Maltodextrins		DHA/ARA
Starches		Soluble fiber/prebiotics
Protein Source		Insoluble fiber
Whole		***Other Considerations***
Human (breast milk)		Osmolality: Renal solute load
Cow's milk		Ca and PO_4 content and ratio
Soy		
Hydrolyzed		
Free amino acid		

ARA, arachidonic acid; DHA, docosahexaenoic acid; LCT:MCT ratio, long-chain to medium-chain triglyceride ratio.

Figure 10-2 Midarm circumference. **A,** Locate the midpoint of the arm with arm bent at a 90-degree angle, and tape at acromion and olecranon processes. **B,** Mark at midpoint. **C,** Make measurement at midpoint with arm hanging loosely.

protein. The initial "moon face" of kwashiorkor is often mistaken for proper nutrition. The child is often edematous, which becomes strikingly apparent after nutritional repletion (Fig. 10-5). Hepatomegaly and mental status changes are common. Skin changes in patients with kwashiorkor include hyper- or hypopigmentation with a scaly, weeping dermatitis that may ulcerate and desquamate (Fig. 10-6). The rash is often more prominent in areas that are chronically irritated (e.g., the infant's groin and areas of peripheral edema) (Fig. 10-7). In marasmic kwashiorkor, both patterns of malnutrition may develop together, resulting in a combination of clinical features.

Failure to Thrive

The term *failure to thrive* is a descriptive term used to depict inadequate weight gain over time, often used when weight for age crosses two percentile isopleths or when weight for age falls below the 3rd percentile for age. As previously stated, caution must be used when weight gain consistently tracks below the 3rd percentile, as this may reflect a normal growth pattern based on standard weight distribution patterns (Fig. 10-8). Most failure to thrive, by Waterlow criteria, is marked by decreased weight for height, with initial sparing of height for age and head circumference for age, with gradual loss in height and head circumference for age as the undernourished state continues. A more accurate description of this abnormal pattern of growth can be classified as inadequate intake, maldigestion, malabsorption, ineffective use of calories, or increased metabolic demand. Table 10-4 lists some of the more common diagnoses associated with failure to thrive. At times, the etiology can be mixed as an underlying diagnosis may be compounded by inadequate intake secondary to its presenting symptoms.

A detailed history is often helpful in narrowing the differential diagnosis. This starts with a dietary assessment including not only the type and amount of oral intake, but also specific behaviors surrounding eating, and in infants, the preparation of formula, as incorrect mixing can lead to decreased caloric intake as well as the potential for electrolyte abnormalities such as hyponatremia. Three-day diet diaries can be helpful in reviewing caloric intake, but are subject to bias after a deficiency of intake is considered. A detailed gastroenterologic review of systems including assessment of appetite, vomiting, and stool output is mandatory as is a general review of systems that may point to a chronic medical illness.

Laboratory testing can serve as (1) a diagnostic tool for defining an underlying condition, (2) a marker for the degree of malnutrition, and (3) a screening tool for specific nutrient or micronutrient deficiencies. A complete blood count can suggest an underlying inflammatory condition, identify iron deficiency or other type of anemia, and serve as a basic immunologic assessment, as infection can be a major source of morbidity in this population. Serum electrolytes may reflect abnormal losses due to diarrhea or excessive vomiting and identify acidosis from an underlying metabolic disease. A 72-hour fecal fat level or fecal pancreatic elastase may depict fat malabsorption. Fecal α_1-antitrypsin and urinalysis can aid in the diagnosis of abnormal protein losses. Analysis of stool for reducing substances may reflect carbohydrate malabsorption. Analysis of amino or organic acids in specific cases can point to metabolic disorders. Diagnosis-specific screens such as a sweat test for cystic fibrosis or tissue transglutaminase IgA antibody for celiac disease can also be useful in the patient with abnormal growth patterns. Decreases in specific proteins can be helpful as a marker of catabolism. Albumin ($t_{1/2}$, 20 to 24 days) is commonly used, although not particularly

Table 10-4	Common Etiologies of Failure to Thrive		
Inadequate Intake	**Inadequate Absorption**	**Increased Caloric Needs**
Caloric deprivation	Celiac disease	Congenital heart disease
Behavioral feeding disorders	Intestinal inflammation	Chronic pulmonary disease
Disorders of swallowing	Fat malabsorption (cystic fibrosis)	Malignancy
Vomiting/reflux	Chronic diarrhea	Renal disease
Anorexia/poor appetite		Genetic disease

Figure 10-3 Marasmus. **A,** Note the profound wasting and sparse hair. **B** and **C,** Note the wasting of subcutaneous tissue over the thorax with prominent ribs and loose skinfolds in the groin. **D** and **E,** Note the loss of subcutaneous fat, profound wasting, loose skinfolds, and sparse hair. *(Courtesy Jonathan Spector, MD, Boston, Mass.)*

Figure 10-4 Gastrointestinal tract injury associated with malnutrition. **A,** Normal jejunal mucosa with tall villi and deep crypts. **B,** Blunted villi lead to chronic diarrhea and malnutrition. Note the lack of increase in crypt depth and lymphocytic infiltrate seen in celiac disease (see Fig. 10-28) and other diseases with active cell turnover.

helpful, to depict the current nutritional status. Transferrin ($t_{1/2}$, 9 days), prealbumin ($t_{1/2}$, 2 days), and retinol-binding protein ($t_{1/2}$, 12 hours) may be more sensitive indicators, although most of these proteins can act as acute-phase proteins and thus are of limited use. Lean body mass may also be assessed by measuring 24-hour urinary creatinine compared with the standard norms for height (creatinine height index). Although laboratory tests can be helpful, they are not mandatory and the decision for testing should be derived from the history and physical examination.

Therapy for malnutrition is twofold. All attempts should be made to treat the underlying cause of the symptoms. As important, nutritional rehabilitation through the provision of sufficient calories for growth should be implemented once malnutrition is recognized. Care must be undertaken when providing nutritional rehabilitation, as one consequence of aggressive therapy is the refeeding syndrome (Table 10-5).

Specific Nutrient Deficiencies

In addition to more general malnutrition states, either excess or deficiencies of specific nutrients, vitamins, and minerals can be seen in isolation or as complicating factors of chronic disease (Table 10-6). For example, fat-soluble vitamin deficiency (vitamins A, D, E, and K) can be found with fat malabsorption or in isolation due to inadequate intake. Vitamin D is essential for normal calcium, phosphorus, and magnesium homeostasis. Vitamin D deficiency may lead to rickets, the inadequate mineralization of growing bones, and osteomalacia. There is growing evidence that it also plays a role in various physiologic functions including immune function, and deficiency has been associated with risk for osteoporosis, heart disease, various cancers, type 1 diabetes, and multiple sclerosis later in life. Classic vitamin D deficiency presents at weight-bearing age and results in poor growth, curvature of weight-bearing bones (Fig. 10-9), widening of epiphyses, and costochondral "rachitic rosary" beading (Fig. 10-10). Craniotabes, or softening of the skull, may be seen in infants. With appropriate vitamin and mineral supplementation, resolution occurs followed by bone remodeling (Fig. 10-11). Common laboratory findings are summarized in Table 9-5. Vitamin D deficiency is especially prevalent in breast-fed infants, infants with darker skin, and infants and children with decreased sun exposure. Poor absorption in children with cholestasis, Crohn disease, cystic fibrosis, and celiac disease and abnormal hydroxylation in end-stage renal disease place these populations at risk as well. In fact, the preponderance of vitamin D

Figure 10-5 Kwashiorkor. This patient has a typical edematous appearance in the periorbital area, extremities, and abdomen.

Table 10-5	Considerations in the Refeeding Syndrome

Physiologic
Rapid increase in insulin
Extracellular movement of ions to intracellular space
Sodium/water retention

Electrolyte Abnormalities
Hypophosphatemia
Hypokalemia
Hypomagnesemia
Hyponatremia
Thiamine deficiency

Monitoring
Daily electrolyte monitoring
Cardiovascular monitoring
Heart rate/blood pressure
Fluid balance

Figure 10-6   Kwashiorkor. **A** and **B,** These infants demonstrate kwashiorkor with "flaky paint" dermatosis, pigmentation changes, and pitting edema. *(Courtesy Jonathan Spector, MD, Boston, Mass.)*

deficiency without rickets places otherwise healthy children and adolescents at risk if they are not consuming the recommended daily allowance in dairy and other vitamin D–fortified foods. Whereas the recommended daily intake was 200 IU/day, the American Academy of Pediatrics has now recommended intake of 400 IU/day to prevent complications of vitamin D deficiency. Other fat-soluble vitamin deficiencies are seen in patients with fat malabsorption such as cholestatic liver disease and cystic fibrosis. Vitamin K deficiency results in prolongation of the prothrombin time and international normalized ratio (INR). PIVKA (elevations of proteins induced by vitamin K absence) may detect subclinical vitamin K deficiency, but are not done on a routine basis. Supplementation of vitamin K either orally, or, in some cases, intramuscularly is indicated in vitamin K deficiency. Vitamin A deficiency can lead to night blindness, xerophthalmia, follicular hyperkeratosis, or Bitot spots. Vitamin E deficiency is marked by absence of deep tendon reflexes and subsequent ataxia. It has also been linked to hemolysis and possible retinopathy of prematurity. Isolated deficiencies of vitamins A and E are rare and

are generally found in the context of fat-soluble vitamin malabsorption. Water-soluble vitamin deficiencies are also uncommon unless unintentionally excluded in the diet. For example, an infant fed goat's milk, instead of breast milk or a cow's milk–based formula, is at risk for folate deficiency. One notable exception is vitamin B_{12}, which requires active uptake in the terminal ileum. Patients with terminal ileum disease or resection are at particular risk of vitamin B_{12} deficiency, which results in a macrocytic anemia (see Chapter 11, Fig. 11-9), hypersegmented neutrophils (see Chapter 11, Fig. 11-10), and/or neurologic findings due to poor myelination of nerve fibers. Neurologic findings when detected early can be reversible. Supplementation is either intramuscular or (more recently) through intranasal mucosal absorption; the latter is generally reserved for adolescents and adults.

Other specific nutritional deficiencies can sporadically occur in the pediatric population, especially when receiving nontraditional diets. Patients on extremely low-fat diets or who are receiving exclusive parenteral nutrition, in which

Figure 10-7   Kwashiorkor. The rash of kwashiorkor is scaly and erythematous and may weep, especially in edematous areas.

Table 10-6	Nutritional Deficiencies with Characteristic Physical Signs
Vitamin/Mineral	**Sign/Symptom**
Calcium, phosphorus, vitamin D	Rickets/osteomalacia
Vitamin A	Night blindness, xerophthalmia, Bitot spots, follicular hyperkeratosis
Vitamin C	Scurvy: bone lesions, bleeding
Vitamin E	Hemolytic anemia, peripheral neuropathy
Vitamin K	Petechiae, ecchymoses
Thiamine (vitamin B_1)	Beriberi: heart failure, increased intracranial pressure
Niacin	Pellagra: dermatitis (sun-exposed areas)
Riboflavin (vitamin B_2)	Angular stomatitis, cheilosis
Vitamin B_6	Anemia, dermatitis, neuropathy
Vitamin B_{12}	Anemia, neuropathy
Folate	Anemia
Iron	Anemia, koilonychia
Biotin	Rash, hair loss
Essential fatty acids	Rash, coagulopathy
Zinc	Rash (acrodermatitis), growth failure, delayed sexual development, ageusia
Copper	Bone changes, hypopigmentation, anemia, neutropenia
Selenium	Cardiomyopathy (Keshan disease)

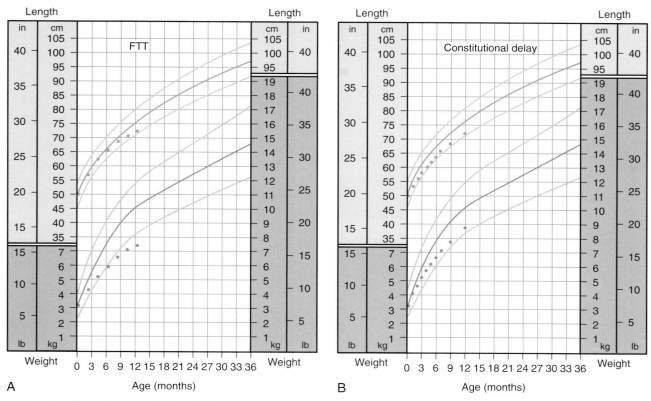

Figure 10-8 Examples of growth curves. **A,** Typical failure to thrive (FTT) with deceleration of weight gain. **B,** Slow growth but at a normal rate consistent with constitutional delay.

standard fat emulsions have been limited/omitted because of concern about cholestasis, can present with essential fatty acid deficiency. α-Linolenic acid (ω-3) and linoleic acid (ω-6) are the essential fatty acids, whereas several others may be considered conditionally essential. Symptoms include a scaly dermatitis and dull, brittle hair and nails. Diagnosis can be suggested on the basis of triene:tetraene ratios. Zinc deficiency encountered in diarrheal diseases and in burns can result in alopecia, diarrhea, and acrodermatitis. Copper, which is often reduced in the diets of patients with chronic liver disease, can present as irritability, bone pain, decreased hair pigmentation, anemia, and neutropenia (Fig. 10-12). Copper deficiency can be diagnosed by serum copper levels and depressed ceruloplasmin. A weeping dermatitis in the perioral, perianal, and eyelid area along with lethargy and malaise has been described in patients with a suspected deficiency in biotin (Fig. 10-13), a conditionally essential amino acid. Further signs and

Figure 10-10 Rickets. Infantile rickets marked by widened wrists **(A)** and enlargement of the costochondral junction ("beading") **(B).** The latter occurred as the result of a rapid growth spurt after liver transplantation.

Figure 10-9 Rickets. Hypophosphatemic rickets marked by obvious bowing of the legs.

Figure 10-11 Rickets. Radiograph of the wrist of a patient with rickets. **A,** Irregularity and widening of the epiphyses in the distal radius and ulna. **B,** With appropriate therapy, remineralization and healing occur.

symptoms of specific nutrient deficiencies can be found in Table 10-6.

GASTROENTEROLOGY

Gastrointestinal symptoms are common in pediatric practice, perhaps second only to respiratory illnesses as a reason for office visits. This section emphasizes the major complaints that bring patients with gastrointestinal (GI) disorders to medical attention, with particular coverage of entities that may be diagnosed by examination.

Reflux

Gastroesophageal reflux (GER) is defined as the passage of gastric contents into the esophagus, when intragastric pressure exceeds the forces that protect the esophagus. As it is not centrally mediated or associated with reverse peristalsis, it is not considered physiologic vomiting. Episodes are generally considered effortless and the refluxate is most often in the form of undigested food, and in infants, curdled milk. GER is a common and usually self-limited condition beginning in early infancy and resolving by 1 to 2 years of age. Symptoms generally begin immediately after feeding but may continue for several hours afterward. GER that does not resolve by 2 years of age or that presents in later childhood more often follows the pattern of adult-onset GER and persists as a chronic condition.

GER associated with one or more concurrent morbidities is often termed *gastroesophageal reflux disease* (GERD). The symptoms often associated with GERD include irritability/fussiness, heartburn, poor weight gain, upper respiratory symptoms, and wheezing (Table 10-7). Apnea and bradycardia have been associated with reflux in the preterm infant, although these episodes usually resolve as an infant reaches term. Sandifer syndrome is described as abnormal posturing and back arching in response to GER and is an uncommon manifestation. Rumination, not typically considered reflux, is the voluntary contraction of abdominal musculature that leads to episodes that manifest similar to reflux. It is generally regarded as a self-stimulating disorder and is more common in adolescence and in various behavioral disorders.

The diagnosis of GER is usually based on clinical symptoms alone. However, diagnostic evaluations may be completed to evaluate for other disorders or to aid when symptoms are not straightforward. An upper GI series is performed to eliminate anatomic abnormalities such as pyloric stenosis, esophageal stricture, duodenal web, or malrotation. Twenty-four hour esophageal pH probe measurements and, more recently, esophageal impedance manometry can confirm the presence of refluxate in the esophagus and help to correlate symptoms with actual episodes of reflux. Impedance manometry has suggested that not all episodes of reflux are acidic in nature. However, infant normative data are lacking, complicating the interpretation of results. Nuclear scintigraphy may be used in isolated cases to evaluate gastric emptying. Esophagoscopy with biopsy can assess esophagitis and can eliminate other complications when chronicity is established such as in eosinophilic or allergic esophagitis and esophageal stricture.

Therapy for GER includes frequent small feedings, maintenance of an upright position after feeds, and frequent burping in infants. This can be accomplished by elevating the head of the crib. Studies have demonstrated fewer reflux events while infants are in the prone position. Because of the known

Figure 10-12 Copper deficiency. **A,** Radiograph of a child with copper deficiency reveals irregular epiphyses with spur formation, cloaking of metaphyses, periosteal new bone formation, and osteoporosis. **B,** After 3 months of intravenous copper, the child demonstrates healing of the metaphyses.

Figure 10-13 Biotin deficiency. **A** and **B,** This child on chronic hyperalimentation developed dermatitis in the perianal, perioral, and eyelid areas along with some thinning of hair. **C** and **D,** The rash has cleared dramatically after 4 days of biotin.

increased risk of sudden infant death syndrome associated with prone positioning, supine positioning continues to be recommended for all infants despite symptoms of reflux. The "infant seat" may worsen reflux by increasing intraabdominal pressure. Thickening feedings with rice or oat cereal (1 tablespoon/ounce) has been shown to decrease the number of vomiting episodes while not affecting the reflux index in infants. Acid suppression with histamine-2 receptor antagonists and proton pump inhibitors has proved both safe and effective in treating reflux in infants and children. The use of prokinetic agents in the management of reflux is controversial and not recommended, as studies have not demonstrated their usefulness. Persistent, complicated reflux may be treated by surgical intervention, most commonly a gastric fundoplication.

Dysphagia

Dysphagia is a symptom that describes difficulty swallowing. Patients with dysphagia report the feeling of the inability to pass esophageal contents into the stomach. When the sensation is in the posterior pharynx or upper esophagus it can be considered a globus sensation. When it is present, one must consider esophageal inflammation or primary dysmotility. More common pediatric disorders associated with dysphagia or the globus sensation include reflux esophagitis with or without stricture, achalasia, eosinophilic esophagitis, and esophageal strictures secondary to caustic ingestions.

Eosinophilic esophagitis is an inflammatory disorder of the esophagus that is a common cause of dysphagia in children. The etiology of eosinophilic esophagitis is not known, although it is generally thought to be the result of an aberrant antigenic immunologic response. Although food antigens are most often suspected, any environmental antigen that traverses the esophagus can lead to its presentation. Similar to other atopic diseases, it is believed that the incidence of eosinophilic esophagitis is increasing. Symptoms can include dysphagia, feeding refusal, epigastric abdominal pain, early satiety, and even food impaction. Symptoms of reflux or esophagitis can complicate the diagnosis. In patients with reflux esophagitis who do not respond to acid suppression, the diagnosis of eosinophilic

Table 10-7	Presentations of Gastroesophageal Reflux
Regurgitation	**Behavioral**
"Spitting," rumination	Dystonic posturing
Emesis	Sandifer syndrome
Failure to thrive	**Respiratory**
Esophagitis	Wheezing, asthma
Irritability	Recurrent pneumonia
Colic	Aspiration
Hiccups	Laryngospasm
Anemia	Apnea
Hematemesis	**Neurologic**
Stricture	Seizure-like episodes
Protein-losing enteropathy	
Occult gastrointestinal blood loss	

Figure 10-14 Eosinophilic esophagitis. These endoscopic pictures of the esophagus demonstrate classic findings of eosinophilic esophagitis, including **A,** linear furrowing of the esophagus and esophageal exudates and **B,** a ringed appearance or trachealization of the esophagus. *(Courtesy Feras Alissa, MD, Pittsburgh, Pa.)*

esophagitis must be considered. The classic appearance of eosinophilic esophagitis on endoscopy is esophageal furrowing and an exudative esophagitis (Fig. 10-14, *A*). Other findings include the formation of concentric rings or "trachealization" of the esophagus (Fig. 10-14, *B*). Histology demonstrates large numbers of intraepithelial eosinophils (>15 to 20 per high-power field) and can show clustering of microabscesses, degranulation, and basal cell hyperplasia (Fig. 10-15). Peripheral eosinophilia can be seen, but is not considered an adequate marker for disease. Treatment includes dietary restriction of the offending antigen when it can be determined, high-dose proton pump inhibitor therapy, and the rapidly metabolized (topical) corticosteroids fluticasone and budesonide. Systemic corticosteroids should be considered only in the most refractory cases or when there is involvement of the stomach and beyond (i.e., eosinophilic gastroenteritis).

Achalasia is an uncommon cause of dysphagia in children often diagnosed by an esophagram (Fig. 10-16) and confirmed by esophageal manometry. Considered a primary dysmotility disorder of the esophagus, it is marked by high pressures of the lower esophageal sphincter (LES) at rest, incomplete relaxation of the LES during swallowing, and uncoordinated peristalsis of the esophageal smooth muscles. Treatment options

include esophageal dilation and/or injection of botulinum toxin into the LES. Both procedures usually need to be repeated when symptoms return. The Heller myotomy is a surgical procedure that is a more permanent treatment.

Accidental caustic ingestions in children, most often alkali in origin, can result in severe esophageal injury, which heals with fibrosis and often results in strictures (Fig. 10-17). The most common long-term symptom of an esophageal stricture is dysphagia. Repeated esophageal dilation is the initial treatment of choice. In severe cases, resection with the creation of an alternate conduit (gastric pull-up or colonic transposition) may ultimately be required. Other causes of dysphagia with or without odynophagia (pain on swallowing) include viral/fungal esophagitis, other primary disorders of dysmotility, and anastomotic stricture or dysmotility subsequent to esophageal atresia repair.

Vomiting

Vomiting is a common symptom in a variety of disorders in childhood. The causes are diverse and range from simple infections, such as streptococcal pharyngitis or acute viral

Figure 10-15 Eosinophilic esophagitis. Histologic specimen from the esophagus demonstrates numerous eosinophils in a microabscess, epithelial thickening, and basal cell hyperplasia.

Figure 10-16 Achalasia. This barium esophagram clearly demonstrates the classic findings of esophageal dilation proximal to the lower esophageal sphincter (LES) and the "bird's beak" appearance of the narrowed LES. *(Courtesy Manisha Harpavat Dave, MD, Plano, Tex; and Ryan Fischer, MD, Pittsburgh, Pa.)*

Figure 10-18 Pyloric stenosis. The giant gastric waves are best seen just after a feeding. Palpation of a gastric olive can sometimes be demonstrated on physical examination.

Figure 10-17 Caustic ingestion. This endoscopic picture of the esophagus is the result of an accidental alkaline ingestion, the most common type of ingestion to cause esophageal burns. Dysphagia and esophageal strictures requiring dilatation are common sequelae of caustic ingestions. *(Courtesy Feras Alissa, MD, Pittsburgh, Pa.)*

gastroenteritis, to more serious ailments such as central nervous system tumors. A broad differential must be considered any time vomiting is the solitary presenting symptom. This section discusses some of the more significant causes of vomiting of primary gastrointestinal illnesses.

Pyloric Stenosis

Hypertrophic pyloric stenosis is due to a narrowing of the pyloric channel secondary to hypertrophy of the pyloric musculature. The etiology of pyloric stenosis is likely multifactorial. Males, most notably first-born males, are more often affected than females, and there has been some evidence of a genetic predisposition. It most often occurs in infants that have reached term. Pyloric stenosis usually presents in infants between 1 and 2 months of age. Symptoms include forceful, projectile, nonbilious emesis, persistent hunger, and eventual weight loss. As symptoms continue, dehydration and a hypokalemic, hypochloremic metabolic alkalosis can be observed on routine laboratory tests. Giant gastric peristaltic waves and the typical firm pyloric olive may be noted on examination (Fig. 10-18). Diagnosis of pyloric stenosis is confirmed by an ultrasound examination that measures the thickness of the pyloric wall and the length of the pyloric channel (Fig. 10-19). Studies have demonstrated that ultrasound has a sensitivity and specificity of nearly 100% in diagnosing pyloric stenosis. In questionable cases, an upper GI barium study may confirm the diagnosis by demonstrating a narrow pyloric channel, called a "string sign" (Fig. 10-20). Correction of pyloric stenosis is completed after metabolic stabilization by pyloromyotomy (see Chapter 17, Fig. 17-36), which is increasingly being done via laparoscopy.

Intestinal Malrotation and Volvulus

Intestinal malrotation is the result of an incomplete rotation of the intestine during embryonic life. Intestinal malrotation causes the intestines not to be properly "fixed" at the mesentery. The resulting "stalklike" mesentery may serve as a focal point for twisting or *volvulus* of the intestine (see Chapter 17, Fig. 17-37). Volvulus presents with the sudden onset of bilious emesis and abdominal pain. Bilious emesis is a hallmark of

intestinal obstruction and should be considered a surgical emergency until proven otherwise. Plain abdominal films may demonstrate paucity of air in the abdomen except for an air bubble in the stomach and one in the duodenum. An upper gastrointestinal series is the "gold standard" for diagnosing a malrotation and volvulus. Classically, the small intestine is rotated to the right side of the abdomen and a narrowing at the site of obstruction has a corkscrew appearance (Fig. 10-21). Under normal circumstances, the C-loop of the duodenum should extend up under the antrum of the stomach and cross the midline. The C-loop of the duodenum not crossing the midline is another radiologic clue of malrotation. Malrotation with an associated volvulus is a surgical emergency, as failure to correct will lead to intestinal ischemia and result in intestinal resection of all compromised bowel.

Intestinal Obstruction

In the neonate as well as older child, there are multiple other causes of intestinal obstruction leading to vomiting. Nonbilious emesis is a feature of upper intestinal obstruction

Figure 10-19 Pyloric stenosis. This ultrasound demonstrates thickening of the pyloric wall and an elongated pyloric channel in an infant with pyloric stenosis.

Figure 10-20 Pyloric stenosis. This typical barium study in a patient with pyloric stenosis demonstrates a "stringlike" pyloric channel.

tube until resolution occurs. Bilious vomiting occurs when an obstruction occurs more distally such as in intestinal atresias. Nonanatomic causes of distal obstruction can occur in cystic fibrosis in the neonate as meconium ileus (see Chapter 16, Fig. 16-28) or as distal intestinal obstruction syndrome (Fig. 10-23), in which there is a fecal impaction at the terminal ileum. The cause of these symptoms is generally thought to be due to aberrant cystic fibrosis transmembrane conductance regulator (CFTR) function in the intestinal lumen, a driving force of intestinal secretion. For further discussion of intestinal obstruction disorders, the reader is referred to Chapter 17.

Other Causes of Vomiting

There are multiple other causes of nonobstructive vomiting that occur in the pediatric population, some of which include inflammation and subsequent pain, which are discussed in subsequent sections. Others are primarily functional disorders that lead to bloating, early satiety, and vomiting. Most are related to delayed or aberrant gastric emptying. Although there are likely multiple factors leading to poor gastric emptying, the most common entity encountered in general pediatric practice is postinfectious dysmotility syndrome. Often triggered by a virus, including Epstein-Barr virus, symptoms may persist for months but generally resolve with time. Those that do not resolve will develop into a phenotype that most resembles postinfectious irritable bowel syndrome. Cyclic vomiting is a condition that generally presents in childhood as cyclic, episodic vomiting with defined symptom-free intervals. Related to migraine headaches, cyclic vomiting usually decreases in interval frequency and resolves over time. As a diagnosis of exclusion, other pathologic entities must be evaluated for by history, physical examination, and perhaps laboratory and diagnostic evaluation.

Abdominal Pain

Abdominal pain may be the most common abdominal complaint of children visiting the pediatrician. Similar to vomiting, the differential diagnosis of abdominal pain is vast and includes intestinal disorders and pain derived from other

proximal to the duodenal biliary sphincter such as occurs in esophageal atresia and gastric/duodenal webs, stenoses, and atresias. In addition, a mass effect from an extraluminal source may lead to obstruction as can be seen in duodenal hematomas, often caused by blunt trauma to the abdomen (Fig. 10-22). In general, duodenal hematomas are managed by supportive care, sometimes including total parenteral nutrition (TPN), or the placement of a transpyloric feeding

Figure 10-21 Malrotation. **A,** An upper gastrointestinal series demonstrating malrotation with the entire small bowel on the right, never crossing the midline, and the colon on the left. **B,** The corkscrew appearance of the duodenum is seen in this patient with malrotation and midgut volvulus. *(Courtesy Stefano Bartoletti, MD, Pittsburgh, Pa.)*

Figure 10-22 Duodenal hematoma. Upper gastrointestinal series demonstrates poor flow through the duodenum **(A)** and mass effect of the hematoma displacing other loops of bowel **(B)**.

abdominal viscera; in addition, it is a general symptom in many other illnesses. Abdominal pain derived from the intestinal tract is generally caused by distention or contraction. On excluding obstruction or anatomic abnormality, it can be conveniently classified as pain derived primarily from mucosal inflammation and as functional pain for which no histologic evidence exists. As all intestinal pain is the result of distention/contraction, an overlap of the two also exists, making diagnosis even more difficult for the physician and more frustrating for the patient and family.

The term *functional gastrointestinal disorder* is used to define several chronic and recurrent gastrointestinal symptoms that do not have an identified anatomic or inflammatory component. Whereas primary dysmotility syndromes such as chronic intestinal pseudo-obstruction may broadly fit this diagnosis, functional gastrointestinal disorders are commonly

Figure 10-23 Distal intestinal obstruction syndrome. Barium enema reveals the cecal obstruction in a child with cystic fibrosis. *(Courtesy Mark Lowe, MD, Pittsburgh, Pa.)*

thought of as symptoms of pain in conjunction with normal motility. The Rome III criteria for pediatric functional gastrointestinal disorders is a symptom-based classification system used to differentiate several subgroups of functional gastrointestinal disorders. Recurrent abdominal pain, irritable bowel syndrome, and functional dyspepsia are a few examples of functional gastrointestinal disorders that cause abdominal pain.

Recurrent abdominal pain, often vague and nonspecific, affects between 10% and 20% of all school-aged children. Typically the pain is episodic, unrelated to meals, and periumbilical in location. In 1958 Apley defined recurrent abdominal pain as three or more episodes of abdominal pain over at least a 3-month time period that interferes with the child's activities of daily living. Multiple studies have demonstrated that less than 5% of these children have an organic disorder. The diagnostic criteria of irritable bowel syndrome (IBS) include abdominal pain or discomfort for at least 12 weeks in the past year along with two of the following three criteria: abdominal pain relieved by defecation, pain associated with change in stool frequency, and pain associated with change in stool form. Other symptoms that support the diagnosis of IBS include bloating, urgency, and the feeling of incomplete evacuation. Functional dyspepsia is defined as chronic or recurrent pain or discomfort located in the upper abdomen. The discomfort is often described as abdominal fullness, early satiety, bloating, belching, or nausea. The symptoms of functional dyspepsia are often aggravated with the consumption of a meal.

The causes of abdominal pain due to inflammation of the gastrointestinal tract are broad and often accompanied by other associated symptoms (Table 10-8). Although pain can be periumbilical or in multiple locations, it may be more localized. Epigastric abdominal pain due to eosinophilic esophagitis and gastroesophageal reflux are two examples discussed previously. Other common inflammatory causes of abdominal pain are discussed below.

Peptic Disease of the Gastrointestinal Tract

Peptic acid–induced gastrointestinal disease should be considered in patients with abdominal pain, especially if it is epigastric or located in the left upper quadrant. Classically described as "burning" in nature, this is not a reliable indicator. In the stomach, peptic disease can be diffuse as occurs in gastritis, isolated as in ulcer disease, or have components of both.

Table 10-8	Clues to Organic Disease in Recurrent Abdominal Pain

Weight loss

Nocturnal pain

Localized abdominal pain

Recurrent emesis

Chronic diarrhea

Heme-positive stools

Abnormal physical examination findings—clubbing, perianal skin tags, abdominal mass

Abnormal screening laboratory test results—decreased albumin, increased ESR/CRP, anemia

CRP, C-reactive protein; ESR, erythrocyte sedimentation rate.

Figure 10-24 Peptic ulcer. Gastric ulcer located in the lower curvature of the stomach. Note the grayish white base of the ulcer crater and the boggy erythematous tissue surrounding the margin of the ulcer. *(Courtesy Feras Alissa, MD, Pittsburgh, Pa; and Cary Sauer, MD, Atlanta, Ga.)*

Acid-induced gastritis tends to occur in the antrum of the stomach and is also a common location for peptic ulcers (Fig. 10-24). Peptic ulcers, a nodular antritis, and duodenal ulcers may signify *Helicobacter pylori* infection (Fig. 10-25). Other types of ulcers, most often shallow and more numerous, can be seen in systemic illnesses such as stress ulcers in critical care patients, general inflammatory conditions such as collagen vascular disease, excessive secretion of acid (Zollinger-Ellison syndrome), and drug therapy such as nonsteroidal antiinflammatory drugs (NSAIDs). Gastritis can occur in other situations, not necessarily primarily mediated by gastric acid. This can occur in eosinophilic gastroenteritis, inflammatory bowel disease, or in some cases nonpeptic irritants such as medicines or bile acids during illnesses with upper intestinal stasis. Upper endoscopy is invaluable in diagnosing gastritis and ulcer disease. Treatment usually involves acid suppression via type-2 receptor antihistamines or proton pump inhibitors. *Helicobacter pylori* infection requires treatment with additional antibiotics. Non–peptic-mediated disease requires additional treatment of the underlying condition. Gastritis that does not respond to optimal acid suppression may benefit from sucralfate.

Diarrhea

Diarrhea in the pediatric patient is most often acute and infectious in etiology. When symptoms persist for more than 2 weeks, chronicity is demonstrated. When determining the cause of diarrheal illness it is usually helpful to determine whether it is acute or chronic; likely infectious or noninfectious; inflammatory or noninflammatory; or osmotic, secretory, or mixed in nature.

Clues to the etiology of diarrhea can be found via stool examination. Stool cultures and examination for ova and parasites can reveal infectious etiologies. Most often, they are obtained after at least 1 week of symptoms, as most viral causes have improved by this time. Of note, *Giardia* infection can present as a more chronic diarrhea. Inflammatory processes can be suggested by the presence of blood in the stool and by some laboratory markers such as anemia, C-reactive protein, or the erythrocyte sedimentation rate, although normal values do not completely exclude inflammation. Fecal calprotectin has been used to mark intestinal inflammation due to inflammatory bowel disease. Fecal leukocytes may be helpful when present, but are also not a sensitive marker for inflammation. Osmotic diarrhea usually improves when the

Figure 10-25 *Helicobacter pylori* gastritis. **A,** Nodular-appearing gastric antrum consistent with *H. pylori*. **B,** Gastric biopsy with inflammatory infiltrate of plasma cells, neutrophils, and occasional eosinophils characteristic of *H. pylori* gastritis. **C,** Steiner silver stain (original magnification, ×400) demonstrates rod-shaped, spiral *H. pylori* bacteria attached to the mucosa. (**A,** *Courtesy Feras Alissa, MD, Pittsburgh, Pa.*)

suspected culprit is removed from the diet. Stool pH can decrease and reducing substances may be present with carbohydrate maldigestion and malabsorption. Random fecal fat is usually not specific for fat malabsorption, although quantitative 72-hour fecal fat can be helpful. Fecal elastase is often used as a marker of pancreatic insufficiency to support a diagnosis of steatorrhea. When stool is watery, fecal electrolytes can suggest a diagnosis of secretory, osmotic, or mixed-type diarrhea.

Malabsorptive Diarrhea

Malabsorption is a common cause of diarrheal illness due to the increased osmotic load placed on the intestine from the malabsorbed substance. When an osmotic diarrhea is suspected, and exogenous sources of osmotically active particles are excluded, malabsorption is a likely cause. One example of an osmotic diarrhea with normal gastrointestinal function is toddler's diarrhea, in which the excessive intake of simple sugars overwhelms the capacity of the normal intestine to absorb them. This type of diarrhea can also exist when non-absorbable sugars or sugar alcohols (sorbitol) are taken in excess.

Malabsorption can occur when there is a deficiency in one aspect of absorption, such as carbohydrate malabsorption in lactose intolerance or sucrose intolerance. Lactose intolerance can be diagnosed by breath test in older individuals and both forms can be detected by disaccharidase analysis of biopsy specimens obtained during endoscopy. Fat malabsorption can be a sign of pancreatic insufficiency often seen with cystic fibrosis. In cystic fibrosis, the pancreas can initially be replaced by fat (Fig. 10-26) and eventually involute.

Malabsorption can also be generalized due to underlying intestinal inflammation or lack of the appropriate surface area such as in congenital enteropathies (tufting enteropathy or microvillus inclusion disease) or the short gut syndrome. Celiac disease is caused by the autoimmune destruction of intestinal villi due to antibodies formed in response to gluten exposure and the mimicry of the gluten component gliadin to the enterocyte protein tissue transglutaminase. The resultant blunting of the intestinal villi (Fig. 10-27) is similar to that found in malnutrition (see Fig. 10-4), although there is more significant lymphocytic infiltrate and crypt hyperplasia in response to the injury. The endoscopic appearance can

Figure 10-26   Early pancreatic changes in cystic fibrosis (CF). This CT scan demonstrates a typical CF-appearing pancreas. The pancreas has been replaced by fat and appears to be absent. *(Courtesy Mark Lowe, MD, Pittsburgh, Pa.)*

initially be noted by a scalloped appearance (Fig. 10-28) and later by a parched-earth appearance as symptoms progress. The classic appearance of malabsorption due to celiac disease is similar to that of malnutrition with failure to thrive, chronic diarrhea, short stature, and wasting of extremities (Fig. 10-29). Serologic testing with tissue transglutaminase IgA antibodies is often used as a screening tool and to monitor disease progression/resolution, although endoscopy is still considered diagnostic. Resolution of symptoms occurs with the removal of gluten from the diet.

Inflammatory Diarrhea

Inflammation is a common component of diarrheal illness. Common causes of infectious diarrhea have a mild inflammatory component, whereas others such as *Clostridium difficile* colitis can show marked inflammation. Autoimmune diseases, or disorders of immune dysregulation such as celiac disease or autoimmune enteropathy, are marked by chronic-type inflammatory infiltrates. Allergic gastroenteritis is marked by inflammation that is largely eosinophilic in nature. When discussing the inflammatory diarrheas, one must include discussion of inflammatory bowel disease (IBD), generally

Figure 10-27   Celiac disease. **A,** Duodenal biopsy from a healthy child demonstrates long villi and normal duodenal architecture. **B,** Duodenal biopsy from a child with celiac disease. Note the flattened villi, lymphocytic infiltrate, and elongated crypts, which are characteristic in patients with celiac disease. *(Courtesy Sarangarajan Ranganathan, MD, Pittsburgh, Pa.)*

Figure 10-28 Celiac disease. Endoscopic picture of the duodenum demonstrates a smooth appearance and scalloping secondary to absent villi in a patient with biopsy-proven celiac disease. *(Courtesy Mark Lowe, MD, and Cary Sauer, MD, Pittsburgh, Pa.)*

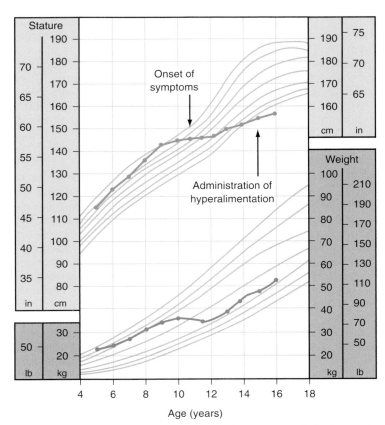

Figure 10-30 Crohn disease. This growth curve demonstrates a decline in growth velocity before onset of disease symptoms and continued poor growth through many exacerbations requiring steroid therapy.

classified as either Crohn disease or ulcerative colitis. The term *undifferentiated* or *nonspecific colitis* can also be included when the pathologic features do not fit clearly into either classification.

The symptoms of inflammatory bowel disease include abdominal pain, weight loss, chronic diarrhea, rectal bleeding, and fever. Children frequently present with growth failure or delayed pubertal development as their sole presenting sign of IBD (Fig. 10-30). Whereas clinical distinctions are at times blurred, Crohn disease is a transmural, or deep, inflammatory process, which accounts for the tendency to form strictures, fistulas, and abscesses (Fig. 10-31). Crohn disease can occur anywhere along the gastrointestinal tract and may include skip lesions. On endoscopy affected bowel has an inflamed "heaped" appearance with deep fissures, cobblestoning, and at times, pseudopolyp formation, although it can also be milder with only aphthous ulcers being apparent (Fig. 10-32).

Perianal signs including abscesses, skin tags, fistulas, and fissures most often occur with Crohn disease (Fig. 10-33). Histologically, the presence of granulomas can distinguish Crohn disease from ulcerative colitis.

Crypt abscesses are often seen in ulcerative colitis and help to distinguish this disorder from many other causes of acute colitis (Fig. 10-34). Ulcerative colitis is also confined to the large bowel. A lead pipe appearance of the colon can occasionally be seen on a plain abdominal film and demonstrated as a featureless colon on contrast enema (Fig. 10-35). Most often, contrast studies show mucosal irregularities, narrowing, or

Figure 10-29 Celiac disease. **A,** This child had a potbelly, vomiting, and weight loss as her major symptoms. Once celiac disease was confirmed, the child was placed on a gluten-free diet. Note the protruding abdomen and wasted buttocks. **B,** After 10 weeks on the diet the improvement is obvious.

Figure 10-31 Crohn disease. **A,** Segmental narrowing of the left colon. **B,** A narrow and irregular terminal ileum. **C,** Stricturing of the duodenum. **D,** Diffuse aphthous ulcers in the stomach of a patient with Crohn disease. *(Courtesy Stefano Bartoletti, MD, Pittsburgh, Pa.)*

Figure 10-32 Crohn disease, endoscopic images. **A** and **B,** Note the deep, linear, ulcerated fissure. **C,** Numerous colonic aphthous ulcers. **D,** A cobblestone appearance of the colonic mucosa.

Figure 10-33   Crohn disease. **A,** The slight raised and erythematous lesion represents a perianal abscess that eventually drained. Note a scar from a previous incision and drainage procedure. **B,** Perianal skin tags are common in Crohn disease and a good clue to diagnosis. **C,** Example of a draining perianal fistula found in a child with Crohn disease. *(Courtesy Feras Alissa, MD, Pittsburgh, Pa.)*

thumb-printing as a sign of inflammation (Fig. 10-36). The endoscopic findings can show generalized friability (Fig. 10-37) and a transition zone to normal colon can sometimes be distinguished.

There are many extraintestinal manifestations of IBD, which can involve almost any organ system. Although many occur at times of active disease, they may also occur at any time or be the presenting symptom of the disease. Osteoarthropathy (clubbing) of the nail beds may be observed in children with IBD. The earliest signs of clubbing are softening and loss of a normal angle at the base of the nail (Fig. 10-38; and see Chapter 16, Figs. 16-2 and 16-3). Many rashes accompany IBD including erythema nodosum (see Chapter 8, Fig. 8-58), erythema multiforme (see Chapter 8, Fig. 8-51), papulonecrotic lesions, and ulcerative erythematous plaques. Perhaps the most specific rash is pyoderma gangrenosum. Initial lesions are papular, then become bullous, and finally are deeply ulcerated and necrotic. The most frequent locations are the cheeks, thighs, feet, hands, legs, and inguinal regions (Fig. 10-39). Other extraintestinal manifestations of IBD include growth failure, delayed menarche, arthritis/arthralgias, ankylosing spondylitis, sacroiliitis, aphthous oral ulcers, uveitis, iritis, and sclerosing cholangitis.

Figure 10-34   Ulcerative colitis. Pathologic image of a colonic crypt abscess in a patient with ulcerative colitis.

Gastrointestinal Bleeding

Visible blood in emesis or stool is always alarming to children and their parents. On occasion, gastrointestinal bleeding is diagnosed by an iron deficiency anemia or through occult blood detection on stool examination. Blood loss in the stool with the association of pain is most often due to underlying inflammation, although larger amounts of blood can cause cramping. As a general rule, blood from an upper gastrointestinal source is black and tarry (melanotic) and becomes brighter red as the source nears the distal gastrointestinal tract. This does not necessarily apply to rapid sources of bleeding. In general, melanotic stools, coffee ground emesis, or hematemesis indicate upper gastrointestinal bleeding, proximal to the ligament of Treitz. Common causes include erosive esophagitis, pill-induced or deep isolated esophageal ulcers (Fig. 10-40), peptic ulcers (see Fig. 10-24), and the various forms of gastritis. Upper gastrointestinal bleeding can be life-threatening in certain situations including bleeding from esophageal varices due to portal hypertension (see Fig. 10-40), or with deep ulcers with exposed vessels (Dieulafoy lesions).

Bleeding from the small intestine can occur with isolated vascular malformations, inflammation, or ulcers, although this is uncommon. Meckel diverticulum presents as painless rectal bleeding due to ectopic gastric tissue leading to ulceration of the contralateral/adjacent small bowel (see Chapter 17, Figs. 17-83 and 17-85). A technetium-99m pertechnetate scan can be valuable in the diagnosis of a Meckel diverticulum (see Chapter 17, Fig. 17-84). The classic triad of colicky abdominal pain, currant jelly stools, and vomiting constitutes the manifestations of intussusception, although seen in only 20% to 40% of children on presentation. Intussusception is most commonly seen in children between the ages of 3 months and 5 years. Older children usually have a "lead point" such as a juvenile polyp, Meckel diverticulum, or thickened bowel associated with inflammation that requires further investigation (Fig. 10-41; and see Chapter 17, Figs. 17-72 to 17-76). Reduction by barium enema or air enema is both diagnostic and therapeutic and simplifies management of this disorder in most instances, although surgery is occasionally necessary. Recurrence of intussusception after reduction is seen in approximately 10% of patients. Bright blood per rectum often indicates loss from the lower gastrointestinal tract. Often, the source of bleeding is self-limited as in anal fissures (see Chapter 17, Fig. 17-78) or isolated juvenile polyps (see Chapter 17, Fig. 17-88). Polyposis syndromes can sometimes be

Figure 10-35 Ulcerative colitis. A lead pipe or featureless appearance to the colon can be suggested on a plain abdominal film **(A)** and visualized on barium enema **(B)** in a patient with ulcerative colitis. *(Courtesy Anna Furr, MD, Portland, Maine.)*

Figure 10-36 Ulcerative colitis. **A,** A narrowing and loss of haustral markings are a sign of colonic inflammation typical of ulcerative colitis. Mucosal irregularities are prominent in the right colon. **B,** Postevacuation barium enema in a patient with ulcerative colitis demonstrates narrowing and irregular borders, indicating colon inflammation.

Figure 10-37 Ulcerative colitis, endoscopic appearance. **A** and **B,** The entire colonic mucosa is inflamed, friable, and granular with obvious exudate and bleeding.

Figure 10-38   Osteoarthropathy (clubbing). Note thickening and loss of the angle at the nail bed in a child with inflammatory bowel disease (see also Chapter 16, Figs. 16-2 and 16-3).

Figure 10-39   Pyoderma gangrenosum. This is a classic, although uncommon, rash associated with inflammatory bowel disease. Initial papulopustules will coalesce to form a deep necrotic lesion.

encountered, especially when there is a strong family history for either a polyp syndrome or polyps early in life.

Persistent bleeding, rapid blood loss, or blood loss leading to anemia requires further evaluation for underlying inflammation or source. Upper and lower endoscopy, depending on the most likely source, can aid in diagnosis. The advent of capsule endoscopy can also aid in the localization of isolated bleeding in the small intestine. Common disorders causing gastrointestinal bleeding are listed in Table 10-9 (see also Chapter 17).

Constipation

Constipation is defined as a delay or difficulty in passing a bowel movement that results in pain and discomfort to the patient. Constipation is usually described as functional or anatomic in origin, although rectal inflammation can also lead to constipation symptoms. Painful defecation during toilet training, illness, or a stressful event often leads to stool-withholding behavior and avoidance of defecation. Overflow incontinence or encopresis is the result of a chronic, distal fecal impaction leading to stretching of the rectal wall and relaxation of the internal anal sphincter. Liquid stool from the proximal colon leaks around the fecal mass, resulting in encopresis. On occasion, major psychopathology is uncovered, especially in the older child, and appropriate intervention is necessary. Bladder dysfunction with urinary incontinence and low-volume/high-frequency voiding may be associated with long-standing constipation.

Examination of the child with constipation usually reveals palpable stool in the descending colon and left lower quadrant. A digital rectal examination is necessary to evaluate stool consistency, the amount of stool present in the rectum, the size of the rectum, and anal tone. A plain film of the abdomen is usually not necessary and adds little to the physical examination but can aid when a digital examination is refused (Fig. 10-42). Rectal prolapse (Fig. 10-43) can occur with excessive straining, and can be seen in association with inflammation or systemic disease such as cystic fibrosis or connective tissue disease.

Figure 10-40   Upper gastrointestinal bleeding. Examples of causes of upper gastrointestinal bleeding, or potential gastrointestinal bleeding. **A,** Erosive esophagitis. **B,** Deep esophageal ulcer. **C,** Esophageal varices. See also Figure 10-24 (peptic ulcer).

Figure 10-41 Intussusception. **A,** A "target lesion" can be seen on this ultrasound demonstrating intussusception. **B,** On occasion, an intussusception can be seen on a plain abdominal radiograph. Note the absence of air beyond the intussusception. **C,** Air enemas are used to both diagnose and reduce an intussusception. **D,** Barium outlines the intussuscepted segment before and after it is reduced. **E,** This is an example of an intussusception seen at laparotomy, necessary when reduction is not successful during a barium or air enema. **F,** A Meckel diverticulum can be a lead point for intussusception. **G,** An intestinal polyp can act as a lead point for intussusception. *(Courtesy Stefano Bartoletti, MD, and Mark Lowe, MD, Pittsburgh, Pa.)*

Table 10-9	Common Causes of Gastrointestinal Bleeding in a Child	
Upper GI Tract	**Lower GI Tract**	
Esophageal varices	Colonic polyps (isolated or polyposis syndrome)	
Pill esophagitis		
Reflux/eosinophilic esophagitis	Anal fissure	
Gastric ulcers	Hemorrhoids	
Gastritis	Intussusception	
Vascular malformations	Meckel diverticulum	
Duodenal ulcer	Colitis (IBD, allergic, infectious)	
Inflammatory bowel disease	Vascular malformations	
	Solitary rectal ulcers	

IBD, inflammatory bowel disease.

Figure 10-43 Rectal prolapse. Rectal prolapse can be seen in children with cystic fibrosis, but is also associated with excessive straining, inflammation, and connective tissue disorders. Most often prolapse self-reduces. When it does not, it requires an urgent surgical consultation. *(Courtesy Mark Lowe, MD, Pittsburgh, Pa.)*

The most commonly evaluated cause of constipation that is not functional in nature is Hirschsprung disease, most often manifesting in infancy. An unprepped barium enema radiographic study can be suggestive of Hirschsprung disease, although rectal biopsy for ganglion cells and acetylcholinesterase stain is necessary for confirmation (Fig. 10-44). In older children, rectal manometric studies may help separate organic from functional disorders. Other anatomic causes of defecation disorders present at birth include imperforate anus which can present in isolation or as part of a cloacal anomaly (see Chapter 17).

PANCREATIC DISEASE

Pancreatic disease is relatively uncommon in the pediatric population, although it can be a source of abdominal symptoms. Congenital anomalies such as annular pancreas, pancreatic divisum, and ductal abnormalities (Fig. 10-45) can be discovered serendipitously during the evaluation for abdominal pain and have been suggested to be a risk factor for pancreatitis. As discussed previously, exocrine pancreatic insufficiency is a common finding in cystic fibrosis (see Fig. 10-26) but generally results in steatorrhea and not abdominal pain.

The most common cause of acute pancreatitis in childhood is idiopathic in origin, although infectious causes, drugs, common bile duct stones, trauma, and malignancy, among other causes, have been implicated. Chronic pancreatitis or recurrent acute pancreatitis episodes can be associated with hereditary forms, especially in the presence of a positive family history. Common presenting symptoms are abdominal pain, usually in the midepigastric area, which can radiate to the back; nausea; and emesis. Symptoms are usually associated with elevation of the pancreatic enzymes amylase and lipase. Chronic recurrent pancreatitis may be more subtle and at times may mimic recurrent abdominal pain. Ultrasound and computed tomography have aided the diagnosis of pancreatitis and the treatment of complications, such as pseudocyst formation (Fig. 10-46).

LIVER DISEASE

Jaundice

The term *jaundice* refers to a yellow discoloration of the skin caused by deposition of bilirubin. *Icterus* refers to discoloration of the sclerae. Both are clinical signs that serum bilirubin is above normal. Determining whether the hyperbilirubinemia is secondary to an elevation in conjugated (direct) or unconjugated (indirect) bilirubin is crucial. Elevated conjugated or direct bilirubin greater than or equal to 2 mg/dL, or greater than or equal to 20% of total bilirubin, signifies a pathologic condition, and further studies are necessary to determine its origin.

A majority of neonatal jaundice is due to an elevation in unconjugated bilirubin. This so-called "physiologic" jaundice is due to increased bilirubin production, inadequate bilirubin excretion, or a combination of the two. The most common causes of neonatal unconjugated hyperbilirubinemia are fetal–maternal blood group incompatibility (ABO or Rh), breast-feeding or breast milk jaundice, hemolysis (glucose-6-phosphate dehydrogenase deficiency, hereditary spherocytosis), and extravascular increased bilirubin due to a cephalohematoma or excessive bruising. Phototherapy is usually the treatment of choice for infants with unconjugated hyperbilirubinemia.

Conjugated or direct hyperbilirubinemia indicates a pathologic condition. The physician must determine the cause of

Figure 10-42 Constipation. This plain film of the abdomen demonstrates a significant amount of stool throughout the colon. Note the dilation of the rectum and colon below the pelvic rim in this child with chronic, functional constipation. *(Courtesy Anna Furr, MD, Portland, Maine.)*

Figure 10-44 Hirschsprung disease. **A,** This barium enema demonstrates a tapered transition zone to a normal-caliber colon that is characteristic of Hirschsprung disease. **B,** This slide is specially stained with acetylcholinesterase. The increased number and size of cholinergic nerves in the lamina propria and muscularis mucosae (stains black) is diagnostic of Hirschsprung disease. *(Courtesy Sarangarajan Ranganathan, MD, Pittsburgh, Pa.)*

the disorder in a timely manner because commencing medical or surgical treatment may affect outcome. The differential diagnosis for neonatal conjugated hyperbilirubinemia and neonatal hepatitis is immense and is usually broken down into intrahepatic and extrahepatic etiologies (Table 10-10). Clues gained during a careful and specific history and physical examination may allow the clinician to narrow the differential diagnosis.

Extrahepatic biliary atresia is the most common indication for liver transplantation in children and a major reason to explore the cause of conjugated hyperbilirubinemia as soon as it is discovered. A timely diagnosis and surgical intervention (Kasai procedure) may prevent hepatic cirrhosis, portal hypertension, and eventual liver transplantation. Extrahepatic biliary atresia may be associated with other congenital abnormalities such as situs inversus viscerum, polysplenia, and other gastrointestinal tract anomalies, such as malrotation (see Fig. 10-21) and vascular anomalies (Fig. 10-47), which may complicate initial surgery and later liver transplantation. It can also present in isolation and is generally thought to be a progressive inflammatory process that can be abrogated by

Figure 10-45 Congenital pancreatic anomaly. This 12-year-old boy had recurrent abdominal pain for 10 years. A retrograde cholangiogram demonstrated an ectatic pancreatic duct. **A,** An operative cholangiogram defined a narrow duct just before entry into the duodenum. **B,** Division of the duct and anastomosis to the jejunum led to complete resolution of symptoms.

Figure 10-46 Pancreatic pseudocyst. Abdominal pain and emesis led to a CT scan in this patient, who had a bicycle handlebar injury 2 weeks earlier. **A,** Septation of the cavity. **B,** Compression of stomach and pancreas by the pancreatic pseudocyst. **C,** Two large pancreatic pseudocysts. *(Courtesy Mark Lowe, MD, Pittsburgh, Pa.)*

Table 10-10	Neonatal Liver Diseases Associated with Conjugated Hyperbilirubinemia
Extrahepatic	Infectious
Biliary atresia	Generalized sepsis
Choledochal cyst	Cytomegalovirus
Spontaneous perforation of bile duct	Herpesvirus
Choledochocele	Enterovirus
Intrahepatic	TORCH infections
Idiopathic neonatal	Endocrinopathies
Hereditary	Hypopituitarism (septo-optic
Alagille syndrome	dysplasia)
PFIC 1, 2, 3	Hypothyroidism
Metabolic	Genetic
Galactosemia	Trisomy 17, 18, 21
Tyrosinemia	Turner syndrome
Cystic fibrosis	Anatomic
α_1-Antitrypsin	Congenital hepatic fibrosis
Bile acid synthetic defects	Caroli disease
Lipid/peroxisomal disorders	
Neonatal iron storage disease	

PFIC, progressive familial intrahepatic cholestasis; TORCH, *to*xoplasmosis, *r*ubella, *c*ytomegalovirus, *h*erpes simplex virus.

Figure 10-47   Vascular anomaly in biliary atresia. The inferior vena cava is interrupted and continues as an azygos vein in this child with biliary atresia. Vascular anomalies are most common in the congenital form of biliary atresia.

restoring biliary flow. Other extrahepatic causes of jaundice in childhood include congenital choledochal cysts, which are surgically correctable and often diagnosed by ultrasound (Fig. 10-48). Extrahepatic causes of jaundice in late childhood and beyond are most often due to biliary stones, which can be a cause of right upper quadrant pain and can be diagnosed via ultrasound with characteristic acoustic shadowing beneath the stone (see Chapter 17, Fig. 17-109).

There have been marked advances in the understanding of intrahepatic cholestatic disorders. The diagnosis of idiopathic neonatal cholestasis can now in some cases be divided into various disorders of the accumulation of bilirubin as well as excretion of the components of bile in the progressive familial intrahepatic cholestasis (PFIC) syndromes. PFIC 1 and 2 can be characterized by low γ-glutamyltransferase (GGT) in comparison with other disorders of neonatal cholestasis. A more common cause of intrahepatic cholestasis is arteriohepatic dysplasia, or Alagille syndrome. Patients with this disorder may have a characteristic face of deeply set eyes and a narrow chin (Fig. 10-49) along with persistent posterior embryotoxon, peripheral pulmonic stenosis or cardiac anomalies, and butterfly vertebrae (Fig. 10-50). Liver histology shows paucity of the interlobar bile ducts. Many patients show variable features of the disorder and prognosis is variable. Over time, patients with disorders of cholestasis can suffer from intractable pruritus due to bile acid accumulation and xanthoma formation as the result of cholesterol deposition (Fig. 10-51).

Figure 10-48   Choledochal cyst. **A** and **B,** Ultrasound and diagram of infant with obstructive jaundice demonstrates cystic structure below the liver. **C,** Intraoperative cholangiogram in the same patient defines the cyst and gallbladder along with hepatic and cystic ducts.

Figure 10-50 Alagille syndrome. These radiographs illustrate defects in the vertebral arches that lead to the butterfly appearance.

Figure 10-49 Alagille syndrome. The child has intrahepatic biliary hypoplasia, butterfly vertebrae, and mild pulmonic stenosis. The father does not have liver disease, but he does have moderate pulmonic stenosis and poor growth. Note the narrow, thin face and pointed chin of both father and child.

Hepatomegaly

Hepatomegaly, or enlargement of the liver, can be seen in isolation or with concomitant splenomegaly. Any assessment of hepatomegaly should also include an assessment of liver span as hyperinflation of the lungs can give the appearance of a large liver on abdominal examination. Isolated hepatomegaly without associated inflammation is often marked by only mild elevations of liver enzymes, although this is dependent on cause. Once hepatomegaly is determined, the cause should be carefully examined and includes the assessment of hepatic congestion due to elevated right-sided cardiac pressures, the abnormal accumulation of intrahepatic substances (such as α_1-antitrypsin, glycogen, lipid, among others), extramedullary hematopoiesis in infancy, or tumors such as hepatoblastoma (see Chapter 17, Fig. 17-145). One chronic hepatic disorder that is associated with minimal elevation of transaminases is congenital hepatic fibrosis, which often occurs with splenomegaly and in conjunction with polycystic kidney disease (Figs. 10-52 and 10-53). As liver function often remains normal, shunting procedures are often the procedure of choice for this condition.

Hepatitis

Hepatitis, or inflammation of the liver, can present as an acute or chronic illness with elevation of transaminases (Table 10-11). Most often, acute hepatitis is associated with either a drug reaction or infection, although some cases are idiopathic. Autoimmune hepatitis, presenting either acutely or as a chronic disease, is associated with autoantibodies and hypergammaglobulinemia. Wilson disease is a disorder of copper metabolism and can present either as chronic hepatitis or during an acute crisis (Fig. 10-54). One notable physical examination finding is Kayser-Fleischer rings, which can be seen on slit-lamp examination of the cornea (Fig. 10-55). Nonalcoholic steatohepatitis (NASH), a consequence of obesity, can present as hepatomegaly due to fat accumulation and is associated with low-grade inflammation.

Chronic Liver Disease

There are many examples of chronic liver disease that can be treated with specific therapies, such as Wilson disease and autoimmune hepatitis. The consequences of chronic liver

Figure 10-51 Xanthomas in chronic liver disease. Characteristic areas in the early stages of disease are pressure points such as the elbows **(A)** and knees **(B)**; later, xanthomas may become generalized **(C)**.

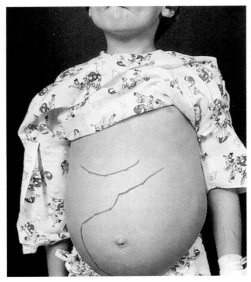

Figure 10-52 Congenital hepatic fibrosis. This clinically well child had hematemesis and hypersplenism with normal liver function studies. Note the massive spleen size and large left lobe of liver. Portosystemic shunting was effective therapy.

Figure 10-54 Wilson disease. Enlarged, firm, nodular-appearing explanted liver from a patient with Wilson disease who underwent liver transplantation.

Figure 10-56 Chronic liver disease/portal hypertension. This child had biliary atresia with good bile flow after a portoenterostomy procedure. Cirrhosis developed late, with physical signs of prominent abdominal veins and ascites.

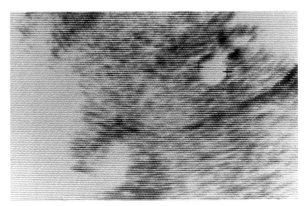

Figure 10-53 Congenital hepatic fibrosis. Ultrasound of the kidney in a patient with congenital hepatic fibrosis reveals a cystic structure.

Figure 10-55 Kayser-Fleischer rings. Kayser-Fleischer rings appear as a brownish discoloration in the posterior part of the cornea, as defined by slit-lamp examination. Early Kayser-Fleischer rings may be seen only by slit-lamp examination and begin at the superior and inferior poles.

Figure 10-57 Spider nevus. The vascular lesion blanches with compression by a glass slide, but it reappears when pressure is released and is a sign of chronic liver disease.

Table 10-11	Hepatitis/Liver Disease Presenting in Older Infancy and Childhood
Viral Hepatitis	***Metabolic***
Hepatitis A, B, C, D (acute or chronic)	α_1-Antitrypsin deficiency
Cytomegalovirus	Cystic fibrosis
Epstein-Barr virus	Wilson disease
Nontypable hepatitis	Nonalcoholic steatohepatitis
Autoimmune Hepatitis	***Drugs***
	Acetaminophen
Biliary Tract Disorders	Anticonvulsants
Choledochal cyst	Chemotherapy
Sclerosing cholangitis	
Cholecystitis	

disease and inflammation can, however, lead to progressive scarring or fibrosis of the liver. As fibrosis progresses to cirrhosis, the liver can involute and become hard and nodular on palpation. Portal hypertension can develop, leading to variceal formation in the esophagus (see Fig. 10-40) and elsewhere. Signs on abdominal examination can include prominent abdominal veins and ascites (Fig. 10-56). Other signs of chronic liver disease include disruptions of the small vasculature including the formation of spider nevi (Fig. 10-57) and intrapulmonary shunting (hepatopulmonary syndrome). Transaminases may remain elevated for some time, but can begin to decrease as hepatocytes are replaced by fibrosis. Synthetic dysfunction occurs and leads to hypoalbuminemia, cholestasis, and clotting abnormalities. In chronic liver failure, treatment is often supportive, with liver transplantation a viable option for therapy.

Bibliography

American Academy of Pediatrics, Committee on Nutrition: The use of whole cow's milk in infancy, *Pediatrics* 91:515–516, 1992.

Balistreri WB, Bezerra JA: Whatever happened to "neonatal hepatitis"? *Clin Liver Dis* 10:27–53, 2006.

Boyle JT: Gastrointestinal bleeding in infants and children, *Pediatr Rev* 29:39–52, 2008.

Butte NF, Hopkinson JM, Wong WW, et al: Body composition during the first 2 years of life: An updated reference, *Pediatr Res* 47:578–585, 2000.

Chiou E, Nurko S: Management of functional abdominal pain and irritable bowel syndrome in children and adolescents, *Expert Rev Gastroenterol Hepatol* 4:293–304, 2010.

Constipation Guideline Committee of the North American Society for Pediatric Gastroenterology, Hepatology, and Nutrition: Evaluation and treatment of constipation in infants and children: Recommendations of the North American Society for Pediatric Gastroenterology, Hepatology and Nutrition, *J Pediatr Gastroenterol Nutr* 43:e1–13, 2006.

DeBrosse CW, Collins MH, Buckmeier Butz BK, et al: Identification, epidemiology, and chronicity of pediatric esophageal eosinophilia, 1982-1999, *J Allergy Clin Immunol* 126:112–119, 2010.

Gold BD, Colletti RB, Abbott M, et al: *Helicobacter pylori* infection in children: Recommendations for diagnosis and treatment, *J Pediatr Gastroenterol Nutr* 31:490–497, 2000.

Hill ID, Dirks MH, Liptak GS, et al: Guideline for the diagnosis and treatment of celiac disease in children: Recommendations of the Pediatric Society for Gastroenterology, Hepatology, and Nutrition, *J Pediatr Gastroenterol Nutr* 40:1–19, 2005.

Jolley CD: Pancreatic disease in children and adolescents, *Curr Gastroenterol Rep* 12:106–113, 2010.

Kahn LU, Ahmed J, Khan S, et al: Refeeding syndrome: A literature review, *Gastroenterol Res Pract* 2011:1–6, 2010.

Kuczmarski RJ, Ogden CL, Guo SS, et al: 2000 CDC growth charts for the United States: Methods and development, *Vital Health Statistics* 11:1–190, 2002.

Leung AK, Sauve RS: Breast is best for babies, *J Natl Med Assoc* 97:1010–1019, 2005.

Sauer CG, Kugathasan S: Pediatric inflammatory bowel disease: Highlighting pediatric differences in IBD, *Gastroenterol Clin North Am* 38:611–628, 2009.

Sinatra FR, Merritt RF: Iatrogenic kwashiorkor in infants, *Am J Dis Child* 135:21–23, 1981.

Sondheimer JM: Office stool examination: A practical guide, *Contemp Pediatr* 7:63–82, 1990.

Vandenplas Y, Rudolph CD, Di Lorenzo C, et al: Pediatric gastroesophageal reflux clinical practice guidelines: Joint recommendations of the North American Society for Pediatric Gastroenterology, Hepatology, and Nutrition (NASPGHAN) and European Society for Pediatric Gastroenterology, Hepatology, and Nutrition (ESPGHAN), *J Pediatr Gastroenterol Nutr* 49:498–547, 2009.

Wagner CL, Greer FR: Prevention of rickets and vitamin D deficiency in infants, children, and adolescents, *Pediatrics* 122:1142–1152, 2008.

HEMATOLOGY AND ONCOLOGY

11

Jean M. Tersak | James D. Cooper | A. Kim Ritchey

HEMATOLOGY

Red Blood Cells

The red blood cell classically is described as a biconcave disk. Red cells evolve from immature forms that scarcely reflect the ultimate stage. Pronormoblasts begin as very large cells with dark blue cytoplasm and a large, centrally located nucleus. As the cell matures, the nucleus becomes pyknotic and is eventually extruded from the cell completely. As the cell begins to make hemoglobin, the cytoplasm undergoes a gradual transformation from dark blue to the eventual pink that is seen on peripheral smears.

A peripheral smear is made with a small droplet of blood on a glass slide. A second slide can be used to smear the blood in a manner that covers one half to two thirds the length of the slide. A well-made smear should not have lines or holes, nor should it reach either end of the slide completely. Commonly, Wright stain is applied after drying to give the cells their characteristic appearance (Fig. 11-1). In general, a normal red blood cell has approximately the same size as a lymphocyte nucleus. Red cells all should be the same relative shape and size, with an area of central pallor that is approximately one third the diameter of the cell (Fig. 11-2). A variety of terms are available to describe the physical properties of mature red blood cells. *Polychromasia* refers to variability in cell color, with *hypochromia* specifically indicating an increased area of central pallor. *Anisocytosis* indicates variability in cell size. *Microcytosis* describes a small cell size, whereas *macrocytosis* refers to large cells. *Poikilocytosis* represents variability in cell shape. The overall number of red blood cells in the circulation cannot be described reliably by the peripheral smear. Laboratory values can also aid in assessing red blood cell morphology. Two of these have wide usage. The mean corpuscular volume (MCV) is a laboratory measure of cell size, and red cell distribution width (RDW) estimates this difference.

The primary function of the red blood cell is to deliver oxygen to the tissues. The effective red cell number commonly is represented by the hemoglobin concentration, in grams per deciliter (g/dL). The oxygen-binding sites of hemoglobin are completely saturated by passage of the RBC through the lungs. As the cells circulate through the systemic capillaries, the hemoglobin releases 25% of its bound oxygen to the tissues. However, the amount of oxygen released in the tissue may be significantly increased under certain conditions (fever, acidosis, level of 2,3-diphosphoglycerate), allowing some compensation for a decrease in hemoglobin. Nonetheless, a progressive decrease in the hemoglobin level eventually leads to tissue hypoxia, which triggers a release of erythropoietin. This induces an increase in RBC production, which brings RBC mass back toward normal values.

Different stages of life and disease states impart different oxygen demands, and therefore hemoglobin levels can vary greatly. In general, full-term newborns are born with relatively high levels of hemoglobin that then fall over the first few months of life. This low point, the physiologic nadir, occurs during the transition in production from fetal to adult hemoglobin. Premature infants may have an earlier, more severe, and more prolonged nadir depending on gestational age. After this time, the average hemoglobin value increases until preadolescence, and by puberty, reaches adult levels. Similarly, the MCV is at a low point after the nadir of hemoglobin, and slowly increases into early adolescence. An estimate of the lower limit of normal for the MCV is 70 femtoliters (fL) plus two times the age in years, from ages 1 to 10 years.

Anemia

Classifications and Symptoms

Increased RBC loss or decreased RBC production can result in an overall decrease in RBC mass below a critical level, leading to anemia. This is the most common abnormality of RBCs, and it is identified as a decreased hemoglobin level. At any given age, anemia is defined practically as a value greater than 2 standard deviations below the mean (Table 11-1). However, physiologically, anemia is best defined as a hemoglobin level that is too low to meet tissue oxygen demands. Conceptually, anemia occurs as a result of one of the following: decreased bone marrow production of red blood cells (RBCs) and reticulocytes (Fig. 11-3), increased destruction of mature RBCs peripherally or as precursors in the bone marrow, or hemorrhage. In addition, a combination of these factors can occur.

Recognition that a child's hemoglobin level is abnormal requires knowledge of age, gender, and race-related normal values. Severe anemia from any cause may elicit symptoms of fatigue; decreased appetite; headache; and, in extreme cases, shock, congestive heart failure, or even stroke. Physical examination of the anemic child may reveal pallor, although in the fair-skinned or dark-skinned child this may be easily missed, unless palmar creases or conjunctivae are also examined thoroughly (Fig. 11-4). Vital signs may be normal, but with severe anemia, tachycardia may be present. In practice, it is common for anemias to be classified on the basis of their cellular morphology, especially size and coloration. The most common scenario encountered in pediatrics is a microcytic anemia due to iron deficiency.

Iron Deficiency

A lack of iron leads to failure of hemoglobin production. Affected children may manifest a peculiar physical finding termed koilonychia, or "spooning" of fingernails and toenails (Fig. 11-5). Glossitis may be observed in iron deficiency and other nutritional deficiencies. Iron deficiency, however, is only a laboratory finding, not a diagnosis. The causes of iron

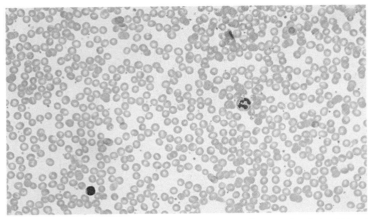

Figure 11-1 Peripheral blood smear: the appearance of a normal peripheral blood smear when viewed under low magnification (×100).

Age	HEMOGLOBIN (g/dL)		MCV (fL)	
	Mean	−2 SD*	Mean	−2 SD*
Birth (cord blood)	16.5	13.5	108	98
1-3 d (capillary)	18.5	14.5	108	95
1 wk	17.5	13.5	107	88
2 wk	16.5	12.5	105	86
1 mo	14.0	10.0	104	85
2 mo	11.5	9.0	96	77
3-6 mo	11.5	9.5	91	74
0.5-2 yr	12.0	10.5	78	70
2-6 yr	12.5	11.5	81	75
6-12 yr	13.5	11.5	86	77
12-18 yr				
Female	14.0	12.0	90	78
Male	14.5	13.0	88	78
18-49 yr				
Female	14.0	12.0	90	80
Male	15.5	13.5	90	80

Table 11-1 Hemoglobin and Mean Corpuscular Volume Values at Various Ages

*Anemia is defined as a value greater than 2 standard deviations below the mean.
Modified from Ianzkowsky P: *Manual of pediatric hematology and oncology,* ed 2, Philadelphia, 1995, Churchill Livingstone.

deficiency must be elucidated through a careful history and physical examination. Although poor nutrition is the most common cause, other causes such as hemorrhage or malabsorption must also be considered. Iron deficiency anemia occurs in infants whose rapidly increasing RBC mass outstrips the dietary iron intake. Because the normal full-term infant has adequate iron reserve to accommodate the increasing RBC

mass through the first 5 months of life, iron deficiency is usually not seen until the second half of the first year of life. It is detected most often in the 10- to 18-month-old child who ingests large volumes of cow's milk and little else. Whole cow's milk not only is deficient in dietary iron but often leads to an enteropathic condition with occult gastrointestinal blood loss, exacerbating the child's iron-deficient status. A second peak of iron deficiency anemia is seen during adolescence in girls.

Figure 11-6 shows a peripheral blood smear of a child with iron deficiency anemia. The RBCs are microcytic and hypochromic. The number of platelets often is increased

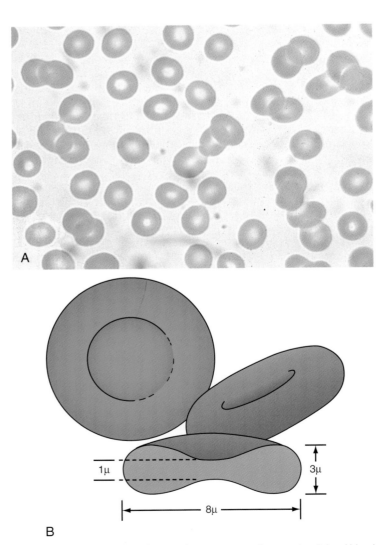

Figure 11-2 Peripheral blood smear: the appearance of a normal peripheral blood smear when viewed under high power (×400). **A,** Biconcave structure of the red blood cell (RBC). **B,** Schematic drawing of an RBC in two views, demonstrating the features of the normal biconcave disk.

Figure 11-3 A, The reticulocyte: a reticulin-stained peripheral blood smear in a patient with a high (18%) reticulocyte count. The darkly stained cells are reticulocytes seen in the peripheral blood of a patient with hemolytic anemia. **B,** High magnification of reticulocytes.

Figure 11-4   Severe anemia. **A,** Pale conjunctiva may be seen in the patient with severe anemia. **B,** Pale palmar creases are also visible in cases of severe anemia. The child in this photograph has a hemoglobin level of 4 g/dL.

(particularly when an enteropathic condition is present), although it may be normal or even decreased. In severe iron deficiency anemia, anisocytosis and poikilocytosis may be prominent. Nonspecific abnormalities of RBC morphology, such as the presence of micro-ovalocytes (see Fig. 11-6) or basophilic stippling (see Fig. 11-8), may also occur. Bizarre RBC shapes are due to a three-dimensional change in structure when viewed in a two-dimensional plane of the light microscope. When viewed in two dimensions, the cells appear ovoid.

The history and physical examination, blood count, and review of the peripheral blood smear may be sufficient for diagnosis in many instances of hypochromic, microcytic anemia. If the evaluation before obtaining a more specific test strongly suggests iron deficiency, a therapeutic trial of iron may be a reasonable approach. However, additional laboratory studies are often indicated. The coexistence of iron deficiency and lead intoxication is well documented, and partial response to iron therapy may indicate concurrent lead intoxication. Securing long-term follow-up of the patient is also imperative. Supplementation with oral iron must continue for approximately 2 months after return of the hemoglobin value to normal to allow for the repletion of body iron stores. The etiology of the iron deficiency anemia also must be addressed to prevent recurrence.

Choosing between specific studies such as serum iron levels and total iron-binding capacity (TIBC) or ferritin and free erythrocyte protoporphyrin (FEP) is often a matter of personal preference. In addition, when the degree of anemia is mild, the results of any combination of tests may be equivocal. Importantly, normal values of ferritin, serum iron, TIBC, and transferrin saturation demonstrate age-related variation.

Ferritin is an acute-phase reactant and may be elevated into the low normal range in a child with a concurrent inflammatory process. However, if ferritin is low, it is diagnostic of iron deficiency. Low transferrin saturation and elevated FEP are also observed in the setting of iron deficiency.

Lead Poisoning

Lead intoxication also leads to microcytic anemia. However, nonhematologic manifestations of lead intoxication, particularly neurologic complications, often dominate the picture. The spectrum of clinical presentations of lead intoxication ranges from vague symptoms of abdominal pain, vomiting, malaise, and behavioral changes to acute encephalopathic conditions, with rapid progression to coma and death. Late physical findings may include papilledema. Significant radiographic changes are also seen in lead intoxication (Fig. 11-7).

Lead intoxication occurs as a result of excessive environmental lead intake. Aerosolized and oral lead-containing environmental contaminants are major sources of lead intoxication. Although clearly a common mechanism in lead poisoning, pica associated with the intake of flaking lead paint represents neither the only nor the prevailing cause of lead intoxication.

Figure 11-5   Spooning of the fingernails occurs in children with severe iron deficiency anemia.

Figure 11-6   Iron deficiency results in a hypochromic, microcytic anemia. This 16-month-old patient had a history of excessive milk intake. Note the marked central pallor of the red blood cells (RBCs) with their small rim of hemoglobin, as well as their small size in comparison with that of the adjacent lymphocyte nucleus. Frequent "cigar cells" can be seen in addition to the hypochromic microcytic RBCs.

Figure 11-7 X-ray findings in lead intoxication. **A,** This hand radiograph of a child with lead intoxication reveals marked linear increases in the density of the metaphyses. These should not be confused with the growth arrest lines that may be seen after a variety of illnesses. **B,** A skull film is shown of a patient with lead intoxication and encephalopathy. Note the split of sutures indicative of increased intracranial pressure. **C,** An abdominal radiograph performed on a child with a history of pica and lead intoxication reveals radiodense, lead-containing paint chips scattered throughout the colon.

The finger-sucking behavior of children in homes where lead paint has become a part of house dust is perhaps a more important factor. A contaminated water supply resulting from old plumbing and deteriorating lead-containing soldered joints can cause lead intoxication in the infant (earlier than the usual at-risk age).

Hematologic abnormalities of lead intoxication are a direct result of the effect of lead on several cellular enzymes involved in heme production. Lead inhibits these enzyme systems, impairing iron use and globin synthesis. Thus despite normal intracellular levels, iron is unable to be incorporated into heme and hemoglobin production fails. Reduced hemoglobin production leads directly to hypochromic, microcytic anemia. Basophilic stippling (Fig. 11-8) is a secondary and inconsistent hematologic manifestation of lead intoxication that occurs as a result of inhibition of yet another RBC enzyme, pyrimidine 5′-nucleotidase. Although basophilic stippling is more prominent in lead intoxication, it is also present in thalassemia and treated iron deficiency. Its presence on the peripheral smear is nonspecific.

Differentiating lead intoxication from iron deficiency can, at times, be difficult. Also, lead intoxication and iron deficiency may coexist, further confusing the diagnosis. Lead poisoning and iron deficiency cause FEP to accumulate in the blood because of the inability to complete the heme biosynthetic pathway through the incorporation of iron into heme. The FEP is elevated in both conditions, although extremely high levels are more common in lead intoxication. Further

testing, such as determination of blood lead level, is necessary to determine the cause of elevated FEP levels. The fact that even low-level lead intoxication may disturb cognitive function underscores the necessity for clinicians to consider this diagnosis.

Figure 11-8 Lead intoxication leads to a hypochromic, microcytic anemia. Prominent basophilic stippling is often seen in cases of severe lead intoxication. However, this finding is not specific for lead toxicity and may also be seen in thalassemia and treated iron deficiency.

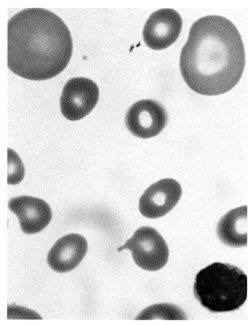

Figure 11-9 Megaloblastic anemia. This peripheral blood smear demonstrates an enlarged red blood cell (RBC, macrocyte) at the *upper left* of the photograph. The RBC is much larger than the normal small lymphocytes in the same field in this patient with megaloblastic anemia.

Figure 11-10 This peripheral blood smear demonstrates the presence of a hyper-segmented polymorphonuclear leukocyte in a patient with phenytoin-induced folate deficiency.

Anemia of Inflammation

Inflammatory diseases, such as chronic infection or collagen vascular disease (particularly juvenile rheumatoid arthritis), may lead to hypochromic, microcytic anemia. Although the symptoms of the child's primary illness usually clarify the diagnosis, there are occasionally cases in which a chronic subclinical infection (particularly of the urinary tract) may go undiagnosed. Differentiating a chronic inflammatory state from other causes of hypochromic, microcytic anemia is usually more easily done on clinical rather than laboratory grounds. One laboratory study that may be of value is serum ferritin determination. Ferritin is decreased in iron deficiency, whereas in chronic inflammatory states it is usually elevated. Also, whereas serum iron is low in both iron deficiency and anemia of chronic disease, TIBC is increased in iron deficiency and decreased in anemia of chronic disease.

Megaloblastic Anemia

Although the etiology of the megaloblastic anemias may vary, common morphologic abnormalities of erythropoietic cells exist. In the bone marrow, the hallmark is the megaloblast, a nucleated RBC with a lacy chromatin pattern and a dyssynchrony of maturation between cytoplasm and nucleus. The morphologic alterations are a direct result of decreased nucleoprotein DNA synthesis compared with cytoplasmic protein synthesis, which stems from a relative decrease in the factors needed in DNA replication, namely folate and cobalamin (vitamin B_{12}).

On the peripheral blood smear, the RBCs are large in size (macrocytes) and display a great deal of variation in their shapes (Fig. 11-9). These macrocytic cells are generally normochromic. In addition, all of the actively dividing marrow cells may become involved in the pathologic process. Neutrophils are the second most likely cells to display morphologic abnormalities. These cells become large and show pathognomonic hypersegmentation of the nucleus (Fig. 11-10). Neutropenia is common. The more severe and prolonged megaloblastic anemias ultimately may lead to moderate thrombocytopenia, with large bizarre platelets on the peripheral blood smear.

Megaloblastic changes in each cell line are shown in Figure 11-11.

Laboratory diagnosis requires the measurement of folate and vitamin B_{12} levels in the serum and RBCs. Because a typical Western diet is unlikely to lead to folate or vitamin B_{12} deficiency, a low level of either should raise questions of altered bioavailability or peculiar diet. Goat milk is folate deficient (although in more recent years many canned goat milk products are folate supplemented), and an infant on a goat milk diet may become folate depleted over time. Fad diets often are not structured thoughtfully and may lead to folate deficiency. Various drugs that decrease folate absorption (phenytoin) or interfere with folate metabolism (methotrexate) may also lead to megaloblastic changes. A pathologic condition of the gastrointestinal tract may cause malabsorption of folate or vitamin B_{12} and secondary megaloblastic changes. This condition may be iatrogenic if a portion of the intestines is removed for medical reasons. Pernicious anemia is a specific cause due to a deficiency of intrinsic factor, which is required for vitamin B_{12} absorption. Glossitis (Fig. 11-12) or angular stomatitis, commonly seen in vitamin B_{12} deficiency, can be helpful physical findings in the diagnostic process.

Pure Red Cell Aplasia

Transient erythroblastopenia of childhood (TEC) occurs in 1- to 4-year-old children and appears 2 weeks to 2 months after a respiratory or gastrointestinal illness. TEC is transient and self-limited, whereas the other forms of red cell aplasia may be chronic. It has been noted that the RBCs in pure red cell aplasia have fetal characteristics, whereas the RBCs of TEC have age-appropriate characteristics (Table 11-2). The cause of TEC remains obscure. TEC may occur after many different viral infections and most likely represents an altered immunity from the infection that affects erythropoiesis. Treatment is supportive and determined by the degree of symptoms.

Non–TEC-acquired pure red cell aplasia is rare in pediatrics. Three types of non–TEC-acquired pure red cell aplasia have

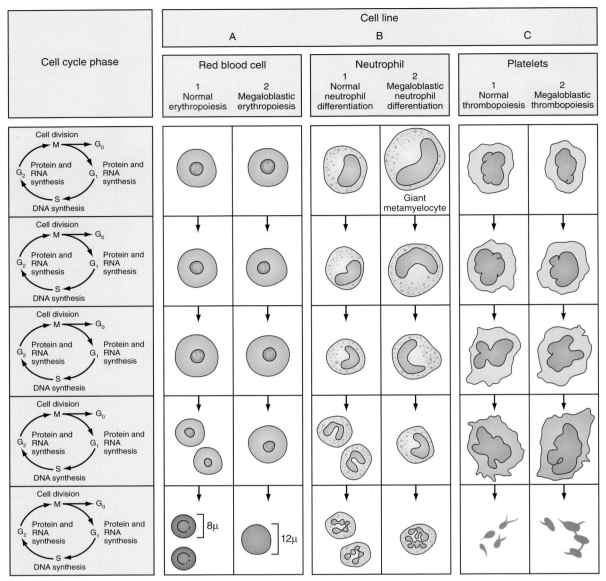

Figure 11-11 Schematic comparison of normal cellular maturation and megaloblastic differentiation of three cell lines. The cell cycle phase is identified to the *left* of the figure. Note that the megaloblastic cells fail to undergo replication of DNA and cellular division at the S and M phases, respectively, leading to large red blood cells, hypersegmented polymorphonuclear leukocytes, and large, bizarrely shaped platelets.

been recognized. Type I has a serum IgG inhibitor of erythropoiesis and high erythropoietin levels. Type II has a low erythropoietin activity level and an erythropoietin IgG antibody. Type III has no anti-erythropoiesis or anti-erythropoietin serum antibodies. Rather, the defect appears intrinsic to the stem cells. Some of these children are preleukemic. Thymoma-associated pure red cell aplasia is extremely rare in children. Drugs, particularly chloramphenicol, have been responsible for a significant percentage of pure red cell

aplasias historically. The peripheral blood smear from a patient with pure red cell aplasia is often nonspecific, and the bone marrow aspirate rarely is more specific. It may demonstrate the vacuolated erythroblasts of the chloramphenicol effect or the multinucleated giant cells indicative of the rare congenital dyserythropoietic anemia.

Hemolytic Anemias

Hemolytic anemias are defined by the premature destruction of red blood cells. This can occur by mechanical, infectious, enzymatic, or immune-mediated mechanisms. Symptoms and severity vary not only among individuals but also between diagnoses. Jaundice, especially scleral icterus, as well as splenomegaly and dark urine can be common presentations during hemolytic episodes. Although all hemolytic anemias may have acute exacerbations, some also feature more chronic phases of red cell breakdown. The history of individual patients, laboratory studies, and blood cell morphology are important factors in making the accurate diagnosis. Treatments can vary; often, splenectomy may be a consideration. However, splenectomy in children is fraught with dangerous sequelae—both infectious risks and vascular injury or thromboses. Some of the most common features are described in Table 11-3.

Table 11-2	Features Differentiating Pure Red Cell Anemia from Transient Erythroblastopenia of Childhood

	DISEASE	
RBC Characteristic	**Pure Red Cell Anemia**	**TEC**
Hemoglobin	Increased fetal	Normal fetal
Cellular antigen	i	I
Mean corpuscular volume	Increased	Normal
RBC enzyme activity	Normal or high	Low

RBC, red blood cell; TEC, transient erythroblastopenia of childhood.

Figure 11-12 A smooth, beefy red tongue may be observed in the physical examination of a patient with vitamin B_{12} deficiency. This patient depended on total parenteral nutrition for several years without vitamin B_{12} supplementation.

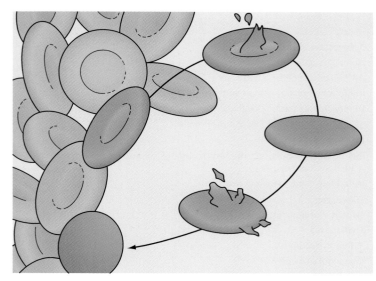

Figure 11-14 A developing spherocyte resulting from the process of repeated membrane fragmentation, loss, and repair.

Hereditary spherocytosis (HS) is the most common cause of genetically determined hemolytic anemia in the white population. HS is transmitted frequently as an autosomal dominant trait, and it is named for the peculiar appearance of the RBCs on the peripheral blood smear (Fig. 11-13). The RBC membrane defect, which most commonly results from inherent cytoskeletal membrane instability due to spectrin deficiency, leads to loss of membrane. Membrane repair occurs, which decreases the normal RBC surface-to-volume ratio; this causes the normal biconcave disk to assume a more geometrically efficient spherical shape (Fig. 11-14). The new morphology creates a less pliable cell. The inability of this new cell to deform during transit through the splenic microcirculation leads to RBC destruction (Fig. 11-15). Osmotic fragility testing,

used commonly in patients with suspected hereditary spherocytosis, is an excellent confirmatory test but is not pathognomonic for the diagnosis.

Hereditary elliptocytosis (HE) is another membrane defect morphologically distinct from hereditary spherocytosis (Fig. 11-16). However, its inheritance and pathophysiology of RBC destruction are similar to that in spherocytosis. In most instances, HE is a mild, well-compensated hemolytic anemia that is clinically insignificant unless splenic hypertrophy develops from another disease process. The elliptocyte form bears only a superficial similarity to that of the ovalocyte of iron deficiency anemia. Unlike those cells, the elliptocytes of HE have normal size, have a normal MCV, and are true elliptocytes. Elliptocytes may also be found in the peripheral blood smear of thalassemia or in megaloblastic anemia—although these findings do not suggest mixed pathologies.

A number of hemolytic anemias are characterized by spiculated RBCs referred to as *acanthocytes* or *echinocytes* (Fig. 11-17). Abetalipoproteinemia generally presents as a neurologic disorder with progressive ataxia, retinitis pigmentosa, fat malabsorption, and the absence of chylomicrons and very low–density and low-density lipoproteins. Acanthocytes develop as a direct result of the alterations of the serum lipids. Altered membrane lipid composition changes the fluidity of the RBC, leading to the abnormal form. Malabsorption of

Figure 11-13 Peripheral blood smear of a patient with hereditary spherocytosis. Note the presence of small, perfectly round cells without an area of central pallor. The mean corpuscular hemoglobin concentration (MCHC) is often increased in this condition but may be normal in some cases. Reticulocyte count is also often elevated owing to the shortened life span of the RBCs and need for increased RBC production relative to individuals without hereditary spherocytosis.

Figure 11-15 Electron micrograph of red blood cells (RBCs) traversing the splenic sinusoids. Note that the RBCs become deformed as they traverse the microcirculation of the splenic sinusoids.

Table 11-3	Common RBC Hemolytic Disorders by Predominant Morphology*

Spherocytes

Hereditary spherocytosis

ABO incompatibility in neonates[†]

Immunohemolytic anemias with IgG- or C3-coated RBCs

Hemolytic transfusion reactions[†]

Severe burns or other RBC thermal injuries

Bizarre Poikilocytes

RBC fragmentation syndromes (microangiopathic and macroangiopathic hemolytic anemias)

Hereditary elliptocytosis in neonates

Elliptocytes

Hereditary elliptocytosis

Thalassemia

(Other hypochromic microcytic anemia)

(Megaloblastic anemia)

Spiculated or Crenated RBCs

Acute hepatic necrosis (spur-cell anemia)

Uremia

Abetalipoproteinemia

Prominent Basophilic Stippling

Thalassemia

Unstable hemoglobin levels

Lead poisoning[‡]

Irreversibly Sickled Cells

Sickle cell anemia

Symptomatic sickle syndromes

Intraerythrocytic Parasites

Malaria

Babesiosis

Bartonellosis

Target Cells

Hgb S, C, D, and E

Hereditary xerocytosis

Thalassemia

(Other hypochromic microcytic anemia)

(Obstructive liver disease)

(Postsplenectomy)

Nonspecific or Normal Morphology

Embden-Meyerhof pathway defects

HMP shunt defects

Adenosine deaminase hyperactivity with low RBC ATP

Unstable hemoglobin levels

Paroxysmal nocturnal hemoglobinuria

Dyserythropoietic anemia

Copper toxicity (Wilson disease)

Erythropoietic porphyria

Vitamin E deficiency

Hypersplenism

*Nonhemolytic disorders of similar morphology are enclosed in parentheses for reference.
[†]Usually associated with a positive Coombs test.
[‡]Disease sometimes associated with this morphology.
Hgb, hemoglobin; HMP, hexose-monophosphate shunt; RBC, red blood cell.
Modified from Nathan DG, Oski FA, editors: *Hematology of infancy and childhood,* ed 2, Philadelphia, 1981, WB Saunders.

Figure 11-16 This peripheral blood smear resulted in an incidental finding of hereditary elliptocytosis in a 3-year-old child. More than 90% of the cells are elliptocytes. The child's only remarkable history was one of neonatal jaundice.

Figure 11-17 Spur cell anemia. The peripheral smear from this patient demonstrates the hematologic findings of acute hepatic necrosis. The anemia associated with the presence of these spiculated cells in the periphery can be severe.

fat-soluble vitamins in abetalipoproteinemia results in vitamin E deficiency, leaving the RBCs subject to oxidative injury. However, despite altered membrane fluidity and vitamin E deficiency, hemolysis in abetalipoproteinemia is mild.

Spur cell anemia is another disorder characterized by acanthocytes. The hemolysis in this disorder, in contrast to abetalipoproteinemia, is brisk. Spur cell anemia develops in the setting of sudden and massive liver injury arising from any cause (e.g., hepatitis with acute yellow atrophy, shock liver, hepatic infarction). The hepatic decompensation leads to increased serum lipid and cholesterol levels, which lead, in turn, to increased RBC membrane cholesterol content, thus altering RBC membrane fluidity. Spiculated cells in lesser numbers can also be seen in uremia and anorexia nervosa, as well as severe malnutrition. Conversely, one of the most frequent causes of spiculated RBCs on the peripheral blood smear is inadequate slide preparation.

Target cells draw their name from their characteristic appearance on the peripheral blood smear. They are often seen as a secondary response to a process that increases the RBC membrane or decreases the RBC content, leading to an increase in the surface-to-volume ratio of the RBCs (Fig. 11-18, *A*). In a dried smear, the excess surface accumulates and bulges outward in the area that is normally the RBC's central pallor, producing the characteristic target cell morphology. Liver diseases of any type, particularly obstructive hepatopathy, are well-known causes of target cell formation. Splenectomy decreases reticuloendothelial remodeling of reticulocytes, removes lipid-loaded RBC membranes, and leads to targeted RBCs. Mechanisms previously discussed that decrease RBC intracellular content, such as hypochromic, microcytic anemia, also induce target formation. In addition, target cells (or more accurately, pseudotarget cells) occur with various hemoglobinopathies. This happens more often in conditions associated with Hgb C, but also with Hgb S, D, and E (Figs. 11-19 and 11-20), because of aggregation of hemoglobin in the central region of the RBC (Fig. 11-18, *B*).

Malaria is the most frequent cause of hemolysis on a worldwide scale. The patient who contracts the disease after being fed on by the tropical *Anopheles* mosquito is parasitized within the RBCs with organisms at the merozoite stage (Fig. 11-21). The parasitization causes a clinical picture of

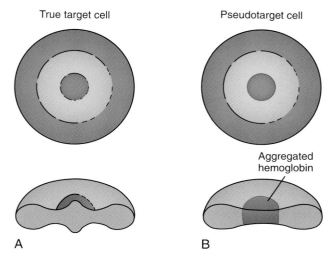

True target cell Pseudotarget cell

Aggregated hemoglobin

A B

Figure 11-18 **A,** Schematic of the morphology of a target cell. **B,** Schematic of the morphology of a pseudotarget cell.

intermittent fever, chills, and jaundice and may lead to encephalopathy, massive hemolysis with hemoglobinuria (blackwater fever), and death. The cause of the hemolysis has been attributed to multiple mechanisms including altered RBC osmotic fragility, membrane loss of negative surface charge, direct injury by the parasite, autoimmunity, splenic pitting, and hypersplenism.

Abnormalities of RBC enzymes may also lead to hemolysis. Although almost any RBC enzymes involved in RBC glycolysis or free radical detoxification via the pentose shunt may be responsible for hemolysis, glucose-6-phosphate dehydrogenase (G6PD) deficiency is by far the most frequent. A second enzyme, pyruvate kinase (PK), when deficient, also leads to a hemolytic state. The blood smears of patients with RBC enzyme deficiency–induced hemolysis are often normal, although occasionally with G6PD deficiency a suspicious morphology may be present (Fig. 11-22). More than 370 variants of G6PD have been identified, for which enzyme activity may be normal, elevated, or severely deficient. G6PD deficiency is transmitted by a sex-linked recessive mode of inheritance.

Figure 11-19 **A,** Peripheral blood smear in sickle cell disease. Note the presence of sickle cells and prominent target cells. A Howell-Jolly body is also present, consistent with auto-infarction and subsequent loss of splenic function. **B,** Schematic of sickle cell and Howell-Jolly body.

Sickled RBC

Howell-Jolly body

A B

Figure 11-20   Peripheral blood smear of a child with hemoglobin SC disease. Sickle cells are seen less frequently in this disease, whereas target cells are more prominent.

Figure 11-22   Peripheral blood smear of a patient with glucose-6-phosphate dehydrogenase (G6PD) deficiency. This patient is experiencing a hemolytic crisis. Note the blister cells with hemoglobin condensed in the remaining (nonblistered) portion of the cell.

Heterozygous females may rarely be affected because of inactivation of the X chromosome according to the Lyon hypothesis or because they are doubly heterozygous. Clinical syndromes may vary as well, with the degree of hemolysis inversely paralleling the level of G6PD activity.

In all instances the hemolysis is due to the intracellular generation of free radicals and peroxides, which fail to be detoxified by the patient with G6PD deficiency. Chronic hemolysis is extremely mild and subclinical in the common types. Triggered hemolysis associated with G6PD deficiency (Mediterranean type) is severe and abrupt and parallels inversely the severe enzyme deficiency. In contrast, triggered hemolysis with G6PD deficiency (A type) may be severe but self-limited when the enzyme deficiency is mild. In addition, some agents that trigger hemolysis with G6PD deficiency (Mediterranean type) may be tolerated by patients with G6PD deficiency (A type). A list of some drugs associated with clinically significant hemolysis in G6PD deficiency is provided (Table 11-4). Research has deemphasized the role of certain drug triggers. In many instances the infection being treated with certain drugs, rather than the drugs themselves, is responsible for the hemolysis.

Pyruvate kinase (PK) deficiency is the second most prevalent enzyme abnormality of the RBC that leads to hemolysis; however, it is a far second, indeed, with 1 case of PK deficiency occurring worldwide for 500,000 cases of G6PD deficiency. Autosomal recessive transmission of the enzyme defect is usually observed in PK deficiency. Like G6PD deficiency, wide clinical variability exists with PK deficiency. Mild, fully compensated hemolytic anemia, as well as severe neonatal hemolysis and hyperbilirubinemia, may occur. Hemoglobin levels range from 6 to 10 g/dL with normochromic anemia with normocytic or macrocytic indices, depending on the degree of reticulocytosis. The reticulocyte count can range from 5% to as high as 90% in the patient who has had a splenectomy. For the subgroup of patients with severe, transfusion-dependent disease, splenectomy may ameliorate or eliminate the need for transfusions. In addition to chronic hemolysis, PK deficiency may have triggered episodes (usually resulting from intercurrent infection).

Direct and indirect Coombs tests, which evaluate the patient's blood for the presence of anti-RBC antibody and complement on RBCs or in the serum, respectively, identify immune-mediated hemolytic anemia. Antibody- and

Figure 11-21   *Plasmodium vivax* malaria. This peripheral blood smear is prepared by the so-called "thick prep" method. *Plasmodium vivax* malaria is seen intracellularly in the red blood cell in the center of the smear.

Table 11-4	Drugs Associated with Clinically Significant Hemolysis in Glucose-6-phosphate Dehydrogenase Deficiency
Antimalarials	Sulfamethoxypyridazine
Pamaquine	Sulfapyridine
Pentaquine	Thiazolesulfone
Primaquine	***Miscellaneous***
Quinocide	Acetylphenylhydrazine
Antipyretics and Analgesics	Fava beans
Acetanilide	Nalidixic acid
Aminopyrine	Naphthalene
Antipyrine	Phenylhydrazine
Sulfa Drugs	Toluidine blue
N-Acetylsulfanilamide	
Salicylazosulfapyridine	

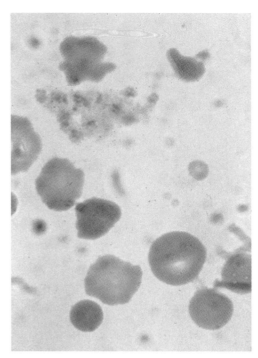

Figure 11-23 Coombs-positive hemolytic anemia. Note the spherocytes and a large red blood cell with polychromasia, indicating the presence of regenerative anemia.

Figure 11-24 Maxillary hyperplasia. Prominent facial bones of a child with sickle cell anemia, due to enlargement of the marrow cavity in this condition of decreased red blood cell survival.

complement-mediated RBC destruction produces spherocytes on the peripheral blood smear (Fig. 11-23). Coombs-positive hemolytic anemia in the newborn most often represents an isoimmune hemolytic anemia. This is caused by a maternal antibody that has crossed the placenta into the neonate, hemolyzing the newborn RBCs. Maternal antibodies form to fetal RBC antigens when fetal blood gains entry into the maternal circulation via a break in placental integrity. Maternal antibodies then cross the placenta and cause fetal RBC hemolysis. In the majority of cases of isoimmune hemolytic anemia, the maternal antibody is directed at ABO or Rh RBC antigens. When Rh antigen is the antibody target, the blood smear does not show spherocytes.

Hemoglobinopathies

Hemoglobinopathies often result in a characteristic and even diagnostic peripheral blood smear. They can be responsible for hemolysis resulting from unstable hemoglobin variants or decreased hemoglobin solubility. Baseline levels of hemoglobin can be much lower in patients with these disorders. Nearly all of the following diagnoses are life-long conditions.

Of the hemoglobinopathies that have altered hemoglobin solubility, none is as well known or as ubiquitous as sickle cell disease. Substitution of valine for glutamic acid at position 6 in the β chain of the hemoglobin molecule leads to the cross-linking of one β chain to a second hemoglobin molecule's β chain when the hemoglobin is in its deoxygenated state. This cross-linkage tips the solubility balance, leading to sickling of the RBC (see Fig. 11-19). Sickle cell disease is by no means exclusive to patients of African origin, with Mediterranean and Middle Eastern peoples also being affected. Sickle cell disease is an autosomal recessive disorder with the heterozygote having a significant but less than 50% proportion of hemoglobin of the sickle cell type. Heterozygous carriers of the sickle cell gene, although suffering a number of difficulties (e.g., poor urine-concentrating ability, occasional episodes of renal papillary necrosis with hematuria), have normal life expectancies and are virtually free of any significant consequences of their heterozygous state.

The clinical signs and symptoms of sickle cell anemia are due to decreased survival and altered rheology of the sickled RBC. As with any chronic hemolytic state, marrow cavity enlargement occurs, leading to maxillary hyperplasia and the so-called sickle cell facies (Fig. 11-24). Sickle cells have altered pliability and lose the ability to deform in the microcirculation (see Fig. 11-15). This leads to tissue infarction and subsequent pain. These vaso-occlusive crises, when occurring in certain locations, give rise to clinical manifestations such as dactylitis (Fig. 11-25), priapism (Fig. 11-26), splenic sequestration, and

Figure 11-25 Dactylitis (hand–foot syndrome). This syndrome, in children with sickle cell disease, primarily affects toddlers. Dactylitis is seen less frequently in older children because the bone marrow of the small bones of the hands and feet loses hematopoietic activity. This loss of marrow activity is due to cortical thickening from increased use of hands and weight bearing by the feet.

Figure 11-26   Priapism in an adolescent with sickle cell disease. Erection had persisted for 12 hours and had become extremely painful for the patient.

skin ulceration. The vaso-occlusive phenomenon may also lead to life-threatening complications of sickle cell disease: overwhelming infection with encapsulated organisms (most often *Pneumococcus*), acute chest syndrome, and stroke. The increased infectious risk in the sickle cell patient has multiple mechanisms, but by far the most important is splenic dysfunction related to congested blood flow and then, ultimately, splenic infarction.

Thalassemia is a term applied to a group of genetic disturbances decreasing hemoglobin production and leading to anemia and/or altered levels of the various hemoglobins in the blood. Thalassemia trait is another cause of hypochromic, microcytic anemia. In patients with β-thalassemia trait, hemoglobin electrophoresis usually reveals an increase in Hgb A_2 and Hgb F, whereas in patients with α-thalassemia trait the findings may be normal. β-Thalassemia major generally presents after the first 6 months of life, at a time when β-chain synthesis increases. Hydrops fetalis may result from α-thalassemia major. Ethnicity may be an important clue in the history: β-thalassemia trait tends to occur in patients of African or Mediterranean descent, whereas α-thalassemia trait tends to occur in patients of African or Asian origin. β-Thalassemia major is largely restricted to people of Mediterranean or Middle Eastern heritage.

β-Thalassemia major (Cooley anemia) causes hypochromic, microcytic anemia that results from ineffective erythropoiesis caused by an imbalance between α- and β-hemoglobin chain synthesis. The peripheral blood smear shows hypochromia; microcytosis; target cells; basophilic stippling; and, often, a large number of nucleated RBCs (Fig. 11-27). β-Thalassemia major is associated with increased marrow activity, which is ineffectively attempting to correct the degree of anemia. The increased marrow activity expands the marrow cavity, producing a characteristic bony hyperplasia evidenced by physical and radiographic findings (Fig. 11-28). Untreated patients with thalassemia major have chronic and severe anemia, marked hepatosplenomegaly, scleral icterus, and listlessness and may have high-output cardiac failure secondary to severe anemia. In addition, malocclusion may occur because of molar hypertrophy. This picture is not usually confused with thalassemia trait, iron deficiency, or lead poisoning.

Although less common than sickle cell disease, anemia associated with hemoglobin C is not rare in the African-American population. As in sickle cell disease, Hgb C disease occurs because of one amino acid change. The change, again

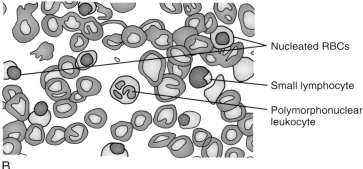

Figure 11-27   Thalassemia major. **A,** This peripheral blood smear of a child with thalassemia major shows hypochromic, microcytic anemia with prominent nucleated red blood cells surrounding the polymorphonuclear cells and lymphocytes. **B,** Labeled schematic of peripheral blood smear.

like Hgb S, is at the sixth position of the β chain but the replacement is a lysine rather than a valine. In its homozygous form, Hgb C disease is a mild disorder characterized by hemolytic anemia and splenomegaly. The tendency of Hgb C to aggregate into precipitates is responsible for the characteristic target (actually pseudotarget; see Fig. 11-18, *B*) morphology of the Hgb C homozygous and Hgb C trait (heterozygous) cells on the peripheral blood smear. Vaso-occlusive phenomena are not associated with this disease, although target cells are formed on the dried peripheral blood smear. However, Hgb C, when paired in a double heterozygous state with Hgb S, results in Hgb SC disease (see Fig. 11-20) and is associated with vaso-occlusive phenomena, although less severe than Hgb SS.

Unstable hemoglobin variants, unlike most hemolytic hemoglobinopathies, rarely have a characteristic morphology, although basophilic stippling and Heinz bodies may be noted on special staining of the peripheral blood (Fig. 11-29). The Heinz bodies represent hemoglobin aggregates that have precipitated intracellularly. RBCs in Heinz body anemia usually are normocytic but may be hypochromic as a result of RBC splenic "pitting" of precipitated hemoglobin. Because the precipitated hemoglobin may be mistaken for reticulum, reticulocyte counts may be spuriously high. Methylene blue staining of RBCs after they have incubated for a few hours can demonstrate the Heinz bodies. Unstable hemoglobinopathies have an autosomal dominant pattern of inheritance, and affected individuals are heterozygotes. A homozygous state would, in most cases, be incompatible with life. Congenital Heinz body hemolytic anemia is an important cause of congenital hemolytic anemia. This condition, although frequently a persistent process in the older infant, has been observed to resolve.

Figure 11-28 **A,** Maxillary hyperplasia resulting from an increased marrow space in a child with thalassemia major. **B,** Skull radiograph of the same patient demonstrates an increased marrow cavity of the skull and facial bones.

The Coagulation System

Platelets mature from megakaryocytes and have a life span of approximately 7 to 10 days. Platelets adhere to the site of injury by connecting to exposed von Willebrand factor on the vessel basement membrane. Subsequently, fibrinogen binding acts as a stimulus for the aggregation of other platelets. Once platelets have gathered at the site of injury, phospholipids on their surface interact with calcium to enable the hemostatic activity of the coagulation cascade. This process is a complex, interconnected series of reactions between enzymes and cofactors that leads to the deposition of fibrin (Fig. 11-30). The extrinsic pathway is activated when exposed tissue factor is contacted by circulating factor VIIa, causing the initial burst of thrombin production. The intrinsic pathway, through feedback mechanisms triggered by thrombin generation, plays an important role in clot propagation and continued fibrin production. Disorders of platelet plug formation commonly present with mucocutaneous oozing or bleeding, whereas disorders of coagulation factors often present with delayed and deeper tissue bleeding due to the ineffective fibrin deposition.

Natural anticoagulants are molecules that help regulate thrombin generation. Through irreversible binding, antithrombin is able to inactivate thrombin and factors VIIa, IXa, Xa, XIa, and XIIa. This reaction normally is quite slow; however, in the presence of heparin, a structural change allows it to act extremely rapidly. Other inhibitors of thrombin include heparin cofactor II, α_2-macroglobulin, and protein Z. Activated protein C (APC), with assistance from protein S, inactivates factors Va and VIIIa. The fibrinolytic pathway produces plasmin, which eventually degrades fibrin. Mediated by tissue-type plasminogen activator (t-PA), plasminogen activator inhibitor (PAI-1), α_2-macroglobulin, and α_2-antiplasmin, the fibrinolytic system also plays important roles in tissue repair, macrophage function, angiogenesis, and tumor invasion.

Questions concerning how, when, and if to test for bleeding disorders are controversial. In many cases, a dental or otolaryngology procedure may be the first challenge of a child's

Figure 11-30 Overview of the coagulation system. *Red and white boxes* represent factors in the clotting cascade. The extrinsic pathway is composed of tissue factor and factor VIIa, whereas the intrinsic pathway features high molecular weight kininogen (HMWK) and factors XII, XIa, IXa, and VIIIa. Both pathways contribute to the conversion of factor X into its activated form (Xa), leading to thrombin generation. Thrombin not only cleaves fibrinogen into fibrin but also upregulates the cascade in several areas to contribute to clot propagation (represented by *blue arrows*).

Figure 11-29 Heinz body preparation. This peripheral blood smear of a 2-week-old infant with brisk hemolytic anemia demonstrates a positive Heinz body preparation. The dark-staining material within two of the red blood cells shows the precipitated hemoglobin that one may see in a condition called *unstable hemoglobin*.

Figure 11-31   A, Petechiae. This infant with severe immune thrombocytopenia has visible petechiae, as well as large ecchymoses. **B,** Purpuric lesions on the oral mucosa or retina are called "wet purpura" and may suggest an increased tendency for major bleeding in the thrombocytopenic patient.

ability to form clots appropriately. A child's personal and family bleeding history are notoriously unreliable as predictors of bleeding disorders. Given the medicolegal risks associated with postprocedural bleeding, however, many practitioners are hesitant to limit their screening practices. If a specific disorder is suggested by a child's presentation, then testing should be targeted toward the most likely diagnosis. Normal values for laboratory studies of coagulation vary from the newborn period through adulthood. Many of the coagulation factors (other than V, VIII, and von Willebrand factor) have reduced levels in infants and gradually increase over the first year of life. As a result, care should be taken when evaluating coagulation studies in pediatric patients. In acute bleeding presentations, an evaluation of surgical or physical causes also should be performed. If the administration of blood products or other hemostatic treatments is not emergently indicated, the performance of pertinent diagnostic tests should be considered first. Transfusions may delay an accurate laboratory diagnosis for days to weeks.

Disorders That Predispose to Bleeding

Bleeding disorders are defined more accurately as an inadequate hemostatic response to tissue injury. The amount of bleeding will depend on the site and degree of tissue injury as well as the severity of the defect in the hemostatic system. Epistaxis serves as a worthwhile example. The nose receives blood from multiple areas and has a rich vascular network (see Chapter 23). Local physical injury and dryness are the most common causes of bleeding. Likewise, infectious or allergic disease can trigger episodes. Whatever the inciting event, however, a child with an intact hemostatic system should be able to control bleeding from the nares with direct pressure, cauterization, or packing. When such conservative measures fail or similar such episodes continue in a recurrent fashion, clinicians should be suspicious that a bleeding disorder may exist. Initial laboratory evaluation of a suspected disorder should follow the same algorithm as that used for preoperative coagulation screening.

Disorders of Primary Hemostasis

The number and size of circulating platelets can be determined by automated or manual methods. Thrombocytopenia is defined as a platelet count less than 150,000 cells/μL. Pseudothrombocytopenia occurs when a normal in vivo platelet count is reported (erroneously) to be low in vitro. This can occur when platelets agglutinate and are bypassed by the automated counter or when very large platelets are misinterpreted as leukocytes. Manual inspection of a peripheral smear

appropriately prepared with a Wright-Giemsa stain will clarify these situations. Platelet size is reported as mean platelet volume, expressed as femtoliters (fL). The presence of large platelets (>7 fL) may be helpful in distinguishing between various platelet disorders.

Thrombocytopenia is the most common hematologic abnormality of neonates. Most commonly, thrombocytopenia in this age group will be secondary to other illnesses, such as sepsis, congenital infections, or necrotizing enterocolitis. In these settings the low platelet count is often a manifestation of disseminated intravascular coagulation. However, thrombocytopenia can be a primary process. Neonatal alloimmune thrombocytopenia (NAIT) is caused by the transplacental passage of maternal antibodies directed against the paternal antigens on an infant's platelets (Fig. 11-31). Incompatibility occurs as commonly as once in every 350 pregnancies (50% will be first pregnancies), although thrombocytopenia develops in far fewer (1 per 1000 to 1500). The thrombocytopenia can be severe and difficult to treat. Intravenous immunoglobulin (IVIG) may be helpful, but the best treatment is the transfusion of maternally donated platelets. Autoimmune thrombocytopenia, on the other hand, results from the passage of maternal autoantibodies. These are far less specific and less likely to cause severe thrombocytopenia. IVIG and corticosteroids have been used as effective treatment.

Idiopathic thrombocytopenic purpura (ITP) is an autoimmune phenomenon characterized by a low circulating platelet count. Most commonly seen in young children, there is a peak incidence from ages 2 to 4 years. ITP is often preceded by a mild viral illness. It also can be a secondary disease process, especially in systemic lupus erythematosus, common variable immunodeficiency, HIV, and hepatitis C. The pathophysiology is complex, but both humoral and cellular immune processes are involved with the generation and then propagation of antiplatelet autoantibodies. Once platelets become coated with IgG, they then are cleared aggressively by tissue macrophages, especially in the spleen.

In general, children with ITP appear well. Symptoms usually are limited to petechiae, epistaxis, and ecchymoses (see Fig. 11-31). Alternatively, a small percentage of children may present with significant mucosal bleeding. In more than half of cases of childhood ITP, the presenting platelet count will be less than 20,000 cells/μL. Review of the blood smear generally reveals large normal platelets but in significantly diminished numbers, and bone marrow aspirate shows prominent megakaryocytes typical of the immune destruction of platelets in ITP (Fig. 11-32). Any signs or symptoms that suggest an alternative diagnosis, such as prolonged fever or

Figure 11-32 Bone marrow aspirate—idiopathic thrombocytopenia (ITP). This bone marrow aspirate shows prominent megakaryocytes consistent with the increased production and immune destruction of platelets in ITP. In children with thrombocytopenia due to decreased production, one would expect megakaryocyte numbers to be decreased.

splenomegaly, should be investigated thoroughly. In the setting of typical ITP, a bone marrow aspiration is not necessary, and there is no evidence to suggest that other diagnostic studies are required.

In most children, the disease is self-limited and outcomes are excellent. Observation alone is a well-accepted treatment option. However, there is a small risk of intracranial hemorrhage, estimated at approximately 1 per 10,000 patients. Corticosteroids are typically used as the primary ITP treatment. Alternatively, intravenous immunoglobulin can be used, or anti-D immunoglobulin (only in Rh-positive patients). Not only do these two medications require intravenous access, but they may also have adverse events or toxicities related to their infusions. Platelet transfusions are of minimal benefit, unless a severe and life-threatening hemorrhage is occurring, and will require two to three times the normal volume. Regardless of the modality of management, a pediatric hematologist should be directing the care of all patients with ITP.

Most of the inherited thrombocytopenias result in moderately depressed platelet counts (50,000 to 100,000 cells/μL) and do not require daily management. However, traumatic injuries, illnesses, or surgical procedures can place these children at risk for bleeding. May-Hegglin anomaly is characterized by macrothrombocytopenia and white blood cell inclusions known as Döhle bodies. Other macrothrombocytopenias are due to autosomally dominant inherited mutations in the *MYH9* gene, which encodes cytoskeletal proteins. Wiskott-Aldrich syndrome (see Chapter 4), on the other hand, is characterized by microthrombocytopenia. This disorder is caused by the X-linked inheritance of mutations and is associated with decreased platelet survival, eczema, and recurrent infections. Treatment of bleeding in inherited thrombocytopenias consists of desmopressin (DDAVP), aminocaproic acid, and platelet transfusions when necessary.

Even when platelets are present in normal amounts, mucocutaneous bleeding due to functional deficits can occur. The most complete test of platelet function is by aggregometry. A sample of patient whole blood or platelet-rich plasma is combined with one of a number of platelet agonist molecules: ristocetin, epinephrine, collagen, ADP, or arachidonic acid. The degree and rate of platelet agglutination are recorded graphically. The various platelet disorders will have unique response patterns to each agonist. Many drugs can affect platelet function temporarily and will make tests of platelet function abnormal. These tests should not be run within

10 days of using such a drug, as the diagnosis of a true disorder could be missed. Other tests can serve as screening evaluations of platelet function, to varying degrees of reliability.

The bleeding time is a surrogate measure of both platelet number and function. At present, this test is not recommended for pediatric patients. Most pediatric hematologists prefer the closure time. The closure time is determined with a cartridge system in which the process of platelet adhesion and aggregation is simulated in vitro. This in vitro testing system provides improved reproducibility, accuracy, and reliability when compared with the standard bleeding time. The test is sensitive to platelet function and von Willebrand factor levels and function. It is important to note that thrombocytopenia and severe anemia will prolong the closure time, making accurate measurements impossible. Although the closure time is more convenient than the bleeding time, its utility as a screening test for coagulation disorders or postoperative bleeding has been poor.

There are several well-known inherited conditions that result in poorly functioning platelets. Glanzmann thrombasthenia was first described in 1918 in a group of patients with normal platelet counts but bleeding symptoms. Subsequently, this abnormality was explained by the inability of platelets to bind fibrinogen and properly aggregate. It is characterized by mucocutaneous bleeding that may begin very early in childhood; epistaxis and, later, menorrhagia are particularly common. Aggregation studies in these patients will show no response to epinephrine, ADP, or collagen but a normal response to ristocetin. Treatment of bleeding usually is accomplished with platelet transfusions; however, repeated transfusions create the risk of anti-platelet antibodies. Bernard-Soulier syndrome also is characterized by recurrent mucocutaneous bleeding but is due to poor binding of von Willebrand factor on the damaged endothelium. Patients also can have a variable thrombocytopenia, although platelets tend to be very large. A diagnosis can be confirmed by review of the peripheral smear and by platelet aggregation studies that show poor response to ristocetin but normal results with other agonists. Treatment can be provided with DDAVP or platelet transfusions.

Drugs and certain disease states can cause temporary impairment of platelet function. Aspirin irreversibly impairs circulating platelets, whereas other nonsteroidal antiinflammatory drugs (NSAIDs) only temporarily inhibit key enzymes. Increased bleeding usually is seen only in patients with an underlying coagulation abnormality, but some patients may be hyperresponsive to the platelet inhibition. Antibiotics, antiepileptics, and psychotropic drugs may also lead to transient inhibitions of platelet function. In addition to medications, systemic illnesses can create an environment in which platelets lose some of their function. Uremia causes platelet inhibition through a variety of mechanisms. The degree of renal failure correlates with prolongation of the bleeding time but not with bleeding.

The primary indication for platelet transfusion is bleeding secondary to thrombocytopenia due to impaired production or a platelet function defect. Antibody-mediated or destructive thrombocytopenias are not usually responsive to platelet transfusion; in such circumstances platelet transfusion is indicated only if there is life-threatening bleeding. Patients can have counts as low as 10,000 cells/μL before a prophylactic transfusion needs to be considered.

Disorders of Secondary Hemostasis

Whatever the cause of coagulopathy, measurement of the PT and aPTT is the first step in clarifying the diagnosis. The prothrombin time (PT), first demonstrated in the 1930s, is a surrogate measure of the coagulation factors involved in the extrinsic and common pathways: VII, X, V, II, and fibrinogen. The PT is typically used to monitor the effects of warfarin therapy or to evaluate for liver disease and vitamin K deficiency. The international normalized ratio (INR) provides standardization of the PT at different laboratories. The activated partial thromboplastin time (aPTT) reflects factors in the intrinsic and common pathways: XII, XI, X, IX, VIII, V, II, and fibrinogen. In addition, the aPTT is affected by prekallikrein and high molecular weight kininogen. Patients who are deficient in factor XII, prekallikrein, or high molecular weight kininogen may have very prolonged aPTT values, although without any evidence of bleeding. The aPTT is less reflective of variations in vitamin K–dependent factors than is the PT; however, it is much more sensitive to the effects of heparin and circulating inhibitors. Both PT and aPTT can be prolonged by deficiencies of factors if levels are less than 30% to 35%.

The most common cause of a prolonged aPTT in children is an inhibitor. The term *inhibitor* can be defined broadly to include anticoagulants, autoantibodies, and lupus anticoagulants. To discern whether a prolonged aPTT is due to factor deficiencies or the presence of an inhibitor, a mixing study can be performed. An abnormal test that corrects is due to deficiencies, whereas those that remain abnormal suggest the presence of an inhibitor. A nonspecific inhibitor, meaning an abnormal mixing study without other hematologic explanation, is a benign and common finding in pediatrics. In this setting, an inhibitor prolongs in vitro clotting times but does not represent a risk factor for bleeding. In children with hemophilia, on the other hand, inhibitors carry different and much more significant implications, as is discussed later.

Hemophilia A is an X-linked bleeding disorder in which patients have a deficiency of factor VIII. Hemophilia B is a similar illness, although with a deficiency of factor IX. Hemophilia A occurs in roughly 1 per 5000 live male births, whereas hemophilia B affects 1 in 30,000. Despite the well-known pattern of inherited mutations in the factor VIII gene, approximately 20% to 30% of patients with severe hemophilia A will not have any affected relatives. Severe hemophilia is usually diagnosed early in the first year of life, especially when a family history is known. Children with mild or moderate degrees of disease may not have bleeding episodes until early childhood. The diagnosis can be suggested by a prolonged aPTT and then confirmed by specific assays for either factor VIII or IX.

The hemophilias are classified by baseline factor level: <1% (1 U/dL) is defined as severe, 1% to 5% (1 to 5 U/dL) as

Figure 11-33 Hemophiliac arthritis. This patient with hemophilia has experienced recurrent hemarthroses. Note the widened joint space on the left knee compared with that of the normal right knee.

moderate, and 6% to 40% (6 to 40 U/dL) as mild. The location, frequency, and type of bleeding episodes relate to the severity of disease. Patients with mild forms of the disease may have bleeding complications only after surgery or major trauma. Those with moderate disease have a higher incidence of minor bleeding and may have bleeding in response to minor trauma or daily activities. Patients with severe hemophilia may have bleeding into joints or muscles with normal daily activities, in addition to minor bleeds and catastrophic hemorrhages from trauma or surgery (Figs. 11-33 and 11-34).

There are selected coagulation disorders that, although rare, may present as part of a larger syndrome. These and other rarely encountered coagulation disorders that are not associated with syndromes should require the input of a pediatric hematologist for management. Some of these rare disorders are listed in Table 11-5. For many, there are no specific treatments available in the United States other than transfused blood products. Fresh frozen plasma (FFP) should be matched to the recipient ABO red cell status, although Rh positivity does not need to be considered. FFP is indicated for patients with significant coagulopathies who are bleeding or require an invasive procedure. Cryoprecipitate, on the other hand, is derived from plasma by thawing FFP and removing the supernatant. This contains concentrated amounts of factors VIII and XIII, von Willebrand factor, and fibrinogen in volumes that, on average, are quite small. In patients with dysfibrinogenemia or hypofibrinogenemia, transfusion of cryoprecipitate is warranted.

Figure 11-34   **A,** Pseudotumor of the femur. This radiographic finding has resulted from recurrent hemarthroses with subsequent bony destruction of the knee and adjacent bony structures. **B,** Note that the opposite knee also demonstrates early destructive changes in the distal femur and joint.

Table 11-5	Rare Bleeding Disorders	
Disorder	**Treatment**	**Notes**
Hypofibrinogenemia	Cryoprecipitate or FFP	Will have very low fibrinogen levels
Dysfibrinogenemia	Cryoprecipitate or FFP	Diagnosed by abnormal reptilase and thrombin times with normal fibrinogen levels
		Usually autosomal dominant inheritance patterns
Factor II (prothrombin) deficiency	FFP or prothrombin complex concentrate	Bleeding usually mild unless after trauma
Factor V deficiency	FFP	Bleeding is usually mild to moderate
		Rarely can be combined with factor VIII deficiency
Factor VII deficiency	Recombinant VIIa	Very rare: 1 per 500,000 in general population
		Very low levels can lead to severe bleeding
Factor X deficiency	FFP or prothrombin complex concentrate	Usually features mild to moderate mucocutaneous and posttraumatic bleeding
Factor XI deficiency	FFP	Autosomal recessive inheritance; most frequently encountered in Ashkenazi Jewish populations
		Bleeding most common after trauma or surgery
Factor XIII deficiency	Cryoprecipitate or FFP	Associated with delayed umbilical cord separation and intracranial hemorrhage with minimal trauma
		Characterized by delayed hemorrhage
PAI-1 deficiency	Antifibrinolytic agents	Bleeding most common after trauma or surgery
		Euglobulin lysis time will be shortened
Antiplasmin deficiency	Antifibrinolytic agents	Mucocutaneous bleeding and hemarthroses
		Symptoms can be similar to those in mild hemophilia
		Euglobulin lysis time will be shortened

FFP, fresh frozen plasma; PAI-1, plasminogen activator inhibitor type 1.

von Willebrand Disease

In the 1920s, Erik von Willebrand described a familial case of mucocutaneous bleeding in Finland. However, it was not until the 1970s that a distinction was made between factor VIII and its carrier, von Willebrand factor. This molecule is synthesized both in endothelial cells and megakaryocytes; patients can have either low, absent, or poorly functioning molecules. von Willebrand disease (VWD) is characterized by excessive mucocutaneous bleeding. It is the most frequently seen inherited bleeding disorder. Its prevalence has been estimated at 1%, although the rate of symptomatic disease is likely closer to 1 per 1000. The diagnosis of VWD begins with three studies. First, the ristocetin cofactor activity measures the function of available von Willebrand factor in plasma. Second, the von Willebrand antigen (VWF:Ag) level measures the amount of von Willebrand factor in the plasma. It also is advisable to ascertain the patient's ABO blood type simultaneously, as patients with type O blood may have VWF:Ag levels lower than the population average. Third, the factor VIII level is measured. Specific testing can be done subsequently to confirm the type of VWD.

Type 1 VWD, the most common, is defined by a partial quantitative deficiency in VWF. It is inherited in an autosomally dominant fashion and usually results in a mild to moderate bleeding risk. The type 2 forms of VWD are uncommon but all feature qualitative defects in VWF or its platelet receptors. Type 2A has poor VWF–platelet adhesion due to decreased levels of large multimers; type 2B leads to increased binding with glycoprotein Ib (GPIb) on platelet surfaces, causing increased clearance of multimers and decreased platelet activity; type 2M involves poor VWF–platelet adhesion without the decrease in large multimers; and type 2N shows decreased binding between VWF and factor VIII, leading to decreased plasma levels of factor VIII. Type III VWD features a near complete deficiency of VWF but is quite rare. Both types 2N and III may lead to musculoskeletal bleeding and can be mistaken for hemophilia A.

DDAVP is a synthetic derivative of antidiuretic hormone and has been studied extensively in the treatment of VWD. Administration of DDAVP will increase plasma concentrations of VWF and factor VIII from endothelial cells. The use of DDAVP, however, is not without toxicities. Most pediatric hematologists now recommend against the use of DDAVP altogether in children younger than 2 years.

Thrombosis in Children

Registries and epidemiologic studies have shown that in the United States, the overall incidence of venous thromboembolism (VTE) is approximately 0.5 to 5 per 10,000 children. There is a bimodal distribution, with a large peak in the newborn period and another in late adolescence. Thromboses often present in the deep veins of an extremity or the vena cava (Fig. 11-35). Much like in adults, thromboses in children often present with pain, swelling, and discoloration. Pulmonary emboli, although less common than in adults, can present with tachypnea, chest pain, tachycardia, and decreased oxygen saturations. Unprovoked pulmonary emboli are rare in pediatrics. Several conditions may underlie or predispose

Figure 11-35 Note the swollen, discolored leg in a child with deep venous thrombosis resulting from protein C deficiency. *(Courtesy R. Kellogg, MD.)*

Table 11-6	Common Thrombophilic Traits and Risk Factors
Thrombophilic Risk/Trait	**Key Principles**
Central venous catheters	• Most common risk factor in pediatric patients • Larger catheter size and smaller vessel lumen increase risk • Risk is increased in hospitalized patients • Routine anticoagulation prophylaxis not recommended
Estrogens (contraception)	• First-generation oral contraceptives (OCPs) have four times the risk • Second-generation OCPs have less; third-generation have more • Risk of thrombosis is multiplied when combined with others
Anti-phospholipid antibodies	• Can be temporary or chronic • Anti-cardiolipin, anti–β2 glycoprotein, and anti-phosphatidylcholine are among most common • Can develop with or without an autoimmune disease • Can lead to catastrophic organ dysfunction
Factor V mutations	• Leiden is most common; followed by Cambridge and HR2 • Makes factor Va resistant to proteolysis by APC • Heterozygotes have two to seven times the risk of thrombosis • Homozygotes have up to 70-fold risk
Protein C deficiency	• Prevalence of heterozygosity is near 1 in 300 • Multiple subtypes of heterozygous states • Unlikely to present with thromboses before puberty • Homozygous deficiencies can present with neonatal purpura fulminans
Protein S deficiency	• Acts similarly to protein C deficiency • Prevalence is near 1 per 33,000 • Risk is increased sevenfold in heterozygous disease • Prevalence of homozygosity is closer to 1 per 1,000,000
Prothrombin gene variant	• Mutation at *G20210A* • Leads to persistence of circulating thrombin • 2% to 3% of white population is heterozygous • Heterozygosity increases risk by threefold
Antithrombin III deficiency	• Gene located on chromosome 1; more than 250 mutations known • Homozygosity not compatible with life • Odds ratio increased 10- to 20-fold in heterozygous states • Thromboses much more common in adults than children • Prevalence varies widely
MTHFR mutations and hyperhomocysteinemia	• Hyperhomocysteinemia can develop in setting of folate or B vitamin deficiency • Can damage endothelium and cause prothrombotic changes • Risk increase by 2.5-fold • Homozygous mutations for G677T have highest risk • Mutation at A1298C confers risk only in compound heterozygotes • Heterozygous mutations do not lead to homocysteine elevation

APC, activated protein C.

children to developing thromboses. Table 11-6 lists some of the most common thrombophilic traits and risk factors. Anticoagulation usually is initiated with unfractionated heparin intravenously or low molecular weight heparin subcutaneously. Both should be performed with the guidance of a pediatric hematologist.

Lemierre syndrome is an example of a thromboembolic disorder often encountered in children. This condition is characterized by jugular vein thrombosis and anaerobic infections in the head and neck region. The occurrence of these thromboses likely is due to a combination of venous stasis, endothelial damage from local inflammation, and an underlying hypercoagulable state (acquired or inherited). Although the syndrome classically has been associated with *Fusobacterium necrophorum*, polymicrobial infections are common in children. Tonsillitis, pharyngitis, mastoiditis, and tooth infections that spread to the pharyngeal spaces can all lead to Lemierre syndrome. Anterior neck disease may present with pain, swelling, and tenderness but posterior compartment disease may

be more difficult to detect until late in its course. Treatment involves targeted antimicrobial therapy and anticoagulation. In severe cases with systemic compromise from septic pulmonary emboli, a thrombectomy of the primary clot may be required.

An increasingly recognized complication of thromboses in children is the postthrombotic syndrome (PTS). This occurs after incomplete recanalization of a vessel that was thrombosed. Pharmacologic anticoagulation as well as the body's natural systems attempt to dissolve a thrombosis and restore blood flow through the vessel. At the same time, however, angiogenic factors are at work to develop collateral vessels around the affected area. If a collateral circulation develops and the primary thrombosis is not recanalized, subsequent blood flow may be more sluggish than normal. Thromboses that persist beyond 6 months of anticoagulation are not likely to resolve. Although PTS does not necessarily confer a risk of subsequent or extended thrombosis, it can produce symptoms over time. Sequelae of PTS, in fact, can mimic the symptoms

Figure 11-36 Disseminated intravascular coagulation (DIC). Peripheral blood smear of a child with meningococcemia and DIC. Note the red blood cell fragments and decreased platelet count.

Table 11-7	Clinical Equivalent of Experimental Disseminated Intravascular Coagulation–Triggering Agents

Gram-negative septicemia

Necrotizing enterocolitis

Shock from any cause

Endothelial damage (virus, bacteria, *Rickettsia*, heat stroke)

Trauma, burns

Ascitic fluid (LeVeen shunt)

Hypoxia-acidosis, severe hyaline membrane disease

Malignancies (acute leukemia, neuroblastoma, rhabdomyosarcoma)

Dead fetal twin

Hemolysis transfusion reaction

Small-for-gestational-age infant (placental infarct)

Purpura fulminans

Localized giant hemangioma

Modified from Corrigan JJ: Disseminated intravascular coagulopathy, *Pediatr Rev* 1:37–45, 1979.

of an acute thrombosis with pain, discoloration, and swelling. These symptoms tend to be transient, intermittent, and recurrent in children. Compression stockings or other local measures are often needed for treatment. Severe and long-standing PTS can lead to venous stasis and ulceration later in life.

Consumptive and Microangiopathic Disorders

Hemolysis of RBCs can result not only from intrinsic abnormalities of the RBCs but also from alterations in the RBC environment. Microangiopathic hemolytic anemia, a hematologic condition of diverse causes, is most often acquired and, rarely, congenital in origin. The hematologic picture is characterized by the presence of burr erythrocytes, schistocytes, helmet cells, and microspherocytes. In almost all cases there is concurrent thrombocytopenia. Additional laboratory studies confirm the presence of intravascular hemolysis including elevated plasma hemoglobin levels, low to absent haptoglobin, and the presence of hemosiderinuria.

Elevated serum fibrin degradation products provide evidence for disseminated intravascular coagulation (DIC). In pediatric patients, infection with shock is by far the most frequent cause of DIC. Regardless of the trigger, production of fibrin in the microcirculation and fibrin deposition in capillaries cause shearing of the RBCs as they cross the capillary beds (Fig. 11-36). In addition to RBC destruction, platelets and clotting factors are consumed. Patients may have petechiae and purpura (Fig. 11-37), or persistent bleeding from venipuncture sites. Table 11-7 lists diseases known to trigger DIC. DIC is also seen in Kasabach-Merritt syndrome when platelet consumption occurs within the endothelial maze of massive strawberry and cavernous hemangiomas (Fig. 11-38).

Microangiopathic changes of the peripheral blood smear may also be seen when RBCs pass through abnormal tissues. Examples of this abnormal physiology include RBC damage in hemolytic-uremic syndrome (HUS) and thrombotic thrombocytopenic purpura (TTP). HUS is a disease of childhood that is characterized primarily by renal insufficiency. TTP is more commonly seen in adults. The patient with TTP experiences neurologic complications in addition to renal abnormalities. These disorders have in common hemolytic anemia, thrombocytopenia, and thrombotic occlusion of the microvasculature of various organs. Scientific evidence indicates that patients with familial occurrence of this syndrome may have a congenital abnormality in the processing of von Willebrand factor.

Figure 11-37 This infant has neuroblastoma and purpuric lesions relating to a tumor-related coagulopathy. Similar lesions may result from other conditions such as severe isolated thrombocytopenia and/or disseminated intravascular coagulation.

Figure 11-38 The hemangiomatous lesion in this patient resulted in Kasabach-Merritt syndrome, in which platelet consumption within the lesion leads to thrombocytopenia.

Table 11-8	Normal Leukocyte and Differential Counts*			
	12 Months	**4 Years**	**10 Years**	**21 Years**
Leukocytes, total	11.4 (6.0-17.5)	9.1 (5.5-15.5)	8.1 (4.5-13.5)	7.4 (4.5-11.0)
Neutrophils, total	3.5 (1.5-8.5) (31%)	3.8 (1.5-8.5) (42%)	4.4 (1.8-8.0) (54%)	4.4 (1.8-7.7) (59%)
Neutrophils, band forms	0.35 (3.1%)	0.27 (0-1.0) (3.0%)	0.24 (0-1.0) (3.0%)	0.22 (0-0.7) (3.0%)
Neutrophils, segmented	3.2 (28%)	3.5 (1.5-7.5) (39%)	4.2 (1.8-7.0) (51%)	4.2 (1.8-7.0) (56%)
Eosinophils	0.30 (0.05-0.70) (2.6%)	0.25 (0.02-0.65) (2.8%)	0.20 (0-0.60) (2.4%)	0.20 (0-0.45) (2.7%)
Basophils	0.05 (0-10) (0.4%)	0.05 (0-0.20) (0.6%)	0.04 (0-0.20) (0.5%)	0.04 (0-0.20) (0.5%)
Lymphocytes	7.0 (4.0-10.5) (61%)	4.5 (2.0-8.0) (50%)	3.1 (1.5-6.5) (38%)	2.5 (1.0-4.8) (34%)
Monocytes	0.55 (0.05-1.1) (4.8%)	0.45 (0-0.8) (5.0%)	0.35 (0-0.8) (4.3%)	0.30 (0-0.8) (4.0%)

*Values are expressed as cells × 10^3/μL. Mean values are given; ranges are in parentheses. Percentage values are for mean values.
From Altman PL, Dittmer DS, editors: *Blood and other body fluids*, Washington, DC, 1961, Federation of American Societies for Experimental Biology.

Heparin-induced thrombocytopenia (HIT) occurs in up to 5% of adult patients who are exposed to heparin, although the incidence in children is significantly less. An initial episode of thrombocytopenia usually occurs approximately 5 to 10 days after exposure to heparin, although repeat episodes can occur within hours. HIT is caused by heparin-dependent antibodies against the platelet factor 4 (PF4) antigen. These IgG antibodies activate platelets that then stimulate coagulation reactions and can lead to a transiently increased risk of thrombosis. Treatment of HIT involves the discontinuation of all heparin (including line flushes), the initiation of alternative anticoagulation, and the avoidance of platelet transfusions.

White Blood Cells

Normal values for total white blood cell (WBC) number and differential counts are age related (Table 11-8). African-American patients may have lower granulocyte counts than white patients of the same age. Leukocytosis and leukopenia are common pediatric problems. In general, these are due to increases or decreases in specific types of WBCs. Most cases of neutrophilia (Fig. 11-39), neutropenia, eosinophilia (Fig. 11-40), lymphocytosis (Fig. 11-41), lymphopenia, or monocytosis (Fig. 11-42) in the pediatric population do not represent primary hematologic disorders. The abnormalities of the blood count often represent the bone marrow response to an associated condition. The pertinent history and physical examination findings related to increases or decreases in WBC numbers are outlined throughout this atlas for various disease states.

Morphologic abnormalities of the granulocytic series, although less common, may provide clues to the diagnosis.

Figure 11-40   Eosinophilia. This patient's blood shows an increased WBC count and increased eosinophils owing to a parasitic infection.

The hypersegmented neutrophil, which may be an early clue to vitamin B_{12} deficiency, has been noted previously (see Fig. 11-10). This needs to be distinguished from familial hypersegmentation by looking at the peripheral smears of family members. On occasion, mature neutrophils may be abnormally large in members of a given family—so-called hereditary giant neutrophils. The Pelger-Huët anomaly (Fig. 11-43) is usually a benign morphologic inherited anomaly, but it is sometimes acquired in adults and generally spurs a search for occult malignancy because of its known association with leukemia and lymphoma. This WBC abnormality has also been described in association with infectious and rheumatologic disorders. Increased numbers of nuclear appendages may also be seen in the neutrophils of patients with trisomy 13 (Fig. 11-44). These, however, may be difficult to distinguish from normal neutrophil "drumsticks," which are nuclear

Figure 11-39   Neutrophilia and increased band forms (left shift). The pattern of a left shift of the white blood cell series is consistent with infection. The peripheral blood smear shows increased neutrophils and band forms in a child with pneumococcal sepsis.

Figure 11-41   Lymphocytosis. An elevated lymphocyte count is seen in the peripheral blood smear of a child with pertussis.

Figure 11-42 Monocytosis. The peripheral blood will often show an increased monocyte count at a time of marrow recovery after significant suppression. In this case the child is recovering from chemotherapy-induced neutropenia.

Figure 11-44 **A,** Nuclear appendages are normally seen in the polymorphonuclear leukocytes of girls. An increase in these appendages is seen in cases of trisomy 13. **B,** Schematic of nuclear appendages.

appendages that occur in 2% to 10% of neutrophils of normal girls.

Toxic granulations, which are prominent azurophilic granules, are another common type of WBC inclusion. They are nonspecific but can be seen in viral and bacterial infections (Fig. 11-45). Toxic granulations must be distinguished from the hereditary dense granulation that may occasionally be present in the neutrophils of normal individuals. Döhle bodies, pale blue inclusions that usually are located peripherally in the cytoplasm of neutrophils, may coexist with toxic granulations. Together with giant platelets, Döhle bodies are seen in patients with the dominantly inherited May-Hegglin anomaly (Fig. 11-46). Large greenish-brown neutrophil inclusions are characteristic of the patient with rare Chédiak-Higashi syndrome (Fig. 11-47). Such granules may appear in eosinophils and basophils as well. WBCs may also acquire inclusions by engulfing particles from their surroundings.

Neutropenia is one of the most common white cell disorders seen in pediatrics. Differing levels of neutropenia, reflected by a diminished absolute neutrophil count (ANC), confer differing risks of infection. Neutropenia can be seen in response to medications, in congenital deficiencies (Kostmann syndrome), or in response to infections. Autoimmune neutropenia develops in response to antibody-mediated destruction of neutrophils. This is generally self-limited and resolves in a matter of months. This is commonly seen in a postinfectious setting. Chronic benign neutropenia has an unclear etiology but can persist for years. Its name can be somewhat misleading, as children are still at risk for severe, and potentially fatal, infections. Cyclic neutropenia, a disorder in which the ANC drops at regular intervals, is extremely rare but can be tested for on a genetic level. During periods of neutropenia, children may develop mucosal ulcerations or breakdown. Children with neutropenia generally do not require isolation or prophylactic antibiotics on a regular basis. However, if febrile, those

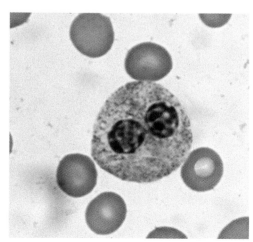

Figure 11-43 Pelger-Huët anomaly. Note the uniform bilobed nucleus of the granulocyte.

Figure 11-45 Döhle body. Toxic granulations and a Döhle body are found in the blood of this child with sepsis. The Döhle body appears as a grayish-blue staining area, which is located at the inferior border of this cell.

Figure 11-46   A, May-Hegglin anomaly. The peripheral blood of individuals with this condition demonstrates Döhle bodies in the white blood cells and giant platelets that may be decreased in number. **B,** Schematic of May-Hegglin anomaly.

children do warrant prompt medical evaluation to rule out a more serious infection. Hormonal stimulation with granulocyte colony-stimulating factor (G-CSF) to increase the ANC usually is required only in settings of severe infections or prominent symptoms.

Atypical lymphocytes are large cells with an irregular plasma membrane that often hug adjacent RBCs. The nucleus of an atypical lymphocyte is also large, and nucleoli may be visible. The abundant cytoplasm is typically basophilic and may contain vacuoles and azurophilic granules (Fig. 11-48). Morphologic subtypes of atypical lymphocytes may occur, but clinically, their recognition is of little use. Although infectious mononucleosis comes to mind when atypical lymphocytes are seen, these lymphocytes are not specific and may be present in many other situations, especially viral illnesses.

Conversely, in some cases leukocytosis may result from an increase in the number of immature rather than mature WBCs of any given cell line (a so-called *shift to the left*). Leukemia (Fig. 11-49) is the prototype, and Figures 11-50 to 11-53 illustrate the varied appearances of blast cells. Figure 11-54 shows a leukemoid reaction, which is characterized by a high WBC count (usually >50,000/mm^3) with an increase in the number of immature myeloid cells. Leukemoid reactions must be distinguished from leukemia. Although this is definitively

accomplished by a bone marrow aspirate, peripheral blood studies can assist a diagnosis. The leukocyte alkaline phosphatase level (LAP score) is increased in leukemoid reaction and decreased in chronic myelogenous leukemia. Patients with Down syndrome may experience a transient leukemoid reaction (transient myeloproliferative disorder) in the newborn period. Additional manifestations of this disorder include hepatosplenomegaly and circulating myeloblasts. Spontaneous remission often occurs. However, 20% to 30% of patients with Down syndrome and transient myeloproliferative disorder develop leukemia within the first 3 years of life.

Histiocytoses

Seborrhea, which is usually a benign finding, may be one of the cutaneous manifestations of *Langerhans cell histiocytosis* (Fig. 11-55). This diagnosis should be considered if the rash is unusually severe or persists despite standard treatment measures. Additional physical examination findings that should

Figure 11-47   Chédiak-Higashi syndrome. Note the neutrophilic inclusion characteristic of this rare disease. *(Courtesy William Zinkham, MD, Baltimore, Md.)*

Figure 11-48   Atypical lymphocyte in the case of infectious mononucleosis. Atypical lymphocytes in the peripheral blood are often observed in patients with infectious mononucleosis. The nucleus is large, and the cytoplasm is abundant. Note that where the cytoplasm of the lymphocyte abuts the red blood cell, the lymphocyte deforms around it.

Figure 11-49 Acute lymphoblastic leukemia—peripheral blood smear. Note the presence of decreased platelets and the absence of normal white blood cells.

Figure 11-52 L3 lymphoblasts. This represents the third morphologic presentation of the lymphoblast. These lymphoblasts are large, deeply staining cells that are often vacuolated. The L3 lymphoblastic cell is characteristic of Burkitt leukemia and lymphoma.

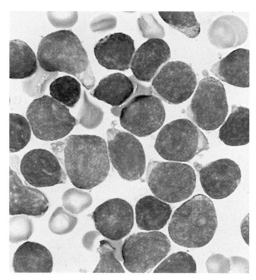

Figure 11-50 Acute lymphoblastic leukemia—bone marrow aspirate. Note the monotonous pattern of the lymphoblastic (L1) cells.

Figure 11-53 Acute myelogenous leukemia. Peripheral blood smear showing an Auer rod (red, rod-shaped figure in the cytoplasm) within a myeloblast of a patient with acute nonlymphocytic/acute myelogenous leukemia.

Figure 11-51 Bone marrow aspirate (L2 lymphoblasts) in another patient with acute lymphoblastic leukemia. These lymphoblasts are larger and more heterogeneous in appearance than L1 lymphoblasts. In addition, the nuclear-to-cytoplasmic ratio is lower, and nucleoli more prominent, than in L1 lymphoblasts.

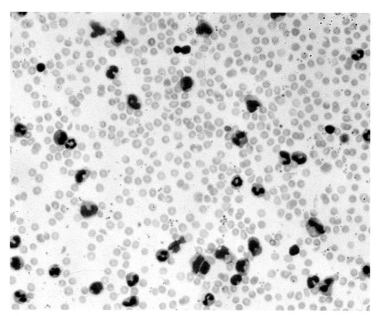

Figure 11-54 Leukemoid reaction. Elevated white blood cell (WBC) count in response to infection. The child whose blood is pictured here was documented to have pneumococcal sepsis with an appropriate WBC response.

Figure 11-55   A, Langerhans cell histiocytosis (LCH). Seborrhea and chronic ear drainage may be presenting clinical features in an infant with LCH. **B** and **C,** Hemorrhagic and papular rashes are also seen in some children with this disease. *(Courtesy P. Gaffney, MD, Pittsburgh, Pa.)*

increase the suspicion for this diagnosis include any erythema of gingival mucosa, organomegaly, or systemic symptoms such as irritability or failure to thrive (see Chapter 8).

Hemophagocytic lymphohistiocytosis (HLH) can be both congenital and acquired. The disorder is best described as reactive in nature, and is due to abnormalities of the antigen-presenting and antigen-processing histiocytes. Its pathophysiology is best thought of as an uncontrolled cytokine storm. This syndrome, when occurring in infants, is often of the familial or genetic type. Hemophagocytosis also can occur in association with systemic infection, underlying malignant disease, or as a manifestation of immune deficiency (Fig. 11-56). Unfortunately, there are no definitive diagnostic tests other than genetic mutation analysis, which can be very time-consuming. In practice, the diagnosis of HLH is based on a variety of clinical criteria. International research studies and consensus panels have led to newly revised suggested criteria (Table 11-9). However, great care is required in making the diagnosis of HLH, as many other systemic illnesses, namely sepsis and liver failure, also can meet several of these criteria in isolation. Prognosis is dependent on the origin as a congenital or acquired variant. The genetic form often leads to rapid clinical deterioration with a guarded long-term prognosis. However, with chemotherapy and bone marrow transplantation, outcomes have improved greatly. In secondary HLH, those individuals who survive their acute process have a more favorable prognosis. Chemotherapy, but not a bone marrow transplant, often still is required.

Bone Marrow Failure

Pancytopenia refers to a reduction in all three formed elements of the blood. In an analogous manner to anemia, pancytopenia is not a single disease entity but rather may result from a

Figure 11-56   Erythrophagocytosis. Numerous red blood cells are engulfed by white blood cell cytoplasm in this peripheral blood smear of a patient with erythrophagocytosis.

Table 11-9	Proposed 2009 Diagnostic Criteria For Hemophagocytic Lymphohistiocytosis
Criteria	**Description**
Any result is diagnostic	Molecular/genetic evidence of HLH or X-linked lymphoproliferative syndrome mutation
If not, three of four must be present	Fever
	Splenomegaly
	Cytopenias of at least two cell lines
	Hepatitis
In addition, at least one of four must be present	Hemophagocytosis on biopsy sample
	Increased ferritin
	Increased soluble IL-2Rα (for age)
	Absent or very decreased natural killer cell function
Other supportive information	Hypertriglyceridemia
	Hypofibrinogenemia
	Hyponatremia

HLH, hemophagocytic lymphohistiocytosis; IL-2Rα, interleukin-2 receptor α.
Adapted from Filipovich AH: Hemophagocytic lymphohistiocytosis (HLH) and related disorders, *Hematology Am Soc Hematol Educ Program* 2009:127-131, 2009.

number of disease processes. Pancytopenia may occur from bone marrow failure or extramedullary cellular destruction (as seen in autoimmune disease, particularly systemic lupus erythematosus) or as a combination of depressed marrow function and increased cellular destruction. When pancytopenia is due to destruction of the formed elements of the blood, invariably there is another underlying disease. On the other hand, the pancytopenia resulting from bone marrow failure can be divided into genetically predisposed marrow failure syndromes and acquired marrow failure syndromes.

Aplastic anemia is marked by peripheral blood pancytopenia associated with bone marrow hypocellularity or acellularity. Acquired aplastic anemia is an immune-mediated disease, although genetic risk factors and environmental exposures likely contribute. Research has resulted in a much deeper understanding of the role that activated T lymphocytes play in presenting hematopoietic cell antigens for destruction. In children, the acuity of presentation in aplastic anemia relates to the degree of pancytopenia. Severe aplastic anemia is classified as a bone marrow sample that demonstrates less than 25% cellularity, in association with peripheral cytopenias in two of the three lineages. The treatment for severe aplastic anemia is either hematopoietic stem cell transplantation (HSCT) or primary immunosuppression.

Pancytopenia is a common presentation for both Fanconi anemia (a chromosomal breakage syndrome) and dyskeratosis congenita (a telomere length disorder). Fanconi anemia, the most frequent of the constitutional marrow failure syndromes, is a familial disorder that also features a variable constellation of congenital anomalies of the skin, skeleton, central nervous system, and genitourinary tract (Fig. 11-57). Fragility of the chromosomes and pancytopenia, however, can occur in the absence of physical anomalies. More uniquely, isolated thrombocytopenia is a common first sign of amegakaryocytic thrombocytopenia and thrombocytopenia–absent radius syndrome (Fig. 11-58). Supportive care with transfusions is an important mainstay for these diseases. Although the hematologic complications of some may resolve over the first year of life, matched-sibling HSCT is the treatment of choice for symptomatic children with many bone marrow failure syndromes.

Figure 11-57 A patient with Fanconi anemia is pictured with her three siblings. This patient had a bone marrow transplant for her underlying condition. Note her diminutive size with respect to her more robust siblings.

ONCOLOGY

Pediatric malignancy is rare when compared with the incidence of cancer in the adult population. However, it remains a significant contributor to the morbidity and mortality of childhood diseases. More than 10,000 new cases of cancer are diagnosed during childhood in the United States each year. The ability to treat and cure childhood malignancies has improved dramatically over the past few decades, which is encouraging. This is due, in large part, to advances made in cooperative group clinical trials, the introduction of novel chemotherapy agents, and improvements in supportive care for the patient receiving chemotherapy. The majority of children with cancer today will be cured. In the year 2010 an estimated 1 in 500 individuals between the ages of 15 and 45 years is a survivor of childhood cancer. Importantly, the

Figure 11-58 A, Child with thrombocytopenia–absent radius syndrome, also known as *TAR syndrome.* **B,** Radiograph of the same patient. Note the absence of the radius.

pediatrician must be involved in monitoring the surviving children and young adults for long-term effects of therapy, a topic addressed in the final section of this chapter.

The initial task of recognizing the signs and symptoms of malignancy usually falls to the pediatrician, family medicine physician, or emergency room physician. The current chapter aims to review clinical presentations that should alert the physician to the possibility of a malignant process. As with most pediatric conditions, the differential diagnosis varies depending on the age of the child. An immediate concern at the time of diagnosis is to prevent any tumor-related complications, including neutropenia due to marrow infiltration or metabolic abnormalities due to increased cell turnover. Signs and symptoms of the most common tumors of childhood are reviewed in a manner that parallels the physical examination. This method may result in some degree of overlap, as many cancers manifest a wide spectrum of presentations that may vary in location within the body. Each tumor subtype is discussed in the context of a region in which it typically presents. For a more detailed description of specific cancers, a more comprehensive text is recommended (see Pizzo and Poplack, 2010, in the bibliography).

Signs and Symptoms

Red flags that signal malignancy may be detected in the course of history taking and physical examination, or in basic laboratory testing. Table 11-10 provides a summary of signs and symptoms that should alert the physician to the possibility of a malignant process. These features may be due to the direct effect of a tumor (e.g., compression or infiltration of an organ). Alternatively, the rapid cell division may lead to metabolic abnormalities including hyperkalemia, hyperuricemia, and hyperphosphatemia with reflex hypocalcemia as a manifestation of tumor lysis. True paraneoplastic syndromes are uncommon in the pediatric population. An example of such a paraneoplastic process occurs in a small percentage of patients with neuroblastoma. Opsoclonus–myoclonus syndrome (random eye movements and myoclonic jerking) tends to occur in patients with low-stage disease and favorable histology of the tumor. Unfortunately, many are left with devastating developmental and neurocognitive deficits that relate to this rare paraneoplastic condition. Even rarer is Kerner-Morrison syndrome, in which the patient experiences intractable secretory diarrhea, hypokalemia, and dehydration. This condition represents the secretion of vasoactive intestinal peptide and has also been described in patients with neuroblastoma.

The child with a new diagnosis of malignancy is sometimes asymptomatic, as may be the case in a child with a palpable abdominal mass. In other cases, nonspecific symptoms may be a prominent finding including fever, weight loss, and/or lethargy. Examples of more specific signs and symptoms in pediatric malignancy include the following: headache and morning vomiting in a patient with a brain tumor; constipation and difficulty voiding in a patient with a pelvic tumor or

spinal cord compression; hypertension in a child with a renal or suprarenal tumor; bone pain and limping in a young child secondary to leukemia or, less commonly, another marrow-infiltrative process.

All of these complaints are more likely to have a cause that is nonmalignant. However, persistence (2 weeks is a reasonable, although not absolute, guideline) or undue severity may give these signs increased significance. Similarly, in the context of a number of predisposing, underlying diseases, malignancy should be considered earlier. Table 11-11 lists examples of inherited cancer syndromes, the cancers to which the affected individuals are predisposed, and the mode of inheritance. Certainly, children with a history of one cancer, by virtue of genetics or as a long-term effect of anticancer therapy, are at greater risk of a second cancer. For example, radiation therapy predisposes to a lifelong increased risk of solid tumors within the radiation field. Cancer in a parent or sibling, although heightening anxiety about the possibility of cancer in a child, is rarely by itself a major predisposing factor. The notable exception is the infant or toddler who has an identical twin with leukemia. In this child the risk of leukemia may be as high as 25%. Retinoblastoma and Wilms tumor are also known to occur with increased frequency in offspring of individuals with these diagnoses.

The clinical findings in the child with malignancy vary greatly depending on the site of origin of the tumor. As mentioned previously, the clinical findings are presented in a regional fashion. Prefacing this is a general discussion of acute lymphoblastic leukemia, the most common cancer of childhood. Every attempt is made to provide a general discussion of individual pediatric cancers through a review of more characteristic physical examination findings. The discussion is not inclusive of all potential manifestations of these diseases. Its intent is to provide a fundamental understanding of the spectrum of malignant diseases of childhood along with the signs and symptoms to alert the physician to their possible presence.

Table 11-11	Inherited Cancer Predisposition Syndromes	
Genetic Syndrome	**Associated Cancers**	**Inheritance**
Ataxia-telangiectasia	Leukemia, lymphoma	Autosomal recessive
Beckwith-Wiedemann syndrome	Wilms tumor, adrenal carcinoma, hepatoblastoma	Autosomal dominant or sporadic
Bloom syndrome	Multiple (epithelial, hematopoietic, lymphoid, connective tissue)	Autosomal recessive
Down syndrome	Acute myeloid leukemia (megakaryocytic: M7)	N/a
Gardner syndrome	Colorectal polyposis and adenocarcinoma, osteoma, soft tissue tumors	Autosomal dominant
Neurofibromatosis type 1	Cutaneous and plexiform neurofibromas, malignant peripheral nerve sheath tumors, gliomas, rhabdomyosarcomas	Autosomal dominant
Neurofibromatosis type 2	Vestibular schwannomas, meningiomas, ependymomas, astrocytomas	Autosomal dominant
Retinoblastoma	Retinoblastoma, sarcomas (including osteosarcoma in radiation fields), melanoma	Autosomal dominant
Xeroderma pigmentosum	Squamous cell and basal cell carcinomas, melanoma, carcinoma of lung, gastric tissue, and brain	Autosomal recessive

Table 11-10	Red Flags of Malignancy	
Pallor, fatigue	Headache, vomiting, lethargy
Petechiae	Lymphadenopathy
Fever without source	Hepatomegaly
Bone pain, limp	Splenomegaly
Weight loss	Abdominal mass
Anorexia	Testiculomegaly

Leukemia

Acute lymphoblastic leukemia (ALL) is the most common cancer of childhood, although acute and chronic myelogenous leukemia also are seen. Symptomatic thrombocytopenia may be the reason a child with leukemia is brought to medical attention. A diminished peripheral count of one or more cell lineages is a common sign at the diagnosis of leukemia. With the initiation of chemotherapy, however, a patient's tumor burden regresses and normal hematopoiesis has an opportunity to resume. Platelet transfusions may be required during episodes of bleeding but are not routinely given as prophylaxis unless the peripheral count is less than 10,000 cells per microliter.

Acute leukemia is the most common cause of malignant replacement of marrow in childhood. The leukemic blast represents a clonal expansion of a cell at a specific stage of lymphoid or myeloid development. Clinical symptoms may include fever, fatigue, pallor, and bone pain as evidenced by limping. ALL accounts for approximately 75% of pediatric cases of acute leukemia. The peak age range is between 2 and 5 years of age. For ALL, an age between 1 and 9 years and a presenting white blood cell count of less than 50,000 remain important indicators of a favorable prognosis. More recent studies demonstrate that the presence or absence of minimal residual disease (MRD) is also an important predictor of the child at increased risk of relapse, and this evaluation tool is becoming a standard aspect of evaluation of the child receiving leukemia therapy. Acute myeloid leukemia (AML) is the other predominant leukemia of childhood, accounting for approximately 20% of cases. The incidence of AML is stable from birth to 10 years of age. There is a slight increase in the number of cases during the teenage years. The finding of pancytopenia, organomegaly, and lymphadenopathy in these conditions relates directly to infiltration of marrow and normal organ tissues with the expanded leukemic clone. As leukemia is a systemic cancer with symptoms of a multiorgan nature, examples of clinical findings are referenced throughout the chapter.

Skin

Morphologic characteristics of cutaneous lesions may allow for the identification of an underlying diagnosis that suggests a predisposition to cancer, such as neurofibromatosis (see Table 11-11). Skin findings also provide a window into bone marrow function through clinical signs such as pallor, indicative of anemia, or bruising and petechiae, suggesting thrombocytopenia. Pallor may be most readily appreciated by examination of the mucous membranes including the conjunctiva and oral mucosa. If the patient is severely anemic, the palmar creases of the hand may also be demonstrably pale. Petechiae may be a normal finding on the face and upper thorax of a patient who has had forceful crying, vomiting, or coughing. Diffuse petechiae, purpura, and oral lesions are more suggestive of the presence of thrombocytopenia or platelet dysfunction (see Fig. 11-37). Bruising also has a typical distribution in childhood and is often prominent on the anterior tibial surfaces of an active child. An abnormal amount of bruising or unusual sites of bruising such as buttocks or back should raise suspicion of abnormal hemostasis. If laboratory studies do not support the presence of thrombocytopenia or a coagulation disorder, the pediatrician must always be careful to consider nonaccidental trauma as the etiology.

Skin rashes may also provide clues to the specific diagnosis. In certain cases, biopsy of the skin may provide diagnostic material, thereby avoiding more invasive procedures. Nodular skin lesions may be observed in both neuroblastoma and in some cases of leukemia (Fig. 11-59). Seborrhea, which is

Figure 11-59 Subcutaneous nodule of neuroblastoma. Skin lesions, which are occasionally seen with leukemia or other solid tumors, may be dark ("blueberry muffin") or skin colored. *(From Pearson H: Tumors of the sympathetic nervous system. In Altman AJ, Schwartz AD, editors:* Malignant diseases of infancy, childhood, and adolescence, *ed 2, Philadelphia, 1983, WB Saunders.)*

usually a benign finding, may be one of the cutaneous manifestations of Langerhans cell histiocytosis (see Fig. 11-55). This diagnosis should be considered if the rash is unusually severe or persists despite standard treatment measures. Additional physical examination findings that should increase the suspicion for this diagnosis include any erythema of the gingival mucosa, organomegaly, or systemic symptoms such as irritability or failure to thrive (see Chapter 8). Melanoma (Fig. 11-60) is extremely rare in childhood. It most likely results from the transformation of pigmented or junctional nevi, and these pigmented lesions should be monitored for any change in size, shape, or regularity of margins. Suspicious lesions warrant biopsy. The biopsy is necessary to determine the diagnosis of a specific skin cancer. Definitive surgery depends on the histologic findings. Squamous and basal cell carcinomas (Fig. 11-61) arise most often in the setting of heritable

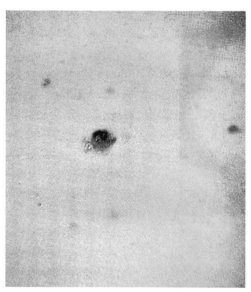

Figure 11-60 Melanoma. In addition to location (see text), suspicious signs of skin lesions include a red-brown-black color that tends to be diffuse at the periphery, crusting, bleeding, pain, or itching.

Figure 11-61   A, Squamous cell carcinoma. **B,** Basal cell carcinoma. This 7-year-old boy received prophylactic cranial radiation as part of his treatment for acute lymphoblastic leukemia 5 years before he developed a second cancer. (**A,** Courtesy J. Zitelli, MD, Pittsburgh, Pa; **B,** from Pratt CB, Douglass EC: Management of the uncommon cancer of childhood. In Pizzo PA, Poplack DG, editors: Principles and practices of pediatric oncology, Philadelphia, 2010, Lippincott Williams & Wilkins.)

diseases, such as xeroderma pigmentosum or basal cell nevus syndrome. These rare cases of pediatric skin cancer are also observed with greater frequency in patients who require long-term immunosuppression, such as recipients of solid organ and bone marrow transplantation.

Head and Neck

Tumors of the central nervous system are the solid tumors most frequently encountered in children. One of the most critical conditions for the clinician to recognize is the patient with increased intracranial pressure, because this is a true oncologic emergency. A typical history might include the occurrence of severe morning headache with associated vomiting. The physical examination may reveal the presence of papilledema or neurologic deficits, such as cranial nerve palsies. Signs and symptoms in the infant may include macrocephaly and a bulging fontanelle due to the absence of fused sutures. Primary or metastatic intracranial tumors may also manifest as seizures or changes in mental status. Most pediatric brain tumors are infratentorial in location. Because these tumors usually arise in the cerebellum, patients may also present with ataxia. Spinal tumors of children may be observed anywhere along the vertebral column. The symptoms of a tumor in this location are caused by compression of the contents of the spinal canal. Pain on percussion over the vertebral column may be an early sign of cord compression and should be actively sought in the child with suspected cancer in this region. Spinal tumors often

have associated weakness, with the affected muscle group corresponding to the level of the lesion. Spinal cord tumors or tumors that press on the cord may present with bowel/bladder dysfunction, paresthesias, or changes in gait.

Clinical presentation varies depending on whether a tumor is supratentorial or infratentorial in location. Supratentorial lesions may present with headache, visual defects, or hemiparesis. Supratentorial lesions are of two major types:
  A. Tumors of the cerebral hemisphere including astrocytoma, ependymoma, glioblastoma, and meningioma (Fig. 11-62, A)
  B. Supratentorial tumors may also originate in the sella or chiasm and include craniopharyngioma, pituitary adenoma, and optic nerve glioma (Fig. 11-62, B)
Common presentations of infratentorial lesions include morning headache and vomiting, sixth nerve palsy, and ataxia. Infratentorial lesions may also be considered in two major categories:
  A. Tumors of the cerebellum including medulloblastoma, astrocytoma, and meningioma (Fig. 11-62, C)
  B. Brainstem tumors including intrinsic pontine gliomas and focal or low-grade brainstem gliomas
It is important to realize that brain tumors are determined to be malignant on the basis of not only histology but also location, given the vital life functions that relate to normal brainstem functioning. Last, developmental delay is a symptom of many brain tumors in the pediatric population.

Figure 11-62   A, Axial T_2 magnetic resonance imaging (MRI) of a child with astrocytoma. **B,** Axial T_2 MRI of a child with craniopharyngioma. **C,** Axial T_2 MRI of a child with medulloblastoma.

Figure 11-63 Leukocoria. Cat's eye reflex, or leukocoria, in a child with retinoblastoma. *(From Abramson D: Retinoblastoma,* CA Cancer J Clin *32:130-140, 1982.)*

Ocular and Otic Findings

Cat's eye reflex, or leukocoria with an absent red reflex, is characteristic of retinoblastoma (see Chapter 19) and should be sought as part of the routine physical examination in the neonate and young child. This is often best appreciated from a frontal photograph of the child (Fig. 11-63) and therefore may be brought to the attention of a physician by a parent. Strabismus (see Chapter 19), particularly when first seen after infancy, may be a sign of an orbital tumor or intracranial pathologic condition and, even if intermittent, merits attention. Proptosis may be observed with several childhood tumors and may represent either a primary tumor or metastatic disease. Orbital rhabdomyosarcoma may present in this way (Fig. 11-64). Langerhans cell histiocytosis (see Fig. 11-55) may also present with a retrobulbar mass and proptosis. The combination of exophthalmos, diabetes insipidus, and bone lesions forms the classic triad that in earlier terminology had been referred to as Hand-Schüller-Christian disease, one of the histiocytosis syndromes. Last, a child with neuroblastoma may present with metastatic disease to the orbit. The resulting condition has been referred to as "raccoon eyes" and is due to ecchymoses in the periorbital area (Fig. 11-65). Heterochromia (Fig. 11-66, *A*), usually a benign entity, may be associated with cervicothoracic neuroblastoma (see also Chapter 19). Aniridia (Fig. 11-66, *B*), or absence of the iris, has a known

Figure 11-65 Raccoon eyes—neuroblastoma. This clinical finding is characteristic of a retro-orbital metastatic tumor in advanced neuroblastoma. This may involve supraorbital or infraorbital areas. "Shiners" resulting from trauma or nonaccidental trauma may be a part of the initial differential diagnosis. *(Courtesy H. Pearson, New Haven, Conn.)*

Figure 11-64 **A,** Retro-orbital rhabdomyosarcoma. This child demonstrates proptosis due to the retro-orbital tumor, as well as a large head due to the presence of increased intracranial pressure. **B,** Rhabdomyosarcoma of the orbit with proptosis shown on axial T_2 FLAIR (fluid-attenuated inversion recovery) magnetic resonance image.

Figure 11-66   A, Heterochromia iridis in an adult. Heterochromia is associated with neuroblastoma. **B,** Aniridia. (**A,** *Courtesy J. Roen, MD, New York.*)

association with malignancy including the WAGR (Wilms tumor, aniridia, genital abnormalities, and mental retardation) syndrome. Aniridia in the infant or toddler should prompt appropriate diagnostic studies.

Chronic otorrhea is seen with Langerhans cell histiocytosis (Fig. 11-67). This diagnosis should be suspected when problems persist despite antibiotics, particularly if additional symptoms are present including skin rash, gingival abnormalities, lymphadenopathy, or organomegaly (see Fig. 11-55). Otorrhea may also be seen with other head and neck tumors, such as rhabdomyosarcoma. Morphologic abnormalities of the ear itself may also provide clues to a diagnosis that may predispose a patient to malignancy. The presence of ear creases or pits may represent a manifestation of the Beckwith-Wiedemann syndrome, in which patients have a known predisposition to hepatoblastoma, Wilms tumor, and other malignancies.

A child with cancer may also present with a lesion of the orofacial region including the jaw and oral and nasal cavities. Inappropriate loosening of the teeth may represent a clinical manifestation of Langerhans cell histiocytosis or Burkitt lymphoma. In the case of African Burkitt lymphoma, an associated jaw mass is also present (Fig. 11-68).

Orofacial Findings

Whereas masses such as the jaw lesion shown in Figure 11-68 are likely to be referred early to an oncologist, intraoral (Fig. 11-69) or intranasal (Fig. 11-70) masses are more likely

to masquerade as nonmalignant lesions, which may forestall correct diagnosis. These may be entirely asymptomatic, or they may cause local bleeding or difficulty swallowing or breathing. Gingival hyperplasia can be seen in children with leukemia, especially the acute myelomonocytic subtype (Fig. 11-71).

Although most physicians look for cervical adenopathy, it is important to remember the other lymph node groups that may be involved by focal or generalized adenopathy in leukemias, lymphomas, or solid tumors. Additional lymph node locations that should be sought during physical examination include supraclavicular, infraclavicular, epitrochlear, inguinal, femoral, and popliteal. Although large, rock-hard nodes that are fixed to the subcutaneous tissue are most convincing for malignancy, texture and size can be misleading. Because Hodgkin disease and non-Hodgkin lymphoma can occur concurrently with or after infectious mononucleosis, a positive monospot test may be a false reassurance. Therefore persistent adenopathy, even in that setting, should be monitored closely. The algorithms for workup of adenopathy and indications for biopsy are reviewed in Chapter 12. Neck examination may reveal abnormalities of the thyroid. Although rare in childhood, a goiter or nodular thyroid with or without bruits may be seen in a patient with thyroid carcinoma.

Chest

External examination of the chest may disclose obvious skeletal or other chest wall masses that may be asymptomatic or associated with pain. Scoliosis has been associated with paravertebral tumors such as thoracic neuroblastoma. A discussion of tumors of muscle or bone origin is presented elsewhere (see the section Musculoskeletal System, later). The pediatric malignancies of this type include rhabdomyosarcoma, Ewing sarcoma, and osteosarcoma. Importantly, these tumors may present as chest wall lesions. However, subsequent discussion in this section provides a more focused review of tumors of the mediastinum. The differential diagnosis of a mediastinal mass depends to a certain extent on location. Tumors of the anterior mediastinum in children and young adults are most commonly lymphomas including both Hodgkin disease and non-Hodgkin lymphoma (Fig. 11-72). Germ cell tumors and, rarely, thymomas may also be seen in this location. Masses of the middle mediastinum and/or hilar adenopathy also most commonly represent lymphoma in childhood. Disease of the lymph nodes within the chest may also indicate the presence of lymphadenopathy secondary to leukemia. The presence of a mediastinal mass in a patient with leukemia is suggestive of T-cell disease and is often associated with a high WBC count and organomegaly. Tumors of the posterior mediastinum are usually of neurogenic origin, including neuroblastoma and Ewing sarcoma. In the case of neuroblastic tumors (e.g., neuroblastoma, ganglioneuroblastoma, ganglioneuroma), calcifications may be present (Fig. 11-73). Parenchymal pulmonary nodules, when tumor related, may be asymptomatic and most commonly represent metastatic solid tumor, such as a sarcoma. Figure 11-74, *A* and *B*, demonstrates plain film and a chest CT scan, respectively, of a patient with pulmonary metastases of osteosarcoma. Pleural effusions may be present when malignant disease occurs in the chest. This is most common in the case of non-Hodgkin lymphoma (Fig. 11-75). Cytology, flow cytometry, and cytogenetics that are performed on pleural fluid may provide diagnostic material with relatively low risk in the patient with compromised respiratory status due to mediastinal disease.

Symptoms of respiratory distress may result from a primary intrathoracic process or may be due to a compromised respiratory effort from an abdominal process, such as an abdominal mass or ascites (Fig. 11-76). Pulmonary findings on physical

Figure 11-67 **A,** Otorrhea in a child with Langerhans cell histiocytosis. **B,** X-ray film showing destruction of the mastoid bone in the same child. (**A,** *Courtesy P. Gaffney, MD, Pittsburgh, Pa.*)

Figure 11-68 Burkitt lymphoma of the jaw in an African child. (*Courtesy I. Magrath, MD, Bethesda, Md.*)

Figure 11-69 Intracranial rhabdomyosarcoma with intraoral extension. The lesion was first detected by the child's dentist and was biopsied by an ear, nose, and throat specialist who did not suspect malignancy.

Figure 11-70 Intranasal glioma. **A,** Normal left nostril. **B,** Intranasal glioma occluding the right nostril. *(Courtesy S. Stool, MD, Pittsburgh, Pa.)*

examination and routine chest radiography allow one to rapidly distinguish an intrathoracic from an intraabdominal process. The superior vena cava syndrome is a true oncologic emergency. It is caused by obstruction of venous return to the heart through the superior vena cava by a mass lesion. Signs and symptoms may include facial swelling and plethora, wheezing, and cough (Fig. 11-77). This syndrome may progress rapidly and lead to cardiorespiratory failure. Emergent intervention with steroid and/or radiation therapy may be required. In caring for the patient with mediastinal disease, one must also pay careful attention to electrolytes and renal function, as patients with non-Hodgkin lymphoma and T-cell leukemia are at high risk of metabolic abnormalities associated with tumor lysis syndrome.

Abdomen

An observant parent may be the first person to detect abdominal swelling or an abdominal mass. This may represent hepatosplenomegaly or a mass of alternative origin. A large abdominal mass may lead to the accumulation of ascites. Superficial venous distention (Fig. 11-78) may signal deep venous obstruction that also relates to the presence of intraabdominal tumor. Patients may also demonstrate lower extremity edema and scrotal swelling in the case of male patients or

Figure 11-71 Leukemic infiltration. This photograph shows a patient with gingival hyperplasia resulting from leukemic invasion of the gums. *(From Bluefarb SM: Dermatology, Kalamazoo, Mich, 1984, Upjohn).*

labial swelling in female patients. The patient may experience respiratory difficulties due to limited chest excursion with inspiration and renal dysfunction due to external compression of the renal vasculature.

The most common malignant cause of hepatosplenomegaly is leukemia or lymphoma, in which case organomegaly is due to infiltration of the involved organs with malignant cells. The abdominal mass may also reflect a primary tumor originating from an intraabdominal organ including the kidney, adrenal gland, liver, or ovaries. Wilms tumor is the most common renal tumor of childhood. The mass arising from the kidney tends to be well encapsulated (Fig. 11-79). It often presents as an asymptomatic abdominal mass. Hypertension may occur as a result of impaired renal blood flow. Hematuria may be observed in approximately 15% of cases.

Children with neuroblastoma and other neuroblastic tumors may also present with an abdominal mass. This tumor may originate from the adrenal gland, resulting in a suprarenal mass. Alternatively, a neuroblastic tumor may originate anywhere along the sympathetic neural pathway. Therefore a paraspinal mass is also a common location for neuroblastoma. Unlike the well-encapsulated lesion of Wilms tumor described previously, neuroblastic tumors often wrap around vital vascular structures in the abdomen, making complete resection difficult (Fig. 11-80). Unlike Wilms tumor, many of the patients will have metastatic disease at the time of diagnosis and may appear more ill. Neuroblastoma has a wide spectrum of presenting symptomatology and prognoses. These are dependent on the patient's age at diagnosis, stage of disease, and biologic features of the tumor. In approximately 85% of cases, this neural tumor secretes excess catecholamines. The measurement of homovanillic acid and vanillylmandelic acid in the urine is an important aid to diagnosis and may be used to monitor disease status.

Non-Hodgkin lymphoma of the abdomen has a wide range of clinical presentations varying from marked retroperitoneal or mesenteric adenopathy to a clinical scenario that mimics an acute abdominal process, such as appendicitis or intussusception (Fig. 11-81).

Hepatic neoplasms are rare in childhood. The two most common hepatic tumors are hepatoblastoma and hepatocellular carcinoma. The former occurs more commonly in young children, with more than 75% of cases reported in children

Figure 11-72   Hodgkin lymphoma. **A,** Chest x-ray demonstrating a large anterior mediastinal mass in a teenage male presenting with Hodgkin lymphoma. **B,** Chest computed tomography (CT) demonstrating the mediastinal mass. **C,** ^{18}F-labeled 2-fluoro-2-deoxyglucose positron emission tomography (FDG PET) demonstrating the metabolically active tissue of the malignancy as intensely bright areas relative to normal tissues.

Figure 11-73   Neuroblastoma. **A,** Supine chest x-ray demonstrating a posterior mediastinal mass in a child with neuroblastoma. **B,** Coronal CT demonstrating extent of paraspinal masses in a child with newly diagnosed neuroblastoma.

Figure 11-74   Metastatic pulmonary nodules. **A,** Chest x-ray of a patient with pulmonary metastases of osteosarcoma. **B,** Coronal chest CT of a patient with pulmonary metastases of osteosarcoma.

Figure 11-75   Malignant pleural effusions. **A,** This chest x-ray shows an abnormal collection of pleural fluid. If malignancy is suspected, the diagnosis can sometimes be made through analysis of the pleural fluid. **B,** Cytology of the pleural fluid obtained by thoracentesis demonstrates large cells, high nuclear-to-cytoplasmic ratios, and fine nuclear chromatin, all features of malignant disease.

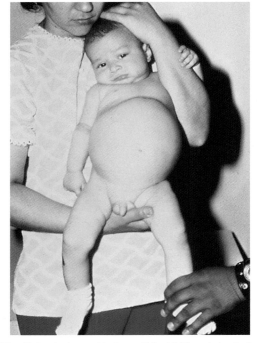

Figure 11-76   Abdominal neuroblastoma. This child has abdominal swelling with hepatosplenomegaly. Further evaluation reveals a diagnosis of neuroblastoma.

Figure 11-77   Superior vena cava syndrome. Discoloration of the face and neck with venous distention. The mediastinal masses that produce these findings often pose considerable anesthetic risk.

Figure 11-78 Intraabdominal tumor. Superficial venous distention may also be seen in cases of extensive intraabdominal tumor. *(Courtesy D. Nakayama, MD, Chapel Hill, NC.)*

Figure 11-79 Axial CT of an abdominal mass originating from the kidney in a child with Wilms tumor.

younger than 3 years of age. Hepatocellular carcinoma usually occurs in older children. An elevated α-fetoprotein level may be observed in both tumors, although it is more often present in cases of hepatoblastoma. The most frequent presenting signs and symptoms for hepatic tumors include an abdominal mass with abdominal distention, anorexia, and weight loss.

A germ cell tumor of the ovary may also present as an abdominal mass. Germ cell tumors develop from the primordial germ cells of the embryo that would normally produce sperm or ova. This group of tumors is discussed further in the next section.

Urogenital Tract

Involvement of the genitourinary system or sacral area by tumor in infancy or childhood often results in the presence of visible abnormalities on physical examination. However, these tumors may also occur in retroperitoneal and intraabdominal

locations. Rhabdomyosarcoma, a tumor of muscle origin, is discussed in greater detail in the following section (Musculo-skeletal System). However, sarcoma botryoides is a particular subtype of rhabdomyosarcoma that most often presents in the genitourinary region. This tumor has a characteristic appearance with its grapelike morphology (Fig. 11-82). Classically, it involves the vagina, but it may also involve the mucosal surfaces of other hollow organs, such as the bladder or, more rarely, the nasopharynx. Sacrococcygeal teratoma is also usually grossly apparent on physical examination (Fig. 11-83). Teratomas are embryonal neoplasms that contain tissues from all three germ cell layers. The sacrococcygeal location is the

Figure 11-80 Neuroblastoma. **A,** Axial CT of an abdominal mass in a child with neuroblastoma. **B,** Coronal CT of a patient with abdominal neuroblastoma, demonstrating the encasement of vital structures and vessels within the tumor.

Figure 11-81 Non-Hodgkin lymphoma of the appendix. Shown is a histologic slide of the appendix, indicating involvement with non-Hodgkin lymphoma. The malignant cells, predominating in the lower half of the slide, are large, with clear cytoplasm and irregularly shaped nuclei.

most common location in childhood. Other sites of origin include the pineal region, mediastinum, retroperitoneum, and ovary and testes. Although teratomas may have benign or malignant elements, nearly 20% of them exhibit malignant features. The sacrococcygeal mass must also be distinguished from a meningomyelocele and other spinal tumors. The primary discussion of Wilms tumor is to be found in the section on abdominal masses (see Abdomen, earlier). As described previously, patients with Wilms tumor may present with asymptomatic hematuria.

Testicular enlargement (Fig. 11-84) may be secondary to involvement by leukemia or lymphoma (in which case bilateral swelling may be seen) or to primary testicular tumors. Primary tumors of the testes and testicular region include germ cell tumors and paratesticular rhabdomyosarcoma. Priapism is a rare complication of chronic myelogenous leukemia

Figure 11-83 Sacrococcygeal teratoma. This teratoma has an external component and is easily visualized on physical examination. The teratoma may contain both benign and malignant elements.

resulting from sludging and mechanical obstruction due to leukemia cells and/or coagulation within the corpora cavernosa.

Abnormalities such as precocious puberty may be caused by a tumor of the central nervous system, gonads (ovaries or testes), or adrenal gland. The inappropriate endocrine-mediated physical examination findings, such as hirsutism, may be the first indication of the presence of a pediatric cancer. Early detection may have an impact on the likelihood of cure, particularly in the case of adrenal carcinomas.

Musculoskeletal System

Bone and joint manifestations of pediatric cancer are relatively common. Arthralgia and full-blown arthritis are well-described presentations of acute lymphoblastic leukemia. Diffuse bone pain, as discussed previously, is also common. Metaphyseal lucencies and growth arrest lines on plain radiographs are often nonspecifically associated with the diagnosis of acute lymphoblastic leukemia (Fig. 11-85). Diffuse osteopenia or lytic bone lesions may also be observed in patients with lymphoid leukemia. Similar lytic lesions and symptoms of bone pain may result from metastatic solid tumor. A rare musculoskeletal finding in the setting of pediatric malignancy is that of hypertrophic osteoarthropathy. This finding has been described in patients with hepatoma, not all of whom have advanced disease at the time of presentation (Fig. 11-86). Hemihypertrophy (see Chapter 9), or relative enlargement of one or more parts of one side of the body, has been associated with the subsequent development of a number of solid tumors including Wilms tumor, adrenocortical carcinoma, hepatoblastoma, and leukemia. Although prospective studies

Figure 11-82 Sarcoma botryoides. A grapelike lesion present in a child with multiple congenital anomalies. The appearance of this lesion is characteristic of the sarcoma botryoides subtype of rhabdomyosarcoma.

Figure 11-84 Testicular mass. This photograph demonstrates unilateral scrotal swelling in an infant with a left testicular mass.

Figure 11-85 X-ray abnormalities in acute lymphoblastic leukemia (ALL). Metaphyseal (**A** and **B**) and growth arrest lines (**C** and **D**) in children with ALL. *(Courtesy J. Medina, MD, Pittsburgh, Pa.)*

have not been performed, a general recommendation is to perform screening abdominal ultrasound every 3 to 4 months until 6 years of age. The finding of hemihypertrophy should be distinguished from hemiatrophy, which is not a predisposing condition. A true mass involving one extremity (see

Figure 11-86 Hypertrophic osteoarthropathy. **A,** Clubbing and **B,** bone lesions in a child with hypertrophic osteoarthropathy secondary to hepatocellular carcinoma not involving the lung. *(Courtesy K.S. Oh, MD, Pittsburgh, Pa.)*

Fig. 11-87, *C*) is not usually confused with hemihypertrophy. Deep vein thrombosis may also result in asymmetry of the extremities. Although this condition may relate to compression from a tumor or the presence of a paraneoplastic syndrome, thrombotic events in childhood usually represent alternative risk factors to thrombosis and are not a consequence of malignancy.

Primary bone tumors most commonly occur in the adolescent age range and should be considered when patients experience persistent pain, even in the absence of objective findings. Osteosarcoma and Ewing sarcoma are the most common bone tumors found in the child and young adult. Osteosarcoma is a primary bone tumor derived from primitive bone-forming mesenchyme (Fig. 11-87). It is characterized by the production of osteoid. The development of osteosarcoma appears to correlate with periods of linear bone growth, as evidenced by its peak incidence during the pubescent growth spurt and the observation that patients with osteosarcoma are taller than average for age. It is usually metaphyseal in location and involves the bones exhibiting the most rapid growth in adolescence including the femur, tibia, and humerus. Ewing sarcoma is the second most common malignant bone tumor (Fig. 11-88). It also has its greatest incidence during the second decade of life. It is an undifferentiated tumor of bone that consists morphologically of densely packed small, round, blue cells. Unlike osteosarcoma, this tumor may also arise from soft tissue, in which case it is termed extraosseous Ewing sarcoma. The characteristic bone lesion is diaphyseal in location. The clinical picture may initially be mistaken as osteomyelitis because of the association of fever in approximately 30% of patients with Ewing sarcoma.

Soft tissue sarcomas represent tumors arising from muscle, connective tissue, and vascular tissue. Rhabdomyosarcoma, a tumor of striated muscle, is the most common soft tissue sarcoma of childhood. This tumor exhibits two age peaks, the first at 2 to 6 years of age and the second at 15 to 19 years of age. Rhabdomyosarcoma may originate in any site of skeletal muscle, and the most frequent presenting sign is the presence of a mass. Rhabdomyosarcoma in children in the younger age peak usually involves the head, neck, or genitourinary

Figure 11-87 Osteosarcoma. **A,** Plain x-ray of the lower extremity in a child with newly diagnosed osteosarcoma. Note the soft tissue swelling, calcification, cortical bone destruction, and new bone formation. **B,** Coronal T_1 with contrast further defines the primary tumor. **C,** Bone scan of a young girl with osteosarcoma to evaluate the primary site for evidence of metastatic disease. Uptake is limited to the site of her primary tumor.

location. Adolescents more commonly develop extremity, truncal, or paratesticular lesions.

Long-term Follow-up of Childhood Cancer Survivors

Over the past several decades, improvements in multimodality therapy have led to markedly improved survival for those who develop cancer as a child or young adult. The 5-year survival rate for childhood cancer is currently in the range of 80% when considering all diseases and stages. This growing population is at increased risk of a variety of long-term sequelae. Therefore, inherent in this improved survival is an obligation to educate survivors who may have been treated as a young child, and to provide monitoring for potential long-term effects of the therapy leading to the cure. Treatment-related factors such as chemotherapy, radiation, and surgery all may lead to

late sequelae. Patient gender, age at the time of treatment, and the presence of additional genetic factors may also play a role. Long-term effects on neurocognitive functioning, cardiovascular and pulmonary symptoms, risk of subsequent malignant neoplasm, infertility, and psychosocial issues in survivors are represented in a growing body of literature. For these reasons, current treatment protocols for childhood cancer place great emphasis not only on improving the cure, but also on decreasing the risk of long-term sequelae.

Recent publications provide a comprehensive overview of the unique medical needs of this population. Because individual health risks depend on the age of the patient at treatment and specific therapeutic modalities used, follow-up evaluations and health screening should be individualized on the basis of treatment history. To improve the systematic follow-up of childhood cancer survivors, the Children's

Figure 11-88 Ewing sarcoma. **A,** Plain x-ray of a child with Ewing sarcoma showing cortical destruction and soft tissue swelling of the diaphysis of the femur. **B,** MRI of the lower extremity further defining the tumor. **C,** Bone scan to evaluate the extent of disease, again limited to the primary site. (*A, Courtesy J. Medina, MD, Pittsburgh, Pa.*)

Oncology Group (COG) organized exposure-based health screening guidelines. These guidelines provide the pediatrician with a framework in which to provide high-quality long-term follow-up care and health supervision for survivors of pediatric malignancy. Ongoing dialog with a pediatric oncology subspecialist will remain an important part of care to allow for communication regarding any changes in follow-up recommendations specific to the childhood cancer survivors under their care.

Bibliography

American Academy of Pediatrics, Section on Hematology/Oncology and Children's Oncology Group: Long term follow-up care of pediatric cancer survivors, *Pediatrics* 123:906–915, 2009.

Favara BE: Hemophagocytic lymphohistiocytosis: A hemophagocytic syndrome, *Semin Diagn Pathol* 9:63, 1992.

Gottschalk S, Rooney C, Heslop H: Post-transplant lymphoproliferative disorders, *Annu Rev Med* 56:29–44, 2005.

Hoffman R, Benz EJ, Shattil SJ, et al, editors: *Hematology: Basic principles and practice*, ed 3, Philadelphia, 2000, Churchill Livingstone.

Lanzkowsky P: *Pediatric hematology and oncology*, New York, 1995, Churchill Livingstone.

Miller DR, Pearson HA, Baehner RL, et al: *Smith's blood diseases of infancy and childhood*, ed 7, St. Louis, 1995, Mosby.

Oeffinger KC, Nathan PC, Kremer LC: Challenges after curative treatment for childhood cancer and long-term follow-up of survivors, *Hematol Oncol Clin North Am* 24:129–149, 2010.

Pizzo PA, Poplack DG, editors: *Principles and practices of pediatric oncology*, 6th ed, Philadelphia, 2010, Lippincott Williams & Wilkins.

INFECTIOUS DISEASE

Marian G. Michaels | Andrew J. Nowalk

In selecting infectious diseases for presentation in an atlas format, we have chosen to emphasize common and serious disorders in which visual findings tend to be prominent. Modes of presentation, patterns of clinical evolution, and spectra of severity are stressed. The following topics are covered: infectious exanthems, mumps, bacterial skin and soft tissue infections, infectious lymphadenitis, bacterial bone and joint infections, and congenital and perinatal infections including pediatric human immunodeficiency virus (HIV) syndrome. Because of their resurgence, we have added sections on tuberculosis and congenital syphilis. This is designed to help practitioners who have seen few, if any, cases during decades of declining incidence to familiarize themselves with their modes of presentation and clinical and radiographic manifestations, thereby assisting earlier recognition and diagnosis.

INFECTIOUS EXANTHEMS

Exanthematous disorders are numerous, commonly encountered, and, because they have many similarities, often a source of clinical confusion. In establishing a diagnosis, the clinician should attend not only to the basic character of the exanthem but also to its mode of spread, its distribution, the evolution of lesions, and the constellation of associated symptoms. In some of these illnesses the presence of a characteristic oral enanthem can be helpful in establishing the diagnosis.

Skin and Soft Tissue Findings in Viral Infections

Along with mumps, three exanthems—measles or rubeola, rubella, and varicella—continue to be regarded as the "usual childhood diseases" worldwide. Although immunization has been responsible for causing a marked decrease in the incidence of measles, mumps, and rubella compared with their incidence in the prevaccine era, cases of measles (and less often mumps) still occur in children who are nonimmunized or in whom the first immunization resulted in inadequate immunity. Although varicella remains a common illness, use of varicella vaccine has decreased its frequency and has modified the skin manifestations.

Rubeola (Nine-Day or Red Measles)

Measles is a highly contagious, moderate to severe acute illness with a typical prodrome and mode of evolution. Prodromal symptoms consist of fever, malaise, dry (occasionally croupy) cough, coryza, and conjunctivitis with clear discharge and marked photophobia (Fig. 12-1, *A*). One to 2 days after onset of prodromal symptoms, a pathognomonic enanthem (Koplik spots) appears on the buccal mucosa (Fig. 12-1, *B*). The lesions consist of tiny bluish-white dots surrounded by red halos, which increase in number and then fade over a 2- to 3-day period. The exanthem is seen first on day 3 or 4, as the prodromal symptoms and fever peak in severity. It is a blotchy, erythematous, blanching, maculopapular eruption that appears at the hairline and spreads cephalocaudally over 3 days, ultimately involving the palms and soles (Fig. 12-1, *C-F*). Once generalized, the rash becomes confluent over proximal areas but remains discrete distally. Older lesions tend to develop a rusty hue as a result of capillary leak and cease to blanch with pressure. Fading commences after 3 days, with clearing 2 to 3 days later. Fine, branny desquamation of the most severely involved areas may ensue. Generalized adenopathy may be present in moderate to severe cases.

During the acute phase of this illness, most patients are quite ill systemically. They are lethargic, have moderate to severe malaise and anorexia, and prefer to be left alone to sleep in a darkened room.

The incubation period for measles is 9 to 10 days, and patients are contagious from approximately 4 days before the appearance of rash until about 4 days after. The attack rate in exposed, susceptible people is greater than 90%. Morbidity is rather high and mortality not uncommon, especially in children of underdeveloped countries. The peak season for measles is late winter through early spring. Potential complications (resulting either from extension of the primary infection or from secondary invasion by bacterial pathogens) include otitis media, pneumonia, obstructive laryngotracheitis, and acute encephalitis. Administration of measles vaccine is highly effective in preventing this disease.

Rubella (German Measles)

Although rubella has little or no prodrome in children, adolescents, like adults, may experience 1 to 5 days of low-grade fever, mild malaise, adenopathy, headache, sore throat, and coryza. Fever, if present at all in young children, is low grade and rarely lasts more than a day. The exanthem is a discrete, pinkish red, fine maculopapular eruption, which, like measles, typically begins on the face and spreads cephalocaudally (Fig. 12-2, *A*). The rash becomes generalized within 24 hours, and then begins to fade, clearing completely by 72 hours. Forschheimer spots, an enanthem consisting of small reddish spots on the soft palate, are seen in some patients on day 1 of the rash and can be helpful in the differential diagnosis (Fig. 12-2, *B*). Adenopathy, often generalized, is a common but not invariable feature. The occipital, posterior cervical, and postauricular nodes tend to be those most prominently enlarged. Arthritis and arthralgias are frequent in adolescent and adult female patients, beginning on day 2 or 3 and typically lasting 5 to 10 days. Large or small joints may be affected.

Many patients infected with rubella do not manifest this typical picture, however, and up to 25% of infected people are asymptomatic yet capable of transmitting the virus to others. In some, the rash may last only 1 day and may involve only the trunk; in others, the exanthem is absent and the patient appears to have pharyngitis or an upper respiratory tract infection. Because infections due to many other viruses including adenoviruses, coxsackieviruses, and echoviruses can produce

Figure 12-1   Rubeola/measles. **A,** During and after the prodromal period, the conjunctivae are injected and produce a clear discharge. This is associated with marked photophobia. **B,** Koplik spots, bluish white dots surrounded by red halos, appear on the buccal and labial mucosa a day or two before the exanthem and begin to fade with onset of the rash. **C-E,** The measles exanthem is a blotchy, erythematous, blanching maculopapular eruption that appears at the hairline and spreads cephalocaudally over 3 days, ultimately involving the palms and soles **(F).** With evolution, lesions become confluent at proximal sites. (*A, C,* and *F, Courtesy Michael Sherlock, MD, Lutherville, Md; **B,** courtesy Robert Hickey, MD, Children's Hospital of Pittsburgh, Pittsburgh, Pa.*)

a rubella-like picture, serologic testing is necessary to establish the diagnosis. Such testing is important if the patient is pregnant or has been in contact with a pregnant woman or if arthritis is a prominent feature, simulating the picture of acute rheumatic fever or rheumatoid arthritis.

The incidence of rubella peaks in late winter and early spring, and the disease is contagious in patients from a few days before to a few days after appearance of the exanthem.

The incubation period ranges from 14 to 21 days. Complications are rare in childhood and include arthritis, purpura with or without thrombocytopenia, and mild encephalitis. The major complication results from spread of the virus to susceptible pregnant women and their fetuses, resulting in congenital rubella syndrome (see the section, Congenital and Perinatal Infections, later). When such an exposure is thought to have occurred, a specimen of blood should be obtained from the

Figure 12-2 Rubella/German measles. **A,** The exanthem of rubella usually consists of a fine, pinkish red, maculopapular eruption that appears first at the hairline and rapidly spreads cephalocaudally. Lesions tend to remain discrete. **B,** The presence of red palatal lesions (Forschheimer spots), seen in some patients on day 1 of the rash, and occipital and posterior cervical adenopathy are findings suggestive of rubella. *(Courtesy Michael Sherlock, MD, Lutherville, Md.)*

pregnant woman as soon as possible for the measurement of antibody. In addition, an aliquot of serum from this blood draw should be frozen for retesting, if necessary. If the sample obtained at the time of exposure is positive for rubella-specific IgG, then the woman was likely to be immune and not at risk. If it is negative, a second sample should be obtained in 2 to 3 weeks and tested concurrently with the remaining aliquot from the initial sample. If this test is negative, a third sample should be obtained at 6 weeks. If antibody is detected in the second or third specimen, infection has occurred and the fetus is at risk.

Varicella (Chickenpox)

Varicella in the normal pediatric host is a relatively benign, albeit highly contagious illness caused by the varicella-zoster virus. A brief prodrome of low-grade fever, upper respiratory tract symptoms, and mild malaise may occur, followed rapidly by the appearance of a pruritic exanthem. Lesions appear in crops and evolve rapidly over several hours. Most patients have three crops, although some may have only one and others may have as many as five. Initial crops involve the trunk and scalp, and subsequent crops are distributed more peripherally; thus the mode of spread is centrifugal. The presence of scalp lesions with the initial crop is often helpful in diagnosing the infection in a patient who presents early in the course of the disease. Lesions begin as tiny erythematous papules that rapidly enlarge to form thin-walled, superficial central vesicles surrounded by red halos (Fig. 12-3, *A*). Vesicular fluid changes promptly from clear to cloudy; then drying begins, resulting in an umbilicated appearance. As the surrounding erythema fades, a central crust or scab is formed, which sloughs after several days. A hallmark of this exanthem is the finding of lesions in all stages of evolution within a relatively small geographic area of skin (Fig. 12-3, *B*). In general, all scabs have sloughed by 10 to 14 days. Scarring usually does not occur unless lesions become secondarily infected. It is important to recognize that in patients with preexisting dermatologic problems, the lesions of varicella, like other viral exanthems, tend to appear first and cluster most heavily at sites of prior skin irritation, such as the diaper area or sites of eczematoid dermatitis (Fig. 12-3, *C* and *D*).

An enanthem is commonly seen and consists of thin-walled vesicles that rapidly rupture to form shallow ulcers (Fig. 12-3, *E*). Other mucosal surfaces may be affected as well. Although skin lesions are pruritic, those on the oral, rectal, or vaginal mucosa and those involving the external auditory canal or tympanic membrane can be painful, necessitating analgesia. Systemic symptoms are generally mild, although

low-grade to moderate fever may be present during the first few days. In most cases pruritus is the child's major complaint. In adolescents and adults the illness is more likely to be severe with prominent systemic symptoms and more extensive exanthematous involvement.

Varicella occurs year-round, with peak incidences in late autumn and late winter through early spring. The period of communicability begins 1 to 2 days before the appearance of lesions and lasts until all lesions have crusted over. The incubation period ranges from 10 to 20 days, with high secondary attack rates in susceptible people. The most common complication in normal hosts is secondary bacterial infection of excoriated skin lesions. Such infection can range from impetigo to cellulitis. Group A β-streptococcal superinfection of varicella lesions can be particularly severe, leading to myositis, sepsis, and purpura fulminans (Fig. 12-4, *A*). Other complications, although rare, include pneumonia, hepatitis, and encephalitis. The onset of these complications is typically heralded by a secondary fever spike concurrent with increase in general systemic symptoms. In patients with encephalitis, an altered level of consciousness along with other signs of neurologic dysfunction occurs. Reye syndrome, an encephalopathy of unclear etiology, is a well-recognized but fortunately rare complication that can occur as a child is recovering from acute varicella. Repetitive pernicious vomiting is followed by an altered level of consciousness in which periods of lethargy alternate with periods of delirium or combativeness.

In the immunocompromised host with deficient cellular immunity, varicella is a severe and often fatal disease with CNS, pulmonary, and generalized visceral involvement. Skin lesions are often hemorrhagic and tend to remain vesicular for a prolonged period of time (Fig. 12-4, *B* and *C*). With potentially immunocompromised children who have not had varicella previously (including those on short-course, high-dose steroids), parents must be forewarned of these dangers and instructed to notify their physician immediately of any possible exposure. This enables the administration of varicella immune globulin product within 96 hours of exposure, thus reducing the severity of illness. If immune globulin is unavailable, some experts recommend prophylaxis with acyclovir starting on day 7 postexposure for high-risk patients.

Herpes Zoster (Shingles)

The varicella-zoster virus, like other herpesviruses, takes up permanent, albeit generally quiescent, residence in its host after initial infection (i.e., varicella). In general, the virus lies dormant in the genome of sensory nerve root cells, but it can

Figure 12-3 Varicella/chickenpox. **A,** The characteristic "dewdrop on a rose petal" is illustrated by this early vesicle on an erythematous base. **B,** The typical features of lesions in all stages of evolution is seen on the trunk of this child. Note the presence of papules, vesicles, and umbilicated and scabbed lesions, all within a small area. **C** and **D,** In this child with underlying eczema, the first crop of vesicles appeared in clusters at sites previously affected by dermatitis. The flexor surface of his arm is covered with numerous discrete lesions, and vesicles are confluent over the plantar surface of his toes and on the balls of his feet. **E,** On mucosal surfaces, thin-walled vesicles may form and rapidly rupture, forming painful shallow ulcers. (**C** and **D,** Courtesy Michael Sherlock, MD, Lutherville, Md; **E,** courtesy Ellen Wald, MD, University of Wisconsin Children's Hospital, Madison, Wis.)

reactivate on occasion. Mechanical and thermal trauma, infection, and debilitation all have been postulated as triggers. Immunosuppression can also predispose to reactivation. In the reactivated form, herpes zoster, lesions consist of grouped, thin-walled vesicles on an erythematous base, which are distributed along the course of a spinal or cranial sensory nerve root (Fig. 12-5). They evolve from macule to papule to vesicle and then to a crusted stage over a few days. Hyperesthesia or nerve root pain may precede, accompany, or follow the eruption and does not correlate with the severity of the rash. Pain, if present at all in pediatric patients, is rarely severe and is generally short-lived, unless a cranial nerve dermatome is involved, in which case pain can be excruciating. Fever and

constitutional symptoms may or may not be part of the picture, but regional adenopathy is common.

Thoracic dermatomes are involved in most patients, followed in frequency by cervical, trigeminal, lumbar, and facial nerve regions. Cranial nerve involvement may produce a puzzling prodrome consisting of severe headache, facial pain, or auricular pain with no evident cause and lasting up to several days before appearance of the eruption. Lesions appear unilaterally on the tonsillar pillars and uvula with involvement of the maxillary branch of the trigeminal nerve; on the buccal mucosa and palate with involvement of the mandibular division; and on the face, cornea, and tip of the nose with involvement of the ophthalmic branch (Fig. 12-5, *D;* and see Chapter

Figure 12-4 Complications of varicella. **A,** Superinfection of this child's lesions with group A β-streptococci led to purpura fulminans. **B** and **C,** Disseminated hemorrhagic varicella. **B,** In the immunocompromised child, skin lesions tend to be hemorrhagic and nearly confluent. **C,** Lesions also evolve more slowly than usual, remaining vesicular for a prolonged period.

Figure 12-5 Herpes zoster (shingles). Dermatomal distribution of lesions is a hallmark of herpes zoster. **A,** Initially discrete thin-walled vesicles on an erythematous base are seen. **B,** Vesicles coalesce over a few days, and lesions then evolve to a crusted stage **(C)**. **D,** Involvement of the ophthalmic branch of the trigeminal nerve produces lesions involving the forehead, eyelids, and nose. (**B,** *Courtesy Michael Sherlock, MD, Lutherville, Md.*)

20, Fig. 20-45). When the geniculate ganglion is affected, vesicles are seen in the external auditory canal in concert with facial paralysis. Although varicella can be transmitted by patients with herpes zoster, contagion is generally less of a problem because most patients have lesions on areas that are covered by clothing and the oropharynx is not involved in most cases.

Adenovirus Infections

More than 40 distinct types of adenoviruses are capable of producing a variety of clinical illnesses including conjunctivitis, upper respiratory tract infections and pharyngitis, croup, bronchitis, bronchiolitis and pneumonia (occasionally fulminant), gastroenteritis, myocarditis, nephritis, cystitis, and encephalitis. An exanthem occasionally accompanies other symptoms, and a variety of rashes have been described. The eruption may consist of discrete, nonspecific, blanching, maculopapular lesions or it may be morbilliform, rubelliform, or, on occasion, petechial. Typically the rash is generalized when first noted. The most readily identifiable clinical constellation consists of conjunctivitis, rhinitis, pharyngitis with or without exudate, and a discrete, blanching, maculopapular rash (Fig. 12-6). Anterior cervical and preauricular lymphadenopathy, low-grade fever, and malaise are common associated findings. The peak season for adenovirus infections in temperate climates is late winter through early summer, and the infection

is maximally contagious during the first few days of illness. The incubation period ranges from 6 to 9 days.

Coxsackie Hand-Foot-and-Mouth Disease

Of the enteroviruses, coxsackievirus group A16 produces the most distinctive exanthem, known as *hand-foot-and-mouth disease*. Patients may have a brief prodrome consisting of low-grade fever, malaise, sore mouth, and anorexia, during which lesions are absent. Within 1 to 2 days, oral lesions and soon skin lesions appear. The former usually consist of shallow, yellow ulcers surrounded by red halos. They are found on the labial and buccal mucosal surfaces, the gingivae, tongue, soft palate, uvula, and anterior tonsillar pillars (Fig. 12-7, *A* and *B*). Early in the illness, small vesicles may be seen on the palate or mucosal surfaces. These enanthematous lesions usually are only mildly painful. The cutaneous lesions begin as erythematous macules on the palmar aspect of the hands and fingers, the plantar surface of the feet and toes, and the interdigital surfaces. On occasion, the buttocks may be involved as well. They evolve rapidly to form small, thick-walled, gray vesicles on an erythematous base (Fig. 12-7, *C-E*), which may feel like slivers, be pruritic, or be asymptomatic. More than 90% of patients with disease caused by coxsackievirus A16 have oral lesions, and about two thirds have the exanthem. In those cases in which the cutaneous manifestations are absent, the process is called *herpangina* (caused by

Figure 12-6 Adenovirus. **A,** This discrete, erythematous, blanching maculopapular rash was generalized when first noted and occurred in association with pharyngitis **(B)** and a nonpurulent conjunctivitis **(C).** (*A and **C,** Courtesy Michael Sherlock, MD, Lutherville, Md.*)

Figure 12-7 Coxsackievirus hand-foot-and-mouth disease. The enanthem of this disorder is characterized by mildly painful, shallow, yellow ulcers surrounded by red halos. These may be found on the labial or buccal mucosa **(A)**, tongue, soft palate **(B)**, uvula, and anterior tonsillar pillars. When oral lesions occur in the absence of the exanthem, the resulting disorder is called herpangina. **C** and **D,** The exanthem of coxsackievirus hand-foot-and-mouth disease involves the palmar, plantar, and interdigital surfaces of the hands and feet and sometimes the buttocks **(E)**. It consists of thick-walled, gray vesicles on an erythematous base. (*D* and *E,* Courtesy Robert Hickey, MD, Children's Hospital of Pittsburgh, Pittsburgh, Pa.)

coxsackieviruses and other enteroviruses) and may resemble early herpes gingivostomatitis. However, coxsackievirus ulcers are less painful and are less often associated with the high fever and intense gingival erythema, edema, and bleeding typical of herpes (see Fig. 12-13).

Coxsackievirus hand-foot-and-mouth disease is highly contagious, with an incubation period of approximately 2 to 6 days. Symptoms last 2 days to 1 week. The peak season is summer through early fall.

Other enteroviral syndromes produced by the coxsackievirus group and by echoviruses include a mild, nonspecific febrile illness with myalgias, headache, and abdominal pain; generalized exanthems that may be maculopapular, vesicular, or urticarial; encephalitis, acute cerebellar ataxia, and myelitis; pleurodynia; myocarditis; hemorrhagic conjunctivitis; and gastroenteritis.

Erythema Infectiosum (Fifth Disease)

Erythema infectiosum is a mildly contagious illness, caused by parvovirus B19, that principally affects preschool and young school-age children. It occurs year-round, with a peak incidence in late winter and early spring. The disorder is characterized primarily by its exanthem. Fever and

constitutional symptoms are unusual. On occasion, headache, nausea, myalgias, and peripheral polyarthralgias are reported. The rash begins on the face, with large, bright red, erythematous patches appearing over both cheeks (Fig. 12-8, *A*). These patches are warm but nontender and have circumscribed borders that are usually macular but may be slightly raised. They are easily distinguished from those of cellulitis and erysipelas (see Figs. 12-34, 12-35, and 12-37) by their symmetry and lack of tenderness, and by the absence of high fever and toxicity. The facial lesions begin to fade on the next day, and a symmetrical, macular or slightly raised, lacy, erythematous rash appears on the extensor surfaces of the extremities (Fig. 12-8, *B*). Over the next day or so, the rash may spread to the flexor surfaces, buttocks, and trunk. Resolution occurs within 3 to 7 days of onset.

Studies have shown that the virus is transmitted primarily by respiratory secretions and that, after transmission, it replicates in red blood cell precursors in the bone marrow. It then may cause a biphasic illness, with fever and nonspecific symptoms accompanied by red blood cell suppression occurring approximately 1 week later, followed by the appearance of the exanthem characteristic of fifth disease 1 to 2 weeks thereafter. Viral shedding ceases before this latter phase. Although red

Figure 12-8   Erythema infectiosum (fifth disease). **A,** On day 1, warm, erythematous, nontender, circumscribed patches appear over the cheeks. These fade on the next day, as **(B)** an erythematous, lacy rash develops on the extensor surfaces of the extremities. (**A,** *Courtesy Robert Hickey, MD, Children's Hospital of Pittsburgh, Pittsburgh, Pa;* **B,** *from Cohen BA, Lehman C, editors:* Dermatlas.org—Dermatology Image Atlas. *Johns Hopkins University [website]. Available from: http://www.dermatlas.org*)

blood cell suppression caused by parvovirus does not result in severe anemia in normal people, it can cause an aplastic crisis in patients with sickle cell disease, other hemoglobinopathies, and other forms of hemolytic anemia.

Roseola Infantum (Exanthem Subitum)

Roseola infantum is a febrile illness that primarily affects children between the ages of 6 and 36 months. The causative agent is human herpesvirus 6. The clinical course begins abruptly with rapid temperature elevation, which occasionally precipitates a febrile seizure. Anorexia and irritability are the major associated symptoms. Examination reveals no source for the fever, which is usually higher than 39°C. Administration of an antipyretic produces only a transient decrease in temperature, which then rises rapidly to its former value. Although most patients do not look toxic, many infants undergo a sepsis workup and lumbar puncture because of the combination of unexplained high fever and marked irritability. Fever and irritability persist for approximately 72 hours, whereupon the fever abruptly subsides. In most cases an erythematous, maculopapular exanthem appears simultaneously with defervescence, but in a small percentage of patients it develops 1 day before or after fever lysis. Lesions are discrete, rose-pink macules or maculopapules that begin on the trunk and then spread rapidly to the extremities, neck, face, and scalp (Fig. 12-9). They may last several hours to a day or two before resolution.

Although cases occur year-round, roseola appears to be more common in late fall and early spring. Secondary cases are uncommon, except in institutional settings. The duration of communicability is unclear, but the incubation period is thought to be 10 to 15 days.

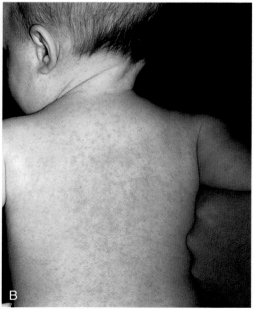

Figure 12-9   Roseola infantum/exanthem subitum. **A** and **B,** The exanthem of this disorder usually appears abruptly after 3 days of high fever and irritability. It is characterized by discrete, rose-pink macules. It may be generalized at first or may start centrally and spread centrifugally. Scalp involvement is prominent.

Infectious Mononucleosis

Infectious mononucleosis is an acute, usually self-limited illness of children and young adults caused by Epstein-Barr virus (EBV). Transmission of EBV can occur by intimate oral contact (i.e., kissing), sharing eating utensils, transfusion, or transplantation. The incubation period usually ranges from 30 to 50 days, although it is shorter (14 to 20 days) in patients with transfusion-acquired infection.

In its most typical form, infectious mononucleosis is characterized by fever, fatigue, pharyngitis, lymphadenopathy, splenomegaly, atypical lymphocytosis, and a positive heterophil antibody response. Nevertheless, most young children with EBV infection do not have classic mononucleosis; instead, they tend to have either a nonspecific illness, which is clinically indistinguishable from other common viral diseases, or, less frequently, subclinical infection.

Clinical Features of Mononucleosis

The illness often begins with a prodrome, which lasts from 3 to 5 days, consisting of fatigue, malaise, and anorexia, often in association with headache, sweats, and chills. Photophobia and edema of the eyelids and periorbital tissues may be noted in some patients (Fig. 12-10, A). The acute phase is usually heralded by a fever, which may show wide daily fluctuations. Pharyngitis and cervical node enlargement then become apparent. The sore throat tends to increase in severity over several days before abating and may be associated with significant dysphagia. Tonsillar and adenoidal enlargement can range from mild to marked, and the tonsillar surface may vary in appearance from one of mild erythema to one of severe exudative inflammation with palatal and uvular edema (Fig. 12-10, B). Halitosis and palatal petechiae are common. Approximately one third of patients show severe pharyngeal manifestations. The anterior cervical lymph nodes are routinely enlarged, and posterior cervical adenopathy is characteristic. In classic cases the adenopathy becomes generalized toward the end of the first week. Involved nodes are firm, discrete, and mildly to moderately tender. Splenomegaly develops in approximately 50% of patients in the second to third week of illness; 10% have associated hepatic enlargement.

An exanthem is seen in 5% to 10% of patients with mononucleosis, although this percentage is greatly increased in patients treated with ampicillin or amoxicillin for pharyngeal or respiratory symptoms. Usually an erythematous maculopapular rubelliform rash, the exanthem can be morbilliform, scarlatiniform, urticarial, hemorrhagic, or even nodular (Fig. 12-10, C and D).

Figure 12-10 Epstein-Barr virus (EBV) mononucleosis. **A,** Eyelid edema is found in 50% of children with infectious mononucleosis. **B,** Severe pharyngotonsillitis is seen in this child, whose tonsils are markedly enlarged and covered with exudate. The uvula is erythematous and edematous. **C** and **D,** In this child with EBV mononucleosis, a diffuse, erythematous, maculopapular rash was part of the clinical picture. Lesions on his face are hemorrhagic and confluent as a result of prior irritation. (He had practiced shaving 2 days before.) Note also the swelling in the region of the tonsillar node and the fact that the child is mouth breathing as a result of adenoidal hypertrophy. (**C** and **D,** Courtesy Michael Sherlock, MD, Lutherville, Md.)

Less common manifestations or complications of mononucleosis include pneumonitis with a pattern of a diffuse, atypical pneumonia; hematologic abnormalities, such as direct Coombs test–positive hemolytic anemia and thrombocytopenia; icteric hepatitis; neurologic disorders, such as acute cerebellar ataxia, encephalitis, aseptic meningitis, myelitis, and Guillain-Barré syndrome; and, rarely, myocarditis and pericarditis. Neurologic and hepatic involvement or widely disseminated disease occasionally can be fulminant, resulting in death. This is particularly true for immunocompromised patients. Other major complications include acute upper airway obstruction resulting from tonsillar and adenoidal hypertrophy and splenic rupture. The latter may occur spontaneously or as a result of minor trauma, repeated palpation, or the increased intraabdominal pressure associated with defecation. Although younger patients are somewhat less subject to the unusual manifestations and complications of mononucleosis, they are more vulnerable to acute upper airway obstruction as a result of tonsillar and adenoidal hypertrophy. This is manifested by mouth breathing, retractions with recumbency, and stertorous snoring and apnea during sleep. Moreover, children younger than 5 years of age who show significant tonsillar and adenoidal enlargement during the EBV infection are more likely to have secondary otitis media and, subsequent to resolution of the acute process, may suffer recurrent bouts of otitis media, tonsillitis, and sinusitis as a result of persistent tonsillar and adenoidal hypertrophy.

Diagnostic Methods

Several laboratory studies may be helpful in suggesting or confirming the diagnosis of infectious mononucleosis. A classic finding is a lymphocytosis with 50% or more lymphocytes and at least 10% atypical lymphocytes. These atypical lymphocytes vary in appearance, in contrast to the monotonous forms seen with leukemia. There is considerable variability, however, in the degree of lymphocytosis and in its timing. Eighty percent or more of patients have mild elevations in liver enzymes early in their disease. Most commonly the diagnosis is confirmed by the finding of heterophil antibodies in the serum toward the end of the first week or at the beginning of the second week of illness. At present, rapid slide tests, of which the Monospot is best known, are the most prevalent method of detecting heterophil antibodies. Although the presence of heterophil antibodies is highly specific for infectious mononucleosis, the sensitivity of the test is limited, in that only about 85% of adolescents, and a much smaller percentage of younger children, with mononucleosis ever show measurable heterophil antibodies. Although EBV infection can be confirmed by measuring specific EBV antibody titers, such studies are usually reserved for patients with severe, prolonged, or atypical heterophil-negative cases of suspected EBV infection. Molecular techniques such as quantitative polymerase chain reaction (PCR) tests are also of value in cases of severe disease or in immunocompromised patients.

Differential Diagnosis of Mononucleosis

In view of the multiple modes of presentation and the wide variability in severity of illness, clinical manifestations, and clinical course, there exists a broad range of differential diagnostic possibilities. In patients presenting with fever and exudative tonsillitis, the principal diagnostic considerations include group A streptococcal pharyngitis, diphtheria, and other viral causes of pharyngitis. If lymphadenopathy and splenomegaly are the predominant features, the differential diagnosis includes cytomegalovirus infection, toxoplasmosis, malignancy, and drug-induced mononucleosis (caused by phenytoin, *para*-aminosalicylic acid, and diaminodiphenylsulfone). In patients with severe hepatic involvement, EBV infection can simulate other forms of viral hepatitis, as well as leptospirosis. Although the history and some aspects of the clinical picture may help in distinguishing one disease from another, specific serologic tests are often required to accomplish this.

Mumps (Epidemic Parotitis)

Mumps is an acute viral illness that preferentially involves glandular and neural tissues. It is rarely seen in the United States since the advent of the MMR (measles, mumps, and rubella) combination vaccine. Although the salivary glands, especially the parotid glands, are the most common sites of clinical involvement, the CNS and other glandular tissues may be affected as well. In up to one third of patients the infection is subclinical. Peak incidence is in late winter and spring. The incubation period is 16 to 18 days, with the disease being contagious in patients from 1 to 7 days before the onset of clinical symptoms and for 5 to 9 days thereafter. Asymptomatic children can also transmit the virus.

Prodromal symptoms consist of fever, headache, malaise, and anorexia. In the typical case these symptoms are followed within 24 hours by the onset of an earache or face pain, which older children can often localize to the region of the pinna. Pain is aggravated by chewing and by stimulation of salivation (in particular, by sour foods). Parotid swelling generally becomes noticeable within the next 24 hours, increases gradually over the ensuing few days, and then abates over a similar period of time. Fever may persist for the duration of swelling but can disappear early in the course. On examination, an area of tender, indurated swelling, extending from the preauricular area through the subauricular space to the postauricular region, can be palpated (Fig. 12-11, *A*). With pronounced enlargement the pinna is pushed up and out (Fig. 12-11, *B*). The gland is indurated and mildly to moderately tender to palpation. The color of the overlying skin is normal. Intraoral examination may reveal erythema and edema of the Stensen duct. Bilateral involvement is usual, although one gland tends to enlarge before the other, and up to 25% of symptomatic patients have unilateral inflammation.

This typical picture is but one of many possible variants of clinical mumps. In some cases the parotid gland is spared and the submental or sublingual salivary glands may be the primary site of involvement. In the former instance, indurated swelling is found below the midportion of the mandible; in the latter case, bilateral submental swelling is seen externally and sublingual swelling is noted intraorally.

Preauricular swelling and induration, the Stensen duct abnormality, and the absence of prominent overlying erythema help to distinguish parotid swelling from cervical adenitis involving the tonsillar node. In confusing cases and in cases in which the submental or sublingual salivary glands are involved, closely simulating adenopathy, the patient can be given lemon juice to sip or a lemon wedge to suck. In patients with mumps, this results in a prompt enlargement of the affected gland and in pain as salivation is stimulated, whereas no such change is seen in patients with adenopathy. In cases of bacterial parotitis, the patient is likely to have high fever and show signs of toxicity. The overlying skin is erythematous, with exquisite tenderness found on palpation (Fig. 12-12). Purulent drainage from the Stensen duct can often be seen when the gland is massaged.

Although it has been estimated that up to 75% of patients with mumps may have cerebrospinal fluid (CSF) pleocytosis, symptomatic meningoencephalitis is seen only in about 10% of patients. CNS symptoms usually follow parotitis but can develop before or even in the absence of salivary gland involvement. There is a wide spectrum in the severity of these symptoms, ranging from isolated headache and malaise with

Figure 12-11   Mumps. **A,** This young boy showed unilateral parotid swelling, which was indurated and moderately tender. Visually it was appreciated best in this view, which reveals swelling anterior and inferior to his left ear. **B,** Bilateral infra- and postauricular swelling (right greater than left) can be appreciated when the patient is viewed from behind. Secondary displacement of the auricle is evident. (**A,** *Courtesy G.D.W. McKendrik, MD;* **B,** *courtesy Michael Sherlock, MD, Lutherville, Md.*)

fever to frank nuchal rigidity with nausea, vomiting, and severe alterations in sensorium. Fortunately, permanent sequelae are rare, although children recovering from severe mumps meningoencephalitis may not return to normal levels of school performance for up to 6 months or a year.

Mumps orchitis is much less common in boys than in men, who have a 20% to 30% incidence. Orchitis usually follows salivary gland enlargement but may occur in its absence. Fever, chills, headache, nausea, vomiting, and lower abdominal pain are prominent and develop with the onset of painful, generally unilateral testicular swelling. Epididymitis is an invariable accompaniment. This process lasts 3 to 7 days.

Oophoritis, seen in an occasional female patient, presents with a secondary temperature spike, nausea, vomiting, and severe lower abdominal pain and tenderness. Involvement may be unilateral or bilateral, and when unilateral and on the right side, it may be indistinguishable from appendicitis. Pancreatitis is an uncommon though potentially severe manifestation. Such patients tend to have sudden onset of excruciating epigastric pain in association with fever, chills, repetitive vomiting, weakness, and prostration. This, too, tends to last for 3 to 7 days. Thyroiditis, mastitis, bartholinitis, and dacryocystitis have been reported in isolated cases as well.

Herpes Simplex Infections

The herpes simplex viruses produce infections that primarily involve the skin and mucous membranes, although in neonates, immunocompromised hosts, and, rarely, normal hosts, infection can result in disseminated disease and CNS involvement. Like other herpesviruses, herpes simplex virus—after producing initial (primary) infection—enters a latent or dormant stage, residing in local sensory ganglia; once latent, the virus can be reactivated at any time, causing recurrent infection. The two distinct serotypes of herpes simplex virus are types 1 and 2. Herpes simplex virus type 1 (HSV-1) is the more common pathogen and can produce a variety of clinical syndromes. In contrast, herpes simplex virus type 2 (HSV-2) is usually a genital pathogen (see Chapter 18), although occasionally it is the source of oral lesions and is the usual agent associated with neonatal herpes (see the section, Congenital and Perinatal Infections, later).

Diagnosis of symptomatic HSV infections can often be made on clinical grounds alone, particularly in cases of primary infection. When the diagnosis is in question, a Giemsa-stained (Tzanck) smear of scrapings obtained from the base of a vesicle (see Chapter 8) usually demonstrates ballooned epithelial cells with intranuclear inclusions and multinucleated giant cells when the lesion is herpetic. Rapid antigen detection tests are more specific and sensitive than Tzanck smears. Viral cultures, obtained by unroofing a lesion and swabbing its base, yield results in 24 to 72 hours. Acute and convalescent titers are less useful and are of no help during recurrences.

Figure 12-12   Suppurative parotitis. This patient had high fever, chills, and marked enlargement of the right parotid gland, which was severely painful and exquisitely tender. The overlying skin is erythematous, and purulent material was seen draining from the Stensen duct. (*Courtesy Sylvan Stool, MD.*)

Figure 12-13 Herpes simplex infections. **A,** Herpetic gingivostomatitis is characterized by discrete mucosal ulcerations and diffuse gingival erythema, edema, and friability in association with fever, dysphagia, and cervical adenopathy. **B,** Numerous yellow ulcerations with thin red halos are seen on the patient's tongue as well. **C,** Thick-walled vesicles on an erythematous base were noted in this child, who showed early findings of intraoral involvement. (**C,** *Courtesy Michael Sherlock, MD, Lutherville, Md.*)

Primary Herpes Simplex Infections

More than 90% of primary infections caused by HSV-1 are subclinical; nevertheless, because the virus is ubiquitous, symptomatic primary infections are common. One of the most prevalent forms of primary infection is *herpetic gingivostomatitis*. Patients with this condition typically have high fever, irritability, anorexia, and mouth pain; infants and toddlers often drool copiously. The gingivae become intensely erythematous, edematous, and friable and tend to bleed easily. Small, yellow ulcerations with red halos are seen routinely on the buccal and labial mucosa, on the gingivae and tongue, and often on the palate and tonsillar pillars (Fig. 12-13, *A* and *B*). Within a short time, yellowish-white debris builds up on mucosal surfaces and halitosis becomes prominent. Thick-walled vesiculopustular lesions may also develop on the perioral skin (Fig. 12-13, *C*). The anterior cervical and tonsillar nodes are enlarged and tender. Symptoms last from 5 to 14 days, but the virus may be shed for weeks after resolution. The illness can vary from mild to marked in severity. Young children with prolonged high fever and intense pain may become dehydrated and ketotic and should be monitored closely and hydrated as needed. The diffuseness of the ulcerations and mucosal inflammation and the intense gingivitis help to distinguish this disorder from herpangina (see Fig. 12-7) and exudative tonsillitis, as well as from other forms of gingivitis.

Patients with primary herpetic infection involving the skin typically present with fever, malaise, localized lesions, and regional adenopathy. The skin lesions generally result from direct inoculation of previously traumatized skin, for example,

at the site of an abrasion, burn, or small cut. Parents, siblings, and playmates with active herpetic lesions (usually cold sores) are often the source, and young children with herpes gingivostomatitis may autoinoculate other body sites with their fingers. The lesions consist of deep, thick-walled, painful vesicles on an erythematous base; they usually are grouped but may occur singly. As they evolve over several days, the vesicles become pustular, coalesce, ulcerate, and then crust over. As a result, the lesions may simulate those of bacterial infection, but the presence of grouped vesicles and the relative sparseness of bacteria on Gram stains of vesicular fluid support the clinical diagnosis of herpes, which can be confirmed by positive findings on Giemsa stain of scrapings from the base of the lesion, rapid viral antigen detection, or viral culture.

Although the virus can infect any area of the skin, the lips and fingers or thumbs (as in *herpetic whitlow*) are the most common sites of involvement (Figs. 12-13 and 12-14). On occasion, the eyelids and periorbital tissues are affected (Fig. 12-15); this can lead to keratoconjunctivitis, which is diagnosed on the basis of finding characteristic dendritic ulcerations on slit-lamp examination (see Chapter 19). Because this complication carries a risk of causing permanent visual impairment, urgent ophthalmologic consultation is indicated whenever there is any suspicion of ocular herpetic infection.

Eczema Herpeticum (Kaposi Varicelliform Eruption)

Patients with atopic eczema and other forms of chronic dermatitis are at risk for a particularly severe form of primary HSV infection and thus should avoid contact with people with active herpetic infections. Parents who have a history of

Figure 12-14 Herpetic whitlow. Grouped, thick-walled vesicles on an erythematous base that are painful and tend to coalesce, ulcerate, and then crust are the typical characteristics of a herpetic whitlow.

Figure 12-15 Ocular herpes may involve only the lids and periorbital skin but can spread to involve the conjunctiva, cornea, and deeper structures, with devastating results.

Figure 12-16   Eczema herpeticum (Kaposi varicelliform eruption). Primary herpes simplex infection in a child with underlying eczema produces crops of hemorrhagic vesiculopustular lesions limited to areas of preexisting dermatitis, which then rupture and crust. **A,** Lesions are seen on the hand of one child and on the face of another **(B).** (**A,** Courtesy Michael Sherlock, MD, Lutherville, Md.)

recurrent herpes and a child with eczema should be instructed to be meticulous about hand washing during periods of reactivation. The illness is heralded by the onset of high fever, irritability, and discomfort. Lesions appear in crops and primarily involve areas of currently or recently affected skin. Typically they evolve to form pustules, which rupture and form crusts over the course of a few days. On occasion, these lesions become hemorrhagic (Fig. 12-16). Multiple crops can appear over 7 to 10 days, simulating varicella. However, the slower evolution of lesions, the tendency of such lesions to become hemorrhagic, their concentration in eczematoid areas, and the persistence of fever and systemic symptoms for as long as 1 week help to distinguish this disorder from varicella. Severity ranges from mild to fulminant and depends in part on the extent of the preceding dermatitis. When the area of involvement is large, fluid losses can be severe and potentially fatal. Accordingly, prompt treatment with intravenous acyclovir is recommended. A significant risk of secondary bacterial infection also exists.

Recurrent Herpes Simplex Infection

As mentioned earlier, after primary infection, HSV becomes latent within the ganglia that lie in the region of initial involvement; reactivation of the latent virus results in localized recurrences at or near the site of previous infection. Fever, sunlight, local trauma, menses, and emotional stress are recognized triggers, and because the mouth is the major site of primary infection, labial and perioral lesions (cold sores) are seen most commonly. Many patients report a prodrome of localized burning along with stinging or itching before the eruption of grouped vesicles. These vesicles contain yellow, serous fluid and often appear smaller and less thick-walled than primary lesions (Fig. 12-17). After 2 to 3 days the vesicular fluid becomes cloudy, and then crusts form. Although fever and systemic symptoms are absent, regional nodes may be enlarged and tender. The localization of the lesions to a small area helps to distinguish them from those of herpes zoster. Prodromal symptoms and discomfort help to distinguish recurrent HSV infection from impetigo and contact dermatitis.

Gianotti-Crosti Syndrome

The eruption of Gianotti-Crosti syndrome, or papular acrodermatitis, although distinctive, often goes unrecognized (or is misdiagnosed). First described in association with anicteric hepatitis B, this exanthem has also been seen with infections due to other viral agents including EBV, coxsackieviruses, parainfluenza viruses, echoviruses, cytomegalovirus, and respiratory syncytial virus. Cases usually occur sporadically but occasionally occur in clusters. Most patients are between 1 and 6 years of age (range, 3 months to 15 years).

A mild prodrome consisting of low-grade fever and malaise is typical and may be associated with generalized adenopathy, hepatosplenomegaly (especially with hepatitis B), upper respiratory tract symptoms, and diarrhea. Within a few days the first of several crops of lesions appears abruptly. The lesions consist of discrete, firm, lichenoid papules with flat tops (Fig. 12-18, A and B) and range from 1 to 10 mm in diameter, tending to be larger in infants and smaller in older children. Papules can be flesh colored, pink, red, dusky, coppery, or purpuric. They are distributed fairly symmetrically over the extremities (including the palms and soles), buttocks, and face, with relative sparing of the trunk and scalp (Fig. 12-18, B), although the upper back may be involved. They tend to remain discrete but can become confluent, especially over pressure points (Fig. 12-18, C), and the Koebner phenomenon may be seen. Pruritus is unusual, and there is no associated mucosal enanthem.

The exanthem often clears within 2 to 3 weeks but can persist for 8 weeks or more. Results of laboratory studies are generally nonspecific; however, liver function tests should be done, and if the results are abnormal, serologic studies for hepatitis B and EBV should be performed.

Figure 12-17   Recurrent herpes labialis (cold sore). After a brief prodrome of burning, these grouped vesicles, filled with yellow fluid, erupted on the child's upper lip.

Figure 12-18 Gianotti-Crosti syndrome. **A** and **B,** Lesions consist of raised lichenoid papules with flat tops that appear in crops and tend to remain discrete. **C,** This child shows the characteristic acral distribution, with lesions involving the extremities and face but with relative sparing of the trunk. **D,** Lesions can become confluent over pressure points such as the knee.

Treatment is symptomatic. Steroid creams are contraindicated because they may make the rash worse.

Skin and Soft Tissue Findings in Bacterial Infections

Streptococcus pyogenes (Group A *Streptococcus*) (Formerly Called Streptococcal Scarlet Fever)

Although most commonly associated with pharyngitis and impetigo, group A β-hemolytic *Streptococcus pyogenes* causes *scarlet fever*, or *scarlatina*. This exanthem is produced by a streptococcal erythrogenic toxin. Streptococcal infections occur year-round, although pharyngitis and scarlet fever have a peak incidence in winter and spring. Transmission requires close contact to permit the direct spread of large droplets, and those with nasal infection are particularly effective sources. The incubation period for scarlet fever ranges from 12 hours to approximately 7 days. The disease is contagious during the acute period, and patients may transmit the organisms during active subclinical infection as well. An average of 50% of family members living with an index case become secondarily infected, and up to half of these have subclinical disease.

Once a severe illness associated with high morbidity and mortality, scarlet fever has become a much milder illness over the past several decades. In classic cases, now seen less than 10% of the time, the patient experiences the abrupt onset of fever, chills, malaise, headache, sore throat, and vomiting; abdominal pain also may be a prominent complaint. Within 12 to 48 hours an exanthem appears and rapidly generalizes, usually beginning on the trunk and spreading peripherally, but sometimes spreading cephalocaudally. The face is flushed with perioral pallor (Fig. 12-19, *A*). The remaining skin becomes diffusely erythematous and is covered by tiny pinhead-sized papules, giving the sunburn appearance of erythroderma. The texture is sandpapery on palpation, and the erythema blanches with pressure (Fig. 12-19, *B*). The skin may be pruritic, but it is not tender. In severe cases, vesicles may form. After generalization the rash becomes accentuated in skin folds and creases, and 1 to 3 days after its appearance, petechiae may appear in a linear distribution along the creases, forming Pastia lines (Fig. 12-19, *C*). Examination of the oropharynx in classic cases reveals large, erythematous and exudative tonsils, along with palatal erythema and petechiae (see Chapter 23). The uvula may be erythematous and edematous as well. The tongue also shows characteristic findings. During the first 2 days it has a white coating through which erythematous papillae project (a "white" strawberry tongue) (Fig. 12-19, *D*). Subsequently the white coat peels, leaving a glistening red surface with prominent papillae (a "red" strawberry

Figure 12-19 Streptococcal scarlet fever. **A** and **B,** In the classic form of this exanthem, the patient has a flushed face, perioral pallor, and a diffuse, blanching, erythematous rash that has a sandpapery consistency on palpation. **C,** Within 1 to 3 days of onset, Pastia lines may be noted. **D,** During the first 1 to 2 days the tongue has a white coating through which prominent erythematous papillae project—a white strawberry tongue. A few days later the white coat peels, leaving the characteristic red strawberry tongue with glistening surface and prominent papillae **(E). F** and **G,** Desquamation occurs in fine, thin flakes as the acute phase of the illness resolves and is proportional to the intensity of the exanthem. **H,** A wide spectrum of severity and manifestations exists. In this child with streptococcal scarlet fever, the rash has a patchy distribution but is accentuated in the axillae and other creases. (*A, B,* and *F, Courtesy Michael Sherlock, MD, Lutherville, Md.*)

tongue) (Fig. 12-19, *E*). Tender cervical adenopathy is noted in 30% to 60% of patients. Without treatment, the rash, fever, and pharyngitis resolve within 1 week; with treatment, improvement is relatively rapid. Desquamation occurs regardless of treatment and begins several days after onset, progressing cephalocaudally (Fig. 12-19, *F* and *G*). The skin is shed in fine, thin flakes (in contrast to the thick flakes that characterize desquamation after staphylococcal exanthems) (Fig. 12-20; and see Fig. 12-22), and the extent of this process is directly proportional to the intensity of the exanthem.

Diagnosis is simple in classic cases, but the wide spectrum of disease severity and of potential manifestations can cause confusion. Fever may be absent or low grade, and malaise may be minimal. Pharyngitis may be mild (without exudate, petechiae, or marked erythema) or absent, even when the throat is the site of infection. In such cases, tongue changes may be absent as well. If streptococcal skin or wound infections are the primary site of infection, the oropharynx is normal. The appearance of the exanthem may vary as well. In some children it is patchy but continues to be most

Figure 12-20   Staphylococcal scalded skin syndrome. **A,** This infant shows evidence of epidermal separation and has numerous ruptured bullae over the inguinal region and thighs. **B,** In this older child, symptoms were mild and only the skin of the face, axillae, and perineum showed signs of epidermal separation. Note the evidence of a positive Nikolsky sign on her upper lip and cheek, the result of wiping her nose. **C,** A denuded area is evident on the upper chest, and thick flakes have begun to form on the face of this infant. Culture of the purulent nasal discharge was positive for *Staphylococcus aureus*. *(Courtesy Michael Sherlock, MD, Lutherville, Md.)*

prominent near skinfolds (see Fig. 12-19, *H*). An occasional child may have diffuse petechiae. Still others may present with fever or nasopharyngitis and urticaria as their initial manifestations. In dark-skinned children, erythema and perioral pallor may be difficult to appreciate and the papules may be larger, thus producing a texture less like that of sandpaper.

Treatment with a 10-day course of penicillin or erythromycin (in penicillin-allergic children) is important for reducing the risk of transmission and preventing rheumatic fever and pyogenic complications, the most common of which include adenitis, otitis, sinusitis, and peritonsillar and retropharyngeal abscesses. Therefore, in patients with fever or nasopharyngitis and urticaria and in children with scarlatiniform eruptions, a screening throat culture for group A streptococci should be obtained, regardless of the presence or absence of other symptoms. Poststreptococcal nephritis, however, is not prevented by antimicrobial therapy.

Staphylococcus aureus

Coagulase-positive *Staphylococcus aureus* are ubiquitous organisms that are carried at any given time by approximately one third of the population. Although the hallmark of staphylococcal infection is the abscess, numerous forms of infection are seen, and at least three distinct generalized exanthematous disorders have now been identified: staphylococcal scalded skin syndrome, staphylococcal scarlet fever, and toxic shock syndrome. In each form the organisms at the primary site of infection release exotoxins, which then produce the characteristic rash. Transmission may occur by means of direct contact with persons who are infected or who are carriers. Sites of carriage include the nose, skin, axilla, perineum, hair, and nails. Spread of infection may also occur through contact with contaminated objects or food. Draining skin lesions, nasal discharge, and contaminated hands constitute particularly important sources of transmission. Traumatic or surgical wounds, burns, insect bites, areas of preexisting dermatitis, viral skin lesions, and prior viral respiratory tract infection all serve as major predisposing conditions.

Staphylococcal Scalded Skin Syndrome

A disorder seen most commonly in infants and young children, staphylococcal scalded skin syndrome is caused by exfoliative toxin-producing *S. aureus*. The primary infection is usually mild, with purulent nasopharyngitis, conjunctivitis, impetigo, and infections of the umbilicus and circumcision sites seen most commonly. Rarely, sepsis, pneumonia, or other

severe invasive staphylococcal infections may precede the onset of the exanthem.

The infecting organisms produce an exfoliative toxin, which is spread hematogenously and causes cleavage of the skin between the epidermis and the dermis. This process may begin within hours or days of the appearance of signs of the primary infection, and typically its onset is heralded by fever and irritability, often accompanied by vomiting. These symptoms are followed by the development of a diffuse erythroderma that spreads rapidly from head to toe and simulates the appearance of sunburn. In contrast to streptococcal scarlet fever, the involved skin is tender, even to light touch. Within 1 to 3 days, thin-walled, flaccid, bullous lesions appear and rupture soon after formation (Fig. 12-20, *A*). Simultaneously, larger portions of the epidermis begin to separate in sheets, and during this phase application of light lateral traction on the skin causes the epidermis to pull away from the dermis, leaving a raw, weeping surface. This separation of the skin in response to stroking is called the *Nikolsky sign* (Fig. 12-20, *B*). After exfoliation the surface gradually dries, forming large, thick flakes (Fig. 12-20, *C*).

A broad spectrum of severity exists for this syndrome. In severe cases the patient appears toxic and in considerable pain. The child may shed large portions of skin, resulting in significant fluid losses that may be accompanied by difficulties with temperature regulation. In mild cases (Fig. 12-20, *B*) toxicity is absent and only localized areas of skin are denuded, with the face and perineum constituting the primary sites of shedding. The causative organism can be isolated from the site of primary infection, but it is absent—at least initially—from the bullae and from sites of skin separation.

Staphylococcal Scarlet Fever

Staphylococcal infection can result in a scarlatiniform exanthem that initially is indistinguishable in appearance from that produced by group A β-hemolytic streptococci. The illness is characterized by fever, irritability, and moderate malaise, followed by the abrupt onset of a generalized erythematous rash, often of sandpapery consistency, with accentuation in the skin creases (Fig. 12-21, *A*). In contrast to the exanthem seen in streptococcal scarlet fever, the involved skin is usually tender, the tongue is normal, and there is no palatal enanthem. Evolution of lesions also differs, in that within 2 to 5 days the skin begins to crack, fissure, and weep, especially in the perioral and periorbital areas and in the skin creases (Fig. 12-21, *B*). It is then shed in large, thick flakes over 3 to 5 days. Local

Figure 12-21 Staphylococcal scarlet fever. **A,** In this patient, nasopharyngitis and purulent conjunctivitis antedated the development of a generalized sandpaper-like rash, which was tender to the touch. **B,** The skin in the periorbital and perioral areas has begun to crack, fissure, and weep serous fluid.

skin and wound infections are common antecedents, and their presence often enables presumptive identification of staphylococci as causative agents early in the disease. However, when nasopharyngitis is the source of primary infection, the picture can be difficult to distinguish from streptococcal infection, especially when strawberry tongue and palatal petechiae are absent. The same may be true if a local infection with lymphangitis is the source. In such cases the tendency for the staphylococcal rash to be tender may be the major clinical distinction. Unless the primary infection is severe enough to warrant parenteral treatment, oral antimicrobial therapy is sufficient.

Toxic Shock Syndrome

Toxic shock syndrome (TSS) is the third syndrome of staphylococcal origin characterized by a generalized exanthem. It is seen in children and adults who have localized infections caused by *S. aureus* and was originally recognized in menstruating females whose vaginas are colonized with toxin-producing organisms. There is a strong correlation with tampon use, indicating that the impedance of normal menstrual flow or the presence of abrasions secondary to use of large bell-shaped tampons may contribute to the development of this syndrome. Patients with nonmenstrual TSS often have a skin lesion, an abscess, or purulent conjunctivitis as the primary focus of infection (Fig. 12-22, *B*).

Staphylococcal TSS begins with a prodrome consisting of low-grade fever, malaise, myalgias, and vomiting. This is followed by an abrupt increase in fever, accompanied by chills, worsening myalgias, repetitive vomiting, abdominal pain, orthostatic dizziness, and weakness. Soon thereafter, patients show a diffuse erythroderma, mimicking a sunburn (Fig. 12-22, *A*). Conjunctivitis with photophobia, oropharyngeal erythema, and a strawberry tongue are common features. Subsequently, severe watery diarrhea, hypotension, and oliguria may become prominent, accompanied by alterations in level of consciousness. This often necessitates massive volume replacement and vasopressor therapy. In severe cases, acute respiratory distress syndrome may develop. Many patients have muscle tenderness and weakness, as well as diffuse abdominal tenderness without peritoneal signs. A small proportion show nonpitting edema of the face, hands, and feet. Over the ensuing days, petechiae and a secondary maculopapular rash may be noted, along with oral ulcerations.

Figure 12-22 Toxic shock syndrome (TSS). **A,** This young boy presented with diffuse erythroderma, fever, chills, myalgias, headache, vomiting, and orthostatic dizziness with mild widening of his pulse pressure. **B,** Examination disclosed an infected puncture wound of the knee, which grew *Staphylococcus aureus*. Although his illness was relatively mild, the association of gastrointestinal symptoms and orthostatic changes suggested TSS, which was confirmed by laboratory studies and by subsequent desquamation **(C).** This begins periungually, and the skin is shed in thick casts. (**C,** *Courtesy George Pazin, MD, University of Pittsburgh Medical Center, Pittsburgh, Pa.*)

Desquamation is routine, usually beginning 1 week after onset of the rash. It is most prominent over the palms and soles and in the periungual areas, and the skin is shed in thick casts (Fig. 12-22, *C*). Removal of any infected source material such as a tampon, and parenteral antimicrobial therapy directed against *Staphylococcus aureus,* are required for effective therapy.

Clinical and laboratory findings in severe cases point toward the existence of diffuse vascular leakage with third-spacing of fluids, electrolytes, and serum proteins. Secondary hypotension and hypoperfusion result in azotemia. Toxin-related hepatic changes may also be noted.

As recognition of TSS has increased, the existence of a wide spectrum of severity has become apparent. Mild cases mimic staphylococcal scarlet fever. Such patients tend to have smaller gastrointestinal losses and less difficulty with fluid shifts and attendant complications. Early recognition of this clinical syndrome and aggressive therapy may often prevent development of shock.

BACTERIAL SKIN AND SOFT TISSUE INFECTIONS

Superficial bacterial skin infections occur with a relatively high frequency in childhood. In most cases the causative organisms are inoculated through a small wound, such as a superficial cut, abrasion, insect bite, or burn. Infection may occur at the time of the injury if the pathogen has colonized the site previously, or it may occur subsequently as the result of scratching, touching, or contamination with dirt. In some cases a preexisting dermatitis sets the stage for secondary infection by breaking down the skin barrier. The risk of infection in patients with preexisting dermatitis must be kept in mind, especially when steroids are prescribed.

Although most superficial infections are relatively minor in severity, diagnosis and proper treatment are important to reduce further spread of infection and to prevent its transmission to others. Deeper skin and soft tissue infections, although less common, have the potential for causing greater morbidity and even mortality. As with superficial lesions, inoculation from an external source is the most common mode of acquisition. In many instances, however, these infections represent metastatic foci of bacteremic spread.

Group A β-hemolytic streptococci and *S. aureus* are the organisms most commonly responsible for skin and soft tissue infections. Both organisms commonly reside in the nasopharynx, and staphylococci routinely colonize the skin, a phenomenon that is less likely with streptococci. Both organisms are transmitted readily by carriers or persons with active nasopharyngeal or skin infections. The fact that each pathogen produces relatively characteristic clinical features can help in their clinical diagnoses. Staphylococci are somewhat more likely to remain localized, stimulating suppuration and tissue necrosis, producing abscesses. Methicillin-resistant *S. aureus* (MRSA) has increased substantially in the community, as well as in health care settings, and cannot be clinically distinguished from methicillin-susceptible strains of *S. aureus.* Conversely, streptococcal infection tends to spread along tissue planes and through lymphatics and thus is more commonly associated with secondary cellulitis, lymphangitis, and regional adenopathy.

Folliculitis

Folliculitis is a superficial infection or irritation of the hair follicles. The scalp, face, extensor surfaces of the extremities, and buttocks are the most common sites of involvement.

Figure 12-23   Folliculitis. The extensor surfaces of the extremities and other hair-bearing areas are the most common sites of this superficial infection of hair follicles. Lesions begin at the base of a hair shaft as erythematous nodules and then evolve to form central pustules with a thin, red rim.

Patients with dry, atopic skin and keratosis pilaris (a condition in which follicles become blocked by keratin plugs) are particularly prone to this problem (see Chapter 8). Additional predisposing factors include seborrhea, excessive sweating, poor hygiene, and topical application of or contact with oils, tars, and adhesives. In each of these situations, obstruction of follicles occurs, setting the stage for inflammation and secondary infection. After occlusion, a superficial erythematous nodule develops around the hair. The lesion then evolves into a thin-walled central pustule with a narrow, red rim (Fig. 12-23). The lesions may itch or burn and subsequently may drain and crust. Although it takes a given lesion 7 to 10 days to heal without treatment, multiple crops may occur. With scratching the infection may spread to other areas, and secondary impetiginous lesions may develop. *Staphylococcus aureus* are the typical pathogens, although other skin colonizers may participate. Oral antimicrobial therapy directed at the staphylococcus and treatment or avoidance of the predisposing condition are the measures indicated to eradicate the process. The frequent involvement of MRSA strains with folliculitis has been reported.

On occasion, the early lesions found in some forms of tinea capitis and tinea corporis may mimic folliculitis, although itching is usually more prominent in fungal infections and the surrounding rim of erythema tends to be wider. Tinea should be suspected, especially if folliculitis is localized to the hairline of the scalp (see Chapter 8). Older lesions, if present, may help in distinguishing between fungal and bacterial infections. Gram stain, potassium hydroxide preparations, and cultures can be useful in evaluating questionable cases.

Impetigo

Impetigo is a superficial infection of the epidermis caused by streptococci, staphylococci, or both. Exposed portions of the body including the face, extremities, hands, and neck are the most common sites of involvement. Lesions teem with organisms and serve as a potential source of transmission to others. In temperate climates the disorder has a peak incidence in summer and early fall because of increased exposure of the body surface to insect bites, injury, and colonization by pathogenic organisms. In warm climates, impetigo is prevalent year-round. Although impetigo has traditionally been considered a streptococcal disease, more recent evidence indicates that *S. aureus* has eclipsed group A streptococci as the predominant cause of impetigo. In patients without preexisting

Figure 12-24 Streptococcal impetigo. This impetiginous lesion has evolved from a papule to a vesicle that ruptured, producing the characteristic honey-colored crust. *(Courtesy Michael Sherlock, MD, Lutherville, Md.)*

erythematous base is revealed. Secondary enlargement and tenderness of the regional lymph nodes are common.

The initial macules of primary staphylococcal impetigo may evolve rapidly to form small, thin-walled pustules (Fig. 12-25, *A*) or the larger flaccid bullae of bullous impetigo (Fig. 12-25, *B*). The latter contain slightly cloudy fluid and are often 1 cm or more in diameter. In either instance the pustules or bullae rupture rapidly, leaving a shallow erythematous base surrounded by a superficial peeling rim (Fig. 12-25, *B*). In patients with more long-standing or combined infection, lesions may crust centrally and enlarge centrifugally. This may result in the formation of a superficial central scab surrounded by a bullous rim or a dried lesion with multiple concentric rings resembling an onion slice (Fig. 12-25, *C* and *D*). Lesions may coalesce over time, and satellite lesions may form around larger primary lesions. Regardless of type, impetigo is frequently pruritic and the patient is stimulated to scratch, thereby spreading the infection to other sites or even inoculating the offending bacteria deeper into the skin.

The possible sources of the causative organisms may be the patient's own skin or nasopharynx or those of another infected person. In patients with facial lesions, the nose is the most likely site of origin. Oral antimicrobial therapy is preferred for eradication and is a particularly important measure if the source of infection is the nasopharynx or if the lesions are extensive, although topical antibacterial therapy with mupirocin is effective for eradicating small numbers of lesions. On occasion, infection with other organisms can simulate the picture of impetiginous lesions. One form of tinea capitis produces lesions identical to those of streptococcal impetigo (see Chapter 8). Hence if small pustules and golden-crusted lesions are seen on the scalp or at the hairline, Gram stain and potassium hydroxide preparations are indicated to ensure the correct diagnosis. *Candida* organisms can produce tiny pustules, which rupture and have a superficial peeling rim,

dermatitis, lesions tend to be localized, but if the child has an antecedent condition, such as eczema, the infection can spread rapidly to involve extensive areas.

In cases of impetigo caused by group A streptococci alone, the lesion begins as a papule and evolves rapidly to become a small, thin-walled vesicle with an erythematous halo. The initially serous vesicular fluid becomes cloudy and the vesicle ruptures, forming a superficial honey-colored crust (Fig. 12-24). If the crust is lifted, a shallow, smooth, weeping,

Figure 12-25 Staphylococcal impetigo. **A,** This infant with staphylococcal diaper dermatitis has multiple small, thin-walled pustules that rupture rapidly and coalesce, leaving a shallow base and a superficial peeling rim. **B,** The various stages of bullous impetigo are evident in this child. Inferiorly an unruptured flaccid bulla is seen with an older lesion above it that has spread outward and crusted peripherally; just above that, another bulla has just ruptured. **C,** In this child with staphylococcal impetigo, older lesions have central crusts with bullous rims that are spreading outward. **D,** The features of long-standing impetigo are seen in this youngster whose lesions are crusted in rings, resembling an onion slice. Note also the smaller satellites surrounding the larger primary lesion.

Figure 12-26   Ecthyma. **A,** In focal ecthyma resulting from the inoculation of group A streptococci, the lesion initially consists of a central vesicle or pustule (that rapidly crusts over) on a painful, indurated, erythematous base. **B,** With progression a deep, widening ulcer forms, as seen in this child after removal of the overlying crust. *(Courtesy Ellen Wald, MD, University of Wisconsin Children's Hospital, Madison, Wis.)*

at times simulating staphylococcal infection in the diaper area. However, in candidal diaper dermatitis, lesions are smaller (1 to 2 mm in diameter), pustules are more evanescent, the inflammation is more diffuse, and the erythema more intense (see Chapter 8) than is the case in staphylococcal impetigo and staphylococcal diaper dermatitis. In confusing cases a potassium hydroxide preparation or Gram stain can be used to clarify the etiology.

Ecthyma

Ecthyma is an ulcerative skin infection that penetrates more deeply than impetigo to involve the dermis. The disorder is most prevalent in tropical climates. Poor hygiene, insect bites, and trauma are the major predisposing factors, accounting for the fact that the lower extremities and the buttocks are the usual sites of involvement. Initially, lesions may resemble impetigo, consisting of a vesicle or a pustule on an erythematous base (Fig. 12-26, *A*), which then ruptures and crusts over. In ecthyma, however, the lesions are painful and the crusts harder, thicker, and more adherent than they are in impetigo, and the surrounding area of erythema is indurated. The ulcerative base beneath the crust gradually deepens and enlarges. Unroofing the crust uncovers a round, deep, punched-out ulcer with raised borders (Fig. 12-26, *B*). The size of the lesions ranges from 0.5 to 3 cm. Without treatment these lesions take weeks to heal, leaving a circumscribed scar.

In most cases ecthyma is the result of direct inoculation of organisms through the skin, with group A β-hemolytic streptococci being the usual pathogen. On occasion, staphylococci or *Pseudomonas* organisms may be the cause; when infecting a small wound, the latter pathogen is more likely to produce a central abscess that exudes a greenish or bluish purulent exudate when its crust is lifted.

Ecthyma gangrenosum is a systemic disease seen predominantly in immunocompromised patients during periods of neutropenia. It is usually caused by septicemia with *Pseudomonas aeruginosa,* during which seeding of organisms results in the appearance of metastatic skin lesions. These begin as pink macules, evolve into hemorrhagic papules, and then necrose centrally to leave a dark eschar on an erythematous base (Fig. 12-27). Subsequently, ulceration occurs, associated with deep necrosis. This metastatic form of ecthyma is distinguished easily from primary cases by virtue of the formation of multiple lesions, the presence of systemic signs of sepsis, and laboratory evidence of neutropenia.

ABSCESSES OF THE SKIN AND SOFT TISSUES

Abscesses are localized collections of purulent material that are buried in a tissue, an organ, or a confined space. They result from the deep seeding of pyogenic organisms, which,

Figure 12-27   Ecthyma gangrenosum. *Pseudomonas* septicemia may result in metastatic ecthymatous lesions that begin as pink macules **(A),** become hemorrhagic **(B),** and ultimately necrose centrally to form a black eschar **(C)**. *(Courtesy Ellen Wald, MD, University of Wisconsin Children's Hospital, Madison, Wis.)*

in the case of abscesses involving the skin and its appendages, are usually coagulase-positive staphylococci. The vast majority of pediatric skin and soft tissue abscesses are caused by *S. aureus*, most commonly methicillin-resistant strains. As the area of inflammation expands outward, central necrosis occurs and the process tends to produce an increase in pressure, with resultant pointing toward the surface or spread along tissue planes with further local tissue destruction. Drainage is essential for healing because the abscess contents provoke a continuing inflammatory response and antimicrobials are generally unable to penetrate to the necrotic center of the lesion. Abscesses of the skin and soft tissues are categorized in part according to the site of involvement and in part according to the structure involved. The types most commonly encountered in childhood are discussed in the following sections.

Paronychia (Periungual Abscess)

A paronychia is a relatively superficial abscess that develops under the cuticle or along the nail fold of a finger or a toe. It occurs when staphylococci and occasionally streptococci gain access through a traumatized hangnail or through lesions created by clipping a cuticle or by chewing on the fingers. On occasion, an ingrown toenail is the predisposing condition; in such cases the nail, which usually was cut improperly, grows laterally into the nail fold, lacerating the soft tissue and setting the stage for infection. In typical cases, erythema, pain, and tenderness develop at the site of injury and are followed rapidly by suppuration (Fig. 12-28). The infection then advances from the portal of entry around the nail fold, and if treatment is delayed, it can burrow beneath the base of the nail, creating a subungual abscess (onychia). On occasion, secondary lymphangitis may develop. Drainage is accomplished readily by undermining the involved portion of the cuticle and nail fold with a scalpel blade. Unless secondary complications have developed, subsequent soaking is usually sufficient to promote healing, although oral antistaphylococcal agents hasten the process.

Abscesses of Skin Appendages

Furuncle

A furuncle, or boil, is a perifollicular dermal abscess that is usually caused by *S. aureus*. It may be the result of extension of superficial folliculitis or of direct inoculation via minor trauma. Hairy areas subject to friction or maceration, as well as the concentrations of sebaceous glands in axilla and inguinal regions, are particularly vulnerable. Skin contact with occlusive agents, such as oils, tars, and adhesives, is another

Figure 12-28 Paronychia. Chewing on a hangnail predisposed this child to the development of a paronychia. Initially, erythema developed near the hangnail and was followed rapidly by suppuration.

common predisposing factor. The incidence of furuncles is much higher in older children and adolescents than it is in younger children.

The lesion begins as a small dermal nodule around a hair follicle, which initially may produce mild discomfort and itching. As it gradually enlarges, pain worsens and is aggravated by touching and motion of the involved area. With expansion, the overlying skin becomes reddened, central necrosis begins to occur, and with increased inflammation and pressure, the infection begins to seek egress. In the case of most furuncles, the abscess burrows toward the surface of the skin, which becomes thinned and shiny as the abscess becomes fluctuant (Fig. 12-29, *A*). Application of warm compresses can hasten this process. At this point, incision and drainage are indicated. Without intervention, spontaneous drainage of bloody purulent material ultimately occurs in most cases and the patient experiences prompt relief of pain (Fig. 12-29, *B*). In areas such as the nape of the neck or upper back, where the overlying skin is thick enough to resist external pointing, the process may take a path of lesser resistance, burrowing outward from the center through the subcutaneous tissues and along fascial planes. If this process is not interrupted by early surgical intervention, the result is a gradual formation of a *carbuncle*, which consists of an extremely painful, exquisitely tender multilocular mass of interconnected dermal and subcutaneous abscesses, with multiple points of partial drainage at the skin surface. Carbuncle formation is often accompanied by fever, chills, and increasing malaise, and there is a

Figure 12-29 Furuncle. **A,** In this well-developed furuncle, the abscess has burrowed to the surface and the skin has thinned centrally and begun to necrose. A wide surrounding rim of erythema and induration exists. **B,** This furuncle, located on the neck of a young infant, had spontaneously ruptured and drained earlier in the day but was beginning to enlarge again. (**A,** *Courtesy Bernard Cohen, MD, Johns Hopkins Hospital, Baltimore, Md.*)

A

B

significant risk of secondary bacteremia. Even with treatment, sloughing and extensive scarring tend to result.

Hidradenitis Suppurativa

In hidradenitis suppurativa, an apocrine gland is the site of infection and abscess formation. Hence localization in these cases is limited to the axillae, perineum, and areolae, and the disorder affects only young people after the onset of puberty. Keratin plugging of apocrine ducts and their hair follicles appears to be a major predisposing factor, and occlusion, maceration, and poor hygiene may exacerbate the problem. The resultant obstruction fosters inflammation and provides a favorable environment for secondary invasion and multiplication of staphylococci and anaerobic bacteria. As the inflammatory process expands, the gland ultimately ruptures and an abscess forms. In contrast to the perifollicular furuncle, this infection is deeper and slower to localize and suppurate. It begins as a firm, mildly tender nodule that enlarges gradually, becoming increasingly uncomfortable and tender to the touch. With further enlargement and suppuration, the lesion(s) point to the surface and drain, although some may rupture subcutaneously. Early diagnosis, incision and drainage of fluctuant sites, institution of a prolonged course of antimicrobial therapy, the wearing of loose-fitting clothing, and adoption of meticulous hygienic practices may bring the problem under control. Delay in diagnosis; inadequate treatment; or, in some cases, recalcitrant disease can result in recurrence or progression with formation of multiple abscesses and sinus tracts, deep fibrosis, and scarring (Fig. 12-30) that ultimately may necessitate surgical excision.

Abscesses of Special Sites

The breasts, scalp, and perirectal areas are three specific sites of abscess formation of particular importance in pediatrics. Breast and scalp abscesses are discussed in the following sections. Perirectal abscesses are described in Chapter 17.

Breast Abscess

Breast abscesses occur within specific age groups among pediatric patients, with incidence peaks in the neonatal and pubertal groups. The incidence is highest in newborns of greater than 31 weeks' gestation at the time of birth, owing in part to physiologic hypertrophy of breast tissue as a result of stimulation by maternal hormones. Colonization of the skin or the nasopharynx with potentially virulent organisms (*S. aureus*, group B streptococci, or coliforms) during birth or in the nursery is another important predisposing factor. Up to 25% of affected infants have overt staphylococcal diaper dermatitis at the time of presentation. Minor local trauma is also thought to be a predisposing factor. Most cases occur during the second or third week after birth, but infection may occur as late as 8 weeks of age. The problem first manifests as swelling and tenderness of the affected breast. Unilateral involvement is the rule. With time, local warmth and overlying erythema become evident and it may be possible to express a purulent discharge from the nipple (Fig. 12-31, *A*). Axillary adenopathy may be present as well. Only 25% of infants have low-grade fever, and other systemic symptoms are uncommon unless treatment is delayed. Depending on the time of presentation, a firm, tender, nonfluctuant nodule may be found on palpation or the mass may be clearly fluctuant, indicating suppuration and necrosis. In the former instance, parenteral antibiotic therapy and close monitoring for progression are indicated. In the latter instance, prompt surgical incision and drainage are required. Broad-spectrum antimicrobial coverage should be provided pending culture results. Commonly recovered organisms include *S. aureus*, *Escherichia coli*, *Salmonella* species, group B streptococci, *Proteus mirabilis*, and mixed flora. Delay in diagnosis and institution of treatment can result in subcutaneous rupture and cellulitic spread with secondary bacteremia (Fig. 12-31, *B*). Delay in surgical drainage of fluctuant lesions can also result in permanent loss of breast tissue, which in girls can produce a cosmetically deforming breast asymmetry that is first noted at puberty.

Breast abscesses may be seen again after puberty. Minor trauma, cutaneous infections, epidermal cysts, and duct blockages appear to be the common antecedent conditions. The clinical picture is similar to that seen in infants. *Staphylococcus aureus* is the usual etiology.

Figure 12-31 Breast abscess. **A,** The typical manifestations of a breast abscess were seen in this neonate—swelling, induration, tenderness, warmth, and erythema. With compression, pus could be expressed from the nipple. **B,** This infant was not brought to the hospital until subcutaneous rupture and extensive cellulitic spread had occurred. She was febrile, toxic, irritable, and listless on presentation.

Figure 12-30 Hidradenitis suppurativa. Obstruction of apocrine ducts and hair follicles predisposes them to infection and suppuration. In this adolescent boy, the process is advanced with multiple abscesses, sinus tracts, and scarring. (*From Cohen B: Atlas of pediatric dermatology, London, 1993, Mosby/Wolfe.*)

Figure 12-32 Scalp abscess. Several days after discharge from the newborn nursery this infant presented with two scalp abscesses and an impetiginous lesion behind the right ear. The surface of the larger abscess is marked by two puncture wounds, which were the site of placement of monitor leads during labor.

Scalp Abscess

As is the case with breast abscesses, pyogenic infections of the scalp are particularly common in the neonatal period. Trauma is the predominant predisposing factor, and in neonates these abscesses commonly develop at sites where scalp leads were inserted for fetal monitoring. In most cases the infection is localized and consists of a tender nodule with overlying erythema (Fig. 12-32). The nodule is commonly fluctuant at the time of presentation, enabling prompt incision and drainage. Staphylococci and coliforms are the major pathogens recovered. Because of the neonate's immunologic immaturity, antimicrobial therapy is also recommended and in most cases can be administered orally. On rare occasions

infection is extensive and takes the form of a necrotizing fasciitis (see later discussion). In these patients and in the rare infant with a localized abscess and systemic symptoms, parenteral broad-spectrum antibiotic treatment (pending culture results) is indicated, in addition to incision, drainage, and debridement. Bacterial scalp abscesses must be differentiated from skin manifestation of herpes neonatorum, which can present at scalp sites as discussed later (see Neonatal Herpes Simplex Infection later in this chapter).

When scalp abscesses are encountered in older children, care should be taken to determine the responsible pathogen. Although staphylococci may be the infecting agent, invasive fungi are more likely to be the responsible organisms. These fungi produce a thick-walled, boggy, multilocular abscess termed a *kerion* (see Chapter 8). Gram stain and potassium hydroxide preparations of purulent contents and of pulled hairs are important, along with fungal culture, because although incision and drainage constitute the treatment of choice for abscesses of bacterial origin, oral antifungal and steroid therapy are indicated for the treatment of a kerion.

Lymphangitis

Inflammation of lymphatic channels is actually a secondary manifestation of infection at a distal site. The phenomenon is the result of invasion of lymphatic vessels by pathogenic organisms, which then spread along these channels toward regional lymph nodes. Group A β-hemolytic streptococci are the most common source of lymphangitis, although overt lymphangitis may also develop in wounds infected by *S. aureus* and *P. aeruginosa*. Clinically, erythematous, irregular linear streaks (which may be tender) are seen extending from the primary site toward the draining regional nodes (Fig. 12-33). The primary site may be an infected wound or an area of cellulitis. Systemic symptoms consisting of fever, chills, and malaise may be present. Without appropriate

Figure 12-33 Lymphangitis. **A,** An insect bite was the source of inoculation of group A streptococci in this child, who subsequently suffered secondary cellulitis and lymphangitis. The erythematous streaks coursing up the leg were tender and slightly indurated. **B,** Three distinct lymphangitic streaks are seen coursing up the instep from an area of cellulitis surrounding a puncture wound of the foot. *Pseudomonas* was the causative organism. **C** and **D,** In this child irregular lymphatic streaks are seen coursing up the arm from a cellulitic area involving the dorsum of his hand.

Figure 12-34   Erysipelas. **A,** This 6-week-old infant had fever, lethargy, irritability, and hypotension in association with erysipelas. The purplish-red lesion was raised, indurated, and tender. The border, although irregular, was sharply demarcated from the adjacent skin. Cultures of blood and tissue aspirate grew group A streptococci. **B,** The sharply circumscribed area of erysipelas on this toddler's leg was pink. On close inspection, one can see that the skin has a peau d'orange quality. **C,** This is seen more clearly in a close-up of an adolescent's forehead. (**C,** *Courtesy James Ferante, MD.*)

antimicrobial therapy, cellulitis may develop or extend and necrosis and ulceration may occur, with the attendant risk of bacteremia. Culture and Gram stain of material from the primary site aid in the selection of antimicrobials; however, presumptive initial therapy is necessary pending culture results as lymphangitis is the prelude to systemic spread.

Erysipelas

Group A streptococci are the source of erysipelas, an unusual and distinctive infection involving a localized area of the dermis and superficial lymphatics. The causative organisms are usually found in the upper respiratory tracts of afflicted patients and are inoculated through a break in the skin barrier. Hematogenous seeding has been postulated in some cases. Systemic symptoms are prominent and precede the appearance of the characteristic skin lesion. The onset is abrupt and is heralded by fever and chills, often in association with nausea, vomiting, and headache. This prodrome is followed by the appearance of an intensely painful skin lesion that consists of a circumscribed, raised plaque that is usually deep purplish-red but that may be red or even pink (Fig. 12-34). The raised border, although irregular, is well demarcated and spreads centrifugally. Red lymphatic streaks may advance ahead of it toward the regional nodes. On close inspection the skin is seen to be edematous and may have a thickened peau d'orange character (Fig. 12-34, *C*). On palpation it is found to be indurated, hot, and exquisitely tender. With evolution, small surface blebs containing yellow fluid may form. The face is the site most commonly involved, with the trunk, neck, and extremities being less frequent areas of localization. Patients may become bacteremic, with the development of metastatic foci of infection. Infants are at particular risk for systemic spread. The clinical picture of erysipelas is so characteristic that streptococcal infection can be presumed and parenteral antimicrobial treatment initiated. Cultures of tissue aspirate from the advancing border of the lesion and cultures of the nose and throat are typically positive for group A streptococci, as are blood cultures in septic patients.

Cellulitis

Cellulitis is an infection of bacterial origin, and subcutaneous loose connective tissue is the primary site of inflammation. With progression, the process extends centrifugally through the subcutaneous tissue and may also ascend to involve the lower dermis. Although cellulitis may develop anywhere on the body, it occurs most commonly on the extremities and face. Three major modes of origin exist:

1. Extension from a wound
2. Hematogenous seeding
3. Extension from a deeper infection

Clinically, cellulitis is characterized by painful, tender, indurated subcutaneous swelling. The overlying skin is smooth, warm, often shiny, and usually erythematous (Fig. 12-35). On occasion, it is pink or has a violaceous hue. In contrast to erysipelas, the margins or borders of both the edema and erythema are indistinct, fading imperceptibly into the surrounding tissues. Before initiation of therapy, rapid extension is the rule. Systemic symptoms can be a sign of more severe disease with hematogenous spread. In such cases, fever, chills, malaise, and headache are typical.

Wound-Related Cellulitis

Extension of infection from an external wound, such as a puncture, laceration, abrasion, or insect bite, is perhaps the most common source of cellulitis, particularly in school-age children and adolescents. Mild local erythema immediately surrounding a wound, an impetiginous lesion, or a pustule may have been noted before the abrupt onset of increased pain and the rapid evolution of subcutaneous inflammation that herald the development of cellulitis. In most cases the primary lesion is readily identifiable at the time of presentation (Fig. 12-35), but in some instances it may no longer be detectable. On occasion, secondary infection of a preexisting dermatitis may result in a cellulitis that spreads with frightening speed (Fig. 12-36). Group A streptococci and *S. aureus* are the organisms recovered most commonly in these circumstances. *Pseudomonas* organisms and mixed flora may be responsible for cellulitis occurring secondary to puncture wounds of the foot (see Fig. 12-33, *B*). Although rapid peripheral spread, overt lymphangitis, and regional adenitis are regarded as highly characteristic of streptococcal infection, this same picture may be seen in patients with cellulitis caused by any of these wound-related pathogens. Fever and other systemic symptoms may be present with wound-related cellulitis but are more likely to occur with cellulitis due to hematogenous seeding or to extension of inflammation from deeper structures. Although MRSA infections are more likely to present with abscess, surrounding cellulitis is not uncommon in these patients.

Figure 12-35 Wound-related cellulitis. **A,** The infected mosquito bite that served as the source of cellulitis in this child can be seen on the left. The area of erythema was indurated and tender. Note that the skin is smooth and the borders fade gradually into the adjacent normal skin. **B,** Mild erythema and edema are evident in the periorbital area of an infant whose laceration from a dog bite had been sutured 48 hours earlier. The edematous areas were indurated and tender. **C** and **D,** This adolescent presented with erythema, edema, and extreme tenderness caused by infection subsequent to ear-piercing. (**C** and **D,** Courtesy Robert Hickey, MD, Children's Hospital of Pittsburgh, Pittsburgh, Pa.)

Hands, feet, and extremities are the most common sites of wound-related cellulitis. This necessitates close assessment and monitoring for further spread and for secondary neurovascular compromise. Inward spread to tendon sheaths of a hand or a foot can have disastrous consequences; hence cellulitis involving these structures must be treated aggressively, and clinical status must be monitored closely. When an extremity is encircled by cellulitis, swelling and increased pressure can result in neurovascular compromise and extensive secondary damage distally if the area is not surgically decompressed.

Gram stain and culture of material obtained from the primary wound may be helpful in identifying the specific pathogen. Blood cultures should be obtained in all patients with systemic symptoms. Prompt treatment is essential to prevent further spread and complications. Antimicrobial therapy often must be selected empirically, pending culture results. Coverage for group A streptococci and MRSA is often indicated.

Major differential diagnostic considerations include angioedema resulting from an insect bite and delayed hypersensitivity reactions to Hymenoptera stings. The former is pruritic and nontender and often has an identifiable central punctum (see Chapter 8); the latter tend to be simultaneously pruritic, painful, and tender (see Chapter 8). Both are unassociated with systemic symptoms or with adenopathy or lymphangitis.

Figure 12-36   This patient with cellulitis of the foot had been receiving topical steroid therapy for contact dermatitis for about 48 hours when he experienced the explosive onset of swelling, redness, and pain. Impetiginous changes are apparent as well. *(Courtesy Michael Sherlock, MD, Lutherville, Md.)*

History of trauma, presence of ecchymotic discoloration, and absence of systemic symptoms all help to distinguish swelling due to injury.

Hematogenous Cellulitis

Hematogenous seeding is another source of cellulitis, particularly in infants and young children. Although young infants may show the sudden onset of sepsis, followed soon afterward by the appearance of cellulitis, older infants, toddlers, and preschool-age children commonly have antecedent upper respiratory tract symptoms. This prodrome is followed by the sudden development of a high fever that begins nearly simultaneously with the appearance of a nondescript area of swelling. Often this swelling is localized in the periorbital region (see Chapter 23), but at times it may be located over the neck or an extremity. The overlying skin rapidly becomes pink, red, or violaceous as the area of edema spreads and becomes indurated. Irritability, anorexia, and signs of toxicity become increasingly marked, in most cases prompting presentation for medical care within 24 hours. *Haemophilus influenzae* type B was once a likely source of this picture, but with widespread use of the Hib vaccine, the incidence of *H. influenzae* cellulitis has plummeted. *Streptococcus pneumoniae*, as well as group B streptococci (in infants younger than 3 months of age), are other responsible pathogens.

Haemophilus influenzae type B appears to be the sole pathogen responsible for cellulitis of the cheek, also termed *buccal cellulitis*. In this form of cellulitis, a type limited exclusively to infants, the swelling, induration, and erythema are located over the midcheek near the mandibular ramus (Fig. 12-37). Localized erythema of the underlying buccal mucosa is a common associated finding. The systemic symptomatology and exquisite tenderness help to distinguish it from "popsicle panniculitis," which results from cold injury. The latter is characterized by the formation of a mildly tender, discrete, indurated, disk-shaped, subcutaneous mass located at the angle of the mouth, with reddish purple discoloration of the overlying skin (Fig. 12-38). Systemic symptoms, induration, and tenderness also help to distinguish hematogenous cellulitis at periorbital and other sites from sympathetic swelling caused by sinusitis, which is nontender and not indurated (see Chapter 23), and from the pruritic nontender angioedema resulting from insect bites (see Chapter 8).

Because of the severity of the illness associated with buccal cellulitis and the inevitability of bacteremia with its attendant risks, expeditious evaluation and treatment are warranted. Blood cultures are positive in a high percentage of patients and may be supplemented by culture of tissue aspirates from the area of cellulitis. High-dose antimicrobial therapy should be administered parenterally, and agents selected that ensure coverage for β-lactamase–producing *Haemophilus* organisms.

Cellulitis Due to Extension of Infection from Deeper Structures

Although less common than the other forms, cellulitis resulting from extension of infection and inflammation from deeper structures may also occur. This possibility necessitates paying close attention to examination of underlying structures in evaluating any patient with evidence of cellulitis. Dental abscesses (see Chapter 20) and acute sinusitis (see Chapter 23) may underlie facial cellulitis. Osteomyelitis may produce secondary cellulitic changes in overlying soft tissues, especially after subperiosteal extension (see Osteomyelitis, later).

Figure 12-37   Hematogenous cellulitis. **A,** A small erythematous patch with indistinct borders appeared on this infant's cheek shortly after the onset of fever, irritability, and anorexia. On palpation it was found to be indurated and tender. Blood culture was positive for *Haemophilus influenzae* type B. **B,** In this toddler, the evolution of buccal cellulitis due to *H. influenzae* was fulminant, resulting in unusually dramatic swelling. (**B,** *Courtesy Kenneth Schuitt, MD.*)

Figure 12-38 Popsicle panniculitis. This older infant, who was fond of popsicles, had bilateral areas of purplish red swelling just lateral to the corners of his mouth. He was otherwise well. On palpation, masses could be appreciated that were mildly tender, discrete, indurated, and disk shaped. These were localized areas of fat necrosis caused by cold injury. *(Courtesy Michael Sherlock, MD, Lutherville, Md.)*

Suppurative lymphadenitis and subcutaneous rupture of skin, scalp, and breast abscesses are other common sources (see Fig. 12-31, *B*). Fever, toxicity, and other systemic symptoms are common with this form of cellulitis. Antecedent history along with the findings on careful examination usually enable identification of this type of cellulitis and recognition of the primary source.

Necrotizing Fasciitis

Necrotizing fasciitis is a severe, deep, necrotizing soft tissue infection, which at a minimum involves subcutaneous tissues and fascial sheaths and often extends to underlying muscle. This process spreads relentlessly along fascial planes, producing edema, vascular thrombosis, and ever-widening necrosis, resulting in extensive soft tissue destruction. Deep surgical and traumatic wounds are major predisposing factors, although injection sites, cutaneous ulcers, abscesses, and omphalitis may serve as the initiating condition. Diabetics with vascular disease are at especially increased risk. The extremities, perineum, buttocks, trunk, and abdominal wall are the most common sites of involvement. Causative organisms include virulent strains of group A β-hemolytic streptococci; *S. aureus*; *P. aeruginosa*; *E. coli*; and mixtures of aerobes, anaerobes, and facultative gram-negative rods.

Moderate to severe systemic symptoms are prominent clinically and, along with fever, usually precede the appearance of cellulitic changes. The local area of inflammation may initially resemble ordinary cellulitis, with nonraised, indistinct margins and localized subcutaneous edema with overlying erythema. However, on careful palpation, it is often possible to appreciate that the edema and induration are deeper and far more extensive than the overlying erythema, and that the induration is unusually firm in consistency. Pain is remarkably severe early on, and often out of proportion to the visible findings. Lesions are exquisitely tender. With progression, the overlying skin itself may become edematous, simulating erysipelas. It will rapidly turn to a patchy grayish-blue, often with surface bullae filled with hemorrhagic fluid. At this point, numbness and decreased sensitivity to pain may be noted centrally. With further evolution, central necrosis or cutaneous gangrene supervenes (Fig. 12-39, *A-C*). If anaerobes are involved,

Figure 12-39 Necrotizing fasciitis. **A,** The extent of cellulitis and tissue necrosis is evident in this child who is recovering from necrotizing fasciitis caused by group A streptococci. On presentation he was thought to have cellulitis but was more ill systemically and appeared much more uncomfortable than would be expected. Furthermore, on presentation the area of induration extended well beyond the overlying erythema. **B,** Necrotizing fasciitis due to *Clostridium septicum* following surgical debridement in a child with presumed cyclic neutropenia. **C,** The same child 1 month later after aggressive surgical and medical management. (**A,** *Courtesy Michael Sherlock, MD, Lutherville, Md.)*

crepitus may become evident clinically or subcutaneous emphysema may be visible on radiographs.

As the localized process evolves, systemic symptoms increase. Signs of poor perfusion, pallor, and mottling are often accompanied by grunting respirations and alterations in level of consciousness including disorientation, obtundation, and seizures. Common laboratory findings in advanced cases include anemia resulting from hemolysis and marrow suppression, proteinuria, hypoproteinemia, hypocalcemia resulting from saponification of necrotic fat, and hyponatremia. Blood and wound cultures are routinely positive.

Mortality ranges from 8% to 70%, depending on the series reported, and morbidity and disfigurement are common in survivors. Delays in diagnosis and inadequate surgical debridement are major factors in cases with poor outcome. Hence early recognition is crucial to ensure appropriate intervention and improve prognosis. This can be particularly difficult in patients with cases resembling ordinary cellulitis that initially abate in response to antimicrobial therapy before worsening. Necrotizing fasciitis should be suspected in any patient with cellulitis (particularly around a deep wound) or omphalitis who has unusually severe pain and systemic symptoms that are out of proportion to local findings. This can enable surgical exploration before advanced skin changes and losses of sensation appear, signaling that necrosis is already extensive. If such changes are present, this process must be presumed. In all cases, findings on examination of frozen sections of biopsy material may confirm the diagnosis. Incision and passage of a probe can also be helpful. If the probe passes easily along fascial planes, the diagnosis is confirmed. Control necessitates wide excision with extensive exposure and debridement of all necrotic tissues in combination with broad-spectrum antimicrobial therapy (guided in part by Gram stain results). Aggressive supportive measures are important as well.

Meningococcal Exanthems

Neisseria meningitidis is capable of producing several clinical illnesses, two of which—acute meningococcemia and chronic meningococcemia (or meningococcosis)—are characterized in part by a generalized exanthem. The organism is carried in the upper respiratory tract of asymptomatic humans who may transmit the organism via droplet spread of respiratory secretions to close contacts. Most people become colonized without clinical disease. Clinical illness is most common in children younger than 5 years of age, with a peak incidence between 6 and 12 months. A secondary peak of lesser magnitude is seen during adolescence and young adulthood. Susceptibility to disease appears to be related to a lack of bactericidal antibody or to a failure to produce antibody in response to infection. Antecedent viral respiratory tract infection can be a predisposing factor.

Although meningococcal infection occurs year-round, the peak season for these illnesses is late winter and early spring. Invasive disease occurs both endemically and epidemically. Persons who have intimate contact with infected patients, such as other members of the same household or persons in "closed communities" such as military barracks, dormitories, or daycare centers, are at highest risk of becoming secondarily infected; and they should receive antimicrobial prophylaxis. The incubation period after exposure ranges from 1 to 10 days, with most clinical cases developing in less than 4 days. Secondary attack rates are highest during epidemic outbreaks. Any mucosal surface is subject to infection, which may remain localized or may serve as the source of invasive disease.

Meningococcal Meningitis and Acute Meningococcemia

The two major invasive forms of meningococcal disease are meningitis and septicemia, which may occur singly or in combination. Patients usually experience a prodromal period

ranging from a few hours to 5 days. During this phase, symptoms of upper respiratory tract infection or nasopharyngitis in association with fever are typical. Patients may also experience lethargy, headache, myalgias, arthralgias, and vomiting. After this, an abrupt change occurs, characterized by increased fever with chills (or occasionally hypothermia), worsening malaise, and progressive lethargy. In the 90% in whom meningitis is the primary manifestation, vomiting, irritability (often with a high-pitched cry in infants), and nuchal rigidity are prominent (Fig. 12-40, *A*). Infants may also have a bulging fontanelle (Fig. 12-40, *B*). Delirium, combativeness, stupor, and seizures may develop in some cases. Although some patients with meningitis also have meningococcemia, cutaneous manifestations, endotoxic shock, and disseminated intravascular coagulation (DIC) are less likely to develop in them than in those without meningeal infection, and mortality is relatively low.

In contrast, approximately 10% of patients show a picture of overwhelming sepsis with little or no laboratory evidence of meningitis. In these patients the abrupt change in the clinical picture just described typically heralds the development of a rash in association with manifestations of shock including mottling, distal coolness with decreased capillary refill or cyanosis, and either widened pulse pressure or frank hypotension. Up to 85% of these patients have cutaneous lesions involving the trunk and extremities. Such lesions may consist of tender pink macules; petechiae, which may be palpably raised; and purpura, which when present is most prominent on the extremities and may progress to form areas of frank necrosis (Fig. 12-41). The combination of purpura and shock is termed *Waterhouse-Friderichsen syndrome* and has been associated in some but not all instances with adrenal hemorrhage and secondary adrenal insufficiency. Evolution may be

Figure 12-40   Meningitis. **A,** Nuchal rigidity and a positive Brudzinski sign are demonstrated. On attempted passive flexion of the neck, the infant grimaces with pain, neck stiffness limits flexion, and the knees and hips are flexed to reduce traction on the meninges. **B,** This infant was also found to have a bulging anterior fontanelle when sitting quietly, reflecting increased intracranial pressure.

Figure 12-41 Meningococcemia. **A,** This youngster manifests the purpuric and petechial rash characteristic of acute meningococcemia. **B,** Petechiae are more apparent in this close-up of an infant. Gram stain of petechial scrapings may reveal organisms. **C** and **D,** Purpura may progress to form areas of frank cutaneous necrosis, especially in patients with disseminated intravascular coagulation (DIC). (**D,** *Courtesy Kenneth Schuitt, MD.*)

fulminant. The prognosis in patients with a short prodrome, fulminant progression, and early appearance of purpuric lesions is particularly poor. More than 60% of such patients have clinical evidence of hypotension and DIC on presentation, and approximately 50% have no leukocytosis or leukopenia, indicating that their immune system has been overwhelmed. Only about 20% of these patients have meningitis. Mortality in such patients approaches 40%, whereas only 3% of those showing slower progression die. Most deaths occur within 24 hours of presentation.

In many cases the diagnosis can be suspected clinically and is confirmed by laboratory findings. Gram-stained smears of petechial lesions and buffy coat preparations often reveal gram-negative diplococci. Cultures of blood, cerebrospinal fluid (CSF), and petechial lesions should be performed unless the severity of illness precludes lumbar puncture. Because of the potential for deterioration, aggressive empiric antimicrobial therapy and vigorous supportive measures should be instituted promptly whenever meningococcemia is suspected.

Among numerous differential diagnostic possibilities are other forms of bacterial sepsis, bacterial endocarditis, Rocky Mountain spotted fever, and various other disorders characterized by thrombocytopenia. Some forms of septicemia caused by gram-negative bacilli initially may be clinically indistinguishable from meningococcal septicemia. Similarly, *Haemophilus influenzae* type B and pneumococcal septicemia may be associated with the development of petechiae, although

in these cases they are not usually palpable. The purpuric lesions of staphylococcal sepsis tend to become pustular early on, and the site of primary infection also helps distinguish infection with this organism. Adenoviral and streptococcal infections may produce petechial rashes but usually do not cause a septic picture. Other clinical characteristics help to identify patients with thrombocytopenia resulting from immune thrombocytopenic purpura, acute leukemia, and mononucleosis; the centripetal mode of spread of the petechial rash of Rocky Mountain spotted fever and the initial distribution and subsequent mode of spread of the lesions of Henoch-Schönlein purpura help to distinguish these illnesses. Differentiation can be particularly difficult in the case of a child presenting with high fever with no source other than that of an upper respiratory tract infection and a petechial rash. These findings may represent early nonfulminant meningococcemia, but they also can be part of the picture of viral illness or another bacterial process; in such cases observation or presumptive therapy may be necessary.

Meningococcosis (Chronic Meningococcemia)

Meningococcosis, a disorder more indolent than acute meningococcemia, is defined as a meningococcal sepsis with a fever of greater than 1 week's duration, without meningitis. On average, symptoms are present for 6 to 8 weeks before diagnosis. In most cases symptoms are intermittent; in all cases they consist of fever and chills (without rigor) and are associated with an exanthem in nearly 95% of cases. The rash waxes and wanes, often in association with the fever. Lesions may consist of tender erythematous, subcutaneous nodules; erythematous macules and papules; or petechiae, occurring singly or in combination. Urticarial lesions are seen occasionally. The feet, legs, upper arms, and trunk are the sites most commonly involved. Mild malaise and myalgias tend to accompany the fever and headache, and arthralgias are also common. In childhood cases swelling of hands, feet, knees, and ankles may occur intermittently, without evidence of warmth or erythema; however, when the legs are involved, the child may refuse to walk.

The diagnosis of meningococcosis can be difficult because early blood cultures are often negative (although children are more likely than adults to have positive cultures) and skin lesions are generally negative for organisms, both on smear and culture. Throat culture is usually negative as well. Leukocytosis is seen with the fever. The sedimentation rate may be normal or elevated. Thrombocytopenia is seen occasionally. Close follow-up monitoring of the clinical course, combined with repeated blood cultures, constitutes the best way to confirm the diagnosis. Of the patients whose infection goes undiagnosed and untreated, approximately one third ultimately suffer severe localized infection (after an average of 10 weeks of illness), with meningitis, carditis, nephritis, and ocular infection occurring most commonly.

SPIROCHETAL RASHES

Lyme Disease

Lyme disease is a multisystem, tick-borne infection caused by the spirochete *Borrelia burgdorferi*. Named for the southeastern Connecticut community where it was first discovered more than 2 decades ago, Lyme disease was originally identified as a cause of chronic arthritis. Subsequent investigation has established the multisystem nature of the illness, which primarily involves the skin, heart, nervous system, and joints.

Transmission of Lyme disease occurs when a person is bitten by an infected *Ixodes* species of tick (deer tick). *Ixodes scapularis* (formerly *Ixodes dammini*) is the most common vector and is found predominantly in the Northeast and Midwestern United States. *Ixodes pacificus* is responsible for transmission in the Western states but is not as commonly infected with *B. burgdorferi*. When not engorged, the tick is about the size of a pinhead. Although the preferred host of *I. scapularis,* and its major reservoir for infection, is the white-footed mouse during the tick's nymph and larval stages, a number of feral animals may harbor *Borrelia*. Most cases occur between spring and fall when the nymph stage of deer ticks is active and people are more likely to be outdoors.

After an incubation period of 3 to 31 days, the distinctive exanthem of Lyme disease, known as erythema migrans, appears in approximately 50% of cases. The rash begins as a red papule or macule at the site of the tick bite and often goes unrecognized. The lesion gradually enlarges (to a median size of 15 cm), forming a large plaque, which tends to clear centrally, giving it an annular configuration (Fig. 12-42).

On occasion, instead of clearing, the central portion develops a bluish discoloration or becomes indurated or vesicular. The exanthem may be warm to the touch, and some patients report mild pruritus, burning, or prickling sensations. Multiple secondary annular lesions or evanescent red blotches, which are smaller than the primary lesion, develop in about 25% of all patients with erythema migrans, representing early disseminated disease (Fig. 12-42, *D*).

Although erythema migrans may be the sole manifestation of early Lyme disease, the exanthem is often accompanied by a flulike constellation of systemic symptoms that are probably the result of early hematogenous dissemination of the causative organism. These symptoms include fever (usually low grade), malaise and fatigue, headache sometimes accompanied by mild meningismus, and myalgias and arthralgias. On occasion, nausea, vomiting, conjunctivitis, pharyngitis, and either regional adenopathy in association with the erythema migrans lesion or generalized adenopathy are seen. Untreated, the erythema migrans lesion gradually resolves over 3 weeks and systemic symptoms often wax and wane over the course of several weeks. With treatment, the rash clears within several days and the systemic symptoms tend to resolve.

Other, less common manifestations of early disseminated disease involve the nervous system and heart. Aseptic meningitis sometimes accompanied by focal neurologic signs and symptoms and unilateral or bilateral facial nerve palsy with or without CSF pleocytosis are the neurologic manifestations seen most often in pediatric patients. Optic neuritis, iritis, and keratitis are unusual. Carditis, characterized by varying degrees of atrioventricular block or myopericarditis, is rare in children.

The arthritis of Lyme disease is a late manifestation, seen in up to 50% of untreated patients. It is pauciarticular, involving large joints, especially the knee. Pain, warmth, and swelling are typical, but overlying erythema is unusual. The initial episode usually lasts about 1 week but can be prolonged. Thereafter, numerous recurrences may be experienced. Rarely, after 1 year, a chronic erosive arthritis may develop. Late neurologic manifestations include encephalitis, encephalopathy, ataxia, radiculoneuritis, and myelitis. The features of this later phase of Lyme disease are probably the result of a combination of ongoing infection and compromise of the patient's immune response.

In patients with erythema migrans, the diagnosis can be made solely on clinical and epidemiologic grounds, even in the absence of a clear history of tick bite. Results of serologic studies generally are not helpful in making a diagnosis during the early stages of the illness. Such studies can be valuable, however, for diagnosing the disease in patients with neurologic, cardiac, or joint manifestations, especially in those with no prior history of a tick bite or erythema migrans. In patients with neurologic complications, both CSF and serum specimens should be submitted for analysis. The interpretation of commercial serologic testing should follow CDC (Centers for Disease Control and Prevention) guidelines for diagnosis of Lyme disease.

Although antimicrobial treatment can be helpful in both early and late stages of the disease, therapy should be initiated as early as possible because it not only hastens resolution of early symptoms but also prevents later complications of the disease.

Rocky Mountain Spotted Fever

Rocky Mountain spotted fever is an acute, potentially life-threatening disease caused by *Rickettsia rickettsii*. These obligate intracellular parasites are transmitted to humans by the bite of an infected tick. Once infected, organisms multiply in host endothelium of small blood vessels and spread hematogenously, resulting in a widespread vasculitis characterized by inflammation and thrombosis with secondary vascular leakage. Because ticks are active during warm months, the peak seasons for this disorder are spring and summer. The incubation period ranges from 2 to 14 days, with an average of 4 to 8 days. Two thirds of cases occur in children younger than 15 years of age. Yearly outbreaks tend to occur in circumscribed geographic areas. Mortality is as high as 5% to 7% and often stems from failure to diagnose and treat the condition in its early phase.

Figure 12-42 Erythema migrans/Lyme disease. **A,** This 2- to 3-cm lesion is just starting to clear centrally. **B,** This larger lesion has formed concentric circles around a central papule. **C,** Central clearing is nearly complete, and within the erythematous border the puncta of two tick bites are evident. **D,** Multiple annular lesions of differing sizes and varying degrees of central clearing are seen in this child with Lyme disease. (*A, Courtesy Sylvia Suarez, MD, Centerville, Va. B, Courtesy Caroline and David Eddy. C, Courtesy Ellen Wald, MD, University of Wisconsin Children's Hospital, Madison, Wis. D, Courtesy J. Carlton Gartner Jr., MD, Alfred I. DuPont Hospital, Wilmington, Del.*)

Onset may be acute or gradual and is characterized by fever and headache. The headache, which may be frontal or generalized, is typically severe, unremitting, and unresponsive to analgesia. Headache may not be a major complaint in very young children, however. Other, less constant symptoms include chills, anorexia, nausea and vomiting, sore throat, abdominal pain, diarrhea, arthralgias, and myalgias. Respiratory symptoms are uncommon. The spleen is enlarged in 30% to 50% of patients, but adenopathy is not prominent. The exanthem is usually noted on or about the third day of illness, but it may appear as late as the beginning of the second week.

In most patients the characteristic appearance and mode of spread of the exanthem are the most helpful clues to clinical diagnosis. The rash begins distally on the wrists, ankles, palms, and soles, usually appearing as an erythematous, blanching, discrete macular or maculopapular eruption. It then spreads centripetally and becomes petechial (Fig. 12-43), although on occasion lesions are petechial from the outset. In some cases the eruption is not prominent and may even be transient, making diagnosis difficult. Conjunctival injection, with photophobia and petechial hemorrhages, often develops simultaneously with the rash. Firm, nonpitting, nondependent edema, beginning in the periorbital region and then generalizing, tends to occur a few days after the onset of symptoms. In severe cases CNS symptoms develop with disease progression and range in severity from restlessness, irritability, and anxiety to confusion, delirium, and coma, with or without seizures and focal neurologic signs. Myocarditis, DIC, renal failure, and cardiovascular collapse are features of advanced disease.

White blood cell counts are normal or low in the first few days and then tend to rise. Thrombocytopenia is common. Other laboratory abnormalities include hyponatremia due to fluid shifts and renal losses, hypoproteinemia resulting from vascular and renal losses and hepatic dysfunction, abnormal liver function tests, and hyperkalemia with increasing cell death.

Because there is no diagnostic test capable of providing prompt definitive results, and because the early institution of antimicrobial treatment is crucial to a favorable outcome, the diagnosis of Rocky Mountain spotted fever must be made on clinical grounds and as early as possible. The diagnosis should be suspected in any child with fever, headache, toxicity, and a centripetally spreading petechial rash, especially when the patient's history suggests or confirms an exposure to ticks in an endemic area. Because of the potentially life-threatening nature of this infection, doxycycline is recommended as the drug of choice regardless of age (despite its usual contraindication in children younger than 8 years). Recovery is the rule if therapy is begun during the first week of illness. If treatment is delayed beyond the first week, however, the outcome may be unfavorable despite the institution of antimicrobial therapy

Figure 12-43   Rocky Mountain spotted fever. **A,** The exanthem characteristic of this disease first appears distally on wrists, ankles, palms, and soles. It may be petechial from the outset, or it may start as an erythematous, blanching, macular, or maculopapular eruption, which then becomes petechial as it spreads centripetally. **B,** In this child the rash has become generalized. Both petechial and blanching erythematous lesions are present. (**A,** *Courtesy Ellen Wald, MD, University of Wisconsin Children's Hospital, Madison, Wis.*)

and vigorous supportive measures. Subsequent serologic confirmation may be made by complement fixation tests or a variety of other assays.

INFECTIOUS LYMPHADENITIS AND ADENOPATHY

Lymph nodes respond to both systemic and local infections with increased cellular multiplication and activity, clinically manifested as enlargement and tenderness. Most often the enlargement is modest and, if biopsied, nonspecific histologic hyperplasia is found. This is termed *reactive adenopathy* and usually resolves without a specific etiology being identified. Nodes usually are 2 cm or less in diameter, and they are discrete, slightly firm or rubbery, and mobile. Discomfort and tenderness are mild. However, in some cases enlargement is marked, inflammation is pronounced, and a specific etiology can be identified on biopsy, a phenomenon termed *adenitis*. If the lymph node itself is infected and not just reacting to distal infection or inflammation, it can be filled with bacteria, neutrophils, and necrotic debris. Nodes usually exceed 2 to 3 cm in diameter, and overlying soft tissues may become edematous, making it difficult to distinguish exact margins. With progression, the overlying skin often becomes erythematous and may become adherent, reducing mobility. Discomfort and tenderness can be severe. Depending on the causative organism, suppuration may occur.

Adenopathy may be generalized or regional, but bacterial adenitis tends to be more localized. Whereas most adenitis is infectious in origin, adenopathy may also be a feature of collagen vascular or neoplastic disease. Malignant nodes are usually firm or hard in consistency but are occasionally rubbery. They are more frequently matted and often appear fixed or poorly mobile. Tenderness is unusual. Depending on the type of malignancy, the adenopathy may be isolated to one region or it may be generalized and associated with hepatosplenomegaly and with systemic symptoms of anorexia, fatigue, weight loss, night sweats, and bone pain. Many of the infectious diseases associated with generalized or cervical adenopathy have been discussed earlier in this chapter. Some

of the distinguishing features of the adenopathy characteristic of these disorders are given in Table 12-1. Neoplastic diseases are discussed in Chapter 11.

In this section we concentrate on the manifestations and causes of focal lymphadenitis. Almost any organism capable of infecting tissue can produce adenitis; hence the number of potential pathogens is large. Assessment is assisted by knowledge of the patterns of lymphatic drainage, the differential diagnostic possibilities of an inflammatory mass in a given region, and the varying clinical characteristics of adenitis produced by individual organisms.

As infection of a lymph node is a secondary phenomenon after drainage of primary infection to a regional node, identification of the primary source will narrow the list of causative organisms. In many instances, close examination of those areas in which lymphatics drain to the affected region reveals the site of inoculation. In all cases, careful history taking concerning prior distal wounds or inflammation and any possible environmental exposures may disclose the identity of the probable pathogen. This can be important for fastidious organisms resulting from unusual exposures.

Superficial Regional Lymph Nodes

Cervical Lymph Nodes

The cervical nodes, being numerous and draining multiple structures, are particularly common sites of acute adenitis (Fig. 12-44). In addition to the upper respiratory tract, the skin of the face, the scalp, conjunctivae, teeth, gingivae, ears, and neck all may serve as primary sites of infection. Nasal and oropharyngeal infections drain to the tonsillar and anterior cervical nodes (Fig. 12-45). Superficial facial infections and facial cellulitis may drain to the anterior cervical chain or to the preauricular or submental nodes. The occipital, posterior cervical, preauricular, and postauricular nodes receive lymphatic drainage from nearby portions of the scalp and thus may become inflamed and enlarged in connection with secondary infection of seborrhea, impetigo, wound infections, tinea capitis, or head lice infestation (Fig. 12-46). Conjunctival infections may result in adenitis of the preauricular node. The

Disorder	Site(s) of Adenopathy	Character of Nodes	Other Features	Laboratory Findings
EBV mononucleosis	Anterior and posterior cervical or generalized	Soft to firm, discrete, mildly to moderately tender	Pharyngitis; splenomegaly (50%); rash (15%); fever, malaise, fatigue	Atypical lymphocytosis; positive Monospot (80% > 4 yr); positive EBV titers; may have abnormal LFTs
CMV infection	Generalized or cervical	Soft to firm, discrete, mildly tender	Fever, malaise, fatigue; occasionally hepatosplenomegaly	Atypical lymphocytosis; abnormal LFTs; urine positive for CMV on culture; CMV titers
Toxoplasmosis	Generalized or cervical	Smooth, firm, mildly tender	Myalgias, fatigue, coryza; occasionally splenomegaly and maculopapular rash	Atypical lymphocytosis (frequent); positive *Toxoplasma* titers
Brucellosis	Generalized or cervical and axillary	Discrete, may be mildly tender or nontender	History of contact with sick farm animal or ingestion of raw milk; afternoon fever and chills; sweats, malaise, headache and backache, arthralgia; splenomegaly; lasts weeks and may become chronic with metastatic abscesses	Normal or decreased WBC count with lymphocytosis; positive cultures and serologic tests
Rubella	Anterior and posterior cervical	Soft to mildly firm, discrete, mildly tender or nontender	Fine, discrete maculopapular rash; Forschheimer spots on palate	Positive rubella titer
Streptococcal pharyngitis	Anterior cervical	Soft to mildly firm, discrete, tender	Pharyngitis or nasopharyngitis; headache, malaise; abdominal pain; may have palatal petechiae and/or scarlatiniform rash	Positive throat culture for group A β-hemolytic streptococci
Herpes simplex	Anterior cervical and submandibular	Soft to mildly firm, discrete, mobile, tender	Gingival erythema, edema, and friability with discrete mucosal ulcers; high fever	Positive viral culture (diagnosis usually made on clinical grounds)
Coxsackievirus herpangina	Anterior cervical	Soft to mildly firm, discrete, mobile, slightly tender	Discrete ulcers on labial mucosa, gingiva, tongue, and tonsillar pillars; may have vesicles on palms and soles	Positive viral culture (diagnosis usually made on clinical grounds)
Adenovirus	Anterior cervical and preauricular	Soft to mildly firm, discrete, mobile, mildly tender	Nonspecific pharyngeal inflammation, occasionally with exudate; may have conjunctivitis	Positive viral culture

CMV, cytomegalovirus; EBV, Epstein-Barr virus; LFTs, liver function tests; WBC, white blood cell.

Figure 12-45   Cervical adenopathy. Bilateral enlargement of the tonsillar nodes in this child was associated with viral pharyngitis.

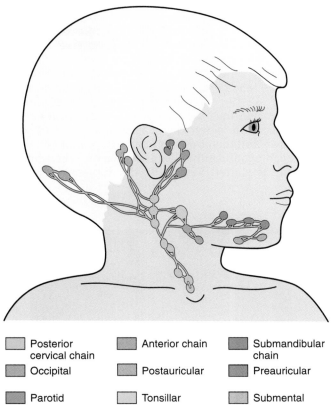

☐ Posterior cervical chain	☐ Anterior chain	☐ Submandibular chain
☐ Occipital	☐ Postauricular	☐ Preauricular
☐ Parotid	☐ Tonsillar	☐ Submental

Figure 12-44   The superficial cervical lymph nodes.

Figure 12-46   Acute postauricular lymphadenitis. This child had folliculitic and crusted scalp lesions and a tender 1.5-cm postauricular node with overlying erythema. The initial suspicion of bacterial infection was not confirmed. A potassium hydroxide preparation and fungal culture identified tinea capitis as the primary process.

teeth, gingivae, and tongue are drained by lymphatics coursing to the submental and submandibular nodes, which can be secondarily involved in cases of dental abscess, gingivitis, and stomatitis. Infections of the external auditory canal and the auricle may drain to the preauricular or postauricular nodes, whereas those involving the neck may affect the anterior or posterior cervical chain.

Although the number of potential causative organisms is high, an individual pathogen can often be implicated by thorough history and physical examination. Differentiation must also be made from other masses that may be present in the cervical region, many of which are congenital and subject to secondary infection, simulating adenitis.

Axillary and Epitrochlear Lymph Nodes

Several anatomic regions drain to the axilla. Those in the anterior pectoral portion drain the breast and chest wall, those in the lateral or midportion receive drainage from the hand and arm (see Fig. 12-51, *C*), and those in the posterior subscapular region drain portions of the back. The epitrochlear node receives lymphatic vessels from the fingers, hand, and skin of the forearm, but it is a much less common site of adenitis than are the axillary nodes. Wound and skin infections, cellulitis, and herpes zoster are major sources of axillary adenitis in childhood.

Inguinal Lymph Nodes

The inguinal lymph nodes are divided into two groups by the Poupart ligament, with those above the ligament called *inguinal* nodes and those below it termed *femoral* nodes (Fig. 12-47; and see Fig. 12-49). The inguinal group receives lymphatics from the external genitalia, anus, umbilicus, lower abdomen and back, buttocks, and upper thigh and may also drain the lower leg. Thus in addition to wound and skin infections, perianal, intraabdominal, and genital infections may serve as sources of inguinal adenitis. The femoral nodes primarily drain the foot and lower leg. The popliteal nodes receive drainage from the foot and lower leg but, like the epitrochlear nodes, are unusual sites of adenitis.

Having contrasted the general features of acute lymphadenitis with those of adenopathy, as well as having discussed the regions of involvement and their likely sources, we now can look at the characteristics of adenitis produced by the various causative organisms.

Figure 12-47   Subacute lymphadenitis of a right inguinal node and left femoral node resulted in dramatic swelling in this toddler. Atypical mycobacteria were found to be causative.

Acute Suppurative Lymphadenitis

Group A β-hemolytic streptococci and *S. aureus* are responsible for causing most cases of acute lymphadenitis. Together they account for up to 80% of cases of cervical adenitis alone. In recent years, staphylococcal infections have surpassed streptococcal infections in frequency. Other than culture of a specimen obtained by needle aspiration, there is no way to distinguish between the two clinically, as the clinical picture for both consists of sudden, painful, and rapid enlargement, usually of a single node. The involved node is firm and exquisitely tender (Fig. 12-48). Within 24 to 72 hours the overlying soft tissue becomes edematous and the skin erythematous. As many as 50% of patients may be febrile, and some appear toxic; bacteremia develops in a small percentage. Left untreated, suppuration occurs during the next several days and is detectable as central fluctuance. Simultaneously, thinning of the overlying skin, which also appears shiny, may be noted as the process points toward the surface (Fig. 12-49). On occasion, the abscess may point inward, rupturing into the soft tissues and dissecting along tissue planes with potentially catastrophic effects. Prompt institution of antimicrobial therapy that empirically covers *S. aureus* can significantly alter this course. When high-dose oral therapy is started before the development of overlying

Figure 12-48   Acute suppurative lymphadenitis. **A,** This youngster was seen within 24 hours of the onset of painful enlargement of the left tonsillar node. Mild overlying edema existed, and the node was markedly tender. **B** and **C,** This boy had massive enlargement of the tonsillar node with overlying edema and mild erythema. The node was exquisitely tender, but there was no evidence of fluctuance. Group A β-hemolytic streptococci grew from his throat culture. The absence of preauricular and postauricular swelling helps to differentiate adenitis of the tonsillar node from parotitis. (**A,** *Courtesy Michael Sherlock, MD, Lutherville, Md.*)

Figure 12-49 Acute suppurative lymphadenitis. Increased pain and erythema, thinning of the overlying skin, and fluctuance on palpation signal that central necrosis has occurred. *(Courtesy Michael Sherlock, MD, Lutherville, Md.)*

cellulitic changes, such changes may be prevented and enlargement halted, followed by regression. Even in patients with swelling and erythema at the start of therapy, the infection may not progress to suppuration. Patients with high fever and toxicity require parenteral treatment, as do children who fail to improve on oral medication. Suppuration necessitates incision and drainage.

Cervical nodes, especially the tonsillar and anterior cervical nodes, are the most common sites of adenitis caused by streptococci or staphylococci. Patients are usually young children, with a peak incidence between 1 and 4 years of age. Many have an antecedent history of rhinitis, often associated with impetiginization of the anterior nares along with anterior cervical adenopathy. Cough, anorexia, vomiting, and fever can be associated findings that may persist or clear before the onset of adenitis. In older children a recent episode of pharyngitis may be reported, and in a small percentage adenitis develops in association with a peritonsillar abscess (see Chapter 23).

Secondarily infected dermatitis, insect bites, impetigo, and wound infections may precede the onset of adenitis in other patients, in which case the node affected depends on the primary site. These infections, as well as cellulitis, are common antecedents of axillary and inguinal adenitis caused by streptococci and staphylococci. Primary sources may be evident at the time adenitis develops, but often have already healed. Although severe tinea capitis may mimic streptococcal and staphylococcal infection in the appearance of the primary lesion and in secondary adenitis, progression to suppuration is unusual. In these patients the occipital and/or postauricular nodes are most likely to be affected (see Fig. 12-46 and Chapter 8).

Although streptococci and staphylococci are the predominant pathogens causing acute lymphadenitis, on occasion anaerobic bacteria including *Actinomyces* are responsible. The vast majority of cases caused by anaerobes are secondary to dental disease including dental abscesses, gingivitis, and stomatitis; as a result, the submental or submandibular nodes are more likely to be affected. On occasion the adenitis appears simultaneously with facial cellulitis stemming from a dental abscess (see Chapter 20).

Actinomycotic adenitis, although unusual, has a distinctive clinical course. Enlargement of the affected node is gradual, and on palpation it is firm and lumpy, has an irregular border, and is mildly to moderately tender. Over time the center blackens and necroses, and a chronic draining sinus may form. Microscopic examination of the discharge discloses characteristic sulfur granules.

Mycobacterial Lymphadenitis

Mycobacterium tuberculosis and nontuberculous or atypical mycobacteria (especially *Mycobacterium avium-intracellulare*) continue to be important causes of lymphadenitis, both in developing and developed nations. Recognition of mycobacterial lymphadenitis is important because its management is considerably different from that for lymphadenitis caused by other bacteria. Both groups of mycobacteria cause similar clinical findings. Nodal enlargement is gradual and persistent. The node is slightly to mildly tender, and initially there is little or no sign of warmth or overlying inflammation (Fig. 12-50, *A*; see also Fig. 12-47). After a few weeks the node becomes adherent to the overlying skin, which in turn becomes thickened and tense, with overlying reddish or reddish purple discoloration (Fig. 12-50, *B* and *C*). Suppuration associated with thinning of the overlying skin may occur several weeks to months after onset and may result in rupture with the formation of a chronically draining sinus. The risk of chronic drainage may be increased if aspiration is attempted. Hence this procedure is not recommended. Although the local clinical findings are similar, there are historic and other differences that can help to distinguish tuberculous lymphadenitis from atypical mycobacterial lymphadenitis.

Tuberculous Lymphadenitis

Children with tuberculosis may be of any age and frequently have a positive history of exposure to an infected adult. Tonsillar and submandibular nodes are common sites of tuberculous lymphadenitis because of the lymphatic extension that occurs from the paratracheal nodes. Supraclavicular nodes are affected as the result of drainage from apical pulmonary lesions. The posterior cervical chain is another common area. Axillary, inguinal, and femoral nodes are more likely sites of enlargement if drainage is coming from a primary skin lesion. The ipsilateral preauricular node enlarges if the conjunctiva is the site of inoculation. Usually a group of nodes in one region is involved if lymphatic spread is the cause. If hematogenous dissemination is the source, involvement is frequently bilateral and may be generalized; in patients with protracted hematogenous dissemination, generalized adenopathy may be present with massive nodal enlargement. The latter usually have systemic symptoms (see the section Tuberculosis, later).

Initially, lymphoid hyperplasia develops as tubercles form, and then necrosis and caseation supervene. Early on, nodes are firm, discrete, and nontender, but with progression they tend to become matted and adherent to the overlying skin, which often becomes discolored, thickened, and scaly (Fig. 12-50, *A-C*). Without treatment, spontaneous drainage ultimately occurs, leaving a draining sinus (Fig. 12-50, *D*).

Chest radiographs reveal findings suggestive of tuberculosis in 75% of patients; the sedimentation rate exceeds 30 mm/hour in up to 80%; and the purified protein derivative (PPD) test is positive, usually with more than 15 mm of induration. Treatment of tuberculous adenitis is pharmacologic, with excision reserved for cases with chronic drainage (see the section Tuberculosis, later).

Adenitis Due to Atypical Mycobacteria

Patients with atypical mycobacterial adenitis are usually younger than 4 years of age and are unlikely to have a history of exposure to tuberculosis. A submandibular, submental, preauricular, anterior cervical, inguinal, or epitrochlear node may be the site of involvement (Fig. 12-50, *E*; and Fig. 12-47). Bilateral adenitis is unusual, generalized adenopathy does not occur, and systemic symptoms are rare. Chest radiographic findings rarely are abnormal; only one third of patients have elevated sedimentation rates; and the PPD test is usually

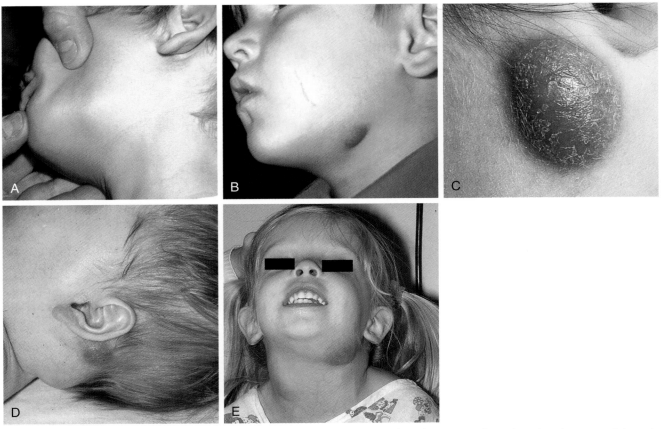

Figure 12-50   Mycobacterial adenitis. **A,** Early in the course of adenitis caused by *Mycobacterium tuberculosis* or atypical mycobacteria, enlargement of the node is gradual, tenderness is mild, and there is little or no sign of warmth or overlying inflammation. **B,** After several weeks the overlying skin becomes thickened, tense, discolored, and adherent to the node. **C,** This preauricular node was fluctuant, indicating suppuration. **D,** *M. tuberculosis* was isolated from the drainage of the postauricular node of this infant, who presented with lymphadenopathy and failure to thrive. **E,** Nontuberculous mycobacteria were isolated from the nodes of this youngster. (*A-C, Courtesy Michael Sherlock, MD, Lutherville, Md.*)

negative or of intermediate reactivity, with induration ranging from 5 to 10 mm. Atypical mycobacteria invariably are resistant to multiple drugs; hence excisional biopsy is generally the treatment of choice. Spontaneous regression does, however, occur over 12 to 24 months, making observation a reasonable course if suppuration or drainage has not occurred.

Adenitis Associated with Animal or Vector Contact

In many children, acute local lymphadenitis results from inoculation of a pathogen by means of an animal scratch or bite, from the bite of an insect vector transmitting a pathogen from an animal host, or from contact with a contaminated animal carcass. In some of these disorders, systemic symptoms are prominent; in others the local adenitis is the primary manifestation.

Pasteurella multocida Adenitis

Suppurative adenitis caused by *Pasteurella multocida* may occur in patients who develop local infection at the site of a scratch or bite inflicted by a dog or cat. Soon after, the manifestations of local infection appear at the primary site (usually within 24 hours), and a regional node enlarges and becomes tender. Overlying swelling and redness are common, and suppuration may occur early. This picture is clinically indistinguishable from that of adenitis due to streptococci or staphylococci, but often *P. multocida* infection can be suspected on

the basis of the history, especially the early onset of symptoms. Axillary and inguinal nodes are the most common sites of involvement.

Cat-Scratch Disease

Although low-grade fever may occur in about 25% of affected patients, adenitis is a primary feature of cat-scratch disease, which is due to a pleomorphic gram-negative bacillus that is seen on Warthin-Starry silver-stained sections of biopsied nodes. *Bartonella henselae* is the causative agent in most cases of cat-scratch disease. Ninety percent have a history of either an antecedent cat scratch or contact with cats, especially kittens. Although inoculation via a cat scratch is the most common means of infection, splinters, puncture wounds, and dog scratches have also been implicated. Incidence is highest in fall and winter in temperate climates, with cases occurring with equal frequency year-round in tropical areas. Most patients are in the 5- to 14-year age range, but family clusters that include younger children and adults have been reported.

Symptoms begin 3 to 30 days after inoculation, with 7 to 12 days being the most common interval. A red papule or series of papules is commonly noted at the site of inoculation (Fig. 12-51, *A* and *B*). Shortly thereafter, one or more regional nodes enlarge, becoming mildly painful and tender (Fig. 12-51, *A* and *C*). Involved nodes are firm, and overlying warmth and mild redness may develop within a few days of enlargement. In order of frequency, axillary, cervical, submandibular, preauricular, epitrochlear, and inguinal nodes have been reported as sites of involvement. In cases involving a

Figure 12-51 Cat-scratch disease. **A,** This boy presented with mildly painful "swollen glands." The left preauricular and tonsillar nodes were enlarged, firm, and mildly tender. An ulcerated papule, evident on his left cheek, was the site of a scratch inflicted by one of his kittens 2 weeks earlier. **B,** A line of papules is seen on the forearm of a 3-year-old at the site of a scratch inflicted by his new kitten 3 weeks before presentation. **C,** Marked enlargement of an ipsilateral axillary node had prompted his visit. The node was firm and only mildly tender. (**A,** Courtesy Kenneth Schuitt, MD.)

preauricular node, associated conjunctivitis is common and points toward conjunctival inoculation as the source. Discomfort generally subsides in 4 to 6 weeks, but the node may remain enlarged or may fluctuate in size for months. Suppuration occurs in about one third of patients.

Diagnosis is made primarily on the basis of history, clinical picture and course, and/or findings yielded by an excisional biopsy specimen. Granulomas with microabscesses are classically seen on histopathology. Warthin-Starry silver stain may reveal organisms suggestive of cat-scratch disease. Treatment is supportive. If lymph nodes are painful, suppurative aspiration can be performed and is preferable to incision and drainage because of concerns that the latter procedure may lead to prolonged drainage and scarring. In protracted or atypical cases, excisional biopsy is suggested. The benefit of antimicrobial treatment in an immunocompetent host remains controversial.

Tularemia

Francisella tularensis most often produces an ulceroglandular syndrome in children, occurring in concert with systemic symptoms. Rabbits, hares, muskrats, and voles serve as endemic sources of this pathogen. Children may acquire disease by handling or skinning dead animals, after an animal bite (especially that of a cat that hunts rabbits), or occasionally from the bite of an insect that serves as a vector for the pathogen. The incubation period ranges from 1 to 21 days. Onset is abrupt and characterized by fever, chills, headache, myalgias, vomiting, and possibly photophobia. Within 2 days, axillary, epitrochlear, or inguinal adenitis is noted, and soon thereafter a painful papule appears distal to the involved node at the site of inoculation. This ruptures in the ensuing day or two, forming a central ulcer with a raised edge. The involved regional node is firm and tender and may be associated with overlying erythema. Generalized adenopathy and hepatosplenomegaly may be noted in some patients, and in the second week of illness a blotchy, erythematous maculopapular rash (or occasionally a vesicular, pustular, or nodosa exanthem) may appear. Without treatment, fever may persist for 2 to 3 weeks and the ulcer may take as long as 1 month to heal. The diagnosis is suggested by history, clinical picture, and course and is confirmed by serologic tests. Streptomycin is the treatment of choice, but intravenous gentamicin is an acceptable alternative.

Bubonic Plague

Now rare in developed countries, bubonic plague, caused by *Yersinia pestis*, continues to sporadically afflict people who live or hunt in areas where infection is endemic in the wild rodent population. Bubonic plague is usually transmitted by flea bite, but on occasion inoculation occurs through a break in the skin as a result of handling an infected carcass. Thus inguinal and axillary nodes are the most common sites of bubo formation. The incubation period ranges from several hours to 10 days and ends with the abrupt onset of high fever, chills, malaise, weakness, and headache. Pain in the area of a regional node precedes rapid nodal enlargement. The node is fixed, firm, and exquisitely tender with overlying edema. Purplish discoloration is common, forming the classic bubo. The inoculation site may appear normal, or it may manifest as a skin abscess. Rapid progression of systemic symptoms occurs, with the patient appearing toxic and apprehensive and often delirious with signs of neurologic dysfunction. DIC and septic shock may supervene if treatment is not instituted promptly. If infection is suspected, the node should be aspirated to obtain material for culture, blood cultures should be performed, and broad-spectrum parenteral antibiotic therapy instituted.

General Approach to Diagnosis of Lymphadenitis

Because of the wide range of pathogens that can produce lymphadenitis, meticulous care must be taken during the clinical assessment. History taking should include questions concerning antecedent and current signs and symptoms, which may include prior wounds such as cuts, bites, punctures, splinters, or scratches distal to the inflamed node. Exposure to other ill persons or to animals, as well as recent travel, should be determined. Questions must also be asked about the presence or absence of systemic symptoms and about the rapidity of the evolution of the adenitis itself. A history of past problems and medication intake is important as well. Physical examination must include precise measurement of the size of the inflamed node, in addition to inspection of overlying soft tissue and palpation to determine contour, consistency, and degree of tenderness. The region drained by the involved node must be inspected for clues as to the probable primary source of infection. Last, close attention should be paid to the child's general status and to other portions of the reticuloendothelial system, such as to other nodal regions, as well as to the liver and spleen.

With the preceding information, the specific pathogen may be evident on clinical grounds alone or the differential diagnostic possibilities may be considerably narrowed, permitting confirmation using a minimum of laboratory tests. Close follow-up is important for all children treated as outpatients, to monitor their clinical course and response to therapy.

BACTERIAL BONE AND JOINT INFECTIONS

Osteomyelitis

The anatomy and physiology of growing bone place children at particular risk for bacterial infection; 85% of cases of osteomyelitis occur in children younger than 16 years of age. In most series the highest incidence has been found to occur in infancy, with a secondary peak between 8 and 12 years of age. Among infants, males and females are affected with equal frequency, but among older children, males predominate at a ratio of 2:1 to 3:1. The advent of antimicrobial therapy and advances in diagnostic techniques has significantly altered the course of the disease and the outcome. Mortality has decreased from 25% in the preantibiotic era to less than 1%; morbidity has declined from 50% to less than 10%.

Staphylococcus aureus is the most commonly identified pathogen in all age groups, followed by β-hemolytic group A streptococci. Gram-negative organisms account for a small percentage of cases. *Salmonella* species are of particular importance in children with sickle hemoglobinopathies, and *Pseudomonas* organisms are often isolated in cases resulting from puncture wounds of the foot. In 15% to 30% of cases no causative organism is identified, often as a result of suppression by prior antibiotic therapy.

An appreciation of the anatomic and physiologic features of bone in general and of growing bone in particular is essential to an understanding of the pathophysiology of osteomyelitis in children. Nutrient vessels enter the diaphysis from the periosteum and extend to the metaphysis (or, in flat and irregular bones, to the area adjacent to the epiphysis), where terminal arterioles form loops and empty into larger sinusoidal veins. This area is one of sluggish, somewhat turbulent blood flow, which is prone to thrombosis and which serves as an ideal site for bacterial deposition in the face of bacteremia. Because they are devoid of phagocytic macrophages, the sinusoidal veins lack defenses against infection. Once bacteria become established within bone, they stimulate an inflammatory response with the formation of exudate. As fluid collects, pressure increases, promoting extension outward and causing further vascular stasis and thrombophlebitis. The resultant ischemia causes local bone necrosis. With further progression, dead bone can form a sequestrum surrounded by purulent material, which becomes inaccessible to antimicrobial penetration.

In infants younger than 8 to 12 months of age, numerous additional factors facilitate extension of infection once it is present. Because the epiphyseal plate has not fully formed, the nutrient arterioles penetrate into the epiphysis; hence rupture of infection into the adjacent joint is common. The cortex of the infant's metaphysis is thin, and the trabeculae are fewer in number, assisting penetration outward to a more loosely attached periosteum, as well as extension toward the diaphysis. Thus infants are more likely to develop subperiosteal abscess, even with early diagnosis (Fig. 12-52). Once the epiphyseal growth plate has formed, it serves as a relatively effective barrier to joint extension, and the frequency of secondary septic arthritis is thereby substantially reduced, although sympathetic joint effusions are not uncommon. An exception to this is hematogenous osteomyelitis involving the proximal metaphysis of the humerus or femur and of the distal fibula, where the synovium of the adjacent joint inserts so as to include the metaphysis within the joint.

Bones become infected through two major mechanisms. Hematogenous spread accounts for most pediatric cases. Areas of rich blood supply and sluggish flow are most vulnerable to bacterial seeding; hence the metaphyseal portions of long bones and the subepiphyseal portions of flat and irregular bones are the usual sites of such involvement. Trauma may be a predisposing factor, by production of small-vessel occlusion with secondary stasis, anoxia, and necrosis. Children with sickle hemoglobinopathies are particularly susceptible to hematogenous osteomyelitis as a result of their vulnerability to bacteremia and sepsis and because of their underlying vascular sludging and infarction.

Figure 12-52   Acute hematogenous osteomyelitis in infancy. **A,** This 1-month-old presented decreased movement of the left arm and prominent swelling of the upper arm and shoulder. On x-ray examination her proximal humerus had a lytic appearance, and the T_2-weighted coronal magnetic resonance image (MRI) shows subperiosteal abscess and bone destruction. **B,** Swelling of the entire leg and foot with overlying erythremia is evident in this 2½-month-old infant, who had rapid extension of osteomyelitis of the tibia.

Spread from a contiguous focus of infection accounts for most remaining cases of osteomyelitis affecting children. Infections of fracture sites, surgical wounds, and puncture wounds, as well as extension of infection from an adjacent site of cellulitis or an abscess, serve as the predisposing conditions, with localization dependent on the original site of injury or infection.

Although important in adults, peripheral vascular disease is rarely a predisposing condition in children. If this does occur in a young person, the patient is usually an adolescent with long-standing diabetes mellitus, and the small bones of the hands or feet are the most common sites of involvement.

In addition to categorization by mode of spread or acquisition, osteomyelitis is further subdivided into acute, subacute, and chronic forms according to duration of symptoms. Of these, the acute form is the most common. The major clinical finding in each form is localized bone pain, which is typically constant, progressively more severe, and exacerbated by movement. Patients commonly report that the pain wakes them from sleep. The overlying soft tissues may appear normal or may be warm, mildly swollen, and occasionally erythematous, but in contrast to cellulitis, these surface findings are often subtle and induration is unusual. Spasm of overlying muscles is often intense, adding to discomfort and the adjacent joint may be held in flexion. Beyond these common features there is a wide range of clinical expression. Appreciation of this spectrum is important to ensure early diagnosis, thus resulting in a more favorable outcome.

Acute Osteomyelitis

Acute Hematogenous Osteomyelitis

In the acute hematogenous form of osteomyelitis, the mode of presentation and the clinical findings are age dependent, although most patients present within 1 week of onset of symptoms.

Infants younger than 6 months of age often present no systemic signs of infection. However, some may have fever and a few may show a frankly septic picture. Early on, irritability and anorexia are the major manifestations. Within a few days, evidence of pain on movement or of decreased use of a limb may be noted (pseudoparalysis). At this time or soon after, localized soft tissue swelling develops. This often extends rapidly to involve the entire extremity, reflecting rapid spread of infection in the underlying bone (Fig. 12-52, B). For the same reason, tenderness is also diffuse. Furthermore, multiple bones may be involved. Careful attention must be given to joint examination because of the high risk of early joint extension and secondary septic arthritis.

In children 8 months to 2 years of age, fever and signs of toxicity are common. A history of antecedent upper respiratory tract or skin infection is present in more than 50% of cases. Systemic symptoms consist primarily of fever and irritability in association with refusal to walk, a limp, or decreased use of an extremity. A small percentage present with more severe systemic symptoms including chills, lethargy, irritability, anorexia, vomiting, and dehydration. At this age children are often unable or unwilling to point to the site of discomfort, but by observation may be found to avoid moving the involved extremity or to hold a particular joint in flexion *consistently*. Soft tissue swelling and warmth may be noted overlying a metaphysis, but this is often subtle or absent in early cases and it is undetectable in cases in which the proximal femur is involved. Comparative circumferential measurements of suspected areas and painstaking care in first eliciting the child's cooperation, and then in palpating for evidence of muscle spasm or point tenderness, are crucial if osteomyelitis

Figure 12-53 Acute osteomyelitis. Fever, hip and thigh pain, and refusal to walk were the chief complaints in this 5-year-old child with osteomyelitis of the proximal femur. On inspection she lay still, holding the left leg externally rotated and flexed at the hip and knee. This same position is also adopted by children with acute arthritis of the hip.

is suspected. Even then, focal tenderness may be difficult to detect early in the course.

Children older than 2 years of age with acute osteomyelitis are sometimes febrile but rarely toxic. They are more likely to indicate a specific site of pain, and point tenderness is generally easy to elicit unless presentation is early. Older patients describe the pain as deep, intense, and constant. Signs of adjacent joint flexion and of nearby muscle spasm are common (Fig. 12-53), but again, overlying soft tissue swelling may be subtle. Unless a sympathetic effusion has developed, the adjacent joint may be passively moved through its full range of motion, although this exacerbates the pain.

If bones other than the long bones of the extremities are the site of infection, the clinical picture can be especially confusing. Osteomyelitis of the pelvic bones may mimic numerous other conditions. Although fever and an abnormal gait are the most common presenting complaints, lower abdominal and groin pain, hip or buttock pain, sciatica, and thigh pain (with swelling) can each be prominent early complaints in individual patients. Often the initial clinical picture is more suggestive of appendicitis, pelvic abscess, or infection of the femur than of pelvic osteomyelitis. To establish the diagnosis, a high level of suspicion and great care in examination are necessary. In patients presenting with abdominal complaints, the absence of rebound tenderness, lesser prominence of gastrointestinal symptoms, onset of pain in the lower abdomen rather than in the periumbilical region, and normal findings on rectal examination can help to distinguish the process from that of acute appendicitis. Furthermore, although most patients have pain on hip motion in one or more planes, range of motion is either normal or only slightly limited, and with careful examination, point tenderness can usually be detected.

Acute Osteomyelitis Due to Contiguous Spread

Acute osteomyelitis resulting from the contiguous spread of infection must be suspected in patients with prior puncture wounds, deep lacerations, surgical incisions, open fractures, abscesses, or cellulitis who experience a sudden onset of increased pain at the wound site. This pain is perceived as deep, severe, and constant and is aggravated by movement. In these cases soft tissue cellulitis is a common associated finding, and fever is usual. If extension of primary soft tissue infection is the source, the patient's condition often may have worsened clinically after a period of improvement in response to antimicrobial therapy or the patient may have failed to show the expected response to therapy.

Diagnostic Methods in Acute Osteomyelitis

Standard laboratory and radiographic studies are of somewhat limited use in the diagnosis of acute osteomyelitis. The sedimentation rate is elevated in the vast majority of patients with osteomyelitis, as well as C-reactive protein % (i.e., C-reactive protein expressed as a percentage of the average level). These markers are helpful primarily in confirming that an inflammatory process is the source of symptoms. White blood cell counts, although sometimes elevated, may be normal in up to 50% of patients and thus are less useful.

Plain radiographic changes lag behind the clinical manifestations and can be subtle. Initial films may be negative (Fig. 12-54, *C*). The first noticeable radiographic change, usually seen about 3 days after the onset of symptoms, is the presence of deep soft-tissue swelling (Fig. 12-54, *A*). In the ensuing days the swelling increases, obliterating fascial planes, and then extends to involve subcutaneous tissues. These soft tissue changes can be difficult to appreciate whenever osteomyelitis involves bones of the trunk or pelvis; however, in cases of pelvic osteomyelitis, clouding of the obturator foramen, distortion of the fascial planes around the adjacent hip, or even displacement of the bladder may be detectable. If a sympathetic joint effusion is present or if rupture into the adjacent joint has resulted in secondary septic arthritis, joint space widening or bony displacement may be evident (Fig. 12-54, *B*; and Fig. 12-52, *A*). Bone changes are not visible radiographically in untreated patients until 10 to 20 days after onset. These changes consist of periosteal elevation followed by focal evidence of bone lysis and, subsequently, by sclerosis or new bone formation at the margins of the lytic lesion (Fig. 12-54, *E*). The radiographic appearance of bone changes

Figure 12-54 Acute osteomyelitis. Radiographic changes lag behind the clinical manifestations in osteomyelitis. **A,** The first noticeable change, occurring about 3 days after onset, is deep soft tissue swelling, seen here adjacent to the metaphysis of the distal tibia on the left. **B,** In this neonate a radiolucency is evident in the proximal metaphysis of the right femur, which is also displaced upward and laterally. On aspiration of the hip, purulent fluid was obtained, confirming the suspicion of rupture of the infection into the hip and of secondary septic arthritis. **C,** This 1-year-old female presented with 4 days of fever and lack of right arm use. Her plain film is normal, but T₁ MRI with gadolinium contrast clearly shows extensive disease in disease **(D). E,** The late changes of a lytic lesion with sclerotic margins are seen in the right femoral metaphysis of this child who was completing his course of therapy. (**A,** *Courtesy Jocelyn Ledesma-Medina, MD;* **B** *and* **E,** *courtesy Rodrigo Dominguez, MD, University of Texas, Houston, Tex.*)

can be significantly delayed in patients who are being treated with an antibiotic for infection at another site, and early diagnosis of osteomyelitis and the institution of appropriate antimicrobial therapy may completely prevent development of these findings.

Technetium scanning provides improved identification and localization of sites of acute osteomyelitis. It can show abnormalities as early as 24 to 48 hours after the onset of symptoms, revealing discrete areas of increased uptake (Fig. 12-55, A-C). The procedure has been particularly useful as a diagnostic adjunct in cases of pelvic and vertebral osteomyelitis in which the mode of presentation simulates the clinical picture of another condition (see Fig. 12-58, C). It can also be helpful in distinguishing osteomyelitis from cellulitis, septic arthritis, and acute bony infarcts. In cellulitis, intense deep soft-tissue uptake with faint diffuse uptake in underlying bone is seen;

in septic arthritis the scan may be normal, or if the condition is accompanied by overlying cellulitis, the scan may show increased periarticular soft tissue uptake; in early infarcts, uptake is decreased. Technetium scans are also helpful in delineating additional areas of involvement in the small percentage of patients with multiple sites. Standard radiographs remain important in identifying fractures and malignancies, which may simulate the appearance of osteomyelitis on bone scans. Awareness that 5% to 20% of children with acute osteomyelitis can have a false-negative bone scan during the first few days is important. The routine use of magnetic resonance imaging (MRI) is increasing as a diagnostic tool in acute osteomyelitis. Findings of increased T$_2$ signal with marrow and surrounding tissue correlate well with the presence of osteomyelitis, and are present well before bony changes occur (Fig. 12-55, C; and Fig. 12-54, D). Imaging with MRI is most

RT ANT LT

Figure 12-55   Technetium scan findings in acute osteomyelitis. This 10-year-old female presented with 3 days of left ankle pain and fever. **A,** A normal plain film of the ankle. **B,** Technetium scan demonstrated increased uptake in the distal tibial metaphysis. **C,** Coronal T$_1$ MRI with contrast showed bone marrow involvement.

useful in resolving cases of pelvic osteomyelitis, where its resolution may help distinguish between joint disease, myositis, and true osteomyelitis. Acute osteomyelitis of the smaller bones comprising the hands and feet is a diagnosis that warrants MRI as the primary imaging modality.

Vigorous attempts must be made to isolate the causative organism in order to optimize therapy on the basis of known sensitivities and a determination of bactericidal levels. Aspiration of the site of maximal tenderness or maximal uptake as revealed by bone scan or MRI can be useful in that it provides material for Gram stain and culture. In cases in which purulent material is obtained, operative drainage should be considered strongly. Even in the absence of exudate, flushing the aspirating needle with culture medium often enables isolation of the causative organism. Blood cultures are positive in more than 50% of patients with acute hematogenous osteomyelitis and should be performed in all suspected cases. The presence of fever on presentation is a strong predictor of a positive blood culture.

Complications of osteomyelitis include secondary septic arthritis with resultant joint damage, epiphyseal injury with long-term morbidity resulting from impaired bone growth, progression to chronic osteomyelitis (now seen in less than 4% of cases), and rarely pathologic fractures. The rate of complications is highest in young infants who often have extensive bone involvement and secondary septic arthritis by the time the diagnosis is made. Care in clinical assessment and aggressive attempts to confirm the diagnosis of acute osteomyelitis as early as possible are as important in ensuring a good outcome and minimizing complications as are adequate antimicrobial therapy and recognition of the need for surgical intervention. Close collaboration between the pediatric physician and orthopedic surgeon is essential to ensure that optimal decisions are made regarding the route and duration of pharmacotherapy and the need for and timing of surgical intervention, if indicated.

Subacute Osteomyelitis

Approximately 10% of cases of hematogenous osteomyelitis have an insidious onset and a subacute course, often characterized by mild to moderate local pain in an extremity, with or without swelling. Fever is unusual, and other systemic symptoms are absent. Typically the patient has had symptoms for a few to several weeks before presentation. In some instances this subacute course appears to be related to partial suppression of the infection by antibiotics that have been administered for infection at another site (such as otitis media or impetigo). In these patients, pain may abate during the period of antimicrobial therapy, only to worsen once they stop taking the medication. On examination, local tenderness is evident and overlying soft tissue swelling may be noted. By the time diagnosis is made, multiple sites are involved in up to 20% of patients.

Although white blood cell counts are usually normal, sedimentation rate and C-reactive protein are elevated in most patients. Blood cultures are rarely positive. Radiographs may show one of several possible findings. In children seen within a few weeks of onset and who have taken antibiotics, radiographic findings may demonstrate early acute osteomyelitis. Other radiographic configurations include an isolated metaphyseal radiolucency surrounded by reactive bone (Brodie abscess); metaphyseal radiolucency with loss or disruption of cortical bone simulating a tumor; an excessive cortical reaction in the diaphysis simulating an osteoid osteoma; or multiple layers of subperiosteal new bone overlying the diaphysis, at times mimicking the appearance of Ewing sarcoma (Fig. 12-56). Although a bone scan is not of great use in distinguishing subacute osteomyelitis from a primary bone tumor,

MRI provides excellent resolution that may clarify the diagnosis. Because of the long course, clinical picture, and uncertain radiographic findings, biopsy is generally required to establish the diagnosis and isolate the causative organism. In the vast majority of cases, *S. aureus* is found. Surgical curettage, immobilization, and antimicrobials are the mainstays of treatment.

Chronic Osteomyelitis

With the advent of antimicrobial therapy and improvements in diagnostic techniques, chronic osteomyelitis has become much less common in developed nations. Delay in diagnosis, inadequate antimicrobial or surgical therapy, and unusually resistant organisms are the major factors now associated with chronic disease. Pathophysiologically, extensive necrosis, sequestrum formation, and decompression caused by fistulization through the overlying soft tissues are characteristic findings (Fig. 12-57). Patients suffer local pain of variable severity and have chronic draining sinuses. Aggressive surgical curettage and long-term antimicrobial therapy are required to achieve resolution, but despite this, permanent functional disability and deformity are not uncommon once osteomyelitis has become chronic.

Juvenile Diskitis and Vertebral Osteomyelitis

Inflammation of intervertebral disk spaces in childhood is a puzzling disorder, in terms of both its pathophysiology and mode of presentation. Before the third decade of life, vascular channels penetrate through the vertebral end-plates and communicate with the intervertebral disk. Thus it is thought that hematogenous spread of organisms to the disk spaces of children is likely, whereas in older patients they may lodge in vascular arcades adjacent to the subchondral plate of the vertebra itself. This factor has been used to explain the higher frequency of diskitis in children and the relative infrequency of acute vertebral osteomyelitis before adolescence. However, differences in the clinical picture, the infrequent isolation of pathogens, and evidence that immobilization alone is effective in treating diskitis—whereas antimicrobial therapy is required in vertebral osteomyelitis—have led to speculation that disk space inflammation may be due to a low-grade viral or bacterial infection.

Known predisposing conditions in adults include urinary tract infections, pelvic inflammatory disease, and bowel and urinary tract surgery; in children they include upper respiratory tract infection, gastroenteritis, and genitourinary infection. The importance of antecedent trauma is unclear. Hematogenous spread may occur through the valveless veins of the Batson plexus or via the vertebral branches of the posterior spinal arteries. In both diskitis and vertebral osteomyelitis, *S. aureus* is the most common pathogen, followed by streptococci, gram-negative enteric pathogens (including *Salmonella* and *Kingella kingae*), and corynebacteria. The lumbar spine and the lower thoracic spine are the most common sites of involvement for both entities.

The clinical picture of diskitis, seen predominantly in children younger than 4 years of age, is dominated by pain and progressive limp. Often, focal back pain that progressively worsens in severity is reported. In a few instances it may be perceived as pain in the flank, abdomen, or hip. It is constant; may be aggravated by sitting, standing, or movement; and is typically worse at night. Very young children may initially be irritable and refuse to walk or even sit. In some cases increased irritability has been noted during diaper changes. Adoption of an abnormal posture is a frequent finding. Most commonly this posture is one of exaggerated lumbar lordosis, but in some cases the lumbar spine may be held stiff and straight. Toddlers may preferentially assume a knee–chest position. Fever is

Figure 12-56 Radiographic findings characteristic of subacute osteomyelitis. **A** and **B,** This 13-year-old boy had a 7-week history of pain and swelling of both ankles. He had been treated with penicillin for presumed rheumatic fever. These radiographs show bilateral soft tissue swelling, multiple metaphyseal radiolucencies in the distal left tibia, and a radiolucency involving the metaphysis and epiphysis on the right. **C,** An extensive area of radiolucency and cortical reaction is seen in the ulnar diaphysis of this youngster. *(Courtesy Department of Pediatric Radiology, Children's Hospital of Pittsburgh, Pittsburgh, Pa.)*

Figure 12-57 Chronic osteomyelitis. Inadequate initial treatment resulted in progression to chronic osteomyelitis in this child. In this radiograph, taken 6 months after the onset of symptoms, a radiodense sequestrum is seen within the metaphyseal radiolucency. The process had also begun to decompress into the soft tissues of the thigh. *(Courtesy Department of Pediatric Radiology, Children's Hospital of Pittsburgh, Pittsburgh, Pa.)*

Figure 12-58   Vertebral osteomyelitis. **A-C,** This 10-year-old boy had a 2-week history of intermittent fever, malaise, and steadily worsening lower back and left hip pain, exacerbated by movement. **A** and **B,** He had an exaggerated lumbar lordosis and extreme limitation of flexion, both standing and sitting. The straight leg raising test also accentuated his pain. **C,** Bone scan revealed selectively increased uptake in the L4 vertebral body. **D,** This 13-year-old girl had an 8-week history of intermittent throbbing pain in her midback with a few days of fever. Pain was worse on arising and in the evening, with prolonged standing and with lying down. She had a markedly elevated sedimentation rate and tenderness to deep palpation in the lower thoracic region. MRI done at the time of biopsy shows fragmentation of the body of T8 with extension of infection into the paraspinous tissues on the right. The biopsy specimen showed that the paraspinous mass consisted of granulation tissue with numerous polymorphonuclear leukocytes and plasma cells and grew *Staphylococcus aureus* on culture. (**C** and **D,** *Courtesy Department of Pediatric Radiology, Children's Hospital of Pittsburgh, Pittsburgh, Pa.*)

often present during the first week or two of symptoms, but it may be absent and is often low grade. Other systemic symptoms are unusual. On occasion, abdominal distention is prominent, raising suspicion of intraabdominal pathology.

Careful examination of the spine may reveal paravertebral muscle spasm with guarding and exquisite focal tenderness, although in some cases tenderness may be vague or absent. Resistance to flexion and extension of the spine is common and in the young may simulate meningeal signs. The loss of normal lumbar lordosis or the presence of local scoliosis may be noted early on. Pain on straight leg raising and hip motion may also be encountered.

The sedimentation rate and C-reactive proteins are elevated unless symptoms have been present for many months, but white blood cell counts are elevated only during the first few weeks. Specific radiographic changes do not appear until 2 to 6 weeks after onset, at which time disk space narrowing becomes evident. In the ensuing weeks, irregularities of the adjacent vertebral end-plates become apparent. A technetium scan can reveal focal increased uptake as early as 1 week after the onset of symptoms. Culture of biopsy specimens of the disk space are commonly negative unless obtained early in the course. Most patients with diskitis improve symptomatically with immobilization alone, and the process appears to resolve after several weeks of casting.

The clinical picture of vertebral osteomyelitis, seen in older children and adolescents, usually is one of insidious onset of progressively worsening back pain that is constant, aggravated by movement, and increasingly resistant to analgesics. Usually fever is absent or low grade. On occasion, the onset is acute, with fever and generalized systemic symptoms accompanying the abrupt appearance of pain. In the rare cases encountered in young children, onset is usually acute and the clinical picture is dominated by abdominal or flank pain, with associated tenderness and often guarding. In some patients, paraspinous or spinous process tenderness, back stiffness, an exaggerated lumbar lordosis, pain on leg motion, or lower

extremity weakness may be noted (Fig. 12-58). Laboratory findings in this setting are similar to those in children with diskitis, with the exception that blood cultures obtained in the acute phase are generally positive. Early radiographic findings are also similar, but frank destructive lesions of the vertebral body develop soon after the appearance of disk space narrowing is noted. Cultures of operative biopsy specimens usually yield *S. aureus*. Antimicrobial therapy is necessary to achieve clinical resolution, and surgical debridement is more likely to be required.

Septic Arthritis

Bacterial invasion of the synovial membrane with resultant septic arthritis is a condition with high potential for long-term morbidity. Release of lysosomal enzymes by neutrophils, abscess formation, the development of granulation tissue, and ischemia resulting from increased intraarticular pressure act in concert to damage the articular surface and promote synovial fibrosis and bony ankylosis. Early diagnosis and treatment are essential to prevent or at least minimize the extent of irreversible damage. This is hindered in many cases, however, by the fact that both the clinical picture and laboratory findings overlap with those seen in patients with viral and other forms of acute arthritis.

Septic arthritis is a disorder primarily affecting young children, with two thirds to three fourths of cases occurring in patients younger than 5 years of age. Males are affected twice as often as females. Ninety percent of cases are the result of hematogenous seeding. Although in most cases the affected joint is the primary site of infection, it is not uncommon for septic arthritis to develop in a child with bacterial meningitis or pneumonia, often manifesting early in the course of treatment. Up to 40% of patients have a history or signs of an antecedent upper respiratory tract infection at the time of diagnosis. This was especially common in cases caused by *H. influenzae* type B, which were frequent before the widespread

Table 12-2	Relative Frequency of Pathogens in Septic Arthritis according to Patient Age		
Neonate	**1 Month to 2 Years**	**2 to 5 Years**	**>5 Years**
Staphylococcus aureus	Group A streptococci	*Staphylococcus aureus*	*Staphylococcus aureus*
Group B streptococci	*Streptococcus pneumoniae*	Group A streptococci	Group A streptococci
Gram-negative enteric pathogens	*Neisseria meningitidis*	*Neisseria meningitidis*	*Neisseria gonorrhoeae*
	Pseudomonas aeruginosa	*Streptococcus pneumoniae*	*Pseudomonas aeruginosa*
	Salmonella species	*Haemophilus influenzae* type B	
	Haemophilus influenzae type B		

Figure 12-59 Septic arthritis. This adolescent boy awoke suddenly at 3 AM with severe left knee pain. By 8 AM he was febrile and had marked swelling with overlying erythema and extreme limitation of movement. Examination of joint fluid revealed gram-positive cocci in chains, with a white blood cell count of 24,000/mm³. Cultures were positive for group A streptococci. (*Reprinted from the Clinical Slide Collection on the Rheumatic Diseases © 1991, 1995. Used by permission of the American College of Rheumatology.*)

use of the Hib vaccine. Streptococcal skin and soft tissue infections may antedate septic arthritis caused by this pathogen. In older children and adolescents, gonococcal urethritis, vaginitis, and cervicitis assume importance as antecedents to hematogenous seeding (see Chapter 18). Prior trauma may also be a predisposing factor and is reported in a significant number of cases. In approximately 10% of patients, the septic arthritis is secondary to rupture of a primary osteomyelitic lesion into the joint space, most often in infants. Direct penetrating injury accounts for a small percentage.

Bacterial pathogens are isolated in 65% to 75% of patients, from either synovial fluid, blood, or both. The relative frequency of pathogens varies considerably with patient age, as shown in Table 12-2. Children with sickle hemoglobinopathies occasionally suffer *Salmonella* septic arthritis, whereas patients with Lyme disease may mimic a septic joint. Failure to isolate an organism can be explained in some instances by suppression caused by prior antibiotic administration.

The joints affected in order of frequency are the knee, hip, ankle, and elbow. The wrist and shoulder are involved less often, with other joints being rare sites of septic arthritis. Only a single joint is affected in more than 90% of patients. *Neisseria gonorrhoeae* is the organism most commonly associated with polyarticular disease, but other pathogens may be responsible, particularly *S. aureus* and *H. influenzae* type B. The hip and shoulder joints, if involved, are particularly prone to damage because clinical signs may be subtle and thus diagnosis is often delayed. Further, because the synovium inserts distal to the epiphysis of the proximal humerus and femur, compromise of the blood supply to the epiphysis is more likely to occur as a result of increased intraarticular pressure.

The typical clinical picture of hematogenous septic arthritis is a young child who presents with fever and signs of toxicity, in association with severe localized joint pain, overlying swelling, and marked limitation in range of motion. Fever may be acute in onset, but the child tends to be seen soon after the onset of joint symptoms. Variations in presentation depend in part on the age of the patient, the joint involved, the causative organism, and the duration of symptoms. Infants and toddlers cannot describe focal pain, and thus present with fever and irritability, the latter aggravated by movement. Refusal to bear weight or decreased use of an extremity may or may not have been noted by the family. When a knee, ankle, wrist, or elbow is involved, local swelling and warmth are usually evident (Fig. 12-59). However, early swelling may be subtle, high fever may make any warmth difficult to distinguish, and surface erythema is often absent. Whenever a hip is involved, swelling and warmth are not evident and pain may be referred to the

knee or thigh. Often the position adopted by the patient is the best diagnostic clue. To minimize intraarticular pressure and pain, the child prefers to lie still with the knee and hip flexed and with the hip externally rotated (see Fig. 12-53). In cases of septic arthritis of the shoulder, subtle swelling may or may not be evident, but the shoulders may not be held at the same level and the arm on the involved side is held against the chest to splint the joint.

Septic arthritis of the sacroiliac joint, which accounts for about 1% of cases, can present a particularly confusing picture, often mimicking hip or intraabdominal disease. Only one third of patients have an acute presentation, the remainder having a subacute course. Buttock and back pain, limp, and fever are the most common presenting complaints. Up to one third of patients complain of unilateral radicular pain. Findings of lower abdominal and rectal tenderness in association with normal hip motion may fool the examiner who fails to recognize that leg and buttock pain necessitate meticulous examination of the lower back. Such an examination reveals tenderness over the involved sacroiliac joint, and pelvic compression replicates the pain, as does hyperextension of the ipsilateral hip with the patient supine and dangling his or her leg over the edge of the table.

Limitation of joint motion and evidence of pain on motion are perhaps the most valuable clinical clues to the diagnosis of septic arthritis. Limitation is usually severe unless presentation occurs early, and motion provokes marked discomfort. Diagnosis can be particularly difficult in neonates and infants, who may be afebrile and often have no systemic symptoms. In such cases, decreased use of an extremity is often the earliest clue. Pain on motion is usually evident, however, even before the appearance of localized swelling.

When septic arthritis results from extension of osteomyelitis into a contiguous joint, distinction between the two processes can be difficult to establish clinically. Focal pain is generally of longer duration, but because most cases occur in infants, this complaint is often unavailable. In older children the hip, shoulder, and ankle are the major sites of this secondary form of septic arthritis. These children usually have a

Figure 12-60   Radiographic findings characteristic of septic arthritis. Although radiographs may be normal early on, joint space widening can be detected. **A,** This infant presented with fever, toxicity, and refusal to move the left leg. Plain film shows capsular swelling and lateral displacement of the proximal left femur. **B,** This 4-year-old boy presented with right hip pain and fever. Coronal STIR (short tau inversion recovery) MRI showed copious fluid in the joint itself. (**A,** *Courtesy Rodrigo Dominguez, MD, University of Texas, Houston, Tex.*)

history of prolonged focal pain, antedating a brief period of respite (due to decompression of the infected bone), followed by the sudden return of pain that is markedly aggravated by joint motion. In the days following a penetrating joint injury, a sudden increase in pain and swelling should prompt immediate suspicion of secondary septic arthritis.

Because of the high cost of delays in diagnosis in terms of morbidity, any child with fever, acute onset of pain, and limited motion of a joint should be presumed to have septic arthritis until proven otherwise. These findings should prompt rapid diagnostic investigation. Plain radiographs with comparison views should be obtained immediately and inspected carefully for signs of joint space widening or capsular distention, although these findings may be absent in early cases. If the hip is the suspected site of pathology, lateral and upward displacement of the femoral head may be noted along with displacement of the gluteal fat lines (Fig. 12-60). Magnetic resonance imaging and bone scans are both useful for evaluating the child with suspected septic arthritis of the sacroiliac joint, and may distinguish between patients with underlying osteomyelitis, pelvic myositis, or true septic arthritis.

Early arthrocentesis should be considered, as examination of joint fluid is the study most likely to yield definitive results. Positive findings on Gram-stained specimens are particularly helpful; cultures are positive in 60% or more of cases. Pleocytosis is common, with two thirds of patients having a white blood cell count of more than 50,000/mm³. Remembering, however, that there is considerable overlap with nonbacterial arthritis in terms of cell counts, differential counts, and protein and glucose levels found on examination of synovial fluid is crucial.

Peripheral white blood cell counts, sedimentation rate, and C-reactive protein level may add suggestive evidence, but again there is overlap with viral arthritis. Up to 20% of patients have white blood cell counts less than 10,000/mm³, although most have a significant leftward shift. The sedimentation rate may be markedly elevated, but is less than 40 mm/hour in half of patients. Blood cultures are positive in up to 40% of cases. As cultures of joint fluid from patients with disseminated *N. gonorrhoeae* infection are often negative, it is

important to culture blood, skin lesions, throat, and cervix or urethra when this agent is suspected.

Diagnosis thus depends on assessment of clinical course, physical findings, and results of multiple laboratory studies. Even with negative findings on Gram stain, empiric antimicrobial therapy selected to cover the most likely pathogens (see Table 12-2) should be started, pending culture results, in patients in whom septic arthritis is deemed likely on the basis of the available findings. As is true of osteomyelitis, collaboration between pediatric and orthopedic colleagues is crucial, for drainage of infected material is essential to ensuring a good outcome.

Any disorder associated with acute arthritis must be considered as part of the differential diagnosis of septic arthritis. In some instances the clinical picture of an obvious viral or vasculitic syndrome enables differentiation. The polymigratory picture of acute rheumatic fever and the much less acute onset of juvenile rheumatoid arthritis help to distinguish these conditions. Adenopathy, visceromegaly, anemia, and radiographic changes help distinguish malignant joint infiltration.

TUBERCULOSIS

After decades of steady decline, tuberculosis has shown a disturbing increase in incidence in the United States in recent years. This appears to be related to a combination of factors: the human immunodeficiency virus (HIV) infection epidemic (which predisposes to the reactivation of prior infection and to the development of active and rapidly progressive disease with new infection); a decline in the services of departments of public health; the rise in the homeless population and of barriers in access to health care; and an increase in the immigration of people from places where tuberculosis is prevalent. Worldwide, famine, war, and natural disasters that create large numbers of refugees; crowded living and working conditions; and sweat shop–type labor practices involving long working hours and the employment of child laborers spawn conditions that favor the acquisition of tuberculosis and its spread. In addition, poor compliance with the lengthy treatment regimens required has led to increased transmission of ever-more-resistant organisms. Those at high risk in the United States include people from ethnic and racial minority groups, especially of low socioeconomic status living in overcrowded conditions in populous urban areas; immigrants and foreign-born adoptees from Southeast Asia, China, Latin America, Haiti, and Eastern Europe; the homeless; migrant workers; elderly persons living in nursing homes; prisoners in correctional institutions; HIV-positive or immunosuppressed people; children in close contact with adults in these groups; and health care professionals. Most are located in seven states—California, Florida, Georgia, Illinois, New York, South Carolina, and Texas (border states or states with large immigrant populations or large pockets of people living in extreme poverty).

Transmission

Tubercle bacilli are transmitted from person to person, with the usual source being aerosolization of organisms from an adult or adolescent with active pulmonary, especially cavitary, disease. Children with primary tuberculous disease rarely transmit infection because they have a relatively small number of organisms, if any, in endobronchial secretions and are rarely able to cough forcefully enough to expel them.

Infants and toddlers living with or in close contact with an infectious adult, and adolescents and young adults helping to care for infectious people are at especially high risk for infection. Thus parents, grandparents, older siblings, nannies and sitters, housekeepers, and boarders are the major sources of transmission to children. Less often, teachers, school bus drivers, coaches, and nurses have been source cases.

The portal of entry in more than 98% of instances is the lung; it is estimated that the inhalation of as few as one to three bacilli in a single aerosolized droplet can result in infection. Rarely a superficial skin or mucous membrane lesion may be the site of inoculation. Congenital infection can occur if a pregnant woman experiences lymphohematogenous spread during gestation or has tuberculous endometritis. Health care professionals are at particular risk when handling specimens of infected secretions or body fluids and contaminated syringes or instruments such as lavage tubes and bronchoscopes.

Pathogenesis

Once the organism has gained entry, there is a silent period of incubation lasting 3 to 10 weeks. The larger the inoculum, the shorter the incubation period and the more severe the signs and symptoms of the primary infection. The end of the incubation period is marked by the development of hypersensitivity to the organism, as manifested by a positive PPD skin test (Fig. 12-61), and can be accompanied by fever of

1 to 3 weeks' duration. During this time, the patient's inflammatory response intensifies in the *primary complex,* which has three components: (1) the primary focus or site at which the bacilli have lodged (usually a subpleural alveolus, which can be at any site in either lung), (2) the inflamed lymphatics that drain the area, and (3) inflamed regional lymph nodes. Macrophages migrate to the primary focus, transform into epithelioid cells, and gather into clusters, forming a tubercle. If the host's immune response is effective, the lesion is walled off and then gradually resolves and disappears. If the host response is less effective, bacilli multiply and the primary focus can caseate centrally. Thereafter, organisms in the lesion can travel along lymphatics to regional nodes, provoking more inflammation along the track and in the nodes. Infection can then spread by way of other lymphatics to more distant nodes—most commonly the paratracheal, anterior cervical, and abdominal nodes. New foci may heal, become dormant with the risk of later reactivation, or progress.

Affected nodes that enlarge and caseate can cause numerous complications. For example, hilar nodes pressing on an adjacent bronchus set up sympathetic inflammation in its wall, leading to partial obstruction as the result of a combination of compression and edema collection. On occasion, the inflammatory process damages the cartilaginous rings, resulting in secondary collapse. In other cases it progresses to perforate the bronchial wall, releasing caseous material into the lumen. This may form an obstructive plug or provoke the formation of granulation tissue. Alternatively, organisms released from the caseous material may then travel through the airways to infect other parts of the lung. Rupture of a caseous subpleural primary focus or node results in pleural effusion. Enlarged caseous subcarinal nodes may compress the esophagus, causing dysphagia, or may rupture into it, producing a bronchoesophageal fistula. Infected nodes can compress the subclavian vein, resulting in edema of the ipsilateral upper extremity, or compress the recurrent laryngeal or phrenic nerves. They may also rupture into the mediastinum, or they may erode into adjacent blood vessels, setting the stage for miliary spread.

The host's ability to mount an effective response to inhibit replication of tubercle bacilli and contain the primary infection depends on several factors. Very young and therefore immunologically immature children, malnourished children, adolescent girls, pregnant women, and immunodeficient or immunosuppressed people are at particular risk for progression of disease. Recent infection, especially pertussis or viral infections such as measles, influenza, and varicella, also increases the susceptibility to tuberculous infection and progression. Genetic selection for resistance in populations living in endemic areas and acquired resistance appears to be somewhat protective.

Figure 12-61   Positive tuberculin skin test. This adolescent boy became infected as a result of living with and helping to care for a grandfather whose chronic "smoker's cough" was ultimately discovered to be a manifestation of chronic cavitary tuberculosis. He had a greater than 15-mm induration. *(Courtesy Kenneth Schuitt, MD.)*

Clinical Forms of Tuberculosis

Infection without Disease

Patients with the latent form of tuberculosis have a positive skin test reaction (see Fig. 12-61) but no clinical signs or symptoms of disease and normal chest x-ray findings. Although many of these children never manifest signs of primary infection, if the infection goes unrecognized and untreated, there is a 10% chance of reactivation of their tuberculosis later in life; thus they serve as a major reservoir. Other patients in this category simply have been identified very early and will go on to suffer clinical disease if treatment is not instituted. Patients with underlying HIV infection have a 10% risk of reactivation each year.

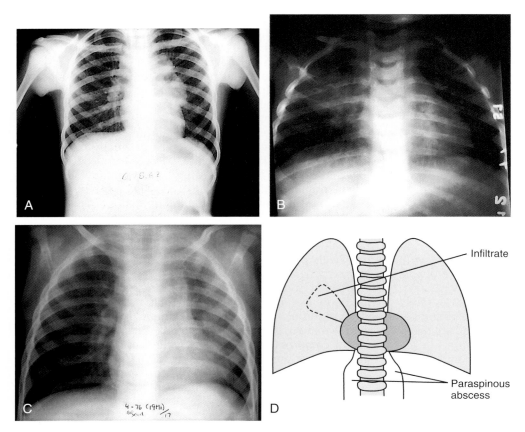

Figure 12-62 Primary pulmonary tuberculosis. **A,** Marked enlargement of hilar nodes without a pulmonary infiltrate is seen in this asymptomatic child. She was tested as part of a contact investigation, and this chest radiograph was obtained because her skin test was positive. **B,** A hazy infiltrate involving a segment of the right upper lobe is seen extending from the hilum to the pleura. This child also has tuberculous spondylitis with a paraspinous abscess, the shadow of which is seen below the diaphragm **(D). C,** In this boy who presented with a pneumonic clinical picture, a hazy infiltrate occupies the entire left upper lobe. (*A and B, Courtesy Jocelyn Medina, MD; C, courtesy Richard Towbin, MD, Children's Hospital of Philadelphia, Philadelphia, Pa.*)

Tuberculous Disease

Patients who have evidence of tuberculosis on chest x-ray or clinical signs and symptoms of pulmonary or extrapulmonary infection are said to have tuberculous disease. The risk of developing disease after infection exceeds 40% for infants, is 24% to 25% for children between 1 and 10 years of age, and is 15% for those between 11 and 15 years of age.

Primary Pulmonary Tuberculosis

The symptoms of primary pulmonary tuberculosis, which are typically insidious in onset, are often attributed to viral illness. Some children have low-grade fever with no apparent source, together with mild anorexia and decreased activity. Others may have associated rhinorrhea, nasal congestion, and pharyngeal erythema and are mistakenly thought to have a viral upper respiratory tract infection. On occasion, erythema nodosum may develop in concert with the fever. Chest examination is generally normal, even in patients with abnormal chest radiographs. Rarely children present with a more dramatic "pneumonic" mode of onset, with high fever, tachypnea, and signs of toxicity. In such cases the clinical findings are those characteristic of lobar pneumonia, with rales, rhonchi, and bronchial breath sounds heard on auscultation and dullness noted on percussion. Patients with either mode of onset tend to show improvement over a few days to a few weeks, although some may be noted to tire easily and be less active than usual. Without specific treatment, some develop low-grade afternoon fevers weeks later that may persist for as long as a few months.

Radiographic findings characteristic of primary pulmonary tuberculosis may be limited to enlarged hilar (Fig. 12-62, *A*) or carinal nodes (seen best on lateral views); faint, cloudy infiltrates that extend to the pleura (Fig. 12-62, *B*); or a lobar infiltrate (Fig. 12-62, *C*) in patients exhibiting the "pneumonic" picture. Infiltrates contain the primary complex and, like it, can be located anywhere in either lung.

Endobronchial Tuberculosis. When enlarged nodes cause bronchial obstruction (usually 3 to 6 months after infection, and most commonly in children younger than 2 years of age), focal hyperaeration or fan-shaped, segmental parenchymal *collapse–consolidation infiltrates* are seen (Fig. 12-63). The latter consist of the primary focus and secondary inflammation and atelectasis. Sometimes narrowing of a bronchial lumen is noted. Infants affected by this endobronchial process often have a harsh, paroxysmal cough that mimics that of pertussis, along with wheezing and rhonchi noted on auscultation. The cough is often worse when the infant is lying supine than when prone. Respiratory distress may be noted during the course of an intercurrent infection. Older children generally have no cough but can manifest the auscultatory findings. With or without treatment, consolidation–collapse lesions can reexpand and resolve; clear with residual calcification of the primary complex and regional node (Ghon complex); or go on to scarring, with progressive contraction of the involved pulmonary segment in association with bronchiectatic changes. Calcification may persist or start resorbing within a few years. On occasion, it progresses to ossification and formation of true bone.

Pleural Effusion. Rupture of a caseous subpleural, primary focus or lymph node can also occur 3 to 6 months after initial infection. This usually occurs in school-age children. The caseous material provokes an intense pleural reaction with the formation of a proteinaceous effusion. This can be localized or generalized. Pleural effusion can also result from hematogenous spread, as well as from direct extension of infection from a subpleural focus. Clinically, development of pleural effusion is heralded by the abrupt onset of fever, chest pain, and shortness of breath and is manifested by decreased chest wall movement and decreased breath sounds, dullness to percussion, and egophony on examination. When the effusion is massive, respiratory distress is evident. Pleural fluid is

Figure 12-63 Progressive primary pulmonary tuberculosis (endobronchial). This 8-year-old girl initially had fever, cough, and mild tachypnea. She was treated with antibiotics for presumed bacterial pneumonia but showed only partial clinical improvement. Repeat radiographs obtained 1 month later showed progression. A purified protein derivative test was then done and was positive. **A** and **B,** She has a collapse–consolidation lesion involving the right lower lobe, with a primary cavity. *(Courtesy Ellen Wald, MD, University of Wisconsin Children's Hospital, Madison, Wis.)*

usually clear or slightly cloudy, greenish yellow, often blood tinged, high in protein, and usually low in glucose. Leukocytes predominate early, lymphocytes later, with counts ranging from 300 to 10,000 cells/mm³. Bacilli are present in small numbers. Radiographs may show clouding of a lower lung field with obliteration of the diaphragm or, in the event of massive effusion, total "white-out" of the lung with mediastinal shift.

Progressive Primary Pulmonary Tuberculosis. Progressive primary pulmonary tuberculosis occurs in infants and young children whose primary focus steadily enlarges, caseates, liquefies, and empties its bacilli-laden contents into a bronchus. The organisms then disseminate through the airways to the rest of the lung, setting up new foci of infection. Clinically these patients have remittent fever, cough, apathy, and malaise, along with anorexia and weight loss. Over time they begin to appear listless and chronically ill. Wet rales may be heard over the site of the primary cavity. Radiographically a small cavity is seen at the site of primary focus, along with a collapse-consolidation lesion (Fig. 12-63) and later diffuse infiltrates. On rare occasions, a large caseous, primary focus can cause a pneumothorax, bronchopleural fistula, or caseous pyothorax if it ruptures into the pleura. Alternatively, it may rupture into the mediastinum, after which caseous material may track upward to the supraclavicular fossa.

Lymphohematogenous Spread and Miliary Tuberculosis

Miliary tuberculosis occurs when bacilli are disseminated from an involved node of the primary complex by means of the bloodstream to distant sites. In some patients this is clinically occult and occurs early during the incubation period or shortly thereafter. Major sites of seeding include the pulmonary apices, spleen, and superficial nodes. In some cases, evidence of resulting metastatic lesions is seen 2 to 4 months later, when the child has a nonspecific illness characterized by

low-grade fever and fatigue, splenomegaly, and generalized adenopathy, sometimes associated with papulonecrotic skin lesions. Others remain asymptomatic, and their metastatic lesions may either remain dormant or reactivate years later.

Acute miliary spread occurs in some patients (usually within 6 months of infection) when a caseous node ruptures directly into a vessel. Organisms in seeded foci may die or set up new foci that are then walled off and become dormant or may progress, expand, and cause further complications. Miliary disease may be detected incidentally in an infant or child who undergoes chest radiography as part of an evaluation for low-grade fever without an apparent source. Other children experience insidious progression of symptoms after intercurrent measles, influenza, or pertussis; still others may have a more abrupt onset of fever, tachypnea, lethargy, and weakness accompanied by hepatosplenomegaly. Within a few weeks, symmetrical tubercles of uniform size are seen throughout the lung fields (Fig. 12-64) and rustling breath sounds can

Figure 12-64 Miliary tuberculosis. Two weeks after miliary spread, this infant's lung fields are symmetrically dotted with tiny tubercles. *(Courtesy Richard Towbin, MD, Children's Hospital of Philadelphia, Philadelphia, Pa.)*

be heard on auscultation. Skin lesions, which may be nodular, purpuric, or papulonecrotic, may appear as well.

A subset of infected children exhibit a process known as *protracted hematogenous spread*, which involves repeated episodes of release of organisms into the bloodstream. These patients have high sustained or spiking fever; leukocytosis (with white blood cell counts up to 40,000/mm³); marked, generalized, nontender adenopathy; and they look quite ill. Within a few weeks, mottled pulmonary lesions of varying size are seen. Polyserositis and multiple bony lesions tend to develop, along with crops of papulonecrotic skin lesions, which form after each episode of seeding.

Extrapulmonary Tuberculosis

Tuberculous Meningitis. After lymphohematogenous or miliary spread, caseous foci may develop in the brain and meninges. Fifty percent of infants and children with miliary tuberculosis go on to develop meningitis. Extension of infection or rupture of one of these foci into the subarachnoid space results in tuberculous meningitis, which usually develops within 3 to 6 months of initial infection in children younger than 6 years of age. The resulting exudate is thick and gelatinous. It infiltrates meningeal and cerebral vessels, causing vasculitis with secondary occlusion and infarction; it impedes CSF flow and resorption, often resulting in a communicating hydrocephalus; and it collects at the base of the brain, impinging on the optic chiasm and the third, sixth, and seventh cranial nerves.

Often preceded by a viral illness or head injury, the onset of symptoms is usually gradual, beginning with anorexia, fever, pronounced apathy, irritability, and emotional lability, often with headache. Within a week or two, drowsiness, vomiting, meningismus, a sluggish pupillary response, and cranial nerve palsies supervene, often accompanied by hyperreflexia and seizures. Confusion, disorientation, dysarthria, tremors, and athetosis are other findings that may be seen during this phase. Untreated, this condition progresses to coma, the syndrome of inappropriate antidiuretic hormone, opisthotonic or decerebrate posturing, the Cushing triad, and death. CSF pressure is usually elevated, and the fluid is clear (although often xanthochromic); cell counts range from 50 to 500 cells/mm³, with leukocytes predominating early and lymphocytes later. The protein content is elevated (often markedly), and glucose levels are usually low. Early diagnosis and the institution of antituberculous therapy can significantly reduce morbidity and mortality, but even with treatment, complications are common in survivors.

Skeletal Tuberculosis. Skeletal tuberculosis is an extrapulmonary manifestation seen in 1% to 6% of children with untreated primary infection; it becomes clinically evident within 6 months to 3 years after the initial infection. Very young children are at greatest risk because of the high rate of blood flow through their growing bones. It can start as a metaphyseal endarteritis subsequent to hematogenous seeding; it can develop by means of extension from lymphatics, especially from a paravertebral node to a vertebra; or it can arise as the result of direct local or hematogenous spread from a neighboring bone.

Formation of granulation tissue and caseation characterize the inflammatory process, which ultimately results in pressure necrosis and the formation of a cold abscess, which can then rupture into an adjacent joint or surrounding soft tissues (see Fig. 12-62, *B*). The vertebrae; bones about the knee and hip; and, in infants, the phalanges are the most common sites involved. Other than the phalanges, involvement of non–weight-bearing bones is unusual. As is often the case with osteomyelitis, a history of antecedent trauma before the onset

of symptoms is frequently obtained. Fever is absent or low grade, unless the lesions develop as part of the process of protracted hematogenous spread. Pain is often relatively mild in comparison with that associated with other forms of bacterial osteomyelitis.

Tuberculous spondylitis usually involves the vertebral bodies of two or more thoracic vertebrae but can affect lumbar vertebrae as well. Clinically, nocturnal pain, manifested by crying in the night and restless sleep; low-grade fever; and later postural change (stiff back, kyphosis) and gait disturbance (with all weight-bearing joints kept slightly flexed) are prominent. Patients with lumbar disease adopt a wide-based stance and gait. Pain may be localized to the back or referred to the chest or abdomen. When cervical vertebrae are affected, pain may be localized to the neck or referred to the occiput or arms; the child may have difficulty holding up the head, and torticollis is often present. On occasion, an opisthotonic posture is adopted. On examination, severe paraspinous muscle spasm, marked limitation of flexion, pain on percussion, and hyperreflexia with clonus may be evident. When there is an associated paraspinous abscess, swelling and fluctuance may be noted adjacent to the site of maximal tenderness. Initially radiographs show slight disk space narrowing; subsequently mild wedging and partial collapse of the vertebral body occur. Later, bony destruction (Fig. 12-65) and ultimately pancake collapse of the vertebral body occur, resulting in kyphotic angulation–Pott disease. Complications include paravertebral, psoas, and retropharyngeal abscesses, as well as neurologic abnormalities secondary to associated spinal cord compression, inflammation, and vasculitis. Because the spinal canal widens caudally, compression is more likely the higher the level of the vertebrae involved.

Involvement of bones about the knee results in pain, stiffness, and limp, which can be intermittent. Limitation of motion varies depending on the extent of associated synovial inflammation. Unilateral thigh or knee pain and limp are the most common modes of presentation of acetabular or proximal femoral disease.

The dactylitis seen in infancy is characterized by painless fusiform swelling of the fingers or toes. Radiographically, affected phalanges, and sometimes metacarpals, initially show fusiform enlargement and increased density. Later, cystic changes are seen.

Tuberculous Pericarditis. Seen in less than 5% of children with progressive pulmonary tuberculosis, tuberculous pericarditis can result from direct invasion of organisms from an adjacent infected lymph node, from rupture of an adjacent

Figure 12-65 Tuberculous spondylitis. Extensive bony destruction of the T12 vertebral body along with mild collapse of T11 is seen. *(Courtesy Jocelyn Medina, MD.)*

primary focus into the pericardial sac, or from lymphatic spread from subcarinal nodes. A hemorrhagic exudate collects and may progress to tamponade. Patients tend to have low-grade fever, anorexia, and rarely chest pain. On examination a pericardial friction rub is usually apparent; with large effusions, heart sounds are diminished and a narrow pulse pressure is noted.

Tuberculous Adenitis. Tuberculous adenitis is discussed earlier in Infectious Lymphadenitis (see Fig. 12-50).

Tuberculosis in Adolescence

Adolescents may suffer a primary infection or experience reactivation of earlier disease. The latter is more likely if the primary infection occurred after 7 years of age. The period of the adolescent growth spurt, especially in girls of low socioeconomic status, is the time when the risk of reactivation or the development of progressive primary disease is greatest. With reactivation, the new lesion develops in the same lobe as that of the old primary complex and tends to remain localized; there is a relatively low risk of hematogenous spread or extension to regional nodes because of prior development of hypersensitization. Affected patients have cough and fever, often accompanied by chest pain, and may exhibit hemoptysis. Anorexia with weight loss and easy fatigability are common. Chest findings may be normal early on, but moist rales may be heard over the apices after cough or on end-expiration. Small round or wedge-shaped infiltrates or linear streaks with mottling may be evident on chest radiograph. This and progressive primary disease can evolve to chronic cavitary disease within a few years if appropriate treatment is not instituted.

With progression, weight loss and fatigue increase and an early-morning cough productive of increasing amounts of sputum becomes bothersome. Daily fevers and night sweats are common, and an appearance of chronic illness supervenes. Wet rales, bronchial breath sounds, wheezing, and dullness to percussion are typical physical findings. Radiographs may reveal mottling, patchy infiltrates, segmental or lobar opacification, and cavitary changes, which may be unilateral or bilateral.

Tuberculin Testing

The "gold standard" of skin testing for tuberculosis is the Mantoux test with 5 tuberculin units (0.1 mL) of purified protein derivative (PPD). This is injected intradermally on the volar surface of the forearm, with the needle bevel up and oriented perpendicularly to the long axis of the arm. After injection, which when done properly raises a wheal, the 27-gauge needle should be left in place for a few seconds to prevent leakage from the injection site. The test should be read by a health care professional 48 to 72 hours later; this is done by measuring the diameter of any induration that develops at the site, again at a right angle to the long axis of the arm (see Fig. 12-61). The test is rarely negative in infected children; anergy is seen only in those who have overwhelming infection or are immunosuppressed and is occasionally seen in a child with an intercurrent viral infection. Use of multiple puncture tests as screening tools should be abandoned because they cannot be standardized. Interpretation of a positive test is based on associated risk factors (Table 12-3).

Case Finding

The most efficient and cost-effective means of identifying infected children is through contact investigation of persons known to be in close contact with an adolescent or adult with

Table 12-3	Interpretation/Risk Factors for Positive Purified Protein Derivative Test
Degree of Induration That Represents a Positive Test	**Risk Factors**
≥5 mm of induration	Known close recent contact with an infected patient
	Immunosuppressed
	HIV positive
	Currently taking steroids
	Chest radiograph showing old healed lesions
≥10 mm of induration	High-risk racial or ethnic group (émigrés from an endemic area)
	Younger than 4 years of age
	Underlying medical condition that increases risk for severe disease (e.g., diabetes, malignancy, chronic renal failure, malnutrition)
≥15 mm of induration	No risk factors

pulmonary tuberculosis. Conversely, if a child is found to be positive, household members and others in close contact should be tested to find the source case.

Because of the low prevalence of tuberculosis in most parts of the United States, routine yearly skin testing is not indicated. However, children from high-risk groups should be tested routinely and all new immigrants should undergo PPD testing.

Diagnosis

Most children with tuberculosis are diagnosed by means of skin testing performed as a result of contact investigations prompted by identification of an infectious adult. Cultures remain essential, for diagnosis and identification of drug-resistant organisms. However, in young children with primary pulmonary tuberculosis, sputum is unavailable for culture; the yield from early-morning gastric aspirates is only about 40%; and the yield from specimens obtained by bronchoscopy is often not much better. Hence cultures of sputum from source-case adults (which have a much higher yield) are often the best means of obtaining organisms and testing their susceptibility to antituberculosis drugs, thereby guiding selection of a treatment regimen.

Other specimens that can be used for cultures include pleural fluid and preferably a pleural punch biopsy specimen from patients with pleural effusion; CSF from patients with meningitis; lymph node biopsy specimens or aspirates from patients with adenitis; bone marrow biopsy or liver biopsy specimens from patients with miliary disease or protracted hematogenous spread; joint fluid or synovial biopsy specimens from patients with tuberculous arthritis; and skin biopsy specimens from patients with cutaneous lesions.

Treatment Principles

Appropriate therapy with antituberculous drugs prevents the development of disease in children who are asymptomatic, halts the progression of disease, and prevents complications. Further, it dramatically reduces the risk of subsequent reactivation. In infectious adults and adolescents, therapy is aimed not only at managing the disease, but also at rendering the person noninfectious as quickly as possible.

Tubercle bacilli thrive in large numbers in the well-oxygenated environment of an open pulmonary cavity but replicate much more slowly, sometimes intermittently, or become dormant in caseous lesions and within macrophages. Naturally resistant organisms are routinely found in patients with large populations of organisms. Therefore agents are selected for their ability to kill organisms in differing environments and to prevent the development of secondary drug resistance. The choice and number of drugs and duration of therapy are determined by the stage and severity of the disease at diagnosis; by epidemiologic data regarding the likelihood of drug resistance; and results of cultures and susceptibility testing, if available. The course of therapy must be lengthy (even with new, shorter regimens) to ensure that slowly growing bacilli are eliminated and to give the patient's own host resistance time to kill organisms that persist, despite therapy. This necessitates close follow-up and the support of health care workers to assist compliance; in some cases, direct supervision of medication administration is necessary.

Children younger than 4 years of age have a high risk for severe disease from *M. tuberculosis*. Accordingly, they should be started on prophylaxis if they have been exposed to an infectious adult, even if their PPD is negative, and kept on it until they are retested 3 months after exposure. Medication can be discontinued if the repeat test is again negative. Children who have a positive PPD without evidence of disease can take a single agent for 9 months. Children with primary pulmonary tuberculosis are treated first with a combination of three drugs for 2 months and then with two drugs to complete a 6- to 9-month course. Those with milder forms of extrapulmonary disease are treated similarly, but for 9 to 12 months. Patients with tuberculous meningitis and those suspected of having resistant organisms are treated initially with four medications, pending the results of susceptibility tests, and treatment is continued for a minimum of 12 months.

Administration of corticosteroids in concert with antituberculosis agents decreases the severity of the inflammatory response and attendant vasculitis and thereby reduces morbidity and mortality in patients with severe complications, such as meningitis, miliary disease with alveolar–capillary block, massive pericardial and pleural effusions, and marked hilar adenopathy that produces respiratory embarrassment.

CONGENITAL AND PERINATAL INFECTIONS

Numerous pathogens that produce relatively mild or even subclinical disease in children and adults can cause severe disease with devastating sequelae in children who acquire such infections prenatally or perinatally. Toxoplasmosis, rubella, cytomegalovirus (CMV), herpes simplex virus (which comprise the TORCH syndromes), and syphilis are well-known sources of pathology. In addition, sepsis, meningitis, pneumonia, and other infections caused by numerous perinatally acquired bacterial pathogens, including tetanus in underdeveloped countries, cause significant neonatal morbidity and mortality, especially in infants born prematurely. Because of the breadth of this subject and space limitations, we have limited discussion to disorders that tend to have distinctive physical findings.

Congenital Toxoplasmosis

Toxoplasma gondii is an intracellular protozoan whose definitive host is the cat. Oocysts are shed in the feces and can survive in soil for years. Infection of humans is acquired primarily from the ingestion or inhalation of oocysts excreted in cat feces or consumption of raw or undercooked meat from animals who acquired infection from oocysts in the soil. On occasion, transmission occurs by means of transfusion or organ transplantation. Although most cases of infection in children beyond the neonatal period are thought to be subclinical, a mononucleosis-like syndrome and cervical adenopathy have been identified as clinical features, and it may well be that in many cases the clinical picture simulates a viral illness and thus the true cause goes unrecognized.

Prenatally acquired infection has the potential to cause serious harm to the developing fetus. In the United States an estimated 1 or 2 per 1000 live-born infants have congenitally acquired toxoplasmosis. Maternal infection during pregnancy results in fetal infection less than 50% of the time, however. The risk of transmission to the fetus increases as gestation advances, but the severity of fetal injury is greater the earlier the infection occurs during pregnancy. Major sites of involvement are the CNS, retina, choroid, and muscles. Seventy percent of congenitally infected infants appear normal at birth, about 10% to 20% are overtly symptomatic, and approximately 10% have detectable chorioretinitis without other abnormalities (see Chapter 19). Infected infants without signs of disease and those with mild chorioretinitis alone are at risk for progressive ocular and, on occasion, CNS involvement if the infection is not diagnosed and treated. In many instances, however, the diagnosis is not suspected until evidence of visual impairment, strabismus, or developmental delay prompts careful ophthalmologic and neurologic assessment.

In symptomatic newborns the classic constellation of hydrocephalus, chorioretinitis, and intracerebral calcifications points toward the diagnosis of congenital toxoplasmosis. However, most often the clinical picture simulates that of other congenital infections, especially cytomegalovirus infection. Affected infants tend to be small for gestational age, may be microcephalic or hydrocephalic, develop early-onset jaundice, have hepatosplenomegaly and diffuse adenopathy, and can have petechial and purpuric lesions or a generalized maculopapular rash. Seizures can occur, and CSF examination may show a pleocytosis with an increased protein content and xanthochromia. Skull radiographs or a head computed tomography (CT) scan may reveal diffuse cortical calcifications (Fig. 12-66), in

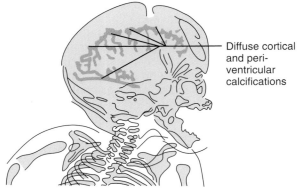

Diffuse cortical and periventricular calcifications

Figure 12-66   Congenital toxoplasmosis. Microcephaly, ventricular dilatation, and cerebral calcifications were prominent findings in this infant with severe congenital toxoplasmosis. *(Courtesy Department of Pediatric Radiology, Children's Hospital of Pittsburgh, Pittsburgh, Pa.)*

contrast to the periventricular pattern seen in infants with congenital cytomegalovirus infection. Interstitial pneumonitis and myocarditis may be prominent features as well. These infants are at high risk of suffering severe neurodevelopmental sequelae, if they survive. Other infected infants may appear normal initially but may rapidly develop signs of neonatal myocarditis with minimal CNS manifestations, although they, too, may have cerebral calcifications, as do many infants with apparently isolated chorioretinitis.

Diagnosis can be confirmed by demonstration of a positive IgM or IgA assay within the first 6 months of life. Double-sandwich enzyme immunoassays or immunoabsorbent assays for *T. gondii*–specific IgM should be used in infants suspected of having congenital toxoplasmosis. Thorough ophthalmologic, auditory, and neurologic evaluations are also indicated. In addition, a head CT scan should be obtained and CSF examined. To halt further and future progression of the disease, all infected infants, whether symptomatic or not, warrant prolonged treatment (up to 1 year) with a combination of pyrimethamine (supplemented with folic acid) and sulfadiazine. This should be instituted and administered in consultation with appropriate specialists.

Congenital Rubella

Widespread use of rubella vaccination has thankfully made congenital rubella a rarity in developed countries. Although normally a benign infection, rubella can lead to severe consequences if acquired in utero. Even if asymptomatic infection occurs in the mother, rubella can be transmitted across the placenta to the developing fetus. The earlier in gestation the infection occurs, the greater the potential for injury. Close to 40% of fetuses infected during the first 8 weeks spontaneously abort or are stillborn, and 25% have gross anomalies noted at birth. Ultimately, 85% of live-born infants infected in the first trimester suffer adverse consequences, as do 35% of those infected between weeks 13 and 16. Infection after 4 months' gestation does not appear to cause disease. The most commonly encountered anomalies are central diffuse cataracts; congenital heart disease (patent ductus arteriosus, pulmonary artery stenosis, pulmonary valvular stenosis); and sensorineural deafness (usually bilateral, occasionally unilateral), seen singly or in combination.

Thus there is a wide range of clinical manifestations. Some infants at risk are normal. Some appear normal at birth but later are found to have hearing loss. Some are small for gestational age and at birth have evidence of congenital heart disease and ocular anomalies, including microphthalmia, glaucoma, cataracts that may be central or diffuse, and pigmented retinopathy (see Chapter 19). Many of these infants develop jaundice within 24 hours of birth and have hepatosplenomegaly and diffuse adenopathy as well. Although usually present at birth, ocular findings may be missed unless a careful ophthalmologic examination is performed.

Ten to twenty percent of live-born infants with congenital rubella show signs of severe disseminated infection at or shortly after birth. In addition to early-onset jaundice, hepatosplenomegaly, and adenopathy, they often have signs of myocarditis with ischemic changes on electrocardiograms, interstitial pneumonitis, thrombocytopenia with petechiae and purpura, and CNS dysfunction that may range from lethargy and hypotonia to frank meningoencephalitis. Radiographs may reveal bony abnormalities consisting of metaphyseal lucencies and irregular epiphyseal mineralization. In some cases a rubelliform rash or a characteristic raised, bluish, papular eruption, termed a *blueberry muffin rash,* may be evident as the result of dermal erythropoiesis (Fig. 12-67, *A*). Most of these severely affected infants are microcephalic, in addition to being small for gestational age. In countries with universal vaccination programs, infants with these findings are more likely to have congenital CMV infection (Fig. 12-67, *B*). Survivors of this "expanded rubella syndrome" are highly likely to be deaf and to have significant psychomotor retardation.

In a small percentage of infants with congenital rubella, delayed manifestations may surface. These include anemia toward the end of the first month; the insidious onset of interstitial pneumonitis; and the appearance of a chronic, generalized rubelliform exanthem at 3 to 4 months of age. Still later, immunodeficiency may be detected. Feeding difficulties, chronic diarrhea, and failure to thrive are common.

Infants with congenital rubella are chronically and persistently infected and tend to shed live virus in urine, stools, and respiratory secretions for up to 1 year. Hence, they should be isolated when in the hospital and kept away from susceptible pregnant women when sent home. Diagnosis can be confirmed by viral culture and specific IgM titers.

Congenital Cytomegalovirus Infection

A ubiquitous virus of the herpesvirus family, CMV infects approximately 1% of all live-born infants while in utero. Infection of the fetus can develop from either primary infection of the mother or reactivation of virus acquired earlier. However, primary infection is believed to be associated with a higher risk for symptomatic disease in the infant. Approximately 10% of infected infants have symptoms at birth. Similar to other TORCH syndromes, findings include small size for gestational age, microcephaly, thrombocytopenia, hepatosplenomegaly, hepatitis, intracranial calcifications (see Chapter 15), chorioretinitis, and hearing abnormalities. Some affected babies can be born with a "blueberry muffin" appearance similar to that of congenital rubella (Fig. 12-67, *A*). Another 10% to 15% of congenitally infected infants may not manifest problems until later in infancy or childhood when they are found to have sensorineural hearing loss and/or developmental delays. Children identified with congenital CMV infection should have routine hearing assessments until 5 years of age, because hearing loss can be progressive.

Neonatal Herpes Simplex Infection

Infants born vaginally to mothers with primary genital herpes simplex infection have a 50% risk of acquiring disease. In contrast, less than 5% born to mothers with recurrent lesions develop herpes neonatorum. Risk of infection increases with prolonged rupture of membranes. Typically the mother is asymptomatic and the infant appears totally normal at birth. Signs of infection may develop any time within the first 4 weeks but usually appear 4 to 8 days postpartum. Infection may be localized to the skin, eye, mouth, or CNS, or it may be systemic. In the latter instance, onset begins with fever or subnormal temperature in association with lethargy, poor feeding, vomiting, and jaundice. The liver and spleen are enlarged and often remarkably firm. Respiratory distress supervenes, followed by a picture that is indistinguishable from that of septic shock with DIC. Approximately three fourths of affected infants have typical herpetic skin or mucosal lesions (Fig. 12-68, *A* and *B*). The scalp and face are the sites most commonly involved (Fig. 12-68, *C*). On occasion, lesions are limited to the conjunctiva or to the oral mucosa. In the absence of these lesions, accurate diagnosis is extremely difficult. The prognosis is relatively good for infants with localized skin, eye, or oral involvement if they are treated promptly with intravenous acyclovir. If untreated, most of these infants will progress to CNS and/or disseminated disease. Mortality

Figure 12-67 Congenital infections. **A,** A newborn with congenital rubella syndrome, including a "blueberry muffin" rash, diffuse petechiae, hepatosplenomegaly, early onset of jaundice, and neurologic depression. **B,** This newborn with severe congenital cytomegalovirus infection was noted to have microcephaly. **C,** CT of the brain of the same infant shows diffuse intracerebral calcifications. (**A,** *Courtesy Michael Sherlock, MD, Lutherville, Md.*)

Figure 12-68 Neonatal herpes simplex type 2 infection. **A** and **B,** Although the child was normal at birth, fever, lethargy, and decreased feeding suddenly developed in this infant at 6 days of age. On examination, multiple grouped vesicular lesions were noted on the trunk and scalp. The liver and spleen were markedly enlarged and firm. He had a fulminant course resembling that of septic shock and died within 24 hours. **C,** Vesicular lesions are found most commonly on the scalp and face, as demonstrated in this infant. (**A** and **B,** *Courtesy Michael Sherlock, MD, Lutherville, Md.*)

of infants with disseminated disease is high, exceeding 50%, but has been reduced by early recognition and systemic antiviral therapy. The survival rate is better in those with localized CNS disease than in those with systemic infection, but severe morbidity results in both.

Less frequently, infections may occur prenatally as a result of ascent from the lower genital tract through ruptured membranes or as a result of maternal viremia. In the event of prenatal acquisition, the infant may die in utero or may be born with jaundice, skin lesions, and signs of systemic infection.

Congenital Syphilis

Initial hopes of eradicating syphilis with the advent of penicillin in the mid-20th century proved to be premature, for as prevalence of disease waned, so did funding for its control programs, and dramatic resurgences occurred in the 1960s and again in the 1980s. Concomitantly, an increase in congenital infection mirrored the rise in incidence of syphilis in women of childbearing age. Fortunately, revitalized control programs once again have decreased the incidence. However, hopes for eradication have yet to be realized, and it remains important for physicians to be able to recognize the clinical manifestations of syphilis. Its congenital form is discussed here. Manifestations in adolescents are presented in Chapter 18.

Women most at risk of acquiring and transmitting syphilis to their infants are young, of low socioeconomic status, have multiple sex partners, and live in an area where syphilis has become endemic. Drug use and the practice of trading sex for drugs substantially increase the risk of acquisition and complicate efforts to trace sexual contacts. Adding to the risk of fetal transmission is the fact that women at greatest risk of acquiring the disease often fail to seek or receive inadequate prenatal care, thus delaying prenatal diagnosis and treatment.

Congenital syphilis results from hematogenous spread of *Treponema pallidum* from an infected mother through the placenta to the developing fetus, resulting in disseminated disease. It appears that risk of transmission to the fetus is greatest when the mother acquires disease during or shortly before pregnancy (i.e., when she is in the primary, secondary, or early latent phase of the disease). Infection early in gestation can result in stillbirth, hydrops fetalis, prematurity, or neonatal death. Live-born infected infants may or may not have obvious signs and symptoms at the time of delivery. Those who do not may develop clinical manifestations during the neonatal period or weeks, months, or even years later if the disease goes undiagnosed and untreated. The earlier the onset, the poorer the prognosis. Although the reasons for delay in symptom onset are not fully understood, it appears that when delivery occurs while the mother is in the incubation period, and is thus seronegative, long-delayed onset is more typical.

Infants who are symptomatic at birth tend to have evidence of intrauterine growth retardation, hepatosplenomegaly, direct and indirect hyperbilirubinemia, Coombs-negative hemolytic anemia, thrombocytopenia, generalized lymphadenopathy (including epitrochlear nodes), and mucocutaneous lesions. These lesions are often vesicular or bullous and ultimately rupture to form superficial crusted erosions or ulcerations. The rash is generalized and includes palms and soles. When skin lesions appear after the first month, they are more likely to be papulosquamous or maculopapular, resembling those of secondary syphilis in older individuals (see Chapter 18). They tend to be oval in shape; pinkish red in color; and distributed predominantly over the back, buttocks, posterior thighs, and soles, although perioral and palmar lesions may be present.

Over time these lesions tend to turn brown in color, and fine desquamation of the palms and soles may be noted (Fig. 12-69, *A* and *B*). Three to four months after delivery, affected infants may develop typical condylomata lata—moist papular or warty lesions around the nose and mouth and in intertriginous areas. Mucosal lesions, termed *mucous patches,* consist of patchy white lesions seen over the palate and other mucosal surfaces. Characteristic snuffles may develop between a week and a few months of age. Affected infants have an increasingly profuse rhinorrhea, in which the nasal discharge can be blood tinged, when there are associated ulcerations of the nasal mucosa. A hoarse cry is commonly seen with snuffles. The nasal discharge, mucosal lesions, and moist cutaneous lesions teem with organisms.

Widespread symmetrical skeletal involvement is seen radiographically in essentially all infants with congenital syphilis (Fig. 12-69, *C* and *D*), although only about 15% have symptoms of pain. Their discomfort is manifested as irritability and pseudoparalysis of Parrot, in which decreased limb movement, especially of the upper extremities, is noted. Osteochondritis, evident on x-ray examination as early as 5 weeks, is characterized by horizontal radiopaque bands often with adjacent lucent lines that are seen in the metaphases, along with irregular demineralization of the lateral aspect, which creates a mottled appearance. In the proximal tibias the medial portion of the metaphyses can be demineralized as well, a phenomenon termed the *Wimberger sign* (Fig. 12-69, *D*). Radiographic evidence of periostitis is generally not seen until about 3 to 4 months of age and is characterized by the formation of one or more layers of periosteal new bone extending along the length of the diaphyses of long bones (Fig. 12-69, *C* and *D*).

CNS involvement is common in infants with full-blown clinical disease but also can be found in some who are otherwise asymptomatic. Accordingly, CSF examination is recommended for all infected infants. Untreated infants can go on to develop meningitis with a clinical picture that simulates that of acute bacterial meningitis. However, CSF examination reveals a monocytosis with moderately elevated protein and a normal glucose level. Chronic meningovascular inflammation may become evident later in the first year. This can progress to fibrosis, resulting in hydrocephalus and cranial nerve palsies (especially of cranial nerves VII, III, IV, and VI) along with regression in developmental milestones. In the second year, progressive cerebral endarteritis may cause focal infarctions with secondary strokelike symptoms and seizures.

All of the symptoms of "early congenital syphilis" just described are the direct result of active infection. Manifestations of "late congenital syphilis" are usually sequelae or stigmata of prior disease activity but can in some instances be due to persistent disease. They may be seen in up to 40% of cases and include the following:

1. Maldevelopment of permanent teeth

   - Hutchinson teeth—the upper central incisors are smaller than normal, barrel shaped, and notched in the center of the incisal surface
   - Mulberry molars—abnormal cusp development results in the formation of multiple peripheral cusps and a central cusp

2. Interstitial keratitis—development of a ground-glass appearance of the cornea and scleral vascularization, which have their onset around puberty

3. Eighth nerve deafness

4. Skeletal stigmata due to sclerotic changes

   - Sabre shin
   - Frontal bossing

Figure 12-69   Congenital syphilis. **A** and **B,** Desquamation of the foot and hand are seen in this infant with congenital syphilis. **C,** This 3-month-old who presented with untreated congenital syphilis had diffuse periosteal reaction of the tibias and generalized demineralization. **D,** Wimberger sign, the osseous destruction of the proximal tibial metaphysis, is seen in another affected infant. (**A** and **B,** Courtesy Pablo Sanchez, MD, and Walid Salhab, MD, University of Texas Southwestern Medical Center; **D,** courtesy Manuel P. Meza, MD, Children's Hospital of Pittsburgh, Pittsburgh, Pa.)

5. Cartilaginous stigmata due to gummatous breakdown and/or ulceration
   - Saddle nose deformity
   - Palatal perforation

6. Clutton joints—painless hydrarthrosis of the knees

7. Rhagades—fissuring of the skin in the perinasal and perioral areas

8. Mental retardation and, more rarely, chronic neurosyphilis with paresis, or less commonly, tabes dorsalis

Testing all pregnant women for syphilis and promptly treating those who are seropositive constitute the mainstay in preventing congenital syphilis. Infants should be further evaluated and treated if the mother did not receive treatment or may have been inadequately treated. The latter should be suspected if a nonpenicillin regimen was used, if there was less than a fourfold decrease in her serum titer after treatment, or if treatment was administered less than 1 month before delivery.

Neonatal Tetanus

Tetanus is an exceptionally painful acute neuromuscular disorder caused by release of a neurotoxic exotoxin by *Clostridium tetani*. The bacterium, a gram-positive anaerobic rod, forms terminal spores that are highly resistant to heat and antiseptics. Prevalent worldwide, the organism is present in the intestines of humans and animals. Accordingly, it is widespread in soil and is found in especially large numbers in the cultivated soil of rural areas fertilized with manure. It is also present in dust and dirt in urban areas. When organisms are inoculated along with dirt or soil into a wound with devitalized or necrotic tissue, they find ideal anaerobic conditions for spore germination. Once they have germinated, spores release two exotoxins: tetanolysin and tetanospasmin. Tetanolysin assists with potentiating infection, and tetanospasmin is one of the most potent neurotoxins known. The toxin diffuses locally, binding irreversibly to presynaptic terminals of lower motor neurons, where it impedes neuromuscular transmission, and, acting on the motor end-plates of nearby skeletal muscle cells, it interferes with contraction–relaxation mechanisms. Additional toxin is believed to spread via the bloodstream and lymphatics to yet other peripheral nerve terminals, and some leaves the inoculum site, traveling via retrograde axonal transport to lower motor neuron cell bodies in the spinal cord and brainstem. There it migrates across synapses to inhibitory interneurons and blocks release of neurotransmitters, thereby suppressing their inhibitory control. Lacking effective inhibition, patients experience persistent muscular rigidity and periodic spasmodic contractions of voluntary muscles, which are extremely painful. The toxin's action on autonomic nerves also results in disinhibition.

Neonatal tetanus is a generalized form of the disorder seen in infants born to unimmunized or inadequately immunized mothers and is usually the result of contamination of the umbilical stump. Cutting the cord with an unclean instrument, application of dirty dressing materials, and/or the cultural practice of placing mud or dung on the stump to hasten cord separation may be the source of the inoculum.

Affected neonates are still seen in significant numbers in more than 50 (mostly underdeveloped) countries worldwide, and neonatal tetanus has its highest incidence in parts of eastern and southern Asia and sub–Saharan Africa. In those areas incidence is highest among the poor, who have little or no access to health care, are poorly educated regarding safe and sanitary birthing practices, and often whose cultures make them suspicious of health care providers and immunizations. Significant underreporting of the disease, especially in remote areas where births and deaths often go unrecorded, makes it impossible to know the exact incidence, but it is estimated to be in the vicinity of 500,000 cases per year. Mortality is high—95% of cases with no treatment and 25% to 90% for infants receiving treatment, depending on its quality.

The incubation period for neonatal tetanus ranges from 3 to 4 days to 2 weeks, with onset of symptoms usually occurring 6 to 7 days after delivery. Initially the baby appears restless and irritable and seems to have difficulty suckling. Within 1 to 2 days, trismus (lockjaw) due to masseter rigidity, dysphagia with drooling, and noisy respirations are noted. These are associated with neck, back, and shoulder stiffness. Subsequently there is rapid cephalocaudal progression of muscular rigidity from neck to back and abdomen, and then the extremities. Opisthotonic posturing is typical, and hands are held fisted and toes fanned out. Orbicularis oris spasm produces the appearance of a sardonic grin termed *risus sardonicus* (Fig. 12-70, A and B). These manifestations are accompanied by fever and the onset of painful tonic or tetanic spasmodic contractions of voluntary muscles, which range from mild to severe, can last a few to several minutes, and can be precipitated by even minimal external stimuli. Masseter, orbicularis, and pharyngeal rigidity make sucking difficult, if not impossible, and significantly impair swallowing. Spasms involving laryngeal muscles and the diaphragm can cause severe respiratory embarrassment. Symptoms of autonomic disinhibition

Figure 12-70 Neonatal tetanus. **A,** This newborn demonstrates the trismus (locked jaw) and fixed smile of risus sardonicus that are typical of tetanus. Note as well the clenched fists and fanned toes. **B,** Viewed from the side, his opisthotonic posturing is more evident. *(Courtesy Jonathan Spector, MD, Boston.)*

include periods of excessive sweating, hypertension, tachycardia, and arrhythmias. Complications include aspiration, atelectasis, pneumonia, fractures of vertebrae and long bones, and respiratory arrest. In survivors, clinical improvement tends to begin about 2 weeks after the onset of symptoms, with a gradual decrease in fever, degree of rigidity and frequency, and intensity of spasms. Resolution then proceeds gradually over the ensuing 6 weeks. Many surviving infants show persistent signs of developmental delay, problems with balance, and some degree of muscle atrophy. Later, when old enough, these children may complain of easy muscle fatigue and cramping.

The diagnosis of tetanus must be made clinically. Laboratory studies are unhelpful.

Successful treatment regimens include the following:
- Prompt administration of tetanus immune globulin to neutralize any free or unbound toxin
- Good local wound care
- Administration of penicillin or metronidazole
- Good supportive intensive care in a dim, quiet room with minimal stimulation
- Neuromuscular blockade and sedation to reduce pain, severity of spasms, and rigidity and to allay anxiety
- Intubation and ventilation as needed for respiratory compromise

- Attention to nutrition, often via total parenteral nutrition
- H₂ blockers to prevent stress ulcers
- Initiation of immunization with tetanus toxoid
- After-care physical therapy

Effective prevention measures in areas where tetanus remains endemic necessitate aggressive outreach immunization campaigns (often to remote areas) aimed especially at women and girls of childbearing age, as well as unimmunized or inadequately immunized pregnant women. These efforts must be combined with carefully tailored and culturally sensitive education programs (to overcome cultural taboos) that emphasize safe and sanitary birthing practices and cord care, as well as conveying the importance and safety of immunizations.

Human Immunodeficiency Virus and Acquired Immunodeficiency Syndrome

HIV-1 is a retrovirus and is the major etiologic agent of acquired immunodeficiency syndrome (AIDS) throughout the world. A second virus, HIV-2, is endemic in West Africa and accounts for the remainder of AIDS cases. HIV is a ribonucleic acid virus that is trophic for CD4⁺ (helper) T lymphocytes, as well as some monocytes, macrophages, and microglial cells of the central nervous system that bear CD4⁺ surface markers. The virus becomes integrated into the host genome and hence persists in the infected individual for life.

More than 9000 children (younger than 13 years of age) in the United States have been reported to the Centers for Disease Control and Prevention (CDC) with AIDS, and more than half of these children have died. Estimates suggest that more than 2 million children worldwide have been infected with the virus. Of these children, the vast majority acquire the virus perinatally from their HIV-infected mothers. This is particularly true in technologically advanced countries, where superb screening procedures are available to ensure the safety of blood supplies. Without intervention, there is a 15% to 30% risk of transmission of HIV from an HIV-infected mother to her offspring. However, in 1994 a large multicenter, randomized, double-blind study proved that maternal-to-child transmission of HIV could be reduced with the use of zidovudine given to HIV-infected women orally during the second and third trimesters, intravenously intrapartum, and to the offspring for the first 6 weeks of life. Subsequent studies using combination therapy with highly active antiretroviral agents were even more successful, preventing almost all vertical transmission of HIV in non–breast-feeding populations. However, these therapies are often unavailable to women in poorer countries of the world because of costs and logistics. Worldwide estimates suggest that 17 million women of childbearing age are currently infected with HIV. Transmission can occur not only during the time of delivery, but also postnatally through breast milk. These staggering figures, along with the problem of accessing these individuals for antenatal and postnatal therapy, tell a sobering story that sorely needs to be addressed.

Blood bank screening procedures introduced in 1985 have virtually eliminated the risk of transmission from exposure to HIV-infected blood products in countries that can afford to use them. Like adults, adolescents acquire HIV through high-risk behaviors, such as unprotected sexual activity and needle sharing. Adolescents account for less than 1% of cases of AIDS reported to the CDC. However, given that it takes an average of 10 years for acquired HIV to progress to AIDS, it is clear that much adult AIDS can be ascribed to HIV infection acquired during the teenage or young adult years. HIV is not transmitted by casual contact with an HIV-infected individual in normal living conditions and school settings. Under unusual circumstances, contact between HIV-infected blood and open skin lesions or mucous membranes of an uninfected individual can result in virus transmission.

The timing of symptom development in untreated HIV-infected children varies. Approximately one third of infants present rapidly in the first months or year of life with one or more of the characteristic AIDS-indicator conditions, suggesting intrauterine infection. The majority of other children infected with HIV present in the first few years of life with a more indolent course, and only a small percentage of children develop symptoms years later akin to what is seen with adults.

HIV-infected infants often present with failure to thrive, developmental delay or loss of developmental milestones, hepatosplenomegaly, lymphadenopathy, candidal skin or mucosal infections (Fig. 12-71), chronic diarrhea, chronic lymphoid interstitial pneumonitis, and recurrent or particularly severe bacterial infections. The last include sepsis, pneumonia, meningitis, abscess, or recurrent episodes of cellulitis, otitis media, and sinusitis. Common pathogens are *S. pneumoniae, H. influenzae, Salmonella, S. aureus,* and gram-negative organisms.

HIV infection is often suspected because of a history of maternal high-risk behaviors or because of a child's clinical presentation. Approximately 50% present with symptoms of HIV infection by the age of 1 year and 82% by 3 years. Increasing attention to testing all women during pregnancy allows for intervention and prevention of perinatally transmitted infection.

Figure 12-71   Child with AIDS. **A,** Oral thrush. **B,** Candidal diaper dermatitis. (**A,** *Courtesy G.B. Scott, MD, and M.T. Mastrucci, MD, Miami, Fla.*)

Figure 12-72 *Pneumocystis jirovecii* pneumonia in a child with AIDS. Note the diffuse bilateral haziness. *(Courtesy G.B. Scott, MD, and M.T. Mastrucci, MD, Miami, Fla.)*

Figure 12-74 CT scan of an infant with AIDS. Note the frontal lobe and basal ganglia calcification and increased ventricular size secondary to cerebral parenchymal volume loss.

Although, as noted earlier, bacterial infections are often seen in HIV-infected infants, opportunistic infections related to defects in cell-mediated immunity also occur. One of the most common of these is *Pneumocystis jirovecii* (formerly *Pneumocystis carinii*) pneumonia (PCP) (Fig. 12-72), which occurs in more than one third of untreated symptomatic HIV-infected children. Other opportunistic infections include *Mycobacterium avium* complex, candidal esophagitis, cytomegalovirus infection, cryptosporidiosis, persistent or disseminated herpes simplex virus, cryptococcosis, and toxoplasmosis and unusually extensive cases of molluscum contagiosum (Fig. 12-73). Of particular note is *M. avium* complex, which may cause fever, weight loss, diarrhea, and abdominal pain.

An especially devastating feature of HIV infection is the encephalopathic condition that leads to developmental delay, loss of developmental milestones, and behavioral alterations. Also seen are pyramidal tract signs, paresis, ataxia, pseudobulbar palsy, and decreased tone. CT scans and MRI studies often show severe brain atrophy with increased ventricular size and calcifications in the basal ganglia and frontal lobes (Fig. 12-74). The course of HIV-related neurologic disease is variable and may be intermittent, static, or relentlessly progressive.

Lymphoid interstitial pneumonitis, leading to chronic interstitial pneumonitis, can be seen in children with HIV (Fig. 12-75). This form of chronic lung disease presents insidiously over the course of several years with cough; wheezing; clubbing of the fingers (Fig. 12-76); hypoxemia; radiologic features of a diffuse reticulonodular infiltrate; and, at times, hilar and mediastinal adenopathy. Children with this condition often have lymphadenopathy, hepatosplenomegaly, parotid gland enlargement, and a longer survival than children who have opportunistic infections.

As with many immunodeficiencies, malignancies also occur in children with AIDS, although at rates significantly lower than in adults. Kaposi sarcoma (Fig. 12-77) and lymphoma have been reported in affected children, particularly in countries with endemic human herpesvirus 8, such as sub–Saharan Africa.

Other clinical manifestations of HIV include diarrhea, hepatitis, pancreatitis, cardiomyopathy (Fig. 12-78), eczema, nephrotic syndrome, and pancytopenia. HIV infection therefore presents with a multitude of clinical pictures. The clinical

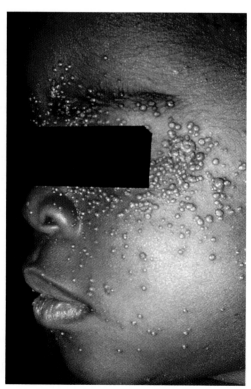

Figure 12-73 Severe molluscum contagiosum in a patient with AIDS. *(Courtesy G.B. Scott, MD, and M.T. Mastrucci, MD, Miami, Fla.)*

Figure 12-75 Lymphoid interstitial pneumonitis in a child with AIDS. Note the diffuse bilateral reticulonodular infiltrates.

Figure 12-76 Clubbing in patient with lymphoid interstitial pneumonitis and AIDS. *(Courtesy G.B. Scott, MD, and M.T. Mastrucci, MD, Miami, Fla.)*

Figure 12-78 Cardiomyopathy in a patient with AIDS. Note the massively increased heart size. *(Courtesy G.B. Scott, MD, and M.T. Mastrucci, MD, Miami, Fla.)*

pattern of disease reflects direct HIV infection, as well as the immune system dysregulation caused by the virus, including evidence of immunodeficiency and autoimmune disease. A variety of immunologic abnormalities occur with HIV infection (Table 12-4).

Diagnosis of HIV infection in children older than 18 months of age is reliably established by detecting serum IgG antibodies to a number of specific HIV antigens, using two assays. The enzyme-linked immunosorbent assay (ELISA) is used as a highly sensitive screening test. Serum reported as positive by ELISA needs to be confirmed by the Western blot assay, which, to be considered positive, must indicate the presence of antibodies against a requisite number of HIV-specific antigens. In rare instances when an HIV-infected child has a B-cell deficiency, detection of viral particles by polymerase chain reaction is recommended even if the child is older than 18 months of age. In contrast, definitive diagnosis in children less than 18 months of age relies on the detection of viral particles. This is because of the ubiquitous presence of passively acquired maternal antibodies (including IgG antibodies against HIV) in newborns of HIV-infected mothers. Accordingly, conventional antibody assays only establish exposure to an infected mother, not true infection of the infant.

Detection of proviral DNA by the polymerase chain reaction (PCR) amplification technique has proved to be a powerful tool in establishing the diagnosis of HIV infection in infants and is relied on early in life. Sensitivity, however, is only about 30% in the first week of life and increases to more than 90% by the end of the first month. A positive test should be confirmed on a separate blood sample. Two negative HIV DNA PCR tests (the first after 1 month of age and the second after 4 months of life) strongly support the absence of mother-to-child transmission. Quantitative HIV RNA amplification can also be used. Conventional p24 antigen detection is not sufficiently sensitive to make it a useful technique in diagnosing HIV infection in infants. HIV culture, although useful, is time-consuming and performed only in specialized research laboratories.

Therapy can be divided into that needed during the evaluation phase of infants born to mothers infected with HIV and that for children conclusively diagnosed with HIV. Zidovudine, as noted earlier, is used for the first 6 weeks of life to attempt to prevent transmission from mother to infant. Trimethoprim-sulfamethoxazole is used as prophylaxis against PCP until a child has had at least two negative HIV PCR tests obtained between 1 and 6 months of age or until the infected child is at least 12 months of age. Children infected with HIV who have CD4+ cell counts less than 15% of total T lymphocytes should remain on PCP prophylaxis. In general, combination antiretroviral therapy is strongly recommended for all infected infants younger than 12 months old and for all symptomatic children. The exact treatment regimens are changing rapidly and are beyond the limits of this chapter.

New therapies for HIV itself and its related complications have changed the prognosis of this disease. Although not a cure, these treatments allow children infected with HIV to grow and develop into relatively healthy toddlers and children and attend school in age-appropriate classes. Accordingly, early diagnosis and aggressive management are critical. Most important, however, is identification and treatment of HIV-infected pregnant women to improve their health and prevent transmission to the newborn altogether.

Figure 12-77 Cutaneous manifestations of Kaposi sarcoma. The purplish hyperpigmented plaques and nodules are characteristic.

Table 12-4	Selected Abnormalities of the Immune System in AIDS
Lymphopenia (more common in adults)	
Decreased helper T lymphocytes (T4)	
Decreased helper-to-suppressor ratio (T4/T8 ratio)	
Decreased T- and B-lymphocyte mitogen responses (pokeweed, phytohemagglutinin, concanavalin A)	
Decreased specific antibody response to antigen	
Increased immunoglobulin levels (IgG, IgD, IgA, IgM, IgG subclasses)	
Deficient serum isohemagglutinin levels	
Positive test for anti-nuclear antibodies	
Positive Coombs test	
Positive circulating immune complex levels	

Bibliography

American Academy of Pediatrics, Committee on Infectious Diseases: *Report of the Committee on Infectious Diseases—Red Book 2009*, ed 28, Evanston, Ill, 2009, American Academy of Pediatrics.

Barton LL, Feigin RD: Childhood cervical lymphadenitis: A reappraisal, *J Pediatr* 84:846–852, 1974.

Barton LL, Friedman AD: Impetigo: A reassessment of etiology and therapy, *Pediatr Derm* 4:185–188, 1987.

Bingham PM, Galetta SL, Athreya B, Sladky J: Neurologic manifestations in children with Lyme disease, *Pediatrics* 96:1053–1056, 1995.

Cherry JD: Newer viral exanthems, *Adv Pediatr* 16:233–286, 1969.

Chesney PJ, Davis JP, Purdy WK, et al: Clinical manifestations of toxic shock syndrome, *JAMA* 246:741–748, 1981.

Clain A: *Demonstrations of physical signs in clinical surgery*, ed 17, Bristol, England, 1986, John Wright-PSG.

Dich VQ, Nelson JD, Haltalin KC: Osteomyelitis in infants and children, *Am J Dis Child* 129:1273–1278, 1975.

Feigin RD, Cherry JD, Demmler-Harrison G, Kaplan S: *Feigin & Cherry's textbook of pediatric infectious disease*, ed 6, Philadelphia, 2009, WB Saunders.

Fleisher G, Ludwig S, Campos J: Cellulitis: Bacterial etiology, clinical features and laboratory findings, *J Pediatr* 97:591–593, 1980.

Hanshaw JB, Dudgeon JA, Marshall WC: *Viral diseases of the fetus and newborn*, ed 2, Philadelphia, 1985, WB Saunders.

Hurwitz S: *Clinical pediatric dermatology*, ed 2, Philadelphia, 1993, WB Saunders.

Krugman S, Katz SL, Gershon AE, Wilfert CM: *Infectious diseases of children*, ed 9, St. Louis, 1992, Mosby.

Lascari AD, Bapat VR: Syndrome of infectious mononucleosis, *Clin Pediatr* 9:300–304, 1970.

Leibel RL, Fangman JJ, Ostrovsky MC: Chronic meningococcemia in childhood, *Am J Dis Child* 127:94–98, 1974.

Long SS, Pickering LK, Prober CG: *Principles and practice of pediatric infectious diseases*, ed 3, New York, 2008, Churchill Livingstone.

Mandell GL, Douglas RG Jr, Bennett JE: *Principles and practice of infectious diseases*, ed 7, New York, 2010, Churchill Livingstone.

May M: Neck masses in children: Diagnosis and treatment, *Pediatr Ann* 5:517–535, 1976.

Nixon GW: Acute hematogenous osteomyelitis, *Pediatr Ann* 5:65–81, 1976.

Rapkin RH, Bautista G: *Haemophilus influenzae* cellulitis, *Am J Dis Child* 124:540–542, 1972.

Remington JS, Baker C, Klein JO, Wilson CB: *Infectious diseases of the fetus and newborn infant,* ed 6, Philadelphia, 2006, WB Saunders.

NEPHROLOGY

13

Demetrius Ellis | Yosuke Miyashita

The manifestations of renal and genitourinary disorders range from readily apparent gross structural abnormalities to subtle abnormalities of the urinary sediment. In this chapter, examples of physical findings, as well as characteristic urinary findings and radiographs, are used to demonstrate the broad spectrum of these disorders in the pediatric population.

ESSENTIALS OF MEDICAL HISTORY AND PHYSICAL EXAMINATION

The medical history and physical examination often provide clues implicating a renal or genitourinary disorder. Congenital but often nonheritable genitourinary disorders are diagnosed with increasing frequency by high-resolution ultrasonography during the second and third trimesters and may include obstructive disorders, such as posterior urethral valves, multicystic dysplasia, polycystic kidney disease, prune-belly syndrome, and renal agenesis. Oligohydramnios and fetal compression signs reflect reduced urine production associated with some of these disorders and may result in early postnatal death as a result of associated pulmonary underdevelopment. Unilateral and, less frequently, bilateral cystic dysplasia is the most common cause of abdominal mass in newborns. A large placenta may be a telltale sign of congenital nephrotic syndrome of the Finnish type, in which severe proteinuria precedes birth. Failure to urinate during the first 24 hours of life should prompt evaluation for obstruction of the kidneys, ureters, or bladder. Urinary tract infection (UTI) should be a consideration in all febrile infants, particularly during the first month, even in the presence of documented sepsis, meningitis, or other sources of infection. Urinary tract anomalies, including vesicoureteral reflux and megaureters distending the abdomen, are common in infants and young children with well-documented UTI. Children with true polyuria or polydipsia, rather than urinary frequency, may have a renal concentrating defect, such as nephrogenic diabetes insipidus, or salt-losing nephropathy, such as nephronophthisis.

Failure to thrive, lethargy, or irritability and recurrent emesis are common manifestations of renal disease in infants and may be associated with metabolic acidosis and other electrolyte disturbances. On occasion, the renal disorder is discovered because of deliberate studies obtained after discovering dysmorphic features, imperforate anus, vertebral abnormalities, fetal alcohol syndrome, or other disorders that have a renal component.

Family pedigrees may facilitate the diagnosis of congenital or heritable disorders such as cystinuria, cystinosis, oxaluria, and polycystic kidney disease and thereby lead to a variety of preventive measures before children become symptomatic. Hypertension in infants without aortic coarctation is most often a result of a renovascular disorder, such as renal venous thrombosis, arterial thrombosis (caused by embolism in patients with ventricular septal defect or patent ductus arteriosus, or a result of umbilical artery catheterization), or renal artery stenosis. Asphyxia at birth or severe dehydration, sepsis, or shock may lead to acute tubular necrosis and oliguric acute kidney injury.

Hypertension in the older child may cause headache, dizziness, recurrent emesis, epistaxis, or visual disturbances. In severe cases secondary congestive heart failure may occur, particularly if there is a history of oliguria, impaired renal function, or glomerulonephritis. Renal and renal vascular disorders account for most cases of hypertension, especially in school-age children and younger. Primary hypertension has become the most common cause in adolescents, often in association with obesity or metabolic syndrome. The presence of café-au-lait spots, neurofibromas, fibrous-angiomatous lesions of the skin, thyroid enlargement, abnormal pulses, or bruits over the renal arteries or major vessels may point to a specific diagnosis.

Gross or microscopic hematuria is the most common reason children are referred to outpatient pediatric nephrology clinics. The medical history is critical to pinpointing the correct cause of hematuria because it facilitates the elimination of a large number of possibilities. These possibilities include complications in the neonatal period necessitating umbilical artery line placement that may result in renal or aortic occlusive disease, bronchopulmonary dysplasia managed with loop diuretics leading to hypercalciuria or nephrocalcinosis, use of medications that lead to tubulointerstitial nephritis or coagulopathies, congenital heart disease leading to subacute bacterial endocarditis with secondary immune complex renal disease or thromboembolic disease, hemophilia, thalassemia, sickle cell disease, and other thrombotic or hemolytic disorders. The social history is particularly important in newborns because it may suggest child abuse, trauma, or Munchausen syndrome by proxy as the cause of the hematuria. Fever without an apparent source and symptoms of frequency, dysuria, back pain, or nocturia may suggest a urinary tract infection (UTI). The presence of hematuria or renal failure in other family members may suggest polycystic kidney disease, whereas a similar history together with neurosensory hearing loss may indicate Alport syndrome. Menarche is at times confused with hematuria.

In children with gross hematuria with or without flank or abdominal pain and absence of urinary casts or significant proteinuria to suggest a glomerulonephritis, a family history of nephrolithiasis or a history of high dietary intake of salt, dairy products, or vitamins suggests hypercalciuria. Apart from hematuria with urinary casts, an acquired glomerulonephritis may be indicated by a history of an antecedent pharyngitis or concurrent infection, pallor, edema, rapid weight gain, arthritis, or arthralgia together with a purpuric or malar rash, which may suggest a diagnosis of Henoch-Schönlein purpura, systemic lupus erythematosus, or petechiae associated with hemolytic uremic syndrome. A history of direct or indirect trauma may explain the hematuria in the active and otherwise healthy adolescent.

Failure to grow in the absence of an obvious nutritional deficit may be a sign of a chronic renal disorder in any child. Evaluation of such a disorder should include a careful urinalysis; complete blood cell count; and measurement of blood urea nitrogen (BUN), serum creatinine, bicarbonate, alkaline phosphatase, calcium, phosphorus, and parathyroid hormone levels.

URINARY SCREENING AND URINALYSIS

Urinalysis

Although the American Academy of Pediatrics (AAP) no longer recommends screening urinalysis, many pediatricians perform this as part of a well-child examination, as a prerequisite to participating in organized sports, or because of medical indications. A carefully performed urinalysis may expedite the diagnosis of various disorders and prevent the performance of unnecessary, costly, and invasive studies. For instance, a child with persistent painless hematuria without microscopic presence of pyuria or bacteriuria need not undergo cystoscopy, voiding cystourethrography, or dimercaptosuccinic acid (DMSA) scan. Alternatively, if such a child also has cellular casts, the diagnostic studies may focus on glomerulonephritis.

The routine urinalysis consists of three basic steps: gross inspection, dipstick screening, and microscopic examination.

Gross Inspection

On gross inspection, the color of urine may be described as clear, yellow, dark yellow, green, brown, tea colored, pink, clear red, grossly bloody, blue, or even black. Smoky, brown, or tea-colored urine is indicative of stagnated blood that has decomposed; the iron component has oxidized in the renal tubules. This commonly occurs in glomerulonephritis. Trauma, kidney stones, urinary tract infections, and strenuous exercise frequently result in frank hematuria. In the absence of hematuria on dipstick screening, numerous natural chromogens and vitamins found in foods, dyes, or medications may alter the normal yellow-amber color of urine imparted by the hemoglobin breakdown product urochrome (Table 13-1).

Most important, one must exclude several medical disorders associated with pigmenturia and chromogens that may influence urine color. Yellow-brown urine may be seen in obstructive jaundice and is due to oxidation of bilirubin to biliverdin; porphyria and urinary porphyrins produce a red urine color; multiple disorders leading to myoglobinuria produce a clear red-brown color; chronic lead or mercury poisoning can also result in red urine color; and conditions leading to hemoglobinuria cause the urine to turn dark brown. Several special conditions in infants and children include the following:

1. "Red diaper syndrome." This is typically the result of a benign condition such as uric acid supersaturation or overgrowth of *Serratia marcescens*.

2. "Black diapers or undergarments." In this disorder, yellow to dark urine becomes black to brown on exposure to air. This condition is also known as alkaptonuria and results from a defect in the enzyme homogentisate 1,2-dioxygenase, which degrades tyrosine, leading to tissue accumulation

Table 13-1	Causes of Urine Color Alteration without Presence of Red Blood Cells

Pink, Red, Cola-Colored, Burgundy

Drug and food ingestion

    Aminopyrine, chronic mercury or lead, benzene, phenolphthalein, phenytoin, carbon tetrachloride, sulfonethylmethane, dinitrophenol, anthocyanin, azo dyes, carotene in carrots, betacyanin in beets, vitamins, blackberries, chloroquine, deferoxamine mesylate, ibuprofen, methyldopa, nitrofurantoin, phenazopyridine, rifampin, Ex-Lax, rhodamine E, sulfasalazine, *Serratia marcescens*, urates (red diaper syndrome)

Dark Brown, Black, Orange

Disease associated

    Hemoglobinuric disorders, alkaptonuria, homogentisic aciduria, melanin, methemoglobinemia, tyrosinemia, obstructive jaundices

Drug and food ingestion

    Alanine, resorcinol, thymol, phenazopyridine (Pyridium), rifampin, warfarin, laxatives, rhubarb

Green

Pseudomonas infection, methylene blue, indicanemia, Hartnup disease, porphyria, drugs (propofol, metoclopramide, cimetidine)

Red Brown

Myoglobinuric disorders, hemoglobinuric disorders, asparagus, B vitamins

Blue

Hartnup disease, tryptophan malabsorption (indigotin, or indigo blue excretion)

and high urinary excretion of the tyrosine byproduct homogentisic acid.

3. "Blue diaper syndrome." This occurs in Hartnup disease (neutral aminoaciduria) and is also seen in tryptophan gastrointestinal malabsorption syndrome, in which indigotin or indigo blue is excreted in the urine.

Screening by Dipstick

The modern dipstick is a marvel of modern biochemistry. Each small square is chemically engineered to be sensitive, specific, and cost-effective for the substance it detects. Despite these advantages, screening by this method has been criticized as being so sensitive that disorders may be suspected in the absence of a pathologic condition, thereby resulting in unnecessary evaluation, costly studies, and anxiety on the part of the child and his or her family. It may also miss significant renal pathology that is not associated with hematuria or proteinuria.

The hematest square contains *o*-toluidine that lyses intact urinary erythrocytes, and the free hemoglobin gives a color reaction proportional to the number of erythrocytes (RBCs) present in the urine sample. The sensitivity of detecting three or more RBCs per high-power field in centrifuged urine ranges from 91% to 100%, with a specificity of 65% to 99%. Free hemoglobin or myoglobin in patients with systemic disorders leading to high plasma concentrations of such pigments also reacts with *o*-toluidine.

Protein is detected by the tetrabromophenol reagent, which relies on the principle that certain pH indicators show a different pH, or pH "error," in the presence of protein as opposed to the absence of protein. This test is particularly sensitive for albumin and less so for other proteins. Hence, significant low molecular weight proteinuria resulting from systemic overproduction or due to insufficient proximal tubular reabsorption in children with tubulopathies may be underestimated or missed by this test.

The nitrite test is often positive in children with UTI because of bacterial pathogen conversion of dietary nitrates. With proven UTI this test has a sensitivity of 35% to 85% and a specificity of 92% to 100%.

The leukocyte esterase test is often positive because of release of this enzyme from neutrophils in individuals with UTI. This test has a sensitivity of 72% to 97% and a specificity of 64% to 82%. In adults and older children (but not in infants) the presence of both positive nitrite and leukocyte esterase tests has both positive and negative predictive values that approach 100%, whereas either test alone has a much lower predictive value for UTI.

Ketones may be detected by the combined presence of sodium nitroprusside and alkaline buffer reagent, which reacts with acetoacetate (diacetic acid) and/or acetone produced by starvation or diabetes mellitus.

Specific gravity (SG), which is a measure of the total solute in urine and depends on both the concentration and molecular weight of solutes, may be quantitated by the N-Multistix SG (Bayer, Elkhart, Ind). Specific gravity contrasts with osmolality, which depends only on the concentration of solutes in urine. The SG square of the dipstick test consists of pretreated electrolytes with a specific association constant (pK_a). Hydrogen ions are released in direct correlation to the concentration of ions in the urine. This causes the pH indicator (bromophenol blue) to turn acidic in direct proportion to the ionic strength of the urine, which in turn corresponds to specific gravity. High urinary protein concentrations give a high SG value by this method. In healthy individuals, about 0.001 unit of SG equals 40 mOsm/kg H_2O. Thus, an SG of 1.010 corresponds to 400 mOsm/kg H_2O, 1.020 equals 800 mOsm/kg H_2O, and 1.030 equals 1200 mOsm/kg H_2O. Children with low fluid intake or dehydration, or those receiving hyperosmolar radiocontrast media, have high SG. Low SG may be found in healthy children with high fluid intake, or in those who are unable to concentrate their urine because of tubulointerstitial disorders or because of inadequate secretion of antidiuretic hormone.

Microscopic Examination

Meticulous examination of the urine sediment begins with centrifugation of 10 mL of freshly voided urine for 5 to 7 minutes at 3000 rpm. Such standardized preparation enables semiquantitative comparison of sequential samples in individual patients and often provides invaluable information concerning the etiology of numerous renal disorders as well as the anatomic location of hematuria or pyuria. Abnormalities commonly encountered on microscopy are shown in Figure 13-1. Dysmorphic RBCs, best seen in uncentrifuged urine by phase microscopy, are usually of glomerular origin as opposed to urologic origin. White blood cells (WBCs) coated with antibody tend to become agglutinated or clumped. Such clumped WBCs are indicative of pyelonephritis or interstitial nephritis rather than cystitis. The presence of several tubular epithelial cells is abnormal.

Scanning of the entire slide may be needed to detect small numbers of casts. Although this is time-consuming, it is a very rewarding practice because the presence of casts is indicative of intrinsic renal injury and may spare the child unnecessary imaging studies. Note that formation of tubular casts is aided by diminished urine flow, high urinary solute concentration, and the hyaline matrix of plasma- and tubule-derived protein in which cells become embedded.

Hyaline casts form on polymerization of Tamm-Horsfall glycoprotein, which is a well-characterized molecule uniquely found in the ascending limb of Henle and distal convoluted tubule. Small quantities of hyaline casts may be found in healthy individuals, but larger numbers of hyaline casts or those containing WBCs or RBCs are considered pathologic. Muddy-brown granular or epithelial cell casts are seen in acute tubular necrosis. Granular casts form from disintegration of cellular elements. These are always pathologic and may be found in most cases of glomerulonephritis. Wide casts may derive from dilated tubules, which occur in individuals with advanced renal disease.

Crystals are best identified in fresh urine that is of near-body temperature. Uric acid crystals and urates are found in urine with a pH below 6.5, whereas phosphates precipitate in urine with a pH above 6.5. Both urates and phosphates precipitate when the urine specimen is refrigerated. Crystals may be found in healthy individuals and in patients with urolithiasis or hyperuricemia, or in individuals with a specific drug intake or poisoning (e.g., ethylene glycol). Exceptions include flat hexagonal crystals, which are pathognomonic of cystinuria.

Hematuria

Isolated gross or microscopic hematuria is probably the most common symptom prompting nephrologic assessment in children. Many such children have asymptomatic microscopic hematuria often detected during routine office visits or physical examinations required before participation in sport activities. Because of the large number of conditions associated with persistent hematuria in children, several algorithms have been devised to aid in the systematic evaluation of this condition (Fig. 13-2).

History and clinical symptoms may point toward trauma, viral or bacterial cystitis, drug-induced hematuria, or other causes. Detection of the most common causes of hematuria, including glomerulonephritis or UTI, can be readily achieved by the finding of cellular casts in a carefully performed examination of the urinary sediment or by appropriate bacterial cultures. Moreover, the absence of red blood cells in a child with positive o-toluidine reagent color change on dipstick testing may lead to the correct diagnosis of conditions associated with rhabdomyolysis or hemolysis. Once these simple measures are undertaken, biochemical techniques are used to investigate renal function and hyperexcretion of metabolites resulting in nephrolithiasis, hemoglobinopathies, or bleeding diathesis, or to perform immunologic assessment of an underlying glomerulonephritis. Measurement of calcium and creatinine concentrations in a single voided urine sample should also be included in the minimal initial assessment of asymptomatic hematuria, because hypercalciuria is found in a large proportion of such children. Identification of possible disorders by such methods may help determine the need for further assessment. Thus, the finding of a nephritic sediment obviates the need for any radiologic procedures, whereas the presence of recurrent well-documented UTIs may be an indication for imaging procedures. In the absence of any physical signs, such as an abdominal mass to suggest Wilms tumor or neuroblastoma, malignancies of the kidney or urinary tract rarely present with isolated gross or microscopic hematuria. Renal ultrasonography coupled with Doppler evaluation of the renal vessels is useful in screening for the presence of tumor, polycystic kidney disease, or renal venous thrombosis in infants. Computed tomography or nuclear magnetic resonance techniques may provide detailed anatomic resolution of such masses.

Invasive cystography or arteriography is rarely necessary in the evaluation of structural lesions underlying isolated hematuria in children. A technetium-99m (^{99m}Tc)-dimercaptosuccinic acid renal scan may disclose renal scars suggestive of chronic pyelonephritis in children with or without vesicoureteral reflux. Last, a renal biopsy may be helpful in making a definitive diagnosis in cases of suspected renal parenchymal disease manifested by hematuria.

Figure 13-1 A, *Left,* Starch granules commonly seen in urine. Notice their variable size (7 to 40 μm), irregular shape with rounded corners, and central indentation. *Right,* "Maltese cross" appearance can be seen with polarized light. Talc particles have a similar appearance. Do not confuse these with lipid droplets seen in children with nephrotic syndrome and lipiduria, which are spherical with clear centers and usually measure less than 7 μm across. **B,** Mites (shown), pinworm ova *(Enterobius vermicularis),* or vegetable fibers and other fecal artifacts may be washed into the urine from the urethra or vaginal introitus. **C,** Tubular epithelial cells in a child with toxic tubulopathy due to amphotericin toxicity. **D,** Transitional epithelial cells arising from the renal pelvis, ureter, or bladder may appear "pear shaped" and can be confused with tubular epithelial cells as seen in **C.** Transitional cells are much larger in size, with smaller distinctive nuclei. These cell types may be found in very small numbers in healthy children. **E,** Yeast hyphae *(arrows)* and leukocytes in an immunosuppressed child. **F,** Wright-Giemsa staining showing eosinophiluria *(arrows)* associated with tubulointerstitial nephritis and acute renal failure in a child with hypersensitivity to methicillin. **G,** Calcium oxalate crystals *(arrows),* usually seen in acid urine, with characteristic octahedral or star-shaped pattern in a child with hematuria associated with hypercalciuria. **H,** Four-sided form of uric acid crystals; other forms include amorphous, six-sided bipyramidal or whetstone crystals. **I,** Coarse granular casts composed of degenerated cellular elements in a child with chronic IgA nephritis. Notice the typical parallel borders and refractivity of casts in general.

ALGORITHM FOR DIAGNOSIS OF HEMATURIA

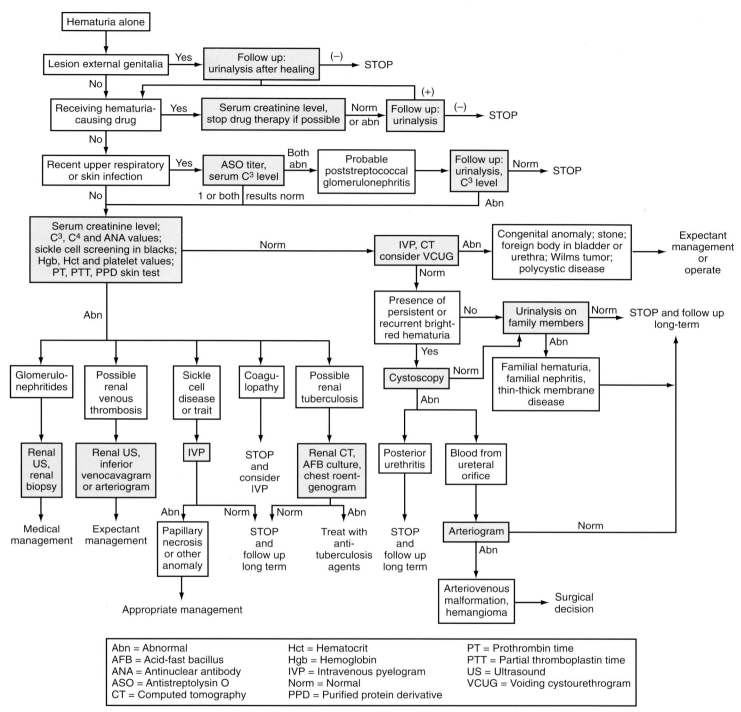

Figure 13-2 Algorithm for diagnosis of hematuria. *(From Brewer ED, Benson GS: Hematuria: algorithms for diagnosis, JAMA 246:877-880, 1981. Copyright 1981, American Medical Association.)*

GLOMERULAR DISORDERS

Nephritis and Nephrosis

In children suspected of having a glomerular disease, the urinary sediment can provide important clues that may expedite the diagnosis and help formulate therapeutic plans. A classic example of nephritic syndrome is that of acute postinfectious glomerulonephritis, in which the urinalysis reveals variable levels of proteinuria; and granular, red (Fig. 13-3) and, less frequently, white (Fig. 13-4) blood cell casts. Acute poststreptococcal glomerulonephritis is the most common and classic example of postinfectious glomerulonephritis, although other preceding infections can cause glomerulonephritis. On the other hand, the urine of children with classic nephrotic syndrome, such as minimal change disease, shows heavy proteinuria (>40 mg/m^2/hour or 1000 mg/m^2/day), free fat droplets and oval fat bodies, and little or no hematuria or other sediment abnormalities.

Acute Glomerulonephritis

Acute glomerulonephritis is characterized by the sudden onset of painless dark, cola- or tea-colored urine; proteinuria; and cellular casts on urine microscopy. Edema, hypertension, and renal insufficiency are common clinical findings and together

Figure 13-3 Red blood cell cast from a patient with poststreptococcal glomerulonephritis. These casts are almost always associated with glomerulonephritis or vasculitis and virtually exclude extrarenal disorders of bleeding.

constitute the nephritic syndrome, which implies the presence of renal inflammation. The most common cause of acute glomerulonephritis in children is acute poststreptococcal glomerulonephritis. This condition follows pharyngitis, otitis media, or pyoderma caused by one of about 10 nephritogenic strains of group A β-hemolytic streptococci. Only about 15% of children infected with these strains manifest clinical symptoms to suggest nephritis. The disorder most frequently affects children ages 4 to 12 years and is more common in males. Both humoral (immune complexes with predilection for glomeruli) and cellular factors have been implicated in the pathogenesis of this disorder. Most symptoms and signs resolve within a few weeks, although microscopic hematuria may last for up to 1 year. Complete recovery of renal function is the rule, with only a few children progressing to renal failure. Other conditions that may present as acute glomerulonephritis include IgA nephritis and Henoch-Schönlein purpura.

In some instances, these disorders may have an aggressive clinical course characterized by oliguria, hypertension, and rapid reduction in glomerular filtration rate, in which case the designation of rapidly progressive glomerulonephritis (RPGN) is given. Renal biopsy in such patients often demonstrates cellular or acellular crescents and inflammatory infiltrates.

In addition to the clinical symptoms, anti-nuclear antibody titer, anti–streptolysin O titer, anti-neutrophilic cytoplasmic antibody titer, serum immunoglobulin concentrations, and C3 and C4 levels are often helpful in differentiating several of the glomerulonephritides. Complement levels are particularly helpful because only a few of these conditions are associated

with depressed levels. The most common of these conditions in pediatrics include acute poststreptococcal glomerulonephritis, lupus nephritis, membranoproliferative glomerulonephritis, and glomerulonephritis associated with chronic indolent infections (ventriculoperitoneal shunt infection, endocarditis, and occult abscess). In poststreptococcal glomerulonephritis, the C3 levels are only transiently reduced and return to normal concentrations within 8 weeks after onset of the renal symptoms.

A typical presentation is that of a child 3 to 10 years of age, whose symptoms during the preceding few days have included mild periorbital edema, headache, and decreasing urine output. The urine is described as being smoky or tea colored. Medical history reveals that 2 weeks earlier the child experienced a febrile illness with painful pharyngitis for which he received no medical attention. Clinical examination reveals a blood pressure of 140/105 mm Hg, mild periorbital edema, and tenderness on palpation of the kidneys. A urinalysis shows the following values: 2+ protein, 3+ blood, and an SG of 1.020. Red blood cell casts (see Fig. 13-3) are seen on urinalysis. Laboratory studies are consistent with mild renal insufficiency and also revealed a protein excretion rate of 1.1 g/24 hours, a low plasma C3 level, and elevated streptozyme and anti-DNase B titers, evidence that strongly implicates a streptococcal infection in the pathogenesis of the glomerulonephritis.

Chronic Glomerulonephritis

White blood cell casts may be seen in the urine sediment of patients with acute or chronic glomerulonephritis, vasculitis, pyelonephritis, and other disorders resulting in tubulointerstitial nephritis. The cast shown in Figure 13-4 occurred in a child with systemic lupus erythematosus whose only symptom was mild back pain. Urinalysis demonstrated 2+ protein, microhematuria, pyuria without bacteria, and red and white blood cell casts. Diagnosis was confirmed by immunologic findings including low serum C3 and C4 levels, high antinuclear antibody titer, and antibodies against double-stranded DNA. Renal biopsy revealed diffuse proliferative lupus nephritis. Several acute glomerular syndromes may progress to chronic glomerulonephritis. In the final stages, many such patients develop hypertension and severe renal failure (uremia). On renal ultrasonography, the kidneys appear small and hyperechoic due to fibrosis.

Henoch-Schönlein Purpura

Three weeks after a respiratory infection, a 2-year-old boy experienced symptoms of generalized malaise, abdominal pain, periorbital edema, and difficulty walking "as if his legs were hurting." One day later he developed an ecchymotic, purpuric rash, the characteristic clinical manifestation of Henoch-Schönlein purpura (HSP). The rash covered the extensor surfaces of the extremities and the buttocks but spared the trunk. Individual lesions faded over 1 week, but new lesions appeared or recurred over several weeks. Other cutaneous manifestations of the vasculitic lesions in this disorder are shown in Figures 13-5 and 13-6.

Some patients initially develop an urticarial-type eruption that subsequently becomes macular or maculopapular. On occasion, younger patients develop an angioneurotic-like edema of the scalp, face, or dorsum of the hands or feet. Of children with HSP, 90% have a prodrome consisting of an upper respiratory infection 1 to 3 weeks before the onset of symptoms, and 80% have melena, hematemesis, and/or arthritis mostly involving the ankles and knees. About half of the patients have renal involvement ranging from simple microscopic hematuria and a variable degree of proteinuria, to oliguria and renal failure. In contrast to adults, use of

Figure 13-4 White blood cell cast from a patient with chronic glomerulonephritis.

Figure 13-5 Older child with severe Henoch-Schönlein purpura vasculitis resulting in cutaneous necrosis just below and anterior to the right malleolus.

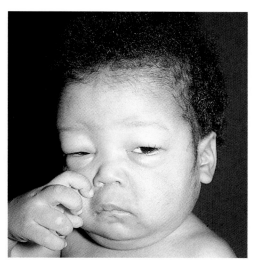

Figure 13-7 Marked eyelid edema in a 2-year-old boy with minimal change disease and nephrotic syndrome. Eyelid edema in any child should prompt the performance of urinalysis, rather than the presumption of allergy.

multiple medications is rarely related to the onset of this condition in children.

There are no distinct biochemical features of this disorder. Leukocytosis and an elevated serum IgA level may be present. In the absence of severe proteinuria, hypoalbuminemia and edema are often a result of protein-losing enteropathy. Platelet counts and coagulation studies are normal. The skin rash is essential for the diagnosis of HSP because the renal abnormalities may otherwise closely resemble a similar disorder known as IgA nephropathy (Berger disease).

Nephrotic Syndrome

Nephrotic syndrome (NS) is defined as any renal disorder resulting in marked proteinuria ($\geq$40 mg/m^2/hour, $\geq$1000 mg/m^2/day, or spot urine protein-to-creatinine ratio > 2.0), leading to hypoalbuminemia, hypercholesterolemia, and edema. Generalized edema and rapid weight gain are characteristic features of this condition, with the former showing a predilection for the eyelids, pleural spaces, abdomen, scrotum, and lower extremities (Figs. 13-7 and 13-8). Although edema usually provokes few complaints, at times it may be disfiguring, and it may produce skin induration and breakdown, or interference with respiratory, genitourinary, or gastrointestinal function. Children with NS rarely have an underlying systemic illness or a history of drug intake and thus are designated as having primary or idiopathic NS. The most common histopathologic entities of noninflammatory glomerular disorders associated with primary NS of childhood include minimal change disease (MCD), focal segmental glomerulosclerosis (FSGS), and membranoproliferative glomerulonephritis (MPGN); membranous glomerulopathy (MGP) is also encountered in older children and in adults. Examples of the pathology of these disorders are depicted in Figure 13-9, A-D.

Lower levels of proteinuria, termed nephrotic-range proteinuria, may also develop in children with acute poststreptococcal glomerulonephritis, HSP, IgA nephritis, or systemic lupus erythematosus, as well as rare patients treated with

Figure 13-6 The typical vasculitic rash of Henoch-Schönlein purpura is evident in the dorsum of the foot of this 15-year-old youngster. He went on to develop rapidly progressive glomerulonephritis and pulmonary hemorrhage that were managed by pulse methylprednisolone.

Figure 13-8 Severe scrotal edema in a 6-year-old boy with nephrotic syndrome.

Figure 13-9   Common pathologic forms associated with idiopathic nephrotic syndrome in children. **A,** Normal glomerular architecture. Notice the lacey appearance of the glomerular basement membrane (GBM) and open capillary loops. **B,** Focal segmental glomerulosclerosis. A few glomeruli (hence focal) may have a segment that is sclerosed as shown in this section stained with hematoxylin and eosin (H&E). Other lesions classified as focal segmental glomerulosclerosis (FSGS) include tip, collapsing, cellular, and "not otherwise specific" forms. **C,** Membranoproliferative glomerulonephritis. This condition is associated with low circulating C3 or low C3 plus nephritic factor, as well as immune complexes seen on immunostaining of frozen renal biopsy sections. Because of proliferation of mesangial cells, the glomeruli are enlarged and often have a lobular accentuation. Mesangial cell interposition leads to characteristic "tram track" or splitting of the GBM as shown in this light photomigrograph. **D,** Membranous glomerulopathy is evident by diffuse thickening of the GBM and associated intramembranous and epimembranous immune deposits.

nonsteroidal antiinflammatory agents and other drugs. Such individuals do not develop the other features of NS.

The clinicopathologic correlation between NS associated with MCD and its favorable response to steroids has become increasingly less important over the past three decades. For example, a landmark multicenter study of childhood NS from 1967 to 1976 (International Study of Kidney Disease in Children, 1978, 1981) found that nearly 80% of all children with NS had MCD (e.g., normal pathology under light microscopy and podocyte foot process fusion seen on electron microscopy), and the chances of undergoing remission by the use of corticosteroids was 93% to 98%. In contrast, FSGS accounted for 5% to 7% of the cases of NS and only 17% to 30% underwent remission after 1 month of treatment with an adequate daily dose of steroids. Also, the same study determined that whereas multiple relapses are common in children with MCD, late resistance to steroids occurred in only 3.3%. More recent experience has challenged this paradigm. The proportion of all children presenting with NS who respond to steroids is perhaps less than 55% regardless of the underlying histopathology, and late resistance to steroids in those with

MCD may exceed 20% of cases. Consequently, over the past 15 to 20 years clinicians use the terms "steroid sensitive" (SSNS), "steroid dependent" (SDNS), and "steroid resistant" (SRNS) to classify individuals with NS, rather than rely solely on the renal biopsy diagnosis to guide management decisions and predict prognosis. It should be noted that in addition to children with SRNS, those with SSNS who develop relapses while still taking steroids, and those with SDNS, have a high likelihood of developing SRNS. In children with SDNS and especially in those with SRNS, treatment often evolves by trial and error.

With the exception of some relatively rare genetic disorders leading to NS, the etiology of idiopathic or primary NS is unknown. Several genetic and acquired derangements in podocytes and their epithelial foot processes lining the glomerular capillaries have been identified, and are collectively known as *podocytopathies*. However, the triggering stimulus of primary NS is unknown. Activation of various immunologic mechanisms, possibly stimulated by infectious agents, is implicated. Several cytokine derangements and vascular permeability factors may also play a role in the development of

Figure 13-10 A graphic representation of the components of the slit diaphragm between two adjacent glomerular podocyte foot processes. The slit diaphragm is a P-cadherin–based adherens junction. Several molecules in this junction interact with the cytoskeleton of the podocytes. Among the known molecules in this interaction are nephrin, podocin, α-actinin-4 (α-act-4), β₁-integrin (β₁), α-dystroglycan (α-DG), β-dystroglycan (β-DG), sodium/hydrogen exchanger regulatory factor-2 (NHERF2), paxillin (P), P-cadherin (P-Cad), synaptopodin (synpo), talin (T), vinculin (V), zonula occludens-1 (ZO-1), and CD2-associated protein (CD2AP). *(Modified from Mundel P, Shankland SJ: Podocyte biology and response to injury,* J Am Soc Nephrol *13:3005-3015, 2002.)*

proteinuria. Regardless of the underlying etiology, both the duration and the magnitude of proteinuria correlate well with the development of renal injury. It is hypothesized that the protein overload overwhelms the capacity of proximal tubular epithelial cells to reabsorb and process proteins escaping the glomerular barrier, resulting in accelerated apoptosis or direct injury to these cells, ultimately leading to interstitial fibrosis. Thus, achieving remission or reducing the amount of proteinuria is a major goal of medical management.

Although genetic mutations of laminin B2 and B3 chain genes and other structural proteins of the glomerular basement membrane can lead to NS, genetic mutations leading to derangements in transcription of several proteins that maintain the structure and function of the slit diaphragm of podocytes are much more common and underscore the importance of this structure as the main barrier to proteinuria (Fig. 13-10). The Finnish-type congenital NS is the prototype of a genetic mutation of nephrin and accounts for 6.25% of children with SRNS. Podocin mutations account for most familial cases of FSGS and of steroid-resistant cases (18%), especially among African-American children. Actinin IV mutations are autosomal dominant and cause a cytoplasmic defect in the podocytes (not in the slit pore diaphragm). African Americans with a form of the specific *MYH9* polymorphism that encodes myosin heavy chain IIA have a much higher risk for developing FSGS in association with human immunodeficiency virus (HIV) infection even during the first few months of life. This may lead to poor association of myosin and actin and disruption of the podocyte cytoskeleton.

However, although genetic mutations point to the importance of aberrant protein transcription in the development of proteinuria and NS, the rising incidence of SRNS and FSGS, especially among African-American children in the United States, suggests an important contribution of environmental rather than genetic influences in triggering primary NS. Thus, acquired and therefore potentially reversible disorders of podocyte function account for the majority of cases of NS. One hypothesis implicates an alteration in the cathepsin L proteolytic pathway of podocytes so as to change cell metabolism and result in proteinuria (Kistler et al, 2010). In fact, a major benefit of cyclosporine use in primary NS may be mediated by direct protection of the podocyte actin cytoskeleton from cathepsin-mediated injury rather than from an immunosuppressive action. Such an understanding may lead to podocyte-targeted therapies. Similarly, deletion of CD2-associated protein (CD2AP), a protein that interacts with nephrin and is essential in maintaining slit diaphragm integrity, leads to NS. Genetic traits may also be important in conferring responsiveness to steroids and calcineurin inhibitors by reversing aberrant mechanisms in podocytes.

Management of SDNS and of SRNS is one of the major challenges in pediatric nephrology today. Management is limited by the lack of clear understanding of the pathophysiology of the underlying disorder and by a dearth of large-scale, placebo-controlled studies. All therapies have potential serious adverse effects. Transplantation has been a successful option in kidney failure; however, in many patients, NS may recur.

Cyclophosphamide has been recommended as the first-line drug for SDNS and for SRNS and is used for a 3-month period. Because a large number of children with biopsy-confirmed FSGS are unresponsive to cyclophosphamide, calcineurin inhibitors such as tacrolimus or cyclosporine are increasingly becoming the first-line drug for FSGS, thereby sparing unnecessary gonadal and other toxicity. Mycophenolate mofetil (MMF) is often added to help maintain remission while allowing reduction of the dosages of steroids and limiting the nephrotoxicity associated with long-term administration of calcineurin inhibitors. Angiotensin receptor blockers and angiotensin-converting enzyme inhibitors are often employed as adjunct antiproteinuric and/or antihypertensive agents in children with SRNS. Plasmapheresis to remove a putative vascular permeability factor has been applied in some individuals with SRNS associated with FSGS, with variable success.

In children with SRNS refractory to the previously described agents, rituximab, an anti-CD20 antibody directed against B cells that may have a regulatory effect on T cells, may be effective. Theoretically, bortezomib, a proteasome inhibitor that may limit antibody synthesis by plasma cells, may also have a benefit in SRNS. However, the efficacy and safety of these agents have not been adequately investigated in the setting of NS.

Steroids are also useful in managing less common causes of NS such as MPGN (see Fig. 13-9, *C*), or steroids alternating with cyclophosphamide for 6 months in adolescents with membranous glomerulopathy (see Fig. 13-9, *D*).

Because agents used to manage NS may have significant short- and long-term toxicity, investigations are currently focusing on the identification of blood and urine biomarkers as "surrogate markers" of the underlying histopathology and steroid resistance, thus permitting the earlier use of other, more effective agents, as well as monitoring of response to treatment. For example, the urine level of CD80 differentiation antigen present in podocytes and in antigen-presenting cells rises in MCD during relapses of NS in children but falls while they are in remission. CD80 is not present in the urine of children with FSGS or in healthy children and may be up-regulated by T cell–derived cytokine interleukin (IL)-13. Serum IgE also increases in children during relapses of MCD. Another study showed a rise in CD19$^+$ lymphocyte count in association with relapses of SDNS or calcineurin-sensitive NS, suggesting an important role of this cell subset in NS.

PEDIATRIC NEPHROLITHIASIS

The diagnosis of nephrolithiasis should be entertained in any child with acute onset of costovertebral angle or abdominal/flank colicky pain. In younger children, renal colic is poorly localized and is often described as diffuse abdominal pain. Small stones may produce no pain and may be detected only after an episode of painless gross hematuria, pyuria, or UTI. Thus, a strong index of suspicion is required on the part of the clinician so that appropriate diagnostic studies are undertaken. Although dietary phytate is a more common cause of endemic stones in the Far East and UTI is more common in Europe, metabolic disorders predominate in children with nephrolithiasis in the United States. Relatively few children pass gravel or stones, and the kind of crystals found in the urine are rarely of diagnostic value. The clinical history and laboratory evaluation often reveal the cause of the stones. Direct chemical analysis of the calculus may also disclose the composition of the stone. One diagnostic approach to pediatric nephrolithiasis is shown in Table 13-2.

The most common calculus found in children consists of calcium oxalate or calcium phosphate followed by uric acid, cystine, and struvite calculi. Calcium calculi frequently occur in children with idiopathic hypercalciuria, which may be manifested by painless microscopic or recurrent gross hematuria for many years before frank nephrolithiasis occurs. Hypercalciuria is found in 35 % of all children evaluated for hematuria. Screening for hypercalciuria may be done with a single voided urine specimen; a fasting calcium-to-creatinine ratio exceeding 0.21 is highly suggestive of this condition, which may then be confirmed by a 24-hour urine collection having calcium content greater than or equal to 4 mg/kg body weight. Children with hyperuricosuria, defined as a uric acid excretion [normalized to glomerular filtration rate: (urine uric acid/plasma uric acid) × plasma creatinine] greater than 0.53 mg/dL in a random urine sample, may have dysuria or pyuria, thereby mimicking UTI. Citrate is an inhibitor of calcium crystallization, and hypocitraturia, defined as less than 400 mg/g creatinine in a 24-hour urine collection, is often found in patients with calcium nephrolithiasis. Table 13-3 shows normal values of both 24-hour urine collection and spot urine samples commonly investigated in patients suspected to have nephrolithiasis and/or nephrocalcinosis.

Table 13-2	Evaluation of Nephrolithiasis

Clinical History

Family history of nephrolithiasis
Immobilization or other protracted illness or stress
High dietary purine intake
Excessive salt or calcium ingestion
Large and infrequent meals
Excessive intake of vitamins or over-the-counter medications
Symptoms of UTI or history of pyelonephritis
Source and calcium content of drinking water
Polyuria or polydipsia

Physical Diagnosis

Band keratopathy and other signs of hyperparathyroidism
Elfin facies and other features of Williams syndrome

Radiologic Studies

Noncontrast helical CT—the most sensitive modality to detect renal or ureteral stone
Ultrasound—especially sensitive in identifying renal calculi, nephrocalcinosis, and radiolucent stones
KUB—for the identification of ureteral stones; radiopaque stones include calcium oxalate and cystine

Urinary Studies

Urinalysis—may reveal pyuria or bacteriuria, inability to lower urinary pH or to concentrate the urine, or flat hexagonal crystals pathognomonic of cystinosis
Urine culture
Screening with cyanide-nitroprusside (cystinosis)
Timed or spot urine collections on two or more occasions*

Biochemical Studies

Creatinine, BUN, electrolytes, total CO_2, albumin, calcium, phosphorus, magnesium, and uric acid; plasma parathyroid hormone levels if indicated
Chemical analysis of gravel or stones

*See Table 13-3 for common urine chemical studies and their normal values.
BUN, blood urea nitrogen; CT, computed tomography; KUB, plain film of kidneys, ureters, and bladder; UTI, urinary tract infection.

Studies report significant increases in incidence of nephrolithiasis in both adults and children. However, assuming that the genetic pool of patients predisposed to hypercalciuria has not changed appreciably, one can speculate that the increase in incidence is due mostly to dietary factors, including high sodium, protein, phosphate and caffeine, and low water intake. The nonabsorptive form of hypercalciuria appears to have an autosomal dominant inheritance underlying a renal tubular defect and net loss of calcium independent of the amount of dietary calcium ingested. The absorptive form may be associated with increased serum concentrations of 1,25-dihydroxyvitamin D resulting in increased fractional absorption of calcium at the intestinal level. Premature infants receiving high dosages of furosemide to control fluid retention associated with pulmonary and cardiac disorders may develop hypercalciuria, nephrolithiasis, and nephrocalcinosis (Fig. 13-11, *A*). Other disorders predisposing to nephrolithiasis include hyperparathyroidism, cystinuria (Fig. 13-12), hyperoxaluria, defects of purine metabolism, and distal (type 1) renal tubular acidosis (see Fig. 13-11, *A-C*). UTIs and obstructive uropathy are also important risk factors in the development of struvite and calcium apatite stones.

Acute management includes pain control, increased hydration to pass the stone, and urologic procedures including extracorporeal shock wave lithotripsy, percutaneous nephrostolithotomy, and ureteroscopy. Indications for urologic procedures include persistent urinary obstruction, unremitting severe pain, struvite calculi, stones that fail to pass after a trial of conservative therapy, and urosepsis. After the acute

Table 13-3	Normal Values for 24-Hour Urine Collection and Spot Urine Samples	

Parameter, Age	24-Hour Sample	Spot Sample (Solute-to-Creatinine Ratio)
Calcium	<4 mg/kg (all ages)	
<12 mo		0.81 mg/mg
1-3 yr		0.53 mg/mg
4-5 yr		0.39 mg/mg
5-7 yr		0.28 mg/mg
>7 yr		0.21 mg/mg
Oxalate	<45 mg/1.73 m² (all ages)	
0-6 mo		260-288 mg/g
7-24 mo		110-139 mg/g
2-5 yr		80 mg/g
5-14 yr		60-65 mg/g
>16 yr		32 mg/g
Uric acid	0.56 mg/dL per GFR	>2 yr: <0.56 mg/dL per GFR
Citrate		
Male	>365 mg/1.73 m²	0-5 yr: 0.42 g/g (for both genders)
Female	>310 mg/1.73 m²	>5 yr: 0.25 g/g (for both genders)
Magnesium	>0.8 mg/kg	>0.13 g/g
Cystine		
<10 yr	<13 mg/1.73 m²	
>10 yr	<48 mg/1.73 m²	
Adults	<60 mg/1.73 m²	

GFR, glomerular filtration rate.
Modified from Hoppe B, Kemper M: Diagnostic examination of the child with urolithiasis or nephrocalcinosis, *Pediatr Nephrol* 25:403-413. 2010.

episode, management can be directed toward prevention of recurrent stones by identifying underlying cause or risk factors. Lifestyle modifications such as increased water intake, reduction of sodium intake, and a low-fat diet may be attempted depending on the urine biochemical abnormality. Use of supplements and medications are also available including potassium citrate to alkalinize urine and to increase urinary citrate, and thiazide diuretics to reduce hypercalciuria.

Renal Vein Thrombosis

Volume depletion secondary to diarrhea or vomiting (Fig. 13-13), hypotension, hypercoagulable or hyperviscosity states (hematocrit more than 65%), or indwelling catheters in the vicinity of the renal veins especially predispose infants to renal vein or intrarenal venous thrombosis. Older children with severe nephrotic syndrome are also prone to this disorder. Among children, 75% of all cases of renal venous thrombosis occur in the first month of life, and 50% of all cases are bilateral. The typical clinical features of renal vein thrombosis are a palpable renal mass in 60% of infants and hematuria and thrombocytopenia, which occur in more than 90% of the patients. Perinatal asphyxia, dehydration, and maternal diabetes mellitus are established risk factors, and hereditary prothrombotic risk factors may also play a role. Renal function may be normal, particularly in unilateral renal vein thrombosis or in bilateral disease that does not result in oliguria. The renal ultrasound is the diagnostic procedure of choice, particularly when coupled with Doppler examination of the renal and adjacent major vessels (Fig. 13-14).

VESICOURETERAL REFLUX

Vesicoureteral reflux (VUR) is an often congenital condition in which the normal valve mechanism of the ureterovesicular junction is impaired, leading to reflux of bladder urine into the ureter or kidneys. VUR is the most common urinary abnormality in children and the frequency of bacterial UTI is second only to otitis media. In a young child with UTI, such reflux of infected urine is a major risk factor for the development of pyelonephritis, renal scarring, and chronic renal damage. VUR is usually discovered after the first or second well-documented febrile UTI. Fluoroscopic voiding cystourethrography (VCUG) is the authors' preferred means for the initial diagnosis and grading of VUR, and radionuclide cystography may be done to monitor the progress of VUR.

The severity of VUR is classified according to the following international grading system (Fig. 13-15):

Grade I—reflux into the ureter only (Fig. 13-16)

Grade II—complete reflux into the ureter, pelvis, and calices without any dilation of the structures (Fig. 13-17)

Grade III—complete reflux with mild dilation or tortuosity of the ureter, and mild dilation of the renal pelvis but only slight blunting of the caliceal fornices (Fig. 13-18)

Grade IV—complete reflux with moderate dilation of the ureter, renal pelvis, and calices; complete obliteration of the sharp angle of the fornices with maintenance of the papillary impressions of the calices (Fig. 13-19)

Grade V—gross dilation and tortuosity of the ureter with gross dilation of the renal pelvis and calices; obliteration of the papillary impressions of the calices (Fig. 13-20)

Figure 13-11   A, Renal ultrasound demonstrates severe nephrocalcinosis in an 8-year-old girl who failed to thrive and showed familial type 1 renal tubular acidosis. Note the multiple echogenic shadows produced by the calcium deposits within the renal parenchyma. **B,** A staghorn calculus in the left renal pelvis of another child with renal tubular acidosis. **C,** Appearance of calculus removed at operation. The shape of the calculus generally conforms to the pelvicaliceal system.

Figure 13-12 A 6-year-old boy, born of a consanguineous marriage, presented with diffuse abdominal pain, oliguria, and mild renal failure. **A,** Plain film of the abdomen showed a slight opacity in the area of the left kidney. **B,** Renal ultrasound demonstrated a distinct shadow produced by the calculus. **C,** An intravenous pyelogram showed the relatively radiolucent stone within the left renal pelvis. Multiple small calculi produced the dilation and partial obstruction of both ureters. **D,** The pathognomonic flat hexagonal crystals found in the urine aided in the diagnosis of cystinuria.

The prevalence of VUR in healthy children is estimated to be between 1% to 3% and 30% to 50% among children with one or more UTIs. Also, VUR is more prevalent among siblings (30% to 35%) and offspring (65%), suggesting a strong genetic component. Renal scarring is fivefold more common with higher grades of VUR and ninefold higher than in those without VUR. As noted in Table 13-4, 80% of VUR resolves spontaneously by 5 years of age, but grade V VUR rarely resolves spontaneously. Hence, given the high rate of spontaneous resolution of VUR, conservative medical management of UTI with trimethoprim prophylaxis may be utilized in children with recurrent UTIs, especially in preadolescents

with grade I to IV VUR. Urology input is especially important in adolescents with grade IV to V VUR.

It has long been hypothesized that recurrent UTIs in young children with VUR lead to renal scarring, hypertension, proteinuria, and renal dysfunction, collectively known as *reflux nephropathy*. The presence of compound renal papillae in infants may predispose to intrarenal reflux of bacteria, resulting in acute tubulointerstitial nephritis (pyelonephritis) and subsequent increased vulnerability to progressive chronic renal injury (Fig. 13-21). Renal scars are best detected by ^{99m}Tc-dimercaptosuccinic acid (DMSA) scan, which is more sensitive than ultrasound and also provides evidence of

Figure 13-13 A 12-year-old boy with ulcerative colitis, who died after a bout of severe diarrhea and dehydration. Apart from dural sinus thrombosis, the left renal vein contained this partially organized clot.

Table 13-4	Spontaneous Resolution Rates for Medically Treated Vesicoureteral Reflux		
Reflux Severity, Laterality, and Age at Diagnosis*	**Percentage Resolved in 5 Years**	**Reflux Severity, Laterality, and Age at Diagnosis***	**Percentage Resolved in 5 Years**
Grade I[†]	92	Bilateral	
Grade II[†]	81	0-24 mo	49
Grade III		25-60 mo	30
Unilateral		61-120 mo	12
0-24 mo	70	Grade IV[‡]	
25-60 mo	51	Unilateral	58
61-120 mo	44	Bilateral	10

*Grade V reflux rarely resolves spontaneously.
[†]No difference by laterality or age at diagnosis.
[‡]Estimates apply only to the time of diagnosis and are not age specific.
From Bundy DG: Vesicoureteral reflex, *Pediatr Rev* 28:e6, 2007.

Figure 13-14 **A,** Renal venous thrombosis. A plethoric 2-day-old infant of a diabetic mother (hematocrit, 75%) was found to have an abdominal mass in the right abdomen on routine physical examination. Laboratory evaluation disclosed hematuria and thrombocytopenia without elevation in blood urea nitrogen (BUN) or serum creatinine concentrations. **B,** Notice the absence of venous pulsations in the lower panel on the Doppler study of the right renal vein while arterial pulsations remained intact. Subsequent serial renal ultrasound studies showed a progressive reduction in the size of the right kidney despite recanalization of the venous thromboses.

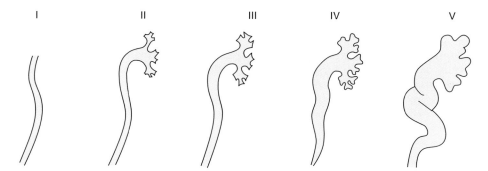

Figure 13-15   Grades of vesicoureteral reflux, schematically presented.

Figure 13-16   Grade I reflux: Cystourethrogram shows reflux only into the ureter.

Figure 13-17   Grade II reflux: Cystourethrogram shows complete reflux into the ureter, pelvis, and calices; no dilation.

Figure 13-18   Grade III reflux: Cystourethrogram shows complete reflux with mild dilation of the ureter and renal pelvis but only slight blunting of the calices.

Figure 13-20   Grade V reflux: Cystourethrogram shows gross dilation of the ureter, pelvis, and calices; obliteration of the papillary impressions of the calices.

pyelonephritis rather than cystitis. However, a renal ultrasound may be done if DMSA scan is not available. Because renal scars are frequently found at the time of diagnosis of the very first UTI, many experts believe that the abnormal appearance on DMSA may represent a focal area of dysplasia that is coincidental with VUR and unrelated to the bacterial infection. Clearly, however, new scars can be seen on prospective imaging for VUR in children with recurrent UTIs, with those less than 2 years of age being at highest risk for this complication. However, only a small fraction of children with VUR develop reflux nephropathy, despite having recurrent UTIs. Genetic variability in mounting an immune response to bacteria or in modulating the level of the inflammatory response is thought to be one of several leading factors proposed to explain interindividual predisposition to renal scarring.

While management is considered important in preventing reflux nephropathy, the management of the child with VUR is controversial. The long-term results (5 to 10 years) of the European arm of the International Reflux Study in Children are summarized by Jodal and colleagues (2006). Children less than 11 years of age, with UTI and nonobstructive grade III to IV reflux managed medically with trimethoprim prophylaxis until reflux improved to grade I, had no difference in the number of UTIs, renal growth, or renal function compared

with children randomly allocated to receive antireflux surgery in addition to trimethoprim prophylaxis. Among 302 children 40 new scars were seen during the first 5 years: 19 in the medical group and 21 in the surgical group. Only 2 further scars were seen among 276 children after 5 to 10 years of follow-up. Children managed medically tended to have higher fever with their recurrent UTIs. Children under 2 years of age had more scars (20%) than those between 2 and 4 years of age (10%); 31 of 40 children were less than 5 years old. These results were similar to those reported by Garin and colleagues (2006) in children ages 3 months to 18 years with grade I to III reflux who were managed for each individual UTI without receiving UTI prophylaxis.

Several prospective multicenter, placebo-controlled, double-blind trials designed to address the effectiveness of antibiotic prophylaxis in preventing UTI and renal injury in the setting of VUR are currently nearing completion. Based on an ad-hoc analysis of the available evidence from these studies, the AAP recently revised the previous Clinical Practice Guidelines in infants with an initial febrile UTI (Pediatrics 128:595-610, September, 2011). The main revisions stem largely from the novel finding that antimicrobial prophylaxis was of no benefit in the prevention of recurrent UTIs and renal injury in febrile infants 2 to 24 months of age with or without grades 1 to 4 VUR. Grade 5 reflux that may require surgical correction or prophylactic antibiotics was present in only 1% of the infants. Consequently, it was concluded that each UTI should be

Figure 13-19   Grade IV reflux: Cystourethrogram shows complete reflux with moderate dilation of the ureter, pelvis, and calices; complete obliteration of sharp angle of fornices.

Figure 13-21   Gross appearance of an inflamed, small-sized kidney with irregular surface due to scarring resulting from recurrent or chronic pyelonephritis associated with reflux nephropathy.

Figure 13-22 High-power view of unspun urine shows several white blood cells and a rod-shaped organism, suggestive of bacterial cystitis.

| Table 13-5 | Sensitivity, Specificity, and Predictive Values of Standard versus Enhanced Urinalysis |

	STANDARD			ENHANCED		
	Cx+*	Cx−†	Total	Cx+	Cx−	Total
Test +	21	5	26	27	2	29
Test +	11	661	672	5	664	669
Total:	32	666	698	32	666	698
Sensitivity		65.6%			84.5%	
Specificity		99.2%			99.7%	
Positive predictive value		80.8%			93.1%	
Negative predictive value		98.4%			99.3%	
Prevalence		4.6%			4.6%	

*Cx+, Culture positive, ≥50,000 cfu/mL.
†Cx−, Culture negative.
From Hoberman A, Wald ER, Perchansky L, et al: Enhanced urinalysis as a screening test for urinary tract infection, *Pediatrics* 91:1196-1199, 1993.

managed expeditiously and appropriately, and that a VCUG is of little value in infants after an initial febrile UTI. Rather than a VCUG, the newer guidelines recommend a renal and bladder ultrasound after the initial treatment of febrile UTI to detect anatomic abnormalities. However, a VCUG may be indicated after a second such infection or if the ultrasound is abnormal. The AAP has also recently recommended that the diagnosis of UTI be based on the finding of pyuria and ≥50,000 colony-forming units per milliliter comprising a single uropathogenic organism in an appropriate urine specimen.

Bacterial Cystitis

Young children whose symptoms include an acute onset of fever, emesis, dysuria, suprapubic pain, and urinary sediment such as that shown in Figure 13-22 should be suspected of having bacterial cystitis. By far, the most common organism cultured from patients with acute or chronic urinary tract infections is *Escherichia coli; Pseudomonas* or *Proteus* organisms are occasionally found, particularly in patients with abnormal genitourinary anatomy.

As noted under Urinary Screening, when the dipstick tests positive for nitrites and leukocyte esterase, both the positive and negative predictive values are nearly 100% accurate in predicting UTI. Also, examination of the sediment after urine centrifugation typically reveals greater than 5 white blood cells along with any number of bacteria per high-power field. Although these are good screening tests in older children with

symptomatic or asymptomatic bacteriuria, they are impractical in infants because of stool contamination, resulting in an increased rate of false-positive results. Screening infants for UTI has been markedly improved with the use of *enhanced urinalysis* utilizing an uncentrifuged urine sample obtained by catheterization or suprapubic aspiration. White blood cells are then counted in a Neubauer hemocytometer (Fig. 13-23), and bacteria are counted in a Gram-stained smear. UTI is then predicted based on the finding of greater than 10 white blood cells per mm³ plus any number of bacteria present in 10 oil fields examined. On the basis of results from the Children's Hospital of Pittsburgh (Table 13-5), enhanced urinalysis is more sensitive (84.5% vs. 65.6%) and has a higher positive predictive value (93.1% vs. 80.8%) than standard urinalysis in predicting UTI in febrile infants.

Although the diagnosis of UTI is established by appropriate urine cultures, the site of infection may not be apparent when considering the child's symptoms or urinalysis findings alone. In severely sick children requiring hospitalization, a DMSA scan (Fig. 13-24) may aid the diagnosis of pyelonephritis in the acute setting. We currently recommend that children with an abnormal DMSA scan undergo standard ultrasonography and VCUG under fluoroscopic monitoring to obtain the best baseline anatomic definition and to assess bladder capacity and emptying. Such studies usually define structural abnormalities leading to obstructive nephropathy or vesicoureteral reflux and are essential in planning the medical and surgical management of these children.

Figure 13-23 Enhanced urinalysis using a Neubauer hemocytometer (original magnification, ×200), showing numerous white blood cells (>10 WBCs/mm³) indicative of a urinary tract infection.

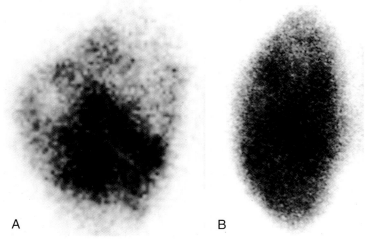

A   B

Figure 13-24 Dimercaptosuccinic acid (DMSA) scan. The image in **A** is abnormal, with numerous filling defects indicative of pyelonephritis, whereas the image in **B** is normal.

Figure 13-25   Newborn with prune-belly syndrome shows the characteristic wrinkled and redundant skin covering the abdominal wall. On palpation, no abdominal muscular tissue or muscular tone could be detected.

DEVELOPMENTAL AND HEREDITARY DISORDERS

Developmental Abnormalities

The number of congenital malformations associated with renal abnormalities is too large to discuss individually in this chapter. Renal abnormalities should be suspected in any child with one or more congenital abnormalities. In this chapter, only a selected number of syndromes are considered in which renal abnormalities are serious, relatively common, and easily diagnosed on the basis of the physical findings.

Prune-Belly Syndrome (Eagle-Barrett Syndrome)

Prune-belly syndrome usually consists of the absence of abdominal musculature, renal and urinary tract abnormalities, and cryptorchidism (Fig. 13-25). Boys are affected more severely and 20 times more frequently than girls. Although there is generally no ureteral obstruction, the ureters are dilated and tortuous, and 75% exhibit reflux. The bladder is enlarged despite low renal pelvic and intravesical pressures. Infection is common because of urinary stasis.

The major determinant of prognosis in these patients is the degree of associated cystic renal dysplasia. Intestinal malrotation is a common associated abnormality; anomalies of the limbs and heart may occur, but these are uncommon. Infertility in males is universal even when it is possible to surgically place the testes into their normal intrascrotal position. Libido and orgasm, however, remain normal. Early orchiopexy may improve the chances for fertility and prevent testicular neoplasia.

Tuberous Sclerosis

Tuberous sclerosis is a neurocutaneous syndrome inherited as an autosomal dominant trait with marked variability of expression. The full syndrome is characterized by myoclonic seizures, mental deficiency, foci of intracranial calcifications, depigmented "ash leaf" cutaneous patches, and pathognomonic skin lesions known as *fibroangiomatous nevi* (adenoma sebaceum). The skin lesion may be present during the first year of life but may go unnoticed until 4 to 7 years of age, when they take the form of discrete yellowish papules distributed along the bridge of the nose and the nasolabial folds (Fig. 13-26). Patients with tuberous sclerosis may have rhabdomyomas and other lesions in many organs and tissues. Tuberous sclerosis is caused by mutations mainly of the tuberous sclerosis complex (*TSC1* and *TSC2*) genes encoding for hamartin and tuberin, respectively. Renal angiomyolipoma is the predominant renal lesion; however, polycystic kidney disease (PKD) may occur because of crossover of the *TSC2* gene, which is contiguous with the *PKD1* gene. Although small asymptomatic cysts are common in autopsy cases of tuberous sclerosis, large renal cysts may be discovered early in infancy

Figure 13-26   This 6-year-old patient with tuberous sclerosis demonstrates characteristic papules distributed across the bridge of the nose and the nasolabial folds. He was originally diagnosed as having polycystic kidney disease because of abdominal distention and bilateral renal enlargement before the onset of any skin lesions.

and suggest the diagnosis of autosomal dominant PKD. Hypertension and renal insufficiency may further confuse the diagnosis. In such instances the diagnosis of tuberous sclerosis is confirmed by family history, the development of other features of the syndrome, and genetic testing.

Imperforate Anus

Because of common embryologic origins and the anatomic proximity of the genitourinary and lower gastrointestinal tracts, children with imperforate anus have a high incidence of genitourinary and lower spinal abnormalities. A high imperforate anus (at or above the levator ani) (Fig. 13-27) is associated with a 50% incidence of genitourinary anomalies, mainly unilateral renal agenesis, neurogenic bladder, or vesicoureteral reflux. In boys, one usually finds a fistulous communication between the blind end of the rectal pouch and the prostatic urethra. In girls, the rectum often communicates with the vagina or posterior fourchette. All children with imperforate anus should undergo evaluation of the genitourinary tract with renal ultrasound and VCUG and must be monitored for UTI.

Posterior Urethral Valves

The most common obstructive lesion of the lower urinary tract in male infants is posterior urethral valves. Such folds traverse the urethra from a point just distal to the verumontanum to the proximal limit of the membranous urethra and obstruct urinary flow with consequent enlargement of the prostatic

Figure 13-27   Imperforate anus. This newborn boy has an absent median raphe and anal atresia. On further study, he was found to have agenesis of the right kidney, severe dysplasia in the left kidney, and a communication of the blind-ended rectal pouch and the prostatic urethra.

Figure 13-28   A, Autopsy findings of a newborn with posterior urethral valves. Notice the marked enlargement and tortuosity of the ureters and the small, thick-walled, muscular bladder. **B,** An antemortem voiding cystoure-throgram shows the markedly dilated proximal urethra typical of this condition.

urethra, hypertrophy of the bladder neck, trabeculation of the bladder, and significant dilation of the upper urinary tract. Infants with posterior urethral valves may experience renal failure and profound electrolyte imbalance. Older children may have abdominal masses, voiding disturbances, or infection. Diagnosis is made radiologically by voiding cystoure-thrography (Fig. 13-28) and confirmed endoscopically. Although urinary diversion is frequently required, some patients can be treated directly by transurethral valve ablation. Surgery is usually successful in achieving urinary drainage, but in many cases associated renal dysplasia may lead to chronic renal failure during infancy or childhood.

Crossed Renal Ectopy

Children with the developmental anomaly of crossed renal ectopy generally have an abdominal mass or hematuria subsequent to minor trauma. Obstruction at the ureteropelvic junction is common. The location of the ectopic kidney may be cryptic, as in the pelvic region, and can be best demonstrated by a renal radionuclide scan. Crossed renal ectopy, renal agenesis, and/or duplication of the collecting system are often found in association with Klippel-Feil syndrome (Fig. 13-29), but have also been associated with cervicothoracic vertebral anomalies and müllerian duct aplasia in girls.

Horseshoe Kidney

Horseshoe kidney results from fusion of the lower renal poles during development (Fig. 13-30). Although generally asymptomatic, patients with horseshoe kidney may have (1) hematuria after trauma to the pelvic area; (2) midline abdominal mass; or (3) ureteropelvic junction obstruction, a common associated finding in this condition.

Figure 13-29   An infant with Klippel-Feil syndrome **(A)** demonstrates a short neck (fused cervical vertebrae) and nonfunctioning right thumb caused by lack of tendons to this digit. Intravenous pyelogram **(B)** reveals crossed renal ectopia of the left kidney, whereas the ureter from the left kidney crosses the midline and inserts into the left side of the trigone.

Figure 13-30 Horseshoe kidney. This excretory urogram was performed as part of the evaluation for gross hematuria after abdominal injury in the child. Notice the unusual and oblong configuration of the collecting system resulting from fusion of the lower renal poles.

Duplication of the Urinary Collecting System

Duplication of the urinary collecting system is one of the most common of all genitourinary abnormalities. It is sometimes familial and more common in girls than in boys. About 30% of the duplications are bilateral (Fig. 13-31) but with much variation in the extent of duplication. This condition occurs when the kidney is penetrated by two separate ureteral buds during nephrogenesis. When present, vesicoureteral reflux usually occurs in the ureter from the lower pole, whereas ureteral obstruction occurs almost exclusively in the ureter from the upper renal segment. Reflux into a duplicated system is unlikely to resolve spontaneously. These associated problems may predispose patients to recurrent infection or hydronephrosis necessitating surgical correction.

Hereditary and Metabolic Disorders

Cystic Kidney Disease

In 1990, Kissane devised a useful classification and overview of the renal cystic disorders of childhood. Only five of the

Figure 13-31 Excretory urogram shows bilateral duplication of the urinary collecting system. This child has recurrent urinary tract infection as the result of vesicoureteral reflux in the ureter from the left lower pole. Ureteral duplication is incomplete on the right side (Y-type).

Table 13-6	Syndromes Associated with Cystic Kidneys	
Syndrome		**Inheritance**
Meckel-Gruber		AR
Jeune thoracic dystrophy		AR
Short rib polydactyly		AR
Zellweger cerebrohepatorenal		AR
Tuberous sclerosis		AD
von Hippel-Lindau		AD
VATER association		NI
Renal-retinal dysplasia		AR
Ivemark		AR
Fryns		AR
Trisomy 21, 13, or 18		—
Oral-facial-digital, type 1		XL
Laurence-Moon-Bardet-Biedl		AR
Kaufman-McKusick		AR
Hypothalamic hamartoma		NI?
Lissencephaly		Variable
Prune-belly		NI?
Ehlers-Danlos		Variable
Branchio-oto-renal		AD
Roberts		AR
DiGeorge		Variable
Smith-Lemli-Opitz		AR
Turner		—
Noonan Caroli		AR

AR, autosomal recessive; AD, autosomal dominant; NI, not inherited; XL, X-linked.
From Zerres K, Volpel MC, Weiss H: Cystic kidneys: Genetics, pathologic anatomy, clinical picture, and prenatal diagnosis, *Hum Genet* 68:104-135, 1984.

most common and most important forms of PKD are presented here. Although autosomal dominant PKD (ADPKD) and cystic renal dysplasia are far more common (1 in 1000 population), autosomal recessive PKD (ARPKD; 1 in 40,000 population) is a much more serious disorder during childhood. Cystic renal dysplasia has no defined inheritance pattern and is often associated with other syndromes. Nephronophthisis, or medullary cystic disease complex, although less common than the other three disorders, is an important cause of end-stage renal disease in childhood. Renal cystic disease may also be an important component of numerous syndromes (Table 13-6) that are not discussed in this chapter.

Polycystic Kidney Disease

Many of the unique features of ARPKD and ADPKD are summarized in Table 13-7. ARPKD typically presents in infancy, although there are childhood and adolescent forms that are less severe. Severe cases can be detected by antenatal ultrasound after 24 weeks of gestation. Severe cases usually present with oligohydramnios, anuria or oliguria, and life-threatening pulmonary hypoplasia. Less severe cases can present with abdominal distention due to enlarged kidneys and renal dysfunction, mainly from tubular dysfunction. Hyponatremia often occurs in infancy and may relate to non-osmotic release of vasopressin, particularly in the setting of pulmonary disease, excessive renal salt wasting, extracellular volume contraction, and inadequate dietary salt replacement. Hypertension is very common even with normal serum creatinine level. Progressive renal failure occurs in a fluctuating course, with initial improvement early in life, with eventual decline to end-stage renal disease.

Congenital hepatic fibrosis is always present in this condition and may predominate over kidney involvement in some patients. Portal hypertension, hypersplenism, and hematemesis are frequent in such patients. In children with ARPKD, the cysts are initially small but can enlarge with age to produce palpable flank or abdominal masses (Fig. 13-32). The preferred imaging technique is ultrasound, but computed tomography (CT) or magnetic resonance imaging (MRI) may visualize cysts

Table 13-7	Autosomal Recessive Polycystic Kidney Disease and Autosomal Dominant Polycystic Kidney Disease	

Clinical Characteristic	ARPKD	ADPKD
Mode of inheritance	Autosomal recessive	Autosomal dominant
Gene	PKHD1 (fibrocystin or polyductin, chromosome 6p21)	PKD1 (polycystin-1, chromosome 16) or PKD2 (polycystin-2, chromosome 4)
Incidence	1:10,000 to 40,000	1:400-1000
Typical age at presentation	Prenatal or infancy	School age to young adulthood
Cyst characteristics	Enlarged echogenic kidneys with no visible or small cysts (microcysts)	Enlarged echogenic kidneys with macrocysts
Extrarenal manifestations	Always with liver disease, many born with pulmonary hypoplasia	Cysts in liver, pancreas, and other organs; brain aneurysm
Outcomes	1-yr survival rate: 85% 10-yr renal survival rate: 71%	Most have few or no symptoms during childhood

ADPKD, autosomal dominant polycystic kidney disease; ARPKD, autosomal recessive polycystic kidney disease.

Figure 13-32 This infant with infantile polycystic kidney disease shows marked abdominal distention and bilaterally enlarged kidneys, as indicated by the outlined area.

better. The pathology of ARPKD kidneys includes cystic dilation localized to the medullary and cortical collecting ducts. This localization is best demonstrated by isolated nephron microdissection (Fig. 13-33). Apart from management of chronic kidney disease, hypertension, and esophageal varices, eventual management may involve nephrectomy, dialysis, and often combined kidney and liver transplantation.

ADPKD, previously known as adult polycystic kidney disease, can be diagnosed in young children. Even within families, there is much variability in the phenotypic expression of clinical course, severity of renal disease, and extrarenal manifestations. With current high-resolution renal ultrasonography, up to 90% of one half of the presumed gene carriers under 20 years of age have detectable cysts. The false-negative ultrasonographic diagnosis for ADPKD in this age group is 8%. Compared with children with less than 10 cysts at the time of diagnosis of ADPKD, those with more than 10 cysts have a similar creatinine clearance but are more likely to complain of flank or back pain or urinary frequency and have a greater incidence of palpable kidneys, inguinal hernias, palpitations, hypertension, and urinary concentrating defect. Pathologically the cysts become very large and asymmetrical and involve all parts of the nephron (Fig. 13-34).

Because of the psychologic and practical implications (insurability, participation in sports), it is recommended that an ultrasonographic or genetic diagnosis be pursued only in

Figure 13-33 **A** and **B,** Cystic areas are apparent in the microdissected nephron tree shown in this photograph. *(Courtesy G. Fetterman, MD, Pittsburgh, Pa.)*

Figure 13-34 Autosomal dominant (adult-type) polycystic kidney disease. Note replacement of normal renal parenchyma by fluid-filled cysts.

Figure 13-36 Bilateral cystic renal dysplasia. Multiple cysts of various size are seen throughout the cortex and medullary regions.

children with suspected ADPKD who manifest hypertension or those participating in contact sports who may be at risk for recurrent gross hematuria that may adversely affect the renal prognosis. Genetic linkage analysis may be done for prenatal diagnosis and family planning purposes or may be limited to individuals with a family history of PKD who are asymptomatic, have a nondiagnostic ultrasound, and wish to donate a kidney.

Except for children with enlarged kidneys and large cysts detected in infancy, renal failure or nephrolithiasis caused by ADPKD rarely occurs in childhood. Similarly, extrarenal manifestations, including rupture of intracranial aneurysm, colonic diverticula, and symptomatic mitral valve prolapse, are rare. Children with acute onset of "thunder clap" headache or neurologic symptoms that suggest impending rupture or compression of an intracranial aneurysm should undergo urgent computed tomography (CT) or magnetic resonance (MR) angiography. Otherwise, screening brain MRI/MRA is recommended only for those with a family history of ADPKD and intracranial aneurysm. Suppression of arginine vasopressin and of aquaporin channels in the uroepithelial lining in the cysts may reduce renal growth and preserve renal function; thus generous water intake is recommended for patients with ADPKD.

Cystic Renal Dysplasia

Pathologically, abnormal renal morphogenesis includes processes leading to both deficient parenchyma (hypoplasia) (Fig. 13-35) and abnormally differentiated parenchyma (dysplasia) (Figs. 13-36 and 13-37). These conditions often coexist and, despite the presence of cysts, the kidneys may be too small to appreciate by bimanual examination (i.e., bracing the flank and back with the fingers of one hand while gradually

producing deep abdominal compression with the other hand). When bilateral, these renal disorders are frequently detected during the first few weeks of life. The infant usually demonstrates poor weight gain, pallor, emesis, and tachypnea. Many of the early symptoms are secondary to metabolic acidosis resulting from renal insufficiency. The amount of urine output bears little relationship to the degree of renal failure as reflected by the serum creatinine level and BUN concentration. Collectively, these conditions constitute the most common cause of chronic renal failure in children.

Patients with renal hypoplasia often have gastrointestinal, central nervous system, cardiac, and pulmonary abnormalities, but other abnormalities of the genitourinary tract are rarely present. Obstruction of the gastrointestinal or genitourinary tract is commonly found in patients with dysplasia. Less common anomalies may include trisomy 21, tracheoesophageal fistula, ventricular septal defect, and lumbosacral dystrophies.

Cystic dysplasia may be a major component of several syndromes with distinct additional malformations (see Table 13-6). Many of these syndromes have defined inheritance patterns. The overall risk for siblings of children with isolated forms of dysplasia or hypoplasia is usually less than 10%, but it may be higher if one of the parents has renal agenesis or a kidney that is affected by the same process. Pediatricians should be aware of several of the more common syndromes described in the paragraphs that follow.

Multicystic Dysplasia

Multicystic dysplasia is the most common cystic disorder in children and the most common cause of abdominal mass in newborns. It is usually unilateral. In typical cases, there is complete loss of the renal architecture, and microscopically there are primitive ducts, fibrosis, and islands of cartilage

Figure 13-35 Unilateral renal hypoplasia/dysplasia. In contrast to the normal right kidney, the left kidney is markedly small. The parenchyma in the upper pole is normal, but microscopic examination of the lower pole showed several morphologic features of dysplasia.

Figure 13-37 A less severe form of multicystic renal dysplasia involving mainly the midportion of the kidney.

representing the distinctive features of dysplasia. This is now most commonly discovered by prenatal sonography, or it may be diagnosed during the neonatal period after palpation of a "lumpy" intraabdominal mass of variable size that often transilluminates. Because atresia of the ureter is usually present, urine output and renal function depend on the presence of bilateral involvement and the degree of associated renal dysplasia. Very large multicystic kidneys can interfere with respiration or produce mechanical intestinal compression. Radionuclide scanning and renal ultrasonography are usually sufficient to establish the diagnosis.

The unaffected contralateral kidney is usually hypertrophied and has normal corticomedullary differentiation and no evidence of obstruction. Obstructive disorders, such as posterior urethral valves, urethral atresia, or ureteroceles obstructing a duplicated ureter draining the upper pole (especially in girls with wetness between episodes of normal voiding), may be associated with morphologic features of dysplasia. Biliary dysgenesis (congenital hepatic fibrosis) rarely has been associated with renal dysplasia.

Because a large percentage of multicystic kidneys spontaneously involute and are rarely the cause of hypertension, infection, or tumor development, the prevailing opinion is that unilateral and asymptomatic multicystic kidneys do not need to be removed. However, correction of any associated obstructive abnormalities that may be present in the contralateral kidney is of vital importance, and therefore patients diagnosed with multicystic dysplasia need a VCUG.

Juvenile Nephronophthisis or Medullary Cystic Disease

Juvenile nephronophthisis (NPHP) and medullary cystic disease share similar morphologic features including autosomal recessive inheritance, prominent tubulointerstitial fibrosis, and cysts that vary in number and size. The cysts are not prominent in most children, prompting the diagnosis of nephronophthisis, particularly if the disorder is autosomally inherited. The cysts usually enlarge with advancing renal failure. Juvenile nephronophthisis accounts for 2.4% of all children with end-stage renal disease in the United States. Polyuria and polydipsia as a result of a concentration defect and, at times, severe salt wasting are prominent clinical features. An ultrasound or abdominal CT scan may reveal normal-sized or small kidneys and loss of corticomedullary differentiation with or without medullary cysts. Hepatic fibrosis is probably the most important manifestation associated with juvenile nephronophthisis. Adults with this disorder have more prominent renal cysts and autosomal dominant inheritance; thus it may be more aptly designated as medullary cystic disease. Genetic testing for NPHP 1 and other associated gene mutations may be done depending on clinical manifestations to confirm this disorder.

Potter Sequence

Potter sequence can occur in any renal cystic or dysplastic disorder severe enough to produce oligohydramnios or anhydramnios. Oligohydramnios leads to a complex syndrome of fetal compression. Although chronic leakage of amniotic fluid may cause oligohydramnios, it most commonly occurs secondary to decreased fetal urine formation because of renal agenesis or severe underlying renal structural disorders. In the extreme example of renal agenesis the virtual absence of amniotic fluid during fetal life leads to pulmonary hypoplasia and fetal compression, which consequently results in abnormal positioning of the hands and talipes and altered facies characterized by abnormally small, posteriorly rotated ears; a small chin; a beaked nose; and unusual facial creases (Fig. 13-38). Such newborns have *Potter syndrome,* and they usually die of respiratory insufficiency secondary to the severe pulmonary hypoplasia and pneumothoraces.

Figure 13-38 Potter facies. This infant with bilateral multicystic dysplasia died at 12 hours of age with pulmonary insufficiency. The altered facies produced by the fetal compression syndrome of oligohydramnios includes small, posteriorly rotated ears, micrognathia, a beaked nose, and wide-set eyes. *(Courtesy T. Macpherson, MD, Magee-Womens Hospital, Pittsburgh, Pa.)*

Alport Syndrome

Alport syndrome, or hereditary nephritis, is typically characterized by recurrent hematuria, progressive renal failure, and neurosensory deafness. It is transmitted by autosomal dominant inheritance with variable penetrance. The majority of affected individuals have abnormal type IV collagen in the glomerular basement membrane as a result of an abnormal X-linked gene present on chromosome 13, known as the *COL4A5* gene. However, a number of mutations have been defined that modify the clinical expression of this disease. The classic clinical presentation is persistent or recurrent hematuria that may be recognized early in childhood. Proteinuria is absent or mild in the early stages of the disease but is invariably present as the disease progresses. The course is commonly one of slowly progressive renal failure, often accompanied by hypertension that is more severe in boys than in girls. The majority of patients with Alport syndrome have neither deafness nor ocular defects, but loss of high-frequency auditory perception occurs in as many as 40% of patients and thus may be used as a clinical marker in family studies (Fig. 13-39).

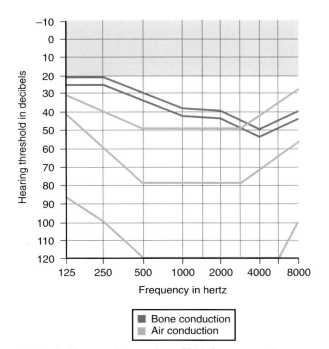

Figure 13-39 In Alport syndrome, a loss of high-frequency auditory perception may be found in 40% of patients. Because the hearing deficit may be most marked at frequencies between 4000 and 8000 Hz, it may be initially detected only by audiometric testing.

Figure 13-40   **A** and **B,** Renal biopsy of a 6-year-old boy with high-frequency hearing loss and persistent hematuria and proteinuria reveals multiple aggregations of foam cells and areas of glomerular sclerosis.

Alport syndrome must be differentiated from the many benign forms of childhood hematuria, including thin glomerular basement membrane disease, and other progressive glomerular disorders. Diagnosis relies on careful family history, genetic testing, audiologic or ocular abnormalities, renal histopathologic features such as the presence of foam cells and glomerular sclerosis on light microscopy (Fig. 13-40), and ultrastructural alterations of the glomerular capillary basement membrane (Fig. 13-41). There is no specific treatment for this disorder; progressive end-stage renal disease is managed by dialysis and renal transplantation.

Hypophosphatemic Rickets

Rickets is a disturbance of growing bone in which defective mineralization of the matrix leads to an abnormal accumulation of uncalcified cartilage and osteoid. Hypophosphatemic vitamin D–resistant rickets is an X-linked inherited disorder that, unlike other forms of childhood rickets, is clinically characterized by normal muscle tone and strength, absence of tetany or convulsions, growth failure, and the predominance of rachitic changes in the lower extremities. The pathogenesis of the disorder is still unclear, but the genetic defect is believed to be an abnormal *PHEX* gene (phosphate-regulating endopeptidase on the X chromosome; Xp22.1). This leads to failure to inactivate undiscovered hormones, termed *phosphatonins,* leading to excessive renal tubular phosphate excretion accompanied by inappropriately normal 1,25-dihydroxyvitamin D synthesis by renal tubular epithelial cells. Biochemical

differentiation consists of hypophosphatemia, normal plasma calcium and bicarbonate levels, normal parathyroid hormone and 1,25-dihydroxyvitamin D levels, and absence of aminoaciduria. The characteristic radiologic features of hypophosphatemic rickets, as in all forms of childhood rickets, include early widening of the spaces between the end of the metaphyses of long bones and an overall decrease in bone density (Fig. 13-42).

The treatment goal is to promote healing of the rickets and to increase growth velocity through normalization of serum phosphorus and alkaline phosphatase concentrations while avoiding hypercalcemia, hypercalciuria, hyperoxaluria, and hyperparathyroidism. These goals are best accomplished by the judicious combined use of oral phosphate and calcitriol. Because nephrocalcinosis and eventually decreased glomerular filtration rate may occur in association mainly with phosphate supplements, sequential biochemical and renal ultrasonographic monitoring is essential in determining the lowest amounts of oral phosphate and calcitriol doses that achieve the treatment objectives while minimizing the complications.

Cystinosis

Cystinosis is an autosomal recessive metabolic disorder caused by mutations in the *CTNS* gene encoding cystinosin protein. It is characterized by the intralysosomal accumulation of cystine in most body tissues. After degrading intracellular protein, the cystinotic lysosomes are unable to transport

Figure 13-41   **A** and **B,** Ultrastructural studies on renal tissue from the same patient as in Figure 13-40 reveal the characteristic lamellation and irregularities of the glomerular basement membrane, diagnostic of Alport syndrome.

Figure 13-42 Hypophosphatemic rickets. Radiograph of the knees of a 2-year-old girl with bowlegs. Note the widened space between the metaphyses and epiphyseal ossification center, cupping and splaying of the metaphyses of the femur and tibia, and an overall decreased density of bone. *(Courtesy M. Goodman, MD, Children's Hospital of Pittsburgh, Pittsburgh, Pa.)*

Figure 13-44 Fabry disease. The small, reddish purple papules are angiokeratomas. This young man had hematuria and minimal proteinuria but no renal insufficiency.

cystine into the cytoplasm because of a defect in cystinosin, which is believed to be the lysosomal carrier–mediated transporter for this amino acid. In its nephropathic form, the disease causes global proximal tubular dysfunction (Fanconi syndrome) and progressive glomerular damage. The clinical manifestations of this renal tubular dysfunction include failure to thrive, renal tubular acidosis, and rickets, which results from persistent urinary losses of bicarbonate and phosphorus. Also associated with this disorder are low molecular weight proteinuria and glucosuria.

Children with cystinosis exhibit a number of common clinical features not obviously related to the renal abnormalities. The majority has blond hair and a fair complexion; this, in association with growth failure and rickets, results in a strikingly similar appearance between unrelated patients. Clinical diagnosis is established by ophthalmologic examination, which detects a characteristic peripheral retinopathy, and by slit-lamp examination, which detects the deposition of crystalline material in the conjunctiva and cornea. Diagnosis is confirmed by the finding of cystine crystals in the bone marrow of affected patients (Fig. 13-43) and by the presence of elevated levels of cystine in fibroblasts or peripheral leukocytes.

Treatment of nephropathic cystinosis consists of correction of the metabolic abnormalities induced by the tubular dysfunction. Patients thus receive carnitine, bicarbonate, phosphorus and potassium supplements, and often thyroxine and vitamin D analogues. The use of cysteamine to cleave cystine

molecules and enhance their efflux from lysosomes has greatly delayed the development of renal failure and extrarenal manifestations of this systemic disorder. Thus, many children nowadays do not require end-stage renal disease therapy until the second decade of life or beyond.

Angiokeratoma Corporis Diffusum (Fabry Disease)

The diagnosis of Fabry disease is usually made in childhood by recognition of its characteristic dermal telangiectasias, especially over the trunk (Fig. 13-44). This is one of the renal X-linked disorders for which prenatal diagnosis is possible through measurement of α-galactosidase (ceramide trihexodase A) in amniotic fluid cells or chorionic villi, or by gene analysis. The absence of this enzyme leads to lysosomal accumulation of an abnormal neutral glycosphingolipid in the vascular smooth muscle of the glomeruli, heart, sympathetic ganglia, and skin. Peripheral nerve involvement results in limb paresthesias and pain. Thrombosis and hemorrhage in these vessels may result in myocardial or cerebrovascular ischemia, and progressive renal failure is usually preceded by hypertension, proteinuria, and hematuria.

Jeune Syndrome

Because many of the children born with Jeune syndrome have severe and usually lethal pulmonary agenesis, the condition is also known as *asphyxiating thoracic dystrophy*. However, many children overcome the early respiratory difficulties and may exhibit a small thoracic cage, brachycephaly, short limbs, abnormal radiologic features of the pelvic bones, and a variety of renal manifestations ranging from mild to moderate glomerular or tubular changes to microcystic renal dysplasia (Fig. 13-45). At the Children's Hospital of Pittsburgh, we have successfully performed renal transplantation in several children with Jeune syndrome and have noticed marked improvement in their growth and bone disease, as well as excellent neurologic and intellectual development.

Denys-Drash Syndrome

Denys-Drash syndrome is characterized by Wilms' tumor, male pseudohermaphroditism, and nephropathy. Because 70% of such children have nephrotic syndrome in the first month of life, they are often misdiagnosed as having congenital or Finnish-type nephrotic syndrome. However, the presence of severe hypertension and ambiguous genitalia facilitates the diagnosis of Denys-Drash syndrome and leads to early bilateral nephrectomy before development of Wilms' tumor. The characteristic glomerular lesion is that of diffuse mesangial sclerosis (Fig. 13-46). This progressive disorder leads to hypertension and hyperkalemia that is disproportionate to the reduction in glomerular filtration rate (hyporeninemic

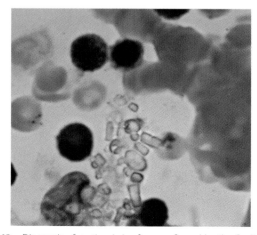

Figure 13-43 Diagnosis of cystinosis is often confirmed by the finding of cystine crystals in bone marrow aspirate from affected individuals, as seen here.

Figure 13-45   Brachycephaly, short stubby fingers, alopecia, and short stature in a 2-year-old girl with Jeune syndrome and moderate renal failure.

Figure 13-46   Distinctive glomerular lesion of diffuse mesangial sclerosis in Denys-Drash syndrome. Notice the spongy and "solid" appearance of the mesangium without proliferative changes and the obliteration of the capillary lumina. Interstitial inflammation and dilated tubules are also apparent.

Alagille Syndrome

The main components of Alagille syndrome, which is also known as *arteriohepatic dysplasia,* are absence of intrahepatic bile ducts leading to cholestatic jaundice, unusual facies, posterior embryotoxon, vertebral defects, and pulmonary artery hypoplasia. Children with this condition have high circulating concentrations of total cholesterol, phospholipids, triglycerides, pre-β- and β-lipoproteins, and elevated apolipoproteins. Thus, large lipid accumulations in the skin and other tissues are common (Fig. 13-47, *A*). Various renal abnormalities have been increasingly appreciated in association with Alagille syndrome. In one report, 18 of 26 such patients had glomerular lesions characterized by mesangial lipidosis. Although severe

hypoaldosteronism). Without bilateral nephrectomies, renal failure occurs at 1 to 4 years of age. Ambiguous genitalia are not a universal feature. The phenotypically female youngster whose biopsy is shown in Figure 13-46 had an XY karyotype and absence of testes, ovaries, fallopian tubes, and uterus on abdominal laparotomy performed at the time of renal transplantation.

Figure 13-47   **A,** Large xanthomatous subcutaneous deposits of cholesterol in the dorsal aspect of the feet of a 5-year-old boy with Alagille syndrome. **B,** Renal failure occurred secondary to diffuse renal arteriolar occlusion in lipid-laden endothelial cells and macrophages. **C,** Striking autofluorescence of the lipids is seen within such occluded vessels.

renal dysfunction is uncommon, children surviving advanced stages of liver failure may also develop severe renal failure. The latter may occur in association with liver failure ("hepatorenal syndrome") or may result from marked occlusion of renal arteries by lipid-laden or foam cells as shown in Figure 13-47, *B* and *C*.

RENOVASCULAR HYPERTENSION

Renal Artery Stenosis

Although only 5% of pediatric hypertension is caused by renal artery stenosis, detection of this abnormality is particularly important because a cure usually can be achieved. The basic pathophysiology of all renovascular hypertension involves activation of the renin–angiotensin–aldosterone system. If a lesion in the minor or major branches of the renal artery significantly decreases renal perfusion pressure, it causes increased renin release from the affected kidney. The high plasma renin activity leads to increases in angiotensin II levels with subsequent increases in total peripheral vascular resistance. This also leads to increased adrenal aldosterone production with resultant renal sodium and water retention and expansion in extracellular fluid volume.

Renovascular hypertension should be suspected in any hypertensive child with the physical finding of high-pitched bruits heard in the flank or abdominal areas or when stigmata of syndromes associated with arterial abnormalities are present (e.g., homocystinuria, Marfan syndrome, neurofibromatosis type 1, and Williams syndrome). Patients with renovascular hypertension may show abnormalities on radionuclide renal scans, Doppler interrogation of the renal arteries, or elevated plasma renin activity. Renal artery angiogram is the diagnostic study, but CT or MR angiograms are usually performed first in patients with suspected renovascular hypertension.

Intrinsic diseases of the renal artery include fibromuscular dysplasia, thrombotic and embolic lesions, aneurysms, arteritis, and arteriosclerosis. The lesions of fibromuscular dysplasia involve multiple areas of stenosis alternating with aneurysmal dilation in the distal two thirds of the main renal artery (Fig. 13-48). Pheochromocytoma and neurofibromatosis may also be associated with renal artery disease. Although difficult to differentiate from fibromuscular dysplasia histologically, the narrowing of the renal artery associated with neurofibromatosis generally begins within 1 cm of the origin from the aorta, distinguishing it from the distal involvement of fibromuscular dysplasia (Fig. 13-49). The majority of pediatric patients with polyarteritis nodosa have renal involvement with hypertension, which leads to arterial lesions characterized by multiple

Figure 13-49 Arteriogram of a 13-year-old patient with neurofibromatosis, mild mental retardation, and a blood pressure of 140/100 shows narrowing of the renal artery close to its origin from the aorta, in contrast to the distal involvement of fibromuscular dysplasia.

thrombi and aneurysms (Fig. 13-50). Such arteriographic findings are diagnostic in the child with hypertension accompanied by weight loss, fever, and systemic manifestations of diffuse arteritis.

Correction of renovascular hypertension caused by intrinsic disease of the renal artery includes surgical revascularization of the kidneys or dilation of discrete stenoses by transluminal angioplasty. Diffuse arteritis, which may cause renovascular hypertension in children with underlying systemic diseases, is treated medically with corticosteroids, immunosuppressives, or anticoagulants depending on the nature of the primary disease process. Young children with bilateral renal artery stenosis together with coarctation of the abdominal aorta represent a challenging management problem. The small-caliber vessels and possible scarring in the vessel walls render bypass or reconstructive surgery a most difficult task. Transluminal angioplasty is also ineffective in many cases. This problem has been successfully managed by staged bypass of the coarctation and autotransplantation of one kidney, followed by autotransplantation of the remaining kidney at a later time.

Hirsutism

Although there are many endocrinologic causes of hirsutism, a number of drugs used in children with renal disorders are capable of producing this condition. Marked hirsutism generally accompanies the use of minoxidil or diazoxide, which are potent antihypertensive agents causing direct relaxation of arteriolar smooth muscle. Cyclosporine, used widely to combat tissue allograft rejection after organ transplantation, has a dose-dependent effect on hair growth, whereas tacrolimus causes

Figure 13-48 Arteriogram of a 12-year-old patient with malignant hypertension shows multiple areas of stenosis alternating with aneurysmal dilation in the distal segment of the renal artery, characteristic of fibromuscular dysplasia.

Figure 13-50 This arteriogram is from a 12-year-old girl with weight loss, fever, abdominal pain, and malignant hypertension. Note the diagnostic features of renal involvement with polyarteritis nodosa, characterized by multiple thrombi and aneurysms.

Figure 13-51   Autonomous hyperparathyroidism and severe renal osteodystrophy in a 6-year-old boy with renal failure caused by posterior urethral valves. **A,** Bossing of the occiput. **B,** Radiograph shows distal femoral and proximal tibial areas, as well as subperiosteal erosion of the cortical bone and active rickets in the epiphyseal ossification centers.

minimal hirsutism. Hirsutism and alteration in body image may be a major determinant of drug compliance, particularly in adolescent patients undergoing organ transplantation.

CHRONIC RENAL FAILURE

Secondary Hyperparathyroidism

Also known as renal osteodystrophy or "renal rickets," secondary hyperparathyroidism is the osseous manifestation of chronic renal failure and results primarily from two major pathologic processes: (1) relative deficiency of 1,25-dihydroxyvitamin D, which leads to impaired mineralization of cartilage and bone, resulting in rickets and osteomalacia; and (2) an excess of parathyroid hormone, which leads to osteitis fibrosa cystica, the classic bone disease of primary hyperparathyroidism. In any given patient each of these pathologic processes may occur with varying severity, giving a wide range of clinical and radiologic presentations. In children, the condition is clinically characterized by growth retardation, bone pain, and deformity of long bones. The radiologic features in children include increased thickness and fraying of the radiolucent zone in the region of growth plates; subperiosteal erosion of the cortices of long bones and phalanges; and changes in bone density

including osteoporosis, osteosclerosis, or coarsening of the trabecular pattern of long bones (Fig. 13-51) or, rarely, brown tumors (Fig. 13-52).

Prevention or treatment of this disorder consists of hormone replacement and aggressive medical control of the mineral imbalance, metabolic acidosis, and malnutrition. When the glomerular filtration rate decreases below 50 mL/minute/ 1.73 m², these children are often begun on commercially available 1,25-dihydroxyvitamin D_3, which is normally synthesized by healthy kidneys. A combination of low-phosphorus diet and calcium carbonate or calcium acetate preparations is given to reduce intestinal absorption of dietary phosphate while simultaneously providing calcium supplementation and intestinal acid–neutralizing capacity, which helps to control the metabolic acidosis and hydrogen deposition in bone.

Anemia of Renal Failure

Severe anemia in chronic renal failure is caused by the inability of the damaged kidneys to secrete sufficient amounts of erythropoietin. In untreated children with end-stage renal failure, the hemoglobin levels are often lower than in adults (5 to 7 g/dL), and severely limit their tolerance of physical activity. Good overall nutrition and replacement of folic acid

Figure 13-52   **A,** This 5-year-old boy with moderate renal failure secondary to obstructive uropathy was admitted for evaluation of loose teeth, marked protrusion of the mandible, and exploration of a radiolucent mandibular tumor. **B,** Surgery was canceled after biochemical evaluation was consistent with renal osteodystrophy. Biopsy revealed a brown tumor resulting from intense osteoclastic activity and bone resorption. Medical treatment resulted in regression of the tumor and the prognathia, bone remineralization, strengthening of the dental ridge, and dental preservation.

Figure 13-53 Facial and radiologic features of the anemia of renal failure and extramedullary erythropoiesis in the same child shown in Figure 13-52. Notice the thickened cranial table with the brushlike projections.

and other erythroactive water-soluble vitamins lost through dialysis treatments only partially obviate the need for blood transfusions. Thus many patients develop the facial features and radiographic appearance of Cooley anemia (Fig. 13-53). Use of recombinant erythropoietin has resulted in a marked improvement in the quality of life while preventing hemosiderosis, allergic reactions, infections, and other risks associated with frequent blood transfusions.

Growth Failure

Growth failure remains a major problem for children receiving dialysis and may persist after successful renal transplantation. Although there is adequate synthesis of endogenous growth hormone and its tissue-active form, insulin-like growth factor-1 (IGF-1), the latter is bound by circulating IGF-1-binding protein-3, which accumulates in chronic kidney disease, thereby decreasing the free form of IGF-1. Recombinant human growth hormone therapy has been extremely efficacious in overcoming this functional resistance and in promoting the growth of such children.

Bibliography

Alagille D, Estrada A, Hadchouel M, et al: Syndromic paucity of interlobular bile ducts (Alagille syndrome or arteriohepatic dysplasia): review of 80 cases, *J Pediatr* 110:195–200, 1987.

American Medical Association, Board of Trustees: Clinical laboratory tests and standards, *JAMA* 255:373, 1986.

Bhimma R: *Acute poststreptococcal glomerulonephritis* (website). http://emedicine.medscape.com/article/980685-overview. Accessed September 2011.

Bradley M, Schumann B: Examination of urine. In Henry JB, editor: *Todd-Sanford-Davidsohn clinical diagnosis by laboratory methods*, Philadelphia, 1984, WB Saunders, p 380.

Brewer ED, Benson GS: Hematuria: algorithms for diagnosis, *JAMA* 246:877–880, 1981.

Committee on Practice and Ambulatory Medicine and Bright Futures Steering Committee: recommendations for preventive pediatric health care, *Pediatrics* 120:1376, 2007.

Committee on Quality Improvement Subcommittee Urinary Tract Infection: Practice parameter: The diagnosis, treatment, and evaluation of the initial urinary tract infection in febrile infants and young children, *Pediatrics* 103:843–852, 1999.

Coulthard MG: Vesicoureteric reflux is not a benign condition, *Pediatr Nephrol* 24:227–232, 2009.

Faul C, Donnelly M, Merscher-Gomez S, et al: The actin cytoskeleton of kidney podocytes is a direct target of the antiproteinuric effect of cyclosporine A, *Nat Med* 14:931–938, 2008.

Fogazzi GB: Crystalluria: a neglected aspect of urinary sediment analysis, *Nephrol Dial Transplant* 11:379–387, 1996.

Frick GM, Gabow PA: Hereditary and acquired cystic disease of the kidney, *Kidney Int* 46:951–964, 1994.

Garin EH, Olavarria F, Garcia Nieto V, et al: Clinical significance of primary vesicoureteral reflux and urinary antibiotic prophylaxis after acute pyelonephritis: a multicenter, randomized, controlled study, *Pediatrics* 117:626–632, 2006.

Gilli G, Berry AC, Chantler C: Syndromes with a renal component. In Holliday MA, Barratt TM, Vernier RL, editors: *Pediatric nephrology*, ed 2, Baltimore, 1987, Williams & Wilkins.

Goldraich NP, Goldraich IH: Update on dimercaptosuccinic acid renal scanning in children with urinary tract infection, *Pediatr Nephrol* 9:221–226, 1995.

Graff L, editor: *A handbook of routine urinalysis*, Philadelphia, 1983, JB Lippincott.

Habib R, Dommergues JP, Gubler MC, et al: Glomerular mesangiolipidosis in Alagille syndrome (arteriohepatic dysplasia), *Pediatr Nephrol* 1:455–464, 1987.

Harms E: Prenatal diagnosis of inborn errors of metabolism with renal manifestations, *Pediatr Nephrol* 1:540–545, 1987.

Hodson EM, Craig JC: Therapies for steroid-resistant nephrotic syndrome, *Pediatr Nephrol* 23:1391–1394, 2008.

Hoppe B, Kemper M: Diagnostic examination of the child with urolithiasis or nephrocalcinosis, *Pediatr Nephrol* 25:403–413, 2010.

International Study of Kidney Disease in Children: Nephrotic syndrome in children: prediction of histology from clinical and laboratory characteristics at time of diagnosis, *Kidney Int* 13:159–165, 1978.

International Study of Kidney Disease in Children: The primary nephrotic syndrome in children: identification of patients with minimal change nephrotic syndrome from initial response to prednisone, *J Pediatr* 98:561–564, 1981.

Jensen JC, Ehrlich RM, Hanna MK, et al: A report of four patients with the Drash syndrome and a review of the literature, *J Urol* 141:1174–1176, 1989.

Jodal U, Smellie JM, Lax H, et al: Ten-year results of randomized treatment of children with severe vesicoureteral reflux: final report of the International Reflux Study in Children, *Pediatr Nephrol* 21:785–792, 2006.

Kaplan BS, Kaplan P, Rosenberg HK, et al: Polycystic kidney disease in childhood, *J Pediatr* 22:867–880, 1989.

Kaplan MR: Hematuria in childhood, *Pediatr Rev* 5:99–105, 1983.

Kim JS, Bellew CA, Silverstein DM, et al: High incidence of initial and late steroid resistance in childhood nephrotic syndrome, *Kidney Int* 68:1275–1281, 2005.

Kissane JM: Renal cysts in pediatric patients: a classification and overview, *Pediatr Nephrol* 4:69–77, 1990.

Kistler AD, Peev V, Forst A-L, et al: Enzymatic disease of the podocyte, *Pediatr Nephrol* 25:1017–1023, 2010.

Lau KK, Stoffman JM, Williams S: Neonatal renal vein thrombosis: Review of the English-language literature between 1992 and 2006, *Pediatrics* 120:e1278–e1284, 2007.

Laufer J, Boichis H: Urolithiasis in children: current medical management, *Pediatr Nephrol* 3:317–331, 1989.

Mayo Clinic Staff: *Urine color* (website). http://www.mayoclinic.com/health/urine-color/DS01026. Accessed September 2011.

McCrory WW: Glomerulonephritis, *Pediatr Rev* 5:19–25, 1983.

Meyers KEC: Evaluation of hematuria in children, *Urol Clin North Am* 31:559–573, 2004.

Mollet G, Ratelade J, Boyer O, et al: Podocin inactivation in mature kidneys causes focal segmental glomerulosclerosis and nephrotic syndrome, *J Am Soc Nephrol* 20:2181–2189, 2009.

Montini G, Hewitt I: Urinary tract infections: to prophylaxis or not to prophylaxis? *Pediatr Nephrol* 24:1605–1609, 2009.

Niaudet P: *Autosomal recessive and dominant polycystic kidney disease in children.* UpToDate (website). http://www.uptodate.com/contents/autosomal-recessive-polycystic-kidney-disease-in-children?source=search_result&selectedTitle=43%7E150. Accessed September 2011.

Niaudet P: Long-term outcome of children with steroid-sensitive idiopathic nephrotic syndrome, *Clin J Am Soc Nephrol* 4:1547–1548, 2009.

Peters CA, Skoog SJ, Arant BS, et al: Summary of the AUA guideline on management of primary vesicoureteral reflux in children, *J Urol* 184:1134–1144, 2010.

Sibley RK, Mohan J, Mauer SM, et al: A clinicopathologic study of forty-eight infants with nephrotic syndrome, *Kidney Int* 27:544–552, 1985.

Smith J, Stapleton FB: *Epidemiology of and risk factors for nephrolithiasis in children.* UpToDate (website). http://www.uptodate.com/contents/epidemiology-of-and-risk-factors-for-nephrolithiasis-in-children. Accessed September 2011.

Strauss J, Abitbol C, Zilleruelo G, et al: Renal disease in children with the acquired immunodeficiency syndrome, *N Engl J Med* 321:625–630, 1989.

Subcommittee on Urinary Tract Infection, Steering Committee on Quality Improvement and Management: Urinary tract infection: clinical practice guideline for the diagnosis and management of the initial UTI in febrile infants and children 2 to 24 months, *Pediatrics* 128:595–610, 2011.

Zerres K: Genetics of cystic kidney disease, *Pediatr Nephrol* 1:397–404, 1987.

14

UROLOGIC DISORDERS

Mark F. Bellinger

Many congenital urologic malformations and acquired disorders, and the results of common urologic surgical procedures, may produce visible or palpable findings on physical examination. Some clinical presentations are unique. In other cases, disorders of varying etiology may present similar signs, symptoms, and physical findings. Differential diagnosis is essential to an appreciation of pediatric urologic disorders.

PHYSICAL EXAMINATION

Items of patient and family history may prove to be important in consideration of the differential diagnosis of urologic disorders. A family history of urinary infection, hydronephrosis, vesicoureteric reflux, cystic kidney disease, compromised fertility, or genital malformation may indicate the presence of heritable urinary anomaly.

Examination begins with a general overview of the patient. Hemihypertrophy, congenital scoliosis, an abnormal gait, facial or external ear deformities, or the presence of multiple congenital anomalies may be associated with urologic disorders. Abdominal examination should begin with inspection for visible masses, followed by gentle palpation. Enlarged kidneys are usually palpable as upper abdominal or flank masses in small children and infants, but may be difficult to appreciate in older children. An enlarged bladder or lesion of gynecologic origin may be palpable as a midline mass arising out of the pelvis. Abdominal masses should be characterized as cystic or solid; smooth, lobulated, or irregular; fixed or mobile; and tender or nontender. The abdominal portion of an abdominoscrotal hydrocele may be palpable in the left or right lower quadrant, and may increase in size when the scrotal component (large hydrocele) is compressed (Fig. 14-1).

The inguinal areas should be examined for palpable gonads. Gonads palpable in the groin are frequently quite mobile and may move during examination from the inguinal canal almost into the scrotum, or lateral to the scrotum toward the perineum. They may also move from a palpable position in the groin to disappear into the abdomen during examination; therefore high testes may be palpable on one examination and nonpalpable on the next. The sensitivity of palpation for detection of inguinal testes and other masses may be increased by the use of soap or lubricant on the examiner's fingers. It may be difficult to palpate an inguinal testis by trying to "pinch" it between the fingers, whereas lubricated fingers gliding over the inguinal canal may easily detect a gonad as it slides beneath the fingers. The best technique is to place the fingers flat, over the inguinal canal and above the level of the internal inguinal ring, and slide them slowly toward the pubis, then over the pubis toward the scrotum and down over the perineum lateral to the upper scrotum. On occasion, a vas and spermatic cord palpable in the groin (most notably where it passes over the pubic tubercle) may end in a small "nubbin" (remnant of an atrophic testis), which may be palpated in the upper scrotum or just above the scrotum. The structures of the inguinal canal should be examined in a similar fashion to detect thickening of the cord structures that may be seen in the presence of an inguinal hernia or communicating hydrocele. Masses in the inguinal canal may also represent an inguinal hernia containing bowel, omentum, or bladder (or ovary in girls, perhaps a testis in a phenotypic female with androgen insensitivity) (Fig. 14-2), communicating hydrocele or hydrocele of the cord, or malignancy of the paratesticular tissues or cord structures (i.e., sarcoma). Inguinal lymphadenopathy is usually detected lateral to the inguinal canal.

Genital examination should include both inspection and palpation. The penis should be of appropriate length and diameter. Penile stretch length can be determined by using a ruler or tongue blade pressed against the pubic symphysis as the penis is gently stretched alongside it and the position of the tip of the glans marked for measurement. A concealed or buried penis may occur after circumcision or may be congenital. In most cases, hidden penises are retractile, in large part due to a thick suprapubic fat pad. Most cases of buried penis will resolve with time, whereas in severe cases the tethering may be due to dysgenetic fascial attachments and will require surgical correction. It may be difficult to determine the difference between the two in younger boys. Penoscrotal fusion or webbing may also cause an anomalous appearance and entrapment of the penis (see Fig. 14-32).

The foreskin should be examined for adhesions to the glans, which may represent merely residual preputial fusion to the glans that will resolve spontaneously, or preputial skin bridges, which can occur after circumcision and require surgical division. The urethral meatus should be examined for size and location. The presence of chordee (ventral penile curvature) or a suggestion of its presence should be noted. The size and degree of development of the scrotum and the location and size of the testes are determined.

Retractile testes should come well into the dependent portion of the scrotum when the room is warm and the patient is relaxed. If it is difficult to determine whether the testes are undescended, retractile, or normal, repeat examination may be helpful. The epididymis should be palpated and examined for tenderness or the presence of masses. The spermatic cords should be examined for the presence of abnormal findings (thickening, masses, varicocele). The cord is most easily examined as it crosses over the pubic tubercle. Male patients should be examined in both the supine position and in the standing position with and without Valsalva maneuver.

In the female patient the introitus should be inspected to confirm a normal size and location of the clitoris, the urethral meatus, the vaginal introitus, and hymenal ring. Labial masses, swelling, or adhesions (fusion) may completely conceal the introitus. Lysis of labial adhesion may be necessary to allow examination of the introitus. Masses protruding from the urethral meatus or located near or originating in the vicinity of the meatus should be noted. Vaginal or urethral discharge, the presence of hymenal tags, or an imperforate hymen may be

Figure 14-1 Bilateral abdominoscrotal hydrocele in an infant. Bilateral large hydroceles extend up the inguinal canals. The *blue dots* on the abdomen mark the upper limits of the abdominal portion of the hydroceles.

Figure 14-2 Androgen insensitivity. Left inguinal testis in an XY phenotypic female with androgen insensitivity.

seen. Posterior displacement of the vaginal introitus with a short or mucosalized perineal body is abnormal. The appearance and position of the anus should be noted. Rectal examination may be performed to assess sphincter tone or to help characterize abdominal or pelvic masses.

The lower back should be examined for hair tufts, clefts, sinus tracts, or other signs of spinal dysraphism. A general neurologic examination and testing of the anal wink, bulbocavernosus reflex, and lower extremity reflexes should be performed, especially if neurovesical dysfunction is suspected. The bulbocavernosus reflex is assessed by a brisk squeeze of the glans penis or clitoris or a tug on an indwelling Foley catheter. A positive response, which indicates an intact sacral reflex arc, is indicated by reflex contraction of the anal sphincter and bulbocavernosus muscle. Absence of the reflex strongly suggests the presence of a sacral neurologic lesion.

ANTENATAL URINARY TRACT DILATION

Detection of urinary tract dilation (hydronephrosis, hydroureteronephrosis, pyelectasis, pyelocaliectasis) in the fetus is common, either during screening for a fetal anomaly or as a serendipitous finding (Fig. 14-3). All fetal urinary tract dilation demands some degree of postnatal evaluation. Most cases of hydronephrosis, even of a significant degree, are not detectable by physical examination of the neonate. Because only the most severe cases present as an abdominal or flank mass, a distended bladder, or generalized increase in abdominal girth and thus lead to immediate uroradiologic evaluation, most questions surround those infants with modest fetal hydronephrosis and a normal postnatal physical examination. All infants with fetal urinary dilation should have postnatal ultrasonography. In severe bilateral cases, ultrasound may be

Figure 14-3 Fetal hydronephrosis. **A,** Fetal ultrasonography performed to assess gestational age reveals bilateral fetal hydronephrosis and a distended bladder. **B,** Voiding cystourethrogram reveals posterior urethral valves and severe bilateral vesicoureteric reflux. BL, bladder; LT, left kidney; RT, right kidney.

Figure 14-4 Postnatal hydronephrosis. **A,** Intravenous pyelogram at 1 month of age shows incomplete left ureteral duplication with hydroureteronephrosis of both ureters. **B,** Intravenous pyelogram at 4 months of age without surgical intervention reveals spontaneous improvement in hydroureteronephrosis. Subsequent diuresis renogram showed equal renal function and prompt washout; the hydronephrosis completely resolved by 2 years of age.

performed urgently, whereas in less severe hydronephrosis, ultrasound examination may best be performed 3 to 10 days after delivery to allow increased urine production to fill out dilated systems that may be relatively decompressed in the immediate postnatal period, especially in a relatively dehydrated infant. When postnatal ultrasound is normal (spontaneous resolution of fetal hydronephrosis occurs in up to 20% of cases) (Fig. 14-4), follow-up ultrasound should be performed at several months and perhaps at 1 year because delayed reappearance of dilation has been reported.

When postnatal hydronephrosis is documented, complete radiographic evaluation is indicated (an exception may be made in very mild cases of pyelectasis in males who may require only limited ultrasound follow-up). If dilation is severe, renal function poor, or coexistent anomalies demand it, evaluation should be performed as soon as possible. Voiding cystourethrography is an integral part of the evaluation of every infant with hydronephrosis and should be the first study performed in all cases to rule out both infravesical obstruction and vesicoureteric reflux (see Fig. 14-3, *B*). Subsequent evaluation by intravenous urography, radionuclide scan, or both may be appropriate to assess function and to document whether true obstruction or mere dilation is present. If the infant is in stable condition (particularly when the lesion is unilateral or moderate in degree with good renal function), radionuclide evaluation should be delayed for 4 to 6 weeks or longer to allow improved glomerular filtration, making studies more accurate. If nonobstructive dilation is documented, long-term follow-up may document gradual resolution of the hydronephrosis in some cases and persistent dilation in others.

POSTERIOR URETHRAL VALVES

Valvular obstruction of the posterior urethra is a common cause of infravesical obstruction in males. Presentation may be associated with prenatal hydronephrosis (see Fig. 14-3), urinary tract infection, incontinence, or renal failure. Although the classic presentation of infants and older children with urethral valves is a diminished urinary stream, few children are actually evaluated because of this symptom. Neonates may present with severe pulmonary hypoplasia and renal failure or with bladder distention and hydroureteronephrosis. Older boys with unrecognized urethral valves may present with symptoms ranging from incontinence to renal failure. Voiding cystourethrography is the key to the diagnosis of urethral valves. In most cases endoscopic fulguration of urethral valves is undertaken (Fig. 14-5, *A-C*). In some cases cutaneous vesicostomy may be indicated, especially in tiny babies in whom

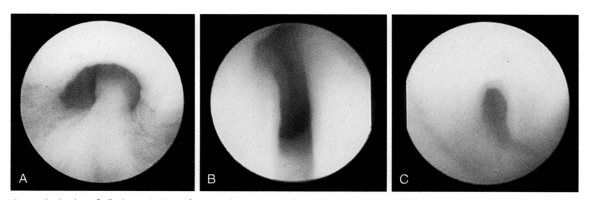

Figure 14-5 Posterior urethral valves. **A,** Endoscopic view of a normal posterior urethra and verumontanum. **B,** Type II urethral valves. The sail-like right and left leaflets are partially disrupted superiorly. **C,** Type III urethral valves. These almost complete iris-diaphragm valves cause a more significant obstruction than type II leaflets.

urethral instrumentation may be problematic. Rarely is upper tract diversion (ureterostomy or pyelostomy) indicated. The ultimate prognosis for renal function depends on the state of the renal parenchyma (whether or not dysplasia is present) and of bladder compliance (poorly compliant bladders with diminished elasticity may fail to allow reflux or hydronephrosis to improve after valve ablation and may be associated with a worse prognosis for continence and renal function).

CRYPTORCHIDISM

Cryptorchidism occurs in approximately 33% of premature and 3% of full-term boys. Observing gradual testicular descent over several weeks in a premature infant is not unusual. Cryptorchidism is associated with many syndromes but rarely with urinary tract anomalies. The exception is true congenital monorchism, which may be associated with ipsilateral renal agenesis. Renal ultrasound is indicated. In most cases of an absent testis, however, spermatic structures are present, which indicate that the testis was formed but subsequently atrophied due to a prenatal event. In these cases, concern for ipsilateral renal agenesis is minimal. Conversely, ultrasound examination of the lower quadrant and inguinal canal to search for a non-palpable testis is not indicated and is a highly unreliable examination. Hypospadias associated with even unilateral cryptorchidism should raise the question of intersex anomalies, and karyotype should be determined in the neonate (Fig. 14-6). When bilateral nonpalpable testes are present in infancy, endocrinologic evaluation (serum follicle-stimulating hormone [FSH], luteinizing hormone [LH], testosterone) may determine whether functional testicular tissue exists. The infant with cryptorchidism should be monitored closely, with hormonal or surgical treatment undertaken at about 6 months of age.

PRUNE-BELLY (EAGLE-BARRETT OR TRIAD) SYNDROME

Prune-belly syndrome has a fascinating constellation of physical findings and occurs almost exclusively in boys at a rate of 1 in 35,000 to 50,000 live births. The triad includes abnormal abdominal musculature (variable degrees of muscular laxity, which may be asymmetrical); abdominal cryptorchidism; and floppy dysmorphic urinary tracts, most with vesicoureteric

Figure 14-6 Intersex. Hypospadias and left cryptorchidism in a neonate found to have mixed gonadal dysgenesis with a mosaic karyotype.

reflux (Fig. 14-7). Plain abdominal radiography demonstrates the bell-shaped thorax and abdomen seen in this syndrome. The typical prune-belly refluxing ureter, with increasing tortuosity in the lower portion, is revealed by voiding cystourethrogram or intravenous urogram. Because of the severe risk of sepsis associated with urinary tract infection, urethral catheterization should be undertaken only with the utmost care to prevent infection and with antibiotic prophylaxis. Megalourethra may be seen. Associated with the syndrome in most patients are prostatic hypoplasia and dimples on the lateral aspects of the knees, which some experts believe are secondary to an exaggerated cross-legged position in utero. Gastrointestinal and cardiac anomalies occur in a proportion of patients, but the factor that most determines longevity is the presence and degree of renal dysplasia.

Figure 14-7 Prune-belly syndrome. **A,** Classic appearance of a wrinkled abdomen in a neonate. In older babies, the belly is less wrinkled and more floppy. **B,** Empty scrotum of the same infant.

Figure 14-8 Patent urachus in a girl with recurrent umbilical drainage and inflammation.

ANOMALIES OF THE URACHUS

The urachus extends from the bladder dome to the umbilicus and is usually a vestigial structure during extrauterine life. Several lesions may result from persistence of the urachus: patent urachus, vesicourachal diverticulum, urachal cyst, and alternating urachal sinus. Many of these lesions go unrecognized for long periods before becoming symptomatic. Patent urachus results when the urachal lumen fails to obliterate and the bladder communicates with the umbilicus (Fig. 14-8). Umbilical drainage, inflammation, or infection may result. Voiding cystourethrography is important in the evaluation of possible urachal disorders and to exclude infravesical obstruction. The differential diagnosis includes persistent omphalomesenteric duct. Urachal cysts may become infected and present in infancy through adulthood with suprapubic or infraumbilical pain, tenderness, a palpable mass, or abdominal wall inflammation (Fig. 14-9). Urinary tract infection with irritative voiding symptoms or sepsis may result. Ultrasonography or computed tomography (CT) may aid in diagnosis. Urachal diverticula are usually clinically inconsequential unless they are large enough to cause urinary stasis and infection. Because unrecognized urachal remnants may be the source of carcinoma in adults, many cases with a poor prognosis due to delayed detection, even asymptomatic urachal lesions, should be excised. Many "urachal" lesions in newborns turn out to be merely localized umbilical granulomas.

HYDRONEPHROSIS

Ureteropelvic Junction Obstruction

Lesions of the ureteropelvic junction (UPJ) are a common cause of hydronephrosis. UPJ obstruction may present as antenatal hydronephrosis, neonatal flank mass, urinary tract infection, or recurrent abdominal pain in the older child and adolescent. In many cases of significant obstruction the kidney may not be palpably enlarged. UPJ obstruction may be documented by ultrasound or intravenous pyelography and confirmed by retrograde pyelography (Fig. 14-10, *A*). Voiding cystourethrography is important, particularly in infants, because vesicoureteric reflux may coexist with UPJ obstruction. In some cases reflux is the primary lesion, with the UPJ kink as a secondary lesion (Fig. 14-10, *B*), whereas in other cases, severe reflux may be the primary lesion with a secondary kink at the ureteropelvic junction, which may or may not prove to be obstructive (Fig. 14-10, *C*). Not all hydronephrotic kidneys are truly obstructed. In borderline cases, radionuclide diuresis renography (Lasix renal scan) (Fig. 14-11) or percutaneous antegrade pressure perfusion studies (Whitaker test) may be necessary to determine whether surgical intervention is warranted. Some dilated but unobstructed infant kidneys spontaneously return to a normal or near-normal appearance with time (see previous discussion).

Figure 14-9 Urachal abscess. **A** and **B,** Views of an infected urachal abscess in a girl with fever and abdominal pain.

Figure 14-10   Ureteropelvic junction obstruction. **A,** Retrograde ureterogram defines obstruction at the ureteropelvic junction. **B,** The coexistence of vesicoureteric reflux and ureteropelvic junction obstruction is seen in this voiding cystourethrogram. **C,** Voiding cystourethrogram demonstrates a nonobstructive kink at the left ureteropelvic junction.

Megaureter

The term *megaureter* is descriptive of a large ureter, with or without intrarenal hydronephrosis (Fig. 14-12). Megaureters may be the result of massive vesicoureteric reflux or obstruction at the ureterovesical junction, or they may be nonobstructive. Experience with neonatal megaureters has shown that many of these lesions, when studied by diuresis renography or Whitaker protocols, are found to be nonobstructive. Some resolve spontaneously. The repair of true obstructive megaureters requires excision of the abnormal distal ureter and reimplantation of the tapered segment into the bladder. A nonrefluxing megaureter is thought to be due to either local neurologic or, more likely, muscular abnormalities of the distal ureter that interfere with normal peristalsis. Megaureters may be discovered on antenatal ultrasonography or present as a source of urinary tract infection. Calculi may form in them.

MULTICYSTIC RENAL DYSPLASIA

Multicystic renal dysplasia (see Chapter 13) is the second most common cause of renal enlargement in the neonate and may be discovered by antenatal ultrasound, serendipitously, or

RENOGRAM

Figure 14-11   Diuresis renogram. The radionuclide is administered, followed by a diuretic. The curves show a normal right kidney (prompt decrease in counts as the radionuclide is washed out of the collecting system) and an obstructed left kidney (only a small fraction of the radionuclide is slowly drained out of the collecting system).

Figure 14-12   Megaureter. Intravenous pyelogram shows a left megaureter with hydroureteronephrosis and a normal right kidney and ureter.

Figure 14-13 Multicystic dysplasia. **A,** Ultrasound examination of a multicystic kidney. **B,** Nuclear medicine scan of a nonfunctional left multicystic dysplastic kidney (posterior view). The top area of contrast represents the right kidney, and the lower one is the bladder.

during the evaluation of an abdominal mass. Multicystic renal dysplasia must be differentiated from hydronephrosis, and the combination of ultrasonography and radionuclide scan is usually diagnostic because, although the ultrasound appearance may be similar, multicystic kidneys rarely function on scan (Fig. 14-13). Because contralateral vesicoureteric reflux is common, some authors believe that voiding cystourethrography should be performed in all patients to detect reflux into the solitary functioning kidney. A large percentage of multicystic kidneys spontaneously involute as determined by follow-up ultrasonography, and it may be that many cases of "congenitally absent kidney" represent unrecognized involution of a multicystic dysplastic kidney. There is still debate about the indications for nephrectomy in these kidneys. The Urology Section of the American Academy of Pediatrics has undertaken longitudinal follow-up of these patients. It appears that the potential for hypertension, infection, and malignancy in these kidneys is small.

SIMPLE RENAL CYSTS

Simple renal cysts were thought to be rare in children until the advent of high-resolution ultrasound technology. They are now frequently detected, albeit much less commonly than in adults, in whom the incidence increases with age. As a result, the traditional admonition to surgically explore all cysts in children has been replaced by a policy of radiographic evaluation similar to that in adults. Simple cysts should be treated as benign. Most renal cysts are discovered serendipitously while evaluating the urinary tract for infection-related symptoms, but large cysts occasionally present as abdominal masses. Radiologic evaluation usually includes ultrasonography, but CT (Fig. 14-14) and even cyst puncture for aspiration and contrast studies may be used to confirm the nature of the cyst. The differential diagnosis includes cystic Wilms' tumor, multilocular cystic dysplasia, duplication anomaly with hydronephrosis, caliceal diverticulum, and adult polycystic disease.

CUTANEOUS URINARY DIVERSION

Although permanent urinary diversion in children is rarely performed in this age of intermittent catheterization and urinary tract reconstruction, temporary diversion still has an important role in difficult situations. Understanding the anatomic relationships of urinary stomas is an integral part of caring for children with diversions.

Cutaneous Pyelostomy. The renal pelvis is marsupialized to the skin (Fig. 14-15). This is an uncommon diversion except

in small infants with severe hydronephrosis and compromised renal function.

End Ureterostomy. A single stoma is created, which usually requires using the distal ureter (Fig. 14-16).

Loop Ureterostomy. A double-barreled stoma is created, allowing access to both the proximal and distal ureter (Fig. 14-17).

Intestinal Diversion. An isolated segment of bowel is interposed between the skin and ureters. The normal continuity of the intestinal tract is restored (Fig. 14-18).

Cutaneous Vesicostomy. This is probably the most commonly created temporary diversion in children, usually in cases of urethral valves, neuropathic bladder, prune-belly syndrome, and occasionally severe vesicoureteric reflux. A vesicostomy is basically a vesicocutaneous fistula, and in the small infant it is simply covered with a diaper (Fig. 14-19).

Appendicovesicostomy. This is a continent diversion intended to allow intermittent catheterization of the bladder when urethral access is difficult (Fig. 14-20). The stoma is frequently concealed in the umbilicus.

Nephrostomy. This percutaneous or operatively placed catheter is a temporary urinary diversion or upper tract access for contrast or manometric evaluations (Fig. 14-21).

Figure 14-14 Simple renal cyst. Shown is computed tomography (CT) of a huge left renal cyst, which presented as a left upper quadrant abdominal mass.

Figure 14-15   Cutaneous pyelostomy.

Figure 14-16   End ureterostomy.

Figure 14-17   Loop ureterostomy. Note double-barreled stoma.

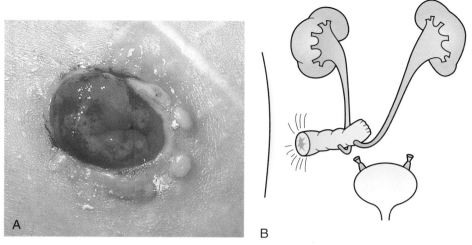

Figure 14-18 Ileal conduit stoma (intestinal diversion).

Figure 14-19 Cutaneous vesicostomy.

Figure 14-20 Appendicovesicostomy.

Figure 14-21   Percutaneous nephrostomy.

EXSTROPHIC ANOMALIES

Classic Exstrophy

Bladder exstrophy occurs in approximately 1 of every 40,000 live births. It predominates in boys and is thought to result from premature rupture of the cloacal membrane. The infant is usually otherwise healthy. Examination reveals a red mucosal surface of varying size on the infraumbilical abdominal wall, which represents the entire bladder opened as a book. On the inferior bladder surface the trigone and ureteral orifices are visible, freely effluxing urine. The penis is epispadiac and lies dorsally tethered against the bladder. When the penis is retracted downward, the entire mucosal surface of the urethra is seen to be splayed open (Fig. 14-22, *A* and *B*). In severe cases the penis may be bifid or rudimentary, and gender may be questionable. The scrotum may be normal or bifid, and testes may be undescended. Inguinal hernias are common. The pubic symphysis is widespread. In girls a hemiclitoris and duplicate vagina are common (Fig. 14-22, *C* and *D*). The delicate bladder surface should be kept moist until urologic consultation is obtained. Prompt upper tract evaluation and neonatal closure are routine. Routine closure in most cases is optimally carried out within 48 hours of birth. When closure is delayed, pelvic osteotomy may be necessary to achieve successful closure.

Cloacal Exstrophy

Cloacal exstrophy is a rare anomaly (1 in 200,000 births). It represents an embryologic mishap similar to that resulting in classic exstrophy, except that rupture of the cloacal membrane occurs before the urorectal septum has completed its descent to separate the hindgut from the bladder. The resulting constellation of anomalies is severe, with long-term survival little better than 50% in most cases. Most children have a large omphalocele, and the majority have myelomeningocele and hydrocephalus. Examination of the exstrophic mucosa reveals that the bladder is divided into two widely separated halves, with a strip of bowel mucosa in the middle (Fig. 14-23). This strip is the ileocecal segment, usually accompanied by a long, prolapsed tubular structure, which is the terminal ileum. Separate orifices enter the appendix (or appendices) and a short,

blind colon. The anus is imperforate. The genitalia are usually hypoplastic with the genital primordia widely separated at either side of the exstrophic cloaca. A female gender assignment is commonly thought to be appropriate because of the extreme difficulty that may be encountered in the creation of a functional phallus in many cases, although gender assignment is now a controversial topic. A multispecialty approach should be taken to the infant with cloacal exstrophy.

Epispadias

Epispadias represents the less severe end of the spectrum of exstrophic anomalies, and has a spectrum of severity. Approximately 55% of patients are boys with penopubic epispadias and urinary incontinence. These boys have a palpably and radiographically widened pubic symphysis and a broad, spade-like penis with the urethra opened fully on its dorsal surface up to the level of the bladder neck. The penis is usually tethered dorsally, and the patient is usually incontinent (Fig. 14-24, *A*). A smaller percentage of boys demonstrate only penile or balanitic (glanular) epispadias. These boys have normal urinary continence. In girls with epispadias (the most rare cases of epispadias), incontinence is usually accompanied by a wide urethra and a bifid clitoris (Fig. 14-24, *B*). The cosmetic appearance of the genitalia in both genders can be improved by genitoplasty, but the larger problem is incontinence, which is accentuated by small bladder capacity. Surgical correction is the rule, and may be performed in stages. Renal ultrasonography and voiding cystourethrography should be performed in all cases.

URINARY RETENTION

Acute urinary retention in infants and children is usually voluntary and associated with severe acute cystitis, urethritis, meatitis (in boys), or vaginitis. Severe constipation may result in urinary retention. In boys, urethral stricture (congenital, traumatic) and meatal stenosis with meatitis (Fig. 14-25, *A*) should be considered. Urethral valves are more likely to cause dysuria or straining without complete retention. Retention in girls is unlikely to be caused by even severe labial adhesions, so uncommon lesions such as a prolapsed ureterocele should

Figure 14-22 Exstrophy. **A** and **B,** Classic bladder exstrophy in a boy infant with a small bladder. **C** and **D,** Bladder exstrophy in a girl. Note the separate openings to each hemivagina.

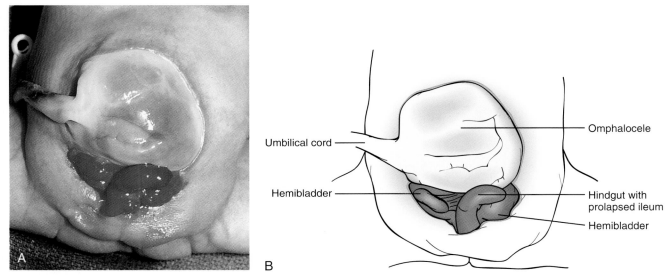

Figure 14-23 **A** and **B,** Cloacal exstrophy.

Figure 14-24 Epispadias. **A,** Penopubic epispadias with incontinence in a boy infant. **B,** Epispadias in a girl reveals a patulous urethra and widespread hemiclitoris.

be considered. Bladder or urethral calculi can also cause retention, and these (Fig. 14-25, *B*) can be diagnosed by a plain abdominal film and ultrasound examination. Pelvic masses (bladder, prostate, or genital rhabdomyosarcoma or other malignancy [Fig. 14-26]; uterine or ovarian masses; hydrocolpos; or hydrometrocolpos) secondary to imperforate hymen or vaginal atresia, sacrococcygeal tumors, or tumors of neural origin may cause retention due to neurologic involvement of the sacral nerve roots or due to bladder neck or urethral compression. Acute neurologic changes associated with spinal cord injury or tumor or transverse myelitis may cause neurogenic retention. Intermittent catheterization may be extremely valuable in managing the bladder until diagnostic evaluations can be completed.

NEUROVESICAL DYSFUNCTION

Neurovesical dysfunction in childhood may be either congenital (meningocele, myelomeningocele, intradural lipoma, diastematomyelia, sacral agenesis) or acquired (trauma, transverse myelitis, spinal cord tumor). Independent of etiology, the evaluation and management of the child with neurovesical dysfunction are extremely important to preserve renal function, prevent renal damage from infection, and provide social continence. Physicians caring for an infant with neurovesical dysfunction should ensure that periodic evaluation of the child's urinary tract is carried out. This evaluation may include radiographic or urodynamic studies, which should be repeated several times during the first year of life or after injury and at least yearly thereafter or as indicated. Danger signs may include infection, fever, or a change in normal pattern of bladder or bowel continence (Fig. 14-27).

Uninhibited bladder contractions and dyscoordinated voiding may be seen in other neurologic conditions, and these may result in bladder dysfunction severe enough to cause not only incontinence or retention of urine but also upper tract deterioration. Multiple sclerosis and other demyelinating diseases are examples. Severe cerebral palsy is frequently associated with incontinence, although upper tract deterioration is uncommon.

Figure 14-25 Urinary retention. **A,** Urinary retention secondary to severe chronic balanitis (balanitis xerotica obliterans). **B,** Urinary retention secondary to an impacted urethral calculus.

Figure 14-26 Bladder rhabdomyosarcoma. Shown is an ultrasound examination of the bladder in a boy who presented with urinary retention. The study reveals polypoid lesions of a botryoid rhabdomyosarcoma, which obstructed the bladder outlet, causing urinary retention.

Figure 14-28 Voiding dysfunction. Voiding cystourethrogram of a boy with Hinman-Allen syndrome shows severe dilation of the prostatic urethra thought to represent urethral valves. Severe bilateral hydronephrosis resulted from vesicoureteric reflux.

NONNEUROGENIC VESICAL DYSFUNCTION

The "nonneurogenic neurogenic bladder," or what is termed *Hinman-Allen syndrome*, is a little-known but important entity that may result in incontinence and renal failure. This syndrome represents a learned disorder of micturition and usually presents as day and night incontinence, fecal soiling, and urinary tract infection. Many of these children display behavioral problems. This syndrome seems to be at the far end of the spectrum of the frequency syndrome of childhood; it, along with its slightly more prevalent and symptomatic cousin, dysfunctional voiding, represent two symptomatic diagnoses seen with increasing frequency by both pediatricians and pediatric urologists. Most children with dysfunctional voiding have some degree of incontinence and fecal soiling. Some have urinary urgency to the point of incontinence, although overflow incontinence from a full bladder may also occur (the lazy bladder syndrome). On occasion, the child may display disordered micturition without symptoms of incontinence and may have only urinary tract infection as a symptom of the dysfunction. In severe cases in which bladder function is severely disordered and detrusor/sphincter dyscoordination is severe, the child's bladder may appear to have the configuration of a bladder that has suffered damage from infravesical obstruction or neurovesical dysfunction (Fig. 14-28).

The diagnosis of dysfunctional voiding is one of exclusion, made after ruling out occult neuropathy such as a tethered spinal cord (CT or magnetic resonance imaging [MRI] scan of the lumbosacral spine) and infravesical obstruction (voiding cystourethrogram and urodynamic evaluation), because the uroradiographic findings often mimic neurovesical dysfunction or obstruction. If child and family are cooperative, bladder retraining using a timed, double-voiding regimen may be effective, frequently augmented with biofeedback. In severe cases, intermittent catheterization may be necessary to reverse hydronephrosis. When renal function is in jeopardy and patient cooperation is minimal, temporary urinary diversion may be appropriate. Many children with this disorder require behavioral or psychological therapy in combination with thoughtful urologic management.

ANOMALIES OF THE MALE GENITALIA

Hypospadias

Hypospadias is a common anomaly that occurs in approximately 1 in 250 male births. The configuration of the urethra varies from mild glanular hypospadias to severe perineal hypospadias with chordee (ventral penile curvature). In describing the appearance of the hypospadiac penis, it is important to refrain from nonspecific terms such as *first-degree* and *minimal*. Proper definition of the anomaly should give an accurate description of the location of the meatus (glanular, coronal, subcoronal, distal shaft, midshaft, proximal shaft, penoscrotal, scrotal, perineal) and the presence or absence of chordee (Fig. 14-29). When hypospadias is associated with cryptorchidism, karyotype should be determined. Voiding cystourethrography is not indicated in hypospadias except in severe lesions or in boys with a history of urinary tract infection. Renal sonography is more likely to be abnormal in boys with proximal hypospadias. Infants with hypospadias should not be circumcised because the dorsal preputial skin may be necessary for urethral and penile reconstruction.

Figure 14-27 Neurovesical dysfunction. Severe bladder trabeculation and vesicoureteric reflux in a child with myelomeningocele.

Figure 14-29 The various forms of hypospadias, revealing location of the meatus. **A,** The typical appearance of the "dorsal hood" prepuce seen in association with hypospadias. **B,** Glanular hypospadias. **C,** Subcoronal hypospadias. **D,** Midshaft hypospadias. **E,** Scrotal hypospadias with bifid scrotum but without chordee. **F,** Perineal hypospadias with chordee.

Repair is usually undertaken at approximately 6 months of age.

Chordee

Chordee (ventral penile curvature) without hypospadias occurs much less frequently than chordee with hypospadias. Chordee may be a minor problem related to skin tethering; may be a result of abnormal development of the urethra and ventral penile structures; or may be due to a congenitally short urethra, in which case surgical correction requires division of the urethra and interposition of a skin tube. If chordee is suspected in the neonate, circumcision should be delayed until examination under anesthesia and artificial erection can determine whether either circumcision or repair is appropriate (Fig. 14-30).

Penile Torsion

Torsion of the penis may be congenital or acquired. Congenital torsion may be severe and related to anomalous development of the corporal bodies, but, most commonly, it is mild and related to dysgenetic subcutaneous fascia (Fig. 14-31). In many cases the ventral median raphe is seen to spiral around the shaft. Most penile torsion is counterclockwise. Acquired torsion may occur after circumcision or hypospadias repair.

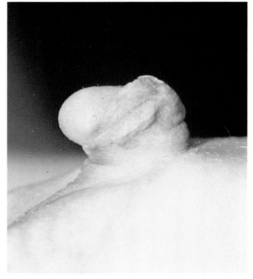

Figure 14-30 Chordee not associated with hypospadias.

Figure 14-31   Mild counterclockwise penile torsion.

Figure 14-33   Buried penis after circumcision.

Webbed Penis

This minor anomaly is easily corrected with a V-Y scrotoplasty (Fig. 14-32), although in many minor cases, circumcision alone is enough to remove the appearance of webbing. Webbing is caused by the transposition of scrotal skin onto the ventral penile shaft at the penoscrotal junction. The ill effects are purely cosmetic in nature.

Buried Penis

Buried penis may occur as a primary finding in the neonate, but it is most common after circumcision (Fig. 14-33). Buried penis is usually the result of a thick suprapubic fat pad; it resolves with normal development. In severe cases, dysgenetic subcutaneous fascial bands bind the penis down. Secondary buried (entrapped) penis after circumcision may be similar to congenital buried penis, and observation may be the rule, although many children will require surgical correction if the phimotic band gradually becomes tighter and voiding is affected.

Postcircumcision Concerns

Meatal Stenosis

Relative meatal stenosis is common after circumcision, secondary to mild recurrent meatitis. Mild to moderate stenosis is usually asymptomatic, but dysuria, strangury, or deflection of the urinary stream may bring the child to a physician's office. Mere examination of the meatus is insufficient to document stenosis, and the urinary stream should be observed for a thin or upward stream or for bulging of the meatus (Fig. 14-34). In many cases referred for evaluation, the urinary stream appears normal and no intervention is necessary. Meatotomy performed in the office under local anesthesia is curative.

Meatal Bridges

Meatal bridges are unusual lesions that appear to result from meatal stenosis in which the ventral aspect of the meatus recanalizes, leaving a bridge of skin across the meatus that may cause dysuria or deflection and spraying of the urinary stream (Fig. 14-35).

Preputial Adhesions and Skin Bridges

Fibrinous adhesions are a result of incomplete retraction of the prepuce during normal development or after circumcision. These adhesions resolve spontaneously with normal hygiene

Figure 14-32   Webbed penis.

Figure 14-34   Meatal stenosis. Observation of the urinary stream in suspected meatal stenosis reveals a full stream, ruling out significant meatal stenosis.

Figure 14-35   Meatal bridge.

Figure 14-37   Penile inclusion cyst after circumcision.

and development. Fibrous adhesions (preputial skin bridges) result when the free edge of the circumcising incision adheres to the glans penis and, if not properly cared for, fuses to the glans. The resulting bridge of skin may cause penile torsion or trap smegma, causing recurrent inflammation or infection (Fig. 14-36). Circumferential skin bridges may be quite disfiguring, and can be challenging to repair without causing scarring of the glans epithelium. Proper instruction on care of the infant penis after circumcision should prevent most of these bridges from forming.

Epithelial Inclusion Cysts

Frequently encountered after circumcision, and usually on the line of the circumcision scar itself, these whitish subcutaneous accumulations of desquamated skin appear as mobile, firm accumulations of white sebaceous material (Fig. 14-37). In some cases, a small tract to the skin may be evident and pressure on the lesion may result in extrusion of a small amount of smegma-like substance, although most of these cysts do not communicate with the skin. Occasionally becoming infected, these cysts apparently result from inversion of small amounts of skin at the time of circumcision. Surgical excision, rather than attempts to drain the cyst, are curative.

Microphallus

Microphallus (micropenis) is a small, normally formed penis more than 2 standard deviations below the mean (<1.9-cm stretch length in neonates) (Fig. 14-38). It is important to

obtain an accurate penile stretch length and corporal shaft diameter by using a rigid ruler placed on the pubic symphysis and stretching the penis to extend the glans as far as possible along the ruler, while not stretching the prepuce. Microphallus is thought to result from failure of normal penile growth after 14 weeks' gestation. Two primary causes of the failure of penile growth may be hypogonadotropic hypogonadism (failure of the hypothalamus to produce gonadotropin-releasing hormone [GnRH]) and primary testicular failure (deficient testosterone production) (hypergonadotropic hypergonadism). Karyotype should be determined. Follicle-stimulating hormone (FSH), luteinizing hormone (LH), and testosterone levels should be measured in addition to a diagnostic human chorionic gonadotropin (HCG) stimulation test to assess testicular function. Evaluation of pituitary–hypothalamic function should be carried out by measurements of serum, glucose, sodium, potassium, cortisol, and thyroid hormone levels, and perhaps an MRI scan to assess the anatomy of the hypothalamus and midbrain. Although a great deal of controversy exists about the long-term outlook for penile growth at puberty and about the appropriateness of female gender reassignment in infancy, most authors suggest a diagnostic trial of testosterone for 3 months before making a final decision about gender assignment. An increasing impetus is toward the male sex of rearing.

Figure 14-36   Preputial skin bridges after circumcision.

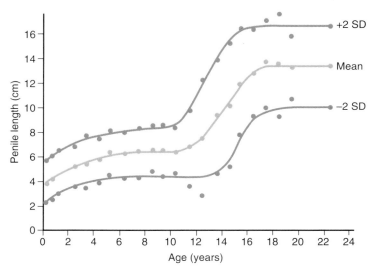

Figure 14-38   Cumulative frequency curves of penile length for age. (*From Lee PA, Mazur T, Danish R, et al: Micropenis. I. Criteria, etiologies, and classification, Johns Hopkins Med J 146:156-163, 1980. © The Johns Hopkins University Press. Reprinted with permission of The Johns Hopkins University Press.*)

Figure 14-39   Diphallus. Both of these penises were functional. Continence was normal.

Figure 14-41   Paraphimosis. Catheterized patient with edematous prepuce proximal to the glans.

Diphallus

Diphallus is a rare entity usually associated with severe deformities of the lower urinary tract and genitalia. Complete evaluation of the upper and lower urinary tract is mandatory. In most cases of diphallus, one penis is dominant in erectile and urethral function, but in some, the bladder is septate or duplicated, and each phallus plays a significant role (Fig. 14-39).

Priapism

Priapism is a persistent, painful erection in which the corporal bodies are firmly erect but the glans is soft (Fig. 14-40). The shaft and preputial skin may become edematous, and the pain of priapism is usually severe. Priapism in children is usually related to an underlying disease state as opposed to the more common idiopathic variety seen in adults. It is most frequently associated with sickle cell disease but may be seen in relation to pelvic malignancy, leukemia, blunt perineal trauma, or secondary to acute spinal cord injury. Sickle cell–related priapism should initially be treated as any other sickle cell crisis, with oxygenation, exchange transfusion, and systemic alkalinization. Surgical therapy may be necessary to irrigate the corpora cavernosa or perform a cavernosal-spongiosal shunt or vascular bypass.

Acute Balanitis and Posthitis

Balanitis (inflammation of the glans) and posthitis (inflammation of the prepuce) are most common in uncircumcised boys with infection from smegma entrapped beneath the foreskin. Usual treatment involves slight dilation of a snug preputial opening, warm baths, and a broad-spectrum antibiotic for a few days if the process is severe. Candidiasis or other causes should be treated appropriately. Whether balanitis or posthitis indicates the need for circumcision is determined on an individual basis once the acute inflammation has resolved.

Paraphimosis

Phimosis describes the inability to retract a tight, scarred prepuce. If a tight prepuce is retracted over the glans to the level of the corona *(paraphimosis),* the constricted ring of skin may act as a tourniquet applied to the distal shaft and glans, and ischemia may result (Fig. 14-41). Treatment may involve manual compression of the glans and edematous prepuce to allow reduction of the tight band. In severe cases when reduction of the paraphimosis cannot be achieved manually, a dorsal slit must be made, surgically dividing the phimotic band. Circumcision may be appropriate after an episode of paraphimosis.

Lesions of the Scrotum and Scrotal Contents

The scrotum is composed of several fascial and muscular layers containing the spermatic cord and its contents, as well as the testes and their appendages. Any layer of the scrotal wall or any of the contents of the scrotum may produce a clinically evident lesion. Each testis is an ovoid structure lying in a vertical plane in its hemiscrotum in which it is quite mobile, moving up and down with cremasteric contraction and relaxation and separated from the contralateral testis and scrotal contents by the fibrous median septum. Posterior and slightly lateral to the testis lies the epididymis, which may be closely applied to the body of the testis or attached by a somewhat longer mesoepididymis. The appendix testis and appendix epididymis are small embryologic remnants attached to the upper anterior testis or head of the epididymis. These structures are not palpable in the normal state and are not constant findings in all boys.

Figure 14-40   Priapism.

Figure 14-42   Median raphe cysts of the perineum and posterior scrotum.

Median Raphe Cysts

Epithelial inclusion cysts of the median raphe of the scrotum and perineum are not rare (Fig. 14-42). Although isolated cysts may be seen, a more common finding is a chain of cysts extending along the midline of the perineum and scrotum. The cysts are filled with white or yellow epithelial debris and are usually asymptomatic, although infection of the cyst contents may occur. The cystic lesions appear to represent infolding of skin during fusion of the labioscrotal folds during formation of the external genitalia. Excision of the median raphe and cysts should be performed carefully in one elongated excision, leaving behind no area of microscopically encysted skin that might subsequently enlarge into a clinically evident cyst.

Acute Scrotum

The acute scrotum is a urologic surgical emergency until proven otherwise. It is most imperative to rule out torsion of the spermatic cord. The most important aspects of evaluating the patient with an acute scrotum are history and physical examination. The nature of the onset of pain and swelling is important, as is a history of dysuria, fever, hematuria, previous urinary tract infection, urethral instrumentation, and scrotal or perineal trauma. Examination of the scrotum starts with the normal testis, while observing the involved testis for its size, location, and anatomic orientation. The skin and wall of the scrotum are examined for edema, inflammation, and fluctuation. Mobility of the testis should be assessed, as should the presence or absence of a cremasteric reflex ipsilateral to the involved testis. Laboratory evaluation includes urinalysis, white blood cell count, and testicular flow scan or color Doppler examination if appropriate. The bottom line is expeditious evaluation with a liberal approach to exploration if the diagnosis is uncertain.

Torsion of the Spermatic Cord

Torsion of the spermatic cord is the most significant condition that must be excluded in cases of scrotal pain and swelling (Fig. 14-43). Because the testis deprived of its normal blood supply has at most a few hours before irreversible injury destroys spermatogenic potential, acute swelling of the scrotum is a diagnostic and surgical emergency until torsion has been adequately excluded as a cause. Torsion may occur at any age.

Antenatal torsion is thought in most cases to represent extravaginal torsion or torsion of the entire scrotal contents including the covering tunics. It occurs during descent of the testis and usually presents at birth as a firm, nontender mass high in the scrotum or at the scrotal inlet. Frequently there is fixation to the overlying skin as a part of the inflammatory response. Although a point of current controversy, the classic teaching has been that these testes are not salvageable and that it is more important for the contralateral testis to have normal scrotal fixation and not be prone to asynchronous torsion. Although "salvage" of a testis after antenatal torsion is unlikely, acute torsion can occur during delivery and may rarely be a reversible situation. Synchronous or asynchronous contralateral torsion may occur. A scrotal mass at birth has been in some centers considered a surgical emergency until proven otherwise. Many pediatric urologists now believe that immediate exploration of both testes should be undertaken to assess viability of the involved testis and, more importantly, to ensure the safety of the solitary surviving testis. Others consider that a firm testis at birth represents an old event, and exploration is not warranted. The risk of general anesthesia must be considered.

Intravaginal torsion (within the tunica vaginalis) may occur at any age. Most patients have acute, painful swelling of the scrotum, and many also have lower abdominal pain, nausea, and vomiting. It is not unusual for a boy to awaken with pain, but torsion can also occur after scrotal trauma or during almost any activity. On occasion, torsion has a much more insidious onset as a dull scrotal pain of subacute nature. Dysuria is usually absent, and urinalysis is normal, but leukocytosis may be noted. Examination may vary depending on the time elapsed after the acute episode. Most patients are uncomfortable. The scrotum early on may appear normal but soon becomes red and swollen, with the testis elevated because of foreshortening of the spermatic cord. The contralateral testis may have more of a transverse orientation than normal, although examination is very unreliable in indicating the presence or absence of a bell-clapper deformity. In the acute stage, a hydrocele may develop. The testis may have an abnormal orientation, with the epididymis located in an abnormal position due to torsion of the cord. The cremasteric reflex is usually absent, and elevating the testis to the pubic symphysis increases pain (negative Prehn sign). When inflammation has progressed, the scrotum becomes a firm, homogeneous mass in which all anatomic landmarks are lost.

If torsion is suspected, attempting to detorse the cord by gentle twisting in either direction may allow the cord to untwist, at least partially. If detorsion occurs, relief of pain is instantaneous. Nuclear blood flow scan or color Doppler ultrasound, if immediately available, may be helpful in many instances. A normal nuclear medicine scrotal scan shows identical flow to both testes (see Fig. 14-43, C). When the scrotum contains an inflammatory process, blood flow is increased on the involved side (see Fig. 14-43, D), whereas in the presence of an acute torsion, blood flow is diminished. A missed torsion, in which the scan is performed several hours or days after torsion occurs, appears as a central area of diminished flow surrounded by a halo of increased activity (see Fig. 14-43, E). Color flow Doppler imaging has proven to be a superior alternative to nuclear medicine imaging in almost all cases of acute or chronic scrotal conditions, offering not only determination of the presence or absence of blood flow to the testis, but also anatomic information about the scrotum and its contents not available in nuclear medicine studies. When torsion of the

Figure 14-43 Intravaginal torsion of the spermatic cord. **A,** Torsion of the spermatic cord. **B,** Surgical exploration and detorsion of the left spermatic cord. The left testis was necrotic. The right testis also shows bell-and-clapper deformity. **C,** Nuclear blood flow scan showing normal flow to both testes. The dark area above the scrotum is the bladder full of radionuclide, which is excreted in the urine. **D,** Nuclear blood flow scan showing increased flow to the right testis resulting from epididymitis. **E,** Nuclear blood flow scan showing the classic bull's-eye configuration of a missed torsion of the right testis.

spermatic cord is diagnosed, immediate surgical exploration is warranted (see Fig. 14-41, *A*).

Torsion of Testicular Appendages

The appendix testis and appendix epididymis are embryologic remnants that are normally undetectable on routine examination. Torsion of an appendix, which can occur in the early pubertal age group, may be difficult to differentiate from torsion of the spermatic cord. Early after the onset of acute scrotal pain, a small tender mass may be palpable on the upper anterior surface of the testis or epididymis (Fig. 14-44, *A*). In light-skinned children, the swollen, dark, infarcted appendage may be visible through the scrotal skin (the "blue dot" sign of Dresner) (Fig. 14-44, *B* and *C*). In later presentations the entire testis and scrotum may become inflamed and indistinguishable from torsion of the spermatic cord. Color flow Doppler examination may indicate increased blood flow, and an enlarged torsed appendage may be visualized.

Epididymitis

Epididymal inflammation may be bacterial or nonbacterial in etiology. True bacterial epididymitis is rare in children. Nonbacterial inflammation may be caused by reflux of sterile urine into the ejaculatory ducts or ectopic insertion of a ureter into the seminal vesicle or vas deferens. In many cases of nonbacterial epididymitis, anatomy is normal and no obvious etiology

is evident. Nonbacterial epididymitis would appear to be more common than bacterial inflammation, or at least is named as a diagnosis related to scrotal swelling in more instances. The clinical presentation of epididymitis may be indolent or acute, as with torsion. Fever often accompanies bacterial epididymitis, and the urinary sediment may reflect infection. Examination of the scrotum in early stages demonstrates a tender, slightly swollen epididymis (Fig. 14-45), but later the entire scrotal contents are replaced by an inflammatory mass. The cremasteric reflex is present, and elevation of the testis on the pubis may relieve pain (Prehn sign). A radionuclide scan or color Doppler examination demonstrates increased blood flow. Ultrasound may show an enlarged epididymis. If torsion of the spermatic cord cannot be excluded, surgical exploration must be carried out promptly. All children with bacterial epididymitis should undergo complete upper and lower urinary tract radiographic evaluation after resolution of the acute process (renal ultrasound and voiding cystourethrography). Scrotal abscess formation may result from bacterial epididymitis. Nonbacterial epididymitis is treated expectantly. Administration of nonsteroidal antiinflammatory medication and limitation of activity to bed rest for 48 hours in cases with severe scrotal swelling usually result in rapid improvement of clinical symptoms.

Undescended Testes

See the earlier discussion in Physical Examination.

Figure 14-44   A, Torsion of appendix testis or epididymis. **B,** Examination of the left hemiscrotum in a case of torsion of the appendix testis reveals a "blue dot" sign. **C,** Operative findings after torsion of an appendix epididymis.

Chronic Scrotal Swelling

Varicocele

A varicocele consists of dilated veins of the pampiniform plexus of the spermatic cord (Fig. 14-46). Varicoceles occur primarily on the left side and may be found before puberty. They may be bilateral. The postulated causes of varicocele vary from hormonal to hydrostatic. The postulated cause of testicular injury from varicocele varies from hormonal deficiencies to temperature effects. Most varicoceles decompress in the supine position. Those that do not decompress or those that present with acute onset on either side may lead

Figure 14-45   Epididymitis.

Figure 14-46   Varicocele.

to concern about lesions in the kidney or retroperitoneum causing obstruction to venous outflow. Most varicoceles are asymptomatic and are noted by the child incidentally or discovered on routine examination. Pain secondary to varicocele is uncommon, but a dull aching may occur in large varicoceles.

Infertility is found in approximately 33% of adults with varicoceles, and because semen analyses are not generally available in children, controversy has arisen over the proper management of adolescents. Ablating varicoceles in adolescents with testicular growth failure ipsilateral to the varicocele, or in those with bilateral varicocele, is common practice. In patients with minimal or no testicular atrophy, observation and serial measurements of testicular volume are indicated, with the option to perform varicocele ablation if ipsilateral testicular growth failure becomes evident.

Spermatocele

Spermatoceles or epididymal cysts are common in adolescents. They are painless cystic masses located in the epididymis (commonly in the upper pole) (Fig. 14-47). They vary in size but are usually less than 1 cm in diameter. They are mobile, transilluminate, and do not vacillate in size, although gradual enlargement may occur. Ultrasound examination may be helpful if the diagnosis is in doubt. Spermatoceles contain sperm and are essentially retention cysts of the epididymis or tubules of the rete testis. Excision is not usually recommended in routine symptomatic cases but may be appropriate for painful or enlarging cysts.

Hydrocele

Hydroceles are fluid accumulations within the tunica vaginalis or processus vaginalis (Fig. 14-48). They may be small or large, are usually painless even if they are large, and may be tense enough to obscure palpation of the testis. They transilluminate. Simple scrotal hydroceles are common in neonates and usually resolve spontaneously over several months. When examining an infant with a huge hydrocele, examination of the lower abdomen should be performed to rule out the presence of an abdominoscrotal hydrocele. The presence of an abdominoscrotal hydrocele may be noted if compression of the scrotal hydrocele causes enlargement of a lower quadrant mass. Ultrasound may confirm this finding. Large hydroceles may present in adolescence without an obvious etiology. In adolescent cases, when the testis cannot be

Figure 14-48 Hydrocele.

palpated, an ultrasound examination should be done to verify that the testis is normal. If the processus vaginalis remains patent, a communicating hydrocele results and may present with periodic increase and decrease in scrotal size. In these cases, thickening of the inguinal spermatic cord may be noted. If a segment of processus vaginalis fails to obliterate, trapping fluid in midcord, a hydrocele of the cord may result. These may also communicate with the peritoneum through a patent processus vaginalis and thus may vacillate in size. When the diagnosis of an inguinal mass is uncertain, imaging (ultrasound or CT) or exploration may be warranted because soft tissue sarcomas may originate from spermatic cord and paratesticular tissues.

Testis Tumors

Malignant tumors of the testis may occur at all ages, from neonate to adulthood. Most testis tumors present as a firm, painless mass within the testis. Large masses may seem to replace the testicular parenchyma. The mass may be smooth or irregular to palpation. On occasion, a sudden enlargement of a tumor or bleeding within the tumor may cause a painful, rapid enlargement of the involved testis. Solid masses within

Figure 14-47 Spermatocele **(A)** and operative appearance of large spermatocele **(B).**

Figure 14-49   Testis tumor. **A** and **B,** Ultrasound examination of two patients with palpable testis tumors.

Figure 14-50   Idiopathic hypertrophy of left labium majus.

the substance of the testis should be considered malignant until proven otherwise. Testicular ultrasound is helpful in the evaluation of testicular masses (Fig. 14-49).

LESIONS OF THE FEMALE GENITALIA

Labial Hypertrophy

Rarely, hypertrophy of one or both labia majora may cause unilateral or bilateral prominence of the labial structure. Herniation of an ovary into the labium should be easily ruled out by physical examination. Vascular or lymphatic malformations must be ruled out in bilateral lesions, but many unilateral cases are idiopathic (Fig. 14-50). Resection of the hypertrophic tissue may be indicated when the lesion appears to be idiopathic.

Labial Adhesion (Fusion)

Labial adhesions (fusions) are common in the prepubertal age group. They represent fusion of the labia minora, postulated to be the result of inflammation of the thin labial mucosa that simply adheres in the midline. Fusion begins posteriorly and may progress until almost complete fusion results (Fig. 14-51). On inspection, the vaginal introitus may be closed with the exception of a small anterior opening. Severe fusion may be associated with dysuria, postvoid dribbling as the urine voided into the vagina drains out, or urinary tract infection. Although most adhesions lyse spontaneously as puberty approaches and

the vaginal epithelium cornifies, problems of hygiene and discomfort bring many girls to the physician for evaluation and treatment.

Labial fusion must be separated mechanically. Lysis may be managed by parents at home, by merely cleansing the introitus in an anterior-to-posterior motion, and applying a petroleum or other ointment to diminish mucosal irritation. Lysis can also be performed easily in the office: merely spreading the labia or mechanically separating the adhesions with an ointment-covered gloved finger will usually suffice. No anesthetic should be necessary. Some practitioners believe that lysis should be followed by the application of estrogen cream to the area for several days to thicken the vaginal mucosa. Unfortunately, many physicians think that the mere application of estrogen will allow the adhesions to lyse. This is untrue. After lysis, simple hygiene should prevent recurrence.

Urethral Prolapse

Prolapse of the urethra occurs almost exclusively in black girls. Its cause is unknown. The presentation is usually bloody spotting, with occasional mild dysuria. Examination reveals a

Figure 14-51   Labial adhesions. Only a small opening remains anteriorly.

Figure 14-52 Urethral prolapse. This is a chronic case in which the initial hemorrhagic nature of the acute prolapse has resolved with observation, leaving a protuberant, edematous urethra.

Figure 14-54 Prolapsed ureterocele. The catheter enters the urethra.

reddened or dark circumferential prolapse of the urethra with an otherwise normal introitus (Fig. 14-52).

Introital Polyps

Small polyps may originate from the urethral meatus or hymenal ring (Fig. 14-53). These usually are thin mucosal tags that cause no symptoms and require no specific treatment. Fleshy polyps or multiple polyps should be examined closely and biopsied to exclude malignancy such as sarcoma botryoides (see Chapter 11).

Prolapsed Ureterocele

Prolapse of a large ureterocele through the urethral orifice should be considered in the differential diagnosis of all interlabial masses in infants and children (Fig. 14-54). Ureteroceles are cystic dilations of the distal ureter, which are located in the bladder or urethra and may prolapse through the urethral meatus as reddened or even necrotic mucosal surfaces. A prolapsed ureterocele, unlike urethral prolapse, does not present a symmetrical orifice but rather presents an

Figure 14-53 Introital polyp. A small polyp of the posterior vaginal fourchette.

Figure 14-55 Ectopic ureter. **A,** A drop of urine exits from the orifice of an ectopic ureter located just below the urethral meatus in the urethrovaginal septum. **B,** Retrograde pyelography of the same ureter reveals a huge, tortuous ureter subtending the upper pole of a right complete ureteral duplication. Heminephrectomy cured the patient's incontinence.

Figure 14-56   Paraurethral cyst.

asymmetrical protrusion through the urethra. Catheterization alongside the prolapse may locate the lumen of the urethra. Prolapse of a ureterocele may be associated with a palpable distended bladder or flank mass (hydronephrosis). Ultrasonography of the bladder and kidneys demonstrates unilateral or bilateral hydronephrosis or hydronephrosis of a segment of a complete ureteral duplication, usually the upper pole of an obstructed renal unit. Voiding cystourethrography with intravenous urography or radionuclide studies and occasionally direct puncture of the ureterocele with contrast injection may be appropriate to define the anatomy of the malformation in a few cases.

Ectopic Ureter

Ureteral ectopia may be associated with a single collecting system or a complete duplication of the collecting system (complete ureteral duplication). In females, an ectopic ureter may drain into the bladder neck, urethra, urethrovaginal septum, vagina, or uterus. Girls with ectopic ureter into the urethra, urethrovaginal septum, or vagina may have a normal voiding pattern but with a continuous dribbling incontinence of small amounts of urine. In some of these girls, a tiny ectopic ureter may be seen to drip urine from the introitus (Fig. 14-55).

Paraurethral Cysts

Cystic lesions of the paraurethral or vaginal mucosa may be found on routine examination and are usually asymptomatic. They rarely cause voiding symptoms and occasionally present in older girls as palpable interlabial masses. Normal mucosa overlies the cyst, which usually displaces the urethral meatus slightly from the midline. Most cysts rupture spontaneously, but aspiration or marsupialization may be necessary (Fig. 14-56).

Congenital Obstruction of the Vagina

Vaginal obstruction may occur as a result of an imperforate hymen, vaginal atresia or septa, or urogenital sinus malformation. Fusion anomalies of the müllerian structures may result in a septate vagina or bicornuate uterus with one obstructed segment. Neonates may have abdominal masses or urinary retention; girls with a didelphic or bicornuate uterus may have pelvic pain or menstrual irregularities at puberty. Examination of the infant may reveal a distended vagina (hydrometrocolpos) with a bulging hymenal membrane. If a vaginal septum or atresia is the cause of the obstruction, external genital examination may be normal and a complete pelvic examination with vaginoscopy may be necessary. Ultrasonography of the pelvis may be helpful, but pelvic CT or MRI scan may give the most anatomic information (Fig. 14-57). All girls with uterine or vaginal anomalies should have imaging of the upper urinary tract, given the high incidence of upper tract anomalies in this group. As a corollary, girls with proven unilateral renal agenesis should be monitored through puberty for the development of müllerian anomalies, commonly uterus didelphys with an obstructed unilateral uterine horn or vagina

Figure 14-57   Hydrometrocolpos. **A,** Sagittal ultrasound of the pelvis in a neonate with a large pelvic hydrometrocolpos secondary to distal vaginal atresia. "M" delineates the mass (hydrometrocolpos), and "BL" defines the anteriorly displaced and compressed bladder. **B,** Catheter drainage of released white mucoid drainage, with disappearance of the pelvic mass.

Figure 14-58 Various causes of genital ambiguity. **A,** Congenital adrenal hyperplasia. **B,** Mixed gonadal dysgenesis. **C,** True hermaphroditism. **D,** Posteriorly displaced urogenital sinus.

ipsilateral to the side of the absent kidney. Pelvic ultrasound examination in the peripubertal period is an effective way to monitor these girls.

AMBIGUOUS GENITALIA

Human genitalia begin as undifferentiated structures that early in gestation are identical in both sexes. The combined effects of genetic, hormonal, and local influences modify the structure and function of the genitalia to produce genital structures appropriate to the gender of the individual (see Chapter 9). When abnormal development occurs, genitalia of indeterminate nature may result. The recognition of abnormal genitalia is the first step in the evaluation of intersex. The combination of hypospadias and bilateral or unilateral cryptorchidism should be considered as representative of intersex until proven otherwise. Examination of the genitalia in suspected intersex cases should include assessment of phallic length and diameter; presence or absence of gonads and their size; assessment of labioscrotal and perineal anatomy; rectal examination; ultrasonography, MRI, or CT of the pelvis; and flush genitogram (urethrogram) to delineate urethral or vaginal structures. A full genetic and endocrine evaluation should be carried out as well (Fig. 14-58).

Figure 14-59 Ambiguous genitalia in a girl with a high imperforate anus.

Figure 14-60   Genital trauma. **A,** Trauma to the glans penis from a falling toilet seat; a common injury that is usually best served by observation unless the urethra is disrupted. **B,** Perineal trauma. The testes were injured, but the urethra was intact. **C,** Scrotal trauma. The testicular tunics were intact, and primary skin closure produced an excellent result.

Genital Ambiguity Associated with Imperforate Anus

The embryologic deformity that produces a high imperforate anus in girls occasionally also influences the formation of the external genitalia by presumed local factors. The end result may be genitalia that appear to be masculinized (Fig. 14-59).

GENITAL TRAUMA

Injury to the genitalia may be the result of minimal trauma or may be a part of multiple trauma. Although genital trauma may not be life-threatening, proper management may be important to the later well-being and psychosocial development of the patient. This is particularly important in children. Trauma to the penis or scrotum should always raise the question of urethral injury (Fig. 14-60, *A*). This is easily ruled out in the emergency department or x-ray department by injecting contrast (intravenous contrast in case of extravasation into vascular structures) through the urethral meatus, using a blunt-tipped syringe or a small catheter. Once urethral injury has been excluded, urethral catheterization can be performed safely. Scrotal trauma mandates critical evaluation of the testes. Scrotal ultrasound may be necessary to rule out

testicular rupture or laceration. When injury is discovered, examination and repair should be performed in the operating room (Fig. 14-60, *B* and *C*). Scrotal and testicular trauma is not uncommon in breech delivery, when the scrotum is the presenting part. Prompt urologic assessment should be sought. Ultrasound examination of the testes may be helpful if massive edema or hematoma precludes thorough examination. If injury is suspected, surgical exploration is the most conservative approach. Trauma to the female genitalia and perineum usually requires examination under anesthesia to allow a complete evaluation of the injury, with concomitant repair when necessary.

Bibliography

Belman AB, Kaplan GW: *Genitourinary problems in pediatrics*, Philadelphia, 1981, WB Saunders.
Gillenwater JY, Grayhack JT, Howards SS, et al, editors: *Adult and pediatric urology*, Philadelphia, 2002, Lippincott Williams & Wilkins.
Lee PA, Mazur T, Danish R, et al: Micropenis. I. Criteria, etiologies, and classification, *Johns Hopkins Med J* 146:156-163, 1980.
Walsh PC, Retik AB, Vaughan ED, et al, editors: *Campbell's urology*, Philadelphia, 2002, WB Saunders.
Williams DI, Johnston JH, editors: *Paediatric urology*, London, 1982, Butterworth.

NEUROLOGY

Rajiv Varma | Shelley D. Williams | Henry B. Wessel

NEUROLOGIC EXAMINATION

The primary objective of the neurologic examination is to assess the functional integrity of the central nervous system (CNS) and the peripheral nervous system (PNS) and to detect and localize any sites of neurologic dysfunction. Techniques and interpretation of the pediatric neurologic examination are based largely on knowledge of normal growth and development. The examination is preceded by a thorough history of the presenting problem including timing and mode of onset; course; and a past medical history that focuses on the antenatal, perinatal, and neonatal periods for possible prior insults (e.g., bleeding, infection, hypoxia, drugs, trauma). Abnormalities of birth weight; the need for resuscitation after delivery; early neonatal problems with hypoglycemia, hypocalcemia, or severe jaundice; and abnormalities in activity or difficulty feeding shortly after birth often serve as red flags. This is followed by a detailed history of behavior; growth and development with attention to evidence of delay, slowing, cessation, or regression of developmental milestones; and any possible association with prior illness or trauma. Obtaining a family history of neurologic, neuromuscular, or developmental problems is also important.

The traditional systematic neurologic evaluation proceeds from assessment of mental status and language functions through evaluation of cranial nerves, gross motor function, muscle strength, gait and station, balance and coordination, sensory systems, and deep tendon reflexes. It is applicable to older children and adolescents without significant modification from the evaluation geared to the adult. Tools essential to the neurologist include the reflex hammer, bright penlight, ophthalmoscope, and stethoscope. For evaluation of the primary sensory modalities of light touch, pain, temperature, and vibration, wisps of cotton, sterile disposable pins, glass test tubes (to hold hot and cold water), and a tuning fork (256 Hz for children and young adults, 126 Hz for older persons) are used. A collection of small, common objects (e.g., coins, buttons, keys) to be identified by feel alone are useful for assessment of cortical sensations of stereognosis. Derangements of primary sensory function may be present with lesions at the level of the nerve roots, plexuses, or peripheral nerves. If a particular area of decreased sensation is identified in part of a limb, careful delineation of its boundaries often suggests root (dermatomal), plexus, or peripheral nerve involvement (Fig. 15-1, *A* and *B*).

Neurologic examination of the younger child requires flexibility and a gentle, staged approach. The first stage consists of observation, much of which can be done while taking the history as the infant sits in the parent's lap or while the toddler or older child plays with toys. The child's level of alertness and interest in people and the environment are assessed. Facies, head shape, body habitus, spontaneous movements, position, and posture are noted, along with spontaneous

vocalizations and quality and pitch of cry in infants. In the child old enough to walk, stance and gait, as well as the ability to run, stoop, and recover; climb onto a stool; and rise from the floor (when developmentally appropriate), are observed. These observations provide a good general impression of the child's developmental level and abilities.

Much of the remainder of the neurologic examination also lends itself to play, and in the second stage of observation a more detailed assessment of mental status, language, handedness, and fine and gross motor skills is performed by engaging the child in play. A selection of rattles, keys, spinning and mechanical toys, dolls, cars, small blocks, noise makers, tennis balls, hand puppets, crayons, and picture books supplement the traditional instruments. If further observation of gait is necessary, the examiner can have the child walk to or with the parent. Children older than 4 years of age love to show what they can do when asked to walk on their heels or toes, hop, or do tandem gait along a line. Pat-a-cake games are popular for testing rapidly alternating movements with young children. Then, with the child comfortable and rapport established, the hands-on examination is initiated with the child still dressed and in the parent's lap. Trying to catch the otoscope light as it is shown over various parts of the body can precede following the light with the eyes and looking at it. For infants and toddlers, following a face or spinning toy is still better for testing extraocular movements (Fig. 15-2). Having a parent jingle keys at the child's eye level and asking the child to look at the sound while looking in the child's eyes assists the ophthalmoscopic examination in older preschool and young school-age children (Fig. 15-3). Asking young children to make faces, stick out their tongues, and blow up balloons is another helpful technique in assessing cranial nerves.

Tone is assessed by observing resistance to passive motion. Then active motion and motion against resistance are checked. Older preschoolers and school-age children love showing their muscles, and push–pull games can be used to test muscle strength, especially when the child's efforts are admired. Deep tendon reflexes can often be tested at this time with only the shoes off. These are normally brisk, or 3+, in the young infant, becoming 2+ by 6 months of age. If directly tapping on the tendon seems upsetting to the child, it may help to place a finger over the tendon to be percussed and tap that. In infants and toddlers, it is often easier to elicit the ankle jerk by placing a finger over the ball of the child's foot and gently dorsiflexing it before percussing the Achilles tendon (Fig. 15-4). Preschoolers and young children love having the examiner express surprise and pleasure when reflexes are elicited.

Finally the parent is asked to help undress the child, and the remainder of the examination proceeds with the parent providing reassurance and assistance as needed. During this stage, head circumference is measured in the infant and toddler, and the head, midline of the neck and back, and skin are carefully examined for abnormalities. Muscles are inspected

Figure 15-1 Cutaneous sensory innervation. The segmental or dermatomal (nerve root) distribution is shown on the left side of the body, and the peripheral nerve distribution on the right side of the body. **A,** Anterior view. **B,** Posterior view. *(Modified from Simon RP, Aminoff MJ, Greenberg DA: Clinical neurology, ed 4, Stamford, Conn., 1999, Appleton & Lange.)*

Figure 15-2 Testing extraocular motion. Older infants and toddlers tend to be captivated by spinning or sparkling toys and readily follow the objects, making it easy to test such motion.

Figure 15-3 Ophthalmoscopic examination. Having a parent hold and jingle keys at the child's eye level and asking the patient to look toward the sound enhances the child's ability to focus, assisting good visualization of the retina in young children.

Figure 15-4 Achilles reflex. Gently dorsiflexing the foot before percussing the Achilles tendon makes it easier to elicit this reflex.

for symmetry, and extremity circumference is measured a set distance from a bony landmark if asymmetry is suspected, and abnormal muscle movements are noted. The appropriate disappearance or persistence of primitive reflexes is determined in infants (see Chapter 3). The Babinski reflex is difficult to elicit and interpret during the first year of life because stroking the sole of the foot may simply stimulate withdrawal or plantar flexion. Using the Oppenheim technique—running the thumb down the medial surface of the tibia—gives a more interpretable response (Fig. 15-5). Evaluation of sensation is difficult in the younger child and is generally limited to appreciation of light touch and pinprick. These may be assessed with minimal discomfort by using a partially unbent paper clip.

Neurologic examination of the newborn is highly specialized. The essential components of the neonatal examination include assessment of gestational age, growth patterns, dysmorphic features, motor tone, postures, spontaneous activity, cry, respiratory patterns, brainstem reflexes, response to bright light, response to noxious stimuli, developmental reflexes, and deep tendon reflexes (see Chapter 2). Normal findings vary with gestational age. The immaturity of the newborn's CNS, with functioning largely at a subcortical reflex level, may

conceal all but the most severe neurologic deficits—hence the often deceptively normal examination of the newborn with hydranencephaly.

The most prevalent neurologic disorders in childhood are related to CNS infection, ingestions, congenital malformations, perinatal insults, trauma (including abuse), progressive neurodegenerative or neuromuscular processes, and metabolic disorders. This chapter concentrates on selected neurologic disorders accompanied by physical signs that can be detected on visual inspection.

NEUROCUTANEOUS SYNDROMES

The neurocutaneous syndromes or phakomatoses are congenital, often inherited disorders with prominent cutaneous and neurologic manifestations. The simultaneous involvement of the skin and nervous system, both derivatives of embryonic ectoderm, suggests that these disorders may be caused by an unknown abnormality of the embryonic epiblast. Although the clinical and pathologic features of the phakomatoses are diverse, these syndromes share a propensity for malformations and hamartomatous tumors of multiple organs. Among the more frequently encountered phakomatoses are neurofibromatosis, tuberous sclerosis, Sturge-Weber syndrome, ataxia-telangiectasia, and linear sebaceous nevus.

Neurofibromatosis 1

Neurofibromatosis 1, or NF-1 (previously known as von Recklinghausen disease), is the most common of the neurocutaneous syndromes and affects about 1 in 3000 individuals. Although usually inherited as an autosomal dominant disorder, up to 50% of cases may be sporadic. Molecular genetic testing for mutations of the *NF1* gene is clinically available. The *NF1* gene has been localized to chromosome 17q. Neurofibromin, its gene product, acts as a tumor suppressor, and its function is altered in affected patients. Characteristic clinical manifestations include multiple hyperpigmented skin macules (café-au-lait spots), axillary or inguinal freckling, multiple skin neurofibromas, and iris hamartomas (Lisch nodules). Associated abnormalities may include optic gliomas; other CNS tumors of glial or meningeal origin; neurofibromas of spinal or peripheral nerves; pheochromocytoma, macrocephaly, and cognitive impairment; and bony abnormalities. Diagnostic criteria for NF-1 are summarized in Table 15-1.

Multiple café-au-lait spots, the most frequently encountered cutaneous abnormality, are brown hyperpigmented macules with smooth margins, usually most numerous over the trunk (Fig. 15-6, *A*; and see Chapter 8, Fig. 8-131, *A-C*). Other abnormalities of cutaneous pigmentation may include axillary or

Figure 15-5 Oppenheim technique for checking the Babinski response. Running the thumb down the medial surface of the tibia produces a more interpretable response in infants and toddlers because it avoids stimulation of a plantar flexion or withdrawal response.

Table 15-1	Diagnostic Criteria for Neurofibromatosis 1

Diagnostic criteria are met if two or more of the following are found:

- Six or more café-au-lait macules >5 mm in greatest diameter in prepubertal children and >15 mm in greatest diameter in postpubertal individuals
- Two or more neurofibromas of any type or one plexiform neurofibroma
- Axillary or inguinal freckling
- Optic glioma
- Two or more Lisch nodules (iris hamartomas)
- A distinctive osseous lesion such as a sphenoid dysplasia or thinning of long bone cortex with or without pseudarthrosis
- A first-degree relative (i.e., parent, sibling, or child) with NF-1, according to these criteria

NF-1, neurofibromatosis 1.

Figure 15-6 Neurofibromatosis 1 (NF-1). Clinical manifestations of cutaneous pigmentary abnormalities. **A,** Most common are multiple café-au-lait spots over the trunk. **B** and **C,** Also seen are axillary freckling and extensive areas of hyperpigmentation. *(Courtesy Michael Sherlock, MD, Lutherville, Md.)*

inguinal freckling or extensive areas of hyperpigmentation (Fig. 15-6, *B* and *C*). Hyperpigmented skin lesions almost always precede neurologic symptoms and often increase in size and number with advancing age. They are not necessarily present at birth and may be inconspicuous in early childhood, becoming more prominent at puberty. Ninety-seven percent of patients with NF-1 have at least five café-au-lait spots by 20 years of age.

Although multiple café-au-lait spots are a clinical hallmark of NF-1, they may also occur as an autosomal dominant trait unassociated with the other features of neurofibromatosis. Genetic investigations in such families have excluded linkage to the *NF1* locus on chromosome 17, indicating a distinctly different genetic association. Multiple café-au-lait spots can be found, as well, in a variety of other conditions (Table 15-2). They are a prominent feature of McCune-Albright syndrome, the additional manifestations of which include skeletal dysplasia and endocrine abnormalities. Those seen in McCune-Albright syndrome are often large and have irregular ("coast of Maine") margins (see Chapter 8, Fig. 8-131, *D*), in contrast to the smooth ("coast of California") borders characteristic of the hyperpigmented lesions of NF-1. Café-au-lait spots also may be encountered in tuberous sclerosis and neurofibromatosis 2 (NF-2) but are seldom prominent. They are present in about 10% of the general population (typically four or less in number) and are not by themselves a sign of disease.

Additional cutaneous manifestations of NF-1 may include extensive plexiform neuromas at the terminal distribution of nerve fibers (Fig. 15-7; and see Chapter 8, Fig. 8-81) or small subcutaneous nodules—neurofibromas—scattered along the course of nerve trunks (Fig. 15-8).

Pigmented hamartomas of the iris, termed *Lisch nodules*, are seen in more than 90% of patients with NF-1 who are older than age 6 years and can be found in nearly one third of younger individuals (Fig. 15-9). They do not occur in the normal population. Although these hamartomas are asymptomatic and do not correlate with the extent or severity of other manifestations, they are helpful in establishing the diagnosis.

Short stature and macrocephaly are common in patients with NF-1, and skeletal abnormalities are found in 51% (Fig.

15-10). Osseous lesions, if present, usually appear in the first year of life. The characteristic findings include the following:

1. Severe angular scoliosis with dysplasia of the vertebral bodies (see Fig. 15-10, *A*)

2. Defects of the posterior superior wall of the orbit

Table 15-2	Conditions Associated with Café-au-lait Lesions
Disorder	**Clinical Features**
Neurofibromatosis	Most common in NF-1, rare in NF-2 (see sections on NF-1 and NF-2 and Table 15-3)
Tuberous sclerosis	See Table 15-4
McCune-Albright syndrome	Polyostotic fibrous dysplasia, precocious puberty, endocrine dysfunction
Watson syndrome	Features of Noonan syndrome (webbed neck, hypertelorism with antimongoloid slant, low-set ears, pulmonic stenosis, low intelligence), plus meets criteria for NF-1
Epidermal nevus syndrome	Verrucous skin lesions, scoliosis, aortic coarctation, mental retardation
Bloom syndrome	Severe intrauterine and postnatal growth retardation, photosensitivity, telangiectatic erythema of cheeks/face
Ataxia-telangiectasia	Ataxia, conjunctival telangiectasia, recurrent sinopulmonary infections
Silver syndrome	Intrauterine growth retardation, hemihypertrophy, syndactyly, triangular facies, premature sexual development
Gaucher disease	Opisthotonos, splenomegaly, cranial nerve dysfunction, regression of motor milestones
Turner syndrome	Short stature, webbed neck, coarctation of aorta, delayed puberty
Fanconi anemia	Aplastic anemia, hyperpigmentation, short stature, mental retardation, congenital anomalies of bone, heart, eye, kidney
Multiple lentigines (LEOPARD) syndrome	Multiple small lentigines, hypertelorism, pulmonic stenosis, cryptorchidism, mild growth retardation, sensorineural deafness

NF-1 and NF-2, neurofibromatosis types 1 and 2.

Figure 15-9 Neurofibromatosis 1 (NF-1). Pigmented hamartomas of the iris (Lisch nodules).

Figure 15-7 Neurofibromatosis 1 (NF-1). Extensive plexiform neurofibroma of the palm. *(Courtesy Michael Sherlock, MD, Lutherville, Md.)*

3. Congenital bowing and thinning of the cortices of long bones and pseudarthrosis of the tibia, fibula (Fig. 15-10, *B*; and see Chapter 8, Fig. 8-131, *B*), femur, or clavicle (see Chapter 6, Fig. 6-77)

4. Disorders of bone growth associated with elephantoid hypertrophy of overlying soft tissue

5. Erosive bony defects produced by contiguous neurogenic tumors

6. Scalloping of the posterior margins of the vertebral bodies corresponding to saccular areas of dilation of the spinal meninges (Fig. 15-10, *C*)

Patients with NF-1 can be affected with various tumors of the brain, spinal cord, and peripheral nerves, although at much less frequency than in patients with NF-2. Optic nerve glioma is the most common CNS tumor and affects 15% of patients with NF-1, usually occurring by age 3 to 6 years. It often presents as progressive visual loss with optic atrophy and tends to be less aggressive than in patients without NF-1.

Figure 15-8 Neurofibromatosis 1 (NF-1). Subcutaneous neurofibroma along the course of a nerve trunk. *(Courtesy of Michael Sherlock, MD, Lutherville, Md.)*

Ependymomas, meningiomas, brainstem gliomas, and astrocytomas also have been reported.

Magnetic resonance imaging (MRI) scans frequently show areas of increased signal intensity on T_2-weighted images of the globus pallidus, brainstem, or cerebellar white matter (Fig. 15-11). These are commonly termed unidentified bright objects (UBOs) and are believed to represent increased fluid within the myelin associated with dysplastic glial proliferation. UBOs do not appear to correlate with neurologic dysfunction. However, their presence helps confirm the diagnosis of NF-1. Computed tomography (CT) seldom demonstrates corresponding abnormalities.

Learning disabilities and behavior problems are common and may affect up to 40% of patients with NF-1. Although their full-scale intelligence quotient is generally lower than that of the general population, severe mental retardation is rare. Approximately 10% of patients with NF-1 have seizures.

A small percentage of patients with NF-1 have dysplasia of the renal or carotid arteries. Renal artery stenosis can cause systemic hypertension, and adult patients with NF-1 may develop pheochromocytoma with concomitant hypertension. Cerebral artery dysplasia can include moyamoya syndrome with abnormal vessels of the circle of Willis, predisposing to cerebral infarction in children and cerebral hemorrhage in adults.

Neurofibromatosis 2

Neurofibromatosis 2, or NF-2 (also known as *bilateral acoustic neurofibromatosis*), is a distinct genetic disorder characterized by autosomal dominant inheritance of bilateral acoustic neuromas with a penetrance of more than 95%. NF-2 occurs in approximately 1 in 50,000 people. It results from a mutation of the *NF2* gene on the long arm of chromosome 22. The *NF2* gene product, merlin or schwannomin, serves to suppress tumor formation, and its dysfunction leads to the common occurrence of CNS tumors in patients with NF-2. Most patients eventually develop bilateral acoustic neuromas (vestibular schwannomas).

Symptoms usually first appear in the teens or early twenties, when pressure on the vestibulocochlear or facial nerve complex results in impaired auditory discrimination, hearing loss, tinnitus, unsteadiness, or facial weakness. Presenile lens opacities, found in half the patients examined, may precede the onset of symptoms referable to acoustic neuroma. Other Schwann cell tumors of cranial nerves, spinal roots, or the spinal cord, as well as multiple CNS tumors of meningeal or glial origin, may develop. Cutaneous manifestations such as

Figure 15-10   Neurofibromatosis 1 (NF-1). Radiographic manifestations of skeletal abnormalities. **A,** Severe angular scoliosis and vertebral dysplasia. **B,** Congenital bowing and pseudarthrosis of the tibia and fibula. **C,** Scalloping of the posterior margins of the vertebral bodies resulting from dural ectasia. *(Courtesy Department of Radiology, Children's Hospital of Pittsburgh, Pittsburgh, Pa.)*

café-au-lait spots, cutaneous neurofibromas, and axillary or inguinal freckling are less common in NF-2 than in NF-1, and Lisch nodules are not typical. Diagnostic criteria for NF-2 are summarized in Table 15-3.

Tuberous Sclerosis

Tuberous sclerosis (TS) is inherited as an autosomal dominant trait. Two genes appear to cause the disorder: *TSC1* located on chromosome 9q and *TSC2* on chromosome 16p. Their gene

Figure 15-11   Neurofibromatosis 1 (NF-1). T_2-weighted magnetic resonance imaging (MRI) demonstrates high signal–intensity areas in the region of the globus pallidus bilaterally. *(Courtesy Division of Neuroradiology, University Health Center of Pittsburgh, Pittsburgh, Pa.)*

products (hamartin for *TSC1* and tuberin for *TSC2*) have tumor suppressor activity, which is dysfunctional in affected patients. Both genes produce similar phenotypes when expressed. Genetic testing is available and currently detects 60% to 80% of cases. Although 1 in 6000 to 9000 people in the population carry a *TS* gene, expression is highly variable and full expression of disease is seen in only 1 in 150,000 members of the population. Most carriers have hypopigmented macules (ash-leaf spots) as their only manifestation. Spontaneous mutation appears to account for the majority of newly diagnosed cases, and in up to 2% of patients without a positive family history, the disorder may be the result of germline mosaicism.

The more prominent features of this neurocutaneous disorder include seizures (96%), mental retardation (60%), intracranial calcification (49%), tumors of various organs (including the brain, heart, liver, and kidneys), and cutaneous lesions. Seizures are the most frequent presenting complaint. Clinical expression can be quite variable even among affected members of the same family. Diagnostic criteria are summarized in Table 15-4.

Table 15-3	Diagnostic Criteria for Neurofibromatosis 2

Bilateral eighth nerve masses seen with appropriate imaging techniques (e.g., CT, MRI)

or

A first-degree relative with NF-2 and a unilateral eighth nerve mass
or two of the following:

- Neurofibroma
- Meningioma
- Glioma
- Schwannoma
- Juvenile posterior subcapsular lens opacity

CT, computed tomography; MRI, magnetic resonance imaging; NF-2, neurofibromatosis 2.

Table 15-4	Diagnostic Criteria for Tuberous Sclerosis

Major Features

Facial angiofibromas or forehead plaque

Nontraumatic ungual or periungual fibroma

Hypomelanotic macules (i.e., ash-leaf spots [≥3])

Shagreen patch (connective tissue nevus)

Multiple retinal nodular hamartomas

Cortical tuber

Subependymal nodule

Subependymal giant cell astrocytoma

Cardiac rhabdomyoma, single or multiple

Lymphangiomyomatosis

Renal angiomyolipoma

Minor Features

Multiple randomly distributed pits in dental enamel

Hamartomatous rectal polyps

Bone cysts

Cerebral white matter radial migration lines

Gingival fibromas

Nonrenal hamartoma

Retinal achromatic patch

"Confetti" skin lesions

Multiple renal cysts

Definite Tuberous Sclerosis

Two major features or one major and two minor features

Probable Tuberous Sclerosis

One major plus one minor feature

Possible Tuberous Sclerosis

Either one major feature or two or more minor features

Modified from Roach ES, Gometz MR, Northrup H: Tuberous Sclerosis Complex Consensus Conference: Revised clinical diagnostic criteria, *J Child Neurol* 13:624–628, 1998.

The characteristic skin lesion of tuberous sclerosis is the angiofibroma *(adenoma sebaceum)*. These are seen as erythematous papules distributed over the nose and malar region of the face (Fig. 15-12). Approximately 40% of children with tuberous sclerosis demonstrate these lesions by 3 years of age.

Hypomelanotic macules with irregular borders, termed *ash-leaf spots,* are another common cutaneous manifestation (Fig.

15-13, *A* and *B*). These generally appear earlier than adenoma sebaceum and may be present at birth. They are detectable by 2 years of age in more than half of affected children. They resemble vitiligo but differ in that they are not completely devoid of melanin. In fair-skinned infants, these nevi may be demonstrable only under Wood lamp light.

Another valuable cutaneous marker is the *shagreen patch,* a plaque of thickened skin with a cobblestone or orange-peel texture often seen on the dorsal aspect of the trunk (Fig. 15-14). Histologically, the shagreen patch is a connective tissue nevus.

Additional dermatologic manifestations of tuberous sclerosis include periungual fibromas (Fig. 15-15) and macular areas of hyperpigmentation. Recognition of the cutaneous features can suggest an etiologic diagnosis in some patients with mental retardation or seizures. Oral examination may reveal pitting of dental enamel.

In patients with tuberous sclerosis, CT scans often demonstrate subependymal nodules seen as intracranial calcifications that appear as multiple scattered areas of increased density adjacent to the walls of the lateral and third ventricles (Fig. 15-16). CT is superior to MRI for demonstration of small calcifications. No relationship has been established between the extent of periventricular calcification and clinical severity as judged by developmental function or seizure frequency. CT may also demonstrate asymptomatic but typical intracranial calcifications in individuals who lack external manifestations of the disorder. This can help identify subclinical cases and improve the accuracy of genetic counseling in affected families.

The characteristic gross abnormality of the brain in TS is the presence of multiple gliotic nodules (hamartomas) of varying size, which constitute the tubers for which this disorder is named. These are located over the convolutions of the cerebral hemispheres and beneath the ependymal lining of the lateral and third ventricles. Heterotopic nodules of identical structure may be found in the cerebral white matter as well. Although cortical tubers are rarely apparent on CT scans, they are readily identified by MRI studies (Fig. 15-17). Severely affected patients have a greater number of cerebral cortical lesions detected by MRI scans, suggesting that MRI may be useful in predicting eventual clinical severity in young children with newly diagnosed tuberous sclerosis. Tumors may arise from cortical or subependymal tubers, complicating the course of the disease by producing increased intracranial

Figure 15-12 Tuberous sclerosis. **A,** This adolescent boy had adenoma sebaceum in a characteristic malar distribution and chin lesions as well. **B,** A close-up view of nasal lesions is shown.

Figure 15-13   Tuberous sclerosis (TS). **A,** An ash-leaf spot is an oval depigmented nevus with irregular borders. **B,** This child with TS has numerous hypopigmented macules over his scalp, and the hair growing from these is hypopigmented as well (a phenomenon termed *poliosis*). *(Courtesy Robin Gehris, MD, Children's Hospital of Pittsburgh, Pittsburgh, Pa.)*

Figure 15-14   Tuberous sclerosis. Shagreen patch. This plaque of thickened skin with a cobblestone texture is distinctive but is one of the less common cutaneous manifestations. *(Courtesy Michael Sherlock, MD, Lutherville, Md.)*

Figure 15-15   Tuberous sclerosis. Periungual fibromas. These nodular lesions can occur singly or multiply in the ungual or periungual areas. *(Courtesy Michael Painter, MD, Children's Hospital of Pittsburgh, Pittsburgh, Pa.)*

Figure 15-16   Tuberous sclerosis. This computed tomography (CT) cut through the foramina of Monro shows the multiple periventricular calcific deposits characteristic of this disorder. *(Courtesy Division of Neuroradiology, University Health Center of Pittsburgh, Pittsburgh, Pa.)*

Figure 15-17   Tuberous sclerosis. MRI demonstrates multiple cortical tubers that appear as areas of increased signal intensity in this T_2-weighted image. The signal abnormalities arise predominantly within the white matter subjacent to the tuber. *(Courtesy Division of Neuroradiology, University Health Center of Pittsburgh, Pittsburgh, Pa.)*

Figure 15-18 Tuberous sclerosis. CT scan demonstrates a large subependymal astrocytoma, which intermittently obstructed the ventricular system, producing episodic symptoms of increased intracranial pressure. *(Courtesy Division of Neuroradiology, University Health Center of Pittsburgh, Pittsburgh, Pa.)*

Figure 15-19 Sturge-Weber syndrome. A nonelevated purple cutaneous vascular malformation, often termed a *port-wine stain*, is seen in a trigeminal distribution, including the ophthalmic division.

Sturge-Weber Syndrome

The cardinal manifestations of Sturge-Weber syndrome are as follows:

1. A vascular malformation or port-wine stain over the face that involves the cutaneous distribution of the ophthalmic division of the trigeminal nerve

2. Ipsilateral leptomeningeal angiomatosis with associated intracranial calcifications

3. A high incidence of mental retardation and ipsilateral ocular complications

The port-wine stain (Fig. 15-19) is usually present at birth and consists of a pink-to-purple macular cutaneous vascular malformation. Only patients with lesions involving the cutaneous distribution of the ophthalmic division of the trigeminal nerve (i.e., forehead and upper eyelid) are at risk for associated neuro-ocular complications (Fig. 15-20). Repeated ophthalmologic and CT or MRI examinations are indicated only in this high-risk group, which has a 10% to 20% incidence of associated intracranial angiomas.

The coincidence of seizures and a facial vascular nevus should suggest the diagnosis of Sturge-Weber syndrome, which can be confirmed by CT scan (Fig. 15-21) or MRI. These scans may be normal at birth but subsequently show

pressure and other symptoms associated with intracranial mass lesions. Up to 80% of patients with tuberous sclerosis develop seizures of variable types that are often difficult to control. Infantile spasms are common and may be the presenting symptom leading to diagnosis. Patients with a history of infantile spasms and those who develop other types of seizures when very young tend to have more severe seizure disorders and poorer cognitive function.

Subependymal giant cell astrocytomas (SEGAs) (Fig. 15-18) can affect 10% of patients with tuberous sclerosis and are clinically manifested by symptoms of obstructive hydrocephalus. The site of obstruction is often at the level of the foramen of Monro in the lateral ventricles. Such patients may present with signs of increased intracranial pressure (headache, vision changes, and/or papilledema), behavior change, or worsening seizure control.

Visceral lesions associated with tuberous sclerosis include cardiac rhabdomyoma, renal angiomyolipomas, pulmonary lymphangiomyomatosis, and hepatic hamartoma. Cardiac rhabdomyomas occur in up to two thirds of patients and may be multiple. They tend to regress over the first few years of life and are usually asymptomatic, although occasionally an affected newborn may have obstructive congestive heart failure. About three fourths of patients with tuberous sclerosis have renal angiomyolipomas, which are often bilateral and multiple. Most remain clinically silent, but tumors greater than 4 cm in size are more likely to be symptomatic and may cause hematuria or proteinuria. Renal disease is the most common cause of death in adults with the disease and may be manifest as flank pain, hematuria, or retroperitoneal hemorrhage. Renal cysts occur earlier and less often than do angiomyolipomas. Rarely, children with tuberous sclerosis can present in infancy with polycystic kidney disease. Chronic renal failure and malignant transformation of renal tumors are rare. Pulmonary lymphangiomyomatosis affects less than 2% of patients, mostly females, and is rare before the adult years. Symptoms include dyspnea, spontaneous pneumothorax, and hemoptysis. Hepatic hamartoma is clinically insignificant.

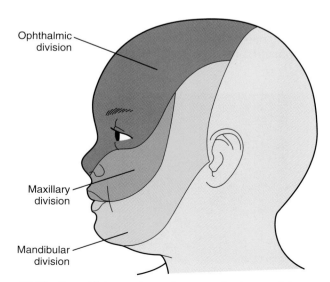

Figure 15-20 Sturge-Weber syndrome. Cutaneous distribution of the division of the trigeminal nerve. Only patients with facial port-wine stains that involve the ophthalmic division are at risk for associated neuro-ocular symptoms.

Figure 15-21   Sturge-Weber syndrome. Although the CT scan is usually normal at birth, findings such as gyriform contrast enhancement, seen here in the left occipital, temporal, and parietal lobes **(A),** and associated hemispheric atrophy **(B)** may be observed as early as 4 months of age. Serpiginous parenchymal calcifications may be found in the older child **(C).** *(Courtesy Division of Neuroradiology, University Health Center of Pittsburgh, Pittsburgh, Pa.)*

areas of gyriform contrast enhancement corresponding to the leptomeningeal angiomatosis. Serial examinations often demonstrate progressive ipsilateral cerebral atrophy. Additional findings may include serpiginous calcifications of brain parenchyma underlying vascular malformations of the pia. These intracranial calcifications are first seen on CT scan but become evident on plain skull films by the end of the second decade.

Associated ocular abnormalities are often encountered. Buphthalmos (corneal enlargement) or a coloboma may be present at birth, and glaucoma frequently develops in infancy or later childhood (Fig. 15-22). Dilated vessels in the sclera, conjunctiva, and retina are common, and angiomatous malformations of the choroid occasionally occur.

The estimated incidence of facial cutaneous angioma is 1 in 5000, and the estimated frequency of the complete syndrome is 1 in 30,000. Among patients with the complete syndrome, seizures occur in 90%, and contralateral hemiparesis eventually develops in one third. Early developmental milestones are often normal, but about 50% develop cognitive difficulties ranging from mild to severe. Behavioral problems are common. Patients with refractory epilepsy are more likely to be more severely delayed. Although most cases are sporadic, genetic determination has not been ruled out. No cases of direct transmission from parent to child have been reported, however.

Klippel-Trénaunay Syndrome

Patients with Klippel-Trénaunay syndrome (KTS) are born with a port-wine stain that is usually located over the lateral aspect of one leg. Less often an arm and a leg may be affected. In rare instances more extensive, even bilateral, involvement is seen. The surface lesion is associated with an underlying vascular malformation, which provides an unusually rich blood supply to soft tissue and bony structures that results in hypertrophy (usually hemihypertrophy) and lymphedema (Fig. 15-23, *A* and *B*). These features are often evident in the newborn, and progressive enlargement occurs during the first

Figure 15-23   Klippel-Trénaunay syndrome. **A,** This infant with KTS is unusual in that he has vascular malformations involving both lower extremities, which extend upward over the lateral aspects of the abdominal wall. **B,** In this view of his feet, one can appreciate a greater degree of hypertrophy on the right.

Figure 15-22   Buphthalmos. Enlargement of the cornea of the right eye is evident. This is one of the associated ocular findings in Sturge-Weber syndrome and should prompt urgent evaluation for associated glaucoma. *(From Booth IW, Wozniak ER:* Pediatrics, *Baltimore, 1984, Williams & Wilkins.)*

Figure 15-24 Ataxia-telangiectasia. Characteristic telangiectases in the bulbar conjunctiva usually develop between 3 months and 6 years of age.

Figure 15-25 Linear nevus sebaceus of Jadassohn. This yellowish-tan, waxy-appearing lesion became elevated at puberty and was associated with seizures and mental retardation.

few years. Most cases are sporadic. However, a few cases have been reported to be autosomal dominant.

Ataxia-Telangiectasia

Ataxia-telangiectasia is a multisystem, autosomal recessive degenerative disorder characterized by ataxia, oculocutaneous telangiectasia, immunodeficiency, and a high incidence of neoplasia. The nature of the basic underlying defect is unknown. Affected individuals are extremely sensitive to ionizing radiation and have defective DNA repair mechanisms. Molecular genetic testing for *ATM* (ataxia telangiectasia mutated), the only gene associated with ataxia-telangiectasia, is clinically available. Ataxia is the usual presenting feature, and the course of the neurologic disturbance is rather stereotypic. Tremors of the head may be seen before 1 year of age, and unsteadiness of gait is evident when the child first walks. Progressive global ataxia and slurred, scanning, dysarthric speech are typical during the early school-age years. Loss of deep tendon reflexes and impairment of position and vibratory sensation are evident by the end of the first decade. Adolescence is marked by choreoathetosis, dystonic posturing, gaze apraxia, and progressive dementia. Nonclassic forms of ataxia-telangiectasia have included adult-onset cases and presentations with early dystonia.

The characteristic cutaneous manifestations of this disorder appear by 6 years of age. Telangiectases first appear on the bulbar conjunctivae (Fig. 15-24) and develop later over the malar regions, ears, antecubital fossae, neck, and upper chest.

Neuropathologic changes are widespread, with the cerebellum being the site of maximal degeneration. Loss of Purkinje and basket cells, thinning of the granular cell layer, and mild changes in the molecular layer are characteristic findings.

Systemic manifestations include major defects in cellular and humoral immunity. Deficiencies of IgA and IgM are characteristic and together with impaired cellular immunity contribute to susceptibility to the recurrent sinus and pulmonary infections that mark this disorder, as well as to the tendency to develop malignancies of the lymphoreticular system (most commonly acute lymphoblastic leukemia or lymphoma) during adolescence or early adulthood (see Chapter 4). Serum α-fetoprotein levels are elevated, which serves as a nonspecific marker. Adult family members of patients, especially mothers, may also be susceptible to malignancy, breast and lung cancer being the most common.

Linear Sebaceous Nevus

The nevus sebaceus of Jadassohn is usually present at birth, manifest as a yellowish-tan, waxy linear lesion (Fig. 15-25) that contains a papillomatous excess of sebaceous glands. This

nevus may be found on the scalp, face, neck, trunk, or extremities. With time, the lesion becomes unsightly. This eventuality and a 15% to 20% risk of malignant degeneration have led practitioners to recommend early surgical excision. Although usually seen as an isolated abnormality in otherwise normal individuals, an association with seizures and mental retardation has been reported. The risk of neurologic abnormalities is greatest when the cutaneous lesion is located in the midfacial area.

Epidermal Nevus Syndrome

Epidermal nevus syndrome is a congenital neurocutaneous disorder in which an epidermal nevus is seen in association with neurologic dysfunction. The latter may include seizures, paresis, mental retardation, and developmental delay. Unilateral hemimegalencephaly with intractable seizures is the commonest CNS abnormality. Disorders of segmentation/migration and multiple other structural CNS anomalies have been reported. Extra-CNS congenital defects may involve connective tissues, especially the skeleton; as well as ocular, cardiac, and genitourinary systems. The skin lesions are hamartomatous (derived from embryonic ectoderm) and characterized by hyperplasia of the epidermis and adnexal structures. They are usually present at birth, although some may appear later in the first year. They appear as raised, often warty hyperpigmented lesions typically in a linear pattern (Fig. 15-26). They may enlarge subsequently but tend to stabilize in size by puberty. Most cases are sporadic, although a small number are autosomal dominant.

Incontinentia Pigmenti

Incontinentia pigmenti is a rare, X-linked dominant syndrome with cutaneous, neurologic, ophthalmologic, and dental manifestations. It is caused by a mutation in the *NEMO* gene.

Neurologic and ophthalmologic problems often become manifest during early infancy and are reported to occur in about 30% of patients. They may include seizures, cerebrovascular accidents, developmental delay, mental retardation, and microcephaly. Cutaneous features are described in Chapter 8 (see Chapter 8, Fig. 8-97).

CENTRAL NERVOUS SYSTEM MALFORMATIONS

Malformations of the CNS are a leading cause of neurologic and developmental disability in infants and children. Although CNS malformations are not necessarily accompanied by external dysmorphic features, disturbances of cranial volume,

Figure 15-26   Epidermal nevus syndrome. **A,** Hyperpigmented verrucous papules are seen unilaterally over the upper arm, trunk, hip, and lumbosacral area of this adolescent boy. He had had a seizure in infancy and was learning disabled. **B,** In this infant, raised hyperpigmented lesions are present on the left face and both sides of the forehead and were associated with intractable seizures. *(Courtesy Robin Gehris, MD, Children's Hospital of Pittsburgh, Pittsburgh, Pa.)*

abnormalities of head shape, and skin lesions overlying the dorsal midline should alert the physician to the possibility of associated CNS dysmorphogenesis.

Macrocephaly

Macrocephaly is defined as a head circumference greater than 2 standard deviations above the mean for age, gender, and gestation. This abnormality can be caused by a myriad of conditions (Table 15-5) including hydrocephalus (excessive accumulation of cerebrospinal fluid [CSF]); intracranial mass lesions (tumors, subdural effusions); thickening or enlargement of the skull (primary skeletal dysplasias); and a true increase in brain substance (megalencephaly). The latter is seen in Soto syndrome, achondroplasia, neurocutaneous syndromes, and certain lipidoses, leukodystrophies, and mucopolysaccharidoses. Primary megalencephaly may occur as a benign familial trait.

Evaluation of the child with a head that is abnormally large or appears to be growing at an excessive rate should include the following:

1. Serial measurements of head circumference

2. Measurement of the parents' head circumferences and exploration of family history for evidence of macrocephaly or neurologic and cutaneous abnormalities

3. Developmental history

4. Careful examination for evidence of increased intracranial pressure, developmental delay, skeletal dysplasia, abnormal transillumination, cranial bruits, ocular abnormalities, or organomegaly

Plain skull radiographs may provide evidence of increased intracranial pressure (see Fig. 15-38), identify intracranial

calcification (Fig. 15-27), or detect primary skeletal dysplasias (Fig. 15-28). CT or MRI scans allow assessment of ventricular size and permit detection of intracranial mass lesions and chronic subdural effusions. CT is the method of choice for demonstrating intracranial calcification and detecting fresh blood.

Hydrocephalus

Hydrocephalus is caused by an imbalance between CSF production and resorption that is of sufficient magnitude to result in a net accumulation of fluid within the ventricular system. Impaired CSF resorption may occur secondary to obstruction of CSF pathways within the ventricular system (noncommunicating hydrocephalus) or as a result of obstruction of the subarachnoid space (communicating hydrocephalus). Hydrocephalus secondary to CSF overproduction is rare but does occur in some cases of choroid plexus papilloma (see Fig. 15-42). Noncommunicating hydrocephalus is often due to aqueductal stenosis or congenital malformations of the fourth ventricle, and it is a common complication of tumors or vascular malformations of the posterior fossa that compress the cerebral aqueduct or obstruct outflow from the fourth ventricle. Causes of communicating hydrocephalus include intracranial hemorrhage, meningitis, cerebral venous or dural sinus thrombosis, and diffuse infiltration of the meninges by malignant cells.

The clinical manifestations of hydrocephalus in infancy are stereotypic. The head is excessively large at birth or grows at an abnormally rapid rate, becoming macrocephalic over the first few months. The forehead is disproportionately large, and the face appears small in relation to the calvarium. The scalp is thin and glistening, and its veins are distended, often becoming strikingly dilated when the infant cries. The anterior fontanelle is large, tense, and nonpulsatile, and the sutures are excessively wide (Fig. 15-29, *A*). Divergent strabismus,

Table 15-5 Causes of Macrocephaly

Early Infantile	Late Infantile	Early to Late Childhood
(Birth-6 Months)	(6 Months-2 Years)	(After 2 Years)
• Hydrocephalus (progressive or arrested) — Induction disorders (congenital malformations) • Spina bifida cystica, cranium bifidum, Chiari malformations (types I, II, and III), aqueductal stenosis, holoprosencephaly • Mass lesions — Neoplasms, A-V malformations, congenital cysts • Intrauterine infections — Toxoplasmosis, cytomegalovirus infection, syphilis, rubella — Perinatal or postnatal infections • Bacterial, granulomatous, parasitic — Perinatal or postnatal hemorrhage • Hypoxia, vascular malformation, trauma • Hydranencephaly • Subdural effusion — Hemorrhagic, infectious, cystic hygroma • Normal variant (often familial)	• Hydrocephalus (progressive or arrested) — Space-occupying lesions • Tumors, cysts, abscesses — Postbacterial or granulomatous meningitis — Dysraphism • Dandy-Walker syndrome, Chiari type I malformation — Posthemorrhagic • Trauma or vascular malformation • Subdural effusion • Increased intracranial pressure syndrome — Pseudotumor cerebri • Lead, tetracycline, hypoparathyroidism, steroids, excess or deficiency of vitamin A, cyanotic congenital heart disease • Primary skeletal cranial dysplasia (thickened or enlarged skull): Osteogenesis imperfecta, hyperphosphatemia, osteopetrosis, rickets • Megalencephaly (increase in brain substance) — Metabolic CNS diseases: leukodystrophies (e.g., Canavan, Alexander), lipidoses (Tay-Sachs), histiocytosis, mucopolysaccharidoses — Proliferative neurocutaneous syndromes: von Recklinghausen, tuberous sclerosis, hemangiomatosis, Sturge-Weber — Cerebral gigantism • Soto syndrome — Achondroplasia — Primary megalencephaly • May be familial and unassociated or associated with abnormalities of cellular architecture	• Hydrocephalus (progressive or arrested) — Space-occupying lesions — Preexisting induction disorder • Aqueductal stenosis — Chiari type I malformation — Postinfectious — Hemorrhagic • Megalencephaly — Proliferative neurocutaneous syndromes — Familial • Pseudotumor cerebri • Normal variant

From Gabriel RS: Malformations of the central nervous system. In Menkes JH, editor: *Textbook of child neurology,* ed 2, Philadelphia, 1980, Lea & Febiger. A-V, atrioventricular.

Figure 15-27 Macrocephaly. Frontal **(A)** and lateral **(B)** radiographs reveal bilaterally symmetrical, paraventricular cerebral calcifications in association with cranial enlargement in an infant with congenital cytomegalovirus infection. *(Courtesy Department of Radiology, Children's Hospital of Pittsburgh, Pittsburgh, Pa.)*

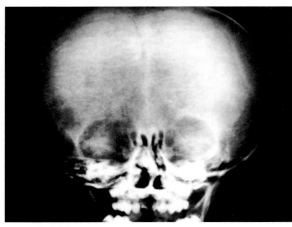

Figure 15-28   Macrocephaly. Plain skull radiographs allow detection of primary skeletal dysplasias. In this case, note the mosaic rarification of the cranial vault and multiple wormian bones characteristic of osteogenesis imperfecta. *(Courtesy Department of Radiology, Children's Hospital of Pittsburgh, Pittsburgh, Pa.)*

abducens nerve paresis, and impaired upward gaze are important ocular findings. With severe hydrocephalus, there may be forced, conjugate downward deviation of the eyes so that the inferior half of the iris is hidden by the lower eyelid, producing the "sunsetting" sign (Fig. 15-29, *B*). Neurologic abnormalities

include developmental delay, persistence of early infantile automatisms, and spasticity and hyperreflexia of the lower extremities. CT or MRI scans demonstrate enlargement of the ventricular system and thinning of the cortical mantle and may provide additional anatomic information concerning the etiology (Fig. 15-29, *C*).

Infantile hydrocephalus must be distinguished from other causes of macrocephaly in infancy such as chronic subdural hematoma, expanding porencephalic cyst, and certain degenerative disorders that may produce abnormal enlargement of the head (see Table 15-5). In premature infants with suspected hydrocephalus, the normally rapid rate of postnatal head growth must be taken into account.

Dandy-Walker Malformation

The Dandy-Walker malformation is a primary developmental abnormality characterized by progressive cystic enlargement of the fourth ventricle beginning early in fetal life. This is accompanied by enlargement of the posterior fossa and upward displacement of the tentorium, torcula, and transverse sinuses. Associated hydrocephalus is almost universal, and may be present at birth or may develop later, during infancy or childhood. Of affected individuals, 60% show signs of hydrocephalus and increased intracranial pressure by 2 years of age.

Clinical manifestations of Dandy-Walker malformation are variable and depend on the severity and rate of progression

Figure 15-29   Infantile hydrocephalus. **A,** Characteristic enlarged head, thinning of the scalp, distended scalp veins, and a full fontanelle. **B,** Paresis of the upward gaze is seen in an infant with hydrocephalus resulting from aqueductal stenosis. Paresis is more apparent on the right. This phenomenon is often termed the *sunsetting sign.* **C,** CT scan demonstrates a dilated ventricular system and thinning of the cortical mantle. (**A,** *From Booth IW, Wozniak ER: Pediatrics, Baltimore, 1984, Williams & Wilkins;* **B,** *courtesy Albert Biglan, MD, Children's Hospital of Pittsburgh, Pittsburgh, Pa;* **C,** *courtesy Division of Neuroradiology, University Health Center of Pittsburgh, Pittsburgh, Pa.)*

Figure 15-30 Dandy-Walker malformation. **A,** Transillumination demonstrates a posterior fossa cyst. Note also the bulging occiput, prominent scalp veins, and enlargement of the head. **B,** CT scan shows a posterior fossa cyst, a small cerebellar remnant, and associated hydrocephalus. (*A, Courtesy Michael J. Painter, MD, Children's Hospital of Pittsburgh, Pittsburgh, Pa.*)

of the associated hydrocephalus. A child with a symptomatic condition often has an unusually prominent bulging occiput in addition to the usual findings of hydrocephalus. In children younger than 1 year of age, transillumination of the skull effectively demonstrates the posterior fossa cyst (Fig. 15-30, *A*). Ataxia, nystagmus, and cranial nerve deficits may also be prominent features.

Plain skull radiographs demonstrate posteroinferior enlargement of the cranial vault, thinning and ballooning of the occipital squama, and upward displacement of the torcula. CT or MRI scans confirm the presence of a large posterior fossa cyst, a small cerebellar remnant, and associated hydrocephalus (Fig. 15-30, *B*).

Hydranencephaly

Hydranencephaly is a severe anomaly of the brain characterized by the absence of the cerebral hemispheres despite intact meninges and a normal skull. Affected children often appear deceptively normal at birth, with little to suggest the presence of a severe brain abnormality (Fig. 15-31, *A*). Because newborns function at a subcortical reflex level, even complete absence of the cerebral hemispheres may not interfere with normal reflexes. However, within the first few weeks of life, developmental arrest, decerebration, hypertonia, and hyperreflexia become apparent in the infant with hydranencephaly. Most of these infants do not live beyond 6 to 12 months, although survival for several years is occasionally reported. Seizures are common, and progressive enlargement of the head may complicate nursing care.

The diagnosis may be suggested if, on transillumination of the skull, the entire calvarium is lit up (Fig. 15-31, *B*). However, severe hydrocephalus and bilateral subdural hygromas may present a similar appearance.

On CT (Fig. 15-31, *C*) or MRI, CSF signal intensity replaces the supratentorial brain parenchyma with sparing of the thalami, brainstem, cerebellum, and choroid plexus. The falx is intact, distinguishing this from holoprosencephaly. A thin rim of cerebral parenchyma is lacking, distinguishing this from severe unshunted hydrocephalus. To distinguish this disorder from massive bilateral subdural hygromas, cerebral angiography is required to confirm absence of the cerebrum.

Microcephaly

Microcephaly is defined as a head circumference more than 2 standard deviations below the mean for age, gender, and conceptual age. Apart from cases resulting from premature closure of the sutures (generalized craniosynostosis), microcephaly reflects an abnormally small brain and can be a symptom of any disorder that impairs brain growth (Table 15-6). The neurologic manifestations range from minor (e.g., poor fine motor skills, mild intellectual impairment) to profound (e.g., decerebration, chronic vegetative state). Diagnostic evaluation should include a family history, prenatal history, a search for associated congenital anomalies, karyotyping, amino acid screening, and serologic studies for intrauterine infection. Plain skull radiographs can detect craniosynostosis, whereas CT scan is useful in identifying intracranial calcifications. MRI is preferred for delineation of recognizable patterns of CNS dysmorphogenesis.

Midline Defects and Occult Spinal Dysraphism

Development of the human nervous system begins early in the third week of gestation with the proliferation of ectodermal cells in the dorsal midline to form the neural plate. By the end

Table 15-6	Causes of Microcephaly
Genetic Defects	***Antenatal Irradiation***
Autosomal recessive defects	***Exposure to Drugs and Chemicals during Gestation***
Autosomal dominant defects	
Disorders of Karyotype	Ethyl alcohol exposure (fetal alcohol syndrome)
Trisomies	Phenytoin exposure
Deletions	Trimethadione exposure
Translocations	Methyl mercury exposure
Intrauterine Infections	***Maternal Phenylketonuria***
Rubella	***Perinatal Insults***
Cytomegalovirus infection	Traumatic
Toxoplasmosis	Anoxic
Congenital syphilis	Metabolic
Herpesvirus infections	Infectious

Figure 15-31   Hydranencephaly. **A,** Patient, age 3 weeks, has a deceptively normal appearance with little to suggest a severe brain abnormality. **B,** Transillumination of the skull lights up the entire calvarium, suggesting the diagnosis. **C,** CT scan demonstrates replacement of the cerebral hemispheres by a large, water-dense cavity with residual islands of brain tissue in regions of the occipital poles and right inferior temporal lobe. *(C, Courtesy Division of Neuroradiology, University Health Center of Pittsburgh, Pittsburgh, Pa.)*

of the fourth week, the neural plate has invaginated and then fused in the midline to form the neural tube. The cerebrum, diencephalon, midbrain, and brainstem develop from the rostral portion of the neural tube. The caudal portion separates from the overlying ectoderm, forming the precursor of the spinal cord, and is surrounded by mesodermal elements destined to form the vertebral bodies and supporting soft tissue structures. Midline spinal cord and vertebral skeletal defects, termed *spinal dysraphism*, result from defective closure of the caudal portion of the neural tube. Abnormal neural tube closure beginning early in the embryologic sequence produces dysraphic states involving both neural and skeletal elements (myelomeningocele [see Chapter 1, Fig. 1-20, *C*]), whereas closure defects occurring later produce congenital anomalies restricted to the posterior elements of the vertebrae (spina bifida occulta).

Occult spinal dysraphism is a defect of intermediate severity in which vertebral anomalies are associated with underlying intraspinal tumors or developmental abnormalities. Its presence is often (although not always) betrayed by cutaneous and subcutaneous abnormalities centered over the midline of the back, such as a hairy patch (Fig. 15-32, *A*), skin tag, port-wine stain, hemangioma, subcutaneous lipoma (Fig. 15-32, *B*), cutis aplasia, or sinus tract (Fig. 15-32, *C*). Infants with atypical dimples or clefts (>5 mm) that are located more than 2.5 cm from the anus also have an increased incidence of underlying malformations, whereas those with simple blind dimples located within the gluteal cleft or within 2.5 cm of the anus do not. Although neurologic abnormalities are commonly associated with the lesions mentioned earlier, they are by no means universal. Figure 15-33 shows a child with

a large lumbosacral hemangioma who did not have any associated neurologic abnormality.

Midline defects are not limited to the caudal portion of the neural tube but can occur over the head and neck as well. Most notably, these include encephaloceles. These may be obvious in their appearance (see Chapter 1, Fig. 1-20, *A*), may have no external findings (see Chapter 23, Fig. 23-36), or may be associated with an overlying scalp lesion such as a vascular malformation (Fig. 15-34).

Because early diagnosis and neurosurgical intervention can prevent the onset and/or progression of neurologic deficits, newborns with midline cutaneous or subcutaneous stigmata and those with atypical dimples or clefts should undergo radiologic screening. Ultrasonography has proved to be the best tool for this purpose before ossification of the posterior vertebral elements (at 3 months) because it not only can detect vertebral defects and spinal anomalies but also can be used to assess cord motion. If this reveals an underlying malformation or anomaly, follow-up MRI and neurosurgical referral are indicated. Common intraspinal lesions include dermoid tumors, intraspinal lipomas (Fig. 15-35), and diastematomyelia (Fig. 15-36).

Although some patients with occult spinal dysraphism may show signs of neurologic dysfunction and talipes equinovarus from birth, most develop symptoms insidiously after a symptom-free interval. Dysfunction usually begins at approximately 3 years of age, but many do not develop problems until school age or adolescence. Presenting complaints may include back or leg stiffness, clumsiness, mild weakness or numbness of the lower extremities, or problems with bowel or bladder dysfunction.

Figure 15-32 Cutaneous and subcutaneous markers of occult spinal dysraphism. **A,** Note the hairy patch over the lumbar region, here associated with diastematomyelia. **B,** The soft subcutaneous mass seen overlying the sacrum of this infant was determined to be a lipoma. **C,** Sacral sinus tract associated with intraspinal dermoid tumor. (*A and C, Courtesy Michael J. Painter, MD, Children's Hospital of Pittsburgh, Pittsburgh, Pa; B, from Cohen BA:* Atlas of pediatric dermatology, *London, 1993, Mosby-Wolfe.*)

Objective findings may consist of decreased tone and decreased deep tendon reflexes in the lower extremities; patchy decreases in sensation; and foot deformities consisting of broadening and shortening, deepening of the arch, and contractures of the toes (see Chapter 21, Fig. 21-110). Symptoms of associated tethering of the spinal cord may be present in infancy, but often their onset is delayed until the child enters a period of rapid growth and develops back, leg, or buttock pain; signs of lower limb spasticity; and, on occasion,

bowel and bladder dysfunction. These symptoms presumably are due to progressive deformation of the tethered cord, which is not free to "ascend" normally within the spinal canal as the rate of linear growth of the vertebral column outpaces that of the spinal cord. Tethering of the spinal cord by an anomalous filum terminale (Fig. 15-37), producing similar signs of progressive neurologic dysfunction, can occur in the absence of associated cutaneous abnormalities, vertebral defects, or intraspinal tumors.

Figure 15-33 Lumbosacral hemangioma. This child has a large lumbosacral hemangioma that extended well below the surface and wrapped around the vertebral column, but regressed promptly and was not associated with any abnormality of the underlying neural or bony structures. (*Courtesy Robin Gehris, MD, Children's Hospital of Pittsburgh, Pittsburgh, Pa.*)

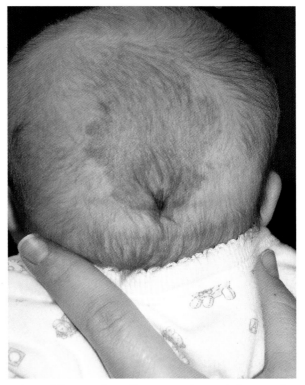

Figure 15-34 Midline vascular malformation with an underlying atretic encephalocele in an infant who had no signs of neurologic dysfunction. (*Courtesy Robin Gehris, MD, Children's Hospital of Pittsburgh, Pittsburgh, Pa.*)

Figure 15-35 Occult spinal dysraphism. CT scan demonstrates an intraspinal lipoma in a child with a subcutaneous lipoma over the lumbar spine.

Figure 15-37 Tethered cord resulting from a tight filum terminale. On myelography, the conus medullaris is pulled down to L3-L4 by a tethered filum terminale, the upper portion of which is thickened. Presenting symptoms included weakness of plantar flexion, eversion of the feet, and bladder dysfunction. *(Courtesy Charles Fitz, MD, Children's Hospital of Pittsburgh, Pittsburgh, Pa.)*

Figure 15-36 Diastematomyelia. This 6-month-old infant had progressive inturning and plantar flexion of the left foot and a slightly deviated gluteal cleft. On myelogram, her spinal cord splits at L1, coursing around a bony spur at L2, then rejoins at L4-L5. She also had complete spinal dysraphism of L2-L4 and partial dysraphism at L1 and L5.

INCREASED INTRACRANIAL PRESSURE

The cranial cavity is occupied by the brain, blood, and CSF. An increase in the volume of any of these compartments, unless accompanied by a concomitant decrease in one or both of the other compartments, results in increased intracranial pressure. Increased intracranial pressure can result from a wide variety of disorders and is itself hazardous. Recognition of associated signs and symptoms permits early diagnosis and prompt intervention to forestall progressive brain injury or catastrophic neurologic deterioration.

Primary Signs and Symptoms

The clinical manifestations of increased intracranial pressure vary with age. In infants, examination of the anterior fontanelle allows reliable assessment of intracranial pressure. In the normal, quiet infant held in an upright or sitting posture, the anterior fontanelle is flat or slightly concave. Under these conditions, an anterior fontanelle that bulges above the contour of the calvaria and that is excessively firm on palpation is always abnormal (see Fig. 15-29, *A*; and see Chapter 12, Fig. 12-40, *B*). Because the cranial sutures are not fused in infants and young children, increased intracranial pressure rapidly produces separation of the bony plates of the skull. In infants, this can be detected by palpation; in older children, skull radiographs may be necessary to identify widened cranial sutures (Fig. 15-38, *A*). Prominent convolutional markings on the inner table of the skull (Fig. 15-38, *B*) are a less useful

Figure 15-38 Findings of increased intracranial pressure that may be seen on standard skull radiographs. **A,** Widening of the cranial sutures. **B,** Prominent convolutional markings on the inner table of the skull (beaten silver skull). **C,** Erosion of the sella turcica, in this case resulting from a craniopharyngioma. (**A,** *Courtesy Department of Neuroradiology, University Health Center of Pittsburgh, Pittsburgh, Pa;* **B** *and* **C,** *courtesy Jocelyn Medina, MD.*)

radiographic sign because they are frequently seen on skull radiographs of normal children. However, when secondary to increased intracranial pressure, they are preceded by suture diastasis and changes in the sella turcica (Fig. 15-38, *C*). An excessive rate of head growth is a prominent feature of chronically increased intracranial pressure in infants and children up to 3 years of age. Associated findings may include frontal prominence and distended scalp veins (see Fig. 15-29, *A*). If the ability to compensate for increased intracranial pressure by expansion of the calvaria is exceeded, other symptoms appear. These may include listlessness, irritability, poor feeding, vomiting, failure to thrive, paresis of upward gaze (see Fig. 15-29, *B*), increased tone, hyperactive stretch reflexes, and a high-pitched cry. Papilledema is uncommon.

In older children and adults the most consistent clinical features of increased intracranial pressure include headache, vomiting, visual disturbances, and papilledema. Headaches are of variable severity. They may be constant or intermittent and generalized or localized to frontal, temporal, or occipital regions. In some, but by no means all cases, they recur on early rising or awakening and are accompanied by vomiting. The headaches may be exacerbated by sneezing, coughing, or straining. Vomiting resulting from increased intracranial pressure is no different from vomiting from other causes. It is seldom projectile and is not necessarily accompanied by headache.

Horizontal diplopia (double vision) secondary to paralysis of one or both abducens nerves is the most common visual disturbance. Initially, double vision may occur only on lateral gaze toward the side of the paretic lateral rectus muscle. This may be intermittent and may not be accompanied by limitation of ocular motility sufficient to be seen by the examiner. With progression, diplopia becomes constant and is present even with the eyes in the primary position, and an internal strabismus results (Fig. 15-39). Selective vulnerability of the sixth cranial nerve to increased intracranial pressure may be explained by its long intracranial course and proximity to rigid structures. Other visual disturbances may include transient obscurations, visual field deficits, and impaired upward gaze.

Sustained intracranial hypertension produces papilledema, a passive swelling of the optic disk (Fig. 15-40). The observation of papilledema in a child with headache, vomiting, or visual disturbances confirms the presence of increased intracranial pressure. The absence of venous pulsations or the presence of associated flame-shaped hemorrhages can help distinguish papilledema from other causes of blurred optic disk margins.

Increased intracranial pressure may be accompanied by changes in personality and behavior, deteriorating school performance, decreased appetite and activity, and alterations in level of consciousness.

Etiologies

Causes of increased intracranial pressure include cerebral edema, mass lesions, trauma, CNS infections, pseudotumor cerebri, and hydrocephalus.

Figure 15-39 Left abducens (sixth cranial nerve) palsy. This boy presented with headaches and diplopia and was found to have papilledema and a left abducens palsy. Note that his left eye cannot move past the midline on left lateral gaze. (*Courtesy Kenneth Cheng, MD, Children's Hospital of Pittsburgh, Pittsburgh, Pa.*)

Figure 15-40 Papilledema. Fundus photograph shows blurring of the optic disk margin, elevation and hyperemia of the optic nerve head, and distention of the retinal blood vessels. (*Courtesy Kenneth Cheng, MD, Children's Hospital of Pittsburgh, Pittsburgh, Pa.*)

Figure 15-41 Cerebral edema. CT performed 24 hours after severe hypoxic–ischemic injury. Note the obliteration of the cerebral ventricles, the loss of gray matter–white matter differentiation, and the homogeneous "ground-glass" appearance. *(Courtesy Department of Neuroradiology, University Health Center of Pittsburgh, Pittsburgh, Pa.)*

Figure 15-42 Choroid plexus papilloma. CT of an infant with excessively rapid head growth. There is an enhancing mass within the body of the left lateral ventricle and associated ventricular enlargement (hydrocephalus) secondary to excessive secretion of CSF by the tumor. *(Courtesy Michael Painter, MD, Children's Hospital of Pittsburgh, Pittsburgh, Pa.)*

Cerebral Edema

Cerebral edema (Fig. 15-41), an expansion of brain volume resulting from an increase in brain content of water and salt, is a response of brain tissue to a variety of insults. Vasogenic cerebral edema results from the alterations in vascular permeability produced by brain tumor, trauma, abscess, and hemorrhage. Cytotoxic cerebral edema, caused by swelling of brain cells (neurons and glia), usually results from infection, hypoxia, ischemia, or toxins.

Intracranial Mass Lesions

Tumors, intracranial hemorrhages, abscesses, and vascular malformations produce increased intracranial pressure by occupying space, causing cerebral edema, obstructing CSF pathways, and altering blood flow.

Intracranial Tumors

Choroid plexus papillomas, by secreting an excess of CSF, cause communicating hydrocephalus (Fig. 15-42). Although astrocytomas and oligodendrogliomas of the cerebral hemispheres (Fig. 15-43) often manifest as seizures or contralateral motor difficulties, symptoms of increased intracranial pressure are the initial manifestations in 37% of cases and are present at the time of diagnosis in 80%. *Pineal region tumors* (Fig. 15-44) frequently obstruct the third ventricle or cerebral aqueduct, producing signs and symptoms of increased intracranial pressure accompanied by *Parinaud syndrome* (impairment of the upward gaze with preservation of the downward gaze and retraction–convergence nystagmus with attempted upward gaze) resulting from compression of the periaqueductal gray (see Fig. 15-29, *B*). *Hypothalamic region tumors* such as craniopharyngioma (Fig. 15-45) manifest as growth retardation or failure of sexual maturation accompanied by visual field defects resulting from compression of the optic chiasm. Hydrocephalus occurs in 25% of cases.

Headache and vomiting accompanied by disturbances of gait and coordination are frequent presenting manifestations of posterior fossa tumors such as cerebellar astrocytoma, medulloblastoma, and ependymoma. Midline tumors involving the cerebellar vermis can produce truncal ataxia (Fig. 15-46, *A*), whereas mass lesions of the cerebellar hemispheres often cause unilateral limb ataxia and horizontal nystagmus

(Fig. 15-46, *B*). The cardinal manifestations of brainstem glioma (Fig. 15-47) are cranial nerve palsies associated with contralateral hemiplegia and ataxia. Increased intracranial pressure is not an early feature.

Brain Abscesses

Brain abscesses (Fig. 15-48) are uncommon in the absence of predisposing factors such as chronic otitis or sinusitis, chronic pulmonary infection, dental abscesses, cyanotic congenital heart disease, or immunosuppression. Unless accompanied by prodromal symptoms of fever, headache, lethargy, and malaise, brain abscesses may be impossible to distinguish from other intracranial mass lesions on clinical grounds.

Intracranial Hemorrhage

Spontaneous intracranial hemorrhage (Fig. 15-49) secondary to rupture of a vascular malformation or arterial aneurysm is rare in the pediatric population. Leakage of small amounts of

Figure 15-43 Hemispheric oligodendroglioma. CT scan of a patient with seizures demonstrates a low-density mass lesion in the right frontal lobe. *(Courtesy Michael Painter, MD, Children's Hospital of Pittsburgh, Pittsburgh, Pa.)*

Figure 15-44 Pineal region tumor. CT scan of a patient with headache, lethargy, vomiting, and paresis of upward gaze shows an enhancing mass lesion in the pineal region and severe obstructive hydrocephalus. *(Courtesy Department of Neuroradiology, University Health Center of Pittsburgh, Pittsburgh, Pa.)*

hematoma frequently suffer no immediate loss of consciousness after the traumatic event. Associated linear skull fractures are less common than in adults, and the source of bleeding into the epidural space is generally ruptured epidural veins rather than lacerations of the middle meningeal artery. Hence the evolution of symptoms is slower, and the typical adult picture of immediate loss of consciousness, followed by a brief lucid interval and then collapse, is not seen until adolescence. Often, persistent lethargy and intermittent vomiting are the only initial signs. On early assessment, some affected children and adolescents demonstrate a slowed reaction time, especially when responding to questions (as if there is a processing delay). Severe headache, papilledema, and localizing signs may not emerge for several hours to days. Once neurologic signs and symptoms appear, they may progress rapidly to coma and death or evolve slowly over several days before producing brainstem compression.

Meningitis

Bacterial meningitis (Fig. 15-51; and see Chapter 12, Fig. 12-40, *B*) produces increased intracranial pressure by causing cerebral edema and impairing reabsorption of CSF. Signs and symptoms are discussed in Chapter 12. Although cerebral edema and intracranial hypertension may complicate the course of viral encephalitis, the usual presentation is with seizures, behavioral change, and altered level of consciousness.

Other Causes

Pseudomotor Cerebri

Pseudotumor cerebri is a syndrome of increased intracranial pressure that occurs in the absence of hydrocephalus or an intracranial mass lesion. The disorder may be associated with the use of certain drugs (e.g., steroids, tetracycline, vitamin A, oral contraceptives); can occur as a complication of otitis media or sinusitis; and can be caused by a variety of endocrine and metabolic disturbances. Another risk factor is obesity. It is also more common in adolescent girls. However, in many instances pseudotumor is idiopathic. The presenting symptom is headache. Papilledema is the rule, and abducens nerve palsy is common (see Figs. 15-39 and 15-40). There may be associated nausea and vomiting, but most children do not appear

blood into the subarachnoid space produces symptoms (e.g., fever, headache, stiff neck) that mimic those of bacterial meningitis. In such cases the correct diagnosis may first be suspected when lumbar puncture yields grossly bloody fluid. The presentation of large subarachnoid hemorrhages is catastrophic, with sudden onset of excruciating headache followed by collapse and evidence of increased intracranial pressure.

Head trauma results in increased intracranial pressure by provoking cerebral edema or causing intracranial hemorrhage. The modes of presentation of *cerebral contusion, subdural hematoma,* and posttraumatic cerebral edema are discussed in Chapter 6. The features of *epidural hematoma* (Fig. 15-50) in childhood, which differ from those encountered in adults, are emphasized here. Infants and young children with epidural

Figure 15-45 Craniopharyngioma. **A,** CT scan shows a large, spherical suprasellar mass, obliteration of the third ventricle, and associated hydrocephalus. **B,** MRI scan provides superior visualization of the anatomic relationship of this tumor with the optic chiasm and hypothalamus. *(Courtesy Department of Neuroradiology, University Health Center of Pittsburgh, Pittsburgh, Pa.)*

Figure 15-46 Cerebellar neoplasms. **A,** Midline ependymoma filling the fourth ventricle and invading the cerebellar vermis. **B,** Glioblastoma of the right cerebellar hemisphere. (**A,** Courtesy Michael Painter, MD, Children's Hospital of Pittsburgh, Pittsburgh, Pa; **B,** courtesy Department of Neuroradiology, University Health Center of Pittsburgh, Pittsburgh, Pa.)

Figure 15-47 Brainstem glioma. This 6-year-old girl had a 2- to 3-month history of personality change, decreased school performance, and intermittent urinary retention and constipation; a 3-week history of ataxia and vague upper back pain; and a 6-day history of severe frontal headache with vomiting after breakfast. She had diplopia secondary to left sixth nerve palsy, nystagmus, right facial weakness, slurred speech, dysphagia with drooling, torticollis, an unbalanced gait with a tendency to list to the left, dysmetria greater on the left, and bilateral papilledema. Her MRI scan showed marked enlargement of the pons resulting from a mass lesion extending into the brainstem and compressing the fourth ventricle, causing hydrocephalus. (Courtesy Charles Fitz, MD, Children's Hospital of Pittsburgh, Pittsburgh, Pa.)

Figure 15-48 Brain abscess. CT scan demonstrates a low-density mass lesion with an enhancing rim and surrounding edema in an immunosuppressed patient with an *Aspergillus* abscess. Bacterial abscesses and neoplasms can present a similar CT appearance. (Courtesy Department of Neuroradiology, University Health Center of Pittsburgh, Pittsburgh, Pa.)

Figure 15-49 Intracranial hemorrhage. Enhanced MRI scan demonstrating a cerebral hemangioma with associated old hemorrhage. (Courtesy Michael J. Painter, MD, Children's Hospital of Pittsburgh, Pittsburgh, Pa.)

Figure 15-50 Epidural hematoma. In this patient, blunt head trauma was followed by vomiting, progressive obtundation, and decreased movement of the left arm and leg. The CT scan showed a large, lens-shaped epidural hematoma over the right hemisphere. (Courtesy Department of Neuroradiology, University Health Center of Pittsburgh, Pittsburgh, Pa.)

Figure 15-51 Bacterial meningitis in an infant with fever; lethargy; nuchal rigidity; and a tense, distended fontanelle. The CT scan shows contrast enhancement of the cortical gyri and ependyma of the lateral ventricles. *(Courtesy Department of Neuroradiology, University Health Center of Pittsburgh, Pittsburgh, Pa.)*

Figure 15-52 Neurocysticercosis. This 12-year-old presented with focal seizures and chronic headaches after recent travel to an endemic area. MRI revealed a small ring-enhancing cyst in the left temporal lobe with surrounding edema, thought to be consistent with neurocysticercosis. *(Courtesy Patricia Crumrine, MD, Children's Hospital of Pittsburgh, Pittsburgh, Pa.)*

acutely ill. Many patients have visual obscurations. Progressive papilledema may lead to optic atrophy, and treatment is essential to prevent loss of vision. Pseudotumor cerebri is a diagnosis of exclusion. A CT or MRI scan must be done to rule out hydrocephalus or a mass lesion. A magnetic resonance venography (MRV) scan with contrast will evaluate for obstruction of venous outflow tracts, which occurs in conditions such as venous sinus thrombosis or jugular vein compression. Examination of the cerebrospinal fluid is unremarkable apart from increased opening pressure.

Neurocysticercosis

Neurocysticercosis is another disorder that can present with signs of increased intracranial pressure. It is the most common CNS parasitic infestation worldwide and is endemic in Mexico; Central and South America; and parts of Asia including China, Africa, and India. Neurocysticercosis is being seen with increasing frequency in developed countries, often in immigrants from or recent visitors to endemic areas. Cerebral cysticercosis occurs when larvae of the pork tapeworm *(Taenia solium)* encyst in CNS tissues. Eating contaminated pork carrying the *T. solium* larvae leads to acquisition of the intestinal tapeworm. Cysticercosis results from fecal–oral transmission of the ova shed by the adult intestinal tapeworm and is often transmitted to affected children by family, household, or community contacts who carry the adult *T. solium* tapeworm. After transmission, hematogenous spread to neural, ocular, or muscular tissues can occur. Seizures are the most common presenting sign of neurocysticercosis and are often accompanied by headache. Less commonly, patients can develop meningitis as a result of inflammatory reactions to ruptured cysts or they may present with signs and symptoms of increased intracranial pressure due to obstruction of CSF pathways by cysts, resulting in noncommunicating hydrocephalus. Findings on neuroimaging vary depending on the stage of development of the organism and range from nonenhancing cysts to ring-enhancing lesions to calcified nodules. Lesions may be single or multiple. Single enhancing cysts are most common in children living in North America (Fig. 15-52).

FACIAL WEAKNESS

The cortical motor center controlling the muscles of facial expression is located in the lower third of the precentral gyrus (Fig. 15-53). Motor fibers arising in the cerebral cortex travel through the corona radiata, internal capsule, and cerebral peduncle into the pons, where the majority decussate to supply the facial (seventh) nerve nucleus on the opposite side. Some fibers, destined to terminate in the portion of the facial nerve nucleus that innervates muscles in the upper half of the face, do not decussate. Thus whereas the portion of the facial nerve nucleus that supplies the lower half of the face receives

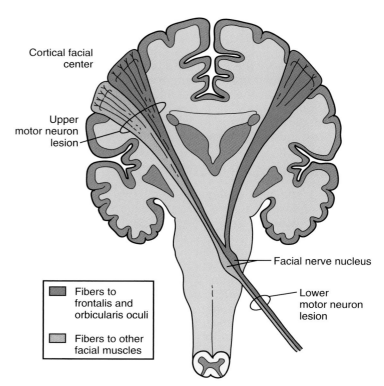

Cortical facial center

Upper motor neuron lesion

Facial nerve nucleus

Lower motor neuron lesion

Fibers to frontalis and orbicularis oculi

Fibers to other facial muscles

Figure 15-53 Central motor control of the facial muscles. The portion of the facial nerve nucleus that supplies the lower half of the face receives predominantly crossed fibers originating from the opposite cerebral hemisphere; the portion that innervates the upper half receives fibers from both cerebral hemispheres. *(Modified from Haymaker W: Bing's local diagnosis in neurological diseases, ed 15, St. Louis, 1969, Mosby.)*

Figure 15-54 Peripheral facial weakness. Flaccid weakness of the entire left face resulting from a lesion of the left facial nerve. **A,** Flattening of the nasolabial fold and inability to retract the corner of the mouth. **B,** Inability to fully close the eye.

predominantly crossed fibers originating from the opposite cerebral hemisphere, the portion that innervates the frontalis muscle and the orbicularis oculi muscle has bilateral supranuclear control.

Peripheral Facial Weakness

A lesion of the seventh nerve nucleus or emergent facial nerve results in flaccid weakness of the entire face on the same side. On the affected side the face is smooth, with flattening of the nasolabial fold; drooping of the corner of the mouth; and inability to smile, frown, retract the corner of the mouth, wrinkle the forehead, or close the eye (Fig. 15-54). Causes of peripheral facial weakness include infection, trauma, hypertension, a cerebellopontine angle mass, tumors of the pons, and acute idiopathic paralysis (Bell palsy).

Central Facial Weakness

With a lesion above the level of the facial nerve nucleus (i.e., an upper motor neuron lesion), there is weakness of the lower part of the face on the opposite side but relative sparing of the upper portion of the face. The ability to wrinkle the forehead (frontalis muscle) and to voluntarily close the eyes (orbicularis oculi muscle) is preserved (Fig. 15-55).

NEUROMUSCULAR DISORDERS

Weakness is the most common presenting symptom of neuromuscular disease. If time is taken to determine the ways in which the weakness interferes with normal activities and uncover the types of tasks that the patient finds difficult, the distribution and severity of muscle weakness can be predicted from the clinical history. Determining the mode of onset and pattern of progression of the symptoms is essential in the differential diagnosis and selection of diagnostic studies. Because many neuromuscular disorders are genetically determined, a complete family history must be obtained.

Essential components of the physical examination of patients with neuromuscular disease include inspection, palpation, percussion, evaluation of deep tendon reflexes, and assessment of muscle strength. Inspection can reveal muscle wasting and atrophy (or, conversely, hypertrophy), abnormal spontaneous activity, and abnormal resting postures. Palpation permits assessment of muscle consistency, determination of muscle tone (with observation of resistance to passive

motion), and detection of muscle tenderness. Percussion is useful in detecting myotonia. Assessment of muscle strength includes individual muscle testing and functional evaluation. The strength of individual muscles is recorded, using a standardized system such as the following:

  0: No contraction
  1: Flicker or trace contraction
  2: Active movement with gravity eliminated
  3: Active movement against gravity
  4: Active movement against gravity and resistance
  5: Normal power

Functional evaluation of muscle strength is accomplished by observing the patient rising from the floor, rising from a chair, stepping onto a stool, climbing stairs, walking on the heels, hopping on the toes, and raising the arms above the head. This evaluation permits rapid detection of proximal weakness of the hips and shoulders and distal weakness of the legs.

Duchenne Muscular Dystrophy

The muscular dystrophies are genetically determined disorders characterized by progressive degeneration of skeletal muscle, usually after a latency period of seemingly normal development and function. The various clinical types of muscular dystrophy are traditionally classified on the basis of patterns of inheritance, distribution of initial weakness, age of onset of clinical manifestations, and rate of progression (Table 15-7).

Duchenne muscular dystrophy, affecting 1 in 3500 male births, is characterized by X-linked recessive inheritance; early onset; symmetrical and initially selective involvement of pelvic and pectoral girdles; pseudohypertrophy of the calves; high levels of activity of certain serum enzymes, notably creatine kinase; and relentless progression leading to wheelchair confinement by adolescence and death from cardiorespiratory insufficiency by age 20 years.

Duchenne muscular dystrophy is caused by a deletion mutation affecting the Xp21 region on the short arm of the X chromosome. Dystrophin, the large cytoskeletal protein normally encoded by this gene locus, is absent from the muscle fibers of patients with Duchenne muscular dystrophy. The precise function of dystrophin in maintaining the integrity of muscle and the mechanism by which dystrophin deficiency produces progressive muscle destruction remain to be determined. Becker muscular dystrophy, an allelic disorder affecting 1 in 30,000 male births, is distinguished clinically by later

Figure 15-55 Central facial weakness. **A** and **B,** Weakness of the left face with relative sparing of the upper portion secondary to a lesion of the right cerebral hemisphere. There is flattening of the nasolabial fold and inability to retract the corner of the mouth, but the ability to close the eye and wrinkle the forehead is preserved. **C** and **D,** CT scans show the depressed fracture of the temporal bone that was responsible for this central facial palsy.

age at onset, slower rate of progression, and longer survival and biochemically by the presence of dystrophin of abnormal molecular weight. Approximately 70% of patients with Duchenne or Becker muscular dystrophy have detectable dystrophin mutations on routine DNA testing of peripheral blood. The remaining 30% are diagnosed by dystrophin analysis of muscle biopsy tissue.

Clinical manifestations of Duchenne muscular dystrophy do not usually appear until the second year of life or later. Early developmental milestones are normally attained, although the first attempts at walking may be delayed. Gait is often clumsy and awkward from the start, and the ability to run is never normally attained. Difficulty in climbing stairs, frequent falls, and progressive difficulty in rising from the floor are early

Table 15-7 Clinical Features of the Muscular Dystrophies

	Duchenne	**Becker**	**Facioscapulohumeral**	**Limb-Girdle**	**Myotonic**
Inheritance	X-linked recessive	X-linked recessive	Autosomal dominant	Autosomal recessive	Autosomal dominant
Age at onset	Early childhood	Late childhood, adolescence	Variable: childhood through early adult life	Childhood to early adulthood	Highly variable
Pattern of weakness	Pelvic girdle, shoulder girdle	Pelvic girdle, shoulder girdle	Face, shoulder girdle	Pelvic girdle, shoulder girdle	Face, distal limbs
Rate of progression	Rapid	Slow	Very slow	Variable	Variable
Associated features	Pseudohypertrophy of calves	Pseudohypertrophy of calves	None	Pseudohypertrophy rare	Myotonia
Systemic features	Mental retardation, abnormal electrocardiogram, cardiomyopathy	Occasional mental retardation	None	None	Frequent mental retardation, heart block, cataracts, premature balding, testicular tubular atrophy, diabetes

Figure 15-56   Duchenne muscular dystrophy. This child, age 5, has difficulty rising from the floor. Unilateral hand support on the knee is required to get erect.

abnormal rotation of the scapulae (Fig. 15-59, *A*). In addition, spontaneous winging of the scapulae may be prominent (Fig. 15-59, *B*).

Weakness of the neck flexors, as evidenced by marked head lag when the child is pulled to sit from the supine position (Fig. 15-60), is an early finding. Enlargement of muscles, particularly in the calves (Fig. 15-61), is a common feature by 5 or 6 years of age. The abnormally enlarged muscles have an unusually firm, rubbery consistency on palpation. Early in the clinical course, this increase in muscle volume may result from true hypertrophy, with muscle strength proportional to bulk. Later, infiltration by fat and connective tissue sometimes maintains this bulk despite loss of muscle fibers. This is called *pseudohypertrophy*.

Charcot-Marie-Tooth Disease

Charcot-Marie-Tooth disease, also known as *hereditary motor-sensory neuropathy type I (HMSN-I),* is an autosomal dominant demyelinating form of peroneal muscular atrophy. DNA studies have distinguished two genetic disorders, HMSN-IA, associated with a gene mutation of chromosome 17, and HMSN-IB, caused by a mutation on chromosome 1. Both share similar clinical features. The onset of symptoms is usually in the second decade, with presenting complaints being foot deformities and gait abnormalities. Often, pes cavus or hammer-toe deformities develop in early childhood long before more overt symptoms appear (see Chapter 21, Fig. 21-109). The clinical picture is quite variable, and because most affected persons do not consult a physician for their neurologic problems, the majority of cases remain undiagnosed. The astute physician considers the diagnosis when a patient who presents with unrelated symptoms is found to have pes cavus or hammer-toes and symmetrical distal weakness.

Muscle weakness and atrophy begin insidiously in the foot and leg muscles. The intrinsic muscles of the foot are often affected first, followed by involvement of the peroneal, anterior tibial, long toe extensor, intrinsic hand, and gastrocnemius muscles. Weakness and atrophy may even spread to the

features. To rise from the floor, the child may at first need only to push with one hand on a knee (Fig. 15-56). However, as weakness of the extensors of the hips becomes more pronounced, rising from the floor becomes increasingly difficult and requires the use of the hands to "climb up the legs" (the Gower maneuver) (Fig. 15-57).

Progressive gluteal weakness leads to the assumption of a compensatory posture characterized by a broadened base, accentuated lumbar lordosis, and forward thrusting of the abdomen (Fig. 15-58). Although weakness of the arms is not a common early symptom, proximal upper extremity weakness is easily detected on clinical examination when the child is lifted with the examiner's hands placed beneath the arms. There is marked laxity of the shoulder girdle musculature associated with upward displacement of the shoulders and

Figure 15-57   The Gower maneuver. This series of diagrams illustrates the sequence of postures used in attaining the upright position by a child with Duchenne muscular dystrophy. **A-C,** First, the legs are pulled up under the body, and the weight is shifted to rest on the hands and feet. **D,** The hips are then thrust in the air as the knees are straightened, and the hands are brought closer to the legs. **E-G,** Finally, the trunk is slowly extended by the hands walking up the thighs. **H,** The erect position is attained.

Figure 15-58 Compensatory posture in Duchenne muscular dystrophy. These brothers, ages 5 and 8, show the progression of compensatory postural adjustments with broadening of stance, accentuated lumbar lordosis, and forward thrusting of the abdomen, all more pronounced in the older boy.

Figure 15-59 Shoulder girdle weakness in Duchenne muscular dystrophy. **A,** This child, age 5, demonstrates weakness and hypotonia of the shoulder girdle musculature. Upward displacement of the shoulders and abnormal rotation of the scapulae are seen when the child is lifted with the examiner's hands under his arms. **B,** Spontaneous winging of the scapulae can be noted in this 8-year-old.

Figure 15-60 Neck muscle weakness in Duchenne muscular dystrophy. This 5-year-old boy has neck flexor weakness. Note the marked head lag when the patient is pulled to sit from the supine position.

more proximal muscles of the leg and forearm. The degree of muscle wasting is often mild; however, in some cases the loss of muscle mass in the distal lower extremities is severe, giving rise to a striking "stork-leg" appearance (Fig. 15-62, *A*). With involvement of the distal upper extremities there may be obvious wasting of the intrinsic hand muscles and development of secondary "claw-hand" deformities (Fig. 15-62, *B*). Deep tendon reflexes are lost first in the gastrocnemius and soleus muscles, and subsequently in the quadriceps femoris muscle and upper limbs. Sensation may be mildly impaired in the distal lower extremities.

Congenital Cervical Spinal Atrophy

Congenital cervical spinal atrophy is a rare disorder that is manifested at birth by dramatic flaccid paresis of the upper extremities (Fig. 15-63, *A*). The presence of congenital flexion contractures suggests chronic denervation that must have

Figure 15-61 Pseudohypertrophy in Duchenne muscular dystrophy. Note the enlargement of the calves in brothers, ages 5 and 8.

Figure 15-62   Charcot-Marie-Tooth disease. **A,** This patient, age 15, with distal muscular atrophy of the lower extremities demonstrates the "stork-leg" appearance. **B,** She also has atrophy of the forearm and intrinsic hand muscles resulting in a "claw-hand" deformity.

occurred in utero and allows this syndrome to be distinguished from injury to the cervical spine or brachial plexuses during delivery (see Chapter 2). Abnormalities in the formation of the transverse palmar creases are present in all cases (Fig. 15-63, *B* and *C*), suggesting an antenatal insult during the first trimester. The disorder is nonprogressive.

Myotonia Congenita

Myotonia congenita is an inherited disorder of skeletal muscle in which muscle stiffness is the only complaint. Autosomal dominant and autosomal recessive forms are related to different mutations of the skeletal muscle chloride channel gene on chromosome 7. The clinical symptoms are rather stereotypic. After a period of inactivity, the muscles stiffen and are difficult to maneuver; however, with continued activity, the stiffness diminishes and movement becomes almost normal. Typically, the child moves clumsily with a stiff, awkward gait and falls often. However, as activity continues, the child begins to walk freely and with adequate "warm-up" can run without difficulty.

Generalized muscular hypertrophy is a frequent finding on examination, with affected children often having an unusually well-developed, athletic appearance (Fig. 15-64). This belies their sedentary habits and physical ineptitude resulting from muscle stiffness. Clinically, myotonia may be demonstrated by observing delayed relaxation of the muscles after sustained voluntary contraction such as clenching of the hand. Myotonia may also be elicited by percussion of the thenar eminence (Fig. 15-65).

THE HYPOTONIC INFANT

Because depression of muscle tone is clinically manifest by paucity of movement, unusual postures, diminished resistance to passive movement, and increased range of movement of joints, the hypotonic infant has been likened to a rag doll. The legs lie externally rotated and abducted, with their lateral surfaces in contact with the bed while the arms are extended at the sides or flexed so that the hands lie beside the head. When the infant is pulled up by the hands from the supine position (traction response), the head falls into extreme

Figure 15-63   Congenital cervical spinal atrophy. **A,** This 2-day-old infant has flaccid paresis limited to the upper extremities and associated congenital flexion contractures. **B,** Wasting and atrophy of the intrinsic hand muscles with flexion contractures of the fingers and poorly developed transverse palmar creases **(C)** were also present.

Figure 15-64 Body habitus in myotonia congenita. This 8-year-old boy demonstrates generalized muscular hypertrophy, giving him a well-developed, athletic appearance.

Table 15-8 | Differential Diagnosis of Hypotonia

Disorders of the CNS	Disorders of the PNS
Chromosome disorders	Spinal muscular atrophies
Trisomy	Congenital polyneuropathies
Prader-Willi syndrome	Transient neonatal myasthenia
Other	Congenital myasthenic syndromes
Other genetic defects	Congenital muscular dystrophy
Static encephalopathies	Myotonic dystrophy
Congenital malformation	Fukuyama-type dystrophy
Perinatal acquired	Other
encephalopathy	Congenital myopathies
Postnatal acquired	Metabolic myopathies
encephalopathy	Systemic illness
Inborn errors of metabolism	Benign congenital hypotonia
Amino acid disorders	
Organic acid disorders	
Urea cycle disorders	
Peroxisomal disorders	
Lysosomal disorders	
Neonatal spinal cord injury	

CNS, central nervous system; PNS, peripheral nervous system.

requires functional integrity of both the CNS and PNS, hypotonia is a common symptom of many disorders affecting the brain, spinal cord, peripheral nerves, and muscles (Table 15-8). Hypotonia also occurs as a nonspecific manifestation of systemic illness. The term *benign congenital hypotonia* is reserved for infants with isolated depression of postural tone that resolves with growth and maturation, usually by 1 year of age. It is often a diagnosis of exclusion.

CHILDHOOD EPILEPSY

The overall incidence of epilepsy follows a bimodal distribution, peaking in children younger than 5 years of age and in adults older than 65 years of age. A classification of epileptic seizures detailed in Table 15-9 divides them into those of focal onset (partial seizures) and those with bilateral cortical representation from the outset (generalized seizures). *Simple partial seizures* have no associated impairment of consciousness and may represent simple motor or sensory phenomena. Patients with *complex partial seizures* experience seizure spread to cortical and subcortical areas resulting in alteration in consciousness. Some partial seizures may secondarily

extension, and the limbs fail to flex to counter the traction (Fig. 15-66, *A*). In horizontal suspension with the chest and abdomen supported by the examiner's hand, the infant with hypotonia drapes limply like an inverted U, and when held under the arms, tends to slip through the examiner's hands (Fig. 15-66, *B*). Because maintenance of normal postural tone

Figure 15-65 Myotonia congenita, delayed muscle relaxation. Percussion of the thenar eminence **(A)** is followed by involuntary opposition of the thumb and visible contraction of the muscles of the thenar eminence **(B)**, which lasts for several seconds.

Figure 15-66   Hypotonic infant. **A,** Abnormal traction response. When the infant is pulled up from the supine position, her head falls into extreme extension and her arms fail to flex to counter the traction applied by the examiner. **B,** When held under the arms, she tends to slip through the examiner's hands.

generalize to contralateral brain areas, with loss of consciousness, often with bilateral convulsive features.

Generalized seizures may be convulsive or nonconvulsive in nature. In children, nonconvulsive generalized seizures often present as absence epilepsy. Other generalized seizures such as tonic, tonic–clonic, atonic, and myoclonic are defined by the type of motor activity observed.

Absence seizures are typically brief in duration (5 to 20 seconds) and are characterized by sudden staring or arrest of activity with abrupt recovery. They are often associated with facial automatisms such as eye flutter, chewing, or ocular supraversion (Fig. 15-67). The incidence of absence epilepsy peaks in children between the ages of 3 and 8 years; however, onset can occur in adolescence. The disorder has a strong genetic predisposition and usually occurs in children who are

otherwise neurologically and intellectually normal. It is often outgrown by late childhood or during adolescence. A typical electroencephalogram (EEG) pattern seen in affected individuals consists of generalized three-per-second spike-and-wave discharges (Fig. 15-68), which can be activated by hyperventilation. Between 40% and 60% of patients with absence seizures go on to experience a generalized tonic–clonic convulsion.

Infantile spasms typically begin before age 2 years, with a peak age at onset between 4 and 6 months. They are classified as flexor, extensor, and mixed flexor–extensor types and are characterized by brief contractions of the neck, trunk, and extremities with the head thrown backward or forward in association with flexion and/or extension of the limbs. They often occur in clusters throughout the day, with greater frequency on awakening or falling asleep. Early in the course of the disorder, they may be mistaken for colic, hiccups, or gastroesophageal reflux. Etiologic origin of infantile spasms is varied and may include metabolic disorders, cerebral malformations, congenital infections, anoxic injury, and neurocutaneous disorders. However, up to 20% of cases are idiopathic or cryptogenic in origin. Tuberous sclerosis is the major single identifiable cause of infantile spasms, accounting for 7% to

Table 15-9	Classification of Epileptic Seizures
Current Terminology	**Other Names**
1. Partial seizures	Jacksonian, adversive, or focal
Simple partial (consciousness not impaired)	motor seizures
Motor signs	
Special sensory (visual, auditory, gustatory, vertiginous, or somatosensory)	
Autonomic	Abdominal epilepsy
Psychic (déjà vu, fear, and others)	
Complex partial (consciousness impaired)	Psychomotor, temporal lobe
Impaired consciousness at onset	
Development of impaired consciousness	
2. Generalized seizures	
Absence (nonconvulsive)	Petit mal
Typical	
Atypical	
Tonic–clonic	Grand mal, major motor
Atonic	Akinetic, drop attacks
Myoclonic	Minor motor
Tonic	
Clonic	
3. Unclassified	Infantile spasms

Modified from Commission on Classification and Terminology of the International League Against Epilepsy: Proposal for revised clinical and electroencephalographic classification of epileptic seizures, *Epilepsia* 22:489–501, 1981.

Figure 15-67   Absence seizure. This 8-year-old girl had a history of brief staring spells reported by teachers and family. Typical absence seizures, recorded during a video electroencephalogram with staring and ocular supraversion lasting under 10 seconds, could be activated by hyperventilation.

Figure 15-68 Absence seizure. This electroencephalographic tracing shows the typical three-per-second (3 Hz) generalized spike-and-wave discharges characteristic of absence seizures.

LP=1.0 HF=38 200 wV 10 S

25% of cases. Patients who have a known underlying disorder and infantile spasms have a higher incidence of developmental impairment than those of unknown cause. Neuroimaging is abnormal in 70% to 80% of affected children. The EEG in patients with infantile spasms often demonstrates a hypsarrhythmia pattern with markedly abnormal background features and multifocal high-voltage epileptic discharges, and it may show a burst–suppression pattern in sleep (Fig. 15-69). The triad of hypsarrhythmia, infantile spasms, and developmental delay is commonly referred to as *West syndrome*. More than 50% of patients with infantile spasms develop other forms of epilepsy later in life.

PAROXYSMAL MOVEMENT DISORDERS OF CHILDHOOD

Paroxysmal (nonepileptic) movement disorders are relatively common in the pediatric population. They are manifest by excessive involuntary movement (dyskinesia) that is episodic and often stereotypic with preservation of consciousness.

Tic

Tics include a wide array of movements and sounds. They are involuntary, sudden, repetitive movements or vocalizations. They typically wax and wane, with old tics being replaced by new ones. Up to 25% of children may have a transient simple tic disorder lasting less than 1 year. The presence of multiple tics lasting longer than 1 year with both vocal and motor varieties fulfills diagnostic criteria for Tourette syndrome. Attention-deficit/hyperactivity disorder, obsessive–compulsive disorder, and learning disabilities are commonly seen in addition to tics in patients with Tourette syndrome.

Shuddering Attacks

Shuddering (shivering) spells are characterized by flexion of the head, trunk, elbows, and knees with adduction of the limbs and are often described as a "chill" or as having a sense of "ice water being poured down one's back." They represent a benign movement disorder often starting in infancy and usually abating in childhood.

Figure 15-69 Infantile spasms. This electroencephalograph tracing shows the hypsarrhythmia pattern consisting of markedly disorganized background and high-voltage multifocal epileptic spikes often found in patients with infantile spasms.

LP=1.0 HF=70 200 wV 10 S

Startle Disease

A startle response is a brief motor response to an unexpected stimulus (auditory, tactile, visual, or vestibular) that readily habituates (e.g., diminishes with repeated exposure). Hyperekplexia (startle disease) is characterized by a nonhabituating, exaggerated startle response to stimuli often followed by a tonic spasm. Affected children often have hypertonia in infancy, feeding difficulties, and apnea. The startle response can be elicited in hyperekplexic patients by tapping on the forehead, nose, glabella, or vertex of the skull. The course of the disease is variable, and cognitive abilities are not affected.

Head Bobbing

Head bobbing consists of jerky head movements at a frequency of two to three cycles per second and resembles that of a doll's head atop a spring. In childhood it may appear as part of spasmus nutans or the bobble-head doll syndrome. Spasmus nutans is a benign disorder of unknown etiology that occurs in early infancy and is characterized by nystagmus (binocular or monocular), head nodding, and head tilt. Neurologic examination is otherwise normal. The syndrome lasts 1 to 2 years and spontaneously resolves. The bobble-head doll syndrome consists of intermittent head nodding and is seen in association with an underlying CNS structural abnormality, often a third ventricular cyst or tumor.

Chorea or Choreoathetosis

Chorea consists of random, brief, rapid, purposeless jerking movements of the limbs, face, tongue, or trunk, whereas choreoathetosis is characterized by slow writhing movements that often are more prominent on one side of the body. Sydenham chorea (St. Vitus dance) is the most prevalent form of acquired chorea in childhood. It is a manifestation of poststreptococcal rheumatic fever and often begins insidiously weeks to months after a streptococcal infection that may or may not have been symptomatic. It is characterized by choreiform movements, emotional lability, and hypotonia. Behavior change, decline in school performance, and anxiety are common associated features. The disorder usually resolves after several months, although recurrences may be triggered by new episodes of streptococcal infection, pregnancy (chorea gravidarum), or oral contraceptive use. Other, less common causes of chorea and/or choreoathetosis in childhood include Wilson disease, Huntington disease, systemic lupus erythematosus, and hyperthyroidism.

Bibliography

Bell WE, McCormick WF: *Increased intracranial pressure in children*, ed 2, Philadelphia, 1978, WB Saunders.

Brooke MH: *A clinician's view of neuromuscular diseases*, ed 2, Baltimore, 1987, Williams & Wilkins.

Chao DH: Congenital neurocutaneous syndromes of childhood. III. Sturge-Weber disease, *J Pediatr* 55:635–649, 1959.

Dubowitz V: *The floppy infant*, ed 2, Philadelphia, 1980, JB Lippincott.

Emery AEH: *Duchenne muscular dystrophy*, ed 2, Oxford, 1993, Oxford University Press.

Enjolras O, Riche MC, Merland JJ: Facial port-wine stains and Sturge-Weber syndrome, *Pediatrics* 76:48–52, 1985.

Fenichel GM: *Clinical pediatric neurology: A signs and symptoms approach*, ed 5, Philadelphia, 2005, WB Saunders.

Goldstein SM, Curless RG, Post JD, Quencer RM: A new sign of neurofibromatosis on magnetic resonance imaging of children, *Arch Neurol* 46:1222–1224, 1989.

Gomez MR, editor: *Tuberous sclerosis*, ed 2, New York, 1998, Raven Press.

Hoffman EP, Fishbeck KH, Brown RH, et al: Characterization of dystrophin in muscle-biopsy specimens from patients with Duchenne's or Becker's muscular dystrophy, *N Engl J Med* 318:1363–1368, 1988.

International League against Epilepsy, Commission on Classification and Terminology: Proposal for a revised classification of epilepsies and epileptic syndromes, *Epilepsia* 26:268–278, 1985.

Martuza RL, Eldridge R: Neurofibromatosis 2, *N Engl J Med* 318:684–688, 1988.

Menkes JH: *Textbook of child neurology*, ed 5, Philadelphia, 1995, Lea & Febiger.

Mitchell WG: Current therapy in neurologic disease: Cerebral cysticercosis in North American children, *Eur Neurol* 37:126-129, 1997.

Osborne JP: Diagnosis of tuberous sclerosis, *Arch Dis Child* 63:1423–1425, 1988.

Paller AS: The Sturge-Weber syndrome, *Pediatr Dermatol* 4:300–304, 1987.

Riccardi VM: Von Recklinghausen neurofibromatosis, *N Engl J Med* 305:1617–1627, 1981.

Riccardi VM, Eichner JE: *Neurofibromatosis: Phenotype, natural history and pathogenesis*, ed 2, Baltimore, 1992, Johns Hopkins University Press.

Roach ES, Gomez MR, Northrup H: Tuberous Sclerosis Complex Consensus Conference: Revised clinical diagnostic criteria, *J Child Neurol* 13:624–628, 1998.

Roach ES, William DP, Laster DW: Magnetic resonance imaging in tuberous sclerosis, *Arch Neurol* 44:301–303, 1987.

Swaiman KF, Ashwal S: *Pediatric neurology: Principles and practice*, ed 3, St. Louis, 1999, Mosby.

Warkany J, Lemire RJ, Cohen MM: *Mental retardation and congenital malformations of the central nervous system*, St. Louis, 1981, Mosby.

PULMONARY DISORDERS

Daniel J. Weiner | Jonathan D. Finder

Respiratory disease is one of the most common reasons that pediatric patients seek medical attention. Signs and symptoms can be subtle, and a careful history and physical examination are always useful in assessment of pediatric patients with respiratory complaints. Diseases of the chest can be divided into two major categories: acquired and congenital. Congenital chest diseases are often symptomatic at all times rather than episodically. A child who has chronic noisy breathing from a congenital vascular ring, for example, is not as likely as the patient with asthma to have intermittent periods of wheezing with long intervals of normal breathing. The spectrum of diseases involving the pediatric respiratory system is primarily dependent on the age of the patient; therefore age must be a primary consideration in the differential diagnosis.

HISTORY

Each pediatric history should include the perinatal history. A history of respiratory distress at birth or intubation, however brief, is important. Prematurity with prolonged need for supplemental oxygen may suggest bronchopulmonary dysplasia with associated structural lung abnormalities. Noisy breathing starting early in life suggests congenital airway obstruction and should be evaluated. Regardless of cause, failure to thrive is a worrisome finding, whereas excellent weight gain in a child with noisy breathing is reassuring.

Distinguishing between constant and intermittent symptoms can be one of the most important means of diagnosing diseases of the pediatric chest. A good "cough history" and "wheeze history" are important and have similar elements. The clinician should inquire about the chronicity of the symptoms; association with feeding; upper respiratory infections; exposures (pets, dust, and especially cigarette smoking are important); and fevers. The effect—or lack thereof—of medications may give important diagnostic information (but may also be confounded by improper administration technique). The nature of the cough is important: wet or dry, paroxysmal or continuous, and staccato (as seen in neonatal chlamydial pneumonia) are important descriptive terms. Post-tussive emesis is a "red flag" to the clinician. The cough that awakens the child at night or keeps the child up much of the night is another worrisome historical finding. Conversely, a persistent cough that disappears in sleep strongly suggests the diagnosis of habit (psychogenic) cough. In pursuing a history of wheeze, it is important to ask the parents or historians what they mean by the term; it may mean "noisy breathing," and it may even be applied to stridor.

In evaluating the infant with frequent episodes of cough and/or wheeze, the clinician should inquire about symptoms and signs of gastroesophageal reflux (GER): food refusal, arching, pain behaviors, frequent spitting, milk or formula found on the bed next to the infant's head in the morning,

recurrent croup, hoarseness, and laryngomalacia. Because reflux is worse when the patient is lying down, symptoms tend to be more prominent at night and during naps.

A family history of atopy including eczema and environmental allergies should be investigated. In inquiring about cystic fibrosis, an autosomal recessive trait, an extended family medical history including grandparents and cousins should be taken. Frequent infections in parents or siblings, particularly those requiring hospitalization, suggest possible immunodeficiency in the family.

Immunization history is essential in identifying patients at risk for pertussis. Often, parents state that the immunizations are up to date, although the child has in fact not had any pertussis vaccinations. Immunization avoidance occurs commonly owing to publicity given to well-disproven theories of immunization-induced autism.

Exercise intolerance is one of the primary symptoms of respiratory disease. The neonate's main output of energy is in feeding, and thus difficulties with feedings should be monitored; toddlers are expected to keep up with peers and/or siblings in play; the school-age child's gym performance should be scrutinized. Wheezing or coughing fits after vigorous exercise can occur in asthma.

PHYSICAL EXAMINATION

Examination of the chest in any uncooperative patient is notoriously difficult, but it can be easily accomplished with patience and a few tricks. The infant or toddler is best examined with his or her shirt off while being held upright in the arms of a parent. The patient should face the parent; this maximizes contact with the parent and allows the patient to feel safe. The room should be at a comfortable temperature. The stethoscope head should be warmed in the clinician's hand or pocket for several minutes before use. The classic four steps in the physical examination—inspection, palpation, percussion, and auscultation—are well applied to the examination of the pediatric chest.

Inspection

Decreased subcutaneous adipose tissue as seen in a patient with cystic fibrosis should be noted. The pattern of breathing should always be evaluated with the child disrobed. Any use of expiratory musculature is abnormal. Suprasternal and intercostal retractions reflect excessive negative pleural pressure and can be seen in normal children with thin chest walls after vigorous exercise. Subcostal retractions are always pathologic and are the result of hyperinflated lungs and a flattened diaphragm pulling inward on the chest wall. In advanced lung disease the use of accessory muscles of inspiration can be noted; the sternocleidomastoid muscle, for example, helps lift the chest (in a "bucket handle" fashion) and increase its anteroposterior diameter, thereby increasing intrathoracic volume. In respiratory muscle fatigue, a pattern of breathing can be observed in which the diaphragm alternates with the intercostal muscles to inflate the lungs. This is known as *respiratory alternans* and is seen as alternating abdominal and chest expansion instead of the usual pattern of simultaneous chest and abdominal expansion. Chest wall deformities such as pectus excavatum or pectus carinatum (see Chapter 17) should be noted.

Palpation

Palpation of the chest can reveal significant findings. The examiner places the hands on either side of the chest as the patient takes a deep breath. The chest should expand symmetrically; asymmetry can be seen in unilateral pulmonary hypoplasia, mainstem bronchial obstruction, and diaphragmatic paresis. Placing fingertips on the upper abdomen just over the insertion of the rectus muscles into the lower rib cage can reveal subtle use of expiratory muscles in children with peripheral (lower) airway obstruction. Similarly, the anterior lower ribs should be assessed with the fingertips. In infants with obstructive lung disease, the lower ribs can be felt to pull inward on inspiration. This is the palpable aspect of a subcostal retraction. With the patient's head in the midline position, the trachea should be palpated at the sternal notch to evaluate for tracheal deviation, as is seen with mediastinal shift. Vocal fremitus should be assessed in patients with suspected pleural fluid accumulation; the vibrations transmitted from the larynx as the child says "99" are diminished when there is an accumulation of air or fluid in the pleural space. Infants and children with tracheomalacia and bronchomalacia often have a palpable vibration in the back. Palpable vibrations in only one hemithorax suggest a partial obstruction of the mainstem bronchus in that hemithorax as seen in bronchomalacia.

Percussion

Percussion of the chest can reveal much more than hyperresonance and dullness over an area of consolidation. Air trapping is the hallmark of small-airway disease and results in a depressed position of the diaphragm. Ordinarily the diaphragm can be found just at or slightly below the tip of the scapula when the patient's arm is at his or her side in children 5 years and younger. In the patient with hyperinflation, the diaphragm is found several fingerbreadths below the scapular tips. This finding, even in the absence of wheezing on auscultation, suggests a lesion of the small airways. An area of consolidation or pleural effusion results in dullness to percussion. Another disorder causing asymmetry of percussion of the two hemithoraces is diaphragmatic eventration, a congenital lesion of the diaphragm in which the diaphragm is replaced with a thin fibrous membrane without contractile properties. Postoperative diaphragmatic paralysis (rarely found after cardiac surgery) can be diagnosed by percussion of the cooperative patient while holding his or her breath at maximal inspiration and at end-expiration.

Auscultation

Auscultation of the pediatric chest requires patience. One often must wait a minute or two for a deep breath in order to appreciate abnormal breath sounds that are not apparent on shallow breathing. Augmenting the expiratory phase with a gentle squeeze of the thorax while listening with the stethoscope may bring out expiratory wheezes.

Abnormal ("adventitial") breath sounds include crackles and wheezes. Wheezes are *continuous* sounds, whereas crackles (formerly referred to as rales) are *discontinuous*. Wheezes and crackles can be inspiratory or expiratory, although crackles are more commonly heard on inspiration and wheezes are more commonly heard on expiration.

Wheezes probably arise from the vibration within the walls of narrowed large- and medium-sized airways. In a patient experiencing an acute exacerbation of asthma, the lungs have wheezes in a range of pitches (described as *polyphonic*) with substantial regional differences in auscultation. Patients with central airway obstruction such as tracheomalacia, on the other hand, have a single pitch of wheeze that sounds the same in all lung fields *(monophonic)* and is heard loudest over the central airway that is obstructed. Foreign bodies can cause a monophonic wheeze that can vary in pitch depending on the degree of obstruction.

Crackles are believed to arise from the popping of fluid menisci within airways. The crackles heard in the lungs of patients with interstitial lung disease have yet to be explained adequately but may arise from the popping open of small airways. Coarse crackles are often audible at the mouth and are a late finding in patients with cystic fibrosis with advanced bronchiectasis. "Rhonchi" refers to the sound made by pooled secretions in the central airways, which can be categorized as harsh, low-pitched central wheezes or coarse, central crackles (depending on the nature of the sounds heard).

Other sounds that can be heard include friction rubs, which are creaking sounds heard during both phases of respiration as inflamed pleural surfaces rub over one another. One of the most important abnormal findings in children is the absence of breath sounds over an area of collapse or consolidation. Phase delay in air entry (such as in unilateral bronchial obstruction) can be detected only with a differential (double-headed) stethoscope (Fig. 16-1).

The notion that the examination of the lungs begins at the fingertips is an important one, as digital clubbing may point to the presence of lung disease. Various stages of clubbing, from mild to severe, are depicted in Figures 16-2 and 16-3. Not all digital clubbing is associated with pulmonary disease (Table 16-1); nonpulmonary causes include cardiac, inflammatory, gastrointestinal, hepatic, and familial, as well as clubbing observed with thyrotoxicosis. Bronchiectasis from cystic fibrosis or from other chronic infectious causes is the major cause of clubbing among all pulmonary diseases. Digital clubbing in any child with a chronic cough or wheezing warrants a thorough evaluation and investigation to determine the underlying disorder.

The astute pulmonologist will carefully examine the remainder of the patient. The examination should also include

Figure 16-1 Differential stethoscope. A differential, or double-headed, stethoscope can be made from a Sprague-Rappaport type stethoscope by adding two chest pieces as shown. This allows for simultaneous auscultation of homologous lung segments. Certain findings can be found only with this stethoscope, including phase delay (typical of foreign body aspiration).

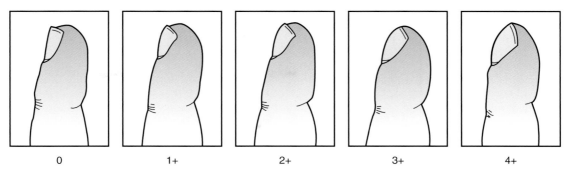

Figure 16-2 Digital clubbing. The 0- to 4-point scale describes the spectrum of digital clubbing as follows: 1+, very mild; 2+, mild; 3+, moderate; and 4+, severe.

evaluation for nasal polyps (see Fig. 16-30), which can be associated with cystic fibrosis, triad asthma, or significant atopy. An increased second heart sound could suggest pulmonary hypertension.

RADIOLOGY

The pediatric chest radiograph is unique in that normal findings may vary with age. The width of the chest on the lateral projection in the chest radiograph of a normal infant (Fig. 16-4) is about the same as the transverse dimension on a frontal projection, and the lungs may appear relatively radiolucent. Further, in contrast with the older child (>2 years of age), the cardiothoracic ratio in the infant normally may be as high as 0.65. The width of the superior mediastinum at this age may also be striking because the thymic shadow is particularly prominent during the first few months of life before the normal process of involution occurs. The normal chest radiograph of an older child (Fig. 16-5) shows the diaphragm on an inspiratory film at the eighth or ninth rib posteriorly (sixth rib anteriorly), a cardiothoracic ratio of 0.5, and pulmonary vessels extending two thirds of the way to the periphery. In most situations a lateral radiograph should accompany the posteroanterior (PA) view because some pathologic findings may be missed on a single projection. For example, a lateral examination yields the best information about the anterior

mediastinum and the tracheal air column and may reveal a small pleural effusion that is unsuspected on the basis of a PA radiograph alone. In combination with the PA view, the lateral projection may help localize an abnormal finding to a particular lobe or segment or document hyperinflation with diaphragmatic flattening (Fig. 16-6). In most situations the chest radiograph taken at full inspiration is most helpful. In the evaluation for bronchial foreign bodies, a comparison of inspiratory and expiratory views (or left and right lateral decubitus films in the younger patient) can help if one lung is unable to empty. In looking for a small pneumothorax, the expiratory film is more helpful because the smaller lung volume allows extrapulmonary air to expand to become more evident.

COUGH

Persistent or recurrent cough represents one of the most common and vexing problems in pediatrics. In most circumstances the tracheobronchial tree is kept clean by airway macrophages and the mucociliary escalator, but cough becomes an important component of airway clearance when excessive or abnormal materials are present, or when mucociliary clearance is reduced, as during a viral respiratory illness. A cough clears airway secretions and inhaled particulate matter through a combination of the high airflow velocities generated during the expiratory phase of the cough and compression of smaller airways, which "milks" the secretions into larger bronchi where they can be eliminated by a subsequent cough. Cough is generally produced by a reflex response arising from irritant receptors located in ciliated epithelia in the lower respiratory tract, but it can be suppressed or initiated at higher cortical centers. One of the most common causes of cough in pediatric patients is the self-limited cough of an acute viral lower respiratory illness or bronchitis that lasts 1 to 2 weeks. The cough that persists longer than 2 weeks is potentially more worrisome. A diag-

Figure 16-3 Digital clubbing in cystic fibrosis.

Table 16-1	Causes of Clubbing
Pulmonary	**Cardiac**
Cystic fibrosis	Cyanotic congenital heart disease
Other bronchiectasis	Subacute bacterial endocarditis
Pulmonary abscess	**Gastrointestinal or Hepatic**
Empyema	Ulcerative colitis
Neoplasms	Crohn disease
Interstitial fibrosis	Polyposis
Pulmonary alveolar proteinosis	Biliary cirrhosis/atresia
Interstitial pneumonitis	**Familial**
Chronic pneumonia	**Thyrotoxicosis**

Figure 16-4 Normal posteroanterior chest radiograph in a 1-month-old infant. *(Courtesy Beverly Newman, MD, Pittsburgh, Pa.)*

Figure 16-6 Posteroanterior chest radiograph demonstrating flattening of the diaphragm due to hyperinflation.

nostic approach to chronic cough is best served by considering the age of the child (Table 16-2).

Several causes of persistent cough are common to all pediatric age groups, such as second-hand cigarette smoke exposure, recurrent viral bronchitis, asthma, gastroesophageal reflux (GER), cystic fibrosis, granulomatous lung disease (e.g., tuberculosis), foreign body aspiration, and pertussis.

Age and Cause

Infancy (Younger Than 1 Year)

Cough starting at birth or shortly afterward may be a sign of serious respiratory disease and must be evaluated assiduously. Cough beginning at this time raises the possibility of congenital infections, such as cytomegalovirus or rubella, which are often associated with other findings, such as hepatosplenomegaly, thrombocytopenia, or central nervous system disease. Pneumonia due to *Chlamydia trachomatis* (Fig. 16-7) generally develops after the first month of life and presents as

an afebrile pneumonitis with congestion; wheezing; fine, diffuse crackles; a paroxysmal cough; and, in approximately 50% of cases, a prior or concomitant inclusion conjunctivitis. Pneumonia caused by *Bordetella pertussis* is a potentially life-threatening illness characterized by severe paroxysmal coughing episodes followed by cyanosis and apnea and is often associated with an inspiratory "whoop." The latter finding may be missing in young infants or those weakened by the recurrent coughing spasms. Newborns and young infants may have apnea as the primary sign of a *B. pertussis* infection. The chest radiograph is nondiagnostic and can be normal or (Fig. 16-8) show perihilar infiltrates; atelectasis; hyperinflation; and, in some cases, interstitial or subcutaneous emphysema.

Figure 16-5 Normal posteroanterior **(A)** and lateral **(B)** chest radiographs of a 6-year-old child.

Table 16-2	Causes of Cough according to Age	
Infancy (Younger Than 1 Year)	Right middle lobe syndrome	
Congenital and Neonatal Infections	Ciliary dyskinesia syndromes	
Chlamydia	Upper respiratory tract disease	
Viral (e.g., RSV, CMV, rubella)	Recurrent viral infection/bronchitis	
Bacterial (e.g., pertussis)	Passive smoke inhalation	
Pneumocystis jirovecii	Gastroesophageal reflux	
Congenital Malformations	Interstitial pneumonitides	
Tracheoesophageal fistula	Pulmonary hemosiderosis	
Vascular ring	**School Age to Adolescence**	
Airway malformations (e.g., laryngeal cleft)	Asthma	
Pulmonary sequestration	Cystic fibrosis	
Other	*Mycoplasma pneumoniae* infection	
Cystic fibrosis	Psychogenic or habit cough	
Asthma	Cigarette smoking	
Recurrent viral bronchiolitis/ bronchitis	Pulmonary hemosiderosis	
Gastroesophageal reflux	Interstitial pneumonitides	
Interstitial pneumonitides	Ciliary dyskinesia syndromes	
Lymphoid interstitial pneumonitis	**All Ages**	
Diffuse interstitial pneumonitis	Recurrent viral illness	
Preschool	Asthma	
Inhaled foreign body	Cystic fibrosis	
Asthma	Granulomatous lung disease	
Suppurative lung disease	Foreign body aspiration	
Cystic fibrosis	Pertussis infection	
Bronchiectasis		

CMV, cytomegalovirus; RSV, respiratory syncytial virus.

Figure 16-8 Pertussis in a 6-week-old infant demonstrates the typical radiographic pattern of perihilar involvement. This child also has right upper lobe atelectasis. *(Courtesy Katie McPeak, MD, Pittsburgh, Pa.)*

A high white blood cell count with a predominance of lymphocytes supports the diagnosis, but unfortunately once the patient has passed through the usually innocent-appearing coryzal stage into the paroxysmal stage, diagnostic tests have a lower yield. Diagnostic approaches to whooping cough include detection of *B. pertussis* DNA by polymerase chain reaction (PCR) and serologic detection of *B. pertussis*–specific IgM or IgA. *Ureaplasma urealyticum* and *Pneumocystis jirovecii* (formerly known as *P. carinii*) have been recognized as causes of pneumonia and persistent cough in this age group.

Congenital malformations, such as tracheoesophageal fistula (Fig. 16-9) and laryngeal cleft or web, can produce

Figure 16-7 Pneumonia caused by *Chlamydia trachomatis* in a 3-month-old infant with inclusion conjunctivitis.

cough via chronic aspiration of gastric contents, milk, or saliva. These anomalies are associated with feeding-related coughing, choking, and occasional cyanosis. Hypoxemia may persist between feedings. Infants with neurologic disorders may have incoordination of swallowing and sucking reflexes that lead to aspiration of milk or gastric contents into the lung. Pulmonary sequestration (in which a portion of the lung is perfused by systemic, not pulmonary arteries) (Fig. 16-10) and bronchogenic cysts (cystic structures arising from the pulmonary epithelium) are rare congenital anomalies that may compress the pulmonary tree or become infected, thereby producing a cough. Aberrant major blood vessels generally cause inspiratory stridor and expiratory wheezing from tracheal compression (Fig. 16-11; see also Fig. 16-25), but a brassy cough may also be observed, as may dysphagia from the associated esophageal compression.

The triad of poor weight gain, steatorrhea, and chronic cough at this age makes cystic fibrosis a strong consideration, and a sweat test at an accredited cystic fibrosis center is mandatory. Asthma (formerly: "reactive airway disease") or bronchial hyperresponsiveness is a common and probably underdiagnosed cause of cough in infancy. Cough or persistent wheezing can be found in these infants, who may have a history of a previous viral lower respiratory illness with or without a family history of wheezing and/or asthma. Babies with GER may have a combination of effortless vomiting; nocturnal cough/wheeze; pain behaviors/arching; hoarseness; laryngomalacia; and, in some cases, poor weight gain. The absence of a history of vomiting ("spitting up") does not eliminate GER as a diagnostic consideration in infants with persistent coughing because occult reflux or microaspiration may induce bronchospasm.

Childhood interstitial lung disease (chILD) refers to a complex and rare group of pulmonary disorders. These disorders usually involve the pulmonary interstitium, but can involve other aspects of lung parenchyma. Although chILD can present in older children, there are several disorders (see later) specific to infancy. The pathogenesis of these disorders is poorly understood.

Causes of chILD are extremely variable and include infections, inhalation injury, chemotherapeutic agents, post–bone marrow transplant lung disease, systemic inflammatory diseases, pulmonary hemorrhage syndromes, structural and growth anomalies, metabolic diseases, and congenital disorders of host defense and of surfactant production. Examples

Figure 16-9 Tracheoesophageal fistula. **A,** Anteroposterior chest radiograph shows feeding tube passing no farther than proximal esophagus; there is an aspiration pneumonitis present. **B,** Lateral view showing the feeding tube in the proximal esophageal pouch with air in the airway, distal esophagus, and intestine. (**A,** *Courtesy Beverly Newman, MD, Pittsburgh, Pa;* **B,** *courtesy Katie McPeak, MD, Pittsburgh, Pa.*)

of chILD that present in infancy include alveolar capillary dysplasia, surfactant B and C deficiencies, ILD associated with *ABCA3* mutations, pulmonary interstitial glycogenosis, neuroendocrine cell hyperplasia of infancy, and follicular bronchitis of infancy.

Patients with chILD may present insidiously with some combination of cough, tachypnea, retractions, exercise intolerance, resting hypoxemia or hypercarbia, or desaturation with exercise; diffuse abnormalities on chest imaging; and crackles and retractions on examination. Growth failure is not uncommon as a complication of these diseases.

The diagnosis of a specific chILD is usually made subsequent to lung biopsy, but this is usually preceded by a variety of less invasive tests (Fig. 16-12) such as a high-resolution computed tomography (CT) scan of the chest, infant lung

function testing, and flexible fiberoptic bronchoscopy with bronchoalveolar lavage. Surfactant disorders (surfactant protein B or C deficiencies, or *ABCA3* mutations) can often be diagnosed by mutation analysis. The prognosis of chILD can be quite variable, with some universally fatal (alveolar capillary dysplasia) or very severe and treatable only by lung transplantation (surfactant protein B deficiency), and some showing gradual improvement over months or years (neuroendocrine cell hyperplasia of infancy).

Preschool

The two most common reasons for a persistent cough in the preschool age group are recurrent viral infections and asthma. The child with asthma may not manifest audible wheezing or dyspnea but rather may have persistent cough, especially with

Figure 16-10 Pulmonary sequestration. **A,** Anteroposterior film shows left lower lobe infiltrate. **B,** Aortic angiogram demonstrates anomalous origin of pulmonary blood supply from abdominal aorta to the left lower lobe in a 7-year-old girl with extralobar sequestration. (*Courtesy Geoffrey Kurland, MD, Pittsburgh, Pa.*)

Figure 16-11   Vascular ring. Barium swallow in a toddler with posterior compression of esophagus and trachea from a vascular ring. *(Courtesy Department of Radiology, Children's Hospital of Pittsburgh, Pittsburgh, Pa.)*

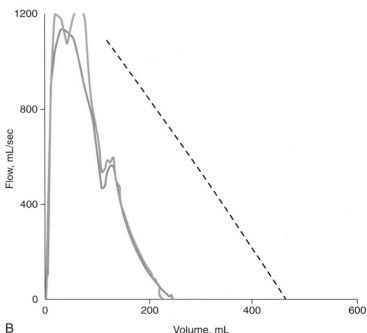

Figure 16-12   Computed tomography scan **(A)** and infant lung function testing **(B)** in a young child with neuroendocrine cell hyperplasia of infancy.

viral respiratory infections, after exposure to noxious inhalants, such as cigarette smoke, or after vigorous activity.

Upper respiratory tract disease and sinusitis have been implicated in the pathogenesis of chronic cough, presumably through the stimulation of pharyngeal cough receptors by upper airway secretions. Parental smoking (passive smoking) itself is a common cause of cough in preschool children. GER more commonly causes cough at a younger age but may appear at any age. The interstitial pneumonitides may also produce a chronic cough in this age group.

An inhaled foreign body in either the tracheobronchial tree or esophagus is an important cause of chronic cough, especially in toddlers. A history of gagging or choking may be absent at this age, physical examination may be unrevealing, and the plain chest radiograph may be normal. Subtle differences in air entry into homologous lung segments, detected with the differential (double-headed) stethoscope (see Fig. 16-1), may be the only indication of a foreign body in the airway. Cough is present in more than 90% of cases; it is usually of abrupt onset, but a quiescent period may occur after inhalation and cough may disappear as irritant receptors adjust to the object's presence. A mobile foreign body may result in the recurrence of cough as new receptors are stimulated by the object. Although inspiratory and expiratory radiography and fluoroscopy are useful in the evaluation of a child with a possible bronchial foreign body, they may be normal and rigid bronchoscopy may be necessary to confirm or disprove the presence of a foreign object (Fig. 16-13). Unilateral air trapping demonstrated by inspiratory and expiratory radiographs (Fig. 16-14, *A* and *B*) (or left and right lateral decubitus films in younger children) strongly suggests an inhaled foreign body.

Suppurative lung diseases, such as cystic fibrosis or bronchiectasis (Fig. 16-15), or deriving from any other causes (e.g., tuberculosis), characteristically result in a chronic cough producing purulent sputum. "Right middle lobe syndrome," commonly associated with enlargement of lymph nodes surrounding the right middle lobe bronchus in tuberculosis, has also been described in asthma and a number of other illnesses and may be associated with chronic cough. Recurrent infection of the middle lobe can ultimately lead to the development of bronchiectasis or fibrosis.

Disorders of ciliary motility (primary ciliary dyskinesia and acquired ciliary dyskinesia) may produce insidious symptoms of chronic productive cough, nasal drainage, recurrent middle ear infections, and fever. Clinical findings include basilar crackles (which can be expiratory) and, later, radiographic changes of recurrent lower lobe infections and bronchiectasis. Repetitive infections occur unless measures such as chest physical therapy, postural drainage, and liberal use of antibiotics are employed. It is now recognized that the classic triad described by Kartagener of situs inversus, sinusitis, and bronchiectasis fits only a limited number of patients because situs inversus occurs in only about half of all patients with primary cilia dyskinesia. Far more common is an acquired ciliary dyskinesia that can follow certain lower respiratory infections (including adenovirus, *Mycoplasma*, respiratory syncytial virus, and influenza). Diagnosis can be made via biopsy of the respiratory epithelium, either from curettage of the nasal

Figure 16-13   Foreign body. Portion of a carrot lodged in the right mainstem bronchus, as seen through a rigid bronchoscope. *(Courtesy S. Stool, MD, Pittsburgh, Pa.)*

Figure 16-15   Bronchiectasis. Bronchogram shows cylindrical bronchiectasis of the left lower lobe in a 5-year-old girl with recurrent pneumonia and chronic cough.

turbinate in the office or from forceps biopsy of the bronchus via rigid bronchoscope under anesthesia. It may also be suggested by a reduced fraction of nitric oxide in exhalate from the nose.

Pulmonary hemosiderosis is a potentially fatal disorder that has been described in association with cardiac or panorganic disease, glomerulonephritis (Goodpasture syndrome), collagen vascular diseases, and as an idiopathic form. Idiopathic pulmonary hemosiderosis (IPH) is a disease of unknown etiology characterized by episodes of dyspnea, cough and/or hemoptysis, cyanosis, fever, and iron-deficiency anemia. Hematemesis or melena may be the only presenting complaint in some patients without symptoms referable to the respiratory tract. As a result of recurrent bleeding episodes, jaundice may be observed, and clubbing develops over time in some patients. Laboratory findings include iron-deficiency anemia and, in a small number of patients, peripheral eosinophilia. Radiographic findings are quite variable, with some patients demonstrating scant transient infiltrates and others showing widespread parenchymal infiltrates that resemble miliary tuberculosis. Hemosiderin-laden macrophages obtained from sputum, gastric washings, or bronchoalveolar lavage suggest the diagnosis, but a lung biopsy is frequently necessary and

will allow the clinician to differentiate vasculitis from capillaritis and assess for iron deposition. A percutaneous renal biopsy or detection of anti–basement membrane antibodies may help in cases of hemosiderosis associated with Goodpasture syndrome.

School Age to Adolescence

Because children are exposed to numerous respiratory viruses during the first several years of school, recurrent viral infection remains an important cause of chronic cough in this age group. Asthma continues to be a consideration in the patient with a chronic cough. Patients in this age group (older than 6 years) can perform pulmonary function tests including bronchodilator responsiveness or bronchial provocation studies to

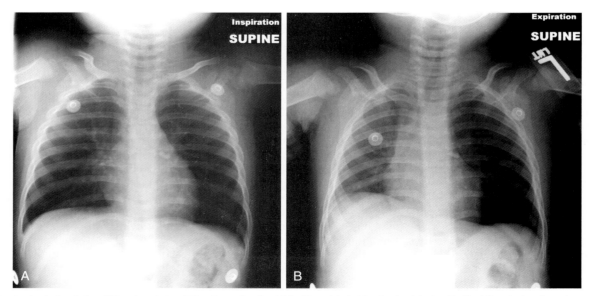

Figure 16-14   Foreign body. Inspiratory **(A)** and expiratory **(B)** radiographs of a child with an inhaled foreign body lodged in the left mainstem bronchus reveal hyperlucency of the left hemithorax and compensatory shift of the mediastinal structures to the right on expiration. *(Courtesy Sameh Tadros, MD, Pittsburgh, Pa.)*

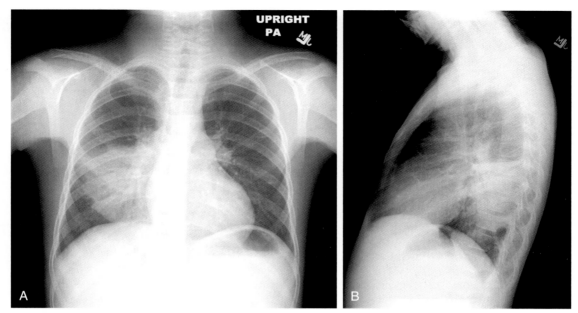

Figure 16-16   Pneumonia. **A,** Posteroanterior view and **B,** lateral view of *Mycoplasma* pneumonia in a 10-year-old boy. Posteroanterior chest radiograph shows right lower lobe (apical segment) involvement of a lobar infiltrative process.

confirm the diagnosis. Other disorders may present with chronic cough at this age including allergic rhinosinusitis, cystic fibrosis, pulmonary hemosiderosis, interstitial pneumonitis, and primary ciliary dyskinesia.

Mycoplasma pneumoniae infection is an important cause of chronic cough among school-age children. In its early stages, the disease is identical to a viral upper respiratory infection with coryza, sore throat, low-grade fever, and malaise. Gradually, the symptoms of lower respiratory involvement emerge and persist. Cough ranges from dry and hacking to one productive of mucoid sputum. On occasion the disease progresses to lobar pneumonia (Fig. 16-16, *A* and *B*) indistinguishable from typical bacterial pneumonia. The cough typically persists for 6 weeks, although it may last for 3 months. Physical findings tend to be minimal, although crackles and wheezing are often noted. The chest radiograph is not diagnostic, and the findings may be either interstitial or bronchopneumonic in character, with predilection for the lower lobes (see Fig. 16-16, *A* and *B*). Often the chest radiograph is normal. Diagnosis of *M. pneumoniae* infection can be made most rapidly by throat swab PCR. Serology is also used, and either paired sera for IgG titer or a single elevated IgM titer can be diagnostic. *Mycoplasma* culture is performed, but the organism is difficult and slow to isolate (taking 60 to 90 days), making this test of little clinical utility.

A psychogenic cough (also called habit cough and cough tic) may be observed after a lower respiratory tract illness. Habit cough may persist for weeks or months after the acute process has subsided. This cough tends to be loud and bizarre in nature and timing; it is often described as "honking" or "barking." This type of cough is short, nonproductive, and nonparoxysmal; it is quite disturbing to family members and classmates, to the point that the child may be excluded from school and other activities. It always disappears with sleep. The cough becomes more obvious with stressful situations or when parents (or physicians) express interest in regarding the cough, and may be decreased by distraction or talking. For this reason, extensive evaluations by medical personnel may merely exacerbate the problem when the diagnosis can be made on the basis of the characteristic quality of the cough and its disappearance in sleep. Demonstrating normal pulmonary function testing and a normal chest radiograph helps to

reassure the parent that other disease has been excluded. Treatment can include speech therapy, distraction, relaxation techniques, and hypnosis.

Cigarette smoking in this age group should also be a consideration, and, unless the rapport between physician and adolescent is particularly strong, the history will likely be unrevealing. Staining of the teeth or fingers or the presence of conjunctivitis may be indirect clues to the underlying cause of the cough. Measurement of exhaled carbon monoxide or carboxyhemoglobin can confirm the exposure.

Evaluation

The history may suggest the underlying cause of the cough (Table 16-3), and, perhaps more importantly, eliciting the cough during the physical examination can help. A wet-sounding (productive) cough suggests suppurative lung disease, such as cystic fibrosis, other forms of bronchiectasis, or ciliary dyskinesia syndromes. The cough in these patients tends to be most severe in the morning because excessive secretions pool in the tracheobronchial tree during sleep. Increased morning cough is also common in patients with

Table 16-3	Characteristics of Chronic Cough and Associated Conditions
Characteristic	**Associated Condition**
Loose, productive	Cystic fibrosis, bronchiectasis, ciliary dyskinesia
Croupy	Laryngotracheobronchitis
Paroxysmal	Cystic fibrosis, pertussis syndrome, foreign body inhalation, *Mycoplasma, Chlamydia*
Brassy	Tracheitis, upper airway drainage, psychogenic cough
After feedings	Pharyngeal incoordination, pharyngeal mass, tracheoesophageal fistula, gastroesophageal reflux
Nocturnal	Upper respiratory tract disease, sinusitis, asthma, cystic fibrosis, gastroesophageal reflux
Most severe in morning	Cystic fibrosis, bronchiectasis
With exercise	Asthma (including exercise induced), cystic fibrosis, bronchiectasis
Loud, honking, or bizarre	Psychogenic cough
Disappears with sleep	Psychogenic cough

sinusitis or increased upper airway secretions from viral infection or allergic rhinitis. A croupy cough may be observed in patients with acute laryngotracheobronchitis, and there may be associated wheezing. A dry or brassy cough is generally seen in patients with larger airway pathology, as in tracheitis or drainage from upper respiratory tract disease; a psychogenic cough may produce similar findings, but this type of cough may be distinguished from the others by its disappearance with sleep. As noted previously, a psychogenic cough is often (but not always) loud, honking, and disruptive. A paroxysmal cough is seen in patients with pertussis syndrome, *Mycoplasma* or *Chlamydia* infection, foreign body inhalation, or cystic fibrosis. A coughing episode associated with feedings suggests pharyngeal incoordination or mass, tracheoesophageal fistula, or GER. Nighttime coughing is noted in cystic fibrosis, asthma, GER, sinusitis, and upper respiratory tract disease. Cough occurring during or shortly after activities suggests exercise-induced asthma, cystic fibrosis, or bronchiectasis.

Examination of the sputum may also be helpful in suggesting the diagnosis. Clear, mucoid sputum containing eosinophils is likely to represent asthma, whereas purulent green sputum is more suggestive of suppurative lung disease, such as cystic fibrosis. A yellow color can be imparted to the sputum by breakdown products of white blood cells; therefore yellow sputum can be seen with bacterial infection (polymorphonuclear leukocytes) or asthma (eosinophils). Blood-tinged sputum can occur in cystic fibrosis, retained foreign body, idiopathic pulmonary hemosiderosis, tuberculosis, bronchiectasis, and some infections. Upper respiratory tract irritation with epistaxis may lead to the mistaken notion that hemoptysis is occurring. Hematemesis may also be mistaken for hemoptysis.

Clinical findings associated with a cough may also point to the nature of the problem. A cough occurring in the presence of poor weight gain and malabsorption makes cystic fibrosis a concern. Cough occurring with wheezing suggests asthma, and if evidence of rhinitis, conjunctivitis, or "allergic shiners" is present, allergic disease may also be a consideration (see Chapter 4). Cough that is worse in the spring and summer months or that occurs only after exercise suggests asthma. Worsening of the cough in winter is consistent with cold-induced bronchospasm or recurrent viral illnesses.

Diagnostic Approach

The approach to diagnosing a patient with persistent cough begins with a complete history in which some of the factors alluded to earlier are targeted (Table 16-4). On physical examination, close attention to nutritional status, associated upper respiratory tract disease, or clubbing of the digits is as important as the examination of the chest. Clubbing of the fingers raises the possibility of cystic fibrosis; any patient with this finding requires a sweat test performed by quantitative pilocarpine iontophoresis at an accredited cystic fibrosis center. On auscultation of the chest, a localized wheeze, particularly if associated with delayed air entry, suggests a foreign body or focal airway lesion leading to narrowing. Inspiratory crackles may be noted in cystic fibrosis, bronchiectasis from other causes, interstitial lung disease, or pneumonia. Crackles are also present during one third to one half of untreated asthma exacerbations, even in the absence of infection.

Most patients with prolonged cough should have a chest x-ray examination. Inspiratory and expiratory radiographs and fluoroscopy may be indicated if inhalation of a foreign body is suspected. A complete blood count (CBC) with differential may suggest the diagnosis in some patients, with eosinophilia seen in allergic disease, lymphocytosis in pertussis and other

Table 16-4	Diagnostic Approach to Cough
Complete history and physical examination
Chest and sinus radiographs
CBC with differential
Pulmonary function tests (including bronchoprovocation tests)
Sweat test (pilocarpine iontophoresis method)
Trial of bronchodilators
Sputum for Gram stain, AFB, and bacterial, viral, and fungal cultures
Quantitative immunoglobulins
Tuberculin skin test/anergy panel
Serologic tests or PCR for *Mycoplasma pneumoniae*
Bronchoscopy
Barium swallow
pH probe or Bernstein test

AFB, acid-fast bacillus; CBC, complete blood count; PCR, polymerase chain reaction.

viral diseases, and an increased proportion of neutrophils in bacterial infections.

Pulmonary function testing can detect lower airway obstruction that may be inapparent on physical examination; improvement in airflow with bronchodilator administration supports a diagnosis of asthma. Certain abnormalities of the shape of the flow–volume loop (see Fig. 16-40) during spirometry can also suggest upper airway pathology (discussed in Diagnostic Techniques, later). In some cases an outpatient trial of inhaled corticosteroids lasting several months or an empiric brief course of oral corticosteroids may serve to confirm the suspicion of asthma. Failure to respond to this regimen suggests that asthma is not the problem, but it could be the result of noncompliance with the prescribed medications. The term *cough-variant asthma* is not used by pulmonologists. This phrase refers to asthma in which cough, rather than wheezing, is the primary symptom. Such patients always have other signs of small-airway obstruction, ranging from hyperinflation evident on percussion of the chest to abnormalities on pulmonary function testing, and as such are diagnosed as having asthma on these grounds.

Examination of sputum with Wright or Gram stain or by cultures may lead to a diagnosis. Eosinophils suggest allergic disease, and polymorphonuclear leukocytes with organisms suggest a bacterial infection.

Quantitative immunoglobulins and immunoglobulin subclasses may be helpful in detecting some immunodeficiencies, and elevated IgE suggests allergic disease. A purified protein derivative (PPD) intradermal skin test placed in conjunction with other antigens of known immunogenicity (e.g., *Candida* or mumps) may be important in some patients. In the appropriate clinical setting, PCR or serologic studies for *M. pneumoniae* are occasionally fruitful. Bronchoscopy may exclude the diagnosis of foreign body or airway malformation as the cause of chronic cough. If foreign body inhalation is likely (based on history and/or physical examination), bronchoscopy is essential and should be performed under general anesthesia with the rigid bronchoscope by a surgeon.

Chest CT may confirm the diagnosis of bronchiectasis and should be performed if surgical removal of the affected segment is contemplated. A barium swallow is useful in patients with suspected tracheoesophageal fistula or primary swallowing disorders. Diagnostic evaluation of suspected aspiration is discussed later. Prolonged monitoring of the pH ("pH probe") in the distal esophagus may confirm the suspicion of GER. In patients suspected of having ciliary dysmotility, a nasal or bronchial ciliary biopsy for examination by light and electron

Table 16-5	Causes of Recurrent or Chronic Stridor
Croup	Pharyngeal or laryngeal masses
Infectious	Papilloma
Allergic/angioneurotic edema, GER	Hemangioma
Laryngomalacia	Laryngocele
Tracheomalacia	Web
Subglottic stenosis	Foreign body
Extrinsic airway compression	Tracheoesophageal fistula
Vascular ring	Vocal cord paralysis
Mediastinal mass	Hysterical or psychogenic
Lobar emphysema	
Bronchogenic cyst	
Foreign body in esophagus	
Thyromegaly	

GER, gastroesophageal reflux.

Figure 16-17 Croup (laryngotracheobronchitis). Radiograph of upper airway shows subglottic narrowing of the trachea, referred to as the "steeple sign." *(Courtesy Beverly Newman, MD, Pittsburgh, Pa.)*

microscopy or a nuclear medicine scan measuring the movement of inhaled radiolabeled particles within the central airways may be indicated.

STRIDOR

A number of clinical entities can produce persistent or recurrent stridor (Table 16-5), and some of these may also be associated with a chronic cough, as described earlier. Stridor is characteristically a harsh inspiratory noise created by obstruction of the larynx or the extrathoracic trachea. With a mild degree of airway narrowing, breath sounds may be normal when the infant or child is at rest, but with any activity that increases tidal breathing (e.g., crying, feeding, agitation), inspiratory stridor may become noticeable.

The most common cause of inspiratory stridor in the pediatric population is infectious croup (acute laryngotracheobronchitis). This disease is most commonly caused by a respiratory virus (parainfluenza, respiratory syncytial, influenza, or rhinovirus), and the patient typically has coryza for 24 to 48 hours before the appearance of croupy cough, hoarseness, and stridor. On occasion, the inflammatory process may spread to the smaller airways and produce wheezing in addition to these symptoms. The "steeple sign" is a characteristic radiographic sign on anteroposterior projections (Fig. 16-17) that may be accompanied by marked dilation of supraglottic

structures, particularly on lateral films. In the majority of patients, serious airway obstruction does not occur and the disease is self-limited. Acute angioneurotic edema is a less common cause of stridor. In most cases it results from an allergic reaction and is potentially fatal. Some children with anatomically normal airways suffer recurrent bouts of stridor, usually in the middle of the night, in the absence of signs of viral infection. Treatment for GER is often helpful in these patients, suggesting that for many, occult GER explains these bouts of recurrent airway obstruction.

The stridor associated with congenital laryngomalacia (Fig. 16-18) generally begins within the first week of life, varies with activity, and is more noticeable in the supine position. Clinical symptoms may suggest the diagnosis, but if severe, bronchoscopic visualization of airway dynamics by flexible bronchoscopy is a safe and reliable method of excluding other causes of stridor. Parents can be reassured that this entity is self-limited, becomes less marked after 6 to 10 months of age, and rarely causes serious problems.

Narrowing of the subglottic region can be congenital or acquired, as in subglottic stenosis associated with endotracheal intubation. Congenital subglottic stenosis improves as

Figure 16-18 Laryngomalacia. A sequence of photographs demonstrates the degree of airway compromise occurring during inspiration in laryngomalacia. The epiglottis is supported by a laryngoscope blade, but the progressive collapse of the other laryngeal structures during inspiration, especially the arytenoid cartilages, is shown clearly. *(From Benjamin B: Atlas of paediatric endoscopy, London, 1981, Oxford University Press.)*

Figure 16-19 Laryngeal papillomatosis. Multiple papillomas involving the larynx are seen in this photograph taken during rigid bronchoscopy. *(From Benjamin B:* Atlas of paediatric endoscopy, *London, 1981, Oxford University Press.)*

the child grows older, but narrowing associated with tracheal intubation may require a tracheostomy, particularly if the infant remains dependent on ventilatory support.

Congenital laryngeal or pharyngeal masses can also produce stridor by obstructing airflow. Laryngeal papillomatosis (Fig. 16-19) is a rare and life-threatening illness that generally presents in the first decade of life. Papillomas can involve the vocal cords, but there may also be widespread involvement of the tracheobronchial tree. Although inspiratory stridor may be observed, hoarseness is a more common presenting feature. Hemangiomas of the larynx or trachea may also produce stridor or a brassy or dry cough. Cutaneous or mucosal hemangiomas noted during the physical examination suggest the possibility of this diagnosis. Laryngeal webs (Fig. 16-20), cysts, and laryngoceles are quite uncommon and are accompanied by respiratory distress, stridor, feeding difficulties, and cyanosis. Diagnosis is made by bronchoscopy. A foreign body in the pharynx or larynx may also cause stridor.

Vocal cord paralysis, either unilateral or bilateral, may be present in the neonatal period, although in the case of unilateral paralysis several weeks may pass before the diagnosis is suspected. A weak or absent cry, hoarseness, inspiratory stridor with or without respiratory distress, and feeding

difficulties are the usual signs of vocal cord paralysis. Bilateral vocal cord paralysis may be seen with hydrocephalus, myelomeningocele, Arnold-Chiari malformation, or other malformations of the brain. Unilateral and bilateral cord paralyses are observed in patients with abnormalities of the cardiovascular system that are accompanied by cardiomegaly (e.g., ventricular septal defect, tetralogy of Fallot) or that cause abnormalities of the great vessels (e.g., vascular ring, transposition, patent ductus arteriosus). The diagnosis is best made by flexible laryngoscopy under minimal sedation so that vocal cord movement can be examined adequately. Because of a strong association of dysfunctional swallow with vocal cord paralysis, a barium swallow should be performed in suspected cases to assess for aspiration.

A bronchogenic cyst (Fig. 16-21, *A* and *B*) in the newborn can cause stridor, as the cyst fills with air after birth and compresses large airways. It can also cause tachypnea, dyspnea, cyanosis, and diminished breath sounds on the affected side. Later, the cyst may become infected, leading to recurrent bouts of fever, cough, and hemoptysis. Finally, an esophageal foreign body may compress the compliant posterior wall of the trachea and produce stridor, cough, and dysphagia.

The diagnosis of psychogenic stridor is generally made during adolescence and is more common in girls. As in psychogenic cough, psychogenic stridor disappears with sleep and is more noticeable with anxiety or when excessive attention is given to the patient. It is the result of adduction of the vocal cords during inspiration.

WHEEZING

Many diseases that produce chronic wheezing in pediatric patients overlap with entities that cause coughing or stridor (Table 16-6). Wheezing is a continuous sound that results from obstruction of airflow in intrathoracic airways. This obstruction can be at the lower trachea or "downstream" in the small bronchi and bronchioles. Wheezes can be heard on expiration or, less commonly, during both phases of respiration. The pitch of the wheeze, the variation in its pitch throughout the lung fields, and an association with hyperinflation as defined by percussion (described earlier) can help differentiate wheezing resulting from obstruction in the small airways (polyphonic) from that in the large airways

Figure 16-20 Laryngeal web. Expiratory view of a laryngeal web, noted at birth in an infant with inspiratory stridor that was exaggerated by crying. The web is seen traversing the area of the glottis. *(From Smalhout B, Hill-Baughan AB:* The suffocating child: bronchoscopy, a guide to diagnosis and treatment, *Ingelheim, Germany, 1980, Boehringer Ingelheim, p. 86.)*

Table 16-6	Causes of Chronic or Recurrent Wheezing
Asthma	Ciliary dyskinesia syndromes
Exercise-induced asthma	Tracheomalacia and/or bronchomalacia
Gastroesophageal reflux	
Hypersensitivity reactions (e.g., ABPA)	Congestive heart failure
	Bronchopulmonary hemosiderosis or Heiner syndrome
Cystic fibrosis	
Aspiration	Endobronchial lesions including localized stenosis
Tracheoesophageal fistula	
Foreign body	Interstitial pneumonitides
Gastroesophageal reflux	Bronchiolitis obliterans
Laryngeal cleft	
Pharyngeal dysmotility	
Extrinsic masses	
Vascular ring	
Cystic adenomatoid malformation	
Lymph nodes	
Tumors	

ABPA, allergic bronchopulmonary aspergillosis.

Figure 16-21 Bronchogenic cyst. **A,** Chest radiograph demonstrates hyperlucency of the left lung. **B,** Magnetic resonance imaging (MRI) of the chest demonstrates a large, centrally located cystic lesion of the left hilum with compression of the adjacent airway. *(Courtesy Beverly Newman, MD, Pittsburgh, Pa.)*

(monophonic). Response to bronchodilator and/or steroids is a useful way of differentiating true asthma (which should improve with these treatments) from wheezing resulting from tracheomalacia or bronchomalacia (which does not improve and may even worsen with bronchodilators). Asthma is the most common cause of wheezing in pediatric patients. Asthma is usually associated with some degree of hyperinflation (air trapping) in the untreated patient younger than 5 years of age. Asthma may take many different forms including typical asthma, exercise-induced asthma, transient wheezing of infancy, and wheezing associated with GER.

A disorder often mistaken for exercise-induced asthma is vocal cord dysfunction. In vocal cord dysfunction, the true vocal cords adduct during inspiration. The adduction of the cords is nearly always of behavioral origin. It results in a sensation of dyspnea, which the patient localizes to the throat—a history inconsistent with asthma. Often the stress of a competitive event brings out this reaction. This diagnosis can be established in the exercise laboratory with the aid of pulmonary function testing. The adduction of the vocal cords can also be demonstrated by flexible nasolaryngoscopy. Despite the psychogenic origin, this disorder is generally best treated by speech therapists; referral to a psychiatrist is rarely necessary.

Increased wheezing in a patient with previously well-controlled asthma should raise the possibility of allergic bronchopulmonary aspergillosis (ABPA). These patients often have an insidious onset of low-grade fever, fatigue, weight loss, and productive cough. Physical findings include expiratory wheezes and bibasilar crackles and, later in the course, clubbing of the digits. Radiographic features of ABPA (Fig. 16-22) include areas of consolidation, atelectasis, and evidence of dilated bronchi radiating from the hila. Diagnosis can be made by positive skin test results with *Aspergillus fumigatus* antigens, elevated total serum IgE levels, elevation of specific IgE, presence of serum precipitins to *Aspergillus* organisms, and isolation of *A. fumigatus* from the sputum culture. Pulmonary function studies may worsen considerably during episodes of ABPA with evidence of increased airway obstruction. A host of hypersensitivity reactions produce extrinsic allergic alveolitis with wheezing. Treatment of ABPA includes prolonged systemic corticosteroids and sometimes antifungal medications.

Other disorders that can provoke wheezing include cystic fibrosis, aspiration events from any cause, and extrinsic masses that compress the airways.

Congenital cystic adenomatoid malformation is a rare cause of extrinsic airway compression in which symptoms generally begin at birth or shortly afterward, as a normal lung is compressed by the lesion with the onset of tachypnea, respiratory distress, and cyanosis. Hydramnios is often noted at birth. Rarely, smaller cysts may be an incidental finding on chest radiography or symptoms may develop after infection of the cysts occurs. The radiographic appearance (Fig. 16-23) is that of single or multiple cystlike areas compressing normal lung, with mediastinal displacement. It is usually confined to a single lobe, and there is no apparent predilection for a particular lobe.

Extrinsic airway compression may produce wheezing or stridor, depending on the site of obstruction. A vascular ring (Fig. 16-24) is much more likely to cause expiratory wheezing than inspiratory stridor (see Chapter 5). Diagnosis can be made by MRI, echocardiography, barium swallow, or bronchoscopy; the last mentioned may demonstrate a pulsatile lesion compressing the trachea. MRI, unlike the other diagnostic choices, delineates the vascular and airway anatomy simultaneously and has become the diagnostic test of choice.

Figure 16-22 Allergic bronchopulmonary aspergillosis. Chest CT of a patient with asthma and allergic bronchopulmonary aspergillosis shows consolidation, atelectasis, and dilated bronchi radiating from the hilum.

Figure 16-23 **A,** Congenital cystic adenomatoid malformation (CCAM). Computed tomography scan of the newborn shows multiple, small air-filled cysts in the left lower lobe. This infant had this diagnosis made by antenatal ultrasound. **B,** Anteroposterior chest radiograph of newborn shows a large air-filled cyst filling most of the right hemi-thorax. Smaller cysts on the right are apparent, although not as well delineated. The right lower lobe is compressed, and the mediastinum is shifted to the left. This infant had this diagnosis made by antenatal ultrasound. (**A,** *Courtesy Sameh Tadros, MD, Pittsburgh, Pa;* **B,** *courtesy Beverly Newman, MD, Pittsburgh, Pa.*)

Barium swallow, which can demonstrate vascular compression, does not delineate vascular anatomy and is no longer routinely indicated for evaluation of vascular ring. Mediastinal masses or, occasionally, enlargement of the thyroid gland may produce tracheal compression and stridor.

Congenital or acquired lobar emphysema usually produces tachypnea and other respiratory symptoms, such as cough, wheeze, intermittent cyanosis, and occasionally stridor. The chest radiograph in lobar emphysema (Fig. 16-25) demonstrates a large, hyperlucent area with few bronchovascular markings and usually compression atelectasis of adjacent lobes. Left upper lobe involvement is most common, but right middle lobe emphysema is also seen. For the infant who is growing well and in whom tachypnea is the primary symptom, or in lobar emphysema associated with a mucus plug, conservative management is indicated. In the symptomatic infant with associated compression atelectasis and/or chronic respiratory distress, resection of the affected lobe is indicated.

Bronchopulmonary dysplasia (BPD, also called chronic lung disease), one of the sequelae of prematurity and its treatment, is associated with recurrent episodes of wheezing, respiratory distress, and tachypnea (see Chapter 2). Otherwise mild respiratory illnesses in these infants with decreased respiratory reserve may progress to lower respiratory tract disease, necessitating frequent hospitalizations. Patients with BPD may develop chronic respiratory insufficiency, pulmonary hypertension, and cor pulmonale. The frequency of wheezing episodes may diminish with age, although it appears that these patients continue to have airway hyperreactivity that is triggered by any number of different insults. GER is common among patients with BPD, as is tracheobronchomalacia. Both of these entities can worsen wheezing in these patients.

Miscellaneous causes of wheezing include idiopathic pulmonary hemosiderosis; aspiration (acute or chronic, described later); endobronchial lesions associated with localized stenosis; and bronchiolitis obliterans. Obliterative bronchiolitis has been described in an idiopathic form, following adenoviral infections or inhalation of toxic agents and in conjunction with other diseases (including rheumatoid arthritis) in adults. Its most common current clinical setting in pediatrics is in the organ transplant recipient. Patients may present initially with fever, cough, or tachypnea and subsequently develop dyspnea and wheezing. Physical findings include wheezing, crackles, and diminished breath sounds. The radiographic pattern (Fig. 16-26) is that of hyperinflation, decreased vascularity, and increased interstitial markings (reflective primarily of increased airway marking) with areas of atelectasis and consolidation. Pulmonary function testing will reveal fixed lower airway obstruction. Complications of adenovirus-induced bronchiolitis obliterans include bronchiectasis, overinflation, recurrent atelectasis, and pneumonia. In many patients the prognosis is poor.

CYSTIC FIBROSIS

Cystic fibrosis (CF) is the most common life-shortening genetic disease among white North Americans, afflicting 1 in 3300 newborns in this group. The incidence in African Americans is approximately 1 in 17,000 and in people of Asian background, 1 in 35,000 to 1 in 50,000. The carrier frequency in the white population is an estimated 1 in 30. CF is a generalized exocrinopathy characterized by the inspissation of abnormally thick and tenacious secretions, principally involving the pancreas and lungs. In the lungs, impaired airway clearance and increased secretions cause obstruction of the airways with retention of bacteria, resulting in chronic endobronchial infection and an inflammatory process that leads to bronchiolitis, bronchitis, bronchiectasis, and bronchiolectasis. The disease is characterized by a gradual decline in pulmonary function. Respiratory disease accounts for the vast majority of deaths in people with CF. In the pancreas, ducts become obstructed by the abnormal secretions, preventing pancreatic enzymes from entering the duodenum and therefore preventing breakdown of dietary fat and protein. The pancreas undergoes autodigestion and is replaced by scar tissue; lifetime deficiency of pancreatic exocrine function results. In 40% to 50% of newborns with CF, enough pancreatic function remains for normal digestion. By 4 to 8 years of age, the proportion of patients with pancreatic insufficiency rises to 85% to 90%, where it remains. The term "pancreatic sufficiency" is used to describe the minority (10% to 15%) of patients with CF with enough pancreatic function to have normal absorption of nutrients (despite having diminished pancreatic function as compared with normal patients). The prognosis for patients

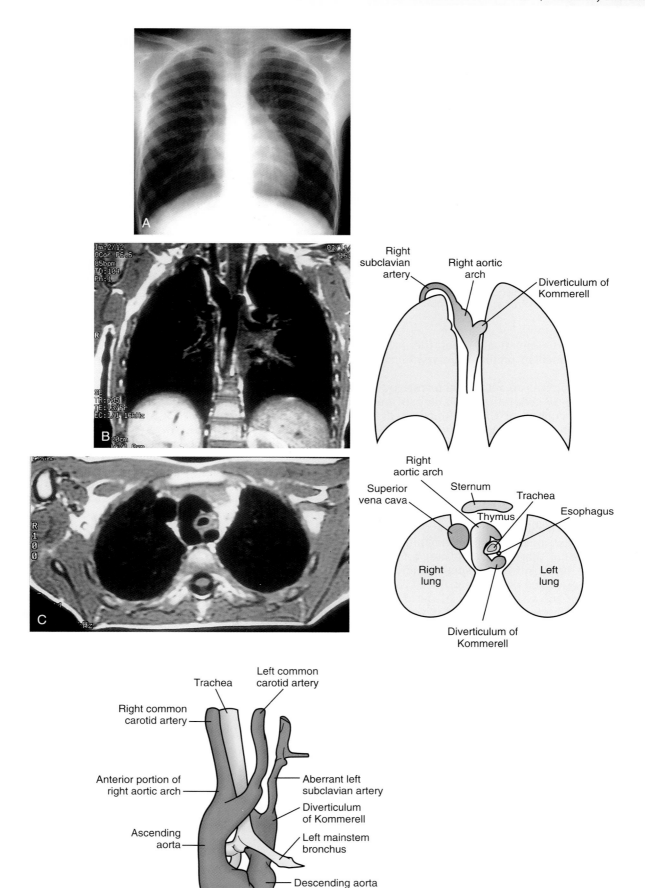

Figure 16-24   Vascular ring. Images depict the vascular ring caused by a right aortic arch with an aberrant left subclavian artery. **A,** Plain chest radiograph demonstrates a right-sided aortic arch, with tracheal deviation to the left. **B,** MRI in the sagittal plane shows the dominant right aortic arch and the remnant of the left aortic arch, called a diverticulum of Kommerell. The aberrant left subclavian artery arises posteriorly from the diverticulum of Kommerell. **C,** MRI of the same patient in the axial plane, demonstrating the vascular ring incarcerating the trachea and esophagus. The ring is completed by the ductus arteriosus, not visible here. **D,** Three-dimensional reconstruction of the vascular anatomy shown in the MRI from the left anterior perspective. *(Courtesy Beverly Newman, MD, Pittsburgh, Pa.)*

Figure 16-25 Congenital lobar emphysema. **A,** Anteroposterior chest radiograph. Left upper lobe shows hyperlucency of the affected globe, atelectasis of the lower lobe, and mediastinal shift. **B,** CT of same patient shows left upper lobe herniating across the midline with compression of structures on the right. *(Courtesy Beverly Newman, MD, Pittsburgh, Pa.)*

with CF has improved dramatically over the past several decades. By 2008 the median predicted survival had risen to 37.4 years of age.

The disease is inherited as an autosomal recessive trait. The protein product of the CF gene—the cystic fibrosis transmembrane conductance regulator, or CFTR—functions as an epithelial chloride channel. Decreased chloride transport and hyperabsorption of sodium across various epithelia result in abnormally viscid and poorly hydrated secretions. Careful cell culture studies have demonstrated a decreased height of the airway surface liquid, which impairs ciliary beating. The most common mutation of the CFTR gene in the North American white population is referred to as *delta-F508*. This mutation is the result of the deletion of three base pairs in the gene and results in a protein missing a phenylalanine residue at amino acid position 508. When genetic testing for CF became available, there was optimism that a small handful of mutations at the CF locus (located on the long arm of chromosome 7) would account for the vast majority of the patients with the disease and lead the way to population-wide screening. This, unfortunately, turns out not to be the case. As of 2010, more than 1700 mutations of this gene had been reported. Thirty-two mutations account for 92% of CF alleles in white

North Americans. In approximately 70% of CF genes delta-F508 is found, and half of North American patients with CF are homozygous for the delta-F508 mutation. Half of the remaining patients are compound heterozygotes, with delta-F508 coupled with another CF allele; the remaining patients have other, non–delta-F508 mutations. A number of investigators have tried to discover genotype–phenotype correlations. The most reliable phenotypic correlate of genotype has been pancreatic function (the compound heterozygote delta-F508/R117H, e.g., usually imparts a pancreatic-sufficient phenotype). Respiratory disease severity has not been well correlated to genotype, and on the basis of variability of disease within families, other modifier genes, as well as environmental factors, apparently play an important role in the clinical expression of CF.

Presentation

CF can present in any number of fashions (Table 16-7). The most common presentation now is without symptoms and by newborn screening (see below). Most symptoms are referable to respiratory or gastrointestinal involvement. Among patients with CF, 5% to 10% present with meconium ileus, which is

Figure 16-26 Bronchiolitis obliterans. **A,** Posteroanterior chest radiograph of 17-year-old with end-stage obliterative bronchiolitis as a complication of bone marrow transplantation for acute myelogenous leukemia. Film demonstrates increased interstitial and airway markings. **B,** CT of same patient demonstrates bronchiectatic changes. *(Courtesy Beverly Newman, MD, Pittsburgh, Pa.)*

Table 16-7 Presentations of Cystic Fibrosis

General	Metabolic
Failure to thrive	Hyponatremic, hypochloremic dehydration
Salty taste to skin	Heat stroke
Gastrointestinal/Nutritional	Metabolic alkalosis
Meconium ileus	Diabetes mellitus
Foul-smelling stools, bloating, abdominal pain	**Respiratory**
Rectal prolapse	Clubbing
Intestinal impaction and obstruction	Asthma
Pancreatitis, acute and chronic	Chronic obstructive pulmonary disease
Hypoproteinemia and edema	Recurrent pulmonary infiltrates
Neonatal hyperbilirubinemia	Chronic cough or sputum production
Cholelithiasis, cholecystitis	Barrel chest
Cirrhosis or portal hypertension	Hemoptysis
Fat-soluble vitamin deficiency (A, D, E, K)	Pneumothorax?
	Cor pulmonale
	Nasal polyps
	Other
	Infertility (males)

Figure 16-28 Meconium ileus. Gross appearance of the thick, tarlike meconium found at laparotomy in meconium ileus.

noted at or shortly after birth. Meconium ileus is a common cause of intestinal obstruction in the newborn; these infants present with abdominal distention, bilious vomiting, and failure to pass meconium stools. Abdominal radiographs show dilated loops of small bowel and a ground-glass appearance in the cecal region, signifying pockets of air within the thick meconium. A barium or water-soluble contrast enema may show a small distal colon (Fig. 16-27). In cases of meconium ileus associated with prenatal rupture and meconium peritonitis, abdominal calcifications may be noted on plain radiographs, and at laparotomy thick, tarlike meconium is found in the terminal ileum (Fig. 16-28). Prolonged neonatal jaundice, generalized edema in a breast-fed or soy formula–fed infant, or hypochloremia with heat prostration are less common presentations of CF in early infancy.

A combination of poor weight gain; loose, foul-smelling, bulky stools; and a voracious appetite are signs and symptoms that most clinicians associate with CF and rarely present a diagnostic problem. Rectal prolapse (Fig. 16-29) may be the presenting feature of CF in about 5% of cases and may recur multiple times. Rarely, the patient may undergo a surgical procedure for the rectal prolapse before the underlying diagnosis is suspected. Rectal prolapse is thought to result from chronic malnutrition, reduced abdominal musculature, and voluminous stools. It does not generally pose problems once the diagnosis has been made and the patient started on supplemental pancreatic enzymes. Gastrointestinal complications of CF include biliary cirrhosis, portal hypertension, hypersplenism, esophageal varices, and clinical evidence of fat-soluble vitamin deficiency.

A chronic productive cough or wheezing in a patient with digital clubbing suggests the diagnosis of CF until proved otherwise. Patients may present with a history of recurrent pneumonia or sinus disease; it is worth noting that the large majority of patients with CF demonstrate pansinusitis radiographically. Nasal polyps (Fig. 16-30) may be a presenting manifestation of CF and are seen in about 20% of patients at some time during the course of the disease. Other initial respiratory presentations are listed in Table 16-7.

The clinical course and severity of the disease vary remarkably. Many patients do not develop signs or symptoms of respiratory disease other than an intermittent, loose cough for years. Other patients have persistent symptoms from early infancy and are rarely without a cough. These patients tend to require frequent visits to the physician and frequent hospitalization and are more likely to have poor weight gain. Virtually all patients develop a loose, productive cough; the sputum may be blood-tinged during acute respiratory illnesses. Hemoptysis occurs in more than half of adult patients with CF and a considerable proportion of adolescents as well. Tachypnea, dyspnea, diffuse crackles, and digital clubbing will develop in most patients. Later, diffuse bronchiectasis, hyperinflation, and a barrel chest deformity are noted. The usual cause of

Figure 16-27 Meconium ileus. Barium enema in a newborn with meconium peritonitis and evidence of a small, unused distal colon (note the small extraluminal calcifications).

Figure 16-29 Rectal prolapse is shown in a toddler not previously recognized as having cystic fibrosis.

Figure 16-30   Cystic fibrosis. Nasal polyps in a patient with cystic fibrosis

death in patients with CF is respiratory failure, often in conjunction with cor pulmonale.

Complications

Complications of CF include hypochloremic metabolic alkalosis, hemoptysis, pneumothorax, pneumomediastinum, hypertrophic pulmonary osteoarthropathy, distal intestinal obstructive syndrome, biliary cirrhosis, pancreatitis, cor pulmonale, and respiratory failure. Among the respiratory complications, massive hemoptysis and pneumothorax with or without pneumomediastinum are potentially life-threatening. Blood streaking of sputum is not uncommon, and massive hemoptysis from rupture of dilated superficial bronchial arteries during chronic suppurative infections may occur in a small percentage of patients. Pneumothorax (see Fig. 16-32, *C*) generally occurs from rupture of bullous lesions created from chronic airway obstruction and presents with acute onset of chest pain and shortness of breath with or without cyanosis. Pneumomediastinum and subcutaneous emphysema may result (Fig. 16-31). Hypertrophic pulmonary osteoarthropathy involving the knees and other major joints occurs in about 5% of patients and is characterized by pain, swelling, and limited mobility of the affected joint.

Figure 16-31   Cystic fibrosis. A teenager with cystic fibrosis, severe respiratory disease, pneumomediastinum, and massive subcutaneous emphysema.

Acute or chronic pancreatitis occurs almost exclusively in patients with pancreatic sufficiency. These patients present with the acute onset of abdominal pain and vomiting and may have recurrent bouts of pancreatitis before the pancreas "burns itself out." Laboratory evaluations reveal elevations of serum lipase and amylase. The differential diagnosis in patients with CF with acute abdominal pain and vomiting includes cholecystitis, appendicitis, and distal intestinal obstruction syndrome. The last is characterized by crampy abdominal pain; constipation; vomiting; and, occasionally, a palpable mass in the right lower quadrant. A history of missed pancreatic enzyme supplements may exist, especially in adolescents.

Excessive loss of chloride and sodium from the salt can lead to hypochloremic metabolic alkalosis in infants who do not receive salt supplementation in their formula, especially during the summer months. This can occur even in the euvolemic state, and if severe, can result in anorexia and vomiting.

Right ventricular hypertrophy and cor pulmonale are findings in the terminal stages of many patients with CF with severe pulmonary disease.

Radiographic Findings

The radiographic and CT findings in CF vary from early hyperinflation and patchy areas of atelectasis to a generalized increase in peribronchial markings with bronchiectasis, parenchymal densities, and large cystic areas noted in severe disease (Figs. 16-32 and 16-33). The Brasfield scoring system is widely used as a means of classifying chest radiographs of these patients. It is based on a 25-point system for findings, such as hyperinflation, linear densities, cystic lesions, atelectasis, and right-sided cardiac enlargement or pneumothorax.

Diagnosis

Diagnosis of cystic fibrosis can be suggested by elevation of serum trypsinogen in the newborn. This test, immunoreactive trypsinogen (IRT), is used as a screening tool in most states as part of the extended newborn screen. Many laboratories will further analyze samples with elevated ITR for common genetic mutations of the CFTR gene. As a result, newborns may be referred to the local CF center having had a genetic diagnosis made before the first visit. Sensitivity of genetic testing for CF varies with ethnic group and remains approximately 92% for the white population with the 87-mutation panel, and 97% to 99% with a comprehensive (1300-mutation) screen. Still, the "gold standard" for initial diagnosis of CF remains the quantitative sweat test. Another advantage of the sweat test is that the results are available the same day, rather than the delay of several weeks with genetic testing. In sweat testing, pilocarpine is driven into the skin with a weak electrical current (iontophoresis) and the resulting sweat is collected with a wristband containing a coiled capillary tube, which wicks the sweat and stores it for analysis. The sweat test must be performed in an experienced laboratory, such as those associated with one of the Cystic Fibrosis Foundation–approved CF centers. Both false-negative and false-positive results are alarmingly common in inexperienced hands. Sweat chloride values of 60 mEq/L or greater are diagnostic of CF. A second sweat test is generally required for confirmation of diagnosis. Sweat chloride values of 40 to 60 mEq/L (or 30 to 60 mEq/L in infants less than 6 months old) are considered borderline and generally require a second test. False-positive values can occasionally occur, but disorders that cause this are readily distinguished clinically from CF. Other entities that elevate sweat chloride include adrenal insufficiency, ectodermal

Figure 16-32   Cystic fibrosis. Typical progression of radiographic changes in cystic fibrosis. **A,** A 2-month-old child with hyperinflation and right middle lobe atelectasis. **B,** A 15-year-old girl with peribronchial cuffing, hyperinflation, and bronchiectatic changes, particularly of the lower lobes. **C,** A 21-year-old man with severe respiratory involvement and an unsuspected right pneumothorax.

dysplasia, nephrogenic diabetes insipidus, hypothyroidism, mucopolysaccharidoses, glucose-6-phosphatase deficiency, hypoproteinemia, and anemia associated with malnutrition. Patients with CF who present with severe malnutrition and edema may have false-negative values on initial sweat tests until their nutritional status improves.

Genetic testing is quite useful in the evaluation of the infant who produces too little sweat for analysis, the patient with borderline sweat chloride, or the patient with normal sweat chloride but clinical features characteristic of CF. Recently, broad testing of the CFTR gene has been offered. It includes all known mutations of both coding and noncoding DNA, which has greatly increased the sensitivity of genetic screening. Mutation-specific therapies have been proposed in CF, and therefore genetic testing of all patients with CF is recommended.

SUDDEN INFANT DEATH SYNDROME

Sudden infant death syndrome (SIDS, also called sudden unexplained death in infancy) is defined as the unexpected death of an infant younger than 1 year of age who has been otherwise healthy and in whom there is no demonstrable pathologic basis for the death as determined by a thorough postmortem examination and death scene investigation. The annual incidence of SIDS in the United States is now approximately 0.5 per 1000 live births. SIDS is the leading cause of death after the neonatal period, with a peak incidence occurring at 2 to 3 months of life and rarely occurring after 6 months of age. Most of these infants die soundlessly during sleep, without any obvious sign of agitation. On occasion, a history of the recent onset of a viral illness may be elicited. SIDS is not a single disease entity but a final common pathway for a number of diseases with early and fatal presentation. Diseases recognized to cause sudden death in infants include the long-QT syndrome (a cardiac conduction defect) and inborn errors of fatty acid oxidation. Accidental or intentional smothering of an infant is usually impossible to differentiate from SIDS at autopsy. The "apnea hypothesis" of SIDS (failure of infants to breathe sufficiently in sleep) has been discarded by the medical community, especially in face of those infants dying of SIDS on home monitors who did not have apnea. Thus the home apnea monitor is of no value in preventing SIDS; even in premature infants with apnea of prematurity, monitoring is of no value after the 44th week of postconceptional life. The true cause of death in most SIDS victims remains unexplained. In SIDS there appears to be a vulnerable period, and other stressors (such as parental smoking, prone

Figure 16-33   Cystic fibrosis. CT scans of a 19-year-old woman with severe bronchiectasis and cystic fibrosis. Thickened airways are seen in longitudinal section through the upper lobes **(A)** and in cross-section in an image from the lower lobes **(B)**.

sleep position, an overheated room, or an unsafe sleep environment) have been shown to increase the SIDS rate. No test can accurately predict which infant is at risk for SIDS. The sleep study (or pneumogram) is of no value in identifying infants at risk for SIDS. Screening electrocardiograms for newborns (looking to identify those with prolonged QTc) have not as yet been recommended by the American Academy of Pediatrics. One intervention that appears to have had an impact on SIDS incidence is the "Back to Sleep" campaign, in which parents are educated to keep their newborn in a supine position during sleep. The rate of SIDS in the United States has declined since the institution of this policy in 1992. Counseling parents to smoke outside the home and car is another important intervention that pediatricians can make.

The term *apparent life-threatening event* (ALTE) was coined to replace "near-miss SIDS." This term refers to an event, witnessed by a parent or caregiver, that is frightening to the observer and that is characterized by some combination of apnea, color change, marked change in muscle tone, choking, or gagging. The observer of an ALTE generally feels that the event would have resulted in the infant's death had he or she not intervened. The role of GER as a major cause of ALTE is controversial, yet anecdotally GER seems to be one of the most common associations with ALTE. In these cases the infant has reflux, laryngospasm, and obstructive apnea. These events are usually associated with forceful respiratory efforts and a color change. Other disorders that can cause ALTE include sepsis/meningitis, inborn errors of metabolism, seizure, pertussis, respiratory syncytial virus infection, congenital cardiac disease, poisoning, and child abuse. Evaluation of an ALTE includes a careful history and physical examination (including funduscopy). Other tests may be necessary based on the history, and could include electrocardiogram; serum electrolytes, glucose, calcium, and ammonia; blood cultures, CBC, and white cell differential; blood gases; and toxicology screen. Evaluation for increased intracranial pressure may include a cranial CT and lumbar puncture when clinically indicated. Studies also include a sleep study that measures respiratory and abdominal wall movement, airflow at the mouth or nose, pulse oximetry and heart rate and, in some cases, pH monitoring of the distal esophagus. Of the above-described studies, the sleep study is usually the least revealing.

APNEA

Clinically meaningful apnea can be defined as the absence of airflow for at least 20 seconds or apnea accompanied by cyanosis or bradycardia. Apnea can be central, obstructive, or mixed. Absence of airflow accompanied by the cessation of chest and abdominal wall movement distinguishes central apnea. Obstructive apnea is the most common form of apnea and is characterized by the lack of airflow at the nose or mouth despite continued respiratory efforts. The first description of it in 1892 in Sir William Osler's *The Principles and Practice of Medicine* (under "chronic tonsillitis") remains the best one: "At night the child's sleep is greatly disturbed; the respirations are loud and snorting, and there are sometimes prolonged pauses, followed by deep, noisy inspirations." Patients with obstructive sleep apnea (OSA) fall into two categories: those with normal upper airway anatomy and those with abnormal upper airway anatomy. The former group includes those with obesity, GER, sickle cell anemia, severe laxity of the supraglottic structures, and marked adenoidal or tonsillar enlargement. The latter group includes patients with Crouzon syndrome, Apert syndrome, Down syndrome, Treacher Collins syndrome, the Pierre Robin sequence, Arnold-Chiari malformation, Prader-Willi syndrome, Möbius

syndrome, and dwarfism. Children with OSA frequently do not have the adult pattern of obesity and daytime hypersomnolence; more often they fail to thrive and may have hyperactivity as a manifestation of inadequate sleep. Diagnosis of OSA requires a sleep study (polysomnogram) in which movement of the chest, movement of the abdomen, heart rate, arterial saturation, and end-tidal CO_2 are measured. Staging of sleep during these studies is important as multiple arousals and/or awakenings may occur in OSA. The arousal-plus-awakening index can quantify the severity of the effects of sleep-disordered breathing on the quality of sleep and help direct management. Cardiac echo and electrocardiogram are indicated in cases of severe OSA because pulmonary hypertension is a common complication. Home apnea monitoring is of no value in OSA because the chest will continue to move, despite absence of airflow. Management of OSA is directed at the underlying disorder (such as tonsillectomy in cases of tonsillar hypertrophy), but cases that result from collapse of the upper airway structures may require constant positive airway pressure administered via nasal mask.

Central apnea may occur in infants with seizure disorders or central nervous system pathology such as Arnold-Chiari syndrome and intraventricular hemorrhage, prematurity, or congenital central hypoventilation syndrome (formerly known as Ondine's curse). Mixed apnea occurs when an obstructive apneic episode is followed by a central pattern of apnea (or vice versa).

Other studies that may be useful in apnea (all types) include ventilatory responses to hypercapnia or hypoxia, a chest radiograph, an electroencephalogram, CT of the brain, pH probe, and/or bronchoscopic evaluation of the airway, particularly in those patients with evidence of obstructive apnea. Laboratory evaluation may include any or all of the following: CBC, arterial or venous blood gases, chest radiography, and electrocardiogram.

ASPIRATION

Penetration of oral or gastric contents into the lungs is a common problem in patients with neurologic impairment. Aspiration can occur in patients with incoordination of swallowing and in neurologically normal patients with severe GER. The terms commonly used to describe these forms are "aspiration from above" and "aspiration from below." Patients with impaired mental status can have both forms of aspiration. Medical treatment of GER and feeding the patient via gastrostomy or gastrojejunal tube may not be sufficient to prevent progressive lung disease in patients who continue to aspirate oral secretions. Ongoing aspiration of saliva leads to progressive injury to the lung and worsening respiratory impairment. Chronic inflammation leads to mixed restrictive–obstructive pulmonary disease (Fig. 16-34) and difficult-to-control asthma. It is chronic aspiration that leads to the premature death that occurs in most children with profound neurologic impairment.

Aspiration can also be present in patients who are intellectually normal but who have delayed gastric emptying and GER. "Microaspiration," which refers to aspiration of tiny, essentially undetectable amounts of gastric contents, can cause intense bronchospasm due to the acidity of the aspirated material. In cats, just 50 µL of 0.1 N hydrochloric acid causes a fourfold increase in airway resistance. Patients with impaired clearance of food from the esophagus (achalasia) can also aspirate during sleep, despite having otherwise normal neurologic status. Aspiration should be suspected in patients with poorly controlled asthma despite aggressive management of asthma, especially in patients with neurologic impairment.

Figure 16-34 Chronic aspiration. Chest radiograph of a 20-year-old with lifelong chronic, severe aspiration shows increased interstitial markings and areas of consolidation–atelectasis.

Determining whether aspiration exists in a patient remains challenging, as there is no gold standard for its diagnosis. For evaluation of swallowing, a barium contrast swallowing study using different consistencies of barium (thin liquid, paste, solid) can determine what consistency of food can be given safely to the patient (Fig. 16-35). It can document where in the swallowing cycle the main pathology resides. Parameters assessed during the modified barium swallow include all of the following: initiation of the swallow (timing and oral control); duration of the swallow; adequacy of the swallow to clear food bolus; presence, amount, and timing of aspiration; protective reactions in response to aspiration; and soft palate control during swallowing. In neurologically impaired individuals, particularly those fed via feeding tubes, the radionuclide "salivagram" is a rapid means of determining whether the patient is aspirating his or her oral secretions. A small radioactive bolus is placed under the tongue, and the patient

Figure 16-35 Aspiration. Barium swallow demonstrating aspiration. Barium has coated the upper airway, outlining the trachea. *(Courtesy Avrum Pollack, MD, Pittsburgh, Pa.)*

is then monitored under a gamma camera. The bolus is then traced: if it enters the lung it bifurcates at the carina; if it enters the esophagus it can be followed into the stomach (Fig. 16-36). The salivagram has the advantages of being physiologic (the patient is not held in an arbitrary position) and requiring no preparation. It results in a low radiation dose to the patient, similar to that of the chest radiogram and a fraction of that used in a barium swallow. The radionuclide gastric emptying or "milk" scan, which uses the same radiation dose as the salivagram, can demonstrate reflux and delay in gastric emptying.

Delayed gastric emptying is important to document because its treatment is essential to the successful treatment of GER. The milk scan is fairly insensitive for aspiration of refluxed gastric contents. When aspiration is strongly considered, flexible bronchoscopy with bronchoalveolar lavage (BAL) for assessment of lipid-laden macrophages (Fig. 16-37) is a useful test. Alveolar macrophages from the BAL fluid are stained for fat. Globules of fat found in a predominance of the macrophages suggest aspiration of food. The sensitivity of the test is unknown, but when moderate or high numbers of macrophages are found, it is believed to be specific for aspiration. Inspection of the upper airway may reveal edema and erythema of the aryepiglottic folds (Fig. 16-38).

DIAGNOSTIC TECHNIQUES

Diagnosis and treatment of children with respiratory complaints may be assisted by the use of pulmonary function tests (PFTs). With appropriate training, and with the technician's patience and encouragement, most children 6 years of age or older can cooperate with simple spirometry and measurements of lung volumes (Fig. 16-39). Interpretation of PFT results in children must take into account variability in performance by children and differences in age, height, weight, sex, and race. In children, PFTs may be useful in establishing the severity of respiratory disease, in guiding the choice of therapy, and in measuring the response to a therapeutic regimen. In some diseases, such as cystic fibrosis or asthma, evidence of increasing airway obstruction may indicate the need to initiate or increase the aggressiveness of therapeutic intervention.

Spirometry is the measurement of airflow after a maximal inhalation (to total lung capacity) and with a rapid and forceful exhalation (to residual volume). The inspection of the shape of flow–volume curves generated during forced expiratory maneuvers is critical for the appropriate interpretation of PFT results (Fig. 16-40). The initial portion of the flow–volume curve is effort dependent, whereas the terminal 25% of the expiratory maneuver is dependent on elastic recoil and airway resistance and is relatively independent of patient effort. A normal-appearing flow–volume curve is shown in Figure 16-40, *A*. With increased airway resistance distal to the central, large airways, the curve becomes concave toward the abscissa (volume axis). This type of concavity therefore suggests obstruction to airflow (Fig. 16-40, *B*). Spirometry can also be used to document reversibility of obstruction after bronchodilator inhalation (Fig. 16-40, *B*). Patients with suspected asthma may develop this configuration of flow–volume curve after bronchoprovocation tests such as inhaled histamine, methacholine, cold air, or after exercise testing.

The restrictive pattern shown in Figure 16-40, *C* demonstrates preservation of expiratory flow function but a reduction in total lung volume. Interstitial lung diseases are among the entities that typically produce this pattern on pulmonary function testing.

Figure 16-36   Abnormal salivagram demonstrates severe aspiration into the lungs at the end of a study. *(Courtesy Martin Charron, MD, Pittsburgh, Pa.)*

The shape of the flow–volume curve may also be helpful in evaluating upper or central airway pathology (Fig. 16-41). Fixed obstruction of the upper airways, as in tracheal stenosis, produces a limitation and plateau of both the inspiratory and expiratory loops of the flow–volume curve. A reduced inspiratory flow and a plateau of the inspiratory loop are suggestive of variable extrathoracic obstruction seen in disorders such as laryngomalacia and vocal cord dysfunction. Chondromalacia of the intrathoracic trachea or major bronchi results in a picture of variable intrathoracic obstruction with reduction and flattening of the expiratory limb because with forceful expiration, pleural pressure exceeds that inside the airway lumen, and the weakened bronchial wall cannot withstand that pressure gradient.

Disease states that affect lung growth would be expected to alter lung volume in addition to airway caliber. These diseases include pulmonary hypoplasia due to severe oligohydramnios or space-occupying lesions (e.g., diaphragmatic hernia or cystic adenomatoid malformation), bronchopulmonary dysplasia, as well as conditions that alter the growth of

the rib cage (thoracic dystrophies, radiation). Plethysmography is based on the principle of Boyle's law. With the subject sitting in a fixed-volume chamber ("box") and breathing with a mouthpiece, a shutter is closed in the inspiratory limb of the breathing circuit. The subject makes small panting maneuvers, resulting in small changes in the volume of the lung and corresponding inverse volume changes in the box. This allows for calculation of the lung volume at which the panting efforts began. The subject usually begins the maneuvers at the end of a breath, and this "resting" lung volume is termed *functional residual capacity* (FRC). A lung capacity is the sum of two or more lung volumes; in the case of FRC, it is the sum of residual volume (RV, the amount of gas remaining in the lung after a maximal exhalation) and expiratory reserve volume (ERV, the amount of gas exhaled from resting lung volume until the lung is empty). In combination with spirometry, other lung volumes and capacities can be calculated (see Fig. 16-39).

The diffusing capacity for carbon monoxide (DL_{CO}) is an integrative measurement that describes the transfer of oxygen

Figure 16-37   Lipid-laden macrophages obtained via bronchoalveolar lavage. If seen in moderate and high numbers, this finding is specific for aspiration of food, either the result of abnormal swallowing or from refluxed gastric contents. *(Courtesy Paul Dickman, MD, Pittsburgh, Pa.)*

Figure 16-38   Gastroesophageal reflux. Endoscopic photograph of the larynx of a patient with severe gastroesophageal reflux. Erythema and edema of the aryepiglottic folds exist. *(Courtesy Robert Yellon, MD, Pittsburgh, Pa.)*

Where:
TLC = IC + FRC
and
TLC = VC + RV

Inspiratory capacity

Vital capacity

Total lung capacity

Tidal volume

Functional residual capacity

Residual volume

Figure 16-39 Schematic representation of lung volumes.

from the alveolus into the red blood cell. This transfer is proportional to the surface area of the alveolar–capillary membrane and to the pressure gradient for carbon monoxide between the alveolus and the blood, and inversely proportional to the thickness of the alveolar–capillary membrane. CO is more soluble in blood than in lung tissue, and it binds rapidly and tightly to hemoglobin in the blood. These properties maintain a diffusion gradient for CO. The patient exhales completely to residual volume and inhales to total lung capacity a gas mixture containing 0.3% carbon monoxide, and holds his or her breath for 10 seconds during which CO diffuses into the blood. The uptake of CO is divided by the partial pressure gradient for CO to calculate $D_{L_{CO}}$. Diseases that decrease the surface area for diffusion (emphysema, pulmonary emboli, resection of lung tissue) or diseases that increase the thickness of the alveolar–capillary membrane (fibrosis, pulmonary edema, proteinosis) would both decrease the diffusing capacity of the lung. Increased $D_{L_{CO}}$ is much less common but can be seen in patients with alveolar hemorrhage, polycythemia, or during exercise (via recruitment of

more pulmonary capillaries). This test may be useful in evaluating patients with diffuse lung diseases or in assessing patients with pulmonary vascular obstruction.

PULMONARY FUNCTION TESTS IN INFANTS

Most of the tests described above have been adapted to infants, with the obvious challenge that maximal efforts cannot be elicited voluntarily. Infants are usually sedated with chloral hydrate, and placed supine with a mask over mouth and nose to measure airflow and pressure at the mouth. These techniques require specialized equipment not available in most pulmonary function laboratories.

The raised volume rapid thoracic compression (RV-RTC) technique is one method that has been used to generate maximal expiratory flow by applying a positive pressure externally to the chest. The infant's lungs are first inflated via the facemask to a predetermined pressure (typically 30 cm H_2O). This results in a lung volume close to total lung capacity. Forced exhalation is achieved with a plastic jacket that

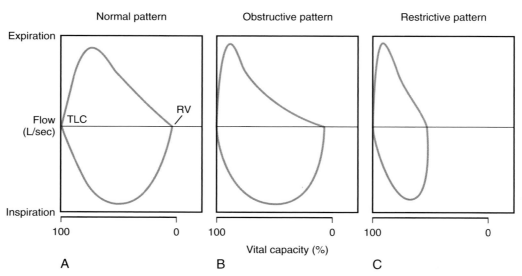

Figure 16-40 Flow–volume curves obtained by spirometry. **A,** Normal configuration of expiratory flow curve. **B,** Reduced expiratory flow rates suggest obstructive airway disease. **C,** Preservation of flow rates with a diminished vital capacity is consistent with restrictive lung disease. RV, residual volume; TLC, total lung capacity.

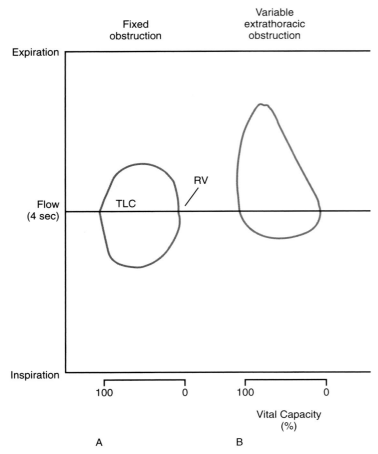

Figure 16-41 Flow-volume curves obtained by spirometry. **A,** Fixed airway obstruction with reduction in inspiratory and expiratory flow rates. **B,** Variable extrathoracic airway obstruction, with reduced peak inspiratory flow rates. RV, residual volume; TLC, total lung capacity.

Table 16-8	Range of Normal Arterial Blood Gas Values by Age		
	pH	**Pco_2**	**Po_2**
Newborn	7.33-7.49	27-41	>60
Infant (<1 yr)	7.34-7.46	26-41	>75
Older child	7.35-7.45	35-45	>75

stridor, unexplained or chronic cough or wheeze, suspected airway malformations or compression, atelectasis, or recurrent pneumonia. To obviate the need for open lung biopsy, flexible bronchoscopy and bronchoalveolar lavage may be particularly useful in immunosuppressed patients with unexplained pneumonia. Flexible bronchoscopy should not be attempted when there is a strong clinical or radiographic suggestion of inhaled foreign body. In these cases, rigid bronchoscopy is the procedure of choice to remove the object. Transbronchial biopsy is performed routinely in patients who have undergone lung transplantation in order to screen for rejection. This technique involves passing biopsy forceps via the suction channel of a bronchoscope under fluoroscopic guidance. It is of occasional usefulness in clinical situations in which the lesion is diffuse, such as interstitial lung disease. Tissue yield is low, and analysis requires an experienced pathologist. Risk of transbronchial biopsy is pneumothorax (approximately 1%) and bleeding.

Arterial blood gas measurements are the standard for assessing gas exchange in critically ill patients. Pulse oximetry and analysis of the CO_2 in exhaled air have become useful noninvasive means of assessing ventilatory status and have been used to avoid routine arterial puncture in both inpatient and outpatient settings. An example is the 16-year-old with Duchenne muscular dystrophy who presents with dyspnea and headache and is found to have an end-tidal CO_2 level of 90 mm Hg, prompting long-term institution of noninvasive ventilatory support. Venous or capillary blood gases can give accurate estimations of pH and Pco_2 but are not used for assessment of arterial Po_2. Normal arterial pH, Po_2, and Pco_2 values are provided in Table 16-8.

Sleep studies are still not widely available for the pediatric population, but they remain an important diagnostic tool. They are useful in the diagnosis of obstructive and central apnea, hypoventilation, and hypoxemia during sleep, all of which can be inapparent on routine testing of the awake patient. Studies vary in complexity from a simple at-home overnight pulse oximetry study to full nocturnal polysomnography with assessment of sleep stage, movement of chest, abdomen, electromyogram of diaphragm, arterial saturation, heart rate, end-tidal CO_2, and eye movements. The "pneumogram" is an abbreviated form of the sleep study in which there is evaluation of chest wall movement, airflow by nasal thermistor (which measures temperature below the nostril), heart rate, and arterial saturation. The pneumogram is insensitive for obstructive apnea, because it does not assess ventilation (as it lacks CO_2 measurement) and does not demonstrate sleep stage or changes in stage with respiratory events, but it is sensitive for central apnea and bradycardia.

encircles the chest and abdomen of the infant, which can be rapidly inflated from a pressure reservoir, generating a full expiratory flow–volume curve. The resultant curves are highly reproducible with values being reported as timed volumes (e.g., the forced expiratory volume in 0.5 second, or $FEV_{0.5}$) in addition to instantaneous flow rates. Lung volumes can also be measured by plethysmographic methods identical to those described previously.

Exercise testing can be a valuable tool to assess the cardiorespiratory fitness of a subject and may provide further information regarding a patient's respiratory reserve in addition to that found during routine PFTs. A progressive exercise study by bicycle ergometry or treadmill can give important information regarding ventilatory effort, heart rate responses, oxygen delivery and uptake, and carbon dioxide production. Evaluation of these parameters may provide information regarding exercise fitness and, if limited, identify whether the limiting factor is ventilatory or cardiac. Like PFTs, exercise testing can be used to assess the severity or progress of disease, evaluate effects of changes in treatment, and provide information about the safety or appropriateness of an exercise program in children with chronic lung disease.

Flexible fiberoptic bronchoscopy can be extremely useful in the diagnosis of lesions of the pulmonary tree and in isolating organisms from patients with pneumonia. Compared with traditional open-tube ("rigid") bronchoscopy, flexible bronchoscopy offers the advantage of better visualization of distal airway segments and upper lobes and allowing the study of airway dynamics during regular tidal breathing. Indications for pediatric flexible bronchoscopy include evaluation of

Bibliography

American Academy of Pediatrics Task Force on Sudden Infant Death Syndrome: The changing concept of sudden infant death syndrome: Diagnostic coding shifts, controversies regarding the sleeping environment, and new variables to consider in reducing risk, *Pediatrics* 116:1245–1255, 2005.

Boucher RC: New concepts of the pathogenesis of cystic fibrosis lung disease, *Eur Respir J* 23:146–158, 2004.

Busse WW, Lemanske RF Jr: Asthma, *N Engl J Med* 344:350–362, 2001.

Chernick V, Boat T: *Kendig's disorders of the respiratory tract in children*, ed 6, Philadelphia, 1998, WB Saunders.

Colombo JL, Hallberg TK: Pulmonary aspiration and lipid-laden macrophages: In search of gold (standards), *Pediatr Pulmonol* 28:79–82, 1999.

Daley KC: Update on sudden infant death syndrome, *Curr Opin Pediatr* 16:227–232, 2004.

Ferber R, Kryger M: *Principles and practice of sleep medicine in the child*, Philadelphia, 1995, WB Saunders.

Finder JD: Understanding airway disease in infants, *Curr Probl Pediatr* 29:65–81, 1999.

Hyatt R, Scanlon P, Nakamura M: *Interpretation of pulmonary function tests: a practical guide*, ed 2, New York, 2003, Lippincott-Raven.

Martinez FD, Morgan WJ, Wright AL, et al: Diminished lung function as a predisposing factor for wheezing respiratory illness in infants, *N Engl J Med* 319:1112–1117, 1988.

Martinez FD, Wright AL, Taussig LM, et al; Group Health Medical Associates: Asthma and wheezing in the first six years of life, *N Engl J Med* 332:133–138, 1995.

Orenstein D, Rosenstein B, Stern R: *Cystic fibrosis medical care*, Philadelphia, 2000, Lippincott Williams & Wilkins.

Orenstein D, Stern R: *Treatment of the hospitalized cystic fibrosis patient*, New York, 1998, Marcel Dekker.

Orenstein SR: Update on gastroesophageal reflux and respiratory disease in children, *Can Gastroenterol* 14:131–135, 2000.

Taussig LM, Wright AL, Holberg CJ, et al: Tucson Children's Respiratory Study: 1980 to present, *J Allergy Clin Immunol* 111:661–675, 2003.

Vaucher YE: Bronchopulmonary dysplasia: an enduring challenge, *Pediatr Rev* 23:349–358, 2002.

SURGERY

Katherine P. Davenport | Timothy D. Kane

17

INTRODUCTION

General pediatric surgery encompasses a wide spectrum of disorders and malformations that overlap with various other medical and surgical specialties. The emphasis of this chapter is on the common conditions that may be seen in general pediatric primary care practices, including some unusual cases.

HEAD AND NECK

Introduction

Most lesions of the head and neck are benign in nature. Lesional location provides essential information about the probable diagnosis. Table 17-1 provides a summary of the common pediatric head and neck lesions by anatomic location. Physical examination and diagnostic imaging studies are important to generate a differential diagnosis and further determine the nature and extent of the lesion. Critical physical examination findings include determination of size, evidence of airway compromise, signs of inflammation, presence of sinus tracts, or ocular involvement.

Computed tomography (CT), magnetic resonance imaging (MRI), and ultrasound (US) have almost completely eliminated plain radiography in the evaluation of lesions of the head and neck. These modalities may better demonstrate details of the bony and vascular structures of the skull base and the cervical spine. Furthermore, underlying brain involvement as either the primary or secondary site may be visualized. Skull and facial films are of limited utility at present. Children with disorders of breathing, swallowing, or phonation require adjunctive endoscopic procedures (nasopharyngoscopy, laryngoscopy, and esophagoscopy) to aid in the diagnosis.

Surgery is often required for head and neck lesions for both diagnostic and therapeutic purposes. Incision and drainage of a cervical abscess may provide a specimen for culture and a means of drainage for resolution. Excisional biopsy is critical to determine the specific pathology of a lesion and to assist with determining the need for further therapies. There are several important conditions of the head and neck in which surgery is unnecessary or may unduly create complications. These include hemangioma, torticollis, and benign reactive adenopathy.

Cervical Lymphadenopathy

Benign reactive cervical lymphadenopathy is the most common mass in the lateral triangle of the neck. These lesions arise as nonspecific hyperplastic responses to infection of the upper respiratory tract (nose, sinuses, ears, mouth, and pharynx) or skin (face and scalp). Typically these nodes are less than 2 cm in size and are rubbery, oval, and isolated. They characteristically occur in children between 2 and 10 years of age. *Streptococcus pyogenes* and *Staphylococcus aureus* are the most common organisms that produce this adenopathy. In most instances, the nodes spontaneously regress after resolution of the inciting infection. Bacterial infection within node(s) may lead to more significant enlargement with increased tenderness, erythema, and ultimately suppuration (Fig. 17-1). Aggressive antibiotic therapy in the early stages of infection may prevent the development of the late suppurative stages that require surgical intervention. Fluctuant masses should be aspirated or incised and drained.

Various clinical presentations may occur with mycobacterial infections including local cervical adenopathy, pulmonary infection, and disseminated disease. The most common form is caused by one of the *Mycobacterium avium-intracellulare-scrofulaceum* (or MAIS) complex, which consists of approximately 15 organisms. These mycobacterial organisms typically produce local cervical disease. Mycobacterial tuberculosis usually presents with pulmonary infection but may rarely have supraclavicular or cervical lymphadenopathy (Fig. 17-2). In contrast, atypical mycobacterial infection usually involves the submandibular, submaxillary, or preauricular lymph nodal regions. Large, firm, immobile, and nontender lymph nodes may arise after inoculation. These may undergo spontaneous breakdown with the development of an abscess and sinus formation. Incision and drainage of fluctuant nodes may lead to a chronically draining sinus.

The differential diagnosis of chronic cervical lymphadenopathy (i.e., nodes that persist beyond 4 weeks) includes cat-scratch disease, atypical mycobacterial infection, and tuberculosis. Cat-scratch disease, a common cause of lymphadenopathy in children, usually develops as a regional nodal enlargement 2 to 4 weeks after inoculation by either a dog or cat. There may be a local reaction to the scratch followed by the evolution of lymphadenopathy, which may persist for several months. On occasion these nodes become suppurative and fluctuant and require surgical drainage. The diagnosis may be made by serologic testing for the antigen or by polymerase chain reaction of nodal tissue. Alternatively, Warthin-Starry, a histochemical silver stain for cat scratch, may identify the *Bartonella* organisms in tissue specimens (Fig. 17-3). Complete resection of the node and any tracts is usually curative. Antimycobacterial therapy is not indicated in most cases of MAIS infection.

Cervical adenitis secondary to *Mycobacterium tuberculosis* infection is usually a manifestation of significant intrathoracic disease and requires aggressive antimycobacterial drug therapy. Surgery is usually unnecessary and should be avoided because of the risk of developing a chronically draining sinus (cervical tuberculosis). Lymphoma may present as painless cervical adenopathy. The absence of antecedent upper respiratory or cutaneous infections, the persistence of nodes beyond 6 weeks, size greater than 2 cm, and firm consistency should raise concern for malignancy. Although cervical adenopathy is more

Table 17-1	Common Lesions of the Head and Neck in Infancy and Childhood	
Region	**Location**	**Common Lesions**
Head	Scalp	Hemangioma, dermoid cyst
	Ear	Preauricular sinus, tag
	Eyebrow	Dermoid cyst
	Base of nose	Meningocele, encephalocele
	Parotid gland	Hemangioma, lymphangioma, rhabdomyosarcoma, lymphoma, mixed tumor, parotitis
Mouth	Tongue	Tongue-tie, macroglossia, lingual thyroid
	Floor of mouth	Ranula
	Cheek and lip	Papilloma, mucocele
	Alveolar ridge	Tooth bud, epignathus
Neck	Midline	Thyroglossal duct cyst, dermoid cyst, submental lymph node, goiter
	Lateral	Branchial cleft cyst or sinus, lymphadenitis, lymphoma, lymphangioma, torticollis

Figure 17-2   The skin overlying a tuberculous lymph node is often discolored and may break down into a chronically draining sinus.

common in Hodgkin disease, non-Hodgkin lymphoma may also present with a cervical mass (Fig. 17-4). Incisional biopsy is diagnostic and mandated when these criteria are met. Other primary malignancies such as neuroblastoma and rhabdomyosarcoma may present as lateral neck masses. Secondary metastases from intraabdominal or head and neck tumors may also occur.

Thyroglossal Duct Cyst and Sinuses

The differential diagnosis for midline neck masses includes thyroglossal duct remnants, dermoid cysts, and lymphadenopathy. During fetal development, the thyroid gland originates at the base of the foramen cecum and descends in the midline along the course of the thyroglossal duct close to the hyoid bone, until it reaches its final destination at the base of the neck. Failure of regression of the thyroglossal duct may lead to cyst formation (Fig. 17-5). These lesions are quite prone to infectious complications and require surgical excision. This excision requires resection of the midportion of the hyoid bone and ligation of the tract leading to the foramen cecum to prevent future recurrence (Fig. 17-6).

Thyroid nodules are common in the pediatric population (Fig. 17-7). However, a greater incidence of malignancy occurs within these lesions in children. Therefore, thorough evaluation and management of these lesions are critical to a favorable outcome. These nodules are twice as common in girls as

boys. They typically present with a midline anterior cervical mass that moves with the thyroid gland. Initial physical examination determines the location of the lesion, as well as the presence of associated lymphadenopathy. In general, clinical findings are unreliable in distinguishing between benign and malignant disease. Although thyroid imaging studies are often indicated, they are rarely helpful in aiding with the diagnosis, unless there is evidence of multiple nodules. A multinodular goiter would suggest nodular Hashimoto disease, which is the most common benign lesion of the thyroid (Fig. 17-8). The utility of ultrasound in distinguishing benign from malignant disease on the basis of a cystic appearance of the lesions is also unhelpful. Furthermore, the utility of fine-needle aspiration cytology in the pediatric population remains an area of considerable debate; reports in the older medical literature suggested a much higher incidence of malignancy in thyroid nodules in children than do current studies. Consequently, there was a much stronger recommendation for surgical excision as the diagnostic procedure of choice. More recent reports have shown that the incidence of benign disease is approximately 20%. Therefore needle aspiration may avert surgical resections for benign disease. Needle aspiration cytology that shows a true malignancy or that has indeterminate pathology should be followed by surgical resection. Total thyroidectomy is recommended for malignant primary lesions; lobectomy

Figure 17-1   Erythema and fluctuance identify the presence of an abscess. An abscess may be present without fluctuance, however, the result of induration from surrounding inflammation.

Figure 17-3   Warthin-Starry silver stain identifies the black-staining organisms associated with cat-scratch disease, seen on examination of an enlarged lymph node.

Figure 17-4 Enlarged lymph nodes in unusual locations, such as in this patient with supraclavicular lymphadenopathy from non-Hodgkin lymphoma, require excisional biopsy to rule out malignancy.

Figure 17-5 Thyroglossal duct cyst produces a firm swelling in the midline of the neck. Its initial manifestation is sometimes a midline cervical abscess.

Figure 17-6 The surgical specimen shows the thyroglossal duct as it courses from the lesion to the hyoid bone (the thicker transverse piece of tissue) **(A)**. The hyoid must be resected to gain access to the tissue that extends to the base of the tongue (foramen cecum), which must be ligated to prevent recurrence **(B)**.

Figure 17-7 Nonfunctioning or "cold" thyroid nodule visualized by thyroid scan **(A)** and magnetic resonance imaging (MRI) **(B)** at surgery was found to be a benign follicular adenoma.

Figure 17-8   Goiter in a 15-year-old girl, resulting from Hashimoto thyroiditis.

Figure 17-10   Thymic cyst extending from the anterior mediastinum on the right into the neck on the left of the photo.

and isthmusectomy are recommended for benign lesions in which cancer cannot be completely ruled out.

Other miscellaneous conditions may occur in the anterior neck, such as midline branchial (cervical) cleft, a linear tract of epithelialized tissue in the anterior midline of the neck that occurs because of aberrant fusion of the branchial arches (Fig. 17-9). In addition, mediastinal lesions such as thymic cyst may present as midline cervical masses (Fig. 17-10).

Branchial Cleft and Arch Anomalies

Cysts and Sinuses

Branchial cleft anomalies give rise to cysts and sinuses in the lateral triangle of the neck. Second branchial cleft anomalies are the most common and typically present as an opening along the lower anterior border of the sternocleidomastoid muscle. These sinuses have their origin in the tonsillar fossa and may travel between the carotid sheath to exit along the border of the sternocleidomastoid muscle. A complete fistula drains through a sinus opening (Fig. 17-11), whereas an incomplete fistula may present as a simple cystic structure in the subcutaneous tissue in the region (Fig. 17-12). Secondary infection of these lesions is common. Excision of the tract to the site of origin in the peritonsillar region prevents recurrence. Other branchial cleft and arch anomalies are less common (Fig. 17-13).

Fibromatosis coli, or fibrous dysplasia of the sternocleidomastoid muscle, is commonly seen in infants and young children (Fig. 17-14). These children present with a mass in the lower neck with tilting of the head and face to the side of the lesion (Fig. 17-15). Parents most often bring their infants in because they are concerned about the possibility of a malignant tumor, whereas older children may present with hemifacial hypoplasia and asymmetry. Early recognition of this condition in infancy and the institution of daily physical therapy may avert surgery and long-term cosmetic deformity. Plagiocephaly and facial asymmetry are the sequelae of untreated deformities.

Scalp and Face Lesions

Scalp

Hemangiomas are benign, congenital, vascular tumors that most frequently arise in the head and neck. These lesions are typically raised above the skin level and may be red or somewhat purple in color. They may blanch on contact. Often hemangiomas may not be present at birth but develop in the first few months of life. Rapid growth and expansion may occur, leading to platelet sequestration and coagulopathy,

Figure 17-9   Midline cervical cleft.

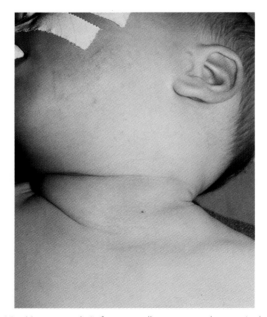

Figure 17-11   Mucus may drain from a small punctum at the anterior border of the sternocleidomastoid, identifying it as the secondary opening of a second branchial cleft fistula. The primary opening lies in the tonsillar fossa.

Figure 17-12 Cartilaginous remnants from the second branchial cleft present as a mobile cyst beneath the anterior border of the sternocleidomastoid **(A)**. In another patient the cyst was infected, producing redness of the overlying skin **(B)**.

known as the *Kasabach-Merritt syndrome*. This condition may be refractory to various medical maneuvers including steroids, radiation therapy, and chemotherapy. Despite significant growth in size during the first year of life, most hemangiomas have a benign course and undergo spontaneous resolution over the first 7 years of life (Fig. 17-16; and see Chapter 8). Surgical intervention is rarely necessary and should be reserved for those patients with impending airway compromise or periorbital involvement. Special consideration must be given to those patients with lesions extending toward the eye or impinging on the airway. Subsequent blindness or airway compromise may be the consequences if intervention is delayed.

Dermoid cysts are congenital lesions that are composed of sequestered hair, skin, and sebaceous structures that occur in areas of embryonic fusion. These lesions are most frequent in the head and neck, but they may arise in other midline sites including the sacral, perineal, and sternal region. They are typically located in the head and neck along the lateral palpebral fissure, occipital scalp, and midline of the neck. Scalp dermoids are often well circumscribed, firm, and fixed to underlying deep structures such as bone, typically arising from the outer bony table of the skull. Midline scalp or back dermoids may have intracranial or intraspinal extension, respectively. They should always be evaluated by MRI before surgical intervention. Dural or central nervous system extension mandates neurosurgical consultation before resection. Treatment for these conditions is surgical (Fig. 17-17).

Face

Several benign remnants of congenital structures may persist at birth, and they raise numerous management considerations. Preauricular skin tags are vestigial cartilaginous remnants that

are removed primarily for cosmetic reasons. In contrast, preauricular pits or sinuses are prone to infectious complications. These anomalies represent epidermal inclusion structures that are related to the embryologic formation of the ear. The sinus may be lined by pilosebaceous structures and exude a sebaceous-like fluid. Complete surgical excision of the sinus and subcutaneous cystic elements is curative. Because most of these lesions are asymptomatic, routine excision should be reserved for those patients who have had infectious complications.

Surgically significant salivary gland pathology is uncommon in the pediatric population. Hemangiomas are the most common benign lesions of the parotid gland in children. As with hemangiomas in other sites, these may not be entirely visualized at birth and may occur over the first few months of life. A small cutaneous birthmark may be the only initial presentation. Rapid growth and significant asymmetry may become apparent (Fig. 17-18). Fortunately, these lesions spontaneously involute with time. In the absence of early complications, surgery, sclerotherapy, or intralesional injection techniques should be reserved until the period after involution. Other causes of parotid enlargement in children include viral (mumps), bacterial (staphylococcal), and mycobacterial (atypical mycobacterial infection or tuberculosis) infections, as well as chronic inflammatory conditions. Treatment specific to these conditions is indicated.

Various intraoral lesions may arise that have surgical significance primarily because of their effects on swallowing, speech, and breathing. Tongue-tie (ankyloglossia inferior) occurs commonly in infancy, usually resolving spontaneously. Some cases persist, and these children may have impaired speech development. Usually a thin membranous structure,

Figure 17-13 First branchial arch fistula, previously diagnosed as an infected lymph node. The location of the secondary opening is near the angle of the mandible.

Figure 17-14 The sternocleidomastoid in a newborn with torticollis may exist as a tight tendon-like cord or may swell and appear as a discrete tumor in the midportion of the muscle, pictured here.

Figure 17-16   Involuting parotid and neck hemangioma. Note the grayish discoloration indicative of resolution.

Figure 17-15   Long-standing torticollis may cause permanent "wry-neck," facial shortening of the affected side of the face, and plagiocephaly.

the frenulum, regresses with feeding. A persistent frenulum may impair speech and feeding. Simple division is therapeutic. Similarly, ranulas may form as pseudocysts in the floor of the mouth. Some spontaneously resolve, whereas a few may become quite large and impair lingual mobility, feeding, speech, and most significantly, breathing. Marsupialization or complete excision is curative (Fig. 17-19).

Lymphangiomas of the floor of the mouth may pose especially challenging management problems (Fig. 17-20). These lesions may cause significant macroglossia that obstructs the airway, requiring tracheostomy. Small vesicular lesions may occur on the lingual surface and exude fluid that may become purulent. Suppurative glossitis may require systemic antibiotic therapy. In addition to airway complications, problems with speech development and mandibular growth may occur. Some authors have proposed partial glossectomy as a therapy. More recent therapies for large intraoral and cervical lymphangiomas extending to the floor of the mouth involve sclerosant injection (hypertonic saline, alcohol, or OK-432) to avoid the morbidity and disfigurement associated with surgery in these areas.

Lingual thyroid is a rare developmental anomaly of the thyroid. Congenital failure of thyroid descent results in

persistence of thyroid tissue at the base of the foramen cecum, giving rise to this problem. At birth infants may present with acute airway obstruction, whereas older children may describe feeling a lump in the throat with swallowing. This condition is often associated with hypothyroidism. Transoral excision requires permanent thyroid replacement because these lesions typically represent the only functioning thyroid tissue in these children.

CHEST

Introduction

Neonatal respiratory distress is rarely of surgical origin. Although medically related conditions such as transient tachypnea of the newborn (TTN) and pneumonia may cause significant symptoms, severe dyspnea, hoarseness, or stridor requires urgent assessment and possible surgical intervention. These latter symptoms should alert the practitioner to the possibility of a problem requiring surgical attention. If the plain radiographs rule out pneumothorax, atelectasis, and pneumonia, the differential diagnosis of these conditions may include proximal obstructive airway lesions, intrathoracic masses, lung bud anomalies (bronchopulmonary foregut malformations), or abdominal masses. For example, infants with a lung bud anomaly such as a cystic pulmonary adenomatoid

Figure 17-17   **A,** Midline scalp dermoid cysts may have intracranial extension and should always be evaluated by MRI before surgery. **B,** The dermoid in this 2-year-old child extends to but not through the dura.

Figure 17-18 Facial hemangioma covering the eye requires medical intervention with prednisone or possibly with propranolol to hasten resolution and avoid loss of sight from amblyopia.

malformation (CPAM) or congenital lobar emphysema (CLE) or, alternatively, an infant with a diaphragmatic hernia may present in a similar manner. Second, a newborn who fails to respond to standard therapy for a presumed pulmonary disorder should be evaluated for a potential surgical etiology. Examples include a premature newborn with tracheoesophageal fistula and esophageal atresia or a neonate being treated for group B streptococcal sepsis who also has a right-sided diaphragmatic hernia.

The clinical evaluation of these patients should include both anteroposterior (AP) and lateral radiographs of the chest. Particular focus should be directed to the soft tissue views of the neck, mediastinum, and airway contour. Fluoroscopic examination provides critical insight into the airway contour and diaphragmatic mobility throughout the respiratory cycle. Esophagogram with either barium or water-soluble contrast may be useful to delineate a vascular ring or mediastinal mass (Fig. 17-21). More invasive studies such as upper airway and esophageal endoscopy may be necessary to elucidate other surgical causes of respiratory distress. Surgical causes of respiratory distress may be subclassified into three major categories: upper airway, intrathoracic, and extrathoracic.

Figure 17-20 **A,** Cervical cystic hygroma. **B,** MRI demonstrates its juxtaposition to the airway structures and vessels in the neck. Acute enlargement at birth secondary to hemorrhage may lead to airway compression.

Upper Airway

The inability of the neonate to breathe orally at birth raises the possibility that an upper airway obstructive lesion may be the source of respiratory distress in this patient population. The newborn infant who is unable to nurse or who has paroxysmal asphyxia (cyclic dyspnea) should undergo a thorough airway and cardiopulmonary evaluation. Lesions involving the upper airway create a characteristic "air hunger" that may

progress to respiratory failure in the neonate. The respiratory difficulties are most marked during the expiratory phase of the cycle, when the airway tends to collapse around the lesion. These infants may be asymptomatic during the inspiratory component of the respiratory cycle, when the airway reaches its greatest diameter. The differential diagnosis for these symptoms should include choanal atresia, esophageal atresia, tracheoesophageal fistula, vocal cord paralysis, nasopharyngeal tumors, oropharyngeal masses, and foreign bodies.

The initial evaluation of infants with presumed airway obstruction should include the passage of a nasogastric tube. Signs of pharyngeal obstruction suggest choanal atresia. This obstruction may be membranous (90%) or bony (10%). Half of these patients may have other forms of associated craniofacial or remote congenital anomalies that require concurrent evaluation and management. Nasopharyngoscopy is diagnostic in most cases. The oral airway must be maintained, and the baby must be fed via gavage feedings until transpalatal repair. Oropharyngeal obstruction may be caused by macroglossia or jaw bony abnormalities. Beckwith-Wiedemann syndrome is associated with lingual hypertrophy and gigantism (Fig. 17-22). Presentation in the newborn should alert the practitioner to the possibility of hypoglycemia secondary to hyperinsulinism. Permanent neurologic sequelae may result from diagnostic delay. Sublingual or lingual lymphangiomas may be associated with massive macroglossia that leads to airway distress. The hypoplastic and recessed mandible associated with Pierre Robin syndrome may cause a normal-sized tongue to fall posteriorly and obstruct the airway (Fig. 17-23).

Figure 17-19 A ranula arises in the floor of the mouth, caused by congenital obstruction of the sublingual duct.

Figure 17-21 Midthoracic compressions into the esophageal barium column identify the presence of vascular ring anomalies (in this case, pulmonary artery sling).

The association of cleft palate and cardiac defects with Pierre Robin syndrome may further exacerbate respiratory distress. Prone positioning of the infant may assist breathing and avert the need for tracheostomy. Alternatively, tracheostomy placement may provide a safer temporizing measure to allow adequate mandibular growth and development and to prevent

Figure 17-22 Beckwith-Wiedemann syndrome. Note hemihypertrophy on the left side, along with the prominence of the tongue. *(Courtesy D. Becker, MD, Pittsburgh, Pa.)*

Figure 17-23 In Pierre Robin sequence, the hypoplastic mandible positions the tongue posteriorly, potentially obstructing the upper airway.

obstruction. Newer techniques of mandibular distraction may avoid the need for prophylactic tracheostomy.

Laryngeal lesions distinctively present with hoarseness, faint crying, or complete aphonia in association with dyspnea. The differential diagnosis for these patients includes laryngomalacia, laryngeal atresia, laryngeal webs, laryngeal clefts, subglottic stenosis, and vocal cord paralysis. Emergency tracheostomy is often indicated in these patients because of the inability to secure an airway, as occurs in laryngeal atresia. Direct airway contamination may occur with feeding in patients with laryngeal clefts because of the communication between the pharynx and the posterior laryngeal defect.

Pharyngeal masses may be another source of upper airway obstruction. These masses include branchial cleft remnants, dermoids, pharyngeal duplications, hemangiomas, lymphangiomas, lingual thyroids, sublingual teratomas, and Zenker diverticula. Large cervical masses such as a cystic hygroma (lymphangioma) (Fig. 17-24) and cervical teratoma (Fig. 17-25) may induce airway compression and cause dyspnea. Antenatal diagnosis of the lesions may indicate a potential airway emergency. The ex utero intrapartum treatment (EXIT) procedure allows time to secure airway control before division of the umbilical cord (Fig. 17-26).

Mediastinum and Diaphragm

Mediastinal masses are uncommon in the pediatric population. The limited space of the thoracic cavity predisposes normal structures to be compressed by space-occupying lesions. Masses in this anatomic region may lead to numerous

Figure 17-24 Large cervical masses like this cervical teratoma diagnosed by antenatal ultrasonography cause prenatal esophageal compression and polyhydramnios. Because of the high risk of upper airway compression at delivery, an ex utero intrapartum treatment (EXIT) procedure is indicated to avoid infant death.

Figure 17-25 **A,** Cervical teratoma at delivery presents airway challenges **(B)** in the perinatal period.

symptoms including cough, dysphagia, dyspnea, and rarely, superior vena cava syndrome. The mediastinal location and the patient's age provide the most critical insight into the diagnosis. The mediastinum may be divided into three major compartments: anterior–superior, middle, and posterior. The location of a mass in any one of these compartments is an important diagnostic feature (Table 17-2). The anatomic boundaries for these compartments include the sternum to the anterior aspect of the trachea and pericardium (anterior); the trachea, major bronchi, and paratracheal structures (middle); and the posterior aspect of the trachea to the spine (posterior). Anterior mediastinal masses typically arise in tissues of thyroid or thymus, and are lymphoid or teratomatous in origin (Fig. 17-27). Middle mediastinal masses are typically tumors or congenital anomalies arising from the tracheobronchial tree, lymph nodes, esophagus, or pulmonary parenchyma. Posterior mediastinal masses are primarily neurogenic tumors or congenital enterogenous lesions (Fig. 17-28).

Esophageal atresia with or without tracheoesophageal fistula is a common cause of airway obstruction. The inability to pass a Replogle (nasogastric) tube into the stomach clarifies this diagnosis. This tube also serves as a sump catheter to drain the proximal pouch and to limit upper airway contamination associated with this anomaly. Infants develop respiratory distress secondary to esophageal obstruction and the tracheoesophageal communication. Neonates with esophageal atresia characteristically have excessive salivation and coughing due to the pooling of secretions in the proximal pharyngeal pouch. Most patients are diagnosed by their inability to tolerate their initial feedings. The diagnosis of congenital esophageal obstruction secondary to esophageal atresia is frequently made on antenatal ultrasonography by the presence of

microgastria, polyhydramnios, and frequent fetal hiccups. Although several major variants of this condition exist, the most common, a blind proximal pouch with a distal tracheoesophageal fistula, occurs in approximately 85% of all patients. Inspired air from the trachea communicates directly to the stomach via a fistulous connection (Fig. 17-29). This leads to gastric distention and retrograde gastroesophageal reflux into the lungs, precipitating respiratory distress. Positive-pressure ventilation by either mask or endotracheal tube should be avoided in these patients before surgery because of the risk of gastric distention and perforation, severe retrograde reflux, and pneumonia (Fig. 17-30). The second most common variant of this condition is pure esophageal atresia, which on plain radiography shows a dilated proximal pouch and a gasless abdomen (Fig. 17-31). On physical examination these infants have a scaphoid abdomen due to the lack of distal air passage into the bowels (Fig. 17-32). Isolated tracheoesophageal fistula without esophageal atresia is the third most common form of this anomaly. These children lack esophageal obstruction and may at times be diagnosed at later ages with symptoms of persistent cough or recurrent pneumonia. Although called an H-fistula, the appearance is more N-shaped with a more proximal communication with the trachea and distal communication into the esophagus. The diagnosis of this variant is made more challenging because of this acute angle of communication between the esophagus and trachea, which inhibits reflux of orogastric contents into the airway (Fig. 17-33).

Congenital diaphragmatic hernia is a common cause of respiratory distress in newborns, occurring with an incidence of approximately 1 in every 4000 live births. Defects in the diaphragm may result either from abnormal fusion of the posterolateral pleuroperitoneal membrane (foramen of Bochdalek) or from defects in formation of the central diaphragmatic muscle (foramen of Morgagni hernia). Diffuse muscular weakness may give rise to diaphragmatic eventration

Figure 17-26 Ex utero intrapartum treatment (EXIT) procedure.

Table 17-2	Mediastinal Masses in Childhood	
Anterior–Superior	**Middle**	**Posterior**
Teratoma including dermoid cyst	Bronchogenic cyst	Neurogenic tumor
Normal thymus	Pericardial cyst	Enterogenous cyst
Lymphoma		Pulmonary sequestration
Vascular malformation		
Thymic cyst		
Cystic hygroma		
Intrathoracic goiter		

Figure 17-27   **A,** A large mediastinal thymic tumor seen on chest radiograph may induce dyspnea, orthopnea, and other pulmonary symptoms. **B,** CT scan demonstrating the anterior mediastinal thymic tumor.

or postcardiac surgical or birth injury to the phrenic nerve. Congenital diaphragmatic abnormalities of the foramen of Bochdalek are the most common form of lesion and are typically left sided in 85% of patients (Fig. 17-34). These defects occur early in gestation, allowing abdominal contents to herniate into the chest. This limits lung expansion and growth, displacing the heart, resulting in pulmonary hypoplasia and persistent pulmonary hypertension. Many of these infants have severe respiratory distress occurring shortly after umbilical cord division. On physical examination there is marked nasal flaring, chest wall asymmetry (larger contralateral hemithorax secondary to lung hyperplasia), displaced heart tones to the side opposite the hernia, and ipsilateral absence of breath sounds with dullness to percussion due to the presence of abdominal viscera in that hemithorax. Plain chest radiography demonstrates intestinal loops within the hemithorax displacing the cardiomediastinal silhouette to the opposite side. Infants with foramen of Bochdalek congenital diaphragmatic hernias have severe respiratory failure secondary to both pulmonary hypoplasia and pulmonary hypertension. Despite aggressive therapy with nitric oxide, high-frequency

oscillatory ventilation, and extracorporeal membrane oxygenation (ECMO), mortality remains approximately 50% (Fig. 17-35).

Diaphragmatic eventration may have a radiographic appearance similar to that of diaphragmatic hernia but usually lacks acute neonatal presentation. Foramen of Morgagni diaphragmatic hernias represent less than 5% of all diaphragmatic hernias. Often they are incidental findings seen on routine radiography obtained for other reasons (typically a cough). Morgagni hernias typically have a sac, which may include the transverse colon, liver, or small bowel (Fig. 17-36). Intestinal incarceration is a rare complication. Cystic pulmonary adenomatoid malformations may be confused with diaphragmatic hernia on plain films and are usually distinguished by the location of the gastric air bubble (Fig. 17-37).

Vascular ring anomalies may be a source of tracheoesophageal compression giving rise to varying degrees of dyspnea or dysphagia. These anomalies originate from persistence of the embryonic aortic arches. Plain film findings demonstrating narrowing of the mediastinal portion of the tracheal air contour suggest the presence of a vascular ring. The diagnosis may be

Figure 17-28   Posterior mediastinal masses include esophageal duplication (illustrated here during left thoracoscopy), neurenteric cysts, extralobar sequestration, anterior myelomeningocele, and neural tumors. Vertebral anomalies coexist frequently.

Figure 17-29   Bronchoscopy visualizes a tracheoesophageal fistula, seen as a posteriorly positioned orifice *(bottom)* in the upper trachea. The carina, seen toward the top of the picture, lies distally.

Figure 17-32 Pure esophageal atresia without distal tracheoesophageal fistula. Esophageal obstruction associated with scaphoid abdomen on physical examination is pathognomonic of pure esophageal atresia.

Figure 17-30 Tracheoesophageal fistula allows air to be forced into the stomach during positive-pressure ventilation by bag and mask or through an endotracheal tube. The stomach may perforate as shown in this patient with a pneumoperitoneum, or ventilation may become suddenly ineffective if a gastrotomy is placed initially during surgical repair.

confirmed by nuclear magnetic resonance imaging (MRI), contrast barium swallow, or endoscopic evaluation of the airway. MRI has replaced aortography for delineating the associated vascular anatomy (Fig. 17-38).

Lung

Lung Bud Anomalies (Bronchopulmonary Foregut Malformations)

Lung bud anomalies (bronchopulmonary foregut malformations) are cystic lung lesions that may induce severe respiratory distress by direct compression of adjacent normal lung tissue. Acute expansion, which may often occur at the time of delivery, may require emergency surgical intervention or the use of high-frequency oscillatory ventilation. This ventilation technique serves as a temporizing means as the infant is prepared for surgery. Congenital cystic anomalies of the lung are the most common cause of respiratory distress in infants and children requiring surgical intervention. These bronchopulmonary foregut malformations have their origin during the early stages of fetal development, between the 3rd and 16th

weeks of gestation. Thus, many of these lesions may be discovered on routine prenatal ultrasound. Progressive enlargement during the first few months of life may lead to acute respiratory distress secondary to compression of normal lung tissue. Smaller or more slowly growing lesions may have a paucity of symptoms. They may go undetected for long periods, before diagnosis by routine chest radiography for infection, dyspnea, or tachypnea. In otherwise normal infants, persistent cough, recurrent bouts of pneumonia, and paroxysmal dyspnea should prompt the primary care practitioner to investigate the diagnostic possibility of an occult congenital cystic lung lesion by plain chest radiography or CT.

Four major bronchopulmonary foregut malformations exist: congenital lobar emphysema (CLE), congenital pulmonary adenomatoid malformation (CPAM), pulmonary sequestration, and bronchogenic cyst. The most common of these, CPAM, results from the proliferation of primordial bronchial structures in the absence of alveoli. CPAMs are subclassified as one of three variants on the basis of their size, shape, and pathologic appearance. Type I CPAM comprises single or multiple cysts greater than 2 cm in diameter and lined with ciliated pseudostratified columnar epithelium. Type I lesions may be difficult to distinguish from diaphragmatic hernias (Fig. 17-39). Type II lesions are small cysts, less than 1 cm in diameter, and lined with cuboidal to columnar epithelium. These lesions are associated with a broad spectrum of congenital anomalies. Type III CPAMs are large benign cysts lined with ciliated cuboidal epithelium or solid masses. These are often fatal and have a high incidence of associated anomalies.

Congenital lobar emphysema is a condition that results from a segment of poorly developed or absent cartilage in the

Figure 17-31 A dilated blind proximal esophageal pouch **(A)** and a gasless abdomen **(B)** are the radiographic hallmarks of pure esophageal atresia.

Figure 17-33 Isolated tracheoesophageal fistula (H-type) as seen here is typically accessed via a cervical approach. The patient's chin is to the left. Blue loops are around the esophagus with the fistula seen as a tubular structure immediately to the left of the esophagus.

Figure 17-34 Congenital diaphragmatic hernia allows intestines to enter the chest in utero.

Figure 17-35 Autopsy specimen of a diaphragmatic hernia illustrates the right lung compression, cardiomediastinal shift, left lung hypoplasia, and visceral herniation through the diaphragmatic defect.

Figure 17-36 A foramen of Morgagni hernia, seen here by laparoscopy as a central tendinous defect in the diaphragm, typically does not present as acute pulmonary distress in the newborn.

Figure 17-37 Macrocystic adenomatoid malformation of the left lung. Large cystic lesions can be mistaken for bowel loops herniating through a diaphragmatic hernia.

Figure 17-38 Posterior view of a three-dimensional reconstruction of an axial MRI scan of a right aortic arch with an anomalous left subclavian artery. Note the close proximity of the anomalous subclavian artery to the esophagus and its potential obstruction of the esophagus. ES, esophagus (yellow); DAo, descending aorta (red); DIV, diverticulum; LSCA and RSCA, left and right subclavian artery, respectively (red); RAA, right aortic arch (red); TR, trachea (white). (*Courtesy Beverly Newman, MD, Children's Hospital of Pittsburgh, Pittsburgh, Pa.*)

Figure 17-39 Macrocystic adenomatoid malformation seen on plain film **(A),** CT scan **(B),** and surgical specimen **(C).**

tracheobronchial tree and leads to lung hyperexpansion secondary to a "check valve effect" and air trapping. Subsequent lung overdistention may lead to respiratory distress, pneumonia, and mediastinal shift. Many of these patients present with symptomatic lesions in the first few weeks of life; however, other patients have a more indolent progression of symptoms over the first 6 months of life. Other patients may remain entirely asymptomatic. The plain radiographic appearance of these patients demonstrates lung hyperlucency and hyperexpansion in the upper or middle lobes (Fig. 17-40). Acute cardiopulmonary decompensation may occur in otherwise healthy patients with this anomaly, due to positive-pressure ventilation such as that which might occur at the time of the induction of general anesthesia for surgery (Fig. 17-41).

Primary pulmonary blastoma is a stromal malignancy of the lung that may present with unilateral hyperinflation, mimicking and possibly confused with lobar emphysema (Fig. 17-42). Pulmonary sequestrations are accessory pulmonary parenchymal tissue that lack direct tracheobronchial communication. These anomalies receive their blood supply from the systemic circulation. They may arise from within the pulmonary parenchyma (intralobar) (Fig. 17-43) or reside separately from normal lung tissue (extralobar) (Fig. 17-44). Although commonly found in the left costophrenic sulcus, sequestrations may be located in either hemithorax or in the abdomen. They may also communicate with other foregut structures in the gastrointestinal tract owing to their shared embryonic origin. Usually asymptomatic and found on routine chest x-ray

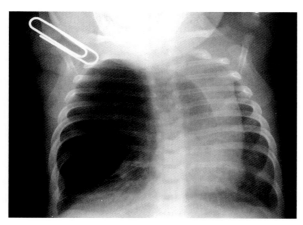

Figure 17-40 Lobar emphysema, usually involving the upper lobes, may become hugely distended and may cause life-threatening respiratory distress.

Figure 17-41 Lobar emphysema may acutely expand with positive-pressure ventilation seen at the time of anesthesia induction. Hyperexpansion of the lobe is clearly apparent at thoracotomy, when lung parenchyma "balloons" into the field.

Figure 17-42   A, Clinical examination of an infant with primary pulmonary blastoma with thoracic asymmetry and hyperinflation. **B,** Anteroposterior chest radiograph demonstrating the unilateral hyperinflation of the left lung and mediastinal shift to the right. **C,** CT scan of the chest showing the pulmonary hyperinflation and tumor mass. **D,** Intraoperative tumor.

or noted as an incidental finding during another thoracic procedure, these lesions may be a source of recurrent intrathoracic infection and should undergo elective resection. Duplex ultrasonography or, more commonly, CT or MRI evaluation may be used in the diagnostic assessment to demonstrate systemic arterial blood supply (Fig. 17-45).

Pneumothorax may occur as a result of thoracic trauma, cystic fibrosis, or spontaneously (Fig. 17-46). Patients may develop acute severe pleuritic chest pain and associated dyspnea. Physical examination findings may demonstrate hyperresonance and diminished breath sounds over the ipsilateral hemithorax. Mediastinal shift, jugular venous distention, hypotension, and diaphragmatic flattening may result from the development of a tension pneumothorax. This requires emergency life-saving needle decompression followed by thoracostomy tube placement. A subpopulation of young patients, usually male and asthenic in build, may present with acute spontaneous pneumothorax. Spontaneous pneumothorax is typically secondary to apical bullous lung disease (Fig. 17-47). The etiology of this condition is unknown. These patients usually require chest decompression by thoracostomy tube placement. Recurrent episodes of spontaneous pneumothorax are an indication for surgical exploration with resection of the apical bullae and either mechanical or chemical pleurodesis.

On occasion, surgical intervention may be necessary in the treatment of pulmonary infections that persist despite aggressive antibiotic therapy (Fig. 17-48). The development of an intrathoracic empyema as a sequela of streptococcal or staphylococcal pneumonia may restrict lung expansion. Surgical intervention may provide the means of diagnosis and the ability to rule out bronchial foreign body obstruction (Fig. 17-49); the capacity to assess for evidence of malignancy; or allow treatment through providing adequate drainage or mechanical pleural clearance. In addition, surgery may provide a means of treatment of chest lesions that may have become secondarily infected (Fig. 17-50). Thoracoscopy with video-assisted thoracic decortication may hasten recovery from pneumonia and these parapneumonic consequences. More recent experience supports the use of chest tube drainage with instillation of fibrolytic therapy (urokinase or tissue plasminogen activator) in the treatment of pediatric empyema.

CHEST WALL

Pectus excavatum ("funnel chest") is the most common congenital chest wall deformity (Fig. 17-51). This condition is characterized by the posterior angulation of the sternum toward the spine and abnormalities of the costal cartilages. Pectus excavatum has a 3 : 1 male predominance. Although

Figure 17-43   Persistent infiltration of the lung parenchyma may indicate an intralobar sequestration, shown here involving the right lower lobe. Also shown is a right diaphragmatic hernia, a frequently associated malformation.

Figure 17-45   Extralobar sequestrations are characterized by the presence of pulmonary parenchyma that lacks tracheobronchial communication and has a systemic blood supply. Angiogram shows systemic blood supply. MRI has supplanted this technique.

Figure 17-44   Thoracoscopic view of an extralobar pulmonary sequestration **(A)**. Thoracoscopic view shows the ligated vessels penetrating the posterior sulcus of the diaphragm **(B)**. Resected extralobar sequestration removed through an enlarged port site **(C)**.

Figure 17-46   This chest film shows typical radiologic signs of tension pneumothorax: mediastinal shift, flattening of the diaphragm, and widening of the intercostal spaces.

often not impressive during infancy, this deformity increases during childhood and adolescence. This chest wall malformation typically causes no cardiopulmonary symptoms or disability. However, there is a subset of patients who will have exercise intolerance, mitral valve prolapse, or gastroesophageal reflux that may be attributable to this deformity. Some debate exists as to the relationship of these symptoms to the defect. Although the psychological implications of this deformity in teenagers relative to their self-esteem may seem to be a more compelling indication for surgical repair, there is evidence that in active patients, improved stamina is achieved after repair of severe pectus excavatum chest wall deformities. A minimally invasive technique, the Nuss procedure, has

Figure 17-47   Thoracoscopic view of apical bullous lung disease. These bullae or blebs may rupture and give rise to spontaneous pneumothorax.

Figure 17-48   Chest film of a child with allergic bronchopulmonary aspergillosis of the right upper lobe, which ultimately required resection.

made the repair of pectus excavatum more appealing to many patients and their families.

Pectus carinatum ("pigeon chest") is a protrusion deformity of the chest wall (Fig. 17-52). This condition represents a spectrum of sternal and midchest anomalies that may give rise to this malformation. Pectus carinatum occurs more commonly in males than females and is usually asymptomatic. Surgical correction of carinatum deformities has been replaced almost completely by nonsurgical chest bracing or compression devices, which are custom fitted and worn by patients for various time periods. Marfan syndrome must be considered in pectus carinatum or pectus excavatum deformities. The coexistence of other conditions such as aortic root abnormalities and ocular lens subluxation should be evaluated in these patients. Poland syndrome is a rare chest wall deformity that consists of a constellation of abnormalities including unilateral agenesis or dysplasia of the rib cage and chondral cartilages, absence of pectoralis major and minor muscles, hand deformities, and breast and areolar defects (Fig. 17-53). Other chest wall deformities include sternal cleft and pentalogy of Cantrell, discussed later (see Abdominal Wall Defects). Ectopia cordis is often complicated by the presence of severe congenital heart disease.

Axilla

Axillary lesions are most often lymphatic in origin. Benign reactive lymphadenopathy secondary to viral or bacterial infections is the most common neck mass. Cystic hygromas or lymphangiomas, also common in the lateral neck, may frequently appear in the axilla. These lesions may exist in continuity with cervical lesions or, more importantly, extend into the mediastinum. Plain chest films or CT scan imaging (preferred) may aid in delineating the anatomy. Hidradenitis, a condition related to the obstruction of sebaceous and sweat glands, commonly presents as an axillary mass that may become superinfected and require surgical drainage.

Breast

Mastitis is a common breast problem of infancy. The evolution of fluctuance or purulence is diagnostic of a breast abscess (see Chapter 12). The presence of this condition requires aggressive antibiotic therapy (sometimes intravenous) and warm compresses. Antibiotics with broad staphylococcal and streptococcal coverage are usually adequate; however, in some cases the addition of gram-negative coverage is necessary.

Figure 17-49 Signs of a radiolucent foreign body are often subtle. Persistent overdistention of the right lung during expiration **(A)** was due to right mainstem bronchial occlusion. Less marked changes are seen during inhalation **(B)**.

Figure 17-50 Large infected bronchogenic cyst in a teenager **(A)** who responded to aggressive antibiotic therapy **(B** and **C)**, and surgical resection **(D)**.

Figure 17-51   Pectus excavatum (funnel chest) seldom creates cardiorespiratory symptoms, but psychological consequences may be severe.

Figure 17-53   Congenital unilateral absence of the anterior ribs, muscle, and soft tissues characterize Poland syndrome, producing its typical appearance pictured here.

Figure 17-52   A, The sternum projects like a keel in front of the anterior chest wall in pectus carinatum (pigeon chest). Like pectus excavatum, pectus carinatum produces no symptoms. **B,** Lateral view of a pectus carinatum.

Restraint relative to invasive procedures, particularly incision, drainage, and debridement, should be maintained to allow spontaneous resolution with medical therapies. Damage to the breast bud may lead to permanent breast asymmetry and deformity in the future. Needle aspiration may be judiciously performed when there is significant concern about the possibility of pus. True abscess formation requires incision and drainage, and families should be warned of the potential long-term ramifications.

Localized breast masses in children are typically benign. In the preadolescent, as early as 6 or 7 years, the development of a firm mobile mass under one areola or both areolae may represent precocious thelarche. This condition may be asynchronous with a pseudotumor appearing several months ahead of the opposite side. Biopsy is never indicated in this scenario because unilateral iatrogenic amastia will result. In adolescents and teenagers, fibroadenomas account for approximately 90% of the reported masses. These smooth and mobile masses are approximately 1 to 2 cm in size. The juvenile variant of this condition may be associated with much larger lesions that cause significant breast asymmetry. The malignant potential of these lesions is low; however, excision is strongly recommended because these lesions do not spontaneously regress. Cosmetic periareolar incisions should be used to excise these tumors. Fibrocystic disease, occurring primarily in older teens and young women, is a breast condition associated with one or more firm, fixed, and ill-defined masses. These masses result from hyperplasia of the fibrous parenchymal tissue of the breast. Variation in the associated symptoms and even the size of these lesions with the phases of the menstrual cycle is a distinctive feature of fibrocystic disease, which is a benign condition. Breast malignancies are rare in the pediatric population. Phyllodes tumors, formerly cystosarcoma phyllodes, are rare fibroepithelial tumors that may be benign but with aggressive local behavior leading to malignancy with a propensity for distant metastases. These tumors may be associated with significant asymmetrical gynecomastia and reach up to 40 cm in size. Surgical evaluation should be sought out early. Routine monthly breast self-examination should be encouraged at puberty in all girls to aid in the detection of significant disease and to avoid undue intervention for benign conditions.

GASTROINTESTINAL

Gastrointestinal Obstruction

Vomiting is the reflex-coordinated response of various stimuli to the central nervous system, resulting in relaxation of the lower esophageal sphincter, increased gastric peristalsis, increased diaphragmatic contractions, and forceful expulsion of gastrointestinal contents. Vomiting is the primary presenting symptom of children with a wide range of conditions from benign responses to minor infectious diseases to the primary manifestation of life-threatening intraabdominal disease. Although the vast majority of children who have this complaint do not have an obstructive lesion, vomiting is the principal symptom of major gastrointestinal obstructive diseases. Distinguishing between self-limited or medical conditions and those that require urgent surgical intervention may be challenging.

The first stage in the assessment is the differentiation of vomiting and regurgitation. Vomiting is the forceful expulsion of gastrointestinal contents, whereas regurgitation is the passive expulsion of enteric contents. The surgical causes of vomiting are typically extrinsic (serosal) inflammatory conditions or intrinsic (mucosal/structural) mechanical lesions. Diagnosis and management are best defined by the patient's age and level of gastrointestinal obstruction. Vomiting associated with fever, abdominal pain, and abdominal tenderness is highly suggestive of peritoneal irritation seen in conditions such as appendicitis. The presence of bilious emesis with or without abdominal distention should raise concern for a mechanical obstruction.

Bilious emesis is a critical finding in the pediatric population. Its presence should always raise a red flag in the evaluation of a vomiting child, especially the newborn or infant. The principal condition of concern is malrotation with midgut volvulus. This typically presents without abdominal distention because the level of obstruction is at or near the ligament of Treitz. Bilious emesis with associated abdominal distention is more characteristic of distal small bowel or colonic obstruction seen in conditions such as intestinal atresias, meconium disease, incarcerated hernias, or Hirschsprung disease. The presence of blood in the stool suggests an associated ischemic process as seen in midgut volvulus, necrotizing enterocolitis (NEC), internal hernia, or intussusception. Finally, the infant or child with a previous history of abdominal surgery, abdominal surgical scars, or abdominal trauma should be suspected of having adhesive small bowel obstruction.

Radiographic evaluation including AP and left lateral decubitus films of the abdomen is often sufficient to generate an adequate differential diagnosis. These studies help identify the presence of dilated bowel loops and/or intraperitoneal free air. In neonates, several common obstructive lesions such as esophageal atresia, pyloric atresia, and duodenal atresia may show no distention. Adjunctive techniques of gastric tube placement and air instillation may provide an air-contrast upper gastrointestinal study in infants with proximal obstructions in whom water-soluble or barium contrast instillation could be hazardous or are contraindicated because of aspiration risks. Upper gastrointestinal contrast evaluation is indicated to rule out malrotation with midgut volvulus in those patients in whom the suspected level of obstruction is in the mid-duodenum or more distal. The presence of scattered abdominal calcifications in the newborn or a calcified pseudocyst indicates in utero bowel perforation and meconium peritonitis (Fig. 17-54).

Distal gastrointestinal obstructions in the newborn period are most indicative of Hirschsprung disease. Before rectal manipulation or examination, these children should undergo a contrast enema. Barium is the preferred contrast medium because of its greater density and improved retention. This is useful for delineating the transition zone on the initial images and retention of material on the postevacuation films. If the transition zone—the region of the bowel where there is a caliber change between proximally dilated and distally decompressed bowel—is not visualized, then consideration should

Figure 17-54 Calcification in an area of meconium peritonitis in the right iliac fossa.

be given to other conditions such as distal ileal atresia, small left colon syndrome, or meconium ileus. Water-soluble contrast may be useful in the latter two conditions by loosening the intraluminal concretions associated with these entities. Meconium ileus is characterized by distal ileal narrowing and obstruction in association with inspissated meconium plugs ("rabbit pellets") and thick putty-like meconium in the more proximal ileum or bowel (Fig. 17-55). Contrast enema may be both diagnostic and therapeutic. Delayed abdominal radiographs in patients suspected of distal bowel obstructions may provide evidence for Hirschsprung disease (particularly at 24 hours postevacuation).

The various causes of gastrointestinal obstruction requiring surgery are organized by age and the level of obstruction. These have been subdivided into two age categories: neonates

Figure 17-55 This plain film shows two signs indicative of meconium ileus: a "soap bubble" mass in the right iliac fossa, produced by the impacted meconium, and distended loops of different diameters, reflecting the gradual distention of the small bowel to the area of obstruction.

and infants to cover the first year of life and toddlers and older children.

Neonates and Infants

A systematic manner by which to subdivide the causes of vomiting is to categorize those with etiologies involving the proximal gastrointestinal tract and those involving the distal gastrointestinal tract.

Nonbilious Emesis

The most common cause of nonbilious emesis in neonates and infants is overfeeding. Gastroesophageal reflux is the second most common cause of vomiting in this group. This condition is associated with the immaturity of the lower esophageal sphincter mechanisms and delayed motility of the gastrointestinal tract. Age-related maturation of these sites leads to complete resolution of this process by 1 year of age in most children. Behaviors related to feeding including overfeeding, too-rapid feeding, inadequate burping, and infant overstimulation may exacerbate the symptoms.

Some patients develop reflux complications related to esophageal or extraesophageal symptoms. These symptoms include pain, bleeding, dysphagia, and failure to thrive secondary to esophagitis. Recurrent pneumonias, otitis media, hoarseness, respiratory distress, and apneic spells may also be related to reflux. Several studies are useful for diagnostic confirmation. Barium swallow with upper gastrointestinal series is quite useful for delineating the anatomy of the esophagus and stomach. It demonstrates pyloric stenosis, malrotation, and the presence of any webs, membranes, or stenoses in these structures. Although this study may show evidence of reflux, it is not a reliable means for the primary diagnosis of reflux (Fig. 17-56). The best methods for diagnosing reflux are esophageal pH probe testing or esophagoscopy with mucosal biopsy. Esophageal pH probe testing is usually performed as an overnight study with a nasoesophageal probe and monitor, which records the frequency and duration of reflux episodes. Distal esophageal mucosal biopsy may represent a more precise diagnostic criterion for clinically significant reflux and may better stratify those patients who would benefit from more aggressive therapies. Liquid-phase gastric radionuclide scintigraphy ("milk scan") may provide evidence of reflux; signal over the lung fields; and quantitative evidence of gastric emptying, an important factor in reflux (see Chapter 16).

Nonoperative and medical strategies are most often adequate to treat patients with reflux. Surgery is reserved primarily for those medically refractory patients with severe complications of reflux disease. The principal strategy of surgery is to strengthen the lower esophageal sphincter mechanism and to repair other associated pathologies that precipitate reflux including hiatal hernia, pylorospasm, and delayed gastric emptying. Laparoscopic fundoplication is the operation of choice and is highly effective at eliminating reflux. The principal side effects are the decreased ability to vomit and a tendency toward the development of postprandial gastric bloating if feedings are initiated too rapidly in the postoperative period.

Hypertrophic pyloric stenosis is a common surgical condition of the newborn period, with an incidence of approximately 1 in every 300 live births in the United States. The etiology is largely unknown. A genetic component to this disease, which occurs rarely in Asians relative to Western European populations, is apparent. Furthermore, approximately 20% of affected male infants and 7% of affected female infants have a relative with pyloric stenosis. Vomiting typically begins during the first or second week of life and becomes progressively projectile. Many babies brought to medical attention have undergone changes in formula because of concerns that their emesis is formula related. Infants often present during the third week of life for surgical evaluation; however, the time of presentation may range from 1 week to 4 months of age. Physical examination findings show evidence of a distended abdomen. Peristalsis of the distended stomach may be visible (Fig. 17-57). The lesion itself is usually palpable in the epigastrium, between the midline and the right midclavicular line, and has the consistency of a small olive. An adequate examination requires a calm infant. Various maneuvers to relax the infant's abdominal musculature assist the physical examination. In the absence of a palpable "olive" on two serial examinations by an experienced examiner, the infant should undergo an abdominal ultrasound or upper gastrointestinal series (Fig. 17-58). The presence of a palpable olive requires no further imaging studies before surgery. The infant needs to be adequately hydrated and have any electrolyte abnormalities corrected before going to the operating room (Fig. 17-59).

Figure 17-56   Fluoroscopic examination of the infant during barium swallow must be of sufficient duration to allow the identification of episodes of reflux (here associated with aspiration into the tracheobronchial tree).

Figure 17-57   Pyloric stenosis may cause epigastric distention by the obstructed stomach. This patient also demonstrates a visible wave of peristalsis, which moves from left to right.

Figure 17-58 Hypertrophic pyloric stenosis. **A,** Ultrasonographic scan of the upper abdomen demonstrates the thickened pyloric muscle, indicated by the cursors. **B,** Barium study of the stomach *(right)* shows thin streaks of barium in the pyloric canal. The hypertrophic pyloric muscle bulged into the gastric antrum produces a "reversed 3" configuration.

Bilious Vomiting without Abdominal Distention

Malrotation is the failure of the midgut (small bowel, right colon, and one third of the transverse colon) to undergo adequate rotation and retroperitoneal fixation during embryonic development. Consequently, the bowel resides on a narrow pedicle (superior mesenteric artery) that is prone to undergo twisting and subsequent volvulus formation. The resulting proximal intestinal obstruction usually occurs in the distal duodenum or proximal jejunum, presenting as bilious emesis. Abdominal distention may not be a component of the early presentation because of the location of the obstruction at the ligament of Treitz and the decompressive nature of the vomiting. The resulting superior mesenteric artery obstruction leads to midgut ischemia and subsequent infarction, if no surgical intervention occurs. Bloody rectal discharge and hematemesis may also occur as the ischemia time increases. Signs of intestinal necrosis may rapidly manifest as abdominal wall edema, cellulitis, distention, and crepitus. Severe short bowel syndrome or death may occur from delayed recognition, diagnosis, and treatment of this important pediatric condition.

Although most patients who present with bilious emesis do not have malrotation with volvulus, the ramifications of diagnostic delay mandate the prompt evaluation of infants who develop these symptoms (Fig. 17-60). Plain radiographs demonstrating gastric distention and duodenal dilatation in the setting of an otherwise nearly "gasless abdomen" should raise suspicions for this condition. The cornerstone of diagnosis is the upper gastrointestinal series, which identifies the contour of the duodenal sweep or C-loop, the location of the ligament of Treitz, and the unobstructed flow of contrast into the jejunum. The most critical of these is the position of the ligament of Treitz, which should be positioned to the left of midline on the AP view and above the level of the pylorus on the oblique view. An abnormally configured duodenal C-loop or a corkscrew appearance to the duodenum with small bowel loops positioned in the right side of the abdomen is diagnostic of disease (Fig. 17-61). Other findings on the upper gastrointestinal series, such as duodenal dilatation, imply obstruction from volvulus or Ladd bands (Fig. 17-62). Barium enema may demonstrate an abnormally placed cecum in the left upper abdomen; it is not an effective diagnostic tool in the acute setting.

Duodenal atresia and duodenal anomalies are important diagnostic considerations in the patient who presents with bilious emesis. Vomiting may occur shortly after birth or at a

Figure 17-59 Laparoscopic view of pyloric stenosis viewing the hypertrophied pylorus **(A)** and pyloromyotomy, demonstrating the serosal incision **(B)**.

Figure 17-60   Malrotation with midgut volvulus without ischemia **(A)**. Malrotation predisposes to volvulus and complete midgut infarction **(B)**.

later time in the setting of annular pancreas, duodenal steno-sis, and duodenal webs. Duodenal atresia is associated with Down syndrome and congenital heart disease in about 30% to 50% of patients. The radiographic appearance of a "double bubble" sign in the newborn is pathognomonic of duodenal obstruction, usually secondary to duodenal atresia (Fig. 17-63). Malrotation without volvulus may be a source of bilious emesis secondary to Ladd bands (lateral peritoneal duodenal attachments), which may partially obstruct the duodenum.

Bilious Vomiting with Abdominal Distention

Small bowel and colonic atresias are the sequelae of intrauterine vascular accidents. These are often late gestational events, and meconium may be present in the bowel distal to the atresia. Therefore early postnatal meconium passage does not

rule out a coexisting atresia. Proximal intestinal atresias are associated with abdominal distention with only a few dilated bowel loops on plain film (Fig. 17-64), whereas distal ileal and colonic atresias are characterized as having multiple dilated bowel loops (Fig. 17-65). The presence of a proximal bowel obstruction in the neonatal period requires no other diagnostic imaging studies before definitive surgery. Contrast studies are critical to differentiate ileal atresia from various other distal obstructions including Hirschsprung disease, meconium ileus, and small left colon syndrome.

Jejunoileal (small bowel) atresias are often isolated conditions, although they may be associated with gastroschisis and meconium disease. The major anatomic variants are subdivided on the basis of whether the bowel and its mesentery are intact. The "Christmas tree" or "apple peel" deformity (type IIIb), named for the spiral appearance of the distal bowel

Figure 17-61   The ligament of Treitz in malrotation is either absent or abnormally located, and the duodenum and small intestine lie on the right side of the abdomen. Duodenal obstruction may be partial (caused by Ladd bands, as seen here) or complete (caused by volvulus).

Figure 17-62   Complete duodenal obstruction from midgut volvulus. Air in the distal gastrointestinal tract fails to rule out complete obstruction from volvulus and distinguishes the diagnosis from duodenal atresia.

Figure 17-63 Swallowed air distends the stomach and proximal duodenum in duodenal atresia, producing the characteristic "double bubble" on plain film. Other contrast studies are unnecessary.

Figure 17-65 Many intestinal loops become distended in patients with ileal atresia (pictured here), making the distinction between this diagnosis and other causes of distal bowel obstruction difficult. Other signs (such as intraperitoneal calcification, indicating meconium peritonitis) and contrast enema are necessary to identify the cause of obstruction.

around the ileocolic or right colic artery, may result in significant bowel loss (Fig. 17-66). Similarly, multiple atresias or the "string of sausages" defect (type IV) may involve an extensive amount of the jejunoileum, leaving little functional mucosal absorptive area. These two conditions put most infants at significant risk of developing short bowel syndrome and long-term, if not permanent, total parenteral nutrition (TPN) dependence.

Meconium disease is the initial presentation of cystic fibrosis in up to 20% of children. The thick viscous meconium in the distal bowel precipitates intraluminal intestinal obstruction. The distal ileum is small, and a microcolon is usually present. Marked proximal jejunoileal dilatation occurs, and the abdomen presents a "soap bubble" appearance on plain radiography (Fig. 17-67). Air–fluid levels are uncommon in this form of intestinal obstruction because of the dense concentration of meconium in the intestinal loops. Contrast enema reveals the presence of a microcolon and inspissated mucus or "rabbit pellets" in the distal ileum. Reflux of contrast proximal to these pellets into dilated bowel may be therapeutic, inducing evacuation of the thick meconium and relief of the obstruction. On occasion, patients with meconium disease may develop an intestinal atresia, volvulus, or perforation with varying amounts of meconium peritonitis. These conditions are referred to as *complicated meconium ileus* and, unlike simple meconium ileus, they always require surgical intervention (Fig. 17-68). Evidence of complicated meconium ileus may be made on prenatal diagnosis or neonatal plain films by

Figure 17-64 Jejunal atresia distends only a few bowel loops proximally, distinguishing it from duodenal and ileal atresia.

Figure 17-66 "Christmas tree" deformity results in proximal jejunoileal atresia secondary to an absent superior mesenteric artery beyond the middle colic branch. The helical appearance of the bowel around the remaining colic vessels gives the characteristic appearance.

Figure 17-67 Meconium ileus presents as a distal small bowel obstruction in the newborn with few air-filled dilated loops due to the meconium-filled bowel loops.

Figure 17-69 The absence of intramural ganglion cells prevents intestinal peristalsis through segments affected by Hirschsprung disease, causing a functional bowel obstruction. The involved segment appears narrow when compared with the distended, obstructed proximal bowel, which possesses normal ganglion cells.

the presence of peritoneal calcifications and ascites. Unsuccessful attempts at contrast reduction of meconium ileus should raise concern for an associated ileal atresia.

Hirschsprung disease, the absence of ganglion cells in the distal rectum, is a common cause of bilious emesis and abdominal distention. Although the classic presentation is that of failure to pass meconium, distal rectal obstruction may also induce vomiting. Plain radiographs of the abdomen in most patients demonstrate marked bowel dilatation. Barium enema studies show proximally dilated bowel (normal) and a nondilated segment (transition zone) juxtaposed to a distal decompressed segment of rectum (Fig. 17-69). A barium study, as outlined earlier, should precede rectal manipulation or enemas, as they may distort the radiographic findings typical of the transition zone and confuse the diagnosis (Fig. 17-70). Suction rectal biopsy performed at the bedside without the need for anesthesia is diagnostic (Fig. 17-71).

Some children escape diagnosis in the first few days or months of life but are plagued by chronic constipation requiring rectal stimulation to evacuate. They may develop chronic symptoms of abdominal distention, growth failure, and

constipation. These patients may also present with an acute life-threatening episode of Hirschsprung-related enterocolitis. These infants or young children develop severe explosive diarrhea, toxic megacolon, and systemic sepsis that may rapidly progress to death. Emergency laparotomy for bowel decompression is mandated. Therapeutic delays secondary to attempts to perform preoperative suction rectal biopsy should be avoided, because of the high attendant morbidity and mortality of this presentation.

Older Infants and Children

Age-specific considerations for the causes of vomiting should direct the diagnostic approaches for children beyond the neonatal and infancy period. Intussusception is a frequent cause of vomiting in toddlers from 6 months to 2 years of age. The etiology of this condition is idiopathic in the majority of children in this age group; however, the presence of a mechanical lead point is more common in older children. Lead points include Meckel diverticula, intestinal polyps, Burkitt or non-Hodgkin lymphoma, intestinal duplication cysts, and seromuscular hematomas secondary to bleeding disorders such as

Figure 17-68 Intense inflammation resulting from free meconium in the peritoneal cavity (meconium peritonitis) may produce visible erythema and edema over the abdominal wall.

Figure 17-70 Barium enema outlines the transition zone between the contracted (aganglionic) rectosigmoid lying distal to the obstructed, but normally innervated, colon. To demonstrate this sign, the examination must be conducted in an unprepped patient who has undergone neither enemas nor digital rectal examination.

C   D

Figure 17-71   Suction rectal biopsy is a bedside procedure **(A)** that provides a small fragment of tissue for pathologic evaluation for ganglion cells **(B)**. A normal suction rectal biopsy with an acetylcholinesterase stain demonstrates a normal band of staining and no giant nerve fibers between the muscular layers **(C)**. Higher power view of a biopsy from a patient with Hirschsprung disease shows darkly staining giant nerve fibers in the muscularis layer (acetylcholinesterase stain) **(D)**. *(**C** and **D,** Courtesy Paul S. Dickman, MD, and Dan Galvis, BS.)*

hemophilia or Henoch-Schönlein purpura. Idiopathic intussusception occurs in the region of the distal ileum and ascending colon. The classic clinical presentation is that of an otherwise healthy infant who presents with paroxysmal bouts of severe colicky abdominal pain associated with drawing his or her legs to the chest, followed by a period of sedation or somnolence. The presentation of this disease may be variable, however. Some children present with unexplained lethargy or seizure-like episodes, causing practitioners to suspect and work up potential neurologic diagnoses such as brain tumors and meningitis. Vomiting or the passage of a bowel movement may be associated with relief of these episodes. The child then resumes his or her typical behavior until another episode occurs. Initially vomiting episodes are nonbilious and likely related to a reflex response mediated by central nervous system mechanisms related to mesenteric traction. As time progresses, the bowel obstruction becomes more complete and the vomiting episodes may become progressively more bilious in nature. Bowel ischemia is typically a late finding in these cases (Fig. 17-72). Most infants are so violently ill that they are brought to medical attention earlier in their course. Mucosal sloughing may occur in the setting of bowel ischemia, producing "currant jelly" stools (Fig. 17-73). Physical examination findings may be notable for a palpable "sausage-shaped" mass located in the right upper quadrant or epigastrium. Consequently, the right lower quadrant may be empty (Dance sign).

The radiographic assessment of intussusception is initially performed with plain films, which in many instances are not helpful. An intussusceptum visualized as a soft tissue cutoff sign or meniscus in the upper or mid-abdomen is diagnostic (Fig. 17-74). Newer techniques using abdominal ultrasonography may have greater sensitivity and specificity than plain radiography. Contrast enema with either barium or air (preferred) may be both diagnostic and therapeutic (Fig. 17-75). Successful reduction is indicated by the prompt and free passage of barium or air into dilated loops of small bowel proximal to the obstruction. The inability to achieve this objective is indicative of a persistent obstruction either secondary to an incompletely reduced intussusception or a second

Figure 17-72   The intestine invaginates into itself in intussusception. The ileum is pulled through the ileocecal valve into the colon, the most common pattern seen in infancy, pictured here.

Figure 17-73   The intussusception—the invaginated portion of bowel—becomes congested and ischemic, leading to the passage of bloody stool mixed with mucus (currant jelly stool).

Figure 17-75   Barium enema confirms the diagnosis by outlining the intussusceptum. The column of contrast can then be used to push the invaginated bowel proximally. Free reflux of contrast into the bowel proximally signals complete reduction of the intussusception.

site of intussusception. These techniques have a low incidence of failure (<10%). Those patients with an incomplete or failed reduction require emergency open or laparoscopic exploration and reduction or resection.

Intussusception may recur within the first 12 to 24 hours after radiographic reduction. Patients with recurrent symptoms should return promptly to the radiographic suite for repeat reduction attempts. Ileoileal or jejunoileal (small bowel) intussusceptions are generally too proximal to be amenable to radiographic reduction; they are typically due to mechanical lead points and require surgery. Postoperative intussusceptions are also located in the small bowel and require operative reduction (Fig. 17-76). Controversy exists regarding the older child who presents with intussusception. Because of the high frequency of a surgical lead point, many favor only diagnostic and nontherapeutic contrast enemas. This is followed by surgical exploration and possible bowel resection.

Internal hernias around postoperative adhesions, amniotic bands, or omphalomesenteric (vitelline) remnants may produce intestinal obstruction. The most common cause of

intestinal obstruction is related to adhesions from previous surgery or abdominal trauma. Often, early preemptive nasogastric decompression may alleviate the symptoms and halt the progression to complete obstruction. Failure of early resolution of the obstruction should prompt emergency exploration. Omphalomesenteric duct remnants, or vitelline bands, may attach to the umbilicus or mesentery, producing a potential site of internal bowel herniation (Fig. 17-77). Rotational anomalies may leave spaces lateral to the duodenum, cecum, and sigmoid colon, giving rise to potential sites of bowel incarceration known as *paraduodenal* or *paracolic hernias*.

Gastrointestinal Bleeding

The evaluation of an infant or child with bleeding from the gastrointestinal tract involves a careful assessment of several important factors and the establishment of a management protocol (Table 17-3). Initially the practitioner must determine whether the episode of bleeding is hemodynamically significant. The next step in the evaluation is to confirm that what appears to be blood is truly blood. Subsequently, the physician should obtain a general idea of the location of blood loss (i.e., upper versus lower gastrointestinal tract) (Table 17-4). Those

Figure 17-74   In some cases the intussusceptum can be seen as a meniscus-shaped mass outlined by air in the colon.

Figure 17-76   Small bowel intussusception typically has a lead point except in patients with postoperative intussusception as shown here. Upper gastrointestinal studies should be avoided in these patients secondary to aspiration risks.

Figure 17-77 Omphalomesenteric remnants, also known as vitelline bands, may produce internal hernias that lead to obstruction.

Table 17-3	Common Causes of Gastrointestinal Hemorrhage	
Site of Hemorrhage	**Patients Younger Than 1 Year**	**Patients Older Than 1 Year**
Upper Gastrointestinal Tract	Gastritis Swallowed maternal blood Peptic ulcer (duodenal and gastric) Malrotation and volvulus	Peptic ulcer Varices
Lower Gastrointestinal Tract	Anal fissure Intussusception Necrotizing enterocolitis Meckel diverticulum Malrotation and volvulus	Colonic polyps Intussusception Meckel diverticulum Infectious diarrhea Inflammatory bowel disease

patients in acute or impending hypovolemic shock require urgent stabilization coincident with diagnostic studies. In cases of more chronic or subacute blood loss, symptoms of anemia, fatigue, and pallor are more common. A thorough history and physical examination in conjunction with serologic, radiologic, and endoscopic studies are critical to ascertain the etiology of the bleeding. The duration, severity (amount), and location of the episode of bleeding are among the most important historical factors. Drug ingestion, exposure to sick contacts, inherited coagulopathies, vitamin deficiencies, or a family history of chronic intestinal disorders may shed further light on the source of bleeding. Severe acute blood loss may be associated with both upper (hematemesis) and lower (hematochezia or melena) bleeding.

Infants

Swallowed maternal blood is a common source of bleeding in the newborn. Most infants have normal vital signs and stable hematocrits. The Apt-Downey test differentiates between maternal and fetal blood in the newborn. A mixture of 1 volume of gastric aspirate and 4 parts of water is centrifuged. The supernatant is removed and mixed at a 4:1 ratio with 1% sodium hydroxide. If the fluid remains pink, the blood has fetal hemoglobin; alternatively, if the mixture turns brown, the blood is from the mother. Hemorrhagic diseases of the newborn may lead to profound upper gastrointestinal bleeding, especially in those infants who fail to receive their perinatal vitamin K injection. This is a rare occurrence because of strict delivery room protocols; however, infants who are unstable or urgently transferred from the delivery room to other institutions may be at greatest risk. Hence the delivery room records for all newborns who present with upper gastrointestinal bleeding should be examined. Nasogastric tube placement or oropharyngeal suctioning shortly after birth may precipitate bleeding that enters the stomach and results in bloody emesis. This typically clears with gastric lavage. Anal fissures are a more benign cause of anorectal bleeding in infants. This may be associated with constipation, hard stools, and anal stenosis (Fig. 17-78).

Table 17-4	Causes of Gastrointestinal Bleeding				
			AGE		
Location	**Appearance**	**Newborn**	**Infant**	**Child**	
Upper gastrointestinal tract	Well	Maternal blood Nasogastric tube Pyloric stenosis Esophagitis	Nosebleeds Nasogastric tube Esophagitis	Nosebleeds Nasogastric tube	
	Ill	Peptic ulcer disease Necrotizing enterocolitis Volvulus	Varices Peptic ulcer disease Medications	Varices Peptic ulcer disease Medications	
Lower gastrointestinal tract	Well	Anal fissure Maternal blood Hemangioma Duplication	Anal fissure Meckel diverticulum Duplication	Anal fissure Juvenile polyp Meckel diverticulum Rectal prolapse	
	Ill	Necrotizing enterocolitis Volvulus Infectious diarrhea	Intussusception Infectious diarrhea Medications Henoch-Schönlein purpura Hemolytic-uremic syndrome	Infectious diarrhea Intussusception Trauma Medications Hemolytic-uremic syndrome Henoch-Schönlein purpura Inflammatory bowel disease	

Figure 17-78 Small tears in the anoderm may bleed, producing small amounts of blood in the stool of healthy infants.

Figure 17-80 Diffuse necrotizing enterocolitis is associated with a patchy distribution of necrosis on the serosal surface of the bowel.

Severe acute gastritis or gastric ulceration may occur in the newborn period and is associated with high morbidity and mortality. These infants often present with hypovolemic shock and free intraperitoneal air (Fig. 17-79). This typically occurs during the first 7 to 10 days of life. Malrotation with midgut volvulus may also present with severe upper gastrointestinal bleeding secondary to either bowel ischemia or sepsis-induced coagulopathy.

Necrotizing enterocolitis (NEC) is the most common abdominal surgical emergency of the newborn period. Although classically an inflammatory condition that presents with abdominal distention, NEC may also precipitate upper or lower gastrointestinal bleeding. Predominantly a condition of premature infants, nearly 15% of cases occur in term infants. The major risk factors in this group include sepsis, low birth weight, congenital heart disease, hyperviscosity syndromes, pulmonary insufficiency, drugs (indomethacin and methylxanthines), and maternal cocaine use. A variant may affect the entire small bowel. The associated pan-necrosis of the small bowel is often referred to as "leopard skin" because of the patchy distribution of necrosis (Fig. 17-80). Numerous etiologic factors have been attributed to the onset of this condition; however, none of them has been solely implicated in the onset of NEC. The patients may have vague symptoms

including abdominal distention, vomiting, increased gastric residuals, and bloody stools. Constitutional symptoms consisting of temperature lability, apnea, and bradycardia, as well as inactivity, are quite common.

On physical examination patients often appear toxic with signs of abdominal distention, edema, and erythema. Apneic and bradycardiac episodes are common. Laboratory values may show neutropenia or leukocytosis, anemia, and metabolic acidosis. Plain radiographs demonstrate pneumatosis intestinalis, the pathognomonic hallmark of the disease. This radiographic finding suggests the subserosal dissection of air and may be linear or cystic (Fig. 17-81). On occasion portal vein gas may be seen, but this may be evanescent. Small, localized collections of air or large amounts of free air that outline the falciform ligament are signs of free intraperitoneal perforation. Pneumoperitoneum, best visualized on the left lateral decubitus film, is an absolute indication for immediate surgical intervention. In general, NEC is managed nonoperatively with intravenous hydration, parenteral antibiotics, nasogastric tube decompression, and suspension of feedings. In addition to perforation, deteriorating clinical status is the other major acute indication for surgery. Despite uneventful recovery from the initial acute-phase disease, some patients develop symptomatic strictures, which require surgical resection (Fig. 17-82).

Toddlers (1 to 5 Years)

Painless rectal bleeding in the toddler should raise concern for the presence of a Meckel diverticulum. Often the bleeding is massive with significant drops in the hematocrit requiring blood transfusion. The initial blood loss is variable and may present as a sentinel bleed that spontaneously resolves, followed by more massive bright red or maroon blood per rectum. Although spontaneous resolution may occur, subsequent episodes of bleeding may be life-threatening. The bleeding results from the ulceration of the ileal mucosa located adjacent to the ectopic gastric mucosa present at the base of the Meckel diverticulum (Fig. 17-83). A technetium-99m pertechnetate isotope scan, called a Meckel scan, identifies gastric mucosa and may be helpful in the diagnosis of disease (Fig. 17-84). During active bleeding the scan may be positive in 85% of patients. False-negative evaluations are common. The use of intravenous pentagastrin or cimetidine may improve the sensitivity of the study. Contrast studies of the distal small bowel

Figure 17-79 The large quantity of free air within the abdomen resulting from a gastric perforation (shown here outlining the edge of the liver) suggests its source.

Figure 17-81 Pneumatosis intestinalis is seen most easily as linear streaks of air outlining the bowel and producing concentric rings when viewed on end. More common, however, is the bubbly pattern seen in the right iliac fossa in this patient, appearing like stool within the lumen **(A)**. In severely affected infants, gas may fill the portal system and produce visible streaks of air on abdominal plain film **(B)**.

(enteroclysis) or colon (barium enema) are of marginal diagnostic utility in this setting and may obscure the scan. Some children must undergo exploratory laparotomy or laparoscopy (Fig. 17-85) to identify the presence of the diverticulum because of the presence of negative studies. Meckel diverticulum may present with obstruction (secondary to volvulus or internal hernia or intussusception) or acute inflammation (diverticulitis) similar to appendicitis.

Esophageal varices are a common source of massive upper gastrointestinal bleeding in children with portal hypertension. Other causes of portal hypertension in children include the presence of extrahepatic portal vein thrombosis or hepatic cirrhosis. Omphalitis, a complication of umbilical venous catheterization in newborns, may precipitate portal vein thrombosis. Children with short bowel syndrome or other chronic intestinal disorders such as intestinal pseudo-obstruction (Fig.

17-86) or microvillus inclusion disease may require chronic parenteral nutrition, which may induce TPN-related liver disease and hepatic failure. One third of patients who undergo a Kasai procedure (portoenterostomy) for biliary atresia develop progressive cirrhosis that leads to variceal bleeding secondary to portal hypertension. Cystic fibrosis, α_1-antitrypsin deficiency, and viral hepatitis are a few of the other common conditions that may induce portal hypertension in children. Upper gastrointestinal endoscopy facilitates direct visualization of the varices in cases of active bleeding and assists therapeutic banding or sclerosant techniques. On occasion, angiography is useful to visualize the anatomy of the portal venous system and its branches. The advent of transjugular intracaval portosystemic shunting (TIPS) has almost eliminated the need for emergency surgical intervention in acutely bleeding esophageal varices.

Vasculitic conditions such as Henoch-Schönlein purpura (HSP) may be a source of lower gastrointestinal bleeding in children. Typically HSP occurs during the postinfectious stage of a major viral or streptococcal illness. Arthralgias and a macular purpuric skin rash in the lower extremities are characteristic of this entity. In both of these presentations, patients may develop intussusception due to the evolution of a

Figure 17-82 In a patient who develops intestinal obstruction during recovery from necrotizing enterocolitis, a colonic stricture must be suspected.

Figure 17-83 The bleeding site in a Meckel diverticulum is typically located on the mucosa of bowel adjacent to the ectopic gastric tissue.

Figure 17-84 A Meckel scan (in which technetium-99m pertechnetate is administered) demonstrates positive uptake in the right lower abdomen.

subserosal mucosal hematoma, which functions as a lead point (Fig. 17-87). The presence of acute renal insufficiency, anemia, pain, and bloody diarrhea is suggestive of hemolytic-uremic syndrome. The triad of azotemia, anemia, and thrombocytopenia confirms the diagnosis. If a coexistent dysentery-like illness is present, then the pathogen should be determined by stool culture or analysis.

Older Children

Benign hamartomatous juvenile polyps most frequently affect children between 2 and 8 years of age. The incidence is approximately 1 in 1000 children. Bleeding is usually painless, low in volume, and found as streaks on the surface of the stool. Two thirds of the bleeding problems are found in the rectum, and 90% are found distal to the sigmoid colon. Many of these lesions undergo autonecrosis and slough into the stool, whereas others may prolapse through the anus (Fig. 17-88). Surgical or endoscopic resection is therapeutic. Patients with Peutz-Jeghers syndrome present with melanotic mucocutaneous pigmentation (Fig. 17-89) and gastrointestinal bleeding due to hamartomatous polyps (Fig. 17-90). These polyps may also cause recurrent episodes of abdominal pain and obstruction. Although most of these polyps are single and rarely present in numbers exceeding 12, a life-threatening variant of this condition, diffuse juvenile polyposis, may present with severe bloody diarrhea, intussusception, rectal prolapse, and protein-losing enteropathy. Total abdominal colectomy is required in these patients.

In contrast to hamartomatous polyps, adenomatous polyps are quite rare as solitary colonic lesions. Children with familial adenomatous polyposis are usually asymptomatic until puberty or late adolescence, when they may develop diarrhea, hematochezia, and anemia. Diffuse adenomatous polyps blanket the colon and may have associated lesions throughout the intestinal tract from stomach to terminal ileum (Fig. 17-91). Surgery is frequently recommended to control recurrent bleeding and failure to thrive and to decrease the long-term high risk of malignancy in these patients.

ABDOMINAL PAIN

The most common surgical emergency of childhood is acute appendicitis. The pathogenesis arises from appendiceal obstruction usually secondary to hyperplasia of submucosal lymphoid tissue or a fecalith. The subsequent development of appendiceal edema, ischemia, gangrene, and ultimately perforation will occur with the passage of time (Fig. 17-92). Despite the classic description of pain originating in the periumbilical region that progressively localizes to the right lower quadrant, the manifestations of appendicitis in childhood are protean. Although the symptom complex typically includes abdominal pain, low-grade fever, and anorexia, some children, particularly those with a retrocecal appendix, have few symptoms and may present days to weeks after their initial episode of appendicitis. These children may present with a localized abscess due to previous perforation and localization by host defense mechanisms. Physical examination findings in most pediatric patients demonstrate tenderness in the right lower quadrant, suprapubic, or lower flank regions that persists or worsens despite hydration and cautious observation. Children with appendicitis are often found lying quietly in bed with their legs flexed at the hips, resisting abdominal palpation. Maneuvers such as coughing, heel-tap, jumping, or even walking may exacerbate the symptoms and are suggestive of peritoneal irritation. Involuntary guarding or muscular spasm overlying the area of peritoneal irritation is a common examination finding that is not masked by mild forms of sedation. A positive psoas or obturator sign is indicative of retroperitoneal appendicitis, which may be associated with few anterior abdominal findings. In general, the routine use of plain abdominal films is unnecessary in the evaluation of the child with abdominal pain. However, the presence of a fecalith in a child with abdominal pain warrants appendectomy, as operative intervention is indicated to avoid progression to perforation (Fig. 17-93). Children with fecaliths in the absence of abdominal pain may undergo elective surgery and/or be followed expectantly.

Perforation occurs due to diagnostic delay that may be related to the nonclassic presentation of acute appendicitis. Symptoms may be confused with gastroenteritis or other

Figure 17-85 Laparoscopic view of a Meckel diverticulum with an apparent vitelline artery **(A)**. Meckel diverticulum at surgery **(B)**.

Figure 17-86 Massive abdominal distention **(A)** and colonic dilatation seen in intestinal pseudo-obstruction may mimic dilatation seen with mechanical obstruction or Hirschsprung disease **(B)**.

Figure 17-87 Henoch-Schönlein purpura causes submucosal and serosal hematomas that may act as a lead point. Note the presence of hematochezia and the diagnostic skin lesions.

Figure 17-88 Juvenile polyps are found most often in the rectosigmoid colon. On occasion they may prolapse through the anus.

Figure 17-89 The characteristic melanotic spots of Peutz-Jeghers syndrome are seen on the lips, buccal mucosa, and anus.

Figure 17-90 Melanotic small bowel polyps characteristic of Peutz-Jeghers syndrome are prone to bleeding or obstruction.

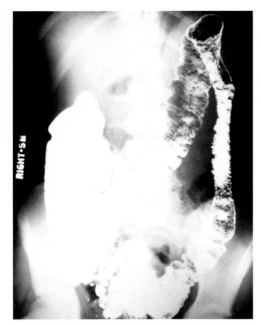

Figure 17-91   Familial adenomatous polyposis. A barium enema study demonstrates multiple small polyps throughout the colon.

Figure 17-93   A fecalith, the round calcification in the iliac fossa, obstructs the appendiceal lumen and initiates inflammatory processes that produce appendicitis.

nonsurgical intestinal illnesses. Perforation leads to either free peritoneal soilage or the development of a localized abscess (Fig. 17-94). Initially, perforation may be associated with the relief of symptoms, which is usually followed by diffuse abdominal tenderness, distention, and rigidity. Patients often appear quite toxic. Alternatively, isolation of the inflammatory process by the omentum and adjacent bowel loops may lead to abscess formation. Patients with localization may appear surprisingly well. Perforation associated with diffuse peritoneal soilage requires surgical exploration for drainage and appendectomy. Localized perforation may be initially managed by the use of intravenous antibiotics with or without percutaneous drainage followed by an interval appendectomy at approximately 6 to 8 weeks after the original presentation. This management approach is associated with fewer perioperative complications and improved outcomes.

Acute appendicitis in the preschool-age child is a clinical challenge for even the most experienced practitioner. Acute abdominal pain is a common presentation of other conditions including otitis media, pneumonia, urinary tract infections, diabetes, sickle cell disease, vasculitis, or enteritis (bacterial

or viral). The difficulties in obtaining a history in this age group, the poor understanding of time, and the challenges of obtaining a reliable physical examination may all contribute to the diagnostic delay. The incidence of perforation exceeds 50%. Unlike older children, these preschoolers seldom wall off their perforation to allow for delayed operative intervention and commonly present with severe peritonitis requiring urgent operative intervention.

The differential diagnosis for appendicitis includes several nonsurgical problems such as gastroenteritis, mesenteric adenitis, constipation, and urinary tract infections, as well as surgical conditions such as Meckel diverticulitis, inflammatory bowel disease (particularly Crohn disease) (Fig. 17-95), and intussusception. Pelvic pathology including ovarian cysts, ovarian torsion (Fig. 17-96), or acute salpingitis with or without associated tubo-ovarian abscess may be readily confused with acute appendicitis, making the negative appendectomy rate much higher in girls than boys. Advancements in radiographic imaging techniques and the increased use of laparoscopy have helped with improving diagnostic accuracy. Cystic ovarian masses represent a wide spectrum of conditions from the simple follicular cyst (see Fig. 17-96) to hormonally active cystic tumors (Fig. 17-97). Large ovarian cysts (>5 cm) that persist for more than 2 to 4 weeks should undergo

Figure 17-92   Laparoscopic view of appendicitis. Note the inflamed, swollen appendix.

Figure 17-94   Perforated appendicitis with a large ring-enhancing abscess seen on CT scan.

Figure 17-95 Findings at laparotomy in Crohn disease reveal petechiae over the serosa of the thickened small bowel, which has mesenteric "creeping fat."

Figure 17-97 A large cystic ovarian tumor removed from a teenage girl with a slowly increasing abdominal girth.

ultrasonography-guided aspiration or laparoscopic fenestration because of their risk of undergoing torsion. Ovarian torsion classically presents with pain out of proportion to the physical examination findings, and typically these patients lack significant gastrointestinal symptoms. Other pelvic masses related to uterine congenital pathology may be a source of abdominal pain (see earlier discussion).

ANUS AND RECTUM

Most congenital anorectal anomalies are clinically apparent at birth. Bilious emesis, poor feeding, abdominal distention, and delayed or absent passage of meconium may herald the presence of a distal obstruction. *Imperforate anus* is the general category assigned to these patients, and it may present as one of three principal anatomic groups. These rectal anomalies are classified on the basis of the position of the rectum and the levator ani muscle complex. Low imperforate anus is associated with the passage of the rectum through the levator ani, and a fistulous tract extends to the perineal region ending in the center of a ridge of tissue on the anus ("bucket handle" deformity) (Fig. 17-98) or anterior to these structures as a perineal fistula (Fig. 17-99). In male infants the fistula may travel in the median raphe of the scrotum, and the meconium may be seen as a string of white or black beads (Fig. 17-100). The prognosis is generally favorable for low lesions because they lie within the levator ani complex. In contrast, high lesions do not pass through the levator ani. A visible fistula does not exist. Most commonly the rectal fistula ends in the

prostatic urethra, bulbar urethra, or bladder neck in males or above the hymen in girls. Meconium is passed with urine via the urethra in males (Fig. 17-101) or transvaginally in females (Fig. 17-102). A variant of high imperforate anus is a cloacal anomaly, which is a complex congenital anomaly in which the urethra, vagina, and rectum share a single perineal opening (Fig. 17-103). The third variant represents intermediate lesions that are partially within the levator ani complex (Fig. 17-104). The surgical management of these lesions is currently undergoing major re-evaluation. However, the classic approach to the care for patients with low lesions is a one-stage repair, or perineal anoplasty (Fig. 17-105). Patients with high and intermediate lesions classically undergo staged repairs with a primary colostomy at birth followed by a perineal pull-through at a later age. Several months after the pull-through they return for their colostomy closure. The prognosis for fecal continence is excellent in patients with low lesions. Because they partially extend into the levator, intermediate lesions also tend to have good outcomes. The prognosis for high lesions is more guarded due in part to the presence of associated congenital anomalies and the quality of the reconstruction (Fig. 17-106).

Rectal prolapse is an uncommon condition that is most often idiopathic in children (Fig. 17-107). The peak incidence of idiopathic rectal prolapse occurs in the second year of life, often precipitated by episodes of diarrheal illnesses, efforts to toilet train, or severe constipation. This process responds spontaneously after the resolution of the acute illness or with dietary and medical manipulations to treat the constipation.

Figure 17-96 **A,** Simple follicular cysts may grow to very large sizes that may fill the cul-de-sac. **B,** Ovarian torsion.

Figure 17-98   A spot of meconium is visible beneath a "bucket handle" bridge of skin in an infant with a low imperforate anus.

Figure 17-100   Low imperforate anus in a male infant. White mucus or black meconium may pass through a perineal fistula from a low imperforate anus into the scrotal raphe.

Nonidiopathic cases are often related to neurologic conditions or chronic diseases. Abnormalities in the development of the muscles of the pelvic floor or the innervation occur in patients with spina bifida and related spinal cord abnormalities. Refractory cases should be evaluated for chronic hookworm infestation with stool evaluations for ova and parasites, which may cause severe tenesmus and straining. Rectal polyps may precipitate prolapse by acting as a lead point for this form of rectal intussusception. Evaluation by contrast enema and sigmoidoscopy are important components of the assessment of children with recurrent episodes. Cystic fibrosis is another common cause of prolapse and should be evaluated in patients with this condition. Surgery is rarely indicated. Circumferential submucosal injections with concentrated dextrose functions as a sclerosant that prevents prolapse from recurring.

Anorectal abscess is a common condition in the first 6 to 10 months of life. The lesions arise from infections of the submucosal crypt glands found along the dentate line. Significant fluctuance requires incision and drainage followed by warm soaks or sitz baths. Recurrent episodes of infection,

although rare, may give rise to a fistula-in-ano or chronically draining sinus (Fig. 17-108). Anal fistulectomy with debridement of the tract is usually curative. Minor degrees of incontinence may complicate this procedure. Chronic recurrent anal fistulas may indicate the presence of Crohn disease, chronic granulomatous disease, or immunodeficiency. Patients with a persistent or refractory condition should be thoroughly evaluated for these entities.

Anal fissure, discussed previously as a cause of gastrointestinal bleeding, is common in young infants. Hemorrhoids are less common in children and typically respond to nonoperative maneuvers.

HEPATOBILIARY SYSTEM, PANCREAS, SPLEEN

Less common causes of abdominal pain in childhood include symptomatic biliary tract disease related to gallstones or choledochal cyst. Children who have a history of hemoglobinopathy (sickle cell disease), chronic hemolysis (spherocytosis), or a strong family incidence of cholelithiasis and who develop colicky right upper quadrant discomfort, epigastric pain, unexplained jaundice, or pancreatitis should undergo ultrasound evaluation for the presence of cholecystitis, cholelithiasis, choledocholithiasis, and pancreatitis (Fig. 17-109). Choledochal cyst is a congenital condition, more common in young girls than boys, that typically presents around 4 years of age with fusiform to cystic dilatation of the common bile duct. Pain from common duct obstruction or acute pancreatitis may be the initial presenting symptom. Surgical excision of the abnormal common duct is indicated in the short term to prevent episodes of pancreatitis and over the long term to eliminate the risk of malignancy (Fig 17-110). Pancreatitis, most often secondary to idiopathic causes in children, may cause abdominal pain in children that may have surgical implications. Initial presentation with hyperamylasemia and hyperlipasemia may progress to the development of a midabdominal mass. These patients should be evaluated for the presence of a pancreatic pseudocyst. Many of these lesions resolve spontaneously and do not require surgical drainage. Pancreatic pseudocysts may also develop after traumatic pancreatic injury (Fig. 17-111).

Diseases of the spleen requiring surgery include hemolytic diseases such as hereditary spherocytosis, hemolytic anemias, asplenism, and occasionally sickle cell disease. Anemia and splenomegaly leading to illness, transfusion requirement, or decreased ability to participate in normal activities of daily living may prompt laparoscopic splenectomy to avoid

Figure 17-99   In male infants, white mucus or black meconium may extend through a low perineal fistula to the midline scrotal raphe to the level of the penis.

Figure 17-101 **A,** No visible external opening forms in high imperforate anus. Absence of the intergluteal cleft is also common, frequently associated with sacral agenesis. **B,** Meconium passes into the bladder or urethra through a rectal fistula and appears in the urine. **C,** Retrograde urethrography demonstrates the rectourethral fistula.

Figure 17-102 A high imperforate anus communicates into the vagina. Meconium is passed through the vagina **(A)**. Vaginoscopy reveals the fistula on the posterior wall of the vagina well above the hymen **(B)**. A bicornuate uterus accompanies rectovaginal fistula in high lesions in girls.

Figure 17-103 Cloacal anomaly is the most complete expression of imperforate anus in girls, with urinary, genital, and intestinal tracts converging into a single cloacal channel that exists as the sole perineal opening.

Figure 17-104 An intermediate lesion passes partially through the levator ani but fails to approach the perineum as closely as low lesions.

Figure 17-105   Anteriorly displaced anus partially within the anal sphincter complex.

Figure 17-106   Bifid scrotum in an infant with imperforate anus is indicative of a high lesion and the likely presence of other anomalies.

Figure 17-107   Although the cause of rectal prolapse is unknown in the majority of cases, all infants should be evaluated for cystic fibrosis.

Figure 17-108   A punctum visible to the left of the anus with a lacrimal duct probe communicates to a crypt in the anal canal by a fistulous tract. Recurrent abscesses arise from a well-formed fistula like this one, an indication for fistulectomy.

complications of splenomegaly or hyperfunction. Preoperative vaccination for pneumococcal, meningococcal, and *Haemophilus influenzae* B organisms is standard. Postsplenectomy oral penicillin prophylaxis (usually until age 21 years) is recommended but controversial in order to avoid overwhelming postsplenectomy sepsis.

ABDOMINAL WALL DEFECTS

Gastroschisis and omphalocele are the two principal congenital abdominal wall defects. Omphalocele arises as a consequence of the embryonic extrusion of the developing midgut from the coelomic cavity into the yolk sac to allow midgut elongation as the abdominal wall expands to accommodate the rapidly growing viscera. Resulting central defects in the medial and lateral wall folds and umbilical ring result in a central abdominal wall deformity. This defect is covered by a sac that has outer amniotic and inner peritoneal layers. The umbilical cord inserts into the sac. This midline defect may be of various sizes from so-called "umbilical cord hernias" to "giant omphaloceles" greater than 10 cm and may exist in the central, epigastric, and hypogastric regions (Figs. 17-112, 17-113, and 17-114). Coexisting anomalies of other midline structures including the heart, sternum, diaphragm, and

Figure 17-109   Ultrasound examination of the right upper quadrant easily demonstrates stones within the gallbladder. An acoustic shadow extends beneath the stone.

Figure 17-110 **A,** Magnetic resonance cholangiopancreatography of a choledochal cyst demonstrating a fusiform dilatation of the common bile duct. **B,** ERCP (endoscopic retrograde cholangiopancreatogram) of a choledochal cyst demonstrating the same irregular mass in the hilum of the liver. **C,** Laparoscopic view of an in situ choledochal cyst with fusiform dilation extending from the hilum to the ampulla. The duodenum is at the southwest corner of the photograph, the liver hilum is in the northwest corner, and the dilated cyst has the Endoloop suture around it.

bladder may occur in 30% to 50% of all patients. Chromosomal anomalies may also be common in this population.

In contrast to omphalocele, gastroschisis is a defect of the right lateral abdominal wall. Although controversy exists as to the distinct etiology, most believe this deformity results from a vascular accident that leads to occlusion of the right umbilical vein with subsequent disruption of the end of the abdominal wall and mild evisceration. The defect is usually small in

Figure 17-111 Pancreatic pseudocysts in the pediatric population most commonly result from blunt traumatic injuries to the abdomen, as occurred in this patient with a handlebar injury.

term infants; however, large amounts of bowel may lie in the amniotic cavity. This anomaly occurs early in gestation, and the bowel is left in contact with the amniotic fluid, which produces an intense inflammatory response or "peel" (Fig. 17-115). This peel is believed to alter bowel motility in the postoperative period, leading to long delays in the return of bowel function. Recent efforts have focused on earlier delivery in the 32- to 34-week gestational age range in order to diminish these deleterious effects on bowel function.

In contrast to omphalocele, gastroschisis is generally not associated with other congenital anomalies. Only 7% to 10% of patients have associated conditions, the most common of which are intestinal atresias. Ischemia due to in utero volvulus, malrotation, or incarceration through the narrow defect may lead to vascular compromise that causes an atresia (Fig. 17-116).

The surgical management of these conditions is similar. In both conditions the goal is the safe primary closure of the defect without creating an abdominal compartment syndrome that leads to pulmonary embarrassment, renal insufficiency, intestinal ischemia, or necrotizing enterocolitis due to either the size of the defect or the rigidity of the bowel. Gastroschisis constitutes a surgical emergency because the exposed bowel may become desiccated or injured. Omphaloceles, which have a protective peritoneal covering, may be managed in a more elective manner. A staged closure must be performed in some patients; this may include placement of a prosthetic Silastic

Figure 17-112   **A,** A small omphalocele with the umbilical cord attached to the apex of the sac. **B,** Giant omphalocele containing liver, stomach, and bowel. Chromosomal and other anomalies, particularly cardiac, are common and should be evaluated in both conditions.

Figure 17-113   Pentalogy of Cantrell is a midline abdominal wall defect (epigastric omphalocele) **(A)** associated with anterior diaphragmatic defect, sternal cleft, ectopia cordis, and congenital heart disease (usually a ventricular septal defect) **(B)**.

Figure 17-114   Cloacal exstrophy consists of an infraumbilical omphalocele with exstrophy of the bladder, in which the bladder is separated into halves by the exposed intestine. Both the proximal and distal loops have prolapsed, producing the "elephant trunk" appearance.

Figure 17-115   In gastroschisis the abdominal defect lies to the right of an intact umbilical cord without a sac, and the intestines are exposed to the amniotic fluid. An inflammatory "peel" develops, which may affect motility.

Figure 17-116 In utero volvulus may complicate gastroschisis. Occurrence of this event early in gestation may lead to intestinal atresia. Extraintestinal anomalies are rare in gastroschisis.

Figure 17-118 Location of commonly found hernias involving the abdominal wall.

silo with daily reductions (Fig. 17-117), and administration of topical desiccants such as silver sulfadiazine (Silvadene), povidone-iodine (Betadine), or merbromin (Mercurochrome). Placement of a prosthetic material such as Gore-Tex (W. L. Gore & Associates, Flagstaff, Ariz) or Surgisis (Cook Surgical, Bloomington, Ind) may provide coverage. These infants have significant postoperative delays in the return of intestinal function and require TPN support for survival.

Umbilicus

The most common condition of the abdominal wall is an umbilical hernia (Figs. 17-118 and 17-119). This results from the failed closure of the fascial ring during the first few years of life. After desiccation of the umbilical vessels and urachus and separation of the umbilical remnant in the first month of life, the umbilical ring typically undergoes closure in the next 2 to 3 years. In some patients this process never occurs. For unclear reasons there appears to be a strong familial and racial predilection for hernia development. This condition has been described as being up to 50 times more common in African Americans than in white populations. Because most of these lesions resolve spontaneously, repair is typically deferred until the fifth birthday. Patients with hernias that are larger than 2 cm in diameter, have a proboscoid or "elephant's trunk" appearance (usually due to a supraumbilical component) (Fig. 17-120), or have a history of incarceration should not have their surgery delayed.

Figure 17-119 Most infants with umbilical hernia undergo spontaneous closure by age 3 to 4 years. Those that persist require repair.

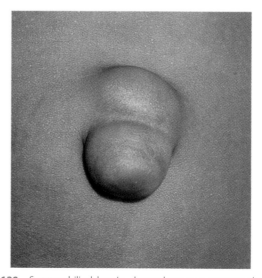

Figure 17-120 Supraumbilical hernia, shown here as a crescent-shaped defect above an umbilical hernia, does not close spontaneously and requires repair.

Figure 17-117 Large abdominal wall defects that cannot be closed primarily may undergo a staged closure with silo placement and daily reductions until the bowel rests comfortably in the abdominal cavity.

Figure 17-121   Omphalomesenteric duct remnant with communication to the umbilicus with meconium exuding from the umbilicus and meconium staining of the abdominal wall **(A)**. Intraoperative view showing omphalomesenteric duct leading from the bowel to the umbilicus **(B)**.

After desiccation of the umbilical remnant, a polypoid mucosal-appearing lesion may persist at the base of the umbilicus. These are most often umbilical granulomas and represent residual hypertrophic granulation tissue at the base of the cord. These are typically managed with topical treatments including alcohol or silver nitrate sticks. Yellow serous or feculent brown drainage from an apparent umbilical granuloma should raise concerns for a patent urachus or persistence of an omphalomesenteric duct sinus. Drainage of yellow serous fluid is suspicious for urine and in the presence of a patent urachus represents the precordial connection between the allantois and the fetal bladder. The persistence of these anomalies raises concern for bladder outlet obstruction and mandates a urologic workup consisting of ultrasound of the bladder and kidney for signs of obstructive uropathy and voiding cystourethrogram. Persistence of an omphalomesenteric sinus may lead to the development of an internal hernia or volvulus (Fig. 17-121). Surgical exploration to ligate the fistula and resect the omphalomesenteric duct remnant is indicated.

Inguinal and Scrotal Disorders

Aberrant descent of the gonads and processus vaginalis gives rise to numerous disorders including hernias, hydroceles, undescended testicles, and testicular torsion (Fig. 17-122). During embryonic development the testicles have their origin at the base of the kidney. Testicular descent leads to an outpouching or evagination of the peritoneal cavity, the processus vaginalis, which follows the gubernaculum into the scrotum. After completion of testicular descent, the processus vaginalis obliterates, separating the scrotum from the peritoneal cavity. Failure of obliteration results in a persistent patent processus that may allow fluid (hydrocele) or intraperitoneal viscera (intestine, bladder, or ovary) to enter the sac (Figs. 17-123 and 17-124). In girls, fusion of the processus vaginalis occurs earlier in embryonic development, which explains their markedly decreased incidence of inguinal hernias. The ovary is typically found in the hernia sac in girls (Fig. 17-125). Clinically, hernias present as bulges in the groin and scrotum (upper labia majora) that increase in size with Valsalva maneuvers including coughing, straining, or crying. Usually the mass reduces spontaneously or with gentle upward manual pressure on the hernia and downward testicular traction. An inability to reduce the mass should raise concerns for incarceration. Alternatively, persistent inguinoscrotal swelling may represent a nonreducible hydrocele or undescended or retractile testicle.

Identification of pediatric hernias on routine physical examination is sometimes difficult. Several provocative maneuvers including induced crying, coughing, gentle abdominal pressure, or other forced Valsalva maneuvers may be helpful. Patients should be examined in both supine and

Normal | Congenital hydrocele | Hydrocele of the cord | Incomplete hernia | Complete hernia

☐ Spermatic cord   ☐ Obliterated processus vaginalis

Figure 17-122   Abnormalities of the processus vaginalis.

Figure 17-123   An incomplete inguinal hernia produces a bulge in the left groin but does not extend into the scrotum.

Figure 17-124 A complete inguinal hernia extends into the scrotum, obscuring the testis.

Figure 17-126 A red, tender hemiscrotum may be due to torsion of the testis with gangrene, a surgical emergency.

upright positions. Despite these attempts, the hernia may not be visualized. The presence of a reliable history and the palpation of a thickened processus vaginalis or "silk glove" sign are adequate evidence to proceed with herniorrhaphy. The "silk glove" sign is the sensation on direct palpation of the spermatic cord as it gently glides between two layers of tissue—"silk." This represents the layers of processus vaginalis or hernia sac. Alternatively, parents may be asked to take a picture of the inguinal region and return when a definite bulge appears. Formerly, herniograms were used to assist in the diagnosis of these difficult cases. However, the attendant complications and risk of pelvic and gonadal radiation have diminished the utility of this study. On occasion other noninvasive studies such as ultrasound have been suggested in these difficult cases.

The presence of an inguinal hernia is an indication for prompt repair. These hernias do not resolve spontaneously and have a high risk of incarceration (up to 30%), the inability to reduce the inguinal hernia into the peritoneal cavity, in the first few months of life. Incarceration may be due to strangulation. Strangulated hernias develop intestinal and/or testicular ischemia with subsequent infarction due to vascular entrapment. Incarceration is associated with severe irritability and emesis. The groin hernia becomes erythematous, edematous,

and tender. Signs of complete intestinal obstruction may occur with associated ileus, emesis, and bloody stools. Systemic sepsis from bowel ischemia may occur.

Acute scrotal inflammation is often a surgical emergency (Fig. 17-126). This may occur not only with incarcerated inguinal hernias but also with other important conditions such as torsion of the testicle, torsion of the appendix testis, testicular trauma, and epididymo-orchitis. Testicular torsion is associated with an acutely tender testicle that may be retracted toward the inguinal region and lie in a somewhat transverse orientation in the scrotum (Fig. 17-127). Torsion of the

Figure 17-127 Twisting of the spermatic cord in testicular torsion pulls the testis proximally, making it lie in a transverse axis. The dark, congested epididymis is seen overlying and to the left of the testis.

Figure 17-125 Ovaries are frequently found in the hernia sac of young girls.

Figure 17-128 The congested, twisted appendix testis contrasts with the normal pale pink testis. If the appendix testis can be identified through the scrotum, scrotal exploration is unnecessary. This torsed appendix testis may appear through the translucent skin as a "blue dot" sign.

appendix testis is associated with the "blue dot" sign, which may be seen through the translucent scrotal skin of infants and young children (Fig. 17-128). This condition does not require surgery if an accurate diagnosis can be made. An antecedent history of testicular injury may assist in distinguishing testicular trauma from an incarcerated hernia. A digital rectal examination is one of the most reliable means of determining whether there is incarcerated hernia in an infant. Transrectal palpation of the internal inguinal ring for the presence of a mass or fullness suggests incarceration. Trans-scrotal transillumination is not always a reliable means of distinguishing between a hydrocele and incarcerated hernia. On occasion the thin-walled dilated bowel may transilluminate, giving the misleading impression that a hydrocele is present. Epididymo-orchitis may be associated with urinary tract symptoms or previous viral or bacterial urinary tract infection.

Hydroceles are most common in infancy and diminish significantly during childhood. They appear as scrotal swellings that may have a diurnal variation in size, often largest in the evening and smaller or absent in the morning. Most hydroceles are isolated to the scrotal region. However, on occasion an isolated inguinal hydrocele may exist that mimics an incarcerated hernia. The classic means of diagnosing hydrocele is by transillumination. Hydroceles that appear at birth are usually noncommunicating and undergo spontaneous resolution over the first year of life. Those that persist beyond 12 to 18 months of age typically have a persistent communication with the peritoneal cavity and need surgical care (Fig. 17-129). Hydroceles may also develop in older children in response to infection or trauma. Persistent hydroceles also require surgical repair. Femoral hernias are uncommon in children (Fig. 17-130).

ABDOMINAL MASSES AND TUMORS

The presence of an abdominal mass in an infant or child mandates a systematic assessment of various factors including the age of the patient, the location of the mass, characteristics of the mass (e.g., firm, cystic, mobile, fixed), and initial diagnostic imaging studies. Although important in other conditions, the history is rarely of major clinical significance in children with abdominal masses because of the protracted presentation of these lesions. On occasion, children may present with acute gastrointestinal or genitourinary tract obstruction. Typically, the physical examination and initial

Figure 17-129 Bilateral congenital hydroceles with buried penis. Groin swellings are absent, distinguishing them from hernias. The fluid collections may fluctuate in size, filling and emptying through a patent processus vaginalis. Spontaneous closure of the processus and absorption of fluid around the testis generally occur, reserving hydrocelectomy for those that persist after age 2 years.

radiographic studies lead to the development of a differential diagnosis that will focus efforts at diagnosis. This serves as a framework from which to further define the nature of the disease.

Location is the most important factor for determining the tissue of origin and behavior of an abdominal mass (Fig. 17-131). Retroperitoneal masses are often solid in nature and fixed to adjacent structures. Intraperitoneal masses that arise from the bowel, mesentery, or omentum are usually cystic and mobile. Dense fibrous adhesions encasing inflammatory lesions may also restrict mobility. Cystic intraabdominal lesions arising from the gastrointestinal or genitourinary tract are usually benign in nature. In contrast, solid intraabdominal lesions are predominantly malignant. Extraabdominal manifestations (metastases and associated congenital anomalies) should always be investigated. Age is the second most

Figure 17-130 Swelling below the inguinal ligament identifies a femoral hernia, extremely rare in childhood.

| Table 17-5 | Possible Diagnoses of Abdominal Masses in Infancy and Childhood |

Region	Organ	Diagnosis
Epigastrium	Stomach	Distended stomach from pyloric stenosis, duplication
	Pancreas	Pseudocyst
Flank	Kidney	Hydronephrosis, Wilms tumor, dysplastic kidney, ureteral duplication
	Adrenal	Neuroblastoma, ganglioneuroblastoma, ganglioneuroma
	Retroperitoneum	Neuroblastoma, ganglioneuroblastoma, ganglioneuroma, teratoma
Lower abdomen	Ovary	Dermoid, teratoma, ovarian tumors, torsion of ovary
	Kidney	Pelvic kidney
	Urachus	Urachal cyst
	Omentum, mesentery	Omental, mesenteric, peritoneal cysts
Pelvis	Bladder, prostate	Obstructed bladder, rhabdomyosarcoma
	Uterus, vagina	Hydrometrocolpos, hydrocolpos, rhabdomyosarcoma
Right upper quadrant	Biliary tract	Cholecystitis, choledochal cyst
	Liver	Hepatomegaly resulting from congestion, hepatitis, or tumor; mesenchymal hamartoma; hemangioendothelioma; hepatoblastoma; hepatocellular carcinoma; hepatic abscess; hydatid cyst
	Intestine	Intussusception, duplication
Left upper quadrant	Spleen	Splenomegaly resulting from congestion, infectious mononucleosis, leukemic infiltration or lymphoma; splenic abscess; cyst
Right lower quadrant	Appendix	Appendiceal abscess
	Ileum	Meconium ileus, inflammatory mass (complicated Crohn disease), intestinal duplication
	Lymphatics	Lymphoma, lymphangioma
Left lower quadrant	Colon	Fecal impaction
	Lymphatics	Lymphoma, lymphangioma

important factor in determining the differential diagnosis of abdominal masses. Table 17-5 summarizes the causes of abdominal masses by age and location.

Plain abdominal radiography often provides basic information in determining the location and potential differential diagnosis of an abdominal mass. Bowel displacement from the pelvis suggests the presence of a pelvic extraluminal mass. In contrast, intraluminal lesions may lead to a small bowel obstruction pattern as seen in meconium ileus, intussusception, or constipation. Calcification seen within the mass on plain film suggests the presence of a malignant lesion such as a neuroblastoma, rhabdomyosarcoma, or teratoma. Ultrasonography is traditionally the initial diagnostic tool of choice in patients with abdominal masses. This modality allows the differentiation of solid versus cystic lesions, a critical first stage of evaluation. Ultrasonography may characterize the lesion as arising within the kidney or in the juxtarenal location. Alternatively, pelvic lesions may also be determined as being cystic or solid in nature (Fig. 17-132). CT allows precise anatomic differentiation of abdominal lesions and the assessment of extraabdominal disease.

CT has become the study of choice by surgeons and other interventionalists in the evaluation of patients with abdominal masses. Because of its utility for assessing extent of local disease, the sites of distant metastases and the character of the lesion, the use of the upper and lower gastrointestinal contrast, in conjunction with intravenous contrast, allows for careful analysis of abdominal and pelvic structures. The presence of bilateral nephrograms and caliceal excretion of contrast is a critical factor if the patient is to undergo a nephrectomy as part of his or her surgical therapy. MRI may be of some utility in patients with abdominal masses; however, in infants this is a somewhat cumbersome study because it is relatively slower and mandates intravenous sedation.

Figure 17-131 Location of commonly found abdominal masses in children. GI, gastrointestinal; MCD, minimal change disease; LLQ, left lower quadrant; RLQ, right lower quadrant.

Liver mass
Choledochal cyst
Benign tumors
Malignant tumors

RLQ mass
Appendiceal abscess
Lymphoma
Ectopic kidney
Ovarian or testicular mass

Lower midline mass
Hydrometrocolpos
Ovarian cyst or tumor
Sacrococcygeal teratoma

Flank
Liver

Flank
Spleen
Gastric

Midline

RLQ   Lower
       midline   LLQ

Flank mass
MCD kidney
Hydronephrosis
Renal vein thrombosis
Neuroblastoma
Wilms tumor
Adrenal hemorrhage

Midline mass
GI duplication
Mesenteric cyst
Omental cyst
Urachal cyst
Meconium pseudocyst
Pancreatic pseudocyst

LLQ mass
Fecal impaction
Ovarian or testicular mass

Figure 17-132 A pelvic neuroblastoma causes compression of the rectum on barium enema study.

Figure 17-134 Posterior urethral valves cause dilation of the bladder and both upper tracts, shown here on anteroposterior **(A)** and lateral **(B)** views of a retrograde contrast study.

Neonates

Neonatal abdominal masses are benign genitourinary lesions in 75% to 80% of cases. The most common abdominal masses are congenital obstructive hydronephrosis and multicystic dysplastic kidney. Congenital hydronephrosis presents as a bulky, smooth, flank mass on physical examination; it is usually secondary to ureteropelvic junction obstruction (Fig. 17-133) and is treated by pyeloplasty to prevent further loss of renal parenchyma or the development of infection. Other genitourinary anomalies such as ureteral duplications and ureteroceles may produce obstructive uropathies that lead to palpable masses. Bilateral flank masses with hydroureteronephrosis may result from posterior urethral valves, the most common cause of distal urinary tract obstruction in boys (Fig. 17-134). Multicystic dysplastic kidney disease often occurs as a unilateral, soft, cystic mass in more than three quarters of cases (Fig. 17-135). Renal vein thrombosis may also present as an abdominal mass in the neonate. This condition is most commonly the result of hyperviscosity syndromes or severe neonatal dehydration (Fig. 17-136). Mesoblastic nephroma, a benign renal tumor that mimics Wilms tumor, is also a common mass that may present in the neonatal period.

Other common abdominal masses in the neonatal period may arise from other genitourinary organs, gastrointestinal structures, or other intraabdominal sites. Ovarian cysts are quite common in the neonatal period. Maternal hormonal stimulation in utero promotes their development, and subsequent withdrawal of this stimulus after delivery leads to their resolution. Congenital vaginal obstruction may also lead to development of a large abdominal mass. Gastrointestinal duplication cysts are often present at birth, but the diagnosis is often not made until later in childhood (Fig. 17-137). Mesenteric and omental cysts are soft, diffuse, and multiloculated lesions that may arise from the omentum or mesentery. These lesions are due to congenital lymphatic obstruction and may be a source of intraabdominal pain secondary to acute hemorrhage (Fig. 17-138). Adrenal masses are common in the newborn and in infancy. These masses may range from the benign mass associated with spontaneous adrenal hemorrhage, perinatal stress, or birth trauma to the malignant neuroblastoma (Fig. 17-139). On occasion, intraabdominal extralobar sequestration may be adjacent to the adrenal gland, suggesting the presence of a malignancy. The most common malignancy of infancy is malignant sacrococcygeal teratoma (Fig. 17-140).

Figure 17-133 The *dashed line* indicates the extent of a flank mass in an infant with ureteropelvic junction obstruction.

Figure 17-135 A multicystic kidney produces a knobby flank mass.

Figure 17-136 Renal vein thrombosis may occur as the result of hyperviscosity syndromes or severe neonatal dehydration.

Figure 17-138 Omental cyst may cause ill-defined episodic abdominal pain.

Toddlers and Young Children

In stark contrast with the neonate, the presence of an abdominal mass in a toddler or young child is almost equally as likely to be malignant as benign. Neuroblastoma, Wilms tumor, rhabdomyosarcoma, hepatoblastoma, and lymphoma are the most common pediatric solid malignancies. Although each may have histologic similarities, they all have distinct differences in behavior and prognosis that are described later.

Neuroblastoma

Neuroblastoma is the most common extracranial malignancy of childhood. The vast majority of patients present before their fifth birthday with extensive locoregional disease (stage 3) or widespread metastases (stage 4). These tumors occur along the embryonic tract of neural crest cell migration and may arise anywhere from the neck to the pelvis. They are typically multilobular and firm retroperitoneal masses that encase vessels and cross the abdominal midline. More than half occur in the adrenal or juxtarenal location (Fig. 17-141). Presenting symptoms may include local pain, abdominal distention, failure to thrive, or paralysis. Several major extraabdominal symptoms including cerebellar ataxia; opsoclonus–myoclonus, also known as *dancing eyes and feet syndrome;* and diffuse, watery diarrhea may be present. Patients may also present with remote neurologic symptoms of paralysis and weakness due to spinal cord invasion or peripheral nerve compression. The prognosis is generally poor (<25% survival). A rare variant of this malignancy known as stage 4-S disease presents with extensive local disease and widespread metastases to bone, skin, and liver in children younger than 1 year of age. Many of these patients will ultimately undergo spontaneous regression with minimal or no therapy.

The radiographic appearance of an intraabdominal neuroblastoma may reveal evidence of an upper abdominal mass with areas of stippled calcifications (Fig. 17-142). CT shows a retroperitoneal mass that crosses the midline with intimate involvement of adjacent vascular structures including the aorta, vena cava and renal vessels, and mesenteric artery. Before CT scanning, intravenous pyelography was the most frequently used modality for diagnosing retroperitoneal masses in children. This has largely been supplanted by the use of ultrasonography and CT scan imaging. A large adrenal or juxtaadrenal neuroblastoma may cause displacement of the kidney, giving a characteristic "drooping lily" sign on intravenous pyelography (Fig. 17-143). The workup of these masses includes an evaluation of the urine for the dopaminergic metabolites vanillylmandelic and homovanillic acid, abdominal and chest CT, technetium scintigraphy (bone scan), and metaiodobenzylguanidine (MIBG) scan. Serologic studies

Figure 17-137 Duplications of the gastrointestinal tract usually arise from the mesenteric border of the bowel and may be cystic **(A)** or tubular **(B)**.

Figure 17-139 Adrenal hemorrhage often results from perinatal stress or birth trauma. The radiographic appearance showing a left suprarenal heterogeneous mass is suspicious for neuroblastoma.

Figure 17-140 Sacrococcygeal teratoma may grow to be fairly large in size, causing in utero growth retardation and/or hydrops fetalis.

Figure 17-141 Adrenal neuroblastoma with signs of local metastasis to retroperitoneal lymph nodes.

including ferritin, neuron-specific enolase, and lactate dehydrogenase have prognostic significance and should be measured in all patients. Newer markers, including TRK-A expression and ganglioside GD_2 expression, may also be useful in determining long-term prognosis.

Wilms Tumor

Wilms tumor is the second most common abdominal malignancy in childhood. Approximately 450 new cases are diagnosed annually in the United States. Most children present before their fifth birthday with a bulky abdominal mass, hematuria, and/or hypertension. Although most children are healthy and asymptomatic at presentation, some children present with severe pain secondary to intratumor bleeding or, rarely, rupture. The physical examination reveals a large bulky tumor in the subcostal region that is usually firm, smooth, immobile, and nontender. Unlike neuroblastoma, at presentation these tumors usually do not cross the midline, nor are there usually signs of metastatic disease. The role of diagnostic imaging is to assess the nature of the tumor, site of origin, contralateral renal function, presence of bilateral disease, extent of local disease (involvement of the renal vessels and/or inferior vena cava), and evidence of metastases. Plain film studies in most tumors may show calcifications, but unlike neuroblastomas these tend to be more linear in appearance

Figure 17-142 **A,** Abdominal examination of a patient with a neuroblastoma, outlining the extent of the palpable tumor. **B,** CT scan of adrenal neuroblastoma with stippled calcifications. **C,** MRI demonstrating inferior displacement of the kidney by the large tumor. The tumor also has calcifications. **D,** Pathologic specimen of the patient's tumor at surgery.

Figure 17-143 Downward displacement of the entire kidney by a left adrenal neuroblastoma leaves the intrarenal collecting system anatomically intact but gives it a "drooping lily" appearance.

Figure 17-144   **A,** Abdominal CT scan of Wilms tumor shows a bulky mass to the right of midline. **B,** Intraoperative Wilms tumor with a large tumor mass involving the kidney.

Figure 17-145   A large hepatoblastoma of the right lobe of the liver. Intravenous urography, CT, and ultrasonography all identified it as a hepatic tumor instead of one arising from the kidney or an adrenal gland.

Figure 17-146   Massive splenomegaly in a patient with a lymphoproliferative disorder. This patient had early satiety and vomiting.

Figure 17-147   **A** and **B,** Laparoscopic views of a symptomatic splenic cyst in an active teenager caused disabling left upper quadrant pain.

Figure 17-148 **A,** Abdominal CT scan showing a large retroperitoneal rhabdomyosarcoma. **B,** Intraoperative view of retroperitoneal rhabdomyosarcoma extending through the mesentery, displacing the small bowel and colon.

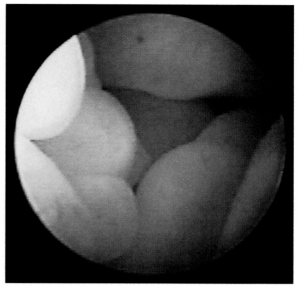

Figure 17-149 Botryoid rhabdomyosarcoma of the bladder has the characteristic "clustered grape" appearance on cystoscopy. Prognosis is usually favorable.

than stippled. CT of the chest and abdomen may answer most of the critical questions important to clinical staging (Fig. 17-144). Signs of tumor extending into the renal veins are of major surgical significance and mandate careful evaluation of the inferior vena cava and right atrium by ultrasound and echocardiography. Evidence of intracaval and right atrial thrombus requires chemotherapy before surgical resection. Lungs, lymph nodes, and the liver are the most common sites of metastasis. Formerly, clear cell sarcoma was considered to be a variant of Wilms tumor but is now believed to be a distinct pathologic entity. Bony metastases are common with this malignancy, and these patients should be evaluated by bone scan.

Hepatic Tumors in Childhood

Hepatic lesions often present in childhood. They may range from benign conditions such as hemangioendothelioma, arteriovenous malformations, mesenchymal hamartoma, and choledochal cysts (see Fig. 17-110). Hepatic tumors may present as bulky masses present in the right upper quadrant or midline that are fixed to the adjacent liver and poorly mobile (Fig. 17-145). Splenomegaly occurs from underlying hematologic diseases such as immunodeficiencies and lymphoproliferation (Fig. 17-146). A splenic cyst may also mimic splenomegaly

before radiographic evaluation. These may be congenital in nature or the result of previous trauma (Fig. 17-147).

Older Children and Teenagers

Soft Tissue Sarcoma

Rhabdomyosarcoma is the most common soft tissue sarcoma of childhood. Although these tumors have histologic features of striated skeletal muscle, they may arise anywhere in the body (Fig. 17-148). Lesions arising in pelvic locations (bladder, vagina, and paratesticular regions) have a nonalveolar histology and a more favorable prognosis (Fig. 17-149). Primary lesions are not confined to the abdominal location but may appear throughout the body. Prognosis depends on the site of occurrence and the histologic characteristics.

Lymphomas

Non-Hodgkin lymphoma may present with abdominal involvement in 25% to 50% of all cases. The peak incidence of occurrence is between 5 and 8 years of age. Most children present with abdominal pain and a palpable mass. These are rapidly growing tumors that may arise from bowel, mesentery, or retroperitoneal structures. Some children may develop an irreducible intussusception requiring surgical resection. These tumors are usually quite responsive to chemotherapy.

Ovarian Tumors

Pelvic tumors in children may also present as lower abdominal masses due to the small, shallow nature of the pediatric pelvis. The differential diagnosis of midline pelvic masses includes ovarian cysts and tumors, hydrocolpos, hydrometrocolpos, and sacrococcygeal teratoma. Ovarian masses may occur in all age groups but are most commonly seen in adolescence. More than 75% of ovarian masses are cystic and benign in nature. Twenty-five percent are solid and may have evidence of malignant changes. Ovarian cysts commonly occur in newborn infants and may be diagnosed prenatally. Many of these resolve spontaneously in the early neonatal period. Large cysts of more than 5 cm in infants are prone to undergo torsion and should be aspirated. Obstruction of the female genital tract by vaginal atresia or imperforate hymen may cause hydrocolpos in infancy

Figure 17-150   A, Imperforate hymen. Accumulated secretions in the vagina and uterus caused bulging of the hymen and a pelvic mass in this newborn. **B,** A pelvic mass arising at the expected time of menarche suggests the presence of an obstructed uterine anomaly, here demonstrated by pelvic ultrasound as an oval mass compressing the bladder anteriorly. Urinary anomalies commonly coexist. BL, bladder.

that may manifest as a large abdominal mass with respiratory embarrassment secondary to diaphragmatic compression. Alternatively, these girls may present at puberty with cyclic abdominal pain, a large pelvic or lower abdominal mass, and the absence of menses (Fig. 17-150). This occurs because of the uterine retention of menstrual products. They may also develop hydronephrosis due to extrinsic vesicoureteral obstruction and coexisting genitourinary tract anomalies, which are quite common in this population.

Inflammatory Masses

Numerous inflammatory conditions that involve intra-abdominal organs may lead to masses. Subsequent to bowel perforations associated with appendicitis, Meckel diverticulitis, or Crohn disease, the omentum and adjacent bowel loops migrate to the area and adhere to the process in an attempt to localize the condition. Development of an abscess cavity with dense fibrosis and capsule formation may mimic a lower abdominal or pelvic tumor. Typically, inflammatory masses are tender and associated with systemic symptoms. Early institution of intravenous antibiotics and percutaneous drainage may lead to earlier resolution of the mass. Children

with ventriculoperitoneal shunts may develop inflammatory pseudocysts, associated with the shunt catheter, that may become secondarily infected. This is often associated with symptoms of fever and abdominal pain. Prompt shunt exteriorization and intravenous antibiotic therapy may allow catheter salvage. Persistent symptoms of sepsis suggest the possibility of an abscess formation or bowel perforation that requires surgical exploration and catheter removal. Crohn disease may present with inflammatory lower abdominal masses or abscesses. These usually respond to aggressive medical management and may respond without surgery. Failure to respond to medical therapies suggests the presence of a stricture, or of a fistula to an adjacent bowel loop or bladder. Upper gastrointestinal contrast studies with small bowel follow-through and barium enema evaluation with reflux into the terminal ileum help delineate the extent of bowel involvement in the process.

Bibliography

Holcomb GW, Murphy JP: *Ashcraft's pediatric surgery*, ed 5, Philadelphia, 2010, WB Saunders.
O'Neill JA, Coran AG, Fonkalsrud E, et al: *Pediatric surgery*, ed 6, St. Louis, 2006, Mosby.

PEDIATRIC AND ADOLESCENT GYNECOLOGY

18

Gina S. Sucato | Pamela J. Murray

Pediatricians and other primary care providers frequently encounter children and adolescents with gynecologic concerns. Patients seek care for prepubertal vulvovaginitis, vaginal discharge, sexually transmitted infections (STIs), menstrual disorders such as dysmenorrhea and abnormal uterine bleeding, as well as other, less common diagnoses. As primary care providers increase their understanding of pediatric gynecology and adolescent medicine, a girl's first gynecologic evaluation may not require a visit to a gynecologist. Accordingly, this chapter emphasizes normal anatomy, techniques of examination, and the conditions most commonly encountered in primary care. Complementary information can be found in Chapter 6 (Child Abuse and Neglect, including detailed illustrations and definitions of genital anatomy, and additional photos of normal and abnormal genital anatomy) and in Chapter 9 (Endocrinology; illustrating Tanner staging and discussing normal, delayed, and precocious pubertal development).

NORMAL FEMALE GENITALIA

Newborn and Prepubertal

In the newborn girl the physical appearance of the genitalia reflects stimulation by maternal sex hormones (Fig. 18-1). Separation of the labia minora reveals thick, redundant hymenal folds that often hide the small central vaginal opening and urethral meatus. The mucosa is moist, vaginal pH is acidic, and a milky discharge (physiologic leukorrhea) is often seen. Vaginal bleeding during the first week of life is common. It is caused by withdrawal of maternal estrogen after delivery, and parents can be reassured that this is normal. Breast development, with palpable breast tissue, engorgement, and less commonly a clear or cloudy discharge, is observed in full-term neonates of both genders (see Chapter 2). Without ongoing stimulation from maternal estrogen, these findings gradually subside over several months. During this period, infants are at increased risk for developing breast inflammation and infection (see Chapter 12). Local trauma, including squeezing, may increase the likelihood of infection.

Similarly, the effect of maternal hormones on the female genitalia gradually disappears; the labia majora lose their fullness, and the labia minora and hymen become thinner and flatter. Separation of the labia minora usually exposes the vaginal opening (Fig. 18-2, *A* and *B*). As the young infant matures, the labia cover less of the vaginal vestibule, particularly when the infant or child is sitting, and thus offer incomplete protection from external sources of irritation. The mucosa has a glistening, reddish pink hue that on first inspection sometimes is mistaken for inflammation by observers unaccustomed to examining prepubertal genitalia. Vaginal pH is now neutral or alkaline, and secretions are minimal.

Physiologic changes also cause variations in the appearance of the hymenal tissues during childhood. During early infancy the tissues are relatively thick and can be redundant into the second year (Fig. 18-3, *A* and *B*). Usually in the first months of life, the hymen becomes thin and translucent, with smooth edges (Fig. 18-2, *A* and *B* and Fig. 18-3, *C-E*). When the child enters puberty, the hymen again thickens under the influence of estrogen.

The shape of the vaginal orifice also varies. Annular (Fig. 18-3, *C*), crescentic (Fig. 18-3, *D* and *E*), and fimbriated (with fingerlike projections around the hymenal rim) hymens are all normal variations. Other irregular shapes occur, such as a teardrop, for example, with the narrow portion formed by an anterior notch to one side of the clitoris. On rare occasions there is a completely imperforate hymen; more commonly there is a septated hymen (Fig 18-3, *F* and *G*), or a fenestrated hymen with small perforations is seen.

From about 6 to 8 weeks of age until puberty the perineum, perivaginal tissues, and pelvic supporting structures are relatively rigid and inelastic. This factor increases the likelihood of tearing as a result of trauma. In addition, before the onset of puberty, the ovaries are positioned above the pelvic brim (Table 18-1). This intraabdominal location accounts for the fact that ovarian disorders in childhood frequently present with abdominal, rather than pelvic, signs and symptoms.

Pubertal

With the onset of puberty the mons pubis begins to fill out and hair begins to grow, typically first in the mid-section. Fat deposition fills out the labia majora. The labia minora thicken, become softer and more rounded, and asymmetry and variations in size and shape become more noticed, particularly in girls who remove their pubic hair.

Girls whose labia minora protrude beyond the labia majora (Figure 18-4 often wonder if their genital appearance is normal. There is no consensus on the diagnostic criteria for labial hypertrophy, but normally the maximal width between the midline and lateral free edge of the labia minora should measure less than 3 to 5 cm. Patients with labial hypertrophy may present with pain, irritation, chronic infection, problems with personal hygiene (e.g., during menses), or problems during sports or sexual activity. Most symptoms can be alleviated by addressing personal hygiene and appropriate choice of clothing to minimize friction. Sometimes use of an antichafe product can help to prevent abrasions. Referral to a surgeon experienced in labioplasty may be considered for a mature, fully developed patient whose symptoms do not respond to conservative management. However, patients should be counseled that surgery can result in scarring, chronic vulvar pain, and dyspareunia. In most cases, reassurance and discussion of the variations in normal anatomy are all that is required.

693

Figure 18-1   Normal appearance of the genitalia in a newborn girl. The labia majora are full, and the thickened labia minora protrude between them. The mucosa is pink, and a milky white discharge is seen, reflecting stimulation by maternal hormones. *(Courtesy Ian Holzman, MD, Mt. Sinai Medical Center, New York, N.Y.)*

Other normal changes during puberty include slight enlargement of the clitoris and increased prominence of the estrogen-responsive urethral mucosa. The hymen also thickens and its central orifice enlarges. The vaginal mucosa thickens and softens and becomes moist and pink as secretions increase and pH levels drop. Perineal and pelvic tissues become more elastic, and the ovaries gradually descend into the pelvis. In the months preceding menarche, physiologic leukorrhea increases and becomes noticeable. It consists of a white discharge containing mature epithelial cells and vaginal secretions stimulated by estrogen (Fig. 18-5). In some girls the unopposed estrogen secretion of puberty stimulates leukorrhea so profuse that it becomes concerning and irritating because the perineum is constantly moist.

The developmental aspects of gynecologic anatomy and physiology are summarized in Table 18-1. There is variation in the range of normal reproductive organ size as seen on ultrasound. Some authors (Garel et al, 2001) have proposed the following as upper values for prepubertal girls: uterine length, 4.5 cm; uterine thickness, 1 cm; and ovarian volume, 4 to 5 mL. The Tanner stages of pubertal development are presented in Chapter 9.

GYNECOLOGIC EVALUATION

Examination of the Prepubertal Patient

Indications

The American Academy of Pediatrics recommends that inspection of the external genitalia be part of every general physical examination. Careful perineal inspection of girls during the first several well-child visits enables early identification of congenital anomalies of the labia and hymen. Anomalies of these external structures are rare, but if present can be associated with anomalies of the urethra and bladder. Evidence of virilization in the newborn, especially when accompanied by hyperpigmentation, should prompt immediate laboratory investigation for evidence of salt-losing adrenal hyperplasia and warrants urgent endocrinology referral.

The proximal vagina, uterus, cervix, and fallopian tubes are derived from the müllerian or paramesonephric ducts and develop concurrently with the urinary tract. Thus girls with renal or urinary tract abnormalities are at greater risk for having associated anomalies of internal genital structures. Ultrasonography has proved very useful in evaluating neonates for suspected upper genital tract anomalies, as these structures are relatively large during the neonatal period because of the influence of maternal hormones and higher levels of gonadotropins. Later in infancy and during childhood, before puberty, they may be difficult to detect because of their small size, although this is less of a problem

Figure 18-2   **A** and **B,** Normal appearance of the genitalia of a 2-year-old girl. The labia majora are flattened, and the labia minora and hymen are thin and flat. The vaginal orifice is easily seen, and the mucosa is thin, relatively atrophic, and red in color. Patient was examined in the semisupine lithotomy position. Visualization was facilitated by use of the labial traction technique **(A),** which involves grasping the labia majora between the thumbs and index fingers and gently pulling them down, laterally and slightly toward the examiner, and by the labial separation technique **(B),** which is achieved by pressing down and laterally on the labia majora with the index and middle fingers on the lower portion of the labia majora.

Figure 18-3 Normal variations in hymenal configuration. **A,** In this young infant, the redundant hymen totally obscures the vaginal orifice. **B,** In a 23-month-old the hymenal folds are redundant and the central orifice is visible. **C,** Annular orifice of a 2-year-old. Note the thin sharp edges of the hymenal membrane. **D,** Crescentic hymenal orifice. **E,** Crescentic orifice with septal remnants at 1 and 5 o'clock. **F** and **G,** Two variations of a septate hymen are seen, one in an infant and another in an older child. See also Fig. 18-7. (*A* and *B,* Courtesy Janet Squires, MD, Children's Hospital of Pittsburgh, Pittsburgh, Pa.; *C,* courtesy John McCann, MD, University of California at Davis, Davis, Calif.; *D, E,* and *G,* courtesy Pat Bruno, MD, Sunbury Community Hospital Center for Child Protection, Sunbury, Pa.; *F,* courtesy Carol Byers, CRNP, Children's Hospital of Pittsburgh, Pittsburgh, Pa.)

with skilled pediatric technicians and radiologists, and more sensitive contemporary equipment. Hence, failure to visualize internal genital structures in prepubertal girls does not equate with agenesis, and in such cases, magnetic resonance imaging (MRI) can clarify the presence or absence of pelvic organs.

Patients who have specific complaints at acute care visits also warrant inspection of the genitalia in addition to abdominal, inguinal, and (when indicated) rectal examination. These complaints include abdominal pain; dysuria, urinary frequency, urgency, incontinence, or enuresis; constipation or encopresis; perineal pruritus, pain, or other abnormal sensation; vaginal discharge or bleeding before menarche; and suspected or acknowledged sexual abuse. (Sexual abuse in the pediatric patient warrants referral to a clinician with the specialized knowledge, skills, and equipment appropriate to this evaluation.) On occasion, colposcopic, radiologic, or internal examination is indicated.

Technique

Whether the patient is being seen for a routine checkup or for a specific problem, the gynecologic portion of the assessment should occur only after establishing rapport to avoid frightening the child. Because parents and health care providers communicate their own comfort levels to children both verbally and nonverbally, a discussion of any parental anxieties and the clinician's self-awareness of his or her own attitudes can facilitate successful examination. The use of pictures and terms or language familiar to the child may further enhance cooperation, but interspersing anatomically correct vocabulary also can be educational.

For routine checkups the task involves simple external inspection. In such instances, after abdominal and inguinal examination, the clinician generally can say to patients old enough to understand, "Now, I need to take a look at your bottom, and you can help me." The desired position for

| Table 18-1 | Developmental Gynecologic Anatomy and Physiology |

	Newborn	**Early Childhood**	**Peripuberty (9-13 Years)**	**Postmenarche (>13 Years)**
Ovarian size and location	Not palpable	Pelvic brim	Within pelvis	1.5 × 2.5 × 4 cm	
Ovarian volume (mL)	0.3-1.7	0.3-1.9	2-8	8-20	
Uterine length (cm)	2.5-4.0	2.0-3.0	3.2-5.4	8.0 (nulliparous) (8 × 5 × 2.5)	
Corpus-to-cervix ratio	3:1	2:1	1:1	2:1-3:1	
Vaginal length (cm)	4	4-5	7-8.5	10-12	
Hymen orifice diameter (mm)	1-4	1-6	5-10	10	
Hymen thickness	Thick	Thin	Thickening	Variable	
Clitoris width (mm)	5	2-5	2-5	5-10	
Clitoris length (mm)	10-15	10-20	10-20	15-20	
Labia minora	Smooth	Smooth, flat	Progressive increase in size and prominence	Tanner stages IV-V completed	
Labia majora	Hairless, prominent	Hairless, thin	Hair growth, labial growth	Separation and differentiation of labia minora and majora	
Vaginal secretions	White or clear, copious	Minimal	White or clear, variable amount, at times profuse	White or clear, variable amount	
pH	5.5-7.0	6.5-7.5	4.5-5.5	3.5-4.5	
Normal flora	Maternal enteric	Nonpathogenic flora including staphylococci and coliforms	Mixed vaginal flora	Lactobacilli dominant	
Hormonal influence	Maternal hormones	Minimal sex steroids	Low and variable levels of endogenous estrogen and androgens	High levels of endogenous cyclic hormones	
Maturation index of vaginal epithelium*				Proliferative[†] phase	Secretory[‡] phase
Parabasal (%)	0	90-100	20-70	0	0
Intermediate (%)	95	0-10	25-50	70	95
Superficial (%)	5	10	10-20	30	5

*Vaginal cells sent in liquid ThinPrep solution (Hologic, Bedford, Mass.).
[†]First half of cycle.
[‡]Second half of cycle.

examination can be explained or demonstrated and the patient shown how to maneuver into it. Drapes generally are unnecessary for toddlers and preschoolers because they are isolating and often perceived as threatening. However, similar to adolescents, school-age children may find drapes helpful in reducing embarrassment.

Young infants can be assessed easily on an examination table after being positioned by the examiner. An older infant, toddler, or preschool child tends to be more relaxed when examined on her mother's lap, with the mother assisting by gently holding the child in either the frog-leg or lithotomy position (Fig. 18-6). School-age children usually can be examined on the table in the frog-leg, lithotomy, or knee–chest position (see Chapter 6). Knee–chest positioning can provide excellent visualization of the hymen and the distal vagina

(Fig. 18-7, *C*), but proper positioning can be challenging; some patients may feel threatened by being examined from behind. An alternative means of achieving visualization of the distal vagina is with the patient supine and performing the Valsalva maneuver (i.e., asking the child to push down as if she were going to pass a stool). This often produces distention of the distal vagina and hymenal orifice, facilitating visualization and atraumatic collection of specimens.

Use of good focused lighting is essential. In the office setting the otoscope provides excellent focused light and low magnification, which is sufficient for most examinations. Since some young children fear it because of prior painful experiences during otoscopy, the patient should be reassured ahead of time that no speculum will be attached and that she will not be forcibly restrained. Preliminary "examination" of the umbilicus may help allay anxiety. Colposcopes and hand-held lenses also provide excellent magnification when available.

Once the patient is properly positioned, visualization of the introitus, hymen, and lower portion of the vagina is facilitated by maneuvers that separate the labia. These maneuvers should be explained first and the child reassured that the examiner is just going to look. If the patient desires or is mildly anxious, she may place her hands beneath the examiner's, or the mother may be enlisted to perform the maneuver. Some girls prefer to separate their labia themselves. The maneuvers include labial separation (see Fig. 18-2, *B*), and labial traction (see Figs. 18-2, *A* and 18-7, *B*). When using a hand-held light (otoscope) a second set of hands (parent or nurse) may be needed to maximize labial separation and focus the light. Care must be taken to ensure that excess traction is not applied during these maneuvers because it can result in painful tearing of labial adhesions, if present.

If the patient is unusually anxious about the procedure and cannot be reassured, the examination should be deferred to a

Figure 18-4 Eleven-year-old patient with hypertrophy of the left labium minus. *(Reprinted with permission from Pardo J, Sola V, Ricci P, et al: Laser labioplasty of labia minora, Int J Gynaecol Obstet 93:38-43, 2006.)*

Figure 18-5 Physiologic leukorrhea. **A,** A milky discharge is seen on the perineum of this normal adolescent. It consists of cervical and vaginal secretions produced in response to estrogen stimulation and can be seen in the newborn, peripubertal, and postpubertal periods. **B,** On microscopy the discharge is found to contain sheets of estrogenized vaginal epithelial cells. Leukocytes are not increased and lactobacilli are the predominant flora.

later date. On occasion, use of an oral benzodiazepine, conscious sedation, or anesthesia may be needed for an adequate evaluation. At no time should a frightened, struggling child be physically restrained and forced to undergo examination; the yield is minimal and the experience physically and emotionally traumatic.

On inspection, the clinician can readily ascertain the presence or absence of pubic hair; note the appearance and configuration of the labia majora, labia minora, clitoris, urethra, hymen, and vaginal orifice; observe the color of the mucosa and the presence or absence of rash or discharge; and often visualize the distal vagina. Vaginoscopy is required only occasionally in the prepubertal child in order to perform a complete evaluation for complaints such as vaginal bleeding with or without evidence of trauma, discharge resistant to routine therapy, a suspected vaginal foreign body, and suspected vaginal tumors. Because of the high potential for inflicting pain, especially if the patient moves suddenly, vaginoscopy generally is best performed under anesthesia or sedation. Some older school-age children may tolerate internal examination by a highly skilled examiner without sedation if preparation is careful. Again, a traumatic experience should be avoided.

Patients with precocious puberty, suspected abdominal masses, suspected vaginal foreign body, and/or abdominal pain should undergo rectal bimanual examination (vaginal bimanual examination is rarely if ever necessary). Use of adequate lubricant, having the child perform a Valsalva maneuver as the finger is inserted into the rectum, and gentle technique reduce discomfort. In most cases this can be accomplished readily in the office. If the patient is unable to cooperate, the procedure should be deferred and an examination under anesthesia considered when warranted on the basis of clinical circumstances or the results of ancillary studies such as sonography or MRI. Computed tomography involves greater radiation exposure and provides poorer resolution of pelvic structures and thus should be used only to provide information not obtainable by other imaging studies.

Specimen Collection

If a prepubertal child with vaginal discharge or perineal or urinary complaints is to be evaluated, it is advisable to ask the family not to bathe the patient or to apply any creams for at least 12 hours before the examination. The patient should always be prepared for the procedure with simple and truthful explanations. Routine bacterial cultures, including those for gonococci, can be collected from any visible discharge on the perineum in the prepubertal child. If no discharge is visible, having her perform a Valsalva maneuver may bring some discharge down to the introitus. If this fails and specimens must be collected because of a history of vaginal discharge, specimens can be collected with little discomfort with a Dacron wire swab; this should also be used to collect *Chlamydia* cultures (required in sexual abuse evaluations), which require superficial epithelial cells from the vaginal wall. Herpes cultures should be obtained from the base of unroofed fresh vesicles or ulcers.

To collect specimens of vaginal secretions for culture, wet mounts, or to evaluate the maturation index of vaginal epithelial cells (see Table 18-1), the Dacron wire swab should be premoistened with sterile nonbacteriostatic saline. Before starting, it is often helpful to allow the patient to handle a moistened swab and touch herself with it. The swab is inserted gently through the vaginal opening, taking care to avoid contact with the hymen, which is exquisitely sensitive. This is most easily accomplished with the patient in the knee–chest position or with use of the Valsalva maneuver. However, if collection is likely to be difficult because of pain or anxiety

Figure 18-6 Optimal positions for perineal inspection of the young prepubertal girl. This patient has skin desquamation subsequent to a streptococcal infection. **A,** Frog-leg position on the mother's lap. **B,** Lithotomy position on the mother's lap.

Figure 18-7   Perineal visualization in various positions and with various techniques of parting the labia (see also Figure 18-2, *A* and *B*). **A-C,** Views of the same child taken on the same day and clearly showing the variations in appearance when using different positions and different techniques to facilitate visualization of the introitus and lower third of the vagina. **A,** Supine frog-leg position. **B,** Supine frog-leg position using labial traction. **C,** knee–chest position. (**A-C,** *Courtesy Mary Carrasco, MD, Mercy Hospital, Pittsburgh, Pa.)*

or because the hymenal orifice is very small, application of a topical anesthetic to the perineal and hymenal area beforehand can be beneficial. Although topical lidocaine preparations work within 5 to 10 minutes, they can produce transient discomfort before the onset of anesthetic action, reducing cooperation in some patients. When time permits, use of a newer topical anesthetic cream (e.g., EMLA or LMX) is an excellent alternative. Dry cotton-tipped swabs should be avoided because they tend to abrade the thin vaginal mucosa of the prepubertal child. Table 18-2 lists the specimens that may be considered in evaluating patients with symptoms of vulvitis, vaginitis, or vaginal discharge.

The newer nucleic acid amplification tests (NAATs) are highly sensitive and specific in detecting *Neisseria gonorrhoeae* and *Chlamydia trachomatis,* and offer the advantage that specimens may be collected from a variety of sites (vaginal wall, urine, urethra, cervix). Product variations necessitate careful adherence to the manufacturer's instructions regarding acceptable collection sites or specimens to ensure optimal results. If forensic evidence is needed, obtaining specimens for gonococcus and *Chlamydia* cultures is advised. In addition, in cases of symptomatic gonococcal infection where there are concerns about antibiotic resistance, a culture with sensitivities may also be desirable to ensure proper antibiotic selection, because sensitivities are not part of NAAT testing. When suspicious of infection with *Trichomonas* in a prepubertal patient, because of a history of sexual abuse, or wet prep findings, a confirmation either by culture incubated in Diamond medium or by NAAT is recommended.

Examination of the Pubertal Patient

Indications

Continuing the practice of routine inspection of the external genitalia at each well-child visit beyond infancy facilitates early diagnosis of any new problems that may arise and allows evaluation of physical growth and secondary sex characteristics that are important to assess during the peripubertal and pubertal periods. This practice also creates an opportunity to discuss normal anatomy and behaviors, including masturbation; to distinguish acceptable from unacceptable (exploitative or abusive) forms of touching; and to help overcome the reluctance of some parents and children to express concerns

about the genitalia. Ultimately, making assessment and counseling a routine part of well-child care may help reduce anxiety and embarrassment for the child when genital or pelvic examinations are required to evaluate medical concerns.

A gynecologic examination should be considered for any patient with a variety of specific complaints and concerns, including those listed in Box 18-1. This examination should include careful inspection of the external genitalia and regional lymph nodes, and palpation of the uterus and adnexa when indicated. In some cases precise assessment of internal pelvic structures may require radiologic imaging. For example, during puberty, if menarche is delayed or menstrual periods are unusually problematic (e.g., excessive pain, unusually irregular flow patterns), ultrasound evaluation can be useful.

Use of a speculum is typically not required but is useful in situations that necessitate visual inspection of the vaginal cavity or cervix, including those listed in Box 18-2. Furthermore, the gynecologic examination is an important part of routine health care for sexually active adolescent girls (Box 18-3), and should be considered at 6-month intervals with greater or lesser frequency depending on behavioral risk factors. In the absence of the above indications, a speculum could first be considered at age 21 years. At this age women should undergo their first cervical cytology screening, using liquid-based cytology or traditional Papanicolaou (Pap) smear, according to recommendations from the Committee on Adolescent Health Care of the American College of Obstetricians and Gynecologists (ACOG, 2010).

Technique

A thorough and directed history precedes the examination. A comprehensive outline is suggested in Table 18-3. Adequate time should be devoted to interviewing the patient alone, which provides an opportunity to ask questions about voluntary and involuntary sexual activity and to explore other concerns that may be difficult to discuss in the presence of a parent. A similar opportunity should be given to the parents to express any particular concerns or worries that they have been reluctant to share in their daughter's presence.

The nature of the initial experience with pelvic examination may greatly affect a young woman's comfort with her body and the ease with which she experiences routine gynecologic care and sexual relations throughout her adult life. Hence, the examiner's approach should be sympathetic, unhurried, and

BOX 18-1

Indications for Gynecologic Examination in Pubertal Patient

ABNORMAL VAGINAL DISCHARGE

PAIN

Pelvic

Perineal

Dysuria

Abdominal (unexplained)

SUSPECTED SEXUAL ABUSE*

CONCERNS WITH PUBERTAL DEVELOPMENT†

No secondary sexual development by age 14 yr

No menarche if start of puberty more than 2 yr ago

No menarche by age 16 yr

Abnormal timing or sequence of pubertal development

Anatomic abnormalities on genital inspection

Increased body hair, severe acne, or masculinization

MENSTRUAL DISTURBANCES

Dysmenorrhea not responsive to standard treatment

Amenorrhea or oligomenorrhea

Abnormal uterine bleeding or polymenorrhea

SEXUAL ACTIVITY

Routine health care for sexually active individual

Sexual contact with partner with a suspected or confirmed STD or related genital symptoms

*See Chapter 6.
†See Chapter 9.
 STD, sexually transmitted disease.

sensitive to the modesty of the patient. When patients have had gynecologic examinations in the past, it is helpful to ask them about their prior experience to avoid repeating any previous emotional or physical trauma.

Young women should be given the choice of being examined with or without an accompanying adult in the room. Some patients, particularly early adolescents, may be conflicted between their extreme modesty and their desire for support from an accompanying friend, partner, or family member. Suggesting that the support person must stay at the head of the table and using drapes that allow visual (eye) contact between patient and examiner is often the most comfortable compromise for younger adolescents. A chaperone

BOX 18-2

Indications for Use of a Speculum during Gynecologic Examination

Pap smear (patients over 21 yr old; earlier in sexually active immune-compromised patients)
Persistent unexplained bleeding
Persistent vaginal discharge
Suspected injury
Suspected foreign body
Suspected anatomic abnormality (e.g., vaginal septum, duplicated cervix)
Sexual assault*

*If assault occurred in the previous 72 hours the patient should be evaluated in a setting equipped to collect and safeguard forensic specimens.

Table 18-2 | Laboratory Investigations for the Evaluation of Gynecologic Complaints

Laboratory Study/ Specimen	Diagnostic Utility
Saline wet mount	Inflammatory cells, yeast, trichomonads, clue cells, lactobacilli, mature and immature epithelial cells, sperm
KOH	Yeast, "whiff test" for bacterial vaginosis (also can be positive with *Trichomonas*)
Vaginal pH	Elevated in bacterial vaginosis (also can be elevated with *Trichomonas*). Obtain from lateral or anterior vaginal wall, not from pooled secretions or saline-diluted specimen
Vaginal specimens	Routine culture (Amies medium without charcoal) for nonvenereal pathogens Culture for enteric bacteria including *Shigella* (Cary-Blair medium) Culture for gonorrhea,* *Trichomonas*, *Chlamydia* (if forensic evidence needed) NAAT for gonorrhea, *Trichomonas, Chlamydia*
Cervical specimens	Culture for gonorrhea* or *Chlamydia* (for forensic evidence); NAAT for gonorrhea or *Chlamydia*
Pap smear/ThinPrep	Squamous intraepithelial lesions; consequences of HPV including precancerous and cancerous lesions; cell maturation index (estrogenization)
Genital ulcer/lesion specimen	HSV culture (if suspect chancroid use moistened swab at base of lesion and transport as rapidly as possible in Amies medium without charcoal; send to reference laboratory to test for *Haemophilus ducreyi*)
Biopsy	Dysplastic, atrophic, or unusual lesions of vulva, vagina, and cervix
Urine specimen	Urinalysis; urine culture; gonorrhea, or *Chlamydia* NAAT
Perianal specimen	Pinworms and eggs: Parent obtains sample during night (or first thing in morning before patient bathes) by pressing firmly over anal area with a pinworm paddle (optically clear polystyrene paddle connected to cap of a transport container) or a 1-inch strip of cellophane tape (which is then affixed to a glass slide)
Serologic tests	Syphilis (RPR and *Treponema*-specific testing), HIV

HIV, human immunodeficiency virus; HPV, human papillomavirus; HSV, herpes simplex virus; NAAT, nucleic acid amplification test; RPR, rapid plasma reagin.
  *Use Amies medium with charcoal.

BOX 18-3

Routine Screening for the Sexually Active Adolescent*

EXTERNAL GENITAL EXAMINATION AND BIMANUAL EXAMINATION

Every 6-12 mo and to evaluate symptoms or exposure to a new partner

SPECIFIC TESTING FOR GC, CT, HIV, AND SYPHILIS

Every 6-12 mo and to evaluate symptoms or exposure to a new partner

WET MOUNT WITH KOH PREPARATION AND VAGINAL PH

Every 6-12 mo and to evaluate symptoms or exposure to a new partner

VERIFICATION OF HISTORY OF VACCINATION FOR HEPATITIS A AND B AND FOR HPV

Every visit until fully immunized

PREGNANCY TEST

Every 6-12 mo and if any history of underprotected sexual intercourse

*See also the following Centers for Disease Control and Prevention website: *Sexually transmitted diseases (STDs)*, www.cdc.gov/std/treatment/default.htm
  CT, *Chlamydia*; GC, gonorrhea; HPV, human papillomavirus.

Table 18-3	Complete History of an Adolescent with Gynecologic Concerns
Category of Information	**Specific Information Required**
General	
Home	Who lives there and quality of relationships; sources of conflict and support
Education/employment	School, grades, curriculum, repeated grades, goals, behavioral or learning difficulties; if working—type, occupational hazards, hours, literacy/numeracy
Activities	Exercise, nutritional content (specifically calcium, iron, fat, fiber, folate), body image, eating behaviors/patterns, peer activities, friends, hobbies
Drugs	Caffeine, tobacco, alcohol, marijuana, crack, cocaine, heroin, hallucinogens, pills, injectable drugs; rehabilitation or treatment history
Suicide	Depression, anxiety, psychiatric treatment, medications, major losses or disruptions, counseling history
Abuse/exploitation	Physical, sexual, or emotional; family, relationship, peer, school, and community violence or exploitation
Obstetric and Gynecologic History	
Menstrual	Menarche (age); cycles (length, duration, quantity of flow, use of pads or tampons); first day of last menstrual period; dysmenorrhea and associated disability; premenstrual symptoms (PMS); abnormal bleeding; mid-cycle pain (mittelschmerz) and spotting; douching; feminine hygiene product use (including scented products and deodorants)
STI	Herpes, gonorrhea, *Chlamydia*, syphilis, PID, pubic lice ("crabs"), HPV (venereal warts), *Trichomonas*, HIV, hepatitis A, B, and C, undiagnosed pelvic pain
Pap	Abnormal results, colposcopy, biopsies, treatments, follow-up
Urologic	Urinary tract infection or kidney problems, enuresis, incontinence, dysuria, urgency, frequency
Vaginal discharge	Color, odor, quantity, duration, pruritus
Vaginal infections	Yeast, bacterial vaginosis, trichomoniasis
Obstetric	Previous pregnancies and outcomes, fertility plans and concerns
Sexual	Last and other recent intercourse and protection; specific HIV risk to self and partners; sexual experience and age at onset; sexual practices, condom use; gender of partners, sexual orientation; number of partners, lifetime and recent; satisfaction with sexual experience; sexual problems with self or partner
Contraceptive	Current and past methods, satisfaction, consistency of use, problems
Past Medical History	Prior sources of care (routine, episodic, and emergency); immunization status including hepatitis A and B and HPV; rubella and varicella status; hypertension; migraines with aura or neurologic signs; thromboembolic events
Medications/Treatment	History of self-treatment with over-the-counter or prescription medications, and any integrative therapies or medications
Family History	Thromboembolic events at an early age or associated with pregnancy or with hormonal contraceptives; disease or death caused by alcohol, drugs, tobacco; gynecologic or obstetric problems; age at childbearing; endocrine problems (especially thyroid); bleeding problems (especially OB/GYN-related bleeding, mucus membrane bleeding, or need for blood transfusion); congenital malformations; mental retardation; reproductive loss

HIV, human immunodeficiency virus; HPV, human papillomavirus; PID, pelvic inflammatory disease; PMS, premenstrual syndrome; STI, sexually transmitted infection.

(such as a nurse) is desirable for all examinations. This should be offered to all patients and is considered standard when the examiner is male, is a trainee, or when there is a history of sexual abuse.

The pelvic examination is done after other components of the physical examination. The patient should empty her bladder beforehand, and a urine specimen can be collected at this time if needed for testing. Raising the head of the examining table 20 to 45 degrees helps relax abdominal muscles and facilitates maintenance of visual contact with the patient. She is then assisted into the lithotomy position at the end of the examination table. During the examination, the examiner should talk to the patient to explain what she or he is seeing and to provide reassurance and education. Maintaining a dialogue throughout the procedure also usually helps the patient relax. Conversation can confirm normal anatomic findings and provide the patient with examples of a correct and comfortable vocabulary describing her reproductive anatomy and function. A hand mirror held by the patient is often useful for similar reasons. Before beginning, the examiner should carefully explain the various parts of the examination: inspection of the external genitalia, speculum examination of the vagina and cervix (with specimen collection), and bimanual palpation. Use of anatomic drawings and/or models can be helpful and educational (Fig. 18-8). Gloves should be worn for both external and internal examinations.

Patient comfort with being touched may be increased by identifying and then touching distal areas first and moving proximally (e.g., knees, thighs, groin, labia, introitus). Next, the external genitalia are inspected. Pubic hair distribution should be noted as should the presence of any nits, lice, skin or vulvar lesions, or vaginal discharge on the perineum. The introital opening is examined and its edges palpated for any

swellings in the regions of the Bartholin glands. Clitoral size is assessed. The urethral opening is then inspected for erythema or discharge. Any purulent material obtained should be cultured for gonorrhea, but swabs used to obtain *Chlamydia* cultures from the urethra and any other sites must have direct contact with the mucosal surface, rather than the discharge itself.

If a speculum examination is required, successful examination depends on adequate patient preparation and use of appropriate instruments. For virginal adolescents, the narrow-bladed Huffman speculum ($\frac{1}{2} \times 4\frac{1}{4}$ inches) is recommended. Although long enough to expose the cervix, its narrow blades are usually inserted easily through the virginal introitus. Most sexually active adolescents can be examined with the straight-sided Pederson speculum ($\frac{7}{8} \times 4$ inches); however, the Huffman speculum should be considered as an alternative for

Figure 18-8 Anatomic drawings are useful for education and to prepare adolescent patients for gynecologic examination.

Figure 18-9 *From left to right:* The Graves speculum is best reserved for large or gravid adolescents; the Pederson speculum is adequate for most sexually active adolescents; the narrow-bladed Huffman is ideal for virginal adolescents.

a first pelvic examination or for particularly anxious patients. The duck-billed Graves speculum ($1\frac{3}{8} \times 3\frac{3}{4}$ inches) is useful in parous patients (Fig. 18-9). Obese patients may require a Graves speculum or a longer Pederson ($1 \times 4\frac{3}{4}$ inches) for adequate visualization of the cervix. Metal speculums are preferred because they are easier to manipulate and are available in a greater range of lengths and widths. If only a single size of disposable plastic speculum is routinely used at a facility, it is important to have a backup supply of smaller metal speculums.

The patient should be shown the speculum and allowed to touch it if she so desires. Patients experiencing their first pelvic examination should be reassured that only the blades of the speculum will be inserted. Comparing the size of an open speculum to a finger or tampon often is reassuring. The patient should be told that she will feel "a sense of pressure," not pain, during speculum insertion and should be reminded to breathe at a regular rate because tensing abdominal or pelvic muscles can produce discomfort and make the examination more difficult to perform.

The examiner may then gently insert the index finger into the vagina to assess the size of the introital opening and to locate the cervix. Vaginal muscle tone can be assessed by asking the patient to "tighten her muscles" around the examiner's finger. Conscious relaxation can be practiced by asking the patient to relax those same muscles and to push her buttocks onto the examining table. Both plastic and metal speculums should be moistened with warm water to increase comfort and ease of insertion. With the index finger partially withdrawn but gently pressing on the vaginal floor, the speculum is inserted over the finger into the vagina, taking care to avoid catching pubic hairs or the labia in the mechanism of the speculum. This is done at an oblique angle along the posterior wall to accommodate the vertical introitus and avoid traumatizing the urethra, which lies above the anterior vaginal wall. Another technique that effectively assists insertion involves using the middle and index fingers to stretch the posterior labial folds down and out before inserting the speculum. With the speculum in place the vaginal walls are inspected for erythema, lesions, and quality and quantity of discharge, and specimens are collected (see Specimen Collection, below).

After specimens have been collected the speculum is removed, and the bimanual (vaginal–abdominal) examination is performed. Water-based lubricant is placed on the two gloved fingers to be used before inserting them carefully through the introitus into the vagina. The examiner should note the size, consistency, position, and mobility of the uterus and check for tenderness on cervical or fundal motion. The adnexa should be palpated for evidence of enlargement or tenderness. After changing the glove on the examining hand, a rectovaginal examination using the index and middle fingers may be performed to confirm an abnormal or uncertain finding on vaginal–abdominal examination, to palpate the cul-de-sac, and to examine a retroflexed uterus.

Once the examination is completed, the patient should be helped out of the lithotomy position, given tissues to wipe away any lubricant or discharge, and allowed privacy to get dressed. At the conclusion of the visit the examiner can present the results of any office-based testing (such as microscopic evaluation of wet mount and KOH preparation). The use of handouts, printed pictures, or line drawings can enhance the patient's understanding of the results (see Fig. 18-8). This is also an opportunity to encourage communication between the young woman and her parent, as appropriate to the circumstance.

Specimen Collection

Adolescents should be advised not to douche or to use tampons or feminine hygiene products before a gynecologic examination. To obtain a vaginal sample for gonorrhea (GC) and *Chlamydia* (CT) NAAT, slide the swab 4 to 5 cm into the vagina and rotate it for 10 to 15 seconds, moistening it against the walls of the vagina. The vaginal pH level can be measured by moistening a cotton-tipped swab on the lateral vaginal wall and rolling it on pH paper (with an appropriate range of pH 3.6 to 6.1). Vaginal pH levels are elevated in bacterial vaginosis and tend to be increased with trichomonal and decreased with candidal infections, respectively. Vaginal secretions should also be obtained with a cotton or Dacron swab and placed in a tube with 1 mL of nonbacteriostatic normal saline for wet mount and potassium hydroxide (KOH) examination. The swabs for GC and CT NAAT and for wet mount may be obtained by the patient ("self-swab") if the patient prefers, and additional examination is not required.

To review the wet mount, a drop of the saline solution containing vaginal secretions is examined under low ($\times$10) and high ($\times$40) power for distribution of epithelial cells, leukocytes, yeast forms, *Trichomonas* organisms, and clue cells. A drop of 10% KOH is added to a second drop of the saline solution. This preparation is immediately "whiffed" for the presence of the acrid odor associated with amines that is found in bacterial vaginosis and often in patients with trichomoniasis. After this, microscopic scanning of the KOH preparation facilitates identification of yeast forms that may be obscured by epithelial cells on the wet mount.

If a speculum examination is required (see Box 18-2), the vaginal pH level is measured by holding pH paper (described previously) against the lateral vaginal wall, away from pooled secretions. Visible vaginal secretions from the posterior vaginal pool should be obtained with a cotton or Dacron swab for wet mount. Before obtaining samples from the cervix, any surface mucus should be gently removed with cotton swabs. Purulent secretions (mucopus) typically turn the swab yellow and may be saved for microscopic examination. The normal nulliparous cervix usually has a small round os (Fig. 18-10). Any cervical lesions seen, such as cysts, warts, polyps, or vesicles, should be noted. An ectropion (or eversion) of the endocervical columnar epithelium onto the cervical surface is common and normal in adolescents (Fig. 18-11). Ectropion should be distinguished from cervicitis, the latter being suggested by erythema, friability, and/or mucopurulent cervical discharge (see Fig. 18-41, *A*).

When a speculum examination is necessary, endocervical swabs can be sent to test for GC and CT as part of routine sexual health care or for the evaluation of pain, bleeding, or cervical discharge. Gonorrhea cultures are obtained by inserting a sterile swab into the endocervical canal and

Figure 18-10 Normal nulliparous cervix. The surface is covered with pink squamous epithelium that is uniform in consistency. The os is small and round. A small area of ectropion is visible inferior to the os. *(Courtesy C. Stevens.)*

rotating it for at least 10 seconds. The swab is then placed immediately into a selective transport or culture medium. Either medium must be at room temperature before inoculation. Gonorrhea-specific media prevent bacterial overgrowth by other species and allow a longer transport time. *Chlamydia* cultures require mucosal surface cells because the pathogen is an obligate intracellular organism. Dacron swabs are placed in the endocervical canal and thoroughly rotated to obtain the necessary cellular material. Wooden swabs are not acceptable for *Chlamydia* tests. NAATs, because of their ability to detect minute quantities of pathogen DNA/RNA, do not require obtaining mucosal cells for either GC or CT.

Cervical cytology (Pap) screening using liquid-based cytology to check for cervical dysplasia (a precursor of cervical cancer) is done by rotating a plastic Ayre spatula

Figure 18-11 Ectropion. Columnar mucosal cells usually found in the endocervical canal have extended out onto the surface of the cervix, creating a circular raised erythematous appearance. Note the normal nonpurulent cervical mucus. This normal variant is not to be confused with cervicitis. *(Courtesy E. Jerome, MD.)*

circumferentially (360°) around the cervical os, including the entire squamocolumnar junction. A sample from the endocervical canal is collected with a cytobrush (or a cotton swab if the patient is pregnant). Each sample is swished in liquid ThinPrep solution according to laboratory protocol. Cervical cytology results can be uninterpretable in the presence of inflammation and bleeding; therefore it is preferable to defer collection until infections are treated and menstrual bleeding has finished. However, concerns about patient follow-up or urgent clinical needs can justify collection of specimens at less optimal times. It should be noted that a number of strains of human papillomavirus (HPV) have been identified as causative in cervical cancer, as well as genital warts. However, currently available vaccines against HPV do not cover all strains associated with cervical cancer. Therefore Pap smears remain indicated for all patients 21 years and older, unless the patient has immune suppression or HIV infection, in which case annual Pap should begin with the onset of sexual activity.

GENITAL TRACT OBSTRUCTION

Labial Adhesions

The most common form of "vaginal obstruction" in prepubertal patients is really a pseudo-obstruction or partial obstruction produced by "fusion" of the labia minora as a result of labial adhesions. On inspection the clinician finds a smooth, flat membrane with a thin lucent central line overlying the introitus. It is postulated that inflammation and erosion of the superficial layers of the mucosa—whether caused by infection, dermatitis, or mechanical trauma—result in agglutination of the apposed labia minora by fibrous tissue on healing. The process typically begins posteriorly and extends forward. In most cases the fused portion is less than 1 cm in length, but on occasion it can extend to cover the vaginal vestibule and rarely the urethra (Fig. 18-12, *A* and *B*). Even when fusion is extensive, urine and vaginal secretions are able to exit through the opening anteriorly. However, some urine may become trapped behind the adhesions after toileting. This may cause further irritation, perpetuating the condition or fostering extension of the adhesions. Although most labial adhesions are asymptomatic, some patients have symptoms of lower urinary tract and vulval inflammation.

If resolution of the fused labia is desired, the condition readily responds to application of estrogen cream along the line of fusion twice daily for 2 weeks followed by nightly application for an additional week. On occasion the course needs to be extended for an additional 2 weeks, or an increased volume of estrogen cream is advised. After the labia have separated, a zinc oxide–based cream should be applied nightly for several months to prevent recurrence. The patient's parent should be informed that topical estrogen may cause transient hyperpigmentation of the labia and the areolae and an increase in breast tissue, but that these changes regress once therapy is completed. An estrogen withdrawal bleed (similar to that seen in the neonate) occasionally occurs. Removal of irritants, treatment of infections, and instructions on good perineal hygiene help prevent recurrence. Nonetheless, refusion can occur, although repeated treatment is not necessary if the child is asymptomatic.

Manual separation of fused labia is painful, traumatic, and frequently followed by a recurrence. Hence this practice should be abandoned. True fusion—adhesions present in the first months of life or adhesions that do not respond to the prescribed therapy—requires further evaluation for abnormalities in gender differentiation or androgen production.

Figure 18-12 Labial adhesions. Agglutination and adhesion of the labia minora, as a result of healing after inflammation, produce the appearance of a smooth flat surface overlying the introitus, divided centrally by a thin lucent line. **A,** In this infant, the fused portion involves the posterior half of the introitus. **B,** In another, the fused area has extended much further anteriorly. (**A,** *Courtesy Carol Byers, CRNP, Children's Hospital of Pittsburgh, Pittsburgh, Pa.;* **B,** *courtesy D. Lloyd, MD.*)

Female Genital Cutting

Female genital cutting (FGC) is another cause of genital tract obstruction seen with increasing frequency by pediatricians, especially those who care for large numbers of patients from Africa, the Middle East, and Asia. This ritual cutting and alteration of female genitalia has no known medical benefits and carries potentially life-threatening short- and long-term health consequences. Figure 18-13, *A-D* illustrates the various types of FGC. Further information about this topic can be found at the World Health Organization website (see Websites, following the bibliography). The World Health Organization is working to eliminate this practice, considering it a human rights violation of girls and women. However, pediatricians who encounter girls who have undergone these procedures must be sensitive both to the complex religious and sociocultural norms that motivate families to practice FGC as well as to the consequences to the individual patient.

Imperforate Hymen

The congenital anomaly referred to as *imperforate hymen* consists of a thick imperforate membrane located just inside the hymenal ring. This is the most common truly obstructive abnormality. It is frequently missed on the newborn examination because of the redundancy of hymenal folds. However, it may become evident by 8 to 12 weeks of age on careful perineal inspection, appearing as a thin, transparent hymenal membrane that bulges when the infant cries or strains. On occasion, young infants have copious vaginal secretions secondary to stimulation by maternal hormones, and as a result of this anomaly they develop hydrocolpos. In such cases the infant may have midline swelling of the lower abdomen (especially noticeable when the bladder is full) that feels cystic on palpation. Perineal inspection reveals a whitish, bulging membrane at the introitus. The cystic mass may also be palpable on rectal examination. In the presence of a neonatal withdrawal bleed or trauma, a hematocolpos may develop. This presents as a red or purplish bulge (Fig. 18-14). Treatment consists of incision of the membrane to allow drainage, followed by excision of redundant tissue.

If her condition goes undetected, the patient with an imperforate hymen usually develops hematocolpos in late puberty. The major complaints are intermittent lower abdominal pain and low back pain, which rapidly progress in severity and duration. Over time difficulty in urination and defecation may develop, and a lower abdominal swelling may become noticeable. The patient has well-developed secondary sex characteristics but has had no menstrual periods. Perineal inspection reveals a thick, tense, bulging membrane, often bluish in color, at the introitus (Fig. 18-15, *A*). A low cystic swelling is palpable anteriorly on rectal examination. Operative incision allows drainage of the accumulated blood and vaginal secretions (Fig. 18-15, *B*) and is followed by excision of the membrane. Other partially obstructive hymenal abnormalities may allow menstrual blood to flow but later cause difficulty inserting tampons or initiating intercourse. Because hymens are not of müllerian origin, imperforate hymens are not associated with other genitourinary abnormalities.

Other forms of genital tract obstruction (Box 18-4) are rare. In most cases early routine genital inspection reveals the absence of a vaginal orifice, enabling early delineation of the anomaly and thus facilitating treatment. Proximal obstructing anomalies may not be apparent on physical examination. If missed in infancy or childhood, partial or complete obstruction can present with a wide range of signs and symptoms, such as those listed in Box 18-5. As noted earlier, ultrasonography is a valuable screening tool in evaluating girls suspected of having genital tract obstruction, bearing in mind its limitations in visualization of internal structures after the neonatal period and before puberty, when they are very small given minimal amounts of estrogen and gonadotropins. When structures are not seen or when further anatomic detail is required, consultation with a radiologist regarding an MRI is recommended.

GENITAL TRAUMA

As mentioned earlier, the genital structures and pelvic supporting tissues of the prepubescent girl are smaller and considerably more rigid than those of adolescent or adult women. This inelasticity significantly increases the risks of tearing with

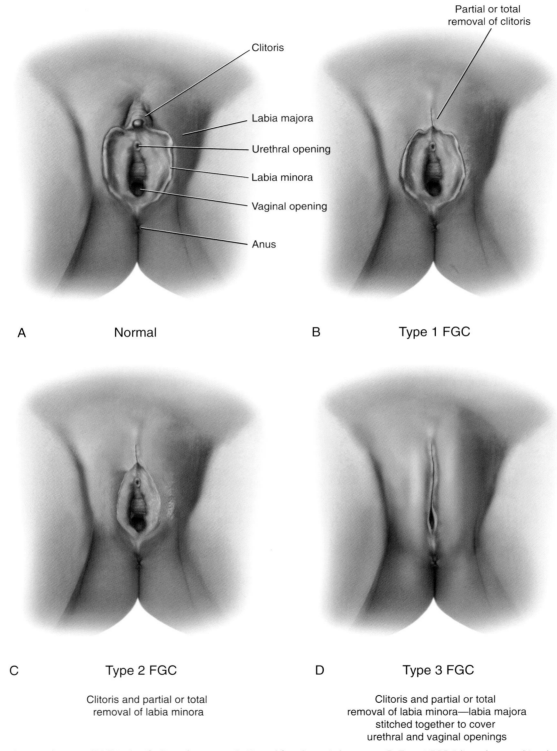

Figure 18-13   Female genital cutting (FGC) is classified into four types. **A,** Normal female genital anatomy. **B,** Type 1 FGC, "clitoredectomy," involves partial or total removal of the clitoris, and/or the skin around it. **C,** Type 2 FGC, removal of the clitoris and labia minora. **D,** Type 3 FGC, removal of the clitoris and labia minora, and labia majora sewn together to cover urethral opening and most of the vaginal opening. Type 4 FGC involves all other alterations including pricking, piercing, incising, or cauterizing the genitalia.

Figure 18-14 Imperforate hymen with neonatal hematocolpos. A dark purplish bulge at the introitus was noted by the mother during a diaper change.

Causes of Genital Tract Obstruction

Labial fusion (underlying endocrine pathology)
Labial adhesions (partial obstruction)
Female genital cutting sequelae
Imperforate hymen
Vaginal atresia (failure to canalize the vaginal plate)
Vaginal (with or without uterine) agenesis, including Mayer-Rokitansky-Kuster-Hauser syndrome (müllerian aplasia); congenital absence of the vagina and uterus
Transverse vaginal septum at the junction of the upper one third and lower two thirds of the vagina
Longitudinal vaginal septum
Androgen insensitivity (testicular feminization syndrome)
Obstructing müllerian malformations, with elements of duplication, agenesis, and/or incomplete fusion
Tumors of the upper and lower genital tracts; other pelvic masses

either blunt or penetrating trauma, and of internal extension of injury, especially in cases of penetrating trauma. Appropriate assessment and management necessitate appreciation of these differences because serious internal injuries of the vagina, rectum, urethra, bladder, and peritoneal structures may underlie deceptively mild external abnormalities. Careful attention must be given to vital signs; abdominal examination; and evaluation of the urethra, hymen, lower vagina, perineal body, and rectum.

Clues to internal extension of injury include hymenal tears, vaginal bleeding and/or vaginal hematoma, tears of the perineal body, inability to urinate or gross hematuria, and abnormal sphincter tone or rectal bleeding. When injuries have extended to involve peritoneal structures, lower abdominal tenderness is seen, and at times is associated with signs of hypovolemia. Direct tenderness may range from mild to marked and may or may not be accompanied by rebound tenderness. On occasion a palpable mass is present. Adolescents, in contrast, are more likely to have contusions than tears and are less likely to have internal extension of injury unless the applied force is very great.

The role of the primary care or emergency physician is to assess the patient's general status and determine the likely extent and cause of the injury. This can be accomplished largely with a good general examination, careful perineal and

Symptoms and Signs Associated with Genital Tract Obstruction

SYMPTOMS

Vaginal, pelvic, or abdominal pain (especially cyclic)
Dysmenorrhea
Urinary tract symptoms
Primary amenorrhea
Irregular vaginal bleeding
Purulent vaginal discharge
Difficulty using tampons
Difficulty initiating intercourse
Dyspareunia

SIGNS

Vaginal, pelvic, or abdominal mass
Hydrocolpos (mucus in vagina)
Hematocolpos (blood in vagina)
Pyohematocolpos (pus and blood in vagina)
Hematometria (blood within the uterus)

Figure 18-15 Imperforate hymen with hematocolpos. This adolescent presented with a 2-month history of intermittent crampy lower abdominal pain, which had acutely worsened. She had well-developed secondary sex characteristics but was premenarchal by history. **A,** Examination revealed midline fullness and tenderness of the lower abdomen and a smooth bulging mass at the introitus. **B,** Incision of the imperforate membrane just inside the hymenal ring allowed the accumulated menstrual blood and vaginal secretions to drain. *(Courtesy D. Lloyd, MD.)*

perianal inspection, rectal examination, and urinalysis. Rectal examination should be deferred in cases of possible anal rape and when anal lacerations are evident on inspection, to prevent further physical and emotional trauma. The physician must be sensitive to the patient's physical discomfort and emotional distress at all times, providing emotional support and appropriate pain control whenever possible. Patients should also be protected from having to undergo multiple examinations, a particular risk with consultation of multiple subspecialists, transfer to other institutions, or in teaching hospitals.

When external inspection suggests that the prepubertal patient's perineal or perianal injuries are more than superficial, internal examination under anesthesia (by a pediatric surgeon or gynecologist) should be arranged. This enables meticulous inspection, wound exploration, and repair under optimal conditions without further traumatizing the child. Some adolescents may be able to tolerate inspection and internal examination as outpatients. However, if injuries are severe or if the postmenarchal patient is too anxious to undergo pelvic examination when indicated, examination under sedation or anesthesia is the better course.

Superficial Genital Trauma

The majority of superficial perineal trauma cases are the result of mild, blunt force incurred via straddle injury, minor falls, or sexual abuse. Patients with accidental injuries that result in pain, swelling, or bleeding are rapidly brought to medical attention. A clear history of the preceding incident (often witnessed) is usually given, and findings fit the reported mechanism of injury. However, accidentally incurred superficial abrasions may not be noticed by parents until the child cries on urination, complains of dysuria, or blood is noticed on the child's underwear or toilet paper. As noted in Chapter 6, victims of sexual abuse may complain of abuse but more often complain of unexplained bleeding or pain with no history of trauma, and the time of presentation is often significantly delayed.

Typical lesions include superficial abrasions, mild contusions, and occasionally superficial lacerations (Fig. 18-16, A-C). The latter are found most frequently at the junction of the labia majora and minora and usually are only 1 to 3 mm deep. Accidental straddle injuries result in the crushing of the perineal soft tissues between the pubis and the object on which the patient falls or bumps herself. Hence these tend to produce abrasions, contusions, or tears in and around the area of the clitoris and the anterior portions of the labia majora and

minora (Fig. 18-16, A and B; and see Fig. 18-18). Minor falls onto or scrapes against sharp objects tend to produce simple perineal and vulval lacerations. As in cases of mild blunt trauma, the junction of the labia minora and majora is the site most frequently involved; however, tears of the labia majora or perineal body are not uncommon. In contrast to accidental injuries, those that result from sexual abuse tend to be more posteriorly located and typically involve tears of the posterior portion of the hymen, the posterior fourchette, or perineal body (Fig. 18-16, C and Fig. 18-17; and see Chapter 6).

Whether blunt or penetrating, when injuries are truly superficial, bleeding, if present at all, tends to be scant. The exception to this is a penetrating injury involving the corpus cavernosum of the labia majora, in which case hemorrhage may be profuse. Patients with superficial injuries may experience mild perineal discomfort and pain on urination, but otherwise are asymptomatic. Most of these injuries can be managed supportively with analgesia, topical bacteriostatic and/or anesthetic ointments, sitz baths, and careful perineal cleansing. Application of the ointment before urinating reduces the severity of dysuria, as does urinating in a tub of water. If urinary retention continues to be a problem, use of a topical anesthetic ointment for a few days may be necessary. Deeper tears of the labia majora necessitate control of bleeding vessels and suturing under anesthesia.

Urethral prolapse and lichen sclerosus et atrophicus may cause bleeding and therefore be mistaken for trauma. See Common Perineal Conditions (later) and Figures 18-28 and 18-29.

Moderate Genital Trauma

Moderately forceful blunt trauma often results in perineal tears and in venous disruption and hematoma formation. Hematomas of the perineum appear as tense round swellings with purplish discoloration, which are tender on palpation (Fig. 18-18). When large, these may cause intense perineal pain. Those located in the periurethral area may interfere with urination. Moderate blunt force can also produce submucosal tears of the vagina and even mucosal separation with resultant vaginal bleeding or vaginal hematoma formation (Figs. 18-18 and 18-19). In some cases the associated external injuries can be deceptively mild (see Fig. 18-19). Vaginal hematomas are the source of significant pain that usually is perceived as perineal and/or vaginal but at times is referred to the rectum or buttocks. Inspection through the vaginal orifice reveals a bluish swelling involving one of the lateral walls. This may also be evident as a tender swelling anterolaterally on rectal examination.

Figure 18-16   Superficial blunt trauma. **A,** Superficial abrasions and bruising are seen anteriorly on either side of the clitoris and urethra in a 3-year-old who presented with dysuria. **B,** In another toddler a superficial abrasion/laceration is seen between the left labia minora and majora after a straddle injury. **C,** These healing superficial abrasions involving the posterior fourchette and perianal area were the result of sexual abuse. *(A and B, Courtesy Janet Squires, MD, Children's Hospital of Pittsburgh, Pittsburgh, Pa.)*

Figure 18-17 Superficial penetrating injury. This infant had a chief complaint of blood spotting on the diaper. Inspection revealed a perineal tear just posterior to the hymenal ring. There was no evidence of internal extension on vaginoscopy under anesthesia. Sexual abuse was suspected.

Figure 18-19 Moderate blunt trauma. This 6-year-old girl had painless vaginal bleeding, which had soaked three sanitary pads in 2 hours. External inspection revealed a superficial tear of the anterior portion of the perineal body, a small hematoma to the right of the introitus, and blood trickling through the vaginal orifice. Examination under anesthesia disclosed a tear of the lateral vaginal wall. Sexual abuse was strongly suspected. *(Courtesy K. Sukarochana, MD, Pittsburgh, Pa.)*

Moderate penetrating injuries result primarily from falls onto sharp objects ("picket fence injury"), rape, sexual molestation with phallus-shaped objects, and occasionally auto accidents. Lesions include perineal tears that extend into the vagina, rectum, or bladder but do not breach the peritoneum. Although many patients have external lacerations that obviously are extensive on inspection (Fig. 18-20; and see Chapter 6), a significant proportion have deceptively minor external injuries. In the absence of associated hematomas, extensive tears may produce little pain. Furthermore, although most such injuries result in moderate bleeding, some patients have remarkably little blood loss.

Whether the mechanism of injury involves blunt force or penetration, internal extension of injury is probable when physical findings include bleeding through the vaginal orifice; a vaginal hematoma; rectal bleeding, rectal tenderness, or abnormal sphincter tone; or gross hematuria or inability to urinate. All such patients warrant exploration and repair in the operating room. This obviates the need for extensive examination in the office or emergency department.

Figure 18-18 Moderate genital trauma. After a straddle injury on a diving board, this 9-year-old girl had vaginal bleeding. Inspection disclosed a hematoma of the anterior portion of the right labia majora, contusions of the clitoris and anterior labia minora, and a hematoma protruding through the vaginal opening. A small superficial laceration is present on the left, between the labia majora and minora. At vaginoscopy under anesthesia a vaginal tear involving the right lateral wall was found. *(Courtesy K. Sukarochana, MD, Pittsburgh, Pa.)*

Figure 18-20 Moderately severe penetrating genital trauma. This youngster fell while roller skating downhill and slid on her bottom for several feet over the sidewalk, tearing her perineum on an object projecting up between two of the cement plates. A laceration involving the right labia majora and minora, extending through the perineal body to the anus, is evident on inspection. The patient complained of only minor discomfort. Examination under anesthesia revealed vaginal and rectal extension of the tear with complete transection of the external anal sphincter. The peritoneum was intact.

Figure 18-21   Severe blunt perineal trauma. After a fall from a second-story window in which she had landed on her bottom, this young child had labial contusions and hematomas, lower abdominal tenderness, and signs of hypovolemia **(A).** The force of the fall ruptured pelvic vessels, resulting in retroperitoneal bleeding that ultimately extended along the anterior abdominal wall **(B).** These photographs were taken several days after the injury. *(Courtesy Marc Rowe, MD, Sanibel, Fla.)*

Severe Genital Trauma

Severe falls from heights onto flat surfaces can produce major perineal lacerations simulating penetrating injury. In addition, they occasionally disrupt the pelvic vessels, mesentery, and intestine, with or without pelvic fracture (Fig. 18-21). Similarly, severe penetrating injury may produce tears that extend through the cul-de-sac, rupturing pelvic vessels and tearing intraabdominal structures. External injuries in these cases usually are extensive and associated with significant bleeding, but on occasion can be deceptively minor in appearance. Children with peritoneal extension of injury complain of lower abdominal and perineal pain, which may radiate down one leg. Abdominal examination should reveal at least mild direct tenderness early on. Later, guarding and rebound tenderness may be noted. Patients with pelvic bleeding ultimately tend to develop signs of hypovolemia, although this may not be evident immediately after the injury. Any patient with clinical signs of peritoneal extension of genital trauma warrants prompt hemodynamic stabilization followed by appropriate imaging, surgical exploration, and repair.

VULVOVAGINAL DISORDERS

Vulvovaginal Complaints in Prepubertal Patients

Strictly defined, the term *vulvovaginitis* denotes an inflammatory process involving both the vulva and the vagina. In practice, however, the term *prepubertal vulvovaginitis* is used less precisely to refer to patients who describe symptoms of dysuria, vulvar pain or itching, or vaginal discharge but who may lack signs of inflammation or who have evidence of only vulvar or vaginal involvement. Vulvovaginal complaints are relatively common in prepubertal girls in part because the labia do not fully cover and thus do not completely protect the vaginal vestibule from friction and external irritants, especially when the child is sitting or squatting. In addition, the unestrogenized vaginal epithelium is thin, relatively friable, and more easily traumatized. Transient irritation without discharge is common in the young child as a result of exposure to chemical irritants and inconsistent hygiene. Frictional irritation and poor aeration are also common and can be exacerbated by obesity. Finally, young children are less careful than older children and adults about cleansing their perineum after toileting and avoiding contamination with stool.

Causes of vulvovaginitis are most easily classified into noninfectious and infectious subgroups, with the latter subclassified into nonsexually and sexually transmitted infections. Table 18-4 presents the most common causes of noninfectious vulvovaginitis with specific historic clues suggestive of each condition. Table 18-5 presents the infectious causes. Nonsexually transmitted bacterial pathogens and the herpes simplex viruses often are spread to the vulvovaginal area from another site (e.g., nose, mouth, throat, skin, or gastrointestinal tract) by the patient's hands. *Candida* organisms, although a common cause of diaper dermatitis, rarely cause vulvovaginitis in the prepubertal child who is no longer wearing diapers. However, children who are receiving systemic antibiotics or steroids, or have underlying diabetes mellitus, may develop dysuria and vulvar discomfort that responds to topical (azole) antifungals. In the prepubertal child, vulvovaginitis caused by sexually transmitted pathogens is almost always acquired through sexual contact (Chapter 6). In contrast to adolescents and adults, prepubertal girls are at little risk for internal extension of vulvovaginal infections (cervicitis and pelvic inflammatory disease) because the unestrogenized genital tract does not support the ascent of infection through the uterus and fallopian tubes.

The evaluation of prepubertal patients with vulvovaginal complaints must include questions related to the following: symptoms experienced including any associated abdominal pain, dysuria, frequency, urgency, or perianal pruritus; symptom duration; a history of any recent respiratory, gastrointestinal, and urinary tract infections; exposure to irritants (Box 18-6); hygiene practices; bowel and bladder habits; type of clothing worn; recent activities (such as daily swimming); and medications and topical agents. When sexual abuse is suspected, a list of the child's caretakers should be obtained along with any history of possible sexual contact (Chapter 6). Developmental, behavioral, environmental, and medical histories all may contribute to a definitive diagnosis and aid in the formulation of a therapeutic plan.

Physical assessment must include determination of the degree of pubertal development, inguinal and abdominal examination, along with careful rectal, perineal, and vaginal inspection. The degree and extent of inflammation and excoriation should be documented. Parents should be encouraged to bring in any available soiled or discolored underwear,

Table 18-4	Noninfectious Causes of Prepubertal and Postpubertal Vulvovaginitis and Dysuria

Condition	Historical Clues
Poor hygiene	Recent toilet independence; infrequent bathing, hand washing, and clothing changes; soiled underwear
Poor perineal aeration	Tight clothing, nylon underwear, tights, and leotards; wet bathing suits; hot tubs; obesity
Frictional trauma	Tight clothing, sports, sand from sandbox or beach play, excessive masturbation or sexual abuse, obesity, hair removal
Chemical irritants	See products listed in Box 18-6
Contact dermatitis	Poison ivy; see also Box 18-6
Vaginal foreign bodies	Wiping habits, excessive masturbation or self-exploration, sexual abuse, use of condoms, tampons, or sex toys
Parasites, insect bites, infestations	Home environment, pets, sandboxes, travel, camping, exposure to woods or beach
Medication-related	Topical steroid or hormone creams, antibiotics, chemotherapy
Generalized skin disorders	History of pruritus, chronic skin lesions, prior diagnosis
Anatomic anomalies	Vesicovaginal or rectovaginal fistula, ectopic ureter, spina bifida, cloacal anomalies, urogenital anomalies
Neoplasms	Discharge, bleeding, bulging abdomen, change in bowel or bladder function, premature puberty
Systemic illness (Stevens-Johnson syndrome, Crohn disease with perineal fistulas and ulcers, toxic shock syndrome)	Prior infection or medication use; tampon use; evidence from other physical findings including rash, failure to gain weight or height, abdominal pain, diarrhea
Pelvic appendiceal abscess	History of anorexia, vomiting, fever, and progression of periumbilical to right lower quadrant pain

Table 18-5	Infectious Causes of Prepubertal and Postpubertal Vulvovaginitis

Nonsexually Transmitted Pathogens	Sexually Transmitted Pathogens
Bacterial Respiratory and/or Skin Pathogens Group A β-hemolytic streptococci Streptococcus pneumoniae Staphylococci Candida species*	**Bacterial Pathogens** Chlamydia trachomatis Neisseria gonorrhoeae Mycoplasma genitalis Ureaplasma species Treponema pallidum
Viral Pathogens Herpes simplex virus types 1 and 2 Epstein-Barr virus (EBV) Varicella-zoster virus	**Protozoa** Trichomonas vaginalis
Gastrointestinal Pathogens Escherichia coli Shigella species Enterobius vermicularis Yersinia species	**Viral Pathogens** Herpes simplex virus types 1 and 2 Human papillomavirus Human immunodeficiency virus (HIV)
	Parasites Phthirus pubis (lice) Sarcoptes scabiei

*Infection rare before puberty.

foreign objects. X-rays of the pelvic area should be ordered selectively when benefit outweighs the risk, and information cannot be obtained without radiation exposure.

Vulvovaginal Complaints in Pubertal Patients

Among sexually active adolescent girls, infectious processes are the major source of vulvovaginal inflammation, and sexually transmitted pathogens are the predominant offending organisms. Estrogenization and maturation of the genital tract alter its pathophysiologic response, favoring upward spread of some infectious processes, particularly those caused by gonorrhea and Chlamydia. As a result, asymptomatic or subclinical upper tract infection, cervicitis, endometritis, and pelvic inflammatory disease are significant concerns after menarche.

Vulvar lesions, vaginal discharge, odor, pruritus, and dysuria are common complaints in adolescents. Irregular or postcoital bleeding, dyspareunia, pelvic pain, and fever may be reported as well. These symptoms are relatively nonspecific and may represent the final common pathway of different causes of irritation, infection, or infestation.

In addition to identification of specific etiologic agents, a major goal of evaluation is to differentiate vulvovaginal or cervical processes from pregnancy (normal or ectopic), from upper tract disease (e.g., pelvic inflammatory disease, adnexal torsion, or cysts), from urinary tract problems, and from intra-abdominal processes (e.g., appendicitis, colitis, endometriosis, chronic constipation, or tumors). Hence a complete gynecologic examination is necessary when evaluating sexually active adolescents with vulvovaginal complaints and should be considered for symptomatic nonsexually active adolescents. Systemic signs and symptoms and abnormalities on bimanual pelvic examination suggest processes involving the uterus and adnexal and/or peritoneal structures. In contrast, isolated vulvovaginal disorders rarely are accompanied by such findings. In most cases, careful history, inspection, office laboratory tests and selected cultures (see Table 18-2), and other tests for infectious etiologic agents (see Table 18-5) provide a

which should be checked for fit, cleanliness, and signs of blood, discharge, stool, and urine. When patients are seen by appointment for vulvovaginal complaints, parents should be asked not to bathe or apply creams to the child for 12 to 24 hours before the evaluation; otherwise, many children with a history of discharge have none when examined.

The presence of a vaginal discharge necessitates specimen collection (see Table 18-2 and Examination of the Prepubertal Patient, earlier). If a vaginal foreign body is suspected, rectal examination and vaginoscopy are indicated in consultation with a practitioner experienced in such procedures. Ultrasonography can be helpful in confirming the presence of some

BOX 18-6

Products That Can Cause Chemical Irritation or Contact Dermatitis

Bubble bath or other bath additives
Harsh or perfumed soaps
Harsh laundry detergents
Dryer sheets or fabric softeners
Talc or other powders
Topical creams or ointments
Shaving or hair removal products
Perfumed or dyed toilet paper
Perfumed sanitary pads and panty liners
Douches or other feminine hygiene products
Urine or stool
Spermicides

| Table 18-6 | Clinical and Laboratory Features of Disorders Causing Vaginal Discharge in Adolescents |

	Physiologic	Candida	Chlamydia	Gonorrhea	Trichomonas	Bacterial Vaginosis	HSV
Appearance of discharge	White, gray, or clear, mucoid	White, curdlike, with adherent plaques	Mucopus at cervix; friable cervix with bloody discharge	Mucopus at cervix; yellow or greenish discharge	Gray, yellow, or green; sometimes frothy; malodorous	Gray, white; homogeneous, thin	Serous
Amount of discharge	Variable	Variable	Variable	Variable	Profuse	Variable	Variable
Vulvar and vaginal inflammation	None or mild with copious leukorrhea	Usual	Not usual	Not usual	Common	Rare	Common with a few to many ulcers
pH of vaginal discharge	≤4.5	≤4.5	Variable	≤4.5	≥4.5	≥4.5	≤4.5
Microscopy	Epithelial cells, few WBCs, lactobacilli	↑WBCs, positive KOH with pseudohyphae and budding yeast in 50% of patients	↑WBCs	↑↑WBCs	↑↑WBCs, motile trichomonads in saline prep in 50% of patients	Few WBCs; positive for clue cells in saline prep	↑↑WBCs
Predisposing or concurrent factors	Secretion of estrogen	Menstruation, broad-spectrum antibiotics, diabetes, local heat and moisture, pregnancy, OCPs, topical steroid or hormone creams, HIV and other immune deficiencies	Sexual activity, other STI	Sexual activity, other STI; symptoms develop during and after menstrual period	Other STI	Previous BV, sexual activity, douching	Stress and local trauma (including shaving)
Other clinical signs and symptoms	None	Itching prominent; may have dysuria or dyspareunia	Urethritis, PID, perihepatitis	Urethritis, PID, perihepatitis, pharyngitis, proctitis, systemic illness, arthritis, tenosynovitis, skin lesions	Vulvar itching and burning prominent; dysuria; pelvic discomfort	Fishy odor; odor increased after unprotected intercourse	Regional adenopathy with primary infection; prodromal and undercurrent itching and pain
Whiff test (acrid amine odor on addition of 10% KOH)	Negative	Negative	Negative	Negative	Sometimes positive	Positive	Negative

↑, increased; ↑↑, markedly increased; BV, bacterial vaginosis; HIV, human immunodeficiency virus; HSV, herpes simplex virus; OCP, oral contraceptive pill; PID, pelvic inflammatory disease; STI, sexually transmitted infection; WBCs, white blood cells.

specific diagnosis on which to base treatment decisions. Some clinical and laboratory features of various etiologic agents of vaginal discharge are presented in Table 18-6.

Physiologic Leukorrhea

Physiologic leukorrhea is a normal phenomenon and not a form of vulvovaginitis. These normal secretions are produced in response to estrogen stimulation and thus are seen in the newborn period and return during the months preceding menarche. Physiologic leukorrhea is clear or milky, relatively thin, odorless, and (usually) nonirritating (see Fig. 18-5, *A*). When dried on underwear, it may appear yellow. Girls near menarche often complain of discharge because they and their mothers are not aware that these new secretions are normal. Furthermore, because of the unopposed influence of estrogen, some pubertal girls experience a transient period of excessive leukorrhea that can be irritating.

Examination reveals normal pubertal development including findings of breast development, presence of pubic hair, and evidence of estrogenization of the labia and distal vaginal mucosa along with the typical discharge. Diagnosis is confirmed by findings on wet preparation microscopy, which discloses estrogenized epithelial cells with no increase in leukocytes (see Fig. 18-5, *B*). As a general guide, there should be no more than one polymorphonuclear leukocyte for every

vaginal epithelial cell. Neither bimanual nor speculum examinations are necessary unless concurrent symptoms or findings suggest other problems. Treatment consists of reassurance and education.

ETIOLOGIES OF VULVOVAGINAL DISORDERS

Noninfectious Vulvovaginitis

Noninfectious vulvovaginitis is common in prepubertal children but occurs less frequently after menarche. Clinical findings vary considerably depending on cause. Although the physical findings often are unimpressive, patient and parental concern with the symptoms may be great. In some patients the vulva and vagina appear normal, whereas in others varying degrees of inflammation or irritation are present, at times accompanied by signs of excoriation. Vaginal discharge is unusual, however, and vaginal cultures grow normal or nonspecific flora (Box 18-7). Individuals with underlying dermatologic disorders may be more susceptible to noninfectious causes of vulvovaginitis. Symptoms are similar for most etiologies: perineal itching or pain, external or contact dysuria, and occasionally, vaginal discharge.

BOX 18-7

Organisms Thought to Constitute Normal or Nonpathogenic Vaginal Flora

AEROBES AND FACULTATIVE ANAEROBES

Branhamella catarrhalis
Candida albicans and other yeasts*
Corynebacterium species
Diphtheroids
Enterococcus species
Escherichia coli
Haemophilus species
Lactobacillus species
Klebsiella species

Mycoplasma species*
Neisseria sicca
Proteus species
Pseudomonas species
Staphylococcus species
Streptococcus species

ANAEROBES

Bacteroides species
Clostridium species
Peptococcus species
Peptostreptococcus species

*Candida species as well as Mycoplasma hominis and Ureaplasma urealyticum can constitute normal flora in asymptomatic women; however, they may be responsible for genital tract infections as well.

Figure 18-22   Poor perineal hygiene. Despite prior cleansing by a nurse for a "clean-catch" urine sample, the initial specimen contained numerous white cells and debris. When the perineum was rechecked, the infant was found to have copious amounts of smegma adhering to the clitoris and labia minora and stool on the posterior perineum. Urine obtained after thorough recleansing was normal.

Treatment consists of removal of the offending agent or causative circumstance along with symptomatic measures. Recommended hygienic practices include providing a sufficient number of opportunities to urinate, using a front-to-back wiping technique, and regular washing with warm water without excessive scrubbing. Products to avoid are listed in Box 18-6. Patients with vulvovaginal inflammation are encouraged to wear loose-fitting clothes and white cotton underwear that is well rinsed after regular washing. Failure to improve should lead to consideration of other etiologies including sexual abuse, and the possibility of nonadherence with treatment. Referral to a clinician with expertise in pediatric gynecologic problems may be indicated.

In prepubertal girls, chronic irritation from any cause may predispose the labia minora to agglutinate, resulting in labial adhesions (see Fig. 18-12 and Labial Adhesions, earlier). Urine trapped behind the adhesions after toileting may cause further irritation, helping to perpetuate the condition or causing adhesions to extend.

Irritation Related to Hygiene Practices

Poor perineal hygiene is one of the most common causes of irritation. Examination typically reveals mild nonspecific vulvar inflammation. Pieces of stool and toilet paper may be seen adhering to the perineum and perianal areas and smegma may be found around the clitoris and labia (Fig. 18-22). Underwear is often soiled. Coliforms tend to predominate on vaginal culture when there is associated vaginal inflammation. In the majority of cases the search for other causes is unrewarding, and symptoms resolve with a regimen of sitz baths and careful cleansing after urination and defecation. Finding a frankly feculent vaginal discharge should lead to the consideration of a rectovaginal fistula.

Pubic hair removal has become increasingly common for women and young girls, sometimes starting shortly after pubic hair first appears. Complications of hair removal are common and include razor burn; contact dermatitis from shaving products; mechanical folliculitis; infectious folliculitis (Fig 18-23) commonly from Staphylococcus aureus, Streptococcus pyogenes, and Pseudomonas aeruginosa; and mechanical spread or trigger of viral infections such as human papillomavirus, molluscum contagiosum, and herpes simplex virus. Mild topical corticosteroids and topical antibiotics can be used to prevent and treat folliculitis. Clinicians who commonly encounter these issues should familiarize themselves with the pros and cons and various methods of pubic hair removal (Trager, 2006).

Maceration Secondary to Moisture and Chafing

Moisture, whether from normal secretions, perspiration, or swimming, when unable to evaporate, promotes maceration and inflammation of perineal tissues. Obesity, wearing tight clothing or tights over nylon underwear, and sitting for long periods in a wet bathing suit or leotard are common predisposing factors to this form of vulvar irritation. Nonspecific inflammation, often with frank maceration, is the predominant physical finding (Fig. 18-24). A history of a chronically wet perineum and the smell of urine on the child's underclothes should lead the clinician to consider the possibility of urinary incontinence, a vesicovaginal fistula, or ectopic ureter. When maceration occurs, secondary infection is common, and some patients have associated intertrigo (irritant dermatitis where opposing skin surfaces touch). Attention to perineal hygiene and drying, weight loss (when appropriate), avoidance of tight

Figure 18-23   Pubic hair removal. After shaving, this 17-year-old girl developed impetigo, a common and highly contagious bacterial skin infection caused by Staphylococcus aureus. It cleared quickly with the use of oral and topical antibiotics. (Reprinted with permission from Trager JDK: Pubic hair removal—pearls and pitfalls, J Pediatr Adolesc Gynecol 19:117-123, 2006.)

Figure 18-24 Maceration secondary to poor perineal aeration. This child's chief complaint was one of dysuria. On examination the inner surfaces of the labia were found to be macerated and mildly inflamed. Adherent smegma is also visible. The child had been wearing tights over nylon underwear.

Figure 18-25 Nonspecific inflammation characteristic of chemical irritant vulvovaginitis.

clothing, use of antichafing products, and treatment of secondary infection are the mainstays of management.

Contact Dermatitis, Allergic Vulvitis

Allergic vulvitis should be considered in patients whose most prominent symptom is pruritus, although scratching and excoriation may result in secondary burning and dysuria. When patients are seen in the acute phase, inspection of the labia and vestibule reveals a microvesicular papular eruption that tends to be intensely erythematous and may be somewhat edematous. Excoriated scratch marks are common. When the process has become chronic, the vulvar skin has an eczematoid appearance with cracks, fissures, and lichenification. Poison ivy is a common cause, as are the exposures listed in Box 18-6.

Chemical Irritant Vulvovaginitis

Many of the agents listed in Box 18-6 can act as chemical irritants. Before toilet training, children whose diapers are changed infrequently may develop irritation caused by ammonia produced when the organisms in stool split the urea in urine. Itching and dysuria are prominent symptoms, and examination usually discloses mild nonspecific inflammation (Fig. 18-25), at times associated with signs of scratching. On occasion, findings are normal. Diagnosis is dependent on a thorough history (see Table 18-4 and Box 18-6).

Frictional Trauma

Frictional trauma may be the source of superficial abrasive changes and, when chronic, may result in lichenification or even atrophic skin changes (Fig. 18-26). Wearing tight clothing, certain sporting activities (especially gymnastics and long-distance cycling and running), sand from sandboxes, and excessive masturbation are the major predisposing factors.

Pelvic Appendiceal Abscess

Girls with appendicitis may develop a purulent vaginal discharge caused by sympathetic inflammation of the vaginal wall. On microscopy the discharge contains numerous leukocytes, epithelial cells, and mixed flora (Fig. 18-27). When the

antecedent clinical course and findings on examination suggest appendicitis, the presence of vaginal discharge may be a secondary finding rather than a sign of a primary genital infection.

Fistulas

Because patients with vesicovaginal fistulas and ectopic ureters have a history of a constantly wet perineum they frequently have symptoms of vulvovaginitis. Nonspecific inflammation and maceration are the predominant physical findings

Figure 18-26 Frictional trauma. This patient's labial skin shows nonspecific thickening and mild irritation. She had a history of recurrent vaginal foreign bodies and was strongly suspected to be a victim of chronic sexual abuse. *(Courtesy K. Sukarochana, MD, Pittsburgh, Pa.)*

Figure 18-27 Sympathetic purulent vaginal discharge. This photomicrograph shows numerous leukocytes and epithelial cells, with mixed flora. The 4-year-old patient had a history of vomiting, anorexia, abdominal pain with marked right lower quadrant and pelvic tenderness, and a purulent vaginal discharge and was found to have a pelvic appendiceal abscess. The vaginal discharge was the result of sympathetic inflammation.

prepubertal patients, and necrotic tumors, which can produce a discharge that is clinically indistinguishable from that of a vaginal foreign body.

COMMON PERINEAL CONDITIONS

Urethral Prolapse

Urethral prolapse is often mistaken for vulvovaginitis or perineal trauma. Dysuria, perineal pain, and bleeding are the most frequent symptoms. The phenomenon is more prevalent among African-American and obese prepubertal school-age girls. Increased intraabdominal pressure often precipitates the prolapse of the urethra through the urethral meatus. Constipation, especially when chronic; coughing; and crying may all contribute. The classic physical finding is a red or purplish red, swollen, and friable piece of tissue lying over the anterior introitus (Fig. 18-28). It often has a doughnut shape and is tender. With optimal positioning and careful visualization, the clinician can see that it encircles the urethral meatus. Because the urethral mucosa is responsive to estrogen, application of

(see Fig. 18-24). Rectovaginal fistulas can also cause vulvovaginal inflammation, but the presence of a grossly feculent vaginal discharge usually makes diagnosis relatively easy. When a rectovaginal fistula is neither congenital nor posttraumatic in origin, or when a perianal fistula is found, inflammatory bowel disease should be considered (Chapter 10).

Vaginal Foreign Body

The hallmark of a vaginal foreign body is the presence of a profuse, foul-smelling, brownish or blood-streaked vaginal discharge. However, some children have a less dramatic presentation with a yellow, mildly purulent discharge. The majority of patients are in the 3- to 8-year-old age group. Some have developmental delay or other psychosocial and behavioral problems. When a prepubertal patient is found to have a vaginal foreign body, it is important to obtain a detailed behavioral history of the child in addition to a family psychosocial history because the problem often is recurrent and may be the result of disturbed behavior by the patient or of chronic sexual abuse.

Wads of toilet tissue, paper, cotton, crayons, and small toys are the materials found most often; however, all types of small objects have been retrieved. There may be a long noninflammatory latency period for inert materials. The objects most commonly found in adolescents are forgotten tampons or retained condoms. Retained tampons or condoms are usually evident by a pungent odor, which may be the presented complaint. Careful visual and manual inspection in the adolescent patient may locate the offending agent. Removal manually or with an alligator forceps is usually curative, but antibiotic treatment may be considered in the presence of a purulent discharge. Suppositories or substances inserted for therapeutic purposes, or objects used in sexual activity may also cause problems. Objects made of hard materials may be palpable on rectal examination. Radiographs are rarely necessary because direct vaginoscopy is almost always required. Results of wet preparation and culture are nonspecific. Vaginoscopy is diagnostic and, when tolerated, it provides access for extraction, which is curative. In the prepubertal age group, it is best accomplished under general anesthesia or conscious sedation.

Major differential diagnostic considerations for a brownish/bloody vaginal discharge are *Shigella* vaginitis, seen in

Figure 18-28 Urethral prolapse. **A,** This child had acute complaints of bleeding and dysuria. The prolapsed urethral mucosa is red, friable, and has a doughnut shape encircling the urethra. **B,** In another patient the prolapsed mucosal tissue is thickened and erythema is less prominent. (**A,** *Courtesy John McCann, MD, University of California at Davis, Davis, Calif.;* **B,** *courtesy Carole Jenny, MD, Hasbro Children's Hospital, Providence, R.I.*)

Figure 18-29   Lichen sclerosus. **A,** The skin overlying the labia majora has become atrophic and appears pale and thin. It is dotted with small, superficial ulcerations. **B,** In this child with complaints of bleeding and pruritus, skin breakdown is evident along with petechial hemorrhages. **C,** A pruritic, atrophic, eroded, hypopigmented patch involving the anogenital skin and mucous membranes in this 5-year-old girl has an hourglass configuration. (*C, From Cohen BA:* Pediatric dermatology, *ed 2, London, 1999, Mosby.*)

estrogen cream twice daily usually results in resolution. Oral analgesics and topical antibacterial and/or anesthetic creams provide symptomatic relief. Treatment of underlying causes reduces the risk of recurrence.

Lichen Sclerosus

Lichen sclerosus is a chronic dermatologic disorder of unknown etiology that involves primarily the perineum and perianal area in prepubertal girls. It begins insidiously, sometimes preceded by perineal itching and occasionally by a mild watery discharge. At first there may be no readily visible signs, and symptomatic treatment is often prescribed to no effect. Eventually small pink or white, flat-topped papular lesions appear on both cutaneous and mucosal surfaces, and these coalesce to form larger plaque-like lesions that may have scaly surfaces. Vesiculation may occur followed by superficial ulceration or excoriation with increased erythema, maceration, and punctate bleeding (Fig. 18-29, *A*). The latter occurs especially when pruritus incites rubbing or scratching (Fig. 18-29, *B*). With progression, the involved epithelium becomes thin, atrophic, and hypopigmented. When both the vulvar and perianal areas are affected, the distribution has been likened to an hourglass or a figure-eight (Fig. 18-29, *C*). On resolution of active lesions, the involved area is characterized by confluent, white, atrophic patches with a shiny surface.

The disorder tends to wax and wane over one to several years, often resolving around puberty. Acute exacerbations, which are often precipitated by local irritation or trauma, respond best to very short-term treatment with an ultra high–potency topical steroid ointment. Although lichen sclerosus is common in prepubertal girls and rare in adolescence, topical hormone preparations have not been found to be effective.

Diagnosis generally can be made on clinical grounds, although some atypical cases may require dermatologic consultation and possibly a biopsy. When ulcerations and bleeding are present, concerns regarding sexual abuse may arise. The pattern and distribution of lesions, their failure to heal rapidly, and the chronicity of the disorder help distinguish it from abrasions and lacerations due to abuse. In vitiligo, which may have a similar distribution when present in the anogenital area, the involved skin is totally devoid of pigment but is otherwise normal (i.e., not atrophic or inflamed) in appearance. In the adolescent lichen planus may present similarly

with white streaks on the vulva, but more typically the rash is violaceous.

Acute Genital Ulcers

The appearance of an acute genital ulcer in a girl can create alarm and distress in both the patient and her parents. The differential diagnosis is broad (Bandow, 2010) and includes infectious and noninfectious causes. Herpes simplex virus (HSV) is the most common infectious cause and both HSV type 1 and type 2 can be spread via nonsexual transmission by caregivers or from autoinoculation. Noninfectious causes include autoimmune or other systemic illness, drug reactions, and aphthous ulcers. A thorough history and physical is warranted, with particular attention to excluding underlying systemic conditions (such as HIV infection, Behçet disease, or Crohn disease) and identifying recent viral infection or other triggering factors such as tight-fitting clothing, sexual activity, or abuse.

When such factors are absent, and lesions are characteristic, vulvar aphthae are a likely cause. The typical location of vulvar aphthous ulcers is the medial labia minora (often on apposing labial surfaces as "kissing" lesions), but other sites include the vagina, introitus, fourchette, labia majora, and perineum. Appearance varies, but aphthous ulcers tend to be deeper than ulcers caused by HSV, and typically appear well demarcated with a necrotic base and ragged margins (Fig. 18-30, *A* and *B*). Lesions may be covered by yellow-gray exudate or by eschar, and surrounding inflammation with or without cellulitis can occur.

Evaluation should include HSV culture, or preferably polymerase chain reaction (PCR) assay, from the lesion, and serum IgG and IgM antiviral capsid antigen for Epstein-Barr virus. Beyond that, a large laboratory workup is rarely informative and should be based on the history and examination, including a comprehensive evaluation for STI when indicated. Bacterial and fungal cultures tend not to yield pathogens and biopsy is rarely indicated.

Vulvar aphthous ulcers are generally self-limited, resolving in 2 to 3 weeks. However, treatment with a topical steroid such as 0.05% clobetasol ointment twice daily for 7 to 10 days is recommended. Patients with milder symptoms can be managed as outpatients with supportive care including sitz baths, barrier agents such as sucralfate, and/or topical anesthetics such as combined lidocaine, epinephrine, and

Figure 18-30 Genital ulcers. **A,** Vulvar aphthous ulcer in a teenage girl. **B,** Vulvar aphthous ulcer with exudate. *(Reprinted with permission from Bandow GD: Diagnosis and management of vulvar ulcers,* Dermatol Clin *28:753-763, 2010.)*

tetracaine. However, pain can be severe and hospitalization may be required with Foley catheterization to manage dysuria, antibiotics to treat associated cellulitis, and narcotics to treat pain.

Families can be reassured by the comparison of vulvar aphthae to common "canker sores" and by the fact that recurrence and long-term sequelae are uncommon. The likelihood of scarring depends on the size and duration of the original lesions. Follow-up should be weekly until resolution and then yearly to monitor for progression to systemic disease such as Behçet disease, which is a systemic disease characterized by recurrent oral aphthae and associated genital, eye, and skin findings.

Infectious Vulvovaginitis

In contrast to most of the primarily noninfectious forms of vulvovaginitis, vaginal discharge is usually a prominent symptom of infectious vulvovaginitis in all age groups. Although a few pathogens produce a fairly characteristic clinical picture, most do not, the symptoms and discharge seen with many pathogens being relatively nonspecific. Furthermore, in the case of sexually transmitted infections (STIs), more than one pathogen may be present. For these reasons, careful attention to specimen collection technique is important.

There are two major subgroups of vulvovaginal infections. In the first subgroup genital involvement is secondary to a systemic infection or the result of transfer of the pathogen from another primary site such as the skin or the respiratory, gastrointestinal, or urinary tract via contaminated fingers or proximity (see Table 18-5). Infection at the primary site may precede or coexist with the genital infection, and in some cases colonization of another site, without overt infection, appears to predispose. This nonvenereal infectious vulvovaginitis is common in prepubertal patients but is rare in adolescents because the mature female genital tract does not support growth of most of these pathogens.

The second subgroup of infectious vulvovaginitis consists of those infections caused by sexually transmitted pathogens (see Tables 18-5 and 18-6). Both prepubertal and postmenarchal patients can have vulvovaginitis when infected with these organisms. After puberty, however, patients can have other clinical presentations as well, including cervicitis, endometritis, and salpingitis. Table 18-6 enumerates the possible clinical features seen in adolescent girls with STI and summarizes other major epidemiologic characteristics and appropriate diagnostic measures.

Regardless of age, the most frequent mode of transmission of STI is sexual contact. The majority of these infections in prepubertal patients are the result of sexual abuse. (see Chapter 6). Hence, when STI is found in the prepubertal child, the possibility of sexual abuse must be investigated. In adolescence, consensual sexual activity is the major mode of infection by sexually transmitted pathogens, although sexual exploitation and abuse remain significant possibilities. These factors necessitate obtaining a confidential history of sexual activity and case finding of sexual partners. The presence of one STI in any child or adolescent should prompt investigation for others because infection with multiple organisms is common (see Genital Infections Caused by Sexually Transmitted Pathogens, later).

Infectious Vulvovaginitis Caused by Nonsexually Transmitted Pathogens

Vulvovaginitis Caused by Respiratory and/or Skin Pathogens

Bacterial respiratory pathogens can cause vulvovaginitis in prepubertal patients, presumably as a result of orodigital transmission. *Streptococcus pneumoniae* and other respiratory flora can cause purulent vaginal discharge, with associated vulvitis and vaginitis, either after or concurrent with upper respiratory tract infection. The respiratory pathogen most commonly identified as a cause of vulvovaginitis is group A

Figure 18-31 Streptococcal vulvovaginitis. **A,** In this child who had acute vulvar pain, dysuria, and discharge, the area of inflammation is sharply circumscribed and extends from the vulva to the perianal area. **B,** In another patient, who presented late in the course of a case of scarlet fever, vulvar inflammation is still evident and desquamation has begun.

β-hemolytic streptococci. This infection may be associated with streptococcal nasopharyngitis or scarlet fever, or it may occur in apparent isolation, although a throat culture is often positive for streptococci even in the absence of pharyngeal or upper respiratory symptoms. Rapid testing for streptococci from the perineal tissues is not approved by the U.S. Food and Drug Administration (FDA), but may be positive in these cases. The onset of vulvovaginal symptoms is abrupt, with severe perineal burning and dysuria. Inspection reveals a sharply circumscribed area of intense erythema involving the vulva, distal vagina, and perianal area (Fig. 18-31, A). The involved skin may weep serous fluid. Most patients have a serosanguineous or grayish-white vaginal discharge, and about one third have vaginal petechiae. Culture of perineal skin and/or discharge is positive. Desquamation ensues with recovery (Fig. 18-31, B; and see Fig. 18-6).

Impetigo and folliculitis may occur in the vulvar area of patients of any age, usually secondary to poor hygiene, excessive sweating, shaving, or mechanical irritation. Simultaneous involvement of the buttocks or other skin sites is common (see Chapter 12). Some young women with increased androgens, children with a familial predisposition to keratosis pilaris, and patients with Down syndrome may be especially prone to develop folliculitis and/or impetigo (see Fig. 18-23).

Systemic viral infections have also been linked to vulvovaginitis in young children. The specific agent is rarely identified and the course is typically self-limited.

Vulvovaginitis Caused by Gastrointestinal Pathogens

Escherichia coli

Escherichia coli is a frequently identified bacterial cause of vulvovaginitis in prepubertal patients. Treatment with cefixime is frequently sufficient to eradicate the symptoms and discharge. Alternatively, culture and sensitivity may guide antibiotic choice.

Shigella

A distinct, although uncommon, form of vulvovaginitis caused by *Shigella* species has been recognized in prepubertal patients. The majority have no overt gastrointestinal symptoms,

although approximately one third have had associated diarrhea. The predominant complaint is one of an acute or chronic vaginal discharge. A greenish brown, often blood-streaked, purulent, and foul-smelling vaginal discharge is seen on inspection, along with vulvar and vaginal erythema. A positive culture is diagnostic, but enteric-specific bacteriologic transport and culture media must be used. A high rate of coinfection with pinworms has been reported.

Pinworms

Intestinal infestation with pinworms (*Enterobius vermicularis*) is associated primarily with perianal pruritus. However, the worms may crawl forward into the vagina, bringing enteric flora with them and depositing eggs. In some cases vaginal infection and discharge may result. Scratching may produce excoriation and secondary dysuria. A history of preceding perianal pruritus generally is elicited. Inflammatory changes are nonspecific. Pinworm ova and/or adult worms may be found on wet mount examination of vaginal secretions (Fig. 18-32). In the occasional patient with associated vaginal discharge, culture is positive for enteric pathogens. When pinworm infestation is suspected despite negative vaginal smears, a perianal sample should be obtained (see Table 18-2). Alternatively, empiric treatment with mebendazole according to standard guidelines may be instituted.

Candida *Vulvovaginitis*

Candida species are one of the more common sources of nonvenereal infectious vulvovaginitis after puberty. This is rare in the healthy prepubertal child. Predisposing factors, common complaints, and clinical features are listed in Table 18-6. Examination of the vulva usually reveals diffuse erythema (Fig. 18-33, A); with chronic involvement, white or pink cobblestoned plaques on an erythematous base may be seen. Excoriations from scratching and satellite lesions on the perineum are also common. In some cases, signs of perianal dermatitis and intertrigo are found.

Thick creamy or cheesy discharge is often present. In adolescents whitish plaques may adhere to the vagina or cervix (Fig. 18-33, B). A KOH or wet preparation confirms the presence of yeast and often an increase in inflammatory cells

Figure 18-32 Pinworms *(Enterobius vermicularis)*. On this wet mount **(A)** a mature worm is shown surrounded by eggs, which are shown more clearly at higher power **(B)**. Patients with intestinal infestation may have vulvovaginal symptoms as a result of scratching and excoriation or migration of the worms into the vagina.

(Fig. 18-33, *C* and *D*). Topical application of an azole antifungal cream into the lower vagina, or single-dose oral fluconazole, is the treatment of choice. Single-dose oral regimens are less efficacious but are simple and may be more reliable when problems with compliance are an issue. In sexually active adolescents, careful consideration must be given to the possibility of pregnancy before prescribing medication. In patients with recurrences, predisposing factors, such as medications and human immunodeficiency virus (HIV) infection, should be considered. An infected male partner with subacute or chronic monilial balanitis rarely may be the source of recurrences in sexually active patients. This infection generally is not transmitted sexually, and treatment of the partner does not decrease recurrence rates.

Other fungal species such as *Torulopsis* may also cause vulvovaginitis. Clinical presentation tends to be similar to that of *Candida*, but under microscopy these organisms do not demonstrate the classic branching morphology seen with *Candida*. They are often more resistant to first-line antifungal agents, and a fungal culture should be obtained in a patient with apparent persistent or recurrent *Candida* infection. This will provide diagnostic specificity and guide the choice of antifungal treatment.

Genital Infections Caused by Sexually Transmitted Pathogens

Sexually transmitted infections (STIs) are an important cause of short- and long-term morbidity in adolescents (see Table 18-6). Although some infections produce relatively specific clinical findings, many are characterized by nonspecific vulvovaginal inflammation with vaginal discharge, or ulcers. Several pathogens can induce two or three different clinical pictures (or a mixed picture) in adolescents. The major characteristics of the most common STIs are listed in Table 18-7. The high frequency of multiple simultaneous infections necessitates comprehensive laboratory evaluation. It is also important to note that the clinical approach differs considerably between prepubertal and postpubertal patients.

Evaluation for Sexually Transmitted Infections

Before menarche, lack of estrogenization inhibits ascent of infection to the upper genital tract, and subclinical lower tract infection is uncommon. As a result, external inspection of the perineum and lower vagina and laboratory evaluation of vaginal discharge samples are sufficient for identification of most pathogens and for institution of therapy. This does not complete the assessment, however, because whenever an STI is identified in a prepubertal patient, sexual abuse must be considered as the probable source. This necessitates urgent referral to a team specialized in the assessment of child sexual abuse. (Chapter 6).

When evaluating postpubertal patients suspected of having an STI, a sexual history obtained in confidence is essential. Although consensual activity is common in adolescence, patients may be victims of sexual abuse, including incest, sexual exploitation, and date rape. Complaints of pubertal patients with STI include vulvar lesions, vaginal discharge, odor, pruritus, perineal discomfort, and dysuria. There may be associated symptoms of pelvic pain, dyspareunia, fever, and irregular bleeding. A number of pathogens, such as herpes simplex, *Trichomonas vaginalis,* and human papillomaviruses, cause inflammation of not only the vulva and vagina but also the cervix. Patients infected with *N. gonorrhoeae* or *C. trachomatis* may be asymptomatic even in the presence of cervicitis. When symptomatic, they may have bleeding, dysuria, or vaginal discharge; or, with ascent of infection to the upper tract, signs of salpingitis, although this too can be clinically silent (see Tables 18-6 and 18-7). *Neisseria gonorrhoeae* and *C. trachomatis* also infect the columnar epithelium of other genital sites, including the Bartholin glands, the urethra, and the rectum.

A complete pelvic examination is desirable when evaluating adolescents for vulvovaginal complaints and possible STIs. At a minimum this includes inspection of the perineum, collection of vaginal samples for microscopy and the laboratory, and a careful bimanual examination. Cervical motion, or adnexal or uterine tenderness, during the bimanual examination suggests the diagnosis of PID (see Pelvic Inflammatory Disease, later). Consideration should be given to use of a speculum to inspect the vaginal walls and to obtain a vaginal specimen for microscopy that is not contaminated by cervical secretions. A speculum also permits examination of the cervix for the presence of mucopurulent discharge, erythema, focal lesions, bleeding, and friability. Some clinicians advocate collection of a urethral specimen that can be pooled with the vaginal or cervical specimen as a way to enhance

Figure 18-33 *Candida* vulvovaginitis and cervicitis. **A,** The vulva is intensely hyperemic, and a thick, cheesy, white discharge covers the urethra, introitus, and hymenal area. **B,** Whitish plaques may be seen on the perineum and vaginal mucosa and occasionally on the cervix in adolescents. **C** and **D,** These low- and high-power wet mount specimens contain pseudohyphae and budding yeast. (**A,** *Courtesy B. Cohen, MD, Johns Hopkins Hospital, Baltimore, Md.;* **B** *and* **D,** *courtesy Ellen Wald, MD, University of Wisconsin Children's Hospital, Madison, Wis.*)

detection. Sexual partners should be evaluated and treated whenever an STI is identified; otherwise, reinfection is probable.

Adolescent girls with asymptomatic cervical infections may serve as silent reservoirs of sexually transmitted pathogens. This phenomenon is quite significant in the epidemiology of STIs. Hence, female partners of men known to have gonorrhea, *Chlamydia,* or nonspecific urethritis should be evaluated and treated appropriately. The patient and partner(s) must be advised to abstain from sexual intercourse until the course of treatment is completed by all. In the case of single-dose regimens, abstinence should be practiced for 7 days after the partners begin treatment. They also should be seen for follow-up in 3 months to test for reinfection, and thereafter at least every 6 months for STI surveillance because of the significant incidence of another (often subclinical) infection.

The importance of aggressive case finding, diagnosis, and treatment of both infected patients and their partners cannot be overemphasized because of the potential for spread to others and major sequelae that include ectopic pregnancy, infertility, and chronic pelvic pain as a result of smoldering or recurrent upper genital tract disease. Finally, it is the clinician's responsibility to provide education regarding STIs. Patients should clearly understand how the disease was contracted and how to prevent recurrence. Use of condoms should be emphasized at every opportunity. Education includes discussion of responsible sexuality, including abstinence, use of contraceptives, and safer sex practices, as appropriate to the patient.

Surface Infestations and Perineal Lesions

Parasitic Infestations

Two parasitic infestations—scabies and pubic lice—may be transmitted via sexual contact. Both produce symptoms of vulvar and inguinal pruritus and irritation accompanied by finding dark specks of parasite feces on underwear or blood caused by excoriation from scratching. Sexual transmission is more likely in adolescents than in young children, who may acquire the parasites by close nonsexual contact. Development of pubic hair is necessary for the acquisition of pubic lice. Meticulous inspection of the pubic area for nits and adult lice ("crabs") may be necessary to discover early infestations. The clinical findings of both disorders are presented in Chapter 8.

Human Papillomavirus

HPV has emerged as the most prevalent sexually transmitted pathogen found in adolescent girls. Genital warts, also called *condylomata acuminata,* are no longer regarded as an isolated nuisance, but rather as one manifestation of a spectrum of lower genital tract diseases caused by HPV. The virus plays a causative role in the development of cervical intraepithelial neoplasia (CIN) and dysplasia (atypical squamous cells of undetermined significance, or ASC-US; low-grade squamous intraepithelial lesions, or LSIL; and high-grade squamous intraepithelial lesions, or HSIL), and similarly carcinoma of the cervix and of other genital tissues in both men and women. Although cervical cytology screening is not indicated in immunocompetent patients under 21, when performed, the presence

Table 18-7	Major Characteristics of the Most Common Sexually Transmitted Diseases and Diagnostic Measures						
	HSV	**HPV**	**HIV**	***Trichomonas***	**Gonorrhea**	***Chlamydia***	**Syphilis**
Clinical findings	May be normal; vulvar vesicles or ulcers, vulvitis, vaginitis, cervicitis	Vulvar, vaginal, cervical, perineal, and perianal condylomata and flat warts	Treatment resistant or unusually severe presentation of *Candida*, HPV, HSV, or molluscum contagiosum	Vaginitis, vulvitis, vaginal and/or cervical petechiae, profuse watery discharge	May be normal; cervicitis, salpingitis, urethritis, occasionally proctitis, pharyngitis; vaginitis and vulvitis in prepubertal girls	Often normal; cervicitis, salpingitis, urethritis, proctitis; vaginitis and vulvitis in prepubertal girls	Primary—vulvar, vaginal, or cervical chancre; secondary—condylomata lata of vulva; generalized exanthem
Incubation period	3-14 d	On average 1-3 mo (variable, up to 2 yr)	Acute flulike viral illness: several weeks; AIDS: variable—up to 10 yr	3-30 d	2-7 d	7-21 d	Primary: 15-90 d; secondary: 6 wk-6 mo; tertiary: 2-20 yr
Infectivity	75%-80% with active infection	60%-70%	Varies with infecting behavior	70%-90% for M/F transmission, less for F/M	100% M/F; 25% F/M	45% M/F	10%, single encounter; 30%, after 1 mo of sexual activity with an infected partner
Duration	Primary outbreak 2-3 wk; recurrent outbreak 7-12 d; latent infection indefinitely	Variable; often, persistent clinical lesions and subclinical infection	Acute infection (2-3 wk); asymptomatic phase (months); symptomatic HIV (months–years); AIDS (months–years)	Self-limiting in many males; persistent in most females until treated	Until treated	Until treated	Primary: 2-6 wk; secondary: 2-6 wk, may recur; tertiary: persists until treated
Recurrence	60% (HSV-1); 90% (HSV-2) within 1 yr	Variable	Persistence	With reinfection	With reinfection	With reinfection	With reinfection
Routine diagnostic techniques	Culture, antigen testing, serology	Inspection	ELISA, Western blot antibody test	Wet prep, NAAT, culture	NAAT, cervical, pharyngeal or rectal culture*	NAAT, culture*	Serology, dark-field microscopy
Antenatal or perinatal transmission	Yes—can cause skin, CNS, and disseminated infection	Yes—can cause laryngeal papillomas and perineal lesions	Yes, and postpartum via breast milk	Yes—may have neonatal vaginal discharge or asymptomatic colonization	Yes—can cause conjunctivitis, septicemia, meningitis	Yes—can cause conjunctivitis and/or pneumonia	Yes, and postpartum via breast milk
Partner evaluation	Inspection	Inspection	ELISA, Western blot antibody test	Antimicrobial treatment	Diagnostic tests as above and antimicrobial treatment	Diagnostic tests as above and antimicrobial treatment	Serologic and clinical, antimicrobial treatment

*In prepubertal girls, culture discharge for gonorrhea, vaginal wall for *Chlamydia*.

AIDS, acquired immunodeficiency syndrome; F/M, female to male; HPV, human papillomavirus; HSV, herpes simplex virus; M/F, male to female; NAAT, nucleic acid amplification test.

of abnormalities on either standard Pap or liquid-based cytology suggests infection with HPV.

Transmission of HPV is usually via sexual contact in adolescents. Passage to neonates during delivery also has been documented and can result in subsequent development of laryngeal papillomata and perineal lesions. Vaginal involvement is uncommon in the prepubertal child, but when present, is often accompanied by a vaginal discharge. The incubation period is variable and ranges from 1 to 24 months (see Table 18-7).

Condylomata may emerge after subclinical, acute, or chronic nonspecific vulvovaginal inflammation incited by the virus. In most cases the lesions are asymptomatic, although pruritus is reported by some patients. However, when the warts are traumatized or become secondarily infected, pain may be a complaint. A rapid increase in warty tissue may be associated with diabetes, pregnancy, or HIV infection.

In general, the warts appear as fleshy, rounded, or ragged papules often located at the posterior edge of the introitus and/or in the perianal region. Lesions may be discrete early on (Fig. 18-34, *A*), but with evolution tend to become confluent (Fig. 18-34, *B*). The warts can also be flat or even clinically unapparent to the naked eye. Although most lesions involve the perineum and perianal areas, vaginal and cervical

involvement are also common in adolescents (Fig. 18-34, *C*). The virus can also infect other mucous membranes, including the anus, urethra, mouth, larynx, and conjunctiva. Clinical diagnosis is made by careful inspection of the external genitalia, vagina, cervix (in adolescents), and perianal areas for visible warts. A negative serologic test for syphilis helps differentiate HPV disease from the condylomata lata of secondary syphilis.

Molluscum Contagiosum

The sharply circumscribed, waxy, papular, umbilicated lesions of molluscum contagiosum, caused by a poxvirus, can be spread as a result of sexual contact, in which case lesions are found predominantly on the labia, mons pubis, buttocks, and lower abdomen. This mode of spread is much more likely in the adolescent than in the young child. The clinical characteristics of molluscum lesions are presented in Chapter 8.

Syphilis

Syphilitic Chancre. Primary syphilis should be considered in any patient with a genital ulcer (Fig. 18-35). Most involve the genitalia, and in women they tend to be found more often on the cervix or vaginal walls than on the labia. Both external

Figure 18-34   Condylomata acuminata. These sexually transmitted viral warts **(A)** tend to be discrete early on, but with evolution become confluent **(B).** Adolescents have a significant risk of developing vaginal and cervical lesions **(C).** (*A* and *C, Courtesy E. Jerome, MD; B, courtesy M. Sherlock, MD, Lutherville, Md.*)

and internal lesions are painless and tend to go unnoticed unless a young woman happens to undergo pelvic examination while they are present. Hence, active syphilis in women often goes undiagnosed until the secondary stage of the disease. Although a single lesion is typical, multiple chancres are seen in some cases. The chancre usually appears 3 to 4 weeks (up to 3 months) after inoculation with *Treponema pallidum* and is accompanied by inguinal adenopathy. Involved nodes are firm, mobile, and nontender. Because atypical lesions are common, all suspicious ulcers should prompt investigation by dark-field examination of scrapings from the base of the ulcer or of material aspirated from an enlarged regional node. Prior application of topical antibiotic ointment to a chancre can give false-negative results with ulcer scrapings. Reagin serologic tests (Venereal Disease Research Laboratory [VDRL] or rapid plasma reagin [RPR]) usually become positive within 1 to 2 weeks after the appearance of the chancre and are uniformly elevated after 1 month. Positive reagin tests should always be confirmed by a serologic test for fluorescent treponemal antibody. Left untreated, chancres heal spontaneously in 3 to 8 weeks, but the infection persists.

Secondary Syphilis. In the absence of early diagnosis and treatment, hematogenous spread occurs approximately 1 to 3 months after the appearance of the primary chancre, whereupon the lesions of secondary syphilis appear. These are accompanied or preceded by generalized adenopathy and often are associated with systemic flulike symptoms of fever, headache, malaise, arthralgia, sore throat, and rhinorrhea.

Figure 18-35   Primary syphilis. The syphilitic chancre begins as an erythematous papule that erodes centrally. It is typically painless and indurated on palpation, with a smooth base and rolled margins *[Courtesy The Centers for Disease Control and Prevention Public Health Image Library (PHIL).]*

The rash generalizes rapidly, has a symmetrical distribution, and involves the palms and soles. The lesions usually take the form of reddish brown maculopapules, although commonly they are papulosquamous (Fig. 18-36, *A*). Follicular and pustular lesions also may be seen, making secondary syphilis the "great mimicker." They range in size from a few millimeters to 1 cm and can be round or oval. On occasion they clear centrally, becoming annular. As in pityriasis rosea, for which the rash is often mistaken, they are frequently oriented along lines of skin cleavage. Moist papules, called *condylomata lata,* are found in the genital folds, gluteal cleft, and over the medial surfaces of the upper thighs (Fig. 18-36, *B*). These papules often resemble small mushroom caps or have a warty appearance with a pinkish gray color and range in size from 1 to 3 cm. Many patients develop an associated patchy alopecia.

Mucosal lesions, termed *mucous patches* (Fig. 18-36, *C*), appear as centrally eroded, grayish white plaques 0.5 to 1 cm in diameter and can be found on all mucosal surfaces. Condylomata lata and mucosal lesions teem with organisms and are thus highly infectious and are ideal sites for obtaining specimens for dark-field examination. Serologic tests are positive at this stage. The rash persists for 1 to 3 months if untreated and then clears spontaneously, marking the beginning of a period of latency in which the organism persists in multiple tissues with the potential for causing tertiary disease years later.

Bartholin Gland Abscess

Bartholin gland abscess presents as a unilateral red, hot, tender mass at the posterior margin of the introitus at the base of a labium majorum (Fig. 18-37, *A* and *B*). It is generally seen in adolescents with gonorrhea, but it can occur in younger patients infected with gonococci, and it is increasingly associated with *Chlamydia.* When such a mass is encountered, material expressed from the abscess should be cultured because other agents such as streptococci and vaginal anaerobes have also been documented as pathogens. A full evaluation for STIs may be necessary for organism identification. Treatment is based on diagnostic testing results. Often incision, drainage, and packing or placement of a Word catheter are required. Less commonly, abscesses can occur more anteriorly, originating in the periurethral or Skene glands.

Lower Tract Disease

A number of STIs that present as vulvovaginitis in the prepubertal patient produce findings limited to the lower genital tract (e.g., vaginitis and cervicitis) in the adolescent. A

Figure 18-36 Secondary syphilis. **A,** This adolescent had flulike symptoms and a generalized papulosquamous eruption involving the palms and soles. **B,** In another patient, the characteristic moist papules of condylomata lata are seen over the vulva and the medial thighs. **C,** Mucosal lesions were also prominent. The systemic symptoms, mucosal lesions, and involvement of palms and soles helped distinguish the eruption from that of pityriasis rosea, with which it is commonly confused. *(A and C, Courtesy Robert Hickey, MD, Children's Hospital of Pittsburgh, Pittsburgh, Pa.; B, courtesy J. Pledger, The Centers for Disease Control and Prevention, Philadelphia, Pa.)*

discussion of these infections follows. Upper tract manifestations are discussed later in Pelvic Inflammatory Disease.

Genital Herpes

Type 2 and, less commonly, type 1 herpes simplex viruses have been confirmed as genital pathogens in both pubertal and prepubertal girls. In adolescents, genital infection is acquired almost exclusively by sexual or intimate contact with infected mucosal surfaces. In postpubertal patients with vulvar herpetic lesions, further evaluation for simultaneous STIs is warranted.

In prepubertal children, vulvar involvement can also result from sexual contact or by spread from another infected site, such as the lips, mouth, or a herpetic whitlow. It can also be acquired from parents with herpes labialis who fail to wash their hands properly before changing diapers or assisting young children with toileting. Most infections are symptomatic, but occasionally infected individuals have no symptoms. An antibody response, with or without symptoms, can be produced within a few days (see Table 18-7).

Patients with primary infection frequently have systemic symptoms of fever, malaise, and myalgia, in addition to severe perineal pain and dysuria. Tender inguinal adenopathy usually is prominent but may not develop for several days. Perineal inspection reveals single or clustered vesicular lesions and/or ulcers on erythematous and edematous bases (Fig. 18-38, *A*). Acute ulcerations are typically covered by yellow exudate and may be extensive (Fig. 18-38, *B*). A copious, foul-smelling, watery yellow vaginal discharge may be seen, as well. Associated sterile pyuria may be a feature. Dysuria may be so severe as to cause acute urinary retention. The ulcerative phase gradually resolves as lesions heal within a period of 14 to 21 days. After primary infection, a persistent subclinical infection is established in the lumbosacral ganglia.

Viral culture of a fresh and ideally vesicular lesion usually is confirmatory within a few days and is the diagnostic test of choice. Serum confirmation of type 1 or 2 infection is possible, but does not influence treatment decisions. Clinical suspicion is the usual indication for initiating antiviral therapy, as the earlier it is begun the more efficacious it is likely to be.

Recurrences are common and generally are milder, of shorter duration, and only locally symptomatic. Possible triggers of recurrence include fever, menstruation, emotional stress, and friction. On occasion, prodromal tingling, pain, burning, or hyperesthesia is noticed in the area where vesicles ultimately recur. The interval between episodes varies widely.

Trichomonas *Infection*

Trichomonas vaginalis is a flagellated protozoan. It has been found in the vaginal discharge of neonates delivered of mothers infected at the time of delivery, but thereafter it tends to be an unusual finding until the peripubertal period. This is thought to be due to the alkaline environment of the unestrogenized vaginal mucosa, which is unfavorable for growth of the organism. Beyond the neonatal period it is acquired almost exclusively by sexual contact, often in concert with other STIs. However, trichomonads can live on warm, moist surfaces outside a living host for up to 45 minutes. Hence, transmission via fomites is possible although infrequent. Although infection can be asymptomatic in adolescents, symptomatic patients have vulvar pruritus, burning, and dysuria, in association with a profuse vaginal discharge that may be watery, yellowish gray, or green. Some affected adolescents may complain of pelvic pain or heaviness.

On inspection the vulva may be hyperemic and edematous, but the degree of inflammation is highly variable. Because the discharge is profuse, it may be present on the perineum (Fig. 18-39, *A*). It pools in dependent portions of the vagina and coats the vaginal walls (Fig. 18-39, *B*). The vaginal mucosa is erythematous, and vaginal tenderness and petechiae may be noted (Fig. 18-39, *C*). This organism does not routinely ascend to infect the upper genital tract.

Diagnosis is confirmed by finding motile trichomonads on microscopic examination of a saline wet mount (Fig. 18-39, *D*), but this may be positive in only 50% to 60% of infections. On close observation, whiplike flagellar movements are noted. Leukocytes are usually present in increased numbers and may surround the organisms, making detection more difficult. Test yield may be increased by warming the saline solution to body temperature, and diluting a densely cellular discharge may make it easier to see the organisms moving. The slide must be examined soon after preparation because drying makes it uninterpretable. A mildly positive whiff test (release of amine odor on addition of 10% KOH to a drop of discharge) is also common. Trichomonads may also be found in urine specimens. An elevated vaginal pH may also support diagnosis. *Trichomonas* can also be diagnosed by culture or NAAT performed on a vaginal swab.

Oral metronidazole is effective for treatment; intravaginal metronidazole does not have sufficient absorption to reach the

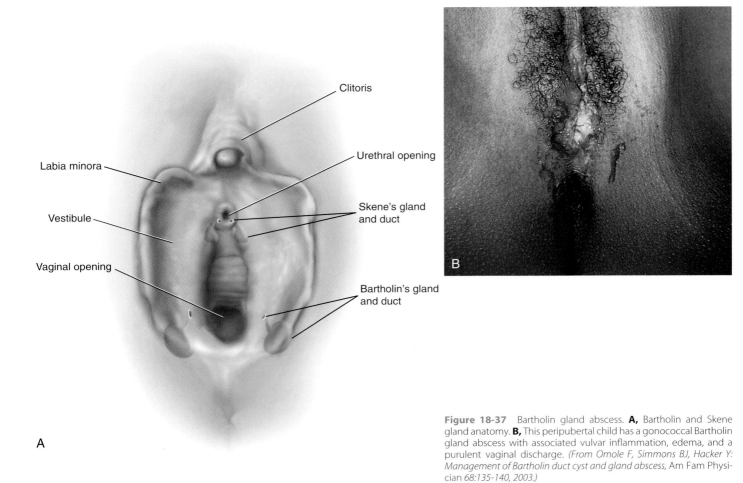

A

Figure 18-37   Bartholin gland abscess. **A,** Bartholin and Skene gland anatomy. **B,** This peripubertal child has a gonococcal Bartholin gland abscess with associated vulvar inflammation, edema, and a purulent vaginal discharge. *(From Omole F, Simmons BJ, Hacker Y: Management of Bartholin duct cyst and gland abscess, Am Fam Physician 68:135-140, 2003.)*

Figure 18-38   Herpes simplex. **A,** This prepubertal child had intense dysuria, perineal pain, and numerous vesicular lesions, a few of which have ulcerated, over her perineum. **B,** The full-blown ulcerative phase of herpetic vulvitis is seen in this adolescent patient.

Figure 18-39 *Trichomonas* infection. **A,** *Trichomonas vaginalis* produces a profuse foul acrid-smelling thin discharge that often is visible on perineal inspection. **B,** In some cases it is homogeneous, and in others it is bubbly as shown here. Vulvar pruritus is often intense. **C,** The vaginal mucosa is inflamed and often speckled with petechial lesions. In adolescents, petechial hemorrhages may also be found on the cervix, resulting in the so-called strawberry cervix. **D,** Microscopic examination of a wet mount reveals motile trichomonads. (*A and **C,** Courtesy Ellen Wald, MD, University of Wisconsin Children's Hospital, Madison, Wis.; **B,** courtesy Harold C. Wiesenfeld, MD, CM, Magee-Womens Hospital of the University of Pittsburgh Medical Center, Pittsburgh, Pa.; **D,** courtesy Jill Huppert, MD, MPH, and Joel Mortensen, PhD, Cincinnati Children's Hospital Medical Center, Cincinnati, Ohio.*)

multiple sites of trichomonal infection, including the urethra and Skene glands. Tinidazole is used when metronidazole fails or organisms are known to be resistant. Sexual partners usually are asymptomatic carriers of small numbers of organisms, but occasionally have symptoms of urethritis. Whether symptomatic or not, they should be treated to avoid subsequent transmission.

Bacterial Vaginosis

Bacterial vaginosis (BV) is a noninflammatory condition that is not sexually transmitted but is associated with sexual activity and STI, and is more common among African-American women and those practicing unprotected sexual intercourse. It represents a disturbance in the vaginal ecosystem with an overgrowth of multiple species of anaerobic bacteria and a corresponding decrease in lactobacilli. The overall concentration of bacteria increases 100-fold. The condition is associated with an increased frequency of preterm labor, and possibly with increased incidence of pelvic inflammatory disease. The major symptom in all age groups is vaginal discharge with a noticeable fishy odor. Adolescents with BV have little vulvovaginal irritation, and the cervix and upper genital tract are spared.

On inspection, discharge is frequently present on the perineum (Fig. 18-40, *A*) and may be seen adhering to the vaginal walls, which do not appear to be inflamed. In general,

the discharge is thin and homogeneous in consistency, grayish white in color, and malodorous. Addition of 10% KOH to a sample of the discharge produces a noticeable amine odor (positive whiff test). A saline wet preparation usually reveals characteristic "clue cells" (Fig. 18-40, *B*). The diagnosis is made clinically by meeting three of the following four criteria: homogeneous white discharge, a positive whiff test, clue cells representing more than 20% of the epithelial cells on a saline wet mount preparation, and vaginal secretions with a pH greater than 4.5. Because BV alone is rarely associated with evidence of tissue invasion, leukocytes should not be seen in increased numbers. If they are, additional pathogens should be sought and are often found. Both oral and intravaginal metronidazole and intravaginal clindamycin are acceptable forms of treatment in the nonpregnant patient.

Gonorrhea

Gonococci are a common cause of treatable bacterial cervicitis in the adolescent and of vulvovaginitis in the prepubertal child. The major complaint is of a purulent vaginal discharge. Before menarche the child may be otherwise asymptomatic, but most experience some degree of vulvar discomfort, pruritus, and/or dysuria. Symptomatic adolescents without upper genital tract extension can have a similar picture. Inspection reveals a profuse purulent discharge that usually is greenish yellow but also can be creamy, yellow, green, or white.

Figure 18-40 Bacterial vaginosis. Overgrowth of multiple anaerobes produces this form of vaginosis. **A,** The major symptom is one of a malodorous homogeneous vaginal discharge. **B,** Characteristic "clue cells" are seen on wet mount and consist of vaginal epithelial cells covered with adherent refractile bacteria. Because the organisms are non-invasive, leukocytes are not increased and mucosal changes are not present. (**A,** *Courtesy Ellen Wald, MD, University of Wisconsin Children's Hospital, Madison, Wis.*)

Inspection of the distal vaginal mucosa in younger children reveals prominent inflammation. In adolescents the vaginal mucosa can appear normal, but the cervix usually is erythematous and friable, with purulent material seen draining through the os (Fig. 18-41, *A*). Patients in this age group may also have objective evidence of urethritis as manifested by erythema, edema, and tenderness of the urethra. Other sites with columnar epithelium are similarly vulnerable to infection. These include Bartholin and Skene glands and the rectum (see Fig. 18-37, *B*).

A Gram-stained smear of the vaginal discharge will reveal large numbers of leukocytes and gram-negative intracellular diplococci (Fig. 18-41, *B*). Cultures or NAATs are used to confirm the infection. Culture is indicated when it is necessary to determine antimicrobial sensitivity and is essential in medicolegal cases. Because simultaneous throat and anal cultures can be positive (despite the absence of anorectal or pharyngeal symptoms) even when the vaginal culture is negative, culture of these sites should be considered when gonorrhea is suspected or confirmed. Both tonsils and the posterior pharyngeal wall should be swabbed in obtaining the throat specimen; the rectal swab should be inserted no more than 1 to 2 cm past the anal orifice to avoid fecal contamination.

Recent studies of women with culture-proven gonococcal cervicitis have shown that concurrent chlamydial infection is present in up to one third. Thus, when purulent cervicitis is found, specific specimens for detection of *C. trachomatis* should also be obtained and treatment for both pathogens

Figure 18-41 Gonorrhea. **A,** Adolescents are vulnerable to ascent of infection and usually have findings of cervical inflammation with mucopurulent discharge. **B,** On Gram stain, the vaginal discharge from the patient in Fig. 18-37, *B* with gonorrhea is found to contain sheets of leukocytes, many of which contain gram-negative intracellular diplococci. (**A,** *Courtesy L. Vontver, MD.*)

begun empirically. Local patterns of bacterial resistance dictate antibiotic choices. Several single-dose oral therapies are usually acceptable for cervicitis. Pharyngeal and anal infection with *N. gonorrhoeae* may also influence antibiotic choice, and current Centers for Disease Control and Prevention (CDC) guidelines should be consulted (see Websites, following the bibliography).

On occasion, patients with gonorrhea may develop disseminated gonococcal infection via hematogenous spread. This phenomenon may occur at any age. It is more common in adolescent girls with asymptomatic (and, therefore, untreated) endocervical infection, in men with asymptomatic urethral infection, and in patients of both genders and all ages with silent anal or pharyngeal infections. It can also be seen in patients with symptomatic vulvovaginitis, cervicitis, or urethritis. In postmenarchal women, systemic symptoms are more likely to develop during a menstrual period.

The clinical picture often has two stages. Initially fever and chills are prominent, and the patient is intermittently bacteremic. During this stage, which lasts 2 to 5 days, polyarthralgias are experienced (involving the knees, wrists, ankles, elbows, and hands) and characteristic skin lesions often appear. The latter begin as small erythematous papules or petechiae that usually evolve to form pustules surrounded by red halos (Fig. 18-42, *A* and *B*). Later, these may necrose centrally. Lesions often contain gram-negative diplococci, which can be seen on a Gram stain, but usually fail to grow on culture. If not diagnosed and treated promptly, patients progress to a second phase, characterized by monarticular arthritis with effusion or tenosynovitis (Fig. 18-42, *C* and *D*).

In up to 50% of these cases, culture of joint aspirates is positive. Specialized techniques to isolate cell wall–deficient organisms further increase culture yield. Myocarditis, pericarditis, endocarditis, and meningitis are other complications of hematogenous seeding.

Chlamydia trachomatis *Infection*

Chlamydia is the most prevalent curable STI causing cervicitis and urethritis, and contributing to upper genital tract disease. Its high prevalence (up to 25%) in adolescent populations and its serious sequelae make its proper diagnosis and treatment an important aspect of adolescent sexual health care. When compared with gonococcal infection, its transmission rate for a single episode of intercourse is lower, but its prevalence is greater and infection persists longer. Of women whose male partners are infected with *Chlamydia*, 45% are infected.

Chlamydiae are slowly replicating obligate intracellular organisms. Diagnosis is confirmed by NAAT on urine or on vaginal or endocervical swabs. Tests of cure are not recommended by the CDC and remain positive for up to 3 weeks after treatment. Reinfection is common and retesting should be considered in 3 months even in the absence of symptoms.

Although most prepubertal girls are asymptomatic, some of those infected with *Chlamydia* may have vaginal discharge and/or bleeding, vulvar pruritus or pain, and vulvar erythema. Symptoms may be intermittent or persistent and coinfection with *N. gonorrhoeae* is common. Adolescent girls may have symptoms of both cervical and urethral infection. Pelvic or abdominal pain, spotting or irregular vaginal bleeding,

Figure 18-42   Disseminated gonococcal infection. **A** and **B,** These pustular skin lesions with red halos are characteristic of disseminated gonorrhea, which can occur at any age. **C** and **D,** Tenosynovitis and monarticular arthritis are commonly seen in association with skin lesions in disseminated disease. Note the signs of effusion in the right knee of the girl shown in **(D).** (**D,** *Courtesy Robert Hickey, MD, Children's Hospital of Pittsburgh, Pittsburgh, Pa.*)

dysuria, and/or vaginal discharge may accompany infection. A picture indistinguishable from that of symptomatic gonorrhea (purulent vaginal discharge, perineal irritation, and findings of cervicitis with mucopurulent discharge) can also be seen (see Fig. 18-41, *A*). Endometritis is common with cervicitis, even in the absence of classic symptoms of pelvic inflammatory disease, and Bartholin duct infections also occur. It is important to note that asymptomatic chlamydial infection in both females and males is common.

On examination of the cervix, the presence of yellowish green mucopus, cervical ectopy, and erythema are all associated with chlamydial infection. Often the cervix is friable, bleeding during the minimal manipulation necessary to obtain specimens. Microscopic evidence of other infections does not decrease the likelihood of *Chlamydia* coinfection and should not deter the practitioner from testing and treating for *Chlamydia* if its presence is suggested by the history or physical findings. As noted earlier, patients commonly have simultaneous infection with gonococci and *Chlamydia*—hence the rationale for testing for both organisms and treating for both when purulent cervicitis is found on examination.

Chlamydia can also produce an acute urethral syndrome in postpubertal patients. Dysuria, urgency, and frequency may be accompanied by physical signs of urethral discharge, meatal redness, and swelling. Pyuria may exist in the absence of bacteriuria. An NAAT for *Chlamydia* can be performed on a urine specimen. Rectal infection exists in both heterosexual and homosexual populations. A rectal swab may be sent for NAAT testing for *Chlamydia*, with the caveat that such testing is not FDA-approved. However, individual laboratories may be approved to perform these tests. Pharyngeal infection is rarely detected. A careful sexual history may reveal extragenital sites of infection, but treatment for infection at these other sites is not known to differ.

Genital Mycoplasmas

Mycoplasma hominis, Mycoplasma genitalium, and *Ureaplasma urealyticum* are the three species of mycoplasma implicated in genital infections. The organisms may be cultured from vaginal specimens of neonates and sexually active women in the absence of disease, but colonization in the prepubertal girl is rare. Mycoplasmas have also been cultured from polymicrobial upper genital tract infections, but it remains unclear whether they are initiators of ascending infections or if they behave as normal bacterial flora accompanying the primary ascending infection of gonorrhea or *Chlamydia* organisms, becoming pathogenic once relocated in the fallopian tubes. Mycoplasmas have also been found to be causative in some cases of acute urethral syndrome. These organisms are not routinely tested for in clinical practice. They are thought to be eradicated by treatments for *Chlamydia*.

Human Immunodeficiency Virus

Acquired immunodeficiency syndrome (AIDS) and other manifestations of HIV infection are discussed in Chapter 12. The adolescent history outlined previously (see Table 18-3) should identify teenagers at risk of acquiring HIV infection. In an attempt to reduce subsequent transmission and to treat infection early, confidential HIV testing is encouraged for all teens at risk of exposure to the virus. The definition of moderate to high risk has been regularly changing as our understanding of the disease, its epidemiology, and treatment opportunities evolves. Reliable sources of such information (e.g., the CDC) should be consulted regularly. From the gynecologic perspective, a number of infections may present differently in the HIV-infected individual (see Table 18-7). Also, cervical cytology screening should be initiated earlier than in immunocompetent individuals.

Pelvic Inflammatory Disease

An important complication of lower genital tract infection in the postmenarchal female is pelvic inflammatory disease (PID). PID results from ascending spread of a cervical infection that may or may not have been symptomatic. The majority of cases of PID are due to mixed anaerobic and aerobic infections, although the classically recognized sexually transmitted pathogens play a critical initiating role. Initiating pathogens implicated include *N. gonorrhoeae, C. trachomatis,* and *M. hominis*. Other organisms, usually considered normal vaginal or enteric flora, are potentially pathogenic when introduced into the upper genital tract. Among these are *Bacteroides* species; other anaerobic gram-positive bacilli and cocci, such as those found in bacterial vaginosis; and aerobes, including streptococcal species, *E. coli, Klebsiella* and *Proteus* species, and *Trichomonas* (see Box 18-7). Women who are immunocompromised or from areas where tuberculosis is endemic may have tuberculosis-associated PID.

Risk factors for developing upper genital tract infection include adolescent age, multiple sexual partners, and previous PID. Because menstruation facilitates ascent of pathogenic organisms from the cervix to the uterus and fallopian tubes, the onset of symptoms often occurs during or shortly after a menstrual period. Long-term morbidity includes an increased incidence of ectopic pregnancy, decreased fertility, and chronic pelvic pain. These sequelae are secondary to tubal occlusion and scarring of pelvic structures. Adverse clinical outcomes and long-term morbidity may be more severe among *Chlamydia*-positive or non-GC/CT patients with PID. Delay in diagnosis and treatment, unusually severe PID, and repeated infection are associated with more severe long-term sequelae. It is estimated that for each episode of PID there is an additional 15% chance of subsequent fertility problems.

The "textbook" picture of acute PID is one of a sexually active female who abruptly develops a high fever and shaking chills in association with intense lower abdominal pain. Nausea and vomiting are common. The patient appears acutely ill and uncomfortable and may have pain on walking, often with a shuffling gait. On examination there is prominent lower abdominal tenderness and guarding, and signs of cervicitis with mucopurulent discharge. Bimanual palpation elicits extreme pain on cervical motion and reveals marked tenderness of the fundus and adnexa. Adnexal enlargement, if present, suggests abscess formation. The erythrocyte sedimentation rate is markedly elevated, and there is a pronounced leukocytosis with a left shift on CBC and differential. This "classic" picture has the highest likelihood of being associated with positive cultures for *N. gonorrhoeae*. It is not the most typical scenario, however. More commonly the onset of symptoms is insidious and the clinical picture more subtle. This is particularly likely with nongonococcal PID. Fever may be absent or low grade; abdominal pain, mild; and blood work frequently is normal. In such cases diagnosis can be particularly difficult, requiring considerable suspicion and a low threshold for obtaining cultures or other tests on the part of the clinician. Lower abdominal, pelvic, and/or cervical motion tenderness and some evidence of lower genital tract inflammation usually are present even in clinically mild cases. A low-grade tubal infection may produce more in the way of adnexal findings and few, if any, uterine signs.

Diagnosis is complicated by the fact that there is wide variation in the severity of the clinical picture. Furthermore, acute salpingitis may mimic a number of other disorders (Box 18-8). The adolescent girl with right lower quadrant (RLQ) abdominal pain is particularly challenging diagnostically. Table 18-8 summarizes clinical findings that may aid in distinguishing among some of the most common causes.

Medical Conditions Manifesting as Acute Right-Sided Abdominal Pain in Adolescent Girls

HEPATIC

Fitz-Hugh–Curtis syndrome
Viral hepatitis (A, B, C, etc.)
Drug-induced hepatitis
Autoimmune hepatitis
Alcoholic hepatitis
Hepatitis secondary to bacteremia
Epstein-Barr virus hepatitis

BILIARY

Acute cholecystitis
Cholelithiasis

INTESTINAL

Inflammatory bowel disease
Irritable bowel syndrome
Constipation
Lactose intolerance

OTHER GASTROINTESTINAL

Subphrenic abscess
Appendicitis
Perforated gastric or duodenal ulcer

PULMONARY

Pneumonia, pleuritis, pleurodynia

RENAL

Acute pyelonephritis or perinephric abscess

GYNECOLOGIC

Pelvic inflammatory disease
Ovarian cyst, torsion, rupture, hemorrhage
Dysmenorrhea
Ectopic pregnancy

Given the variability of the clinical picture in PID, minimal diagnostic criteria have been developed. These include lower abdominal or pelvic pain, and cervical motion or uterine or adnexal tenderness. Although adding additional criteria such as fever, leukocytosis, and abnormal vaginal microscopy may increase the specificity of the diagnosis, this also increases the risk of missing PID and delaying treatment. Because of the potentially devastating long-term sequelae of PID, aggressive, empiric broad-spectrum antimicrobial therapy is warranted. Treatment should include antibiotics that cover the common organisms in accordance with current CDC recommendations (see Websites, following the bibliography).

Indications for hospitalization and parenteral therapy from the outset include the following: suspected abscess, toxicity, inability to take and retain oral medication, and concurrent pregnancy. Admission is also advisable when the exact diagnosis is unclear, or when poor compliance is likely. When initial outpatient treatment is elected, it is mandatory that the patient be reexamined within 24 to 72 hours to document clinical improvement and to confirm compliance with antibiotic use. If on follow-up it is found that there has been no significant clinical improvement, the patient should be admitted for parenteral medication. In addition to antibiotic resistance, failure to improve promptly on therapy, whether oral or parenteral, raises the possibility of complications such as abscess formation; development of a tubo-ovarian complex; or a missed diagnosis such as ectopic pregnancy, miscarriage, or appendicitis. As noted earlier, sonography is useful in evaluating masses and suspected tubo-ovarian abscesses. Laparoscopy may be necessary when surgical conditions are suspected or parenteral medical treatment fails.

Perihepatitis (Fitz-Hugh–Curtis Syndrome)

Perihepatitis, presenting as right upper quadrant (RUQ) pain, is seen as a complication of PID in 5% to 20% of cases. In these instances, the inflammatory process probably ascends from the fallopian tubes along the paracolic gutters to the RUQ, resulting in inflammation of the liver capsule and adjacent peritoneum. The clinical picture is one of moderate to severe pleuritic RUQ pain, which may be referred to the right shoulder, and is associated with fever, chills, nausea, and vomiting. Although the pain can develop simultaneously with pelvic symptoms of PID, in the majority of cases, it may have its onset in the course of an asymptomatic ascending lower

Ultrasonography has proved to be a useful diagnostic tool in many such cases, although it is usually normal in most cases of PID. Optimal imaging of the pelvis and adnexa is achieved with a transvaginal probe. Most of the time, an abdominal probe will be sufficient to provide diagnostic information. Figure 18-43 illustrates ultrasound findings related to ovarian cyst and torsion.

Figure 18-43 Ultrasound findings in the diagnosis of pelvic or abdominal pain. **A,** This image shows an abnormal amount of fluid in the cul-de-sac released from a ruptured ovarian cyst in a 15-year-old with left-lower-quadrant and midline pelvic pain. **B,** In a 12-year-old girl with a 4-day history of colicky right-lower-quadrant pain, ultrasound demonstrates a single large abnormal cyst and multiple small physiologic cysts. Operative diagnosis was right ovarian torsion.

Table 18-8	Pertinent Clinical Characteristics of Disorders Causing Right-Sided or Lower Abdominal Pain in Adolescent Girls			
	PID	**Ovarian Torsion**	**Ovarian Cyst**	**Ectopic Pregnancy**
Location and quality of pain	Mid- and lateral pelvis, usually bilateral; can be vague, dull, crampy, or sharp	Unilateral RLQ or LLQ, colicky	Usually asymptomatic, but may have colicky RLQ or LLQ pain	Lateral pain, colicky, ± uterine cramping
Onset	With GC rapid With *Chlamydia* gradual over days to months	Sudden	Gradual, although rupture or hemorrhage are associated with acutely increased pain	Gradual with sudden exacerbation
History	Unprotected sexual intercourse, previous PID or STI, multiple partners, patient in first half of menstrual cycle	± History of previous episodes of similar pain with resolution, increased ovarian size (anatomic variation predisposes)	Mid-cycle or luteal phase, physiologic rupture causes mittelschmerz, with pain for 24-48 h	Amenorrhea (75%), ± pregnancy signs and symptoms
GI symptoms	Nausea, vomiting, anorexia may be present	Vomiting with onset of pain (25%)	Rare	GI symptoms secondary to pregnancy or severe vomiting secondary to rupture and peritonitis
Masses	Occasional; if present, consider tubo-ovarian abscess or ectopic pregnancy	Usually present, increased size secondary to edema	Often palpable if not physiologic cyst	Adnexal mass palpable in 50% of cases
Physical examination and laboratory findings	Cervical motion and adnexal tenderness, clinical and lab evidence of cervicitis; vaginal bleeding; ± discharge; ± RUQ pain; perihepatitis; ± cervical NAATs for gonorrhea and/or *Chlamydia*	Tender adnexa, ± guarding or peritoneal signs	Unilateral cystic adnexal mass, x-ray rules out dermoid	Normal uterus; unilateral or bilateral adnexal tenderness; positive pregnancy test in most, but inadequate β-hCG rise/48 h after implantation; drop in Hct with rupture
Ultrasound findings	Usually normal, tubo-ovarian complex in 10%-15%	Unilateral ovarian enlargement; solid ovarian mass, ± compromised blood supply on Doppler	Cyst > 3 cm, ± fluid in cul-de-sac frequent incidental finding on ultrasound	Tubal mass, vaginal probe enhances detection
	Inflammatory Bowel Disease	**Appendicitis**	**Irritable Bowel/Constipation**	**Dysmenorrhea**
Location and quality of pain	LLQ, crampy	Periumbilical cramping changing to RLQ cramping or sharp pain	LLQ, crampy or colicky	Suprapubic, mid-abdominal, lower back, dull cramping
Onset	Gradual over weeks to months with exacerbations	Gradual over hours to days	Long history of GI symptoms over months to years	Periodic, evolving over hours; close to onset of flow
History	Weight loss or growth failure, fatigue, rashes, arthritis, fever	Usually no prior pain	± Constipation or diarrhea, distention common, positive family history, symptoms increase with stress	Increasing severity 1-3 yr after menarche
GI symptoms	Increased stool frequency, nocturnal stools, sometimes bloody diarrhea	Vomiting may follow onset of pain, anorexia	Long intermittent history of constipation, ± diarrhea	Diarrhea, flatulence, vomiting not uncommon with start of menses
Masses	Unusual, except with chronic complicated disease	Rare	Feces	None
Physical examination and laboratory findings	Rectoabdominal tenderness, hematologic abnormalities, positive for stool heme	↑ WBCs, fever, evolving peritoneal signs	Occasional tender colon, usually normal	Normal
Ultrasound findings	Normal	Appendix frequently visible	Normal	Normal

Note: Table 18-8 is designed not only to aid the clinician in distinguishing between disorders that present with abdominal pain in adolescent girls, but also to enhance recognition of the fact that a complaint of abdominal pain must be taken seriously and evaluated carefully.

↑, increased; ±, positive or negative; GC, gonococcus; GI, gastrointestinal; β-hCG, β subunit of human chorionic gonadotropin; Hct, hematocrit; LLQ, left lower quadrant; NAAT, nucleic acid amplification test; PID, pelvic inflammatory disease; RLQ, right lower quadrant; RUQ, right upper quadrant; STI, sexually transmitted infection; WBCs, white blood cells.

genital tract infection, or later in the course of a partially treated infection. In many of these patients upper abdominal pain is so severe that the patient is relatively unconcerned about milder degrees of lower abdominal and pelvic discomfort.

On examination, RUQ tenderness and guarding are the major physical findings and peritoneal signs may be present. Gynecologic examination in most instances discloses findings of purulent cervicitis and PID. *Neisseria gonorrhoeae* and *C. trachomatis* are the major pathogens associated with this syndrome. When nongonococcal in origin, the predisposing salpingitis may be silent. Patients with Fitz-Hugh–Curtis syndrome have minimal if any abnormalities of liver function tests. Although usually not necessary, ultrasound examination

of the right upper quadrant should demonstrate a normal liver, biliary tree, and gallbladder. Laparoscopic findings of purulent and fibrinous inflammation of the capsule and hemorrhagic areas of adjacent parietal peritoneum are diagnostic, but laparoscopy is rarely indicated for this condition. Major differential diagnostic considerations are listed in Box 18-8 and Table 18-8.

PREGNANCY

The birth rate for 15- to 19-year-old adolescents in the United States, approximately 42 per 1000, is the highest in the industrialized Western world. Because most of the pregnancies are unintended, adolescents may deny the possibility of their condition for extended periods to themselves, their parents,

Table 18-9	Signs and Symptoms of Pregnancy

First Trimester (6-12 Weeks)	Second Trimester (12+ Weeks)
Amenorrhea	Increased size of breasts, abdomen, waist
Light, irregular vaginal bleeding	Increased weight and clothing size
Syncope or fainting	Increased vaginal discharge
Fatigue	Increased skin pigmentation
Urinary frequency	Congestion of vaginal mucosa
Mood swings	
"Morning" sickness	
Nausea and vomiting	
Food cravings	
Increased facial oil gland activity ("glow")	
Elevated body temperature	
Chloasma (dark facial pigmentation)	
Nasal stuffiness or mucous membrane congestion	

Table 18-11	Causes of False-Positive and False-Negative Urine Pregnancy Tests

False-Negative Test	False-Positive Test
Too early (commonly) or too late (rarely)	Molar pregnancy
	Malignancies (gynecologic and other)
Adulterated urine	Postpartum and postabortion (up to 4 wk)
Ectopic pregnancy (rarely negative, almost always positive)	Chinese herbal medications
	Hematuria or proteinuria*
Impending or missed abortion (rarely negative, almost always positive)	Midcycle LH surge*
	Perimenopausal* (LH elevation)
Dilute urine	Premature ovarian failure* (LH elevation)

*Can occur with less sensitive over-the-counter urine pregnancy tests.
LH, luteinizing hormone.

and others. This delay is associated with decreased options and increased complications of pregnancy and neonatal morbidity. Vaginal bleeding or spotting in early pregnancy may falsely reassure a young woman that she is not pregnant, and minimal weight gain (whether voluntary or involuntary) may further facilitate denial. Some of these patients may present with substitute (not pregnancy-related) or peripheral chief complaints. Among these are pelvic, abdominal, or back pain; vomiting and dehydration; constipation; urinary complaints; and urinary tract infection. Phlebitis; rupture of membranes; symptoms of gestational diabetes; or secondary problems of fatigue, insomnia, or headache ultimately bring some of these patients to medical attention. With or without denial, at the time of presentation the teenager or her parent may suspect pregnancy. Interviewing the patient and parent separately may facilitate a complete and accurate history.

Considering the frequency of teenage pregnancy and the tendency of individuals to have alternative chief complaints, practitioners who care for adolescents should be familiar with the signs, symptoms, and methods of diagnosing pregnancy. Signs and symptoms of pregnancy are outlined in Table 18-9. A chronology of laboratory and clinical findings during pregnancy is presented in Table 18-10.

Home pregnancy tests are variable in sensitivity. Some are identical to and as sensitive as office laboratory enzyme-linked immunosorbent assays (ELISAs), and others may not give a positive result on a first-morning specimen until 14 to 21 days after conception. False-positive and false-negative results are encountered infrequently; causes for both are listed in Table 18-11. In particular, false positives are not caused by foods or drugs, but can occur in certain medical situations including up to 4 weeks after an abortion. Pregnancies are dated from the last normal menstrual period and not from conception, which typically occurs 2 weeks later. This is not well known by the public and should be explained to minimize confusion, facilitate decision-making, and clarify paternity.

ACKNOWLEDGMENT

The authors gratefully acknowledge Holly Davis for all of her work on previous versions of this chapter as well as for contributing all the photographs not otherwise attributed.

Table 18-10	Laboratory and Clinical Correlations of Pregnancy

Gestation*	Serum hCG (MIU/mL)	Signs, Symptoms, and Significant Events
1		Last menstrual period
2		
3	5 (24 h postimplantation)	Conception followed by implantation
4	70-100	Missed period
5	>250	Pelvic ultrasound detects pregnancy; breast changes—tender, swollen; nipples—sensitive, dark
6	>1000	Nausea, morning sickness; softening of lower corpus
7		Bluish color of cervix; softening of cervix; cardiac motion detectable on ultrasound
8	>10,000	
10	100,000 (peak)	
12		Fundus palpable at pelvic brim; fetal heart tones detectable with Doppler
14		Decrease in early signs and symptoms
16	10,000; false negatives may occur in second and third trimesters	Fundus palpable midway between pelvic brim and umbilicus; fetus visualized by x-ray; perception of fetal movement
20		Fundus palpable at umbilicus

*Weeks from last menstrual period.
hCG, human chorionic gonadotropin.

Bibliography

American College of Obstetricians and Gynecologists (ACOG): ACOG Committee opinion no. 463: Cervical cancer in adolescents: Screening, evaluation, and management, *Obstet Gynecol* 116:469–472, 2010.

Bandow GD: Diagnosis and management of vulvar ulcers, *Dermatol Clin* 28:753–763, 2010.

Berenson AB: Appearance of the hymen at birth and one year of age: A longitudinal study, *Pediatrics* 91:820–825, 1993.

Berenson AB, Heger AH, Hayes JM, et al: Appearance of the hymen in prepubertal girls, *Pediatrics* 89:387–394, 1992.

Braverman PK, Breech L: Clinical report—gynecologic examination for adolescents in the pediatric office setting, *Pediatrics* 126:583–590, 2010.

Emans SJ, Laufer MR, Goldstein DP: *Pediatric and adolescent gynecology*, ed 5, Philadelphia, 2005, Lippincott Williams & Wilkins.

Garel L, Dubois J, Grignon A, et al: US of the pediatric female pelvis: A clinical perspective, *RadioGraphics* 21:1393–1407, 2001.

Hammerschlag MR, Guillen C: Medical and legal implications of testing for sexually transmitted infections in children, *Clin Microbiol Rev* 23:493–506, 2010.

Hatcher RA, Trussell J, Nelson AL, et al, editors: *Contraceptive technology*, ed 19, New York, 2007, Ardent Media.

Holmes KK, Sparling PF, Stamm WE, et al, editors: *Sexually transmitted diseases*, ed 4, New York, 2008, McGraw-Hill.

Paradise JE, Campos JM, Friedman HM, et al: Vulvovaginitis in premenarchal girls: Clinical features and diagnostic evaluation, *Pediatrics* 70:193–198, 1982.

Pokorny SF, Stormer J: Atraumatic removal of secretions from the prepubertal vagina, *Am J Obstet Gynecol* 156:581–582, 1987.

Reddy J, Laufer MR: Hypertrophic labia minora, *J Pediatr Adolesc Gynecol* 23:3–6, 2010.

Sanfilippo JS, Lara-Torre E, Edmonds K, et al, editors: *Clinical pediatric and adolescent gynecology*, New York, 2009, Informa Healthcare.

Trager JDK: Pubic hair removal—pearls and pitfalls, *J Pediatr Adolesc Gynecol* 19:117–123, 2006.

Websites

American College of Obstetricians and Gynecologists: www.acog.org
Center for Young Women's Health: www.youngwomenshealth.org

Centers for Disease Control and Prevention: *Sexually transmitted diseases (STDs)*, www.cdc.gov/std/treatment/default.htm

North American Society for Pediatric and Adolescent Gynecology: www.naspag.org/

Society for Adolescent Health and Medicine: www.adolescenthealth.org

World Health Organization: *Classification of female genital mutilation*, www.who.int/reproductivehealth/topics/fgm/overview/en/index.html

OPHTHALMOLOGY

Kenneth P. Cheng | Albert W. Biglan

Infants and children may be affected by conditions not seen in adults, and the examination techniques and treatments that they may need frequently require subspecialty care. More than 50 years ago pediatric ophthalmology became established as a distinct subspecialty of Ophthalmology. Common problems include refractive errors, strabismus, amblyopia, infections, and trauma. Other problems encountered include ocular complications of systemic disease, developmental and genetic conditions, and neoplasms affecting the globe and orbits.

ANATOMY OF THE VISUAL SYSTEM

The visual system is conveniently separated into three principal parts: the globe and surrounding structures (Fig. 19-1), the visual pathways, and the visual or calcarine cortex.

The eyelids provide protection for the globe and assist in even distribution of the tear film over the cornea to provide a clear, undistorted optical surface. The crystalline lens complements the cornea's refracting power with its ability to adjust the focal length of the optical system so that incoming light from objects at any distance may be clearly imaged on the retina. During the first 2 to 3 months of life, children develop the ability to focus on images at any range (accommodation). Light is focused on the macula, the portion of the retina responsible for the central field of vision (Fig. 19-2). The retina contains the photoreceptors, rods and cones, which convert light energy into an electrical nerve response. The fovea centralis is the center of the macula; it has the greatest concentration of cones and is responsible for detailed, colored central visual acuity.

Nerve fibers emanate from the ganglion cell layer of the retina and coalesce to form the optic nerve. The right and left optic nerves pass from the orbits and join together to form the optic chiasm. Nerve fibers from the nasal retina decussate at the chiasm and are directed toward the contralateral side of the brain. Fibers from the temporal retina travel without crossing at the chiasm to the ipsilateral visual cortex (Fig. 19-3). From the optic chiasm the fibers form the optic tracts and synapse in the lateral geniculate nucleus in the midbrain. From there the optic radiations, one on each side of the brain, travel posteriorly to the visual cortex above the cerebellum.

The decussation of nerve fibers at the chiasm and integration in the visual cortex are responsible for binocular vision and the formation of the visual field. For example, if an object is seen off to the person's left, the image is received by the nasal retina of the left eye and the temporal retina of the right eye. Similarly, if the object is off to the person's right, the image falls on the nasal retina of the right eye and the temporal retina of the left eye. The temporal retina images objects in the contralateral visual field, and the nasal retina images objects in the ipsilateral visual field. Because of the decussation of nasal retinal fibers, the right visual cortex receives images from the left side of the visual field and the left visual cortex receives images from the right side of the visual field.

Lesions of the visual pathways produce predictable patterns of visual field loss; for example, a left homonymous hemianopsia (loss of the left side of the visual field) is produced by a lesion of the right occipital cortex. Detection of a visual field defect that respects or does not extend across the vertical midline of the visual field indicates pathology posterior to the optic chiasm (within the intracranial portion of the visual system). Visual field defects that involve both the right and left sides of the visual field in one or both eyes indicate either retinal or optic nerve pathology or lesions to both sides of the intracranial visual system. Because of the anatomy of the optic chiasm, compressive lesions of the chiasm (e.g., pituitary tumors) produce visual field defects involving the left side of the visual field of the left eye and the right side of the visual field of the right eye (bitemporal defects).

The visual field can be arbitrarily divided into the central field of vision and the peripheral field. The macula is responsible for the central field. A physiologic blind spot is found about 10 to 15 degrees temporal to central fixation (the fovea) and represents the area of the visual field that corresponds to the optic nerve head (optic disc). Precise measurement of the visual field of each eye can be obtained in a cooperative child or adult, using a Goldmann visual field perimeter or an automated visual field device. This test requires steady fixation and concentration. In young children, it is impractical to attempt this tedious measurement. In a patient unable to cooperate for a formal visual field test, the fields are assessed by observation of the child's eyes fixating on small targets brought into the peripheral field of vision in each quadrant of the visual field. Visual fields may also be assessed by a confrontation method, in which the child fixates on the examiner's nose and is asked to identify the examiner's fingers as they are slowly brought into each quadrant of the visual field from the periphery.

EVALUATION OF VISION

Selection of a test to measure a patient's visual acuity depends on the patient's age, cooperation, and level of development. The evaluation of vision in a young infant or nonverbal patient requires the use of the fixation reflex. This reflex develops during the first month or two of life. Although almost all 2- to 3-month-old infants can fixate and follow a face or bright object quite well into all fields of gaze, it is not necessarily abnormal for this milestone not to be present until 6 months of age. The level of vision can be estimated by the quality and intensity of the fixation response. If the visual acuity is normal, central fixation is steady and maintained on objects. If visual acuity is profoundly decreased, the quality of fixation may be wandering in nature, poorly maintained, or eccentric. Central, steady, maintained fixation equates to visual acuity of 20/200 or better. Eyes with unsteady or wandering fixation usually have visual acuity decreased to the 20/800 range (Fig. 19-4).

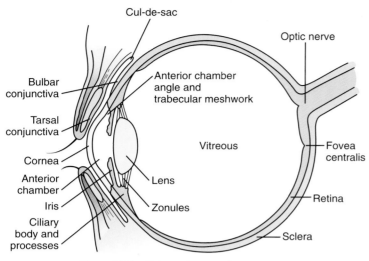

Figure 19-1   Globe and surrounding structures.

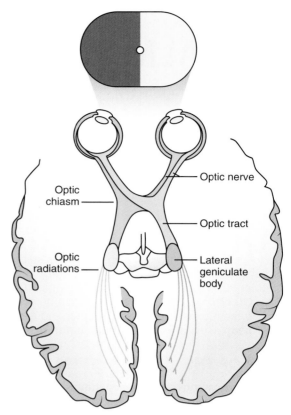

Figure 19-3   Visual field and visual pathways.

The visual pathways coalesce in the visual cortex. Electrical impulses in the visual cortex produced by light stimulation of the retina can be measured by placement of sensitive electrodes on the overlying scalp. This is termed the *visual evoked potential* or *response* (VEP or VER). The pattern visual evoked potential uses an alternating checkerboard stimulus, which can be controlled to produce a pattern of checks that may be increased or decreased in size. This test can be used to estimate visual acuity in preverbal or nonverbal children. Caution must be used in interpreting this test, however, because children and adults with known 20/20 vision can voluntarily suppress the visual evoked response. In addition, children who have significant decreases in their visual acuity may have a visual evoked response that overestimates the visual acuity.

Nonverbal infants or children may have their grating visual acuity measured with Teller Acuity Cards (Stereo Optical, Chicago, Ill.). This test is based on a child's reflex to move the eyes or head toward a pattern of alternating black-and-white stripes of increasing frequency rather than neutral gray of the same brightness.

The Allen object recognition cards, simple pictures of common objects, are useful for assessing visual acuity in a 2- to 3½-year-old child who cannot comprehend the illiterate or tumbling E game or recognize Snellen letters. To perform this test, the child is taught what the pictures are, and then one eye is occluded and picture cards are individually presented at increasing distances until the patient recognizes the cards at 20 feet or fails to recognize the cards (Fig. 19-5). Recognition of the cards at a distance of 20 feet equates to a visual acuity of 20/30. The farthest distance at which the cards can be recognized is noted, and the visual acuity is quantitated as that distance over the denominator of 30 (e.g., 5/30, 15/30, 20/30). This is a measurement of recognition visual acuity. Although use of isolated targets is not ideal for detection of amblyopia, the test can be quickly and easily taught to apprehensive or shy young children and comparison of vision between the eyes detects most cases of amblyopia and other defects in visual acuity.

The LEA symbols are another set of object recognition visual acuity cards. These have the advantage of having five symbols on each card, and the child identifies the symbol in the middle of the card. Presentation of several letters at a time is a more accurate measurement of visual acuity, due to a phenomenon termed *crowding*. Amblyopic eyes recognize letters or symbols better if they are presented in isolation or one at a time rather than if four or more are presented together on lines above and below one another. The difference may be as much as one or two lines of visual acuity (e.g., 20/30 isolated symbol visual acuity reducing to 20/40 or 20/50 when measured with a Snellen letter chart). Many different visual acuity tests are calibrated using different letters and symbols or groups of symbols.

The Sheridan-Gardiner or HOTV visual acuity tests are easy to administer and more accurately measure visual acuity in 4- to 6-year-old children who are beginning to read letters. In the HOTV test the letters H, O, T, and V are individually presented on cards, and the child matches the letter with a corresponding letter on a card that is held on the lap (Fig. 19-6).

Figure 19-2   Normal fundus. Posterior pole with normal optic disc and retinal vasculature. The macula is visualized as an area of increased pigmentation temporal to the optic disc. The retinal vessels surround but do not go through the macula. The fovea centralis or center of the macula is maintaining fixation on the end of a vertical fixation target.

Figure 19-4   Test for central fixation. **A,** An alert child seated on her mother's lap with one eye covered. The child is content to fix and follow with the normal left eye. **B,** The cover (in this case, fingers) is then transferred to the left eye. The child becomes disturbed, pushes the hand away, and moves her head to see. This suggests that the visual acuity in the right eye is not as good as the acuity in the left eye.

Another commonly used test to measure the visual acuity of 3½-year-old children is the "E game." The child is presented with the letter E in decreasing sizes and rotated in an up, down, right, or left orientation, and the child indicates the direction of the crossbars of the E by pointing.

The gold standard for measurement of visual acuity is the presentation of a full line of letter optotypes. This presentation is best achieved with a wall chart or by projection of the letters onto a standardized reflective surface.

Discussion of visual acuity measurements should include whether the visual acuity has been measured without correction of refractive errors or whether any refractive error present has been corrected with glasses or contact lenses (best corrected visual acuity). To differentiate an organic problem of the visual system from simple refractive error, the best corrected visual acuity provides the most useful information. If correction of the patient's refractive error with glasses is not available an approximation of corrected visual acuity may be made by having the patient look through a pinhole. The pinhole prevents indirect rays of light, which need to be refracted by the optics of the eye, from entering the eye, so that the effects of refractive errors in the eye are minimized. Patients demonstrate the pinhole effect when they squint in order to see better. If the patient's visual acuity improves when looking through the pinhole a refractive error is present. If it does not improve then another cause for the decrease in vision is likely.

Normal values for best corrected visual acuity depend on the patient's age. A child at 6 months of age should have a visual acuity of 20/60 to 20/100. A child who is 3 years old can be expected to have an acuity in the range of 20/25 or 20/30, using the E game or a recognition target test. With further maturation, a 5- to 7-year-old child should have visual acuity of 20/20 to 20/25 as tested with a full-line presentation of Snellen letters. If the best corrected visual acuity is less than 20/20 in a child older than 8 years of age, investigation for the cause of the decrease in visual acuity should be made.

It is recommended that vision screening be conducted as part of well-child care at regularly scheduled intervals in the pediatrician's or family practitioner's office. In infancy the fixation and following response of each eye to a fixation target should be recorded. Beginning at age 3, quantitation of visual acuity using Allen cards, the E game, an HOTV chart, or other preliterate vision test should be completed. Later, a Snellen or letter chart visual acuity test should be performed by the office

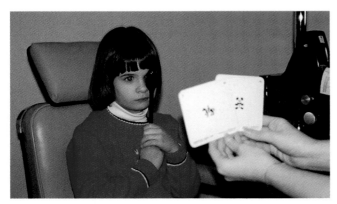

Figure 19-5   Visual acuity testing with the Allen object recognition cards. Recognition of each figure at a distance of 20 feet is equivalent to a visual acuity of 20/30. The visual acuity is quantitated as the number of feet at which each figure may be recognized over 30 (e.g., 5/30, 15/30, 20/30).

Figure 19-6   The Sheridan-Gardiner visual acuity test presents letters of decreasing size to a child who matches the figure presented to one on a card held on his or her lap. This test provides an accurate assessment of visual acuity for children who have not yet mastered reading the alphabet.

staff or physician, and the results should be recorded as part of the patient's medical record. Most importantly, the visual acuity should be equal in both eyes. Further evaluation of a young child is prompted if the patient is cooperating well and the visual acuity is less than 20/40 with letters, or less than 15/30 measured with Allen visual acuity cards, in either or both eyes.

Some state laws require that vision screenings be performed in school at 1- to 2-year intervals. In a child 6 years of age or more, referral to an ophthalmologist is indicated if the vision is less than 20/30 in either eye. If appropriate vision screenings are passed in the primary care physician's office, school, or preschool, and there is no family history of hereditary eye disease or other suspicion or risk factor for eye disease present, comprehensive examination of the child's eyes by an optometrist or ophthalmologist is not necessary.

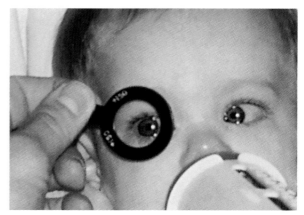

Figure 19-7 Retinoscopy. The examiner is viewing light emanating from the retina through the retinoscope. A lens is held in front of the patient's eye to neutralize refractive errors.

REFRACTIVE ERRORS

Decreased visual acuity is most commonly the result of a refractive error in the eye. This may be due to variation in the curvature of the cornea or lens or variation in the axial length of the eye. Determination of the refractive state of the eye is part of a comprehensive ophthalmic evaluation. In children, an objective measurement of the refractive error is best obtained by using eyedrops that temporarily inhibit accommodation (cycloplegia) and cause pupillary dilation (mydriasis). Cycloplegic–mydriatic agents such as cyclopentolate or tropicamide are instilled, and 30 minutes later accommodation is temporarily paralyzed and the pupil is dilated. A retinoscope is used to project a beam of light into the eye and illuminate the retina. The light is then reflected back to the examiner through the patient's pupil and optical system. The focus of the reflected light is neutralized by placement of appropriate lenses in front of the eye, and the refractive error of the eye is accurately and objectively measured (Fig. 19-7).

Low levels of hyperopia (farsightedness) in the range of +1.50 to +2.00 diopters are normal during childhood and are easily compensated for by the focusing mechanism of the lens (accommodation), so glasses are not necessary. The amount of hyperopia normally increases until 5 years of age and then decreases. Under normal circumstances, emmetropia, or no refractive error, is achieved around adolescence. If excessive axial growth, that is, elongation, of the eye occurs, myopia (nearsightedness) develops. A patient's refractive error

is for the most part genetically predetermined. The effect that environment has on refractive error is not completely understood.

The optical image formed by a hyperopic eye is in focus behind the retina (Fig. 19-8, *C*). By changing the shape of the lens with accommodation, the image can be brought into focus on the retina and glasses may not be required. If a large amount of hyperopia is present (+4.00 diopters or more), fatigue; headaches; asthenopia; and blurring of vision, especially at near, may occur. Hyperopia greater than +5.00 or +6.00 diopters may cause ametropic amblyopia. When this occurs, glasses are prescribed to correct the child's refractive error so that focused images stimulate the development of normal vision. If large hyperopic refractive errors are not treated by 6 to 8 years of age, the resultant amblyopia may be irreversible. The optic discs in eyes with large degrees of hyperopia may have an appearance simulating papilledema (pseudopapilledema) (Fig. 19-9).

Myopia is most commonly caused by an increase in axial length of the eye with respect to the optical power of the eye (see Fig. 19-8, *B*). Children who are myopic can see near objects clearly; objects at distance are blurred and cannot be brought into focus without the aid of glasses or a contact lens. Wearing glasses for myopia does not change the growth of the eye and,

REFRACTIVE ERRORS

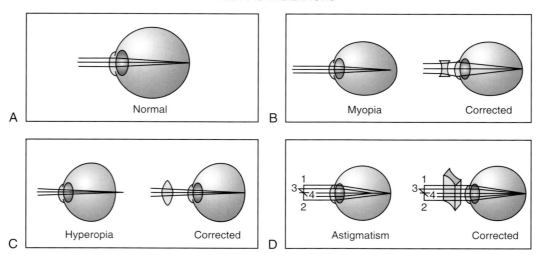

Figure 19-8 In the normal or emmetropic eye **(A)**, light from a distant object is focused on the retina. In a myopic eye **(B)**, it is focused in front of the retina; in a hyperopic eye **(C)**, it is focused behind the retina; and in an astigmatic eye **(D)**, light in different meridians is brought to focus either in front of or behind the retina.

Figure 19-9 Pseudopapilledema in a hyperopic child. Vessels are normal sized; small vessels are continuously visible at the disc margins because there is no edema of the nerve fiber layer. There are no hemorrhages or exudates.

football its characteristic shape. Bulky masses in the lids such as chalazions or hemangiomas may compress the cornea and induce astigmatic refractive errors.

Anisometropia refers to the condition in which one eye has a different refractive error than the other. Usually the eye with the least amount of hyperopia or refractive error is the dominant or preferred eye. The fellow eye may be suppressed and develop amblyopia because the development of the visual system is being stimulated by a sharp focused image from one eye and a less focused image from the other eye. The magnitude of the amblyopia depends on the magnitude of the anisometropia and the age at which it developed. Anisometropia may occur with hyperopia, myopia, astigmatism, or a combination of these refractive errors. If the degree of anisometropia is large, the optical properties of the required correcting lenses produce a difference in image size between the two eyes, *aniseikonia,* which may be difficult for the patient to tolerate.

STRABISMUS

Misalignment of the visual axes is referred to as *strabismus.* Strabismus occurs in 1% to 4% of the population and may be congenital or acquired. It may occur on a hereditary basis, most commonly without a clearly defined inheritance pattern. In the majority of childhood strabismus the misalignment of the eyes is not caused by a specific cranial nerve or extraocular muscle dysfunction. In some cases, strabismus may be caused by cranial nerve paralysis or neuromuscular disorders (myasthenia gravis).

Voluntary and reflex movement of the eyes is mediated via the extraocular muscles. These muscles are coordinated in their saccadic and pursuit movements by centers in the frontal and occipital areas of the cerebral cortex with modification by the cerebellum. Saccades are voluntary movements used to move the eyes to the object of regard. These are rapid eye movements. Pursuit or following movements are used to track or follow moving objects. These are slow eye movements.

contrary to popular belief, does not promote the resolution or progression of the myopia. Bifocals and cycloplegics may have a small effect on slowing the progression of myopia, but no treatment is currently available to reverse or stop the progression of myopia.

Myopia may be present at birth but usually develops with growth spurts that occur between 8 and 10 years of age. The amount of myopia present usually increases until growth is completed after adolescence.

High degrees of myopia ranging from −8.00 to −20.00 diopters may be associated with systemic conditions such as Stickler and Ehlers-Danlos syndromes, which are associated with connective tissue defects and increased axial length of the eye. Myopia is inherited as a multifactorial trait. High myopia with extreme lengthening of the globe may be associated with retinal thinning, peripapillary pigment crescents, staphylomas (a focal area of bulging of the posterior globe wall), and decreased macular function with poor visual acuity. The optic nerve may appear to enter the eye at an angle (Fig. 19-10). High myopia has an increased incidence of retinal detachment, especially after direct trauma to the eye or concussive head trauma.

In astigmatism the refractive power of the eye is different in different meridians (see Fig. 19-8, *D*). This produces a blurred retinal image for objects at both distance and near. Astigmatism occurs when the cornea, lens, or retinal surface has a toric shape rather than a spherical one. This may be likened to the two different radii of curvature that give a

The third, fourth, and sixth cranial nerve nuclei, located in the brainstem, are the centers responsible for innervating the extraocular muscles. In addition to innervation of the inferior oblique, medial, inferior, and superior recti, the third cranial nerve is responsible for innervation of the levator muscle, pupillary constriction, and accommodation of the lens. The fourth cranial nerve provides innervation to the superior oblique muscle, and the sixth cranial nerve supplies the lateral rectus muscle (Fig. 19-11). When one or more of the cranial nerves are paretic, the action of the innervated muscle is decreased, leading to a deficit in the duction or movement

Figure 19-10 High myopia. Thinning of the retinal pigment epithelium produces a tessellated fundus appearance. In eyes with moderate or high myopia a temporal crescent adjacent to the optic disc is frequently present, and the optic disc may have an anomalous tilted appearance.

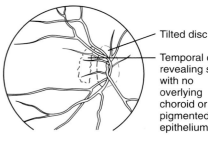

Tilted disc

Temporal crescent revealing sclera with no overlying choroid or pigmented epithelium

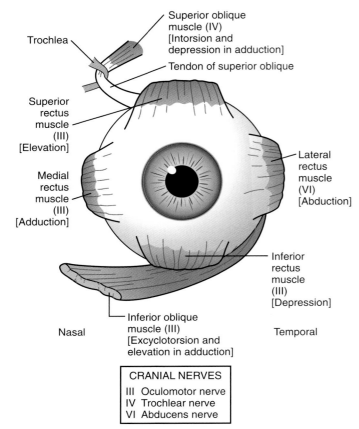

Trochlea

Superior oblique
muscle (IV)
[Intorsion and
depression in adduction]

Tendon of superior oblique

Superior
rectus
muscle
(III)
[Elevation]

Medial
rectus
muscle
(III)
[Adduction]

Lateral
rectus
muscle
(VI)
[Abduction]

Inferior
rectus
muscle
(III)
[Depression]

Inferior oblique
muscle (III)
[Excyclotorsion and
elevation in adduction]

Nasal

Temporal

CRANIAL NERVES
III Oculomotor nerve
IV Trochlear nerve
VI Abducens nerve

Figure 19-11 Innervation (in parentheses) of extraocular muscles and their primary actions [in brackets].

of the eye into the field of action of the muscle. The muscle having a function of movement in the opposite direction is no longer balanced, producing strabismus.

An abnormal head posture may be a sign of strabismus in patients with cranial nerve dysfunction or nystagmus. These postures are observed in children who have good binocular function. Head postures are used to compensate for double vision caused by horizontal, vertical, or cyclovertical muscle palsies. For example, in a patient with a right sixth nerve palsy the abduction of the right eye is deficient. The adducting force of the medial rectus is not balanced, and the eye is in a relatively adducted or esotropic position. The patient then manifests a head turn to the right to allow the right eye to be in a position where less abducting force is required, allowing both eyes to fixate together. In a patient with nystagmus, a head posture may be used to place the eyes at the null point, or direction of gaze where the amplitude of nystagmus is the least. In cases of torticollis, if the head posture is present while the patient is sleeping, the cause of the head posture is unlikely to be ophthalmologic in nature. Conversely, if a patient's head posture goes away when either eye is occluded, it suggests that the cause of the head tilt or turn may be related to a problem of ocular alignment or strabismus. Head turns may sometimes be seen when the vision in one eye is much worse than the other.

Versions

Eye movements are tested by moving the eyes right, left, up, down, up and right, down and right, up and left, and down and left. This tests the function of each extraocular muscle and its counterpart or yoke muscle in the fellow eye. *Versions* refer to movement of both eyes together in conjugate gaze. A

duction is the movement of a single eye. Normal version movements should be present by 4 months of age.

Vergence movements consist of convergence or divergence of the eyes. Vergences are well established by 6 months of age. Convergence of the eyes, coupled with accommodation and miosis of the pupil, is referred to as the *near response*. Convergence assists alignment of the eyes at near.

A strabismus deviation that changes in size or magnitude in different gaze positions is termed *incomitant*. Strabismus deviations that remain the same in all gaze positions are termed *comitant*. Strabismus caused by cranial nerve paralysis is incomitant.

Phorias and Tropias

If strabismus is present, it may be manifest (i.e., a tropia) or held latent by sensory fusion (i.e., a phoria). When the fusion of a patient with a phoria is interrupted by placing an occluder in front of one eye, the eye seeks its position of rest and deviates so that the visual axes of the two eyes are no longer both aligned on the point of fixation. When the eye is uncovered and binocular vision is re-established, the fusion response assists in the realignment of the eyes on the object of regard. A phoria may produce symptoms of fatigue, blurring, or movement of objects. When a phoria breaks down into an intermittent tropia, there may be a symptom of intermittent double vision or *diplopia*. Phorias, especially if large, may become symptomatic at times of fatigue, stress, or illness.

A tropia is a constant or intermittently present ocular deviation. The fusion mechanism is unable to maintain alignment of the eyes on an object of fixation. Young children with tropias develop suppression of the tropic eye as a natural response to avoid diplopia. Older children or adults who acquire a tropia (e.g., from an acquired cranial nerve palsy) have diplopia as a symptom of the misalignment of their visual axes. The deviation present in a tropia may occur in one or all positions of gaze, depending on the cause of the tropia.

Phorias and tropias are classified according to the pattern of the eye deviation. The prefixes *eso-* and *exo-* classify horizontal strabismus. *Hyper-* and *hypo-* are used for vertical deviations, and *incyclo-* and *excyclo-* for torsional deviations.

Esodeviations

An esodeviation is a convergent deviation of the eyes. The deviation may be latent, a phoria (esophoria), or it may occur as a manifest deviation, a tropia (esotropia). Common esodeviations seen in children are infantile esotropia, accommodative esotropia, esotropia resulting from sixth cranial nerve palsy, and Duane syndrome.

Infantile Esotropia

The most common cause for an esodeviation presenting in infancy is infantile, or congenital, esotropia (Fig. 19-12). In this condition the esotropia is seen at birth or very early in infancy. On occasion a family history of infantile esotropia exists. The angle of esodeviation is large and constant. Abduction may be deficient due to contraction of the medial rectus muscles, and differentiation from sixth nerve palsy may be difficult. Cross-fixation is usually present, with the adducted right eye used for vision to the left and the adducted left eye used for vision to the right. Abduction of an eye is checked by occluding the contralateral eye and quickly encouraging fixation movements while holding the head. Doll's head maneuvers may also be used to test abduction of the eyes. Children with this condition usually do not develop much amblyopia and maintain good visual acuity in both eyes

Figure 19-12 Infantile esotropia with asymmetrical corneal light reflexes.

Figure 19-13 Dissociative vertical deviation (DVD), an upward and outward drifting of the right eye. Covering the fixating left eye in the cover–uncover test causes the deviating right eye to move into alignment with the left eye. The covered left eye remains straight and no hypodeviation or exodeviation of the left eye is seen when the cover is removed. This differentiates DVD from a tropia.

whether they are treated or not. There are no associated neurologic or systemic abnormalities.

The esodeviation present in infantile esotropia requires surgical correction. After correction, the ocular alignment is frequently unstable, with further surgery commonly required later in life no matter how early surgery is performed or how well aligned the eyes are after surgery. Inferior oblique overaction and dissociated vertical deviations frequently develop later in childhood or adolescence. Inferior oblique overaction is seen as an elevation of one or both eyes in adduction. Dissociated vertical deviation (DVD) (Fig. 19-13) is an upward and outward "floating" movement of one or both eyes that becomes more prominent with fatigue or inattention. A DVD may be elicited on examination by covering one eye and watching its position as the eye is covered. These patients do not experience diplopia. Patients with infantile esotropia also commonly develop accommodative esotropia, with a need for glasses later in childhood. While excellent visual acuity and alignment of the eyes are most commonly achieved with treatment, the development of high levels of binocular function (stereopsis) is usually not obtained.

Accommodative Esotropia

Accommodative esotropia most commonly presents as an acquired strabismus at 2½ to 5 years of age. Family histories of hypertropia, anisometropia, esotropia, and amblyopia are very common. The presence of uncorrected hyperopia causes the patient to accommodate or focus to obtain clear visual acuity. With accommodation, the synkinetic near response, which includes miosis, accommodation, and convergence of the eyes, occurs. If the fusion mechanism is unable to diverge the eyes to compensate for the excessive convergence accompanying the need to accommodate to correct for the patient's hyperopia, esotropia results.

If an esodeviation is associated with a modest degree of farsightedness, treatment of the hyperopia optically with glasses is indicated. In patients with purely accommodative esotropia, this measure alone may completely correct the deviation (Fig. 19-14). Frequently, especially if the esodeviation has been left untreated for a long period of time, a residual esodeviation will remain. This is a partially accommodative esotropia. Surgical correction may be recommended for these patients. Some patients have straight eyes for some time with their glasses in place and decompensate to partially accommodative or nonaccommodative esodeviations later.

In patients with accommodative esotropia, the eyes are straight with their glasses on and esotropic when they are removed. Frequently, if the patient is only moderately hyperopic in the preferred fixating eye, the patient will say that he or she can see just as well or perhaps better without their glasses. The glasses are not prescribed necessarily to improve visual acuity; rather, the glasses are intended to decrease the accommodative effort and to decrease the esotropia.

In another form of accommodative esotropia, the ratio between accommodative convergence and accommodation (AC/A ratio) may be abnormally high, producing excessive convergence when focusing on near objects. In high AC/A ratio accommodative esotropia, the esodeviation with near vision is greater in magnitude than it is with distance vision (Fig. 19-15). These patients may be treated with a bifocal, which gives them additional hyperopic correction for near, decreasing their accommodative effort at near and decreasing the near esodeviation.

Nonaccommodative Esotropia

Children may develop an esodeviation that is present without any relationship to the patient's refractive error (Fig. 19-16). Correction of the hyperopia with glasses does not improve the esotropia in these patients. These nonaccommodative esodeviations may be associated with poor vision, trauma, prematurity, aphakia, or high myopia. Nonaccommodative esotropia may also develop when accommodative esotropias are left untreated.

Figure 19-14 Accommodative esotropia. **A,** Esotropia. **B,** Glasses have corrected the patient's hyperopia, and the esotropic eye is now straight.

A

B

Figure 19-15   High AC/A ratio accommodative esotropia. **A,** This child with hyperopia has an esotropia when fixing at distance, and a larger angle esotropia in the near range. **B,** When glasses are prescribed to correct the hyperopia the eyes straighten at distances. **C,** The near esotropia remains. **D,** When bifocals are used, the near esotropia is corrected.

Other Causes of Esotropia

Unilateral or bilateral sixth cranial nerve palsy causes deficient abduction and an esodeviation. In sixth nerve palsy the esotropia increases with gaze directed toward the side of the palsy (gaze incomitance). Other signs of the nerve paralysis that may be more difficult to detect include the extent and speed of abduction of the eye. Patients may display a head turn toward the side of the palsy to hold the involved eye in adduction and maintain binocular vision. Sixth cranial nerve palsies in children may be associated with increased intracranial pressure, trauma, tumor, or antecedent viral illness. In benign or "postviral" and traumatic cases the lateral rectus function may return gradually and fully over a 6-month period. In idiopathic cases, if improvement does not occur, if the deviation increases, or if a gaze palsy develops, suspicion should be raised that a tumor, most commonly pontine glioma, may be the cause for the sixth nerve paralysis.

Duane syndrome is a congenital unilateral or bilateral defect characterized by inability to abduct an eye. This may be accompanied by an up or down shoot of the eye and narrowing of the lid fissure on attempted adduction. In attempted abduction the palpebral fissure widens. Duane syndrome is caused by a malformation of the cranial nerve nuclei producing co-innervation of the medial and lateral rectus muscles. The lateral rectus muscle does not contract with abduction and paradoxically co-contracts along with the medial rectus on adduction. The co-contraction with adduction causes a retraction of the globe and the lid fissure narrowing. Patients with Duane syndrome may be esotropic and have a head turn toward the involved side analogous to those seen with a sixth cranial nerve palsy. The changes in lid position and vertical deviations help to differentiate the two conditions (Fig. 19-17).

Pseudostrabismus

Pseudostrabismus is seen in infants with prominent epicanthal folds, closely placed eyes, and flat nasal bridges. Asymmetry of the lids or nasal bridge may also produce pseudostrabismus. When these facial features are present, the white of the sclera between the cornea and inner canthus frequently may be obscured, giving the optical illusion that the eyes are esotropic (Figs. 19-18 and 19-19). Parents and caretakers frequently report subtle esodeviations that worsen with gaze to the right or left. This is frequently pointed out in photographs in which careful examination shows the eyes to be in slight

Figure 19-16   The girl in **(A)** shows nonaccommodative esotropia, an esotropia that could not be corrected with glasses. Surgery was performed, and the 1-week postoperative photograph in **(B)** shows normal ocular alignment with symmetrical corneal light reflexes.

Figure 19-17 Left Duane syndrome. **A,** Right gaze. While the left eye is noted to move into adduction, retraction of the globe is noted along with narrowing of the palpebral fissure. The globe retraction and lid changes are due to co-contraction of the medial rectus and lateral rectus muscles on the involved side. **B,** Fixation target directly in front of patient. The patient is noted to maintain a slight left head turn to keep both of the eyes on the fixation target. The resting position of the affected left eye is slightly in adduction. If the patient's head is forced out of the slight left head turn, the left eye would become slightly esotropic. **C,** Left gaze. The affected left eye is seen to have an absence of abduction resulting from aberrant innervation of the lateral rectus muscle with no contraction in left gaze.

right or left gaze. Observation of symmetrical corneal light reflexes or cover testing confirms or excludes the presence of a true deviation.

Exodeviations

When the visual axes are divergent, an exodeviation is present (Fig. 19-20). Many children with exodeviations have family histories of strabismus. Exodeviations may also occur with vision loss in one eye (sensory exotropia) and cranial nerve paralysis (third nerve palsy). An exodeviation may be controlled by fusion (exophoria), be manifest intermittently (intermittent exotropia), or be constant (exotropia).

Intermittent exodeviations become manifest with fatigue, daydreaming, or illness. Patients with exodeviations frequently squint one eye in bright light, but they typically do not experience diplopia. They may complain of images jumping as they switch fixation or of discomfort at night or when tired. Patients with intermittent exotropia usually do not have amblyopia, or it may only be mild. One third of cases improve spontaneously. Treatment of intermittent exotropia consists of glasses to correct refractive errors, patching, and surgery.

If there is poor vision in one eye, the decreased visual stimulation may produce a sensory deviation. Generally speaking, if the onset of decreased vision occurs after the age of 4 years, an exodeviation will occur; however, if sensory input to the eye is decreased before the age of 2 years, an esodeviation usually occurs. Because young children do not complain of monocular vision loss, especially if congenital or with onset during infancy, sensory strabismus is frequently the presenting sign of vision-limiting pathology of the retina or optic nerve.

Exodeviations may be simulated in patients with widely spaced eyes (hypertelorism) or in those whose maculae are temporally displaced, as may occur in retinopathy of prematurity. When the macula is displaced temporally, the eye rotates outward to align its visual axis on the fixation target. The term *positive angle kappa* is used to describe this condition (Fig. 19-21).

Convergence Insufficiency

Convergence insufficiency describes an exodeviation in which the size of the deviation is greater in the near range than at distance. Most frequently, there is an exodeviation at near only

PSEUDOSTRABISMUS

The eyes appear to be esotropic but they are not. The appearance of esotropia is due to the presence of a wide and flat nasal bridge, prominent epicanthal folds, and decreased intraorbital distance.

The pupillary light is centered. Cover testing shows no movement of eyes.

In left gaze, the white of the sclera is covered by the inner canthal tissue. It appears as if the right eye is esotropic but the light reflex remains centered in the pupil.

The same may be true for right gaze.

Figure 19-19 The characteristics of pseudostrabismus are illustrated.

Figure 19-18 This infant has pseudostrabismus, caused by a flat nasal bridge, epicanthal folds, and closely placed eyes.

Figure 19-20 Exotropia, a divergent deviation of the eyes.

Figure 19-22 Left third nerve palsy with ptosis and an inability to elevate and adduct the eye.

and no distance deviation. This may cause symptoms of discomfort while reading and possibly intermittent double vision at near range. To test for convergence insufficiency, the child is asked to fixate on a target with detail as it is brought progressively closer. Normally the child should be able to converge to a point 10 cm from the nose. If the eyes converge, and then break their alignment and diverge at a distance greater than 10 cm from the eyes, the patient should be evaluated for convergence insufficiency. With cover and uncover testing an exodeviation will be seen at near fixation and it will be smaller or not seen at distance fixation. Treatments include glasses and in some cases convergence exercises and therapy.

Third (Oculomotor) Cranial Nerve Palsy

The third cranial nerve innervates the medial rectus muscle. In third nerve paralysis the action of the lateral rectus muscle, innervated by the sixth cranial nerve, is unopposed and produces an exodeviation. The third nerve also innervates the superior and inferior recti; the inferior oblique muscles; the levator palpebrae superioris, which elevates the lid; the ciliary muscle, which is responsible for accommodation of the lens; and the iris sphincter muscle, which produces miosis of the pupil. In the presence of a complete third cranial nerve palsy, the eye assumes a down and outward position, the eyelid is ptotic, and the pupil is enlarged (Fig. 19-22). Elevation of the eye with forced eyelid closure (the Bell phenomenon) is typically absent in patients with a third cranial nerve palsy (Fig. 19-23). The most common causes for acquired third nerve paralysis in children are trauma and tumor. A third nerve palsy may also occur as a congenital defect.

Vertical Deviations

Isolated vertical misalignment of the eyes is uncommon. Vertical deviations may occur in only one field of gaze, or they may be comitant and equal in all fields of gaze. Vertical

ANGLE KAPPA

Positive angle kappa produces an appearance of exotropia. This appearance is caused by a temporal displacement of the fovea, usually due to cicatricial changes of the retina after retinopathy of prematurity.

The left eye appears exotropic.
Cover testing shows no movement of the eyes.

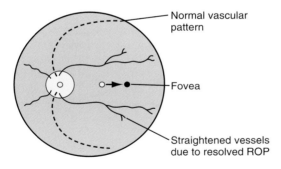

Temporal retinal cicatricial changes after resolution of stage 3 ROP have caused the fovea to be displaced temporalward.

Angle kappa

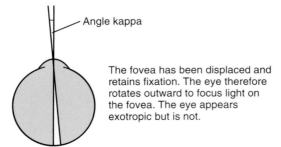

The fovea has been displaced and retains fixation. The eye therefore rotates outward to focus light on the fovea. The eye appears exotropic but is not.

Figure 19-21 Angle kappa. ROP, retinopathy of prematurity.

THIRD CRANIAL NERVE PALSY

A patient with left third cranial nerve palsy will not have a Bell phenomenon on the affected side. The forced opening of tightly closed eyelids will reveal an upward, slightly outward movement of the eye under the closed eyelids (normal Bell response). The patient with a third cranial nerve palsy cannot elevate or adduct the eye. The eye, when opened or under forced eyelid closure, is not elevated.

Figure 19-23 Third cranial nerve palsy.

Figure 19-24 Left fourth nerve palsy with an inability to depress the involved eye in adduction. Abnormal head posture is common with a head tilt away from the side of the fourth nerve palsy, as is overaction of the direct antagonistic inferior oblique muscle, seen as an elevation of the affected eye in adduction (gaze to the opposite side).

Figure 19-26 Brown syndrome, an inability to elevate an eye in adduction resulting from an abnormality of the superior oblique tendon.

deviations may have a cyclotorsional component and be associated with a head tilt or head posture to eliminate double vision. All patients with torticollis should be evaluated for cyclovertical muscle palsies.

The most common cyclovertical deviation is due to a palsy of the fourth cranial (trochlear) nerve (Fig. 19-24). Fourth nerve palsies in children occur congenitally or secondary to head trauma. The eye is excyclorotated, and the head is tilted to the shoulder opposite the side of the paretic nerve and superior oblique muscle. Other features are elevation of the eye and difficulty depressing the eye in adduction (Fig. 19-25). Patients with fourth nerve palsies have diplopia in the contralateral field of gaze, especially up and away from the paretic side. Patients with congenital palsies may not always

recognize this diplopia. Some facial asymmetry, especially of the cheek and jaw line, is usually seen in congenital cases as the children age. Examination of candid photos will typically display head postures that usually are not noticed by family members.

Brown syndrome describes an isolated motility disorder in which there is an inability to elevate the eye when it is adducted (Fig. 19-26). This may be caused by a congenital anomaly of the superior oblique tendon, or it may be acquired as an idiopathic inflammation or tenosynovitis of the superior oblique tendon. Acquired cases may be persistent, resolve spontaneously (sometimes over many years), or respond to nonsteroidal antiinflammatory drugs.

Abnormalities of extraocular muscle innervation rarely cause vertical deviations. Double elevator palsy is an inherited unilateral or bilateral condition in which there is hypotropia and limitation of elevation of the involved eye. To achieve binocularity, patients tilt their chins up and position their heads back. Ptosis is frequently present.

Additional causes of vertical deviations include myasthenia gravis, thyroid ophthalmopathy, chronic progressive external ophthalmoplegia, orbital fractures with muscle entrapment (most commonly the inferior rectus entrapped within a blowout fracture of the orbital floor), and orbital disease with intraorbital masses.

Tests for Strabismus

Although gross observation may detect the majority of cases of strabismus, pseudostrabismus will lead frequently to unnecessary referrals. More significantly, smaller angle deviations may be missed, leading to delays in treatment if further tests for strabismus are not employed by the primary care physician.

The type and degree of ocular misalignment may be estimated using the corneal light reflex test, or Hirschberg method. The patient fixates on a penlight held at 1 m. Using the pupil edge as a point of reference, the light reflections between the two eyes are compared for symmetry; if the light reflex is displaced temporally in one eye compared with the reflex seen in the other eye, an esotropia is present. If the light reflex is displaced nasally in comparison with the other eye, an exodeviation is present (Fig. 19-27). Although observation of the corneal light reflexes is more sensitive and specific than gross observation alone, a more accurate method of detecting misalignment of the eyes is cover and uncover testing.

The cover test requires vision in each eye and use of a target that stimulates accommodation. Cover testing is performed while the patient maintains fixation on targets at 6 m and at 1 m because some types of strabismus produce misalignment of the eyes that is present only at either distance or near. The cover–uncover test is used to detect phorias. This test is

Figure 19-25 Right inferior oblique overaction. In primary (straight ahead) gaze **(A)** and right gaze **(B)** the eyes are well aligned. In left gaze **(C)** the right eye is elevated or hypertropic because of overaction of the right inferior oblique.

HIRSCHBERG TEST
FOR OCULAR ALIGNMENT

A penlight is held 1 meter from the eyes.
The pupillary light reflex is observed and its
relationship to the center of the pupil is noted.

Normal corneal light reflex
The reflexes are symmetrical and slightly
displaced nasally to the center of the pupils.

Left esotropia
The reflex is displaced temporally to
the center of the pupil.

Left exotropia
The corneal light reflex is displaced
nasally to the center of the pupil.

Figure 19-27   Hirschberg test for ocular alignment.

performed by placing a cover over one eye to disrupt fusion or binocularity. As the cover is removed, the previously covered eye is observed. If the eye does not move, both eyes are aligned on the object at that distance; orthophoria is present. If the eye deviates while covered and then moves to regain fusion and assumes fixation as the cover is removed, a phoria exists. The test is then repeated, covering and uncovering the other eye (Fig. 19-28).

The second component of the cover test is performed by covering one eye and observing the movement of the other eye. If neither eye moves as the eyes are alternately covered, the eyes are both aligned on the fixation target and the term *orthophoria* is used. No deviation is present in this case. If a tropia and a fixation preference are present, a fixation movement of the deviating uncovered eye occurs when the preferred fixating eye is covered; when the cover is transferred back, the previously deviating eye again deviates behind the cover (Fig. 19-29). If a deviation is well controlled by fusion (a phoria) and is small in size, it may be safely observed if there are no symptoms and the fundus is normal. When a tropia is present, either constantly or intermittently, after 3 months of age, the patient should be referred to an ophthalmologist. Ophthalmologists use prisms along with cover testing to measure the size of strabismic deviations.

Amblyopia

Amblyopia is present when there is a decrease in vision in one or both eyes and all potential organic causes (refractive errors, media opacities, structural abnormalities) for the decrease in vision have been corrected or excluded. Amblyopia may be caused by the absence of stimulation of the immature visual system by a focused retinal image or by strabismus and the resultant suppression of one eye. Visual deprivation

amblyopia may be caused by a corneal opacity, a dense cataract, vitreous opacity (hemorrhage or inflammation), or high refractive error (Fig. 19-30).

In anisometropic amblyopia an image is clearly focused on the fovea of one eye, but in the other eye the image is out of

HETEROPHORIAS

Normally, both eyes appear to be aligned and centrally fixed.

Exophoria

Cover one eye—that eye deviates away from the other eye.

The cover is then removed—the now uncovered eye returns
to a central position.

The same procedure is then performed on the other eye.

Esophoria

Cover one eye—that eye deviates toward the other eye.

The cover is then removed—the now uncovered eye returns
to a central position.

The same procedure is then performed on the other eye.

Hyperphoria

Cover one eye—that eye deviates superiorly.

The cover is then removed—the now uncovered eye returns
to a central position.

The same procedure is then performed on the other eye.

Figure 19-28   The cover–uncover test for heterophorias.

HETEROTROPIAS

In esotropia, one eye is deviated toward the other. Note that the corneal light reflex is not centrally placed.

Cover the esotropic eye—there is no movement of either eye.

The cover is then removed—again, there is no movement of either eye—no proof of tropia.

The other eye is now covered—as a result, that eye becomes esotropic and the formerly esotropic eye moves to a central position to take up fixation.

If the cover is removed and no eye movement occurs, this indicates that the eyes have equal visual acuity or fixation. This also indicates a relative absence of amblyopia.

If the cover is removed and both eyes move so that the original fixing eye is again centrally fixed and the originally esotropic eye is again esotropic, this indicates that there is amblyopia present. In this case, the patient's left eye is amblyopic.

The same maneuvers can be used to determine the presence of exotropia (outward deviation), hyper- and hypotropia (upward and downward deviation), and cyclotropia (rotary displacement).

Figure 19-29 The cover–uncover test for heterotropias.

focus. The blurred retinal image is suppressed by the child's immature visual system, and that eye is affected by amblyopia. In anisometropic amblyopia, most commonly one eye is more hyperopic than the other. Because both eyes must accommodate the same amount, the less hyperopic eye is preferred and the more hyperopic eye has the blurred image and develops the amblyopia. With high hyperopia or astigmatism affecting both eyes, bilateral ametropic amblyopia may occur if the child does not or cannot accommodate to produce a focused retinal image to stimulate the visual system with either eye. These patients have decreased vision in both eyes. In children with strabismus, the image from the deviating eye is suppressed by the brain as an adaptation to avoid diplopia and the deviating eye develops strabismic amblyopia. Patients often have both strabismus and anisometropia simultaneously as causes for their amblyopia.

The severity of the visual loss produced by amblyopia is determined by the nature of the visual deprivation; the age at onset; and its consistency, severity, and duration. Amblyopia is treated by removing the cause of the amblyopia, if possible, and by forcing use of the affected eye to stimulate the development of the vision from that eye. In bilateral ametropic amblyopia, the appropriate glasses are given as treatment. In strabismic or anisometropic amblyopia, appropriate glasses are given, and the preferred, nonamblyopic eye is penalized to force the use of the amblyopic eye. An occlusion patch placed over the preferred fixating eye is commonly used as treatment.

Other methods of treatment are optical via the eyeglass prescription and pharmacologic, with atropine drops placed in the nonamblyopic eye to prevent accommodation in that eye. This forces the use of the amblyopic eye for reading and near vision.

Amblyopia responds most rapidly and completely to treatment begun early in life. The visual system has developmental phases and if certain levels of visual acuity are not reached early in life the amblyopia present is unlikely to respond completely to treatment. Treatment is more difficult and less effective after 8 years of age but remains possible in older children, especially if they have no history of previous treatment.

DISEASES OF THE EYES AND SURROUNDING STRUCTURES

Eyelids and Adnexa—Anatomy of the Eyelid

The eyelid is composed of skin and its related appendages, glands that contribute to the tear film, and muscular structures permitting the eyelid to open and close (Fig. 19-31). Conditions affecting the eyelid are related to these anatomic structures.

Telecanthus refers to an increase in the distance between the inner canthus of each eye (Fig. 19-32). Telecanthus can be due to the hereditary transmission of facial features or midline embryonic defects, or it can be related to a syndrome such as blepharophimosis, or Komoto syndrome (Fig. 19-33). This inherited syndrome consists of telecanthus, epicanthus inversus (a skinfold projecting over the inner angle of the eye and covering part of the canthus, arising from the lower lid skin), blepharophimosis (horizontal shortening of the lid fissure), and ptosis. *Hypertelorism* refers to an increase in the distance between the nasal walls of the orbits. This is usually associated with telecanthus.

Blepharoptosis, or ptosis, is a unilateral or bilateral decrease in the vertical distance between the upper and lower eyelids (palpebral fissure) because of dysfunction of the levator muscle (Fig. 19-34). Congenital blepharoptosis is frequently transmitted as an autosomal dominant trait with variable penetrance. Congenital ptosis may be either unilateral or bilateral. Other causes for blepharoptosis include ocular inflammation, chronic irritation of the anterior segment of the eye, chronic use of topical steroid eye drops, third nerve palsy, and trauma. Ptosis may be severe enough to cause visual deprivation and amblyopia if the visual axis is occluded. Children with even mild degrees of congenital ptosis should be referred for evaluation because they have a higher than normal incidence of strabismus and anisometropic amblyopia than the general population. In congenital ptosis the eyelid position may improve somewhat from that observed early in infancy, but after that it tends to remain stable or worsen only slightly over time.

The Marcus Gunn, or jaw-winking, phenomenon is caused by a misdirection of the motor division of the fifth cranial nerve to the ipsilateral levator muscle of the eyelid (Fig.

AMBLYOPIA·

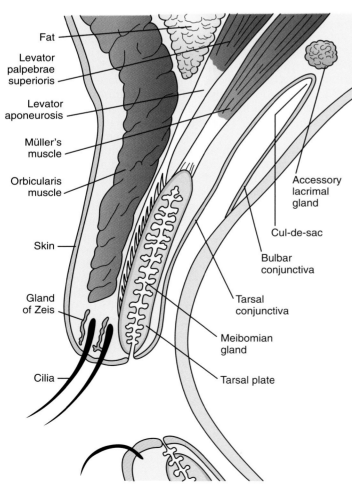

Ametropic
(bilateral)

Strabismic

Deprivation

Anisometropic

Figure 19-30   Amblyopia is produced either by the absence of a focused retinal image (ametropic, deprivation, or anisometropic) or by suppression of a diplopic image (strabismic).

Figure 19-31   Eyelids and adnexa. Cross-section of the eyelid.

Fat

Levator palpebrae superioris

Levator aponeurosis

Müller's muscle

Orbicularis muscle

Skin

Gland of Zeis

Cilia

Accessory lacrimal gland

Cul-de-sac

Bulbar conjunctiva

Tarsal conjunctiva

Meibomian gland

Tarsal plate

19-35). With jaw movement to the ipsilateral side the eyelid droops, and when the jaw is moved to the contralateral side, the eyelid elevates. The eyelid winks with chewing or feeding. This is a benign phenomenon and no further neurologic or systemic evaluation is required. Surgical treatment is not indicated unless the associated ptosis warrants it. Most patients learn to control the winking by avoiding the inciting jaw movement.

Trichiasis is the term used to describe misdirected eyelashes that irritate the cornea or conjunctiva. It can be caused by chronic inflammation of the eyelids, entropion (inturning of the eyelid), eyelid trauma, or inflammatory conditions with scarring of the conjunctiva such as Stevens-Johnson syndrome.

Districhiasis describes a condition in which there is an accessory row of eyelashes (cilia) along the posterior border of the eyelid (Fig. 19-36). Eyelid eversion or ectropion frequently coexists because of defects in the tarsal plate. This condition is inherited as an autosomal dominant condition, but it may also be a sequela of severe ocular inflammation.

Entropion is an inverted eyelid with the lashes rubbing against the conjunctiva or cornea. This may be present at birth or occur with severe blepharospasm, inflammation, or trauma. If severe, abrasion of the cornea by the lashes can cause permanent corneal scarring (Fig. 19-37).

In epiblepharon a skinfold extends over the lid margin and presses the lashes against the globe. It is commonly observed during the first year of life (Fig. 19-38). The lower lid is more commonly affected in the white population, and both the upper and lower lids may be affected in Asian infants. This defect usually corrects itself spontaneously by 1 year of age. In Asians the problem may be persistent. Corneal abrasion usually does not occur because of the soft texture of the infant's eyelashes or when it is the shaft of the eyelash rather

Figure 19-32 Normal adnexal measurements.

Figure 19-33 Komoto syndrome, a combination of blepharophimosis, ptosis, epicanthus inversus, and telecanthus.

Figure 19-34 Unilateral congenital ptosis with lid covering pupil.

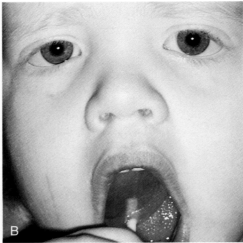

Figure 19-35   Marcus Gunn jaw-winking ptosis. **A,** The ptotic lid position. **B,** Elevation and a wide-open lid with movement of the jaw.

than the tip of the lash that touches the cornea. However, surgical correction may be required if it is persistent and causing corneal abrasion; conjunctival injection, epiphora, and photosensitivity are symptoms in more significant cases.

Ectropion is an outward rotation of the eyelid margin. If severe, ectropion can lead to problems of corneal exposure. Ectropion may be congenital or caused by any condition (trauma, scleroderma), causing the eyelid skin to contract and evert the eyelid (Fig. 19-39). Ectropion may occur after seventh cranial nerve palsy with paralysis of the facial musculature.

Congenital eyelid colobomas are defects or notches in the eyelid margin caused by failed fusion of embryonic fissures early in development. These may be isolated defects or associated with conditions such as Goldenhar syndrome (Fig. 19-40). Goldenhar syndrome consists of eyelid colobomas, corneal–limbal dermoids, vertebral anomalies, and preauricular skin tags.

Ankyloblepharon is a fusion of the upper and lower eyelid margins. This may range from a few thin strands of tissue to complete fusion of the lids. The majority of cases are mild, isolated anomalies and no further evaluation is required. Treatment is by separating the lids, by simple eyelid opening if only threadlike strands are present, or with scissors if necessary.

Children may frequently have a low-grade inflammation of the eyelid margin, chronic blepharitis, caused by *Staphylococcus* infection of the oil glands of the lid margin. Blepharitis may be associated with seborrhea or allergies and occurs commonly in children with Down syndrome. Symptoms include crusting of the lashes, itching, light sensitivity, and irritation of the lids. The lashes may be matted and adherent in the morning. If the condition is chronic and severe, thickening of the eyelid and misdirection of the eyelashes to such a point that they may invert and irritate the cornea or conjunctiva may occur (Fig. 19-41). Complications include ulceration of the lid margin, abscess or hordeolum formation, chronic conjunctivitis, and keratitis (corneal irritation and inflammation).

A hordeolum is an inflamed gland of Zeis at the base of the cilia (Fig. 19-42). This produces painful swelling and erythema of the eyelid. These lesions are commonly called *styes*. Infection, frequently with *Staphylococcus,* may occur. Some discharge may be seen. Rarely, preseptal cellulitis may occur as a complication.

A chalazion is a chronic granulomatous inflammation of the meibomian glands within the tarsal plate. Painless swelling and redness of the eyelid result from distention of the gland and the inflammatory response caused by the retained glandular secretions. The gland may spontaneously rupture either to the conjunctival surface or externally to the skin (Figs. 19-43 and 19-44). Spontaneous resolution may occur; however, tissue reaction may persist and leave a firm mass within the lid.

The mainstay of treatment of hordeolums and chalazions is frequent application of warm compresses. Topical antibiotics may be used, as well as systemic antibiotics if secondary infection or cellulitis appears to be present. Some patients may be affected by multiple, recurring lesions. Surgical excision of the lesions may be required if chronic or inflamed in order to prevent drainage through the skin surface with scarring of the skin or possible permanent loss of lashes if the lid margin is severely affected.

Primary herpes simplex infection may affect the periocular skin and eye (Fig. 19-45). This is characterized by small skin vesicles, affecting the conjunctiva or cornea frequently unilaterally, with an associated mild conjunctivitis and punctate keratitis. Although self-limited, herpes simplex should be treated with topical antivirals to prevent scarring from keratitis. Systemic antivirals may also be used, and if given early, they may reduce the number and duration of lesions. Recurrence or reactivation unfortunately is not prevented by treatment of the primary infection. Chronic systemic treatment may be employed if recurrences are frequent.

Varicella produces eyelid swelling and vesicular skin eruptions, usually without subsequent scarring. Conjunctival vesicles and keratitis may also occur, and topical antibiotics are

Figure 19-36   Distichiasis, a double row of lashes. One row, directed toward the cornea, arises from the meibomian gland orifices. The second row is directed outward in the normal position.

Figure 19-37   Congenital entropion of the right upper lid. The lid is inverted, and the lashes and skin rest on the corneal surface. **A,** The eyelid is propped up with a cotton-tipped applicator, displaying the area of skin inverted against the eye. The povidone-iodine prep solution has not coated the affected area of the lid. **B,** With the upper lid everted and the lids held widely open, extensive corneal scarring caused by the abrasion from the inverted skin and lashes is seen.

Figure 19-38   Epiblepharon. The eyelashes are rotated inward against the globe.

Figure 19-39   Ectropion of the left lower lid resulting from scleroderma. The lower eyelid skin has become contracted, causing eversion of the lower eyelid.

Figure 19-40   Goldenhar syndrome with eyelid coloboma and corneal–limbal dermoid.

Figure 19-41   Blepharitis. Thickened lids with crusting of the lashes.

Figure 19-42   Acute hordeolum of the eyelid (pointing externally) with swelling, induration, and purulent contents.

Figure 19-43   Chalazion. Usually, but not always, painless. The lesion may point externally to the skin side or internally to the underside of the lid.

Figure 19-44 Chalazion of the left lower lid, pointed internally. A pyogenic granuloma consisting of a vascularized mound of conjunctival tissue has developed over the chalazion because of spontaneous rupture of the chalazion under the palpebral conjunctiva with a hypertrophic healing response of the conjunctiva.

Figure 19-46 Infestation of the eyelashes with the crab louse *Phthirus pubis*. The lid margin has a crusty appearance because of the presence of adult organisms and eggs adherent to the eyelashes. The salivary material of the parasites results in toxic and immunologic reactions that cause itching and burning of the eyes.

indicated to prevent secondary bacterial infection. Systemic antivirals may shorten the course and severity of the outbreak if given very early in the course of infection. Herpes zoster is uncommon in children. If present, zoster should be treated as early in its course as possible in order to promote healing and to prevent zoster-associated hyperesthesias. A lesion on the tip of the nose indicates involvement of the ophthalmic division of the maxillary nerve and possible involvement of the eye with keratitis, uveitis, and glaucoma.

Another common eyelid lesion found in children is caused by *molluscum contagiosum* (see Chapter 8). Molluscum is characterized by elevated, 1- to 2-mm umbilicated lesions of the eyelid skin. If the lesions involve the eyelid margin, they may cause an associated keratoconjunctivitis. Molluscum should be considered in the differential diagnosis of chronic conjunctivitis.

Phthiriasis—infestation of the lashes with the crab louse *Phthirus pubis*—manifests as a crusty appearance of the lid margin. Closer inspection reveals egg cases and the adult louse (Fig. 19-46). Ophthalmic ointment, almost any type, suffocates the organisms. Phthiriasis may also produce chronic conjunctivitis, and the lashes should be carefully examined in cases of chronic recurring conjunctivitis.

Lacrimal Gland and Nasolacrimal Drainage System

Reflex tears are produced by the lacrimal gland, whereas the basal secretion of tears comes from the accessory lacrimal glands (Fig. 19-47). Secretions from the glands of Zeis and the

meibomian glands contribute to the tear film. During the first month of life the eye remains moist, but reflex tearing, or tearing resulting from emotion, does not occur until the second month of life or early in infancy.

Disorders of the lacrimal gland are rare in children. Acute dacryoadenitis may occur with viral infections, most frequently mumps (Fig. 19-48). Chronic diseases such as sarcoid, Hodgkin disease, leukemia, and mononucleosis may produce lacrimal gland swelling with a palpable mass in the upper outer portion of the orbit.

Figure 19-45 Primary herpes simplex infection involving the periocular area. Primary infection is frequently associated with a mild diffuse keratoconjunctivitis; dendritic corneal lesions are uncommon in primary infections.

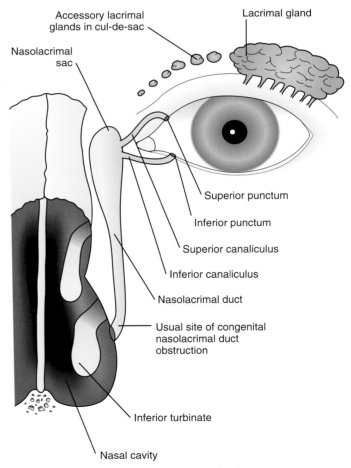

Figure 19-47 Lacrimal secretory and collecting system.

Figure 19-48 Dacryoadenitis. The lacrimal gland has become swollen and inflamed and is visible beneath the lateral aspect of the upper eyelid. The swelling is frequently accompanied by symptoms of pain and tenderness.

Figure 19-50 Congenital nasolacrimal sac mucocele presents shortly after birth as a bluish mass below the medial canthal tendon.

The tears are drained from the eye by the superior and inferior puncta, which connect to the superior and inferior canaliculi (see Fig. 19-47). The canaliculi may unite into a common canaliculus before they enter the nasolacrimal sac, or they may enter the sac separately. The medial canthal tendon is anterior and superior to the nasolacrimal sac. Disorders of the lacrimal sac are then seen primarily inferior to the medial canthus unless there is an overlying cellulitis. The sac is connected to the nasolacrimal duct, which is located in the nasal bone. The distal portion of the nasolacrimal duct enters the nasal antrum beneath the inferior turbinate.

Stenosis or obstruction of the nasolacrimal duct is present in 30% of newborns (Fig. 19-49). The obstruction is usually caused by a membranous obstruction of the nasolacrimal duct. Obstruction may also be caused by the inferior turbinate within the nose. Signs include tearing and mucopurulent discharge, which usually begins 3 to 5 weeks after birth. The absence of conjunctival injection differentiates this condition from conjunctivitis. A helpful diagnostic technique is to apply gentle pressure over the nasolacrimal sac to cause reflux of tears and mucopurulent material from the sac. Spontaneous resolution of the obstruction is common before 6 to 8 months of age. If the obstruction has not cleared by this age, spontaneous resolution is much less likely and the patient should be referred for probing of the nasolacrimal duct. If left past 13 months of age, the recurring infections may cause scarring and stenosis of the nasolacrimal duct, which may require more complicated procedures for treatment.

If both the nasolacrimal duct and the canaliculi entering the sac are obstructed at birth, a bluish firm mass may be present or develop in the area of the nasolacrimal sac

(congenital nasolacrimal sac mucocele or dacryocele) (Fig. 19-50). These patients should be referred promptly because of the risk for development of infection and cellulitis. Other congenital defects of the nasolacrimal collecting system include absence of the puncta or accessory puncta with fistulas from the nasolacrimal sac to the overlying skin.

Obstruction of the nasolacrimal system may also occur secondary to infections such as viral conjunctivitis, trachoma, tuberculosis, or fungal infections. Dacryocystitis, an infection and inflammation of the lacrimal sac and passages, may spread to the surrounding tissues, producing a periorbital cellulitis. Acute dacryocystitis is usually due to bacterial infection (Fig. 19-51).

Conjunctiva

The conjunctiva is a mucous membrane that covers the posterior aspect of the eyelids. It is reflected into the cul-de-sac and extends onto the globe, where it fuses to the sclera at the corneal scleral limbus. The conjunctiva has goblet cells that contribute mucin to the tear film. When the eyelids are closed, the oxygen supplied by the blood vessels of the conjunctiva is responsible for maintaining oxygenation of the cornea. *Conjunctivitis* refers to inflammation of the conjunctiva. Infections of the conjunctiva may be bacterial or viral.

The etiology of neonatal conjunctivitis is related to the time of onset. Neonatal conjunctivitis occurring within the first day or two of life is usually due to the use of Credé prophylaxis for gonococcal ophthalmia neonatorum. One percent silver nitrate solution may cause a mild chemical conjunctivitis that

Figure 19-49 Nasolacrimal duct obstruction. Mucopurulent discharge and tearing (epiphora) are present.

Figure 19-51 Acute dacryocystitis caused by bacterial infection of the nasolacrimal sac associated with nasolacrimal duct obstruction. The infection of the nasolacrimal sac has spread to the surrounding tissues, producing a cellulitis.

Figure 19-52 Ophthalmia neonatorum, a hyperacute bacterial conjunctivitis, with thick purulent discharge and red swollen lids.

Figure 19-54 Papillary conjunctivitis of bacterial or allergic origin.

spontaneously resolves within 1 or 2 days. This is essentially never seen now in the United States, as erythromycin ointment has completely replaced the use of silver nitrate. Neonatal conjunctivitis occurring 2 to 4 days after birth and accompanied by a copious purulent discharge, either with or without corneal involvement, may be caused by gonococci (Fig. 19-52). All cases of neonatal conjunctivitis are emergencies and must be evaluated by an ophthalmologist. Aerobic, anaerobic, and viral cultures must be obtained because corneal involvement, particularly with gonorrhea, may lead to corneal scarring or perforation. With *Pseudomonas* infection corneal perforation may occur within hours of presentation. Infectious neonatal conjunctivitis occurring after 8 days (but before 2 weeks) and accompanied by a watery discharge is often due to chlamydiae. Other common pathogens include *Staphylococcus, Streptococcus,* and *Enterococcus.* Conjunctivitis is usually contracted after early rupture of membranes or during passage through the birth canal.

The conjunctiva has a limited variety of responses to infection or inflammation. Inflammation of the conjunctiva results in the formation of follicles or papillae. A follicle is an aggregate of lymphocytes with an avascular center and a peripheral vascular network (Fig. 19-53). Newborns seldom develop follicles because lymphoid tissues have not yet developed. Viral infections frequently lead to follicular reaction.

Papillae are small, raised nodules with a central vascular core (Fig. 19-54). They may be located on the tarsal surface of the upper and lower eyelids. Papillae may become large, measuring 1 to 2 mm in diameter if inflammation is chronic. Papillae are the conjunctiva's response to bacterial or allergic conjunctivitis. Giant papillae may be produced by the continuous irritation caused by contact lens wear. Differentiation of a follicular response from a papillary response is frequently difficult, and differentiating viral conjunctivitis from bacterial conjunctivitis without cultures is not always definite.

Bacterial conjunctivitis may be acute or chronic. Acute conjunctivitis is painful, with lid edema and keratitis. The bulbar conjunctiva swells (chemosis) and becomes hyperemic (injection). Corneal ulceration may occur as a complication. Children with viral conjunctivitis frequently develop secondary bacterial conjunctivitis. Acute bacterial conjunctivitis is usually due to staphylococcal, pneumococcal, or *Haemophilus* infections. Mucopurulent discharge is associated with tearing, and the eyelids may be stuck together on awakening (Fig. 19-55).

Chronic bacterial conjunctivitis results from bacterial toxins of *Staphylococcus aureus; Proteus* organisms; *Moraxella* organisms; or, in Third World countries, trachomata. A foreign body sensation may be experienced, and the eyes may be hyperemic with a chronic, mucopurulent or watery discharge. Papillary hyperplasia and thickening of the conjunctiva may also occur.

Viral conjunctivitis is usually caused by various strains of adenovirus (Fig. 19-56). Signs include copious tearing with a watery or thin mucopurulent discharge, conjunctival redness, and preauricular lymph node enlargement. Viral conjunctivitis is self-limited and usually resolves in 7 to 10 days depending on the viral strain. Viral conjunctivitis is highly contagious. Certain strains of adenoviral conjunctivitis may cause epidemic keratoconjunctivitis (EKC), which produces corneal involvement with a punctate keratitis that progresses to subepithelial infiltrates (Fig. 19-57) as an immunologic reaction. Patients are contagious only early in their course. Because of the corneal involvement, symptoms of photophobia are more pronounced, and when subepithelial infiltrates are present patients complain of glare and decreased visual acuity. Symptoms in EKC may last from weeks to months. The infiltrates eventually resolve spontaneously. Steroids may alleviate symptoms; however, they prolong the overall course.

Figure 19-53 Follicular conjunctivitis of viral origin.

Figure 19-55 Acute bacterial conjunctivitis. Copious amounts of mucopurulent discharge have made the upper and lower eyelids adherent to each other. Chemosis of the upper and lower lids may also make opening of the eyelids difficult.

Figure 19-56 Viral conjunctivitis with hyperemia and a watery discharge.

Figure 19-58 Conjunctival phlyctenule. A raised area of conjunctival infiltration and localized infection is commonly seen at the corneal–scleral limbus. The center of the lesion is clear or white and may ulcerate. Phlyctenules may also occur elsewhere on the bulbar or tarsal conjunctiva or on the cornea. *(Courtesy Robert Arffa, MD, Pittsburgh, Pa.)*

Allergic conjunctivitis occurs as a hypersensitivity response to dust, pollens, animal dander, or other airborne allergens. The eyes exhibit copious tearing, itching, and photophobia. The eyelids and palpebral conjunctiva are hyperemic and edematous (see Chapter 4). The development of extensive chemosis of the conjunctiva may be sudden and rapid. The conjunctiva may swell to protrude between the eyelids or obscure part of the cornea over the course of hours. A similar rapid development of chemosis may occur with viral conjunctivitis. Simple treatment with cold compresses usually leads to improvement over several hours, and there are no significant sequelae. If the symptoms produced by allergic conjunctivitis are mild, no treatment is required because the child may object more to the use of the drops than to the discomfort of the disease. Allergic conjunctivitis may become chronic with repeated exposure to the allergen. In cases of chronic allergic conjunctivitis, the conjunctiva becomes pale and boggy and demonstrates a papillary reaction. Rare complications include keratitis in advanced cases called limbal vernal keratoconjunctivitis.

Phlyctenular conjunctivitis is the result of a cell-mediated hypersensitivity reaction (Fig. 19-58). Phlyctenular lesions are small, pinkish-white vesicles or pustules in the center of hyperemic areas of the conjunctiva. These lesions may occur at the limbus; on the conjunctiva; or, more rarely, on the cornea. Phlyctenulosis most commonly occurs in association with chronic staphylococcal infection. Symptoms consist of itching, tearing, and irritation. A mucopurulent discharge may occur if secondary infection is present. Patients with corneal phlyctenulosis have more severe symptoms of pain, light sensitivity, and tearing.

Subconjunctival hemorrhages may occur spontaneously, or they may be secondary to coughing episodes, Valsalva maneuvers, or trauma (Fig. 19-59). These appear as striking bright red discolorations underneath the bulbar conjunctiva. The size and configuration of the hemorrhage depend on the amount and location of the blood between the conjunctiva and the globe. The size of the hemorrhage is not indicative of the severity of an injury, and the hemorrhage itself does not have any visual significance. Spontaneous resolution occurs over the course of several weeks.

Cornea

Developmental anomalies of the cornea include sclerocornea, Rieger syndrome, microcornea, and corneal dermoid.

Sclerocornea, present at birth, is a rare condition in which the cornea is white and resembles sclera. Rieger syndrome, a variant of anterior segment dysgenesis, is a dominant hereditary disorder that affects development of the anterior segment of the eye. Features include hyperplasia of the iris stroma, pupillary anomalies, anomalies of the trabecular meshwork, and early-onset glaucoma. Microcornea, whether an isolated anomaly or associated with glaucoma, cataracts, iris abnormalities, or anterior segment dysgenesis, is present when the horizontal corneal diameter is 9 mm or less (Fig. 19-60).

The developmental abnormalities mentioned necessitate further tests to exclude glaucoma. If the anterior segment of the eye is severely disorganized, the cornea is opaque, or glaucoma exists, surgical reconstruction and repair are indicated. The prognosis for vision is guarded for severe cases.

Corneal dermoids occur at the limbus (junction between the cornea and sclera); grow slowly, if at all; and may encroach on the visual axis or cause high degrees of astigmatism

Figure 19-57 Subepithelial infiltrates of epidemic keratoconjunctivitis (EKC) caused by adenovirus. The beam of the slit lamp is used to demonstrate corneal subepithelial infiltrates (small white opacities). Only certain strains of adenovirus produce subepithelial infiltrates, which are immune reactions to the viral antigens. These may persist for months, causing symptoms of glare and blurring of vision.

Figure 19-59 Subconjunctival hemorrhage secondary to blunt ocular trauma.

Figure 19-60 Unilateral microcornea and microphthalmos.

(Fig. 19-61). They are composed of fibrolipid tissue containing hair follicles and sebaceous glands. Corneal dermoids may occur as isolated anomalies or they may be associated with syndromes such as Goldenhar syndrome.

The cornea is also involved in many systemic diseases. Hurler syndrome, a mucopolysaccharidosis, produces clouding of the cornea. The cornea, clear at birth, develops an opacification by 2 to 3 years of age. Pigmentary retinopathy and optic atrophy also develop.

Cystinosis, seen in the early months of life, involves the deposition of L-cystine in the cornea. This may be seen as a subtle haze of the cornea. Slit-lamp examination is necessary to clearly visualize the corneal deposits (Fig. 19-62). The deposits cause pain, photophobia, and decreased vision.

Corneal inflammations are associated with bacterial, viral, mycotic, and allergic diseases. Infectious corneal ulcers usually occur only in the setting of some compromise of the corneal epithelium (e.g., with traumatic corneal abrasion; foreign bodies; exposure keratitis; or contact lens wear, especially sleeping with lenses in place). In the abusive contact lens patient a corneal ulcer may be sterile and caused by the improper use of the lenses. A red, painful eye in a patient with a history of contact lens wear must be evaluated by an ophthalmologist. Infectious corneal ulcers are caused by the invasion of bacterial organisms into the corneal stroma (Fig. 19-63). If the visual axis is involved, scar formation may permanently affect visual acuity. Corneal perforation can occur rapidly in some infections, particularly *Pseudomonas,* and can result in loss of the eye. Bacteria commonly involved include staphylococci, pneumococci, *Moraxella* organisms, *Pseudomonas aeruginosa, Escherichia coli,* and *Klebsiella pneumoniae. Acanthamoeba* and *Fusarium* infectious corneal ulcers in

L-cystine crystals in cornea

Figure 19-62 Cystinosis of the cornea with deposition of L-cystine crystals in the corneal stroma.

A

B

Figure 19-63 Bacterial corneal ulcer. **A,** The conjunctiva displays a marked inflammatory response with injection, most prominent in the quadrant nearest the corneal ulcer. The ulcer is visualized in the slit beam as a small white infiltrate of the corneal stroma. There is an overlying epithelial defect. **B,** The epithelial defect is easier to visualize after the application of fluorescein dye. The dye is taken up by the corneal stroma in the area of the epithelial defect. The areas fluoresce with cobalt blue light illumination.

Figure 19-61 Corneal–limbal dermoid, often associated with Goldenhar syndrome.

Figure 19-64 Herpes simplex keratitis. Infection of the corneal epithelium with herpes simplex virus produces a pattern of fluorescein staining that resembles a neuronal dendrite. The surrounding area may be hazy because of epithelial and stromal edema and infiltration. Conjunctival injection is typically present.

Figure 19-65 Congenital glaucoma. The right cornea is hazy and opaque due to corneal edema. Breakdown of the corneal epithelium has caused ocular irritation, and the conjunctiva is slightly injected. Epiphora is present because of reflex tearing caused by the pain of epithelial breakdown and increased intraocular pressure.

contact lens patients have been recognized and frequently lead to severe vision loss and the need for corneal transplantation. Appropriate smears and cultures are obtained, and treatment is started as soon as possible for corneal ulcers.

Herpes simplex may be transmitted from active herpes in the maternal birth canal, or it may result from direct contact with infected individuals. Primary herpes is a unilateral condition that occurs as a blepharoconjunctivitis or as vesicular lesions of the eyelids with regional lymphadenopathy. A few weeks after infection, half of all patients develop a punctate or typical dendritic keratitis (Fig. 19-64). This is best seen using fluorescein stain and a cobalt blue filter over a penlight.

Recurrent herpes keratitis occurs in 25% of infected individuals. The lesions may have a typical appearance of branching dendrites. Recurrences may be complicated by stromal keratitis, keratouveitis, and anesthesia of the cornea. Stromal disease is a serious complication that reduces visual recovery because of corneal vascularization and scarring. Patients with a history of herpes keratitis must be evaluated by an ophthalmologist for any unexplained episode of conjunctival injection.

Anterior Chamber

The term *anterior chamber* refers to the fluid-filled space between the cornea and the iris diaphragm. The aqueous fluid is optically clear. It provides nutrition for the corneal endothelial surface. The aqueous fluid is secreted by the ciliary processes. It passes through the pupil to the anterior chamber and leaves via the trabecular meshwork in the periphery of the anterior chamber angle where the iris meets the cornea and sclera.

Glaucoma

The incidence of infantile or congenital glaucoma is approximately 1 in 12,500 births. The inheritance of congenital glaucoma is multifactorial; parents of an affected child have a 5% chance of having another child with glaucoma, and an affected parent has a 5% chance of having a child with congenital glaucoma. Two thirds of all patients are male. Glaucoma can present at birth, but more commonly, clinical signs develop during the first several weeks or months of life. An embryonic defect in the development of the trabecular meshwork or filtration area of the eye has been hypothesized as the cause.

Infants with glaucoma have corneal edema, which gives the cornea a hazy or cloudy appearance. Corneal edema may produce an irregular corneal light reflex or dull the red reflex. Initially, the edema may be limited to the epithelium, but stromal edema may follow (Fig. 19-65). As this increases, the

Descemet membrane may rupture and produce Haab striae (Fig. 19-66).

A break in the Descemet membrane may produce a corneal opacity, or, if edema is not present, it may be visualized against the red reflex as a line when viewed with a slit lamp or direct ophthalmoscope. Breaks in the Descemet membrane can produce irregular astigmatism. Glare from the scatter of light produced by the epithelial and stromal edema is responsible for photophobia and blinking. Breakdown of the corneal epithelium may produce pain, squinting, and blepharospasm.

In children younger than 2 years of age, an increase in corneal diameter frequently accompanies increased intraocular pressure (Fig. 19-67). An infant's horizontal corneal diameter is normally 9.5 mm; this increases over the first 2 years of life to a normal corneal diameter of 11.5 mm. Small increases in corneal diameter may be recognized first as asymmetries in the corneal diameter between the two eyes. In addition to enlargement of the corneal diameter, chronic elevated intraocular pressure may also enlarge the entire eye. This produces an increase in axial length and a myopic shift in the refraction. A rapid increase in myopia may be a sign of glaucoma. The

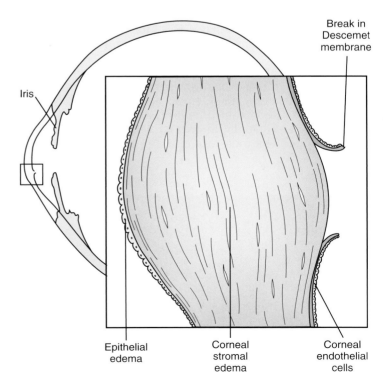

Figure 19-66 Haab striae (breaks in Descemet membrane).

Figure 19-67   Congenital glaucoma. This patient has corneal diameter asymmetry resulting from glaucoma in the left eye. The horizontal corneal diameter is 11 mm in the right eye and 13.5 mm in the left eye. The entire left eye has become enlarged, and the axial length is greater than normal. The increase in axial length of the left eye has produced a myopic refractive error.

Figure 19-69   Typical unilateral iris coloboma in an otherwise normal left eye.

anterior chamber in infancy is shallow when compared with that of older children. An anterior chamber that is deeper than normal is a sign of congenital glaucoma.

Epiphora, or tearing, is a sign of glaucoma and is differentiated from nasolacrimal duct obstruction by the presence of rhinorrhea. When the nasolacrimal duct is obstructed, rhinorrhea is absent. Nasolacrimal duct obstruction is also accompanied by recurrent discharge and infections, whereas glaucoma has clear epiphora only.

The optic nerve damage caused by elevated intraocular pressure is reflected in the degree of enlargement of the optic cup (Fig. 19-68). Asymmetry of the cup-to-disc ratio between the eyes or an increase in the cup-to-disc ratio to greater than 0.5 is a possible sign of glaucoma. In infants and young children the intraocular pressure may be elevated for a prolonged period of time before optic disc cupping occurs. Enlargement of the optic cup is reversible to an extent in infants and young children but is permanent when older. Enlargement of the optic cups without glaucoma may be inherited; examination of family members for comparison may be of value.

Elevation of intraocular pressure (IOP) is the hallmark of congenital glaucoma. Normal IOP in infants and young children is less than 20 mm Hg. Pressures greater than 25 mm Hg strongly suggest glaucoma.

Accurate measurement of pressure is difficult in children. An estimate of the IOP may be obtained by palpating the globes with the fingertips over closed eyelids. More precise measurements are obtained with instruments that require anesthetizing and coming in contact with the cornea. These procedures and decisions regarding the management of IOP

may require an examination that is conducted with sedation or under general anesthesia. Unfortunately, some anesthetic agents alter IOP.

Glaucoma may occur with congenital ocular malformations such as aniridia or mesodermal (iridocorneal) dysgenesis, in systemic syndromes, or after trauma. Sturge-Weber syndrome, neurofibromatosis, Lowe syndrome, Rubinstein-Taybi syndrome, and congenital rubella syndrome are associated with congenital glaucoma. Patients with chronic uveitis frequently develop glaucoma, and 8% to 25% of children with congenital cataracts, especially those with microcornea or microphthalmia, develop glaucoma at some point in life.

Iris

A coloboma results from failed fusion of the embryonic fissure of the optic cup (Fig. 19-69). The defect is usually inferior and nasal in location, and it may involve any ocular structure, most commonly the iris.

Colobomas occur either as isolated defects or in association with systemic syndromes. Iris colobomas occur in the CHARGE association, cat-eye syndrome, Rieger syndrome, and the facioauriculovertebral anomalies. Isolated colobomas may be inherited as a dominant trait.

Aniridia, an apparent absence of the iris, is caused by failure of the mesoderm to grow outward from the iris root during the fourth month of gestation. The pupil appears the same size as the cornea, and iris structures are present as only rudimentary findings (Fig. 19-70). A fibrovascular membrane can form between the rudimentary iris and the trabecular meshwork and cause glaucoma. Hypoplasia of the macula occurs in patients with aniridia, and visual acuity may be decreased to the 20/400 level. Associated defects include corneal opacities, lens dislocations, and cataracts. Affected patients have photophobia and nystagmus.

Figure 19-68   Glaucomatous optic atrophy. In glaucoma, excavation extends to the disc edge in contrast to the physiologic cupping that may be seen in myopia, where a normal rim of tissue exists. Retinal vessels emerge from under the cup edge.

Figure 19-70   Aniridia. Iris structures are present only as rudimentary findings, and the red reflex fills the entire corneal diameter. The edge of the lens is visible peripherally, and early cataractous lens changes are present centrally.

Figure 19-71 Persistent pupillary membranes. Hyperplasia of the mesoderm of the anterior layer of the iris has caused iris strands to become adherent to the anterior lens surface. The lens is clear. These are usually visually insignificant; however, if a plaque is present at the attachment site it may block the visual axis. The pupil may be smaller or less reactive than normal.

Figure 19-73 Juvenile rheumatoid arthritis. Band keratopathy, a deposition of calcium, is seen as white scalelike deposits present on the anterior corneal surface. The pupil is not round because of the presence of posterior synechiae and adhesions between the iris and lens; a cataract is present.

An autosomal dominant inheritance pattern is present in two thirds of all patients with aniridia. Approximately 1 in 70 patients with sporadic aniridia will have Wilms tumor, and 90% of these will occur before age 3. Other genitourinary defects and mental retardation may occur, and many of these patients have chromosomal abnormalities (11p-).

Persistent pupillary membranes are caused by hyperplasia of the mesoderm of the anterior layer of the iris and are a frequent finding in children born prematurely (Fig. 19-71). Instead of terminating at the pupillary margin, iris strands with accompanying blood vessels encroach on the pupillary space or adhere to the anterior lens surface. They are rarely visually significant and, especially in the premature infant, the iris strands frequently spontaneously release from the lens surface with pupil dilation.

Heterochromia iridis, or asymmetry in the color of the iris, is visually insignificant. It may occur as an isolated finding. Heterochromia may develop in congenital Horner syndrome when the affected infant has light-colored irides. As the child ages, the iris in the unaffected eye may darken while the eye with Horner syndrome retains its lighter color. Heterochromia may also occur secondary to inflammation or after intraocular surgery or ocular trauma. Trauma may cause the affected iris to become darker than the fellow iris as late as many years after the incident (Fig. 19-72).

The iris may provide signs that aid in the diagnosis of systemic conditions. Patients with neurofibromatosis may have multiple small melanocytic iris nevi, called *Lisch nodules,* on the surface of the iris (see Chapter 15). These may be identified with magnification provided by the direct ophthalmoscope or by slit-lamp examination. They are of no

visual significance. Other ocular findings associated with neurofibromatosis include plexiform neurofibromas of the lids, thickened corneal nerves, congenital glaucoma, and optic nerve gliomas producing optic atrophy.

In chronic anterior uveitis or iritis, for example in association with sarcoidosis or juvenile rheumatoid arthritis, the iris may be affected by adhesions between the papillary border and the lens (posterior synechiae) or between the peripheral iris and the cornea (anterior synechiae). Posterior synechiae cause the pupil to be less reactive in the area of the synechiae and cause the pupil to lose its round shape (corectopia) (Fig. 19-73).

Patients with juvenile xanthogranuloma, usually younger than 1 year of age, may develop unilateral asymptomatic fleshy, yellowish-brown tumors on the surface of the iris (Fig. 19-74). These vascular lesions bleed easily and may produce a spontaneous hyphema.

Figure 19-72 Horner syndrome (right side) with iris heterochromia. The right upper lid is slightly ptotic, and the right lower lid is slightly higher. Anisocoria is present. The right pupil is smaller than the left. The iris on the side affected by Horner syndrome may be lighter in color than the iris of the fellow eye.

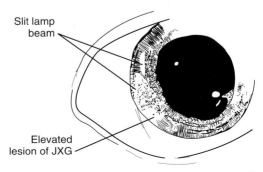

Figure 19-74 Juvenile xanthogranuloma (JXG). The ocular lesion of JXG is visualized as a fleshy, yellowish-brown tumor on the surface of the iris. The lesions are vascular, bleed easily, and can cause spontaneous hyphemas.

Brushfield spots are found in patients with Down syndrome. The spots consist of tiny areas of normal iris stroma that are surrounded by rings of mild iris hypoplasia. Brushfield spots give the iris a speckled appearance. They are of no visual or pathologic significance.

Lens

The lens may be affected by developmental, hereditary, syndrome-related, inflammatory, metabolic, or traumatic conditions. This can result in the development of a cataract, an opacification of the crystalline lens that may be either partial or complete. The lens may also be dislocated from its supporting zonules or subluxated.

Cataracts

Leukocoria refers to the white pupillary reflex seen when there is a light-colored intraocular mass or structure visible in the papillary space. Many conditions of variable severity and prognosis produce leukocoria (Table 19-1). Examination with a penlight, the plus lens of a direct ophthalmoscope, or by slit-lamp biomicroscopy helps to differentiate lens opacification (cataract) from other causes of leukocoria.

Congenital or infantile cataracts may be unilateral or bilateral, and the extent of opacification may be complete or partial (Fig. 19-75). Bilateral cataracts usually arise early in infancy and, if not treated early, may produce severe visual deprivation accompanied by poor fixation and nystagmus. Visually significant unilateral cataracts can cause severe deprivation amblyopia and strabismus. When abnormalities of the red reflex are detected, early referral for treatment is critical for successful visual rehabilitation. Although visually significant bilateral cataracts have gross signs of poor visual development, monocular cataracts may not have grossly visible signs for many months or years, until the cataract is obvious or a sensory strabismus develops.

Opacification of a child's lens may be due to heredity (autosomal dominant), chromosomal disorders (trisomy 13, 18, and 21) (Fig. 19-76), inflammation (iritis and uveitis), infection (TORCH), metabolic disorders (galactosemia and disorders of calcium and phosphorus metabolism), exposure to toxins, vitamin deficiencies (vitamins A and D), systemic syndromes with cataracts (Table 19-2), ocular conditions producing retinal detachment, radiation exposure, and trauma. Roughly one third of pediatric cataracts are hereditary, one third syndrome or disease related, and one third attributed to other or undetermined causes.

The presence of ocular anomalies frequently identifies a developmental defect as being the cause for the cataract. Microphthalmia, the globe being smaller than normal, may be caused by ocular disease or inflammation, or it may be present as a developmental defect (see Fig. 19-60). Eyes with persistent hyperplastic primary vitreous (PHPV) are usually microphthalmic, sometimes only mildly so, and frequently have visually significant cataracts, as well as vision-limiting retinal or optic nerve abnormalities.

Figure 19-75   Complete cataract with no view of the red reflex or retina.

The morphology of the lens opacification may provide a clue to the cause of a congenital cataract if opacification is not complete. During development, the lens cells lay down fibers that grow out from the peripheral lens to the anterior and posterior lens surfaces. These form sutures. Because of this, the gestational age at the time of cataract development determines the location of the opacity. For example, the nuclear cataracts of rubella syndrome (Fig. 19-77) indicate infection early in gestation, whereas a zonular or lamellar cataract represents an insult to the lens occurring later in lens development.

Small central opacities on the anterior or posterior poles of the lens, termed *polar cataracts*, are developmental abnormalities that typically remain stable and rarely affect vision (Fig. 19-78). Lamellar or zonular cataracts have a normal, transparent central nucleus; an affected lamellar zone; and a clear outer layer of cortex. Riders or radial extensions are frequently present (Fig. 19-79). Zonular cataracts may be autosomal dominant, associated with vitamin A and D deficiency, or follow hypocalcemia. Multicolored flecks may be seen in hypoparathyroidism or myotonic dystrophy, and an oil droplet configuration is seen in galactosemia (Fig. 19-80).

If a child has no history of trauma, the family history is unremarkable, the general physical examination fails to suggest a systemic syndrome or chromosomal abnormality, and ocular examination does not help to determine the cause of a cataract, then a focused laboratory evaluation to determine the cause of the cataract may be undertaken. The most common metabolic disorders causing congenital cataracts are hypoglycemia and hypocalcemia. Examination of the urine for reducing substances is performed, and, if positive, laboratory evaluation for galactosemia and galactokinase deficiency should include blood tests for galactose and galactose 1-phosphate uridyl transferase. Examination of the urine for

Table 19-1	Differential Diagnosis of Leukocoria
Angiomatosis retinae	Persistent hyperplastic primary vitreous
Cataracts	Retinal detachment
Coats disease	Retinal dysplasia
Colobomas	Retinoblastoma
Congenital retinal fold	Retinopathy of prematurity
High myopia	Toxocariasis
Incontinentia pigmenti	Uveitis
Medulloepithelioma	Vitreous hemorrhage
Myelinated nerve fibers	

Figure 19-76   Spokelike cortical cataract of Down syndrome. The lens opacification does not affect the visual axis and is visually insignificant. Lens opacification such as this may rapidly progress and produce visual loss, or it may remain unchanged for years. Snowflake cortical opacities may also be seen in Down syndrome, and typically do not progress over the years.

Table 19-2	Syndromes Associated with Cataracts
Albright hereditary osteodystrophy	Kniest syndrome
Alport syndrome	Lazier syndrome
Cat-eye syndrome	Laurence-Moon-Bardet-Biedl syndrome
Cerebro-oculo-facial-skeletal syndrome	Lowe syndrome
Chondrodysplasia punctata (Conradi-Hünermann syndrome)	Marinesco-Sjögren syndrome
	Marshall syndrome
Cockayne syndrome	Myotonic dystrophy
Congenital ichthyosis	Osteogenesis imperfecta
Conradi syndrome	Patau syndrome (trisomy 13)
Craniofacial syndromes (Apert and Crouzon syndromes)	Progeria
	Roberts syndrome
Down syndrome (trisomy 21)	Rothman-Thomson syndrome
Edward syndrome (trisomy 18)	Rubinstein-Taybi syndrome
Hallgren syndrome	Smith-Lemli-Opitz syndrome
Hallermann-Streiff syndrome	Stickler syndrome
Ichthyosis	Turner syndrome
Incontinentia pigmenti	Zellweger syndrome

Figure 19-78   Anterior polar cataract. This type of lens opacity is a developmental abnormality that in most cases remains stable and rarely affects vision.

protein and amino acids identifies patients with Lowe (oculocerebrorenal) syndrome, and a urine nitroprusside test diagnoses homocystinuria. Screening tests for congenital TORCH infections and syphilis should also be performed.

Positional abnormalities of the lens may occur. A partial dislocation of the lens is referred to as *subluxation.* A dislocated lens, called *ectopia lentis,* may cause a profound decrease in vision by producing a large refractive error and amblyopia. Ectopia lentis may be unilateral, bilateral, inherited or sporadic, or it may be due to trauma (Fig. 19-81).

Simple ectopia lentis is a bilateral, symmetrical condition with an autosomal dominant inheritance pattern. Bilateral superotemporal lens dislocation is present in 50% to 80% of patients with Marfan syndrome, although this may not occur until the teen or adult years. Ninety percent of patients with homocystinuria have an inferior lens dislocation, and patients with Weill-Marchesani syndrome may have dislocation of their microspherophakic lenses.

Uvea

Inflammation of the uveal tract (iris, ciliary body, and choroid) has many potential causes including infections (toxoplasmosis, herpes zoster and simplex, and Lyme disease), collagen vascular disease (most frequently juvenile rheumatoid arthritis and sarcoidosis), and trauma. In the majority of children the etiologic agent cannot be determined. Advanced retinoblastoma may also present with signs that suggest uveitis.

Involvement of the anterior segment alone (iritis or anterior uveitis) may produce pain, ciliary injection (conjunctival redness in the circumlimbal area), tearing, photophobia, and decreased vision. Synechiae, adhesions between the iris and lens or peripheral cornea, may produce corectopia, an abnormally shaped pupil. Inflammatory reaction in the anterior chamber may be viewed with the aid of a slit lamp as inflammatory cells and fibrin or protein (flare) in the aqueous fluid. With the high magnification of the slit lamp, inflammatory cells may be seen floating in the aqueous fluid much like dust is seen in bright sunlight shining through a window. If marked, this may give the eye a dull or glassy appearance (Fig. 19-82). Clumps of inflammatory cells may adhere to the posterior corneal surface, forming keratic precipitates (KPs). Inflammatory nodules may also be seen on the surface of the iris or at the border (Busacca and Koeppe nodules) in chronic uveitis.

Iritis, which is milder in degree, may be present without signs or symptoms; children with juvenile rheumatoid arthritis should have periodic screening ophthalmic examinations. Children with polyarticular disease should be examined annually, and those with positive anti-nuclear antibodies and pauciarticular disease, who are more likely to develop ocular complications, should be examined three or four times per year to detect and treat the uveitis before complications of cataracts, glaucoma, and macular edema develop (see Chapter 7).

Pars planitis, or intermediate uveitis, is an idiopathic, bilateral inflammation of the pars plana or pars ciliaris portions of the ciliary body. Symptoms include light sensitivity, "floaters," and blurring of vision. Inflammatory cells in the anterior vitreous can make visualization of the retina with the direct ophthalmoscope difficult. If the inflammation is severe, it may produce leukocoria. No diagnostic laboratory tests are

Figure 19-77   A microspherophakic cataractous lens in rubella syndrome.

Figure 19-79   Lamellar cataract with riders, surrounded by a clear cortex.

Figure 19-80 Cataract of galactosemia. Early lens changes cause the nucleus of the lens to have an "oil droplet" configuration resulting from the accumulation of dulcitol, a metabolic product of galactose, within the lens. The resultant osmotic gradient draws water into the lens, producing the opacification. Early lens changes in galactosemia are reversible.

Figure 19-82 Iritis. Conjunctival injection is most marked immediately around the cornea (ciliary flush).

available in pars planitis, and the diagnosis is made on the basis of characteristic findings and by exclusion. Most cases are self-limited; however, chronic courses with exacerbations and remissions may produce visual loss resulting from cataracts, glaucoma, optic nerve inflammation, and cystoid macular edema. Retinal detachment because of membrane formation and phthisis bulbi may occur in advanced cases (Fig. 19-83).

Posterior uveitis (inflammation of the posterior vitreous, retina, and/or choroid) can be caused by infection, but frequently the precise cause is undetermined. Infection of the retina by protozoa, fungi, and viruses may produce an intense inflammatory response in the vitreous, rendering it hazy or opaque. Leukocoria may be produced if the vitreous is cloudy or if extensive retinal involvement is present.

Vitreous

Vitreous Hemorrhage

Trauma, be it penetrating, concussive, or the result of shaken baby syndrome, is the most common cause of vitreous hemorrhage. Vitreous hemorrhage may occur with hemorrhagic disease of the newborn (hypoprothrombinemia), thrombocytopenia, or in advanced stages of retinopathy of prematurity. Patients with a subarachnoid hemorrhage may develop vitreous hemorrhage (Terson syndrome), and vitreous hemorrhage may also occur in patients with leukemia.

Blood in the vitreous, if located centrally or posteriorly, may be visible with the direct ophthalmoscope. If the vitreous is liquid, the hemorrhage may appear to float inside the eye (Fig. 19-84). Blood in the vitreous may produce leukocoria as it organizes and becomes yellow and then gray in color. Vitreous hemorrhages may resolve spontaneously or, if extensive, require surgery. Vitreous hemorrhages that are slow to resolve in young children may cause amblyopia.

Retina

Developmental Abnormalities

Colobomas

Retinal colobomas are caused by a defect in closure of the embryonal fissure of the optic cup. They may occur unilaterally or bilaterally. Large colobomas are manifest as an absence of the retina and choroid with or without marked excavation of the optic disc (Fig. 19-85). A ring of pigment usually exists around the coloboma. Leukocoria may be produced by the yellowish-white reflection of the underlying sclera, and the red reflex may be seen as flashing from red to white as the eye moves to produce a reflex from normal areas of retina to the area of the coloboma. Using a direct ophthalmoscope, an occasional vessel may be seen bridging the area of the coloboma. The coloboma and retina are at a different plane of focus when visualized with the ophthalmoscope.

Colobomas may occur in otherwise normal eyes or in association with microphthalmia or retinal detachment. If the optic disc and macula are not involved, central visual acuity may be normal. In these eyes there is a peripheral visual field defect corresponding to the area of retinal involvement. Usually the patient is asymptomatic if the optic disc and macula are not involved. Colobomas may be inherited as isolated anomalies, or they may be associated with chromosomal defects (trisomy 13) or other syndrome-related entities (CHARGE association).

Myelinated Nerve Fibers

Before birth, myelination of the optic nerve begins in the central nervous system, progresses peripherally, and usually stops at the optic disc before birth. Myelination may continue beyond the optic disc to include the retinal nerve fiber layer as a relatively benign, isolated, congenital abnormality. Once present, the changes are permanent; however, there is no

Figure 19-81 A traumatic, dislocated cataractous lens.

Figure 19-83 Yellow cyclitic membrane behind a clear lens in a soft phthisic eye.

Figure 19-84 Vitreous hemorrhage. Dispersed red blood cells in the vitreous have made it hazy. The diffraction of light causes blurred vision. Fluid levels are often visible, and collections of blood may appear to float within the eye, variably blocking vision and causing symptoms of seeing cobwebs or large floating spots.

Figure 19-86 Myelinated nerve fibers. Myelination of the optic nerve fibers may continue beyond the optic disc to include the retinal nerve fibers. This is visible as yellowish-white, flame-shaped patches oriented with the retinal nerve fibers. Myelinated nerve fibers may produce the clinical sign of leukocoria. A blind spot is present, corresponding to the area of myelination, but it is symptomatic only if the macula is affected.

progression or worsening of the condition. Myelinated fibers are oriented with the retinal nerve fibers and are easily seen with the direct ophthalmoscope as yellowish-white, flame-shaped patches overlying the sensory retina and choroid (Fig. 19-86). The macula is rarely involved, and normal vision is usually present, although scotomas corresponding to the areas of myelination may be found on visual field examination.

Persistent Hyperplastic Primary Vitreous

PHPV occurs as a unilateral defect in the involution of the primary vitreous during the seventh month of gestation. No systemic associations exist. Eyes with PHPV are usually microphthalmic to varying degrees. PHPV may be associated with cataracts, intraocular hemorrhage, glaucoma, and retinal detachment. Many eyes with mild changes of PHPV may have good visual acuity after cataract surgery and visual rehabilitation; however, retinal or optic nerve abnormalities, if present, may limit vision. These rehabilitated eyes remain at risk for the development of glaucoma later in life. Eyes with advanced PHPV can become phthisical secondary to retinal or ciliary body detachment (Figs. 19-87 and 19-88).

Albinism

Albinism refers to conditions involving deficiencies of melanin in the skin or eye (Fig. 19-89). The loss of pigmentation may be isolated to the eye (ocular albinism), be generalized to the skin and eye (oculocutaneous albinism), or occur in conjunction with a systemic syndrome such as Chédiak-Higashi or Hermansky-Pudlak syndrome.

Ocular albinism may occur as an X-linked or autosomal recessive trait, and spontaneous mutations are frequent. Photophobia is a common symptom. Mild decreases in cutaneous pigmentation are frequent. Patients have iris transillumination defects in which the red reflex is seen through multiple

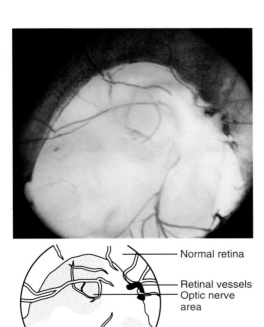

Figure 19-85 Coloboma of optic nerve, retina, and choroid. The yellowish-white sclera is visible, and retinal vessels can be seen coursing through the coloboma.

Figure 19-87 Persistent hyperplastic primary vitreous presenting as a dense fibrovascular retrolental mass with microspherophakia, microphthalmia, and elongated ciliary processes.

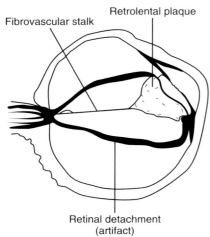

Retrolental plaque

Fibrovascular stalk

Retinal detachment
(artifact)

Figure 19-88 Pathologic section of persistent hypoplastic primary vitreous. *(Courtesy B.L. Johnson, MD, Pittsburgh, Pa.)*

punctate defects in the iris. Absence of pigment in the retinal pigment epithelium layer of the retina makes the fundus appear a lighter yellowish-orange color than usual. The choroidal vasculature, usually hidden by the retinal pigment epithelium, is visible. The macula and fovea are hypoplastic, and visual acuity is decreased to a degree dependent on the absence of pigment and the development of the macula and fovea. The visual acuity may be only mildly affected or, in patients with marked nystagmus, the vision may be severely limited (Fig. 19-90). Ocular albinism is a frequent cause of sensory nystagmus in infancy.

Ocular pigmentary abnormalities may also occur in a milder form, albinoidism. Such patients have iris transillumination

Figure 19-90 Ocular albinism. The fundus has little pigmentation and the choroidal vasculature is readily visible. The macula is poorly developed, producing decreased visual acuity.

defects, fundus hypopigmentation, and photophobia. Their maculae, however, are less severely affected or are normal. Because of this, nystagmus is uncommon and visual acuity is normal or only minimally reduced. Albinoidism is inherited as an autosomal dominant trait with incomplete penetrance.

Coats Disease (Retinal Telangiectasis)

Coats disease occurs unilaterally in boys younger than 18 years of age. The most common age at diagnosis is between 8 and 10 years. Peripheral retinal vessel telangiectasia and aneurysmal dilation lead to extensive areas of exudation, giving the retina a yellowish-white appearance, which may produce leukocoria (Fig. 19-91). The macula is a common site for exudate to collect, and when this is present, visual loss is profound. Treatment is by cryotherapy or laser photocoagulation of the retina; success depends on the degree of macular damage present.

Retinitis Pigmentosa

Retinitis pigmentosa (RP) is a pigmentary retinopathy characterized by visual field loss, night blindness, and a depressed or extinct electroretinogram. Symptoms of visual loss may be present in childhood but usually do not become apparent until the second or third decade of life. Poor night vision is the earliest symptom, followed by progressive loss of peripheral visual field and, finally, loss of central vision. Many different

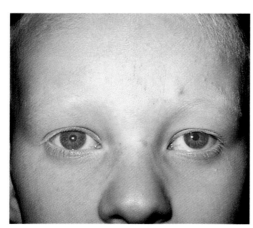

Figure 19-89 Albinism, characterized by white hair, pale skin, and translucent irides.

Figure 19-91 Coats disease. Peripheral telangiectasia along the course of the retinal vasculature leads to exudation, giving the retina a yellowish-white appearance. If the exudate extends to the posterior retina leukocoria may be present.

Figure 19-92 **A,** Retinitis pigmentosa, characterized by retinal pigment deposition, narrow arterioles, and a pale disc. **B,** Early fundus signs of retinitis pigmentosa. The optic disc has a waxy pallor, and the retinal arterial system is sclerotic. In children, pigmentary changes may not be as advanced or as noticeable as in adults.

diseases are characterized by pigmentary retinopathy, and the presentation, progression, and extent of visual loss vary widely. In general, disease within pedigrees has similar clinical characteristics. Unfortunately, treatment for the overwhelming majority of patients is not available at this time. Gene testing for some variations of RP is now available.

The retinal pigment epithelial changes include deposition of pigment in a perivascular pattern. Pigment deposition in the midperipheral retina gives a characteristic "bone spicule" pattern late in the course of the disease (Fig. 19-92, *A*). Early in the disease, the optic nerve may have a waxy pallor and the retinal arteries may be attenuated (Fig. 19-92, *B*).

Systemic disease entities are associated with RP. Patients with sensorineural hearing loss should be examined for the associated presence of retinitis pigmentosa (Usher syndrome and Hallgren syndrome). Renal diseases including Fanconi syndrome, cystinuria, cystinosis, and oxalosis may be associated with pigmentary retinal changes, as may the mucopolysaccharidoses, Refsum disease, and syphilis.

Retinal Detachment

Trauma is the most common cause of retinal detachment in children. Leukocoria occurs when the detached retina is in apposition to the lens or when significant scarring (proliferative vitreoretinopathy) is present. Retinal detachments, if large and located posteriorly, may be viewed with the direct ophthalmoscope as elevations of the retina (Fig. 19-93). The detached retina may move or undulate with eye movement.

Symptoms of retinal detachment, which all patients with a history of blunt trauma to the eye should be advised of, include photopsias (flashing lights); floaters (caused by vitreous hemorrhage); and changes in vision, including blurring of vision or the sensation of a veil or curtain obscuring part of their vision.

Retinopathy of Prematurity

Retinopathy of prematurity (ROP) is characterized by abnormalities in the developing retinal vascular system. Mild forms affect the peripheral retina at the junction between the vascularized and immature avascular retina. These changes can be observed only with an indirect ophthalmoscope and scleral depression. Severe forms produce fibrovascular proliferations that extend into the vitreous (stage 3 disease), which may lead to traction resulting in poor macular development (temporal macular drag) or detachment of the retina (stages 4 and 5 disease) (Fig. 19-94). A white fibrovascular mass may occupy

Figure 19-93 Retinal detachment. The inferior retina is detached, and a demarcation line between the attached and detached retina is visible. Fluid beneath the detached sensory retina shifts with movement of the eye and causes the detached retina to move or undulate with movement of the eye.

Temporal tugging of the retinal vessels

Normal retina

Figure 19-94 Retrolental fibroplasia with temporal drag of the disc.

the retrolental space (retrolental fibroplasia) and produce leukocoria.

In 75% of patients, ROP is bilateral and symmetrical. The majority of patients have only mild forms of the disease (stages 1 and 2 disease), and these patients do not have significant visual sequelae. Advanced ROP primarily affects the ill, premature infant whose birth weight is less than 1250 g. Treatment by laser photocoagulation, and most recently by intravitreal injection of vascular endothelial growth factor (VEGF) inhibitors, to reduce the progression of the disease and the risk of visual loss, is indicated when advanced disease is present, and programs to screen neonates at risk for developing this condition are necessary. All low-birth-weight infants, regardless of the development of ROP, are at higher risk than the general population for strabismus, amblyopia, and refractive errors and should have comprehensive examinations at about 1 year of age.

Retinitis and Retinochoroiditis

Inflammation of the retina and choroid is most commonly the result of viral, protozoal, fungal, or bacterial infection. The final common pathway for recovery or resolution of retinal inflammation is the production of a pigmented chorioretinal scar. The characteristics and location of these scars are frequently, but not always, suggestive of a diagnosis. In many cases, however, isolated chorioretinal scars do not suggest any particular disease and they are frequently of no visual significance.

A rare cause of retinochoroiditis is sympathetic ophthalmia. Sympathetic ophthalmia occurs after a severe injury of one eye, the "exciting" eye, followed by a latent period and the development of uveitis in the uninjured eye, the "sympathizing" eye. Sympathetic ophthalmia may occur as early as 10 days after the original injury but may also have a delayed onset years after the incident. Sympathetic ophthalmia is an autoimmune disorder, and treatment is by immunosuppression, both topically and systemically produced.

TORCH Infection

Toxoplasmosis

Toxoplasmosis, a protozoal infection, causes disease in several forms, depending on whether the infection is congenital (and when it is acquired during pregnancy) or acquired. Infants congenitally infected may have widespread involvement resulting in fetal death if maternal infection occurs in the first or early in the second trimester. If infection occurs in the third trimester effects may include chorioretinitis and encephalomyelitis, but the pregnancy will likely be viable. Of neonates severely affected by toxoplasmosis, 80% have retinochoroiditis. Congenital disease may also occur in inactive and recurrent forms, the effects of which may be limited to retinitis alone. Toxoplasmosis may also be acquired, the incidence worldwide being extremely high with increasing age. Ocular involvement includes papillitis, retinitis, and iritis and is usually bilateral. The retinal lesions are frequently asymptomatic and are found incidentally as inactive pigmented chorioretinal scars.

Inactive lesions may reactivate at any time throughout life, with active inflammation developing adjacent to areas of scarring. This is seen as a white fluffy response that may extend into the vitreous overlying the lesion (Fig. 19-95). Patients with lesions close to the macula or optic nerve should be wary of any visual changes and patients, especially those too young to report visual changes, should be screened for reactivation of their disease.

Figure 19-95 Toxoplasmosis. Acute, recurrent, chorioretinal inflammation may occur adjacent to pigmented scars.

Rubella

Exposure to rubella virus during the first trimester of pregnancy results in an intrauterine infection manifested as congenital rubella syndrome. Ocular findings include microphthalmia, microcornea, corneal opacification, anterior uveitis, iris hypoplasia, nuclear or complete cataracts, and glaucoma. The retinopathy of rubella syndrome is a diffuse "salt and pepper" retinopathy that develops early in childhood and does not affect vision. The pigmentary changes may be similar in appearance to those of syphilis, retinitis pigmentosa, and Leber congenital amaurosis (Fig. 19-96).

Cytomegalovirus

Cytomegalovirus (CMV) infection produces a bilateral retinochoroiditis manifested as multiple, yellowish-white, fluffy retinal lesions (Fig. 19-97). Hemorrhage is a prominent feature. Other ophthalmic manifestations include microphthalmia, uveitis, cataracts, optic disc atrophy, strabismus, and nystagmus.

Figure 19-96 Pigmentary retinopathy in rubella syndrome.

Figure 19-97 Cytomegalovirus (CMV). Retinitis, with hemorrhages and perivascular yellowish-white exudates secondary to cytomegalic inclusion disease.

Figure 19-98 Toxocariasis. The retinal lesion appears as a white elevated mass with surrounding pigmented scar formation.

CMV retinitis may be an opportunistic infection occurring in patients who are immunosuppressed because of immunodeficiency disorders or who are receiving immunosuppressive drugs. Retinal inflammation, edema, and hemorrhage may be extensive and rapidly progressive in these patients.

Herpes Simplex Virus

Herpes simplex virus infection may involve the anterior segment of the eye, with conjunctivitis, keratitis, and iritis or, especially when disseminated in the perinatal period, a retinochoroiditis may develop. Retinal involvement with disseminated herpes simplex virus is severe, with extensive inflammatory reaction producing yellowish-white exudates and retinal necrosis. Ocular involvement occurs in roughly 13% of herpetic infections in newborns. Herpetic retinitis may occur in normal individuals but is more common in the immunosuppressed.

Syphilis

Congenital syphilis may cause bilateral chorioretinitis, resulting in a salt-and-pepper fundus appearance. Differentiation of the retinopathy of congenital syphilis from retinitis pigmentosa may be difficult. Syphilis may also cause interstitial keratitis, anterior uveitis, glaucoma, and optic nerve atrophy.

Toxocariasis

Toxocara canis larvae infect children from 2 to 9 years of age. When the eye is involved, a white, elevated chorioretinal granuloma develops (Fig. 19-98). Chronic unilateral uveitis with opacification of the vitreous overlying the granuloma may occur. Inflammation in ocular toxocariasis occurs only after the infecting organism dies. Externally, the eye does not appear to be inflamed. With extensive inflammation, fibrotic preretinal membranes may develop and produce retinal detachment. Differentiation from retinoblastoma may be difficult. Calcification of the lesion is rare in toxocariasis as opposed to retinoblastoma. The diagnosis is confirmed by enzyme-linked immunosorbent assay for *T. canis* on blood or intraocular fluid.

Bacterial Endocarditis

Cotton-wool spots frequently develop in patients with bacterial endocarditis and septic emboli. These represent infarction of the nerve fiber layer of the retina and appear as white, irregular lesions with indistinct borders. Cotton-wool spots may be seen in any condition that produces retinal ischemia,

such as hypertension and diabetes, or in patients with acquired immunodeficiency syndrome. Intraretinal hemorrhages occur with septic emboli and are flame shaped or dot-blot in nature. If the hemorrhage has a white center from the accumulation of leukocytes, the term *Roth spot* is used. Roth spots are not specific for bacterial endocarditis. They may occur in leukemia or shaken baby syndrome (Fig. 19-99). Conjunctival petechiae may be present as a sign of septic emboli.

Emboli to the eye may cause a central or branch retinal artery obstruction. Occlusion of the central retinal artery causes a sudden profound loss in vision, loss of the pupillary direct light reflex, absence of venous pulsations, and the development of a cherry-red spot in the fovea. Edema and opacification of the ganglion cell layer surrounding the fovea make the fovea stand out as red to produce this sign (Fig. 19-100). Treatment must be provided virtually immediately with the episode; treatment at later times is of limited effectiveness.

Leukemia

Patients with acute lymphoblastic, myelogenous, or monocytic leukemia may develop flame-shaped intraretinal hemorrhages. These are usually extensive and visible with the direct

Figure 19-99 Shaken baby syndrome. Multiple retinal hemorrhages are present in the posterior fundus. There are small flame-shaped hemorrhages within the nerve fiber layer that follow the pattern of the retinal vessels. More extensive areas of hemorrhage have broken through to the preretinal space and are seen as areas of blood that obscure the retina. A Roth spot, that is, a hemorrhage with a white center, is visible just above the optic disc. The white reflection from the camera flash is visible because of dispersed red blood cells within the vitreous.

Figure 19-100 Central retinal artery occlusion. A cherry-red spot is visible in the fovea. This sign is due to edema and opacification of the ganglion cell layer of the retina surrounding the fovea.

ophthalmoscope. The presence of hemorrhage is not correlated with anemia or thrombocytopenia. Leukemic infiltration may also occur in the retina as a perivascular infiltrate in the choroid or in the optic disc, producing disc swelling and a papilledema-like appearance. Leukemic involvement of the orbit may be difficult to distinguish from bacterial orbital cellulitis.

Diabetes

The most common ocular finding in young diabetic patients is transient lenticular myopia. This occurs in patients who have had a rapid rise in blood glucose level. Sorbitol accumulates within the lens as a metabolic product. This increases the lens osmolarity and causes the lens to swell, producing myopia. After the blood sugar level returns to normal, myopia may continue to persist for several days or even weeks, with gradual spontaneous resolution. Children with diabetes may rarely develop cataracts.

The earliest sign of background diabetic retinopathy is the presence of microaneurysms (tiny discrete red spots). Small retinal hemorrhages, cotton-wool spots, venous dilation, and hard exudates (small, discrete, yellow lesions) may also be seen. The occurrence of background diabetic retinopathy is related to the duration and control of the diabetes. Young children appear to have a protective effect from diabetic retinopathy, and changes are seldom diagnosed until years after puberty; however, yearly screening examinations are recommended for juvenile diabetics. Proliferative diabetic

retinopathy seen in adults essentially does not occur until after puberty.

Sickle Cell Retinopathy

The ocular abnormalities of the sickle hemoglobinopathies are caused by intravascular sickling, hemostasis, and thrombosis. Retinal findings occur in the peripheral fundus and cannot be visualized with a direct ophthalmoscope, necessitating screening and detection by an ophthalmologist. Retinal vascular complications occur most frequently in patients with hemoglobin (Hgb) SC disease and S–thalassemia disease. Patients with sickle cell disease (Hgb SS) are less frequently affected, their decreased hematocrit providing protection to the retinal vasculature. Rarely, patients with the milder hemoglobinopathies, AS and AC, may have retinal findings.

Retinal findings may be divided into nonproliferative and proliferative changes. Proliferative changes include arteriolar occlusions that lead to arteriovenous anastomosis, causing areas of retinal nonperfusion. Neovascularization occurs at the edge of these areas of nonperfusion, in the form of a gossamer vascular network (a sea fan), and often leads to vitreous hemorrhage, traction, and retinal detachment (Fig. 19-101, A). The disease process is similar to that seen in retinopathy of prematurity. Proliferative changes of sickle retinopathy should be treated by laser photocoagulation.

Nonproliferative changes include refractile or iridescent deposits, black sunburst lesions, and salmon patch hemorrhages. Refractile deposits are sequelae of old reabsorbed hemorrhages. Sunburst lesions are areas of perivascular retinal pigment epithelial hypertrophy and pigment migration (Fig. 19-101, B). Salmon patch lesions represent areas of intraretinal hemorrhage. Parafoveal capillaries and arterioles may become occluded and produce decreased visual acuity in sickle cell retinopathy. Segmentation of the conjunctival blood vessels produces comma-shaped capillaries ("comma sign").

Permanent vision loss from sickle cell retinopathy is rare in the pediatric age group.

Metabolic Diseases

The mucopolysaccharidoses are syndromes caused by inherited defects in the lysosomal enzymes that degrade acid mucopolysaccharide. All of the mucopolysaccharidoses are transmitted as autosomal recessive traits except type II (Hunter), which is X-linked recessive. A common ocular finding is retinal pigmentary degeneration, which closely resembles retinitis pigmentosa. Optic atrophy also occurs, as does corneal clouding resulting from stromal infiltration.

The sphingolipidoses are caused by a deficiency of the lysosomal enzymes responsible for the degeneration of sphingolipids. Tay-Sachs disease (GM_2 type I gangliosidosis) and

Figure 19-101 Sickle cell retinopathy. **A,** Neovascularization or growth of fragile blood vessels into the vitreous in the midperipheral retina. The white fibrous tissue present is due to the proliferation of fibroglial elements. This produces traction on the retina, which may subsequently lead to retinal detachment. **B,** The black sunburst lesions are areas of perivascular retinal pigment epithelial hypertrophy with pigment migration. This finding is an example of nonproliferative change.

Figure 19-102   Tay-Sachs disease. Because the parafoveal area has many retinal ganglion cells and the fovea has none, the fovea retains its oranges-red color but is surrounded by retina that is whitish in color. This produces the cherry-red spot in the macula.

Figure 19-103   Leukocoria. The patient's left eye has a white pupillary reflex produced by reflection of light from a retinoblastoma. Leukocoria is the most common presenting sign (60%) of retinoblastoma.

Niemann-Pick disease are the two most common sphingolipidoses. Sphingolipids accumulate in the retinal ganglion cells, giving a whitish appearance to the retina. Because the parafoveal area has many retinal ganglion cells and the fovea none, the fovea has its normal oranges-red color, whereas the retina peripheral to the fovea is white. This produces a "cherry-red spot" in the macula (Fig. 19-102).

The mucolipidoses are caused by abnormal glycoprotein metabolism. Mucolipidoses have clinical findings of some of the sphingolipidoses and some of the mucopolysaccharidoses. The ocular findings include corneal epithelial edema, retinal pigmentary degeneration, macular cherry-red spots, and optic atrophy.

Cystinosis, caused by a defective transport mechanism for cystine within the lysosomes, leads to intralysosomal accumulation of cystine. Only patients with the nephritic type of cystinosis develop retinal changes, which include salt-and-pepper changes of the retinal pigment epithelium and areas of patchy depigmentation with irregularly distributed pigment clumps. These changes do not produce loss of vision. Photophobia is due to the accumulation of corneal crystals, which may occur in all types of cystinosis and may be extreme, producing a functional blindness. Treatment of the corneal crystallization with topical cysteamine drops is effective if used on a frequent and long-term basis. The cystine crystals redevelop if the drops are discontinued.

Retinoblastoma

Retinoblastoma is the most common intraocular malignancy of childhood. It occurs with a frequency of between 1 in 14,000 and 1 in 20,000 births. The most common age of diagnosis is between 1 and 1½ years, with 90% of cases presenting before 3 years of age. The most common presenting signs of retinoblastoma are leukocoria (60%) and strabismus (22%) (Fig. 19-103). One third of cases are bilateral. The tumor may present as an elevated, round, white, or yellow mass (Fig. 19-104). Retinoblastoma may be multicentric, with several tumor masses arising within the same eye. Seeding into the vitreous may occur, producing a cloudy vitreous. A frequent feature of retinoblastoma is the presence of calcification within the mass.

Great advances have occurred in the understanding of the genetics of retinoblastoma. Retinoblastoma may be transmitted in an autosomal dominant inheritance pattern. Of patients with the disease, 60% have a family history of retinoblastoma. Penetrance is high (60% to 90%) but incomplete. Sporadic cases occur as either somatic mutations in 75% of patients or germinal mutations that may be passed on to the

offspring of affected patients. These sporadic cases are usually unilateral, and the hereditary forms are usually bilateral; however, a patient with a unilateral tumor may have heritable disease. The gene for retinoblastoma has been identified, and it is possible to determine which patients with unilateral tumors have the hereditary form of the disease and which patients do not. Patients who have the heritable form of the disease, with the deletion of the retinoblastoma gene, may develop tumors of the pineal gland (trilateral retinoblastoma) and have a markedly increased risk of secondary tumors (osteogenic sarcoma).

Untreated, retinoblastoma is virtually 100% fatal. The treatment of retinoblastoma is advancing rapidly, and many eyes, even those with extensive tumor that were previously enucleated, may be saved by combinations of local treatment (laser, thermal, and plaque radiation) and chemotherapy.

Optic Nerve

The optic nerve relays information from each eye to the brain. Its function is assessed by measuring visual acuity, visual fields, color vision, and the pupillary response. Visualization and assessment of the morphology of the optic disc with a direct ophthalmoscope can provide valuable information regarding the function of the nerve.

Color Vision

Change in color vision, particularly the ability to perceive red, is an early feature seen in disorders that compromise the function of the optic nerve. Patients may complain of subjective changes in color perception, or they may demonstrate defects in color vision on objective tests.

Figure 19-104   Retinoblastoma. The tumor mass of retinoblastoma is usually elevated and yellow or white in color. Dilated feeding vessels of the tumor may be visible. Seeding into the vitreous from the tumor may produce a cloudy vitreous.

An easy test to assess color vision is to compare color perception between the two eyes. The patient is asked to look at a red object first with one eye, then with the other, and is asked whether it is more red with one eye or the other. A subjective desaturation of red in one eye is an indication of dyschromatopsia and a potential optic nerve disorder. If the patient reports that the object is only 50% as red with one eye compared with the other, the results would be recorded as a red desaturation of 50%. In children it is valuable to present the object to the "normal eye" first with the question "If this is $1 of red, how much red is it now?" and offering a comparison with the fellow eye. A similar comparison may be performed for brightness by shining a light first into one eye and then into the other. The sense of brightness is also decreased in the presence of optic nerve disease. Formal assessment of color vision is performed using color plates such as the Hardy-Rand-Rittler or Ishihara color plates. Patients with heritable congenital color vision defects are equally affected in both eyes. Patients with asymmetrical optic nerve disease (optic neuritis, tumor, toxic optic neuropathy) have asymmetrically decreased color vision, especially for the red hues.

Pupils

Assessment of the pupils for size, shape, position, and reactivity is an important part of the neurologic and ophthalmic evaluation. Neurologic abnormalities that affect the pupil include defects of the afferent pathway (the optic nerve and visual system), the parasympathetic pathway (for pupillary constriction), and the sympathetic pathway (for pupillary dilation).

Afferent Pupillary Defects

In a normal patient, shining a penlight into one eye causes both pupils to constrict. Pupillary constriction in the illuminated eye is the direct response, and the constriction in the fellow eye is the consensual response. The pupils are normally equal in size even if one eye is blind; each eye receives equal pupillary innervation.

The swinging flashlight test is used to assess optic nerve function (Fig. 19-105). If the optic nerve function is decreased on one side an afferent pupillary defect (APD) is present. Another term for this is *Marcus Gunn pupil*. A penlight is used to illuminate one eye and then the other. If both eyes have equal afferent input, then illumination of either eye should produce equal constriction of the pupils. Normally, after shining a light into one eye, the response is initial constriction of both pupils followed by a small dilation (release). The light is then swung quickly to the fellow eye; a small release may be seen as the light crosses between the eyes and then both pupils should constrict to the same degree as previously seen. When there is a decrease in afferent input (nerve function) on one side (e.g., a monocular optic neuritis), both pupils do not constrict as much when the light is shown into the affected eye compared with the other eye (i.e., both eyes display a relative dilation compared with their size when the normal side was illuminated). The critical observation is that when the affected eye is illuminated, a gradual dilation of the pupils occurs as compared with the response when the normal eye is illuminated. Having the patient maintain fixation on a distant object is important because accommodation causes constriction of the pupils and may lead to misinterpretation of the findings. This test is applicable even if one iris and pupil are of abnormal size or shape or nonreactive (e.g., after intraocular surgery, trauma, or synechiae from uveitis). The normal pupil is observed when the light is shown into either eye, and if there is a greater constriction of it when the light is shown into one side compared with the other, an APD is present.

MARCUS GUNN PUPIL

To perform test:
Shine a bright light into each pupil for about 3–4 seconds. Alternate back and forth. Look for pupil to dilate, instead of constrict, with light.

Left eye has decreased vision due to retinal lesion or optic nerve lesion.

VA OD 20/20   VA 20/400

Both pupils constrict equally because of consensual response.

Both pupils dilate on illumination of eye with afferent defect.

Figure 19-105   Swinging flashlight test.

An APD indicates disease affecting the optic nerve or retina. Unilateral or bilaterally asymmetrical optic nerve disease always causes a relative APD. Mild optic nerve disease with minimal or no objectively measurable decrease in visual acuity still produces an APD, whereas a retinal defect must severely affect the macula or large areas of the retina to produce an APD. Afferent pupillary defects are not seen with dense cataracts, refractive errors, cortical lesions, or functional visual loss. Dense amblyopia may produce a subtle APD.

Anisocoria

Lesions of the parasympathetic or sympathetic system, if unilateral or asymmetrical, cause pupillary constriction or dilation and produce pupils that are unequal in size, termed *anisocoria*. Pupillary involvement in third nerve palsy is usually accompanied by ptosis and disturbances in ocular motility. In cases of brainstem herniation and basilar meningitis, however, pupillary dilation may be the only sign of third nerve palsy. Pharmacologic mydriasis may occur with minimal exposure to atropine, cyclopentolate, or other parasympatholytic agents (e.g., accidental exposure to some pesticides). Pharmacologic testing with 1% pilocarpine is useful for differentiating pharmacologic mydriasis from third cranial nerve palsy; pupillary constriction occurs in third nerve palsy and does not occur with pharmacologic mydriasis. Pharmacologic miosis occurs with echothiophate iodide or pilocarpine.

A lesion at any point along the sympathetic pathway for pupillary constriction results in Horner syndrome. The classic triad of findings includes ptosis, miosis, and anhidrosis on the affected side. The anisocoria of Horner syndrome is more apparent in dim illumination, and the affected pupil shows a lag in dilation on dimming of the lights. The light and near pupillary reactions are intact. The anisocoria of Horner syndrome is best examined with the patient fixating on a distance object and observing both pupils as a bright light is alternately turned on and off. With the light on, both pupils will be miotic and some anisocoria may be observed. Immediately on dimming of the light in Horner syndrome one pupil will dilate more slowly than the other and the magnitude of the anisocoria will be observed to increase (dilation lag). As the light remains dimmed the magnitude of the anisocoria may decrease but it will still be greater than that observed when the light was bright. A ruler or pupil gauge with circles or half circles or different diameters is useful as a reference to accurately determine the pupil sizes. Paresis of Müller muscle of the lid leads to the mild upper lid ptosis seen in Horner syndrome. The lower eyelid on the affected side may rest 1 mm higher than the fellow lid (upside-down ptosis), and the narrowed palpebral fissure gives the appearance of enophthalmos (see Fig. 19-72). Anhidrosis of the ipsilateral side of the body, side of the face, or forehead may be present, depending on the site of the innervation defect. Anhidrosis of the forehead may be assessed by lightly rubbing a smooth plastic ruler across the forehead skin. If the ruler moves smoothly, anhidrosis is present because small amounts of perspiration will cause the ruler to stick and have a jerking motion. A characteristic of congenital Horner syndrome is the development in later childhood or adolescence of iris heterochromia, with the affected iris being lighter in color.

The sympathetic pathway for pupillary constriction involves three neurons. The location of first-order neuron lesions is in the brainstem and spinal cord, examples being cervical trauma or demyelinating disease. Preganglionic or second-order neuron lesions occur within the chest or neck (e.g., neuroblastoma arising in the sympathetic chain). Congenital Horner syndrome, which is most often idiopathic but sometimes produced by birth trauma to the brachial plexus, may also cause a second-order neuron lesion. Third-order neuron lesions, postganglionic in reference to the superior cervical ganglion, are usually benign; however, extracranial or intracranial tumors of the nasopharynx or cavernous sinus may produce such lesions. More common causes for a postganglionic Horner syndrome are migraine variants such as cluster headache. Pharmacologic testing with hydroxyamphetamine drops can differentiate a third-order lesion from a first- or second-order lesion. With a third-order lesion the pupil does not dilate because the nerve's norepinephrine stores are depleted. With a first- or second-order lesion the nerve's norepinephrine stores are normal and pupillary dilation occurs with instillation of the drops. Unfortunately, hydroxyamphetamine eyedrops are not readily available. With causes for Horner syndrome ranging from benign idiopathic lesions and migraine to life-threatening malignancy, patients with newly diagnosed Horner syndrome without convincing histories suggesting benign etiologies require evaluation with imaging of the head, neck, abdomen, and thorax.

Physiologic Anisocoria

Approximately 10% to 20% of the population has a perceptible anisocoria without any abnormal pathologic condition. The degree of anisocoria may vary from day to day, but usually the difference in pupil size is 1 mm or less. Physiologic anisocoria may be congenital or acquired and it may be permanent or resolve. The hallmark of physiologic anisocoria is that the magnitude of anisocoria remains the same in bright and dim illumination; however, in some cases the anisocoria may be slightly more apparent in dim light than in bright light, thereby simulating Horner syndrome. Differentiating physiologic anisocoria from Horner syndrome may be difficult, especially in a moving infant. In physiologic anisocoria, dilation lag is not observed. Pupils with physiologic anisocoria dilate after the instillation of 4% cocaine drops, whereas a Horner pupil fails to dilate. Apraclonidine 0.5% causes a reversal of

the anisocoria in Horner syndrome, but it cannot be used in infants, in whom differentiation of physiologic anisocoria from Horner syndrome is most often necessary, as extreme lethargy and unresponsiveness may occur in infants with apraclonidine use.

Adie Tonic Pupil

A lesion of the postganglionic parasympathetic innervation of the pupil, most commonly due to viral infection, causes Adie tonic pupil. Initially the pupil will be dilated and the anisocoria is greater in bright illumination. The response of the pupil to light is sluggish, with segments of the iris constricting slowly. Miosis with near fixation is normal initially but later also becomes tonic with slow constriction and slow redilation. Denervation hypersensitivity is present and the diagnostic test for Adie pupil is instillation of dilute 0.125% pilocarpine, which causes papillary constriction. Adult females are more commonly affected, but varicella is a cause in children.

Optic Neuritis

Inflammation of the optic nerve may occur either as a papillitis, referring to the intraocular form in which optic disc swelling is present, or as a retrobulbar neuritis, in which the optic disc appears normal and inflammation of the optic nerve occurs posterior to the globe. Vision loss may be sudden, progressive, profound, and accompanied by complaints of pain in or behind the eye, which may be accentuated by movement of the eyes. An afferent pupillary defect is present if the condition is unilateral or if it is bilateral and asymmetrical. Visual fields usually show a cecocentral scotoma, an area of vision loss located in the central visual field.

The optic disc, if affected, may show swelling of the peripapillary nerve fiber layer and elevation. Small vessels at the optic disc margin may hemorrhage or become obscured by edema. The appearance in bilateral disease may be impossible to differentiate from the optic disc swelling present with increased intracranial pressure.

Optic neuritis in children is frequently bilateral and may be idiopathic or follow nonspecific viral prodromes or infection with mumps, measles, chickenpox, or meningoencephalitis. Collagen vascular disease, particularly systemic lupus erythematosus and sarcoidosis, may be associated with optic neuritis. Syphilis and tuberculosis also cause optic neuritis. Visual acuity in idiopathic optic neuritis gradually improves 1 to 4 weeks after onset and usually returns to normal over several months. Episodes may be recurrent. Associations with demyelinating disease occur but less frequently than in adults.

Papilledema

Increased intracranial pressure (ICP) is transmitted to the optic nerves via the cerebrospinal fluid within the subarachnoid space and causes papilledema. The axoplasmic flow from the retinal ganglion cells to the cells in the lateral geniculate nucleus is blocked and causes the optic disc to swell. The degree of disc swelling may be asymmetrical; however, increased intracranial pressure rarely causes papilledema in only one eye. Ophthalmoscopic signs include blurring of the disc margin and disc edema. The disc may be hyperemic because of telangiectasia of the superficial capillaries on the disc, and small hemorrhages may appear on the disc margin (Fig. 19-106). Visual acuity is normal unless hemorrhage and edema involve the macula. Patients may complain of transient obscurations of vision. The visual fields may show an enlarged blind spot, and the pupillary response and color vision are normal.

If increased intracranial pressure is chronic, elevation of the optic disc may persist but the hemorrhages and exudates seen in the acute phase resolve. When the condition is prolonged,

Figure 19-106   Acute papilledema. The disc edges are blurred, and the physiologic cup may be obscured due to the disc swelling and edema of the adjacent nerve fiber layer. Intraretinal hemorrhages and exudates may be present.

Figure 19-107   Optic atrophy. The optic disc is flat, pale, and yellowish-white in color.

optic nerve atrophy and vision loss occur. If intracranial pressure is normalized, it may take 6 weeks for papilledema to resolve and the optic disc to normalize. Patients may have elevated intracranial pressure without developing papilledema, and thus the absence of papilledema does not rule out increased ICP.

Pseudopapilledema

Pseudopapilledema occurs as an anomaly of the optic disc and in eyes with high hyperopia or optic disc drusen (see Fig. 19-9). The disc is not hyperemic, the vessels at the disc margin remain visible, and there is no nerve fiber layer swelling. There may be anomalous branching and tortuosity of the retinal vessels, and the physiologic cup is usually absent. The disc borders may be irregular. Hemorrhages, exudate, cotton-wool spots, and venous congestion do not occur. Spontaneous venous pulsations are an indication that the disc swelling is pseudopapilledema and not caused by increased intracranial pressure; however, they are not present in 20% of the normal population, and therefore their absence does not indicate that the disc swelling is necessarily true papilledema. Central visual acuity is normal.

Optic Disc Atrophy

Optic nerve atrophy is present if the optic disc does not have its typical reddish-orange color. Initially the disc becomes more yellow in color, gradually developing more pallor. The lamina cribrosa may become visible with enlargement of the optic cup, leaving a "pinholed" appearance (Fig. 19-107). As the disease process continues, the disc eventually becomes more pale and eventually white in color, visual acuity decreases, and visual field defects emerge. If the optic atrophy is markedly advanced and the disc is very pale and accompanied by a sluggish papillary response then poor visual acuity may be easily predicted, but if the atrophy is mild accurate prediction of the visual acuity is difficult.

Optic atrophy may occur as a sequela of papilledema, optic neuritis, compressive lesions of the optic nerve or chiasm, tumors of the optic nerve (most commonly glioma in association with neurofibromatosis), trauma, hereditary retinal disease, or glaucoma. Optic atrophy may also be inherited as a recessive or dominant trait. Atrophy may occur as a component of a generalized neurologic condition, such as Behr optic atrophy with cerebellar ataxia, hypotonia, and mental retardation. Leber optic neuropathy occurs in late adolescence or early adulthood, with acute disc edema being rapidly followed by progressive bilateral optic atrophy.

Developmental Anomalies of the Optic Nerve

Developmental anomalies of the optic nerve include colobomas, tilted discs, and optic nerve hypoplasia (see Figs. 19-9, 19-10, and 19-85). The level of visual acuity is related to the type and extent of the defect. Although profound abnormalities certainly have a significant effect on visual acuity, it is difficult to estimate the effect that more minor anomalies, especially optic nerve hypoplasia, may have on vision.

Hypoplasia of the optic nerve occurs either unilaterally or bilaterally. The optic disc is smaller than normal and commonly a surrounding, partial or complete, yellowish-white ring that corresponds to the scleral opening for a normal-sized optic nerve is visible. The term *double ring sign* is used to describe the ring with its surrounding pigment crescent. The retinal vessels are normal in size but may appear crowded as they leave the optic disc (Fig. 19-108). The pattern of vessel branching is typically abnormal. Visual acuity is related to the degree of hypoplasia, and an afferent pupillary defect may be present if the degree of involvement is asymmetrical. Optic nerve hypoplasia is associated with midline central nervous system abnormalities including absence of the septum pellucidum (de Morsier syndrome). Children with optic nerve hypoplasia should be examined for abnormalities in pituitary and hypothalamic function. Optic disc hypoplasia is frequently seen in patients with fetal alcohol syndrome (FAS) (48%). Increased tortuosity of the retinal vasculature may also exist in patients with FAS.

Orbit

Clinical signs of orbital disease are proptosis, restriction in ocular motility, compression of the optic nerve producing optic disc swelling, changes in refraction, and retinal striae. Retinal striae appear as radial lines on the retinal surface and are caused by compression of the posterior portion of the globe.

Orbital disease or trauma may cause orbital asymmetry with displacement of the globe (Fig. 19-109). Posterior (enophthalmos) or anterior (exophthalmos) displacement of the globe in orbital disease may be subtle. Comparison of the position of the globes in relation to the lateral orbital rims, looking for asymmetry, is a valuable clinical test, with subtle differences most easily visualized by viewing the patient from above. The Hertel exophthalmometer is an instrument used to compare the position of the globes in relation to the lateral orbital rim (Fig. 19-110). Palpation of the globes over closed eyelids, gently retropulsing the globe into the orbit, may reveal

Figure 19-108 **A,** Optic disc coloboma. Disc is excavated and has potential for only poor visual acuity. **B,** Optic nerve hypoplasia. A pigment crescent surrounds the hypoplastic nerve. This corresponds to the scleral opening for a normal-sized optic nerve and is termed the *double ring sign* in this patient with ocular albinism. The pattern of the retinal vasculature is also abnormal, as is the retinal pigmentation. **C,** Optic disc hypoplasia. The disc is small with abnormal features. The surrounding larger ring around the disc corresponds to the normal-sized sclera opening for the disc.

the character of an orbital mass and is helpful in assessing proptosis caused by orbital cellulitis. Ocular versions are tested, looking for restrictions in motility. Other adjuncts to the clinical examination include B scan ultrasonography, computed tomography (CT), and magnetic resonance imaging (MRI) of the orbit. Although CT is particularly valuable in the examination of bony lesions and in the assessment of orbital fractures, the radiation exposure with fine-cut orbital CT is significant, and this must be taken into consideration in children.

The most common orbital disease in childhood is infectious cellulitis (see Chapter 23). Capillary hemangioma and lymphangioma are the most common benign primary orbital tumors of childhood. Orbital capillary hemangiomas present shortly after birth, enlarge over the first 6 to 12 months of life, have a period of stability between 1 and 2 years of age, and then begin to regress. Systemic steroids have been the mainstay of treatment, but more recently the use of propranolol has been shown to be very effective. Lymphangiomas may involve the conjunctiva, lids, or orbit. These tumors may rapidly enlarge during upper respiratory tract infections. Sudden enlargement may occur after hemorrhage within the lesion.

Rhabdomyosarcoma is the most common primary orbital malignancy in childhood. This tumor should be a consideration in any child between the ages of 7 and 8 years who has rapidly progressing unilateral proptosis. The tumor mass may be palpable in the upper eyelid area, or it may be located deeper in the orbit.

The most common metastatic lesion to the orbit in childhood is neuroblastoma. This tumor presents with an abrupt onset of proptosis and ecchymosis that may be bilateral (Fig. 19-111). Metastasis in neuroblastoma typically occurs late in the course of the disease, when the primary tumor can easily be detected in the abdomen.

Dermoid and epidermoid cysts are relatively common. These benign masses are usually located anterior to the orbital septum but may extend posteriorly into the orbit. These cysts present as smooth, painless, freely movable round or oval masses and are usually located in the lateral brow area, adjacent to the zygomaticofrontal suture (Fig. 19-112). They may, however, be found near any bony suture. If these lesions can be palpated around their entire extent, no neuroimaging studies may be necessary; however, if they are palpated as extending posterior to the orbital rim, imaging is indicated to exclude extension into the intracranial space or a diagnosis of encephalocele. These cysts contain dermal and epidermal elements that have become isolated from the skin during the course of embryonic development. If ruptured by trauma, an intense inflammatory reaction occurs. Because of this reaction, surgical excision of these lesions is indicated before potential trauma when the child learns to walk.

Optic nerve gliomas are tumors that occur in children younger than 10 years of age. At least one third of children have a history of neurofibromatosis. The presenting sign may be loss of vision or painless proptosis. An afferent pupillary defect and optic atrophy are usually present. Papilledema may also occur. Strabismus may be present because of decreased visual acuity (Fig. 19-113).

Figure 19-109 Blowout fracture of inferior orbital wall with dislocation of the zygoma.

Figure 19-110 The Hertel exophthalmometer measures the anterior-to-posterior distance from the corneal surface to the lateral orbital rim. A base measurement, the distance between the two lateral orbital rims, is recorded to help obtain repeatable instrument placement. Progression or regression can be determined by serial measurements.

Figure 19-111 Neuroblastoma. Neuroblastoma metastatic to the orbit may present with an abrupt onset of unilateral or bilateral proptosis and ecchymosis of the eyelids. Neuroblastoma is the most common lesion to metastasize to the orbit in childhood.

Plexiform neurofibromas are also seen in association with neurofibromatosis. They occur within the orbit or within the upper lid tissue and cause a fullness and ptosis of the lateral portion of the eyelid, leading to an S-shaped upper lid deformity.

Orbital pseudotumor is a unilateral or bilateral orbital inflammatory process affecting the structures within the orbit. Children with pseudotumor have signs of headache, fever, lethargy, orbital pain, proptosis, lid erythema, conjunctival injection, and restricted ocular motility causing diplopia. The extraocular muscles and their tendons may be thickened. Orbital pseudotumor is a benign condition; however, recurrent tumor with scarring and fibrosis may cause restriction of ocular motility. Optic nerve atrophy may occur in extreme cases. Orbital pseudotumor must be differentiated from leukemia. The most common form of leukemia that affects the orbit is acute lymphoblastic leukemia.

OCULAR TRAUMA

In the evaluation of children with orbital or periocular trauma, serious ocular injury must be presumed even if only minimal external signs exist. Presumption of serious injury not only gives the examiner a heightened awareness of the possibilities for serious injury but also signals initiating precautions to protect the eye from further damage. For example, if there is any suspicion that the eye has sustained a penetrating wound by a projectile, a shield must be placed over the eye to prevent any pressure from being placed on the eye to avoid expulsion of intraocular contents. Before any evaluation or manipulation of the patient, an assessment of visual acuity must be performed if possible. This provides information regarding the severity and nature of the trauma and records information that may be of medicolegal importance. If a patient is not able to

Figure 19-113 Optic nerve glioma. Its presence may cause a gradual onset of painless proptosis. Children seldom complain of monocular visual loss, and the discovery of a profound loss of vision may be the presenting sign of an optic nerve glioma. In children, optic nerve gliomas are benign lesions that may, however, extend to the optic chiasm or intracranially.

undergo a formal measurement of visual acuity, the fixation response can be recorded or the patient's ability to count fingers can be recorded. If the patient is able to read but use of an eye chart is impractical in the emergency room setting, the patient's ability to read anything available and the distance that they are able to read from should be recorded. This kind of assessment can be translated to a visual acuity measurement if necessary.

The anatomy of a laceration of the eyelid dictates the measures required for repair. The presence of orbital fat indicates penetration of the septum and entrance into the orbit. In addition, evaluation of the laceration must include the degree of involvement of the lid margin, loss of tissue, injury to the medial and lateral canthal tendons (suggested if there is displacement or deformity of the medial or lateral canthus), and injury to the canaliculi of the nasolacrimal drainage system (Fig. 19-114). Each of these injuries requires a special technique for repair.

Patients who have sustained blunt orbital trauma should be evaluated for a fracture of the orbital floor or the medial wall of the orbit. Signs of injury include enophthalmos, diplopia, restricted gaze, and paresthesias in the distribution of the infraorbital nerve (midface and cheek below the eye). Exophthalmos may occur if there is significant orbital swelling or hemorrhage. Fractures may be isolated to the floor, or they may extend to the orbital rim (Fig. 19-115). The orbital rim should be palpated for discontinuity suggesting fracture and

Figure 19-112 Dermoid cyst. These cysts present as smooth, painless, mobile, subcutaneous, round or oval masses. Dermoid cysts are most frequently located in the lateral brow area adjacent to the zygomaticofrontal suture. Although benign, if they are ruptured by trauma, an intense inflammatory reaction with scarring in the area may occur.

Figure 19-114 Canalicular laceration. This patient experienced a laceration of the upper canaliculus. Simple apposition of the wound edges in this case will not approximate the cut ends of the canaliculus and chronic epiphora will result. Silicone tubes are used to splint the canaliculus during the healing process.

Figure 19-115 Blowout fracture of the right orbit (coronal CT scan). Protruding through the fracture in the orbital floor into the maxillary sinus is orbital fat. The inferior rectus muscle is potentially entrapped within the fracture site.

Figure 19-117 A Desmarres lid retractor may be used to gently open the eyelids of an uncooperative child, or in cases of trauma or preseptal cellulitis in which lid swelling makes opening of the lids for globe examination difficult.

displacement. If subcutaneous air or orbital emphysema is present, the fracture has permitted communication with the sinuses. Intraorbital edema or hemorrhage within the extraocular muscles may also restrict ocular motility. Extraocular muscle entrapment, most frequently the inferior and medial rectus muscles (Fig. 19-116), produces gaze restrictions and diplopia.

Conjunctival lacerations may be accompanied by subconjunctival hemorrhage, which may suggest far more serious injury than that actually present. On the other hand, a small laceration of the conjunctiva may be present in association with a penetrating injury of the sclera and globe. The history and circumstances of the injury must be considered in determining the likelihood of serious injury and the extent of the evaluation necessary because traumatized uncooperative young children may need to be sedated for complete evaluation. If there is extensive subconjunctival hemorrhage and edema and other physical findings and history to suggest a significant possibility for scleral rupture or penetrating injury, surgical exploration of the subconjunctival space may be indicated.

The use of a topical anesthetic such as tetracaine or proparacaine anesthetizes the cornea and conjunctiva and permits a close examination for foreign bodies. A Desmarres lid retractor may help exert gentle pressure to open the lids of uncooperative children or if swelling of the lids makes examination difficult (Fig. 19-117). The lids may also be everted over a cotton swab to inspect the underside of the eyelid (Fig. 19-118). The presence of a foreign body under the upper eyelid causes vertical epithelial abrasions on the underlying corneal surface (Fig. 19-119). Corneal abrasions cause extreme pain, foreign body sensation, and photophobia. The use of sodium fluorescein dye applied to the conjunctival cul-de-sac and examination with a cobalt blue filtered light aid in the detection of a superficial epithelial abrasion. The dye stains areas that are missing epithelium. When possible, examination should be conducted with magnification as provided by a slit lamp or magnifying glass. If the history and examination do not prompt significant concern for a retained foreign body, small corneal abrasions do not necessarily require referral for further evaluation. Such lesions may be treated with topical antibiotic drops or ointment, observing significant improvement in signs and symptoms in 24 hours and complete resolution in 48 hours. Patching of the eye to keep the lid completely closed promotes healing of the epithelium and may make the eye more comfortable. Pain and foreign body sensation will persist until the epithelial abrasions have healed completely.

Blunt trauma to the eye may cause iritis or an anterior uveitis. Patients complain of dull eye pain and light sensitivity. Signs of iritis include miosis of the pupil, tearing, and ciliary injection. With severe blunt trauma, the iris may be avulsed

Figure 19-116 Blowout fracture of the right orbit. The inferior rectus is entrapped in the fracture site, leading to the inability to depress the right eye.

Figure 19-118 The upper eyelid may be easily everted by placing a cotton swab at the upper edge of the tarsal plate, just above the lid crease. The lashes are then gently grasped and pulled anteriorly away from the globe and upward to evert the lid over the cotton swab. The tarsal conjunctiva may be inspected for the presence of a foreign body.

Figure 19-119 Corneal abrasions stained with fluorescein dye and viewed under blue light. The abrasions appear green in the area of corneal epithelial loss where the dye is absorbed.

Figure 19-121 A complication of hyphema is corneal blood staining. This patient's left cornea has an area of brown staining inferiorly because of the prolonged presence of blood, especially when glaucoma or increased intraocular pressure is also present, within the anterior chamber.

from its insertion (iridodialysis) or the iris and ciliary body may be avulsed (cyclodialysis). Tears of the pupillary sphincter may also occur, enlarging the pupil, and are a sign that further evaluation should be conducted. If iritis has been present for a few days or if more severe, synechiae may be present and cause the pupil to be misshapen or poorly reactive to light. Eyes with a history of blunt trauma may have sustained damage to the anterior chamber angle (traumatic angle recession) and glaucoma may develop years after the incident. Periodic screening by intraocular pressure measurement is indicated.

An injury to the globe may cause bleeding from the small vessels of the peripheral portion of the iris or the ciliary body. Blood in the anterior chamber is called a *hyphema*. While the red blood cells are dispersed throughout the aqueous fluid, vision may be dramatically decreased. The blood may remain fluid and shift with changes in head position, or it may clot. Blood, which is heavier than aqueous fluid, usually settles out in the inferior portion of the anterior chamber (Fig. 19-120). Complications of a hyphema include rebleeding, glaucoma, and blood staining of the cornea (Fig. 19-121). Increased intraocular pressure increases the risk of developing blood staining. The opacification of the cornea may resolve over several months. In children, this may cause amblyopia. Hyphemas are serious injuries that require evaluation by an ophthalmologist. The majority of hyphemas resolve over 4 to 5 days with only observation and reduced activity.

Immediate or delayed opacification of the lens, that is, cataract formation, may occur with penetration of the lens capsule or with blunt trauma alone. Blunt trauma may disrupt the lens zonules and dislocate the lens (see Fig. 19-81).

All eyes receiving significant trauma must have an examination of the fundus. Blunt trauma may cause a macular hole or a rupture of the choroid. A choroidal rupture is visualized as a white concentric ring, around the optic disc, where the underlying sclera has become visible (Fig. 19-122). Retinal tears or detachment may follow trauma, and the clinician's index of suspicion should take into account the history of the trauma and the presence of symptoms (photopsia, floaters, and visual changes). Patients with high myopia are at greater risk for retinal detachment after blunt trauma. Retinal tears and detachments after trauma may occur either immediately or in the subsequent weeks after the injury. Patients should be advised of the symptoms of retinal detachment and told to seek immediate ophthalmologic care should they develop.

Trauma may produce retinal hemorrhages that are limited to the retina or that extend into the vitreous. Crushing injury to the chest may raise intrathoracic pressure, with transmission to the retina causing hemorrhages. Purtscher retinopathy includes retinal hemorrhages, cotton-wool spots, retinal edema, and fat emboli. Terson syndrome is the transmission of subarachnoid hemorrhage to the optic nerve and disc, and results in vitreous and retinal hemorrhages. Infants with shaken baby syndrome may have extensive intraretinal hemorrhages accompanying their intracranial injuries, and the severity of intraocular hemorrhage may, but does not always, correlate with the severity of intracranial injury.

In cases of penetrating injury to the eye, the key to examination is to be brief and gentle so as not to complicate the

Figure 19-120 Hyphema. Red blood cells within the anterior chamber have settled into the inferior anterior chamber angle.

Figure 19-122 Blunt trauma to the eye has caused a rupture of the choroid. This is visualized as white concentric rings around the optic disc where, beneath the retina, the choroid has separated, making the underlying sclera visible.

injury by causing expulsion of intraocular contents. Immediately after identifying an ocular injury as penetrating, further examination should be limited and conducted in the operating room under general anesthesia. Topical medications should not be applied to the eye, and the eye should be protected at all times with a shield. Penetrating injuries caused by projectiles or foreign bodies may produce subtle findings. In cases in which the index of suspicion is high, appropriate evaluation may include plain film x-rays or imaging studies including CT or MRI. If the potential intraocular foreign body is metallic, MRI scanning is contraindicated.

Bibliography

American Academy of Pediatrics Committee on Practice and Ambulatory Medicine, Section on Ophthalmology: Eye examination and vision screening in infants, children and young adults, *Pediatrics* 98:153–157, 1996.
Brodsky MC: *Pediatric neuro-ophthalmology*, ed 2, New York, 2010, Springer.
Handler SM, Fierson WM, Section on Ophthalmology; Council on Children with Disabilities; American Academy of Ophthalmology; American Association for Pediatric Ophthalmology and Strabismus; American Association of Certified Orthoptists: Learning disabilities, dyslexia, and vision, *Pediatrics* 127:e818–e856, 2011.
Levin AV, Christian CW: The eye examination in the evaluation of child abuse, *Pediatrics* 126:376–380, 2010.
Levin AV, Wilson TW: *The Hospital for Sick Children's atlas of pediatric ophthalmology and strabismus*, ed 1, Philadelphia, 2007, Lippincott Williams & Wilkins.
Nelson LB, Olitsky SE: *Harley's pediatric ophthalmology*, ed 5, Philadelphia, 2005, Lippincott Williams & Wilkins.
Raab EL, editor: *2010-2011 Basic and clinical science course (BCSC), Section 6: Pediatric ophthalmology and strabismus*, San Francisco, 2010, American Academy of Ophthalmology.
Section on Ophthalmology American Academy of Pediatrics; American Academy of Ophthalmology; American Association for Pediatric Ophthalmology and Strabismus: Screening examination of premature infants for retinopathy of prematurity, *Pediatrics* 117:572–576, 2006.
Tasman W, Jaeger EA, editors: *Duane's clinical ophthalmology*, Philadelphia, 2009, JB Lippincott.
Taylor D, editor: *Pediatric ophthalmology*, ed 2, Boston, 1997, Blackwell Scientific Publications.
Traboulsi EI: *A Compendium of inherited disorders and the eye*, ed 1, New York, 2006, Oxford University Press.
Trobe JD: *The physician's guide to eye care*, ed 3, San Francisco, 2006, American Academy of Ophthalmology.
von Noorden GK, Campos EC: *Binocular vision and ocular motility: Theory and management of strabismus*, ed 6, St. Louis, 2001, Mosby.
Yanoff M, Sassani JW: *Ocular pathology*, ed 6, St. Louis, 2008, Mosby.

ORAL DISORDERS

Brian Martin | Heather Baumhardt | Alene D'Alesio |
Mamoun M. Nazif | David H. McKibben | Holly W. Davis

ASSESSMENT TECHNIQUES

Because oral and oropharyngeal problems and disorders are common and cause a wide variety of symptoms, a thorough oral examination is an essential component of a complete physical examination, enabling the practitioner to make appropriate diagnosis without undue delay.

Key elements of the oral/dental history include the following:

1. Timing of eruption and exfoliation of primary teeth, timing of eruption of permanent teeth, and any problems encountered

2. Brushing and flossing frequency and technique

3. Dietary habits including frequency of bottle-feeding and breast-feeding in infancy; whether infants and toddlers are put to bed with a bottle; time of weaning; frequency of carbohydrate intake; and possible symptoms of eating disorders in adolescence

4. Current source of dental care and frequency of visits

5. Current history of symptoms: oral pain, redness, swelling, drainage, headaches, abdominal pain, decreased appetite (especially for chewy foods)

6. Problems with bite or occlusion

7. History of dental problems and/or orofacial trauma and their treatment

8. Family history of dental problems or disorders

A systematic approach to the examination of a child's dentition is essential and should include assessment of the following:

1. Facial symmetry and balance

2. Lip seal at rest position

3. Occlusion (bite) and tooth alignment

4. Mandibular excursion in lateral, vertical, and anterior/posterior planes

5. Integrity of enamel, presence of caries

6. Appearance of gingivae from both labial-buccal and lingual sides

7. Condition of the other oral soft tissues: tongue, palate, mucobuccal folds, and sublingual spaces

Successful examination requires close visual inspection of the face; palpation of suspected areas of abnormality; and systematic inspection of the dentition, its supporting structures, and the oral soft tissues. This can be challenging with young children, but patience and a gentle, even playful manner can be of great help. At least initially, young children should be allowed to sit on the parent's lap. Toys, puppets, and a rubber glove blown up into a balloon can serve as useful distractions. Drawing a face on a tongue depressor and giving it to the child to hold, as well as letting the child look in the dental mirror, are good ways to introduce these basic instruments and make them less threatening. If an otoscope is being used as a light source in a medical office setting, letting the child "blow out the light" is another good introductory game, as is demonstrating the examination on the parent or examiner. Then the examiner can gradually begin the hands-on assessment. In younger children, a "lap exam" may be a useful way to examine an apprehensive child (Fig. 20-1). The parent places the child in their lap, facing them, and the child's head reclines into the examiner's lap. It is important to have the parent hold the child's hand during the examination. A lap examination is not advised if the mother is pregnant, as the child may accidentally kick the mother. If cooperation cannot be achieved despite these measures, immobilization in a papoose board may be necessary. With older children, examination of the patient in the supine or semirecumbent position with good lighting assists visualization and may be more practical.

Use of a tongue depressor may be necessary to ensure direct visual access to all intraoral areas, and a dental mirror can be quite helpful, especially in assessing the lingual surfaces of the anterior teeth and gingiva and the buccal surfaces of rear molars. Extra effort and patience may be required to ensure that the mucobuccal folds, sublingual space, lingual surface of the anterior teeth, and anterior palate are adequately visualized.

The special aspects of the history and physical assessment of dental and orofacial trauma are detailed in Trauma to the Dentition, later in this chapter.

NORMAL ORAL STRUCTURES

The oral cavity, including the teeth, gingiva, and periodontal ligaments, is in a constant state of evolution during infancy and childhood. From the early teething stage, through the eruption and exfoliation of the primary dentition, and finally to the eruption of all permanent teeth, the oral cavity provides one of the most visible signs of development.

To assist understanding of this chapter and communication when consulting dentists, a review of basic terminology is in order. Each tooth is composed of an outer protective enamel layer; an inner layer of dentin consisting of tubules, which are thought to serve a nutritional function; and a central neurovascular core termed the *pulp*. The roots of the teeth are anchored in the sockets of the alveolar processes of the mandible and maxilla by an encompassing periodontal membrane or ligament. The neurovascular supply to the root apex also passes through this structure. The bony processes between the teeth are referred to as the *interdental septae* (Fig. 20-2).

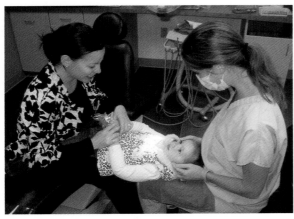

Figure 20-1   Oral examination of a toddler. A lap examination is a useful way to examine a young or anxious child. The patient is able to hold the parent's hand and see the parent during the examination.

After eruption, the visible portions of teeth are referred to as the *crowns,* and the interface between them and the gingiva is termed the *gingival crevice.* Finally, the portions of the gingiva located between teeth are called *interdental papillae.*

Oral Cavity in the Newborn

The lips of an infant reveal a prominent line of demarcation at the vermilion border. The mucosa may look wrinkled and slightly purple at birth, but within a few days it exhibits a drier appearance, with the outer layer forming crusty "sucking calluses." This callus formation affects the central portion of the mucosa and persists for a few weeks to a few months.

The maxillary alveolar arch is separated from the lip by a shallow sulcus. In the midline the labial frenulum extends

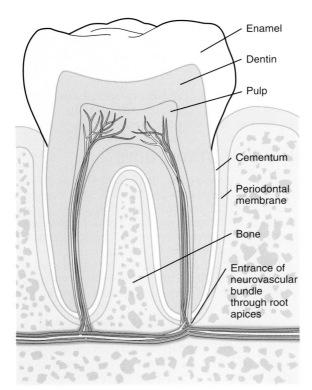

Figure 20-2   Diagrammatic representation of a molar shows the enamel, dentin, and pulp; the cementum; the periodontal membrane; the entrance of the neurovascular bundle through the root apices; and the bony supporting structures.

posteriorly across the alveolar ridge to the palatine incisive papilla. Two lateral miniature frenula are also evident. The alveolar ridge peaks anteriorly and gradually flattens as the ridge extends posteriorly, forming a pseudoalveolar groove medial to the ridge along its palatal side. This flattened appearance is seen in young infants and gradually disappears with the growth of the alveolar process and the formation and calcification of posterior tooth buds. The mandibular alveolar ridges also peak anteriorly and flatten posteriorly. The mandibular labial frenulum connects the lower lip to the labial aspect of the alveolar ridge. Careful visual inspection and palpation of the ridges should confirm the presence and location of tooth buds. Anterior tooth buds are located on the labial side of the alveolar ridges, whereas posterior tooth buds are often located closer to the crests of the alveolar ridges. Palatal morphology and color are variable. The tongue and the floor of the mouth differ only slightly from those of older children.

Primary Dentition

Development of the alveolar bone is directly related to the formation and eruption of teeth, and normal patterns of dental development occur symmetrically. Eruption times and sequence may be extremely variable, but typically at approximately 6 months of age, the mandibular central incisors erupt. This stage is often preceded by a period of increased salivation, local gingival irritation, and irritability. These symptoms may vary in intensity, but they respond well to oral analgesics and usually subside when the primary tooth erupts into the oral cavity. Other symptoms such as fever or diarrhea have never been proven to be directly related to teething. The lower incisors are soon followed by the maxillary central incisors and the maxillary and mandibular lateral incisors (Fig. 20-3). By the end of the first year, all eight anterior teeth are usually visible. At 2 years, all primary teeth have erupted with the exception of the second primary molars, which erupt shortly thereafter. By the age of 3 years, the full primary dentition is typically present and functional (Fig. 20-4).

Any variation in the time and sequence of eruption in an otherwise normal infant may call for early dental referral. In most instances, careful observation is the best course of action. For example, delayed eruption of primary teeth for up to 8 months is occasionally observed, and if seen in the absence of other abnormalities may be a normal variation. Delayed dentition can be a feature of moderate to severe cases of failure to thrive, where it is seen in association with and is a visible reflection of delayed bone age. More rarely, delayed eruption is associated with Down syndrome, hypothyroidism, hypopituitarism, achondroplastic dwarfism, osteopetrosis, rickets, or chondroectodermal dysplasia. A significant

Figure 20-3   Early primary dentition. The mandibular and maxillary central and lateral incisors are the first to erupt.

Figure 20-4 Full primary dentition. By age 3, all 20 primary teeth have erupted.

Figure 20-6 Abnormal eruption patterns frequently occur in the early mixed dentition phase. One example is shown here, with eruption of the permanent central incisors behind the primary teeth.

variation affecting a single tooth or only a few teeth should be carefully investigated as well.

Spacing (extra space between teeth) during this stage is normal and desirable and often indicates that more space is available for the larger permanent teeth. The completed primary dentition establishes a baseline that dictates to a great extent the future alignment of permanent teeth and the future relationship between the maxillary and mandibular arches.

During most of the primary dentition stage, the gingiva appears pink, firm, and not readily retractable. A well-defined zone of firmly attached keratinized gingiva is present, extending from the bottom of the gingival sulcus to the junction of the alveolar mucosa. Rarely, local irritation may develop into acute or subacute pericoronitis, with elevated temperature and associated lymphadenopathy (see Fig. 20-50). Topical and/or systemic therapy may be required for treatment; however, lancing the gingiva to relieve such symptoms is not usually indicated.

Mixed Dentition

The mixed dentition stage of development begins with the eruption of the first permanent molars at about 6 years of age and continues for approximately 6 years. During this period, the following teeth erupt from the gums in sequence: mandibular central incisors, maxillary central incisors, mandibular lateral incisors, maxillary lateral incisors, mandibular cuspids, maxillary and mandibular first premolars, maxillary and mandibular second premolars, maxillary cuspids, and mandibular and maxillary second molars (Fig. 20-5).

The mixed dentition during this stage undergoes certain physiologic changes including root resorption followed by exfoliation of primary teeth, eruption of their successors, and eruption of the posterior permanent teeth. During the period of root resorption of primary teeth, and for several months after the eruption of permanent teeth, the teeth are relatively loosely embedded in the alveolar bone and more vulnerable

to displacement by trauma. Other minor complications may occur during resorption and exfoliation of primary teeth and eruption of permanent teeth. Gingival irritation can occur as a result of increased mobility of primary teeth but usually disappears spontaneously when the tooth is lost or extracted. Two transient deviations of eruption pattern may occur: the mandibular incisors may erupt in a lingual position behind the primary incisors ("double teeth") (Fig. 20-6), and the maxillary incisors may assume a widely spaced and labially inclined position ("ugly duckling" stage). Finally, the occlusal surfaces of newly erupted permanent teeth are relatively "rough" (see Figs. 20-5 and 20-43), assisting plaque accumulation that increases the risk of staining, gingivitis, and formation of caries.

Early Permanent Dentition

The stage of early permanent dentition marks the beginning of a relatively quiescent period in dental development. Activities are limited to root formation of a few permanent teeth and the calcification of the third molars. By this time the length and width of the dental arches are well established (Fig. 20-7); however, the jaws undergo a major growth spurt during puberty that alters their size and relative position. The gingiva begins to assume adult characteristics, becoming firm and pink in color, with an uneven, stippled surface texture and a thin gingival margin. Puberty is occasionally associated with gingivitis, thought to be secondary in part to hormonal changes (Fig. 20-8). The gingivae become mildly edematous and erythematous and bleed with brushing (the common chief

Figure 20-5 Mixed dentition. This transitional stage from primary to permanent dentition begins at age 6 and lasts for about 6 years.

Figure 20-7 The earliest stage of permanent dentition begins with the eruption of the 6-year molars and central incisors. The cuspids and second molars are the last to erupt.

Figure 20-8   Gingivitis during puberty. The gingival tissues are mildly erythematous and edematous, and they tend to bleed easily with brushing. Hormonal changes and inattention to careful dental hygiene are thought to be contributory.

complaint). Inattention to careful dental hygiene may also contribute to development of this disorder, which necessitates good oral hygiene for control.

In Figure 20-9 the primary and permanent dentition are presented diagrammatically.

HARMFUL ORAL HABITS

Thumb and Finger Sucking

Children often develop sucking habits, using the thumb, finger(s), or objects. Thumb and finger sucking begins antenatally and is considered a normal behavior pattern. However, if the habit persists beyond the late primary dentition stage of dental arch development (5 years), the extrinsic forces applied by the sucking action can produce pathologic changes in the child's normal arch growth. These deviations range from minor, reversible changes to gross malformations in the dental arches that produce significant anterior open bites and/or posterior crossbites. The degree of change depends on the duration, frequency, and intensity of the sucking habit (Fig. 20-10).

Bottle and Pacifier Habits

The forces produced by prolonged use of bottles and pacifiers can first cause dental malocclusions and may, if the habit persists, worsen the resulting deformity with the involvement of adjacent jaw structures. Usually, if the child is weaned from the bottle and pacifier by the age of 12 months, no permanent changes in bite development can be expected. The longer any force is applied, however, the greater the risk that the distortion in the dental arches and adjacent bony structures will not self-correct (Fig. 20-11).

Thus the use of bottles and pacifiers should be discouraged by the age of 12 months. After this age, changes in the oral structures have been noted with prolonged use and are more likely to be permanent. Counseling parents during the neonatal period not to put their infants to bed with a bottle, but rather to hold them during all feedings, is probably one of the best ways to prevent later difficulties with weaning. Such practices also prevent the development of nursing bottle caries (see Fig. 20-42).

Therapy

Clinical management of harmful oral habits should be customized to the child's age. Obviously, harsh measures to discourage digit sucking in a 2-year-old are not justified and may be counterproductive. Children who receive frequent criticism for thumb sucking are probably more likely to cling to the habit

than are those whose families ignore it. However, when the habit persists beyond a reasonable age, calm discussions with the child concerning feelings related to the sucking and the physical damage possible if it continues often produce the desired results. When a child has expressed a strong will to cease sucking but is unable to accomplish this goal without help, appliance therapy by a dental professional may be indicated. Referral for oral evaluation and consultation is appropriate after the child has passed the appropriate age of the behavior pattern involved (e.g., older than 5 years of age for digit-sucking habits or 12 months for pacifiers).

NATAL AND NEONATAL ABNORMALITIES

Teeth

Teeth that are present in the oral cavity at birth are called *natal teeth*, whereas those erupting during the neonatal period (30 days after birth) are called *neonatal teeth*. The incidence of natal teeth has been reported to be approximately 1 in 2000 births. Although seen in normal infants, this anomaly is more frequent in patients with cleft palate (Fig. 20-12) and is often associated with the following syndromes: Ellis–van Creveld syndrome, Hallermann-Streiff syndrome, and pachyonychia congenita. The majority, about 90%, of such teeth are true primary teeth, but occasionally they are supernumerary. Some are abnormal, with either hypoplastic defects or poor crown or root development. Natal teeth may cause feeding problems for both the infant and mother. Ulceration of the ventral surface of the tongue by sharp tooth edges (Riga-Fede disease) may develop if natal teeth remain in the oral cavity. This condition is usually transient, but in persistent cases symptomatic treatment or extraction of such teeth may be indicated. Most normal-appearing natal teeth can be retained, but those that are supernumerary, abnormal, or very loose may have to be removed.

Gingival Cysts in the Newborn

Gingival cysts of the oral cavity are small, single or multiple superficial lesions that are formed by tissues trapped during embryologic growth and occur in about 80% of newborns. They are asymptomatic, do not enlarge, seldom interfere with feeding, and usually exfoliate within a few weeks.

Three types of cysts exist:

1. *Epstein pearls* are keratin-filled cystic lesions lined with stratified squamous epithelium. They appear as small, white lesions along the midpalatine raphe and contain no mucous glands (Fig. 20-13).

2. *Bohn nodules* are mucous gland cysts, often found on the buccal or lingual aspects of the alveolar ridges and occasionally on the palate. They are multiple, firm, and grayish white in appearance. Histologically they show mucous glands and ducts (Fig. 20-14).

3. *Dental lamina cysts* are found only on the crest of the alveolar mucosa. Histologically, these lesions are different because they are formed by remnants of dental lamina epithelium. They may be larger, more lucent, and fluctuant than Epstein pearls or Bohn nodules and are more likely to occur singly (Fig. 20-15).

Congenital Epulis in the Newborn

Congenital epulis is a benign, soft tissue tumor seen on the alveolar mucosa at birth or shortly after. It is usually found on the anterior maxilla as a pedunculated swelling (Fig. 20-16)

Figure 20-9 Artist's illustrations of the primary and permanent dentition. **A** and **B,** The numbers represent the average age of eruption for the teeth, indicated in months for the primary teeth and years for the permanent dentition. **C** and **D,** The names of specific teeth in the primary and permanent dentition are shown. **E** and **F,** Tooth numbers diagram: Primary teeth are lettered A-J from *upper right* to *upper left* and K-T from *lower left* to *lower right*. Secondary teeth are numbered 1-16 from *upper right* to *upper left* and 17-32 from *lower left* to *lower right*.

Figure 20-10   Changes in the bite often occur as the result of prolonged digit sucking. This child's upper arch has been narrowed, and an anterior open bite is developing.

Figure 20-11   A 2-year-old with a prolonged pacifier-sucking habit has severe deformity of the alveolar arches and teeth caused by the extrinsic force of the pacifier-sucking action.

Figure 20-12   A natal tooth associated with cleft palate. Extraction is necessary only if it is of abnormal morphology or causes feeding difficulties.

Figure 20-13   Gingival cysts. The small, whitish cystic lesions seen along the mid-palatine raphe are called *Epstein pearls.*

Figure 20-14   Gingival cysts. The firm, grayish-white mucous gland cysts on the buccal aspect of the alveolar ridges are called *Bohn nodules.*

Figure 20-15   Dental lamina cyst. These cysts are found on the alveolar ridge and usually occur singly.

but may appear on the mandible or occasionally on both jaws. The mass is firm on palpation, and the overlying mucosa appears normal. Histologically, sheets of large granular cells are seen. Differential diagnosis should include rhabdomyoma and melanotic neuroectodermal tumor of infancy. The lesion is amenable to conservative surgical excision, and recurrence is infrequent.

Melanotic Neuroectodermal Tumor of Infancy

Melanotic neuroectodermal tumor of infancy is a benign yet aggressive tumor, developing during the first year of life and often found on the anterior maxilla in association with unerupted or erupted teeth. It often bulges and destroys the alveolar bone, thus displacing the associated primary tooth. The tumor mass is grayish blue, firm on palpation, and spherical in shape (Fig. 20-17). Careful surgical removal is effective, and recurrence is unusual.

Figure 20-16   Congenital epulis. This 4-day-old patient has a benign tumor of the anterior maxilla.

Figure 20-17 Melanotic neuroectodermal tumor. This benign but locally aggressive tumor of the anterior maxilla has produced elevation of the lip and displaced a primary tooth.

DEVELOPMENTAL ABNORMALITIES

Soft Tissue Abnormalities

Geographic Tongue (Benign Migratory Glossitis)

Geographic tongue (benign migratory glossitis) is a painless condition characterized by inflamed, irregularly shaped areas on the dorsum of the tongue that are devoid of filiform papillae. Lesions are red, slightly depressed, and bordered by a whitish band (Fig. 20-18). Spontaneous healing followed by the formation of similar lesions elsewhere on the tongue results in a migrating appearance. The etiology is unknown; however, a strong association with stress and allergies is suspected. Although benign, the course of this disorder may be prolonged for months, and it may recur.

Abnormalities of the Frenula

During embryonic life, the maxillary labial frenulum extends as a band of tissue from the upper lip over and across the alveolar ridge and into the incisive (palatine) papilla. Postnatally, as the alveolar process increases in size, the labial frenulum separates from the incisive papilla and becomes relatively smaller. With the eruption of primary and later permanent teeth, the frenulum attachment moves apically and further atrophies as a result of vertical growth of the alveolar process. The developmental gap (diastema) between the maxillary central incisors tends to close with the full eruption of the maxillary permanent canines. On occasion the maxillary frenulum fails to atrophy and the diastema persists (Fig. 20-19).

Figure 20-19 Large diastema (excessive spacing) between the front teeth secondary to an inferiorly positioned maxillary frenulum.

The mandibular midline frenulum only rarely maintains a lingual extension and therefore only rarely causes a diastema between the mandibular central incisors.

The lingual frenulum extends almost to the tip of the tongue in early infancy and then gradually recedes. On occasion, ankyloglossia (tongue tie) is seen (Fig. 20-20), but this is rarely associated with feeding or speech difficulties. Various surgical procedures have been advocated to correct this condition. In general, frenulectomy is seldom indicated and should be recommended only after appropriate justification. Congenital anomalies may include an enlarged frenulum, labiolingual frenulum extensions, or supernumerary frenula as seen in orofaciodigital syndrome (Fig. 20-21).

Gingival Hyperplasia

Generalized gingival hyperplasia is a fairly common nonspecific pathologic entity. This disorder is frequently a complication of drug therapy, as it is seen in patients given phenytoin and cyclosporine. Gingival hyperplasia may also be idiopathic or genetically transmitted as in familial fibromatosis. Differentiation of various types of hyperplasia must be based on thorough physical evaluation and appropriate medical history. Histopathologically, it is impossible to differentiate among

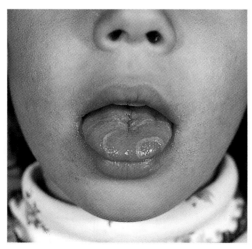

Figure 20-18 Characteristics of benign migratory glossitis (geographic tongue), which is a chronic and often recurring condition affecting the filiform papillae of the tongue. Lesions are red, slightly depressed, and bordered by a whitish band.

Figure 20-20 Ankyloglossia. This extremely short lingual frenulum with a high insertion point on the gingival margin is an indication for surgical intervention.

Figure 20-21   Multiple hyperplastic frenula are seen in this patient with orofaciodigital syndrome. These frenula interfered with the eruption of teeth, causing rotation and crowding.

Figure 20-23   Eruption hematoma. A bluish, fluid-filled, fluctuant swelling can be seen over the crown of an erupting maxillary cuspid. The lesion resolved without treatment when the tooth erupted.

these various disorders; therefore the final diagnosis and recommendations for therapy should be based on all available clinical data and an appropriate dental consultation.

Phenytoin-induced Gingival Hyperplasia

The administration of phenytoin over a period of time frequently causes generalized hyperplasia of the gingiva (Fig. 20-22, *A* and *B*). The gingiva may become secondarily inflamed, edematous, and boggy, especially if proper oral hygiene is not practiced. The severity is often related to the degree of local irritation, stemming from poor oral hygiene, mouth breathing, caries, or poor occlusion (alignment). Because hyperplasia tends to recur after surgical excision, gingivectomy is usually reserved for those patients whose overgrowth interferes with function and for those whose therapy has been discontinued.

Cyclosporine-induced Gingival Hyperplasia

Cyclosporine has been used primarily to treat patients after organ transplantation. The drug has been demonstrated to directly increase cellular growth of gingival fibroblasts. It also increases the production and retention of collagen. Further, this agent's immunosuppressive action may predispose gingival tissues to invasion by microorganisms, thereby increasing

inflammatory changes. Although meticulous oral hygiene reduces inflammation, it has no significant effect on the degree of hyperplasia.

Fibromatosis Gingiva

Fibromatosis gingiva, a rare, genetically determined condition, may be clinically evident at birth and in such instances may prevent or slow subsequent dental eruption. The clinical manifestations include the generalized presence of firm fibrous tissue that extends around the crowns of involved teeth. Inflammation, when present, is usually secondary. Surgical excision of excessive tissues is usually indicated, but recurrence is a possibility.

Idiopathic Gingival Hyperplasia

Different types of patients, often with significant systemic illnesses or syndromes, may manifest generalized gingival enlargements. These may primarily involve the gingival tissues or may sometimes be related to underlying thickening of cortical bone, which causes gingival hyperplasia by impeding dental eruption. Each of these cases must be evaluated individually for possible etiology and appropriate treatment.

Eruption Cysts (Eruption Hematoma)

An eruption cyst is a fluid-filled swelling, nontender in the majority of cases, over the crown of an erupting tooth. When the follicle is dilated with blood, the lesion takes on a bluish color and is termed an *eruption hematoma* (Fig. 20-23). Although the eruption cyst is a superficial form of dentigerous cyst, it rarely impedes eruption. Surgical exposure of the crown is seldom necessary. Rarely, such a cyst may become secondarily infected. In such cases, patients complain of headache or facial pain and the cyst is tender on palpation. Incision and drainage are required typically when infection has developed.

Mucocele and Ranula

A mucocele is a painless, translucent or bluish lesion of traumatic origin, most often involving minor salivary glands of the lower lip (Fig. 20-24). The lesion may alternately enlarge and shrink. The treatment of choice is surgical excision of the lesion and the associated minor salivary gland.

A simple ranula is a retention cyst in the floor of the mouth that is confined to sublingual tissues superior to the mylohyoid muscle. It appears clinically as a bluish, transparent, thin-walled, fluctuant swelling (Fig. 20-25). Herniation of the ranula through the mylohyoid muscle results in a cervical or plunging ranula that becomes more apparent in the oral cavity with the muscle contraction associated with jaw opening. Simple incision and drainage of the ranula is not an acceptable treatment because healing is followed by recurrence. Marsupialization by suturing the edges of the opened cystic wall to

Figure 20-22   Phenytoin-induced gingival overgrowth. **A,** A typical gingival response (hyperplasia) to chronic phenytoin ingestion. Similar gum changes can result from cyclosporine therapy. **B,** Severe overgrowth. The firm, hyperplastic gingival tissues have completely covered the posterior teeth and are interfering with mastication.

Figure 20-24 A mucocele on the lower lip, with the characteristic translucent coloration secondary to fluid retention.

the mucous membrane is the recommended treatment. The plunging ranula must be removed in its entirety along with the associated salivary gland to avoid recurrence.

Salivary Calculus (Sialolithiasis)

Formation of a salivary calculus is rare in the pediatric population, but when it does occur it may affect either the Wharton duct or Stensen duct (Fig. 20-26, *A*). Partial obstruction of the duct results in pain and enlargement of the gland, especially at mealtime. Although palpation of the stone may be possible, dental radiographs confirm the diagnosis and give appropriate information about its size and location (Fig. 20-26, *B*). Larger salivary stones wedged within the ducts may cause localized irritation and secondary infection. If the calculus cannot be manipulated through the duct, surgical intervention may be necessary.

Hard Tissue Abnormalities

Hyperdontia and Hypodontia

Variations in tooth number include both hyperdontia and hypodontia. Supernumerary teeth occur in about 3% of the normal population, but patients with cleft lip and/or cleft palate and cleidocranial dysplasia have a significantly higher incidence. The most common site is the anterior palate (Fig. 20-27). Supernumerary teeth may have the size and morphology of adjacent teeth or may be small and atypical in shape. They may erupt spontaneously or remain impacted. Early consideration of removal is justified because of complications such as impeded eruption, crowding, or resorption of permanent teeth; cystic changes; or ectopic eruption into the nasal cavity, the maxillary sinus, or other sites (Fig. 20-28).

Congenital absence of teeth is more often seen in the permanent dentition than in the primary. Most frequently missing are third molars, second premolars, and lateral incisors.

Figure 20-26 Salivary calculus. **A,** This sialolith obstructing a salivary duct is observed in the floor of the mouth. **B,** A dental radiograph of the sublingual space reveals the size and location of the salivary calculus.

Hypodontia is frequently associated with several ectodermal syndromes such as anhidrotic ectodermal dysplasia and chondroectodermal dysplasia (Fig. 20-29).

Alterations in Tooth Size and Shape

Teeth that are smaller or larger than normal are termed *microdonts* and *macrodonts,* respectively. These teeth are genetic anomalies. They are clinically significant when a discrepancy in tooth size and dental arch length results in severe crowding or spacing of the teeth. Size abnormalities are often localized to one tooth or to a small group of teeth (Fig. 20-30).

Variations in shape also result from the joining of teeth or tooth buds. Fusion is the joining of two tooth buds by the dentin. Concrescence is the joining of the roots of two or more teeth by cementum. Gemination (twinning) results from the incomplete division of one tooth bud, resulting in a large crown with a notched incisal edge and a single root (Fig. 20-31).

Hypoplasia and Hypocalcification

Numerous local and systemic insults are capable of causing the enamel defects of hypoplasia and hypocalcification. The most common etiologic factors are local infection such as an

Figure 20-25 Ranula. The bluish, fluctuant swelling in the floor of the mouth is a retention cyst associated with trauma to a salivary duct.

Figure 20-27 Hyperdontia. Erupted supernumerary tooth lingual to the maxillary central incisor in the deciduous dentition.

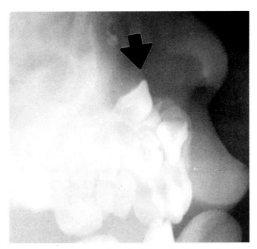

Figure 20-28   Supernumerary nasal tooth. A lateral radiograph of the maxilla shows a supernumerary tooth *(arrow)* erupting through the floor of the nasal cavity in a child with cleft palate who had recurrent epistaxis.

Figure 20-30   A microdont can be seen on this panoramic radiograph near the second molar. Microdonts are often seen in the maxillary lateral incisor region.

abscessed primary tooth, which, when not diagnosed and treated promptly, may damage the enamel of its developing permanent counterpart. Other causes include systemic infections with associated high fever, trauma (such as intrusion of the primary tooth), and chemical injury, of which excessive ingestion of fluoride is an example. Other etiologic factors include nutritional deficiencies, allergies, rubella, cerebral palsy, embryopathy, prematurity, and radiation therapy. Hypocalcification results from an insult during mineralization of the tooth and is seen as opaque, chalky, or white lesions (Fig. 20-32). Hypoplasia results from an insult during active matrix formation of the enamel and clinically manifests as pitting, furrowing, or thinning of the enamel (see Fig. 20-33).

Heritable Defects of Enamel and Dentin

Amelogenesis Imperfecta

Amelogenesis imperfecta is the term used to describe a group of genetically determined defects that involve the enamel of primary and permanent teeth without affecting dentin, pulp, or cementum. Although the types of amelogenesis imperfecta are numerous, the major defect in each is hypoplasia, hypomaturation, or hypocalcification. The hypoplastic type results in thin, pitted, or fissured enamel (Fig. 20-33). Hypomaturation manifests as discolored enamel of full thickness but decreased hardness that tends to chip away slowly, exposing the underlying dentin. Radiographic evaluation demonstrates the decreased density of enamel. In the hypocalcified form the enamel is chalky, variable in color, and quickly erodes (Fig.

20-34). Depending on the type of amelogenesis imperfecta, inheritance may be autosomal dominant, autosomal recessive, or X-linked.

Dentinogenesis Imperfecta

Dentinogenesis imperfecta results in dentin defects and is usually inherited as an autosomal dominant trait. The most common manifestation is opalescent dentin, which may be associated with osteogenesis imperfecta (see Chapter 21). Because of variable phenotypic expression, teeth may be blue, pinkish-brown, or yellowish brown in color and have an opalescent sheen (Fig. 20-35). In any given patient, individual teeth may be variably affected. Despite normal enamel morphology, patients tend to have relatively rapid attrition or wearing down of the crowns, although the rate of wear can be quite variable. The roots are shortened, and the pulp chambers are calcified. Primary teeth are more severely affected than the permanent teeth, although permanent teeth are prone to develop enamel fractures, which can chip or flake off.

DISCOLORATION

Three major types of tooth discoloration are frequently observed: (1) discoloration from stains that adhere externally to the surfaces of the teeth (extrinsic); (2) discoloration from various pigments that are incorporated into the tooth structure during development (intrinsic); and (3) intrinsic discoloration secondary to hereditary defects, which was discussed previously.

Figure 20-29   Hypodontia. The congenital absence of teeth is seen in this patient with hereditary ectodermal dysplasia. This phenomenon may be an isolated anomaly or a manifestation of several syndromes.

Figure 20-31   Radiograph demonstrates gemination (twinning), the incomplete division of a tooth bud resulting in a tooth with a large, notched crown and a single root.

Figure 20-32 Hypocalcification. This 6-year-old patient exhibits early signs of hypocalcification of his permanent molars. Chalky white spots indicate poor calcification of the enamel.

Figure 20-34 Amelogenesis imperfecta, hypocalcified type. The enamel defects result in discoloration and erosion caused by errors in the mineralization stage of tooth development and secondary staining.

Extrinsic Discoloration

Extrinsic discoloration is limited primarily to patients with poor oral hygiene, those receiving certain medications, those who heavily consume stain-containing foods or drinks, or those who smoke or chew tobacco or other substances. It occurs more often at certain locations, especially on the gingival third of the exposed crown. Diagnosis requires appropriate medical, dental, and dietary histories with emphasis on oral hygiene, food and drug intake, and tobacco habits. Treatment includes scaling, dental prophylaxis and polishing, and the practice of regular oral hygiene. The use of abrasive toothpaste can cause excessive wear of the enamel and should be avoided.

Brownish-black stain on the lingual surfaces of anterior and posterior teeth is most common among young children who are taking liquid oral iron supplements and among adolescents who are smokers and tea drinkers. Green stain on the labial surfaces of the anterior maxillary teeth is common among children with poor oral hygiene. The source is usually chromogenic bacteria and fungi (Fig. 20-36). Oranges-red stain is unusual, but when it does occur it can be found around the gingival third of the exposed crown. This stain often results from antibiotic intake, which causes a temporary shift in the oral flora.

Intrinsic Discoloration

Intrinsic discoloration is usually induced during the calcification of dentin and enamel by excessive levels of the body's natural pigments such as hemoglobin and bile or by pigments introduced by the intake of chemicals such as fluorides or tetracyclines. On occasion, isolated intrinsic discoloration occurs as a result of pulpal necrosis, pulpal calcification, or internal resorption.

Hepatic Discoloration

Generalized intrinsic discoloration of primary teeth is seen in patients with advanced hepatic disease associated with persistent or recurrent jaundice and hyperbilirubinemia (Fig. 20-37). The intensity of discoloration varies and may be related to the severity of the disease. Color ranges from brown to grayish-brown and usually has no clinical significance unless it is associated with significant hypoplasia of the dentition.

Discoloration due to Tetracycline

Teeth stained as a result of tetracycline therapy may vary in color from yellow to brown to dark gray. Staining occurs when the tetracycline is incorporated into calcifying teeth and bone. The enamel and to a greater degree the dentin that are calcifying at the time of intake incorporate tetracycline into their chemical structures. The severity of discoloration depends on the dose, duration, and type of tetracycline administered. The initial yellow or light brown pigmentation tends to darken with age (Fig. 20-38). Tetracyclines readily cross the placenta, so staining of primary teeth is possible if tetracycline is taken during pregnancy. Therefore tetracycline should not be prescribed to pregnant women or to children younger than 10 years of age.

Discoloration due to Erythroblastosis Fetalis

Children born with congenital hemolytic anemia caused by rhesus (Rh) factor incompatibility may exhibit distinct discoloration of their primary teeth as a result of the deposition of bilirubin in the dentin and enamel during primary tooth development. The color ranges from green to blue to orange. No treatment is indicated unless discoloration is associated with

Figure 20-33 Amelogenesis imperfecta, hypoplastic type. This process results in generalized pitting of the enamel.

Figure 20-35 Dentinogenesis imperfecta. The bluish, opalescent sheen on several of these teeth results from genetically defective dentin. This condition may be associated with osteogenesis imperfecta.

Figure 20-36 Extrinsic discoloration. The green stain seen on the gingival third of the incisors is associated with poor oral hygiene.

Figure 20-38 Tetracycline discoloration. The severe discoloration seen in this patient is the result of tetracycline administration at a time when calcification of the permanent teeth is occurring.

significant hypoplasia or hypocalcification. The permanent dentition is usually not affected.

Discoloration due to Porphyria

Porphyria, a hereditary disturbance of porphyrin metabolism, may produce a distinct reddish or brownish discoloration of the primary and permanent teeth secondary to deposition of porphyrin in developing teeth (Fig. 20-39).

Isolated Intrinsic Discoloration

Teeth with necrotic pulps develop an opaque appearance with discoloration ranging from light yellow to gray (Fig. 20-40; and see Fig. 20-47, *B*). Such teeth may develop abscesses, periapical cystic lesions, or chronic fistulas. Pulpal calcification (Fig. 20-41) is often associated with a localized yellow discoloration. Internal resorption manifests clinically as a pink discoloration secondary to loss of dentin thickness.

CARIES

The interaction of microorganisms, especially *Streptococcus mutans,* and fermentable carbohydrates results in acid demineralization of susceptible enamel. Caries are seen as yellowish-brown to gray defects in the enamel surfaces of affected teeth (Fig. 20-42). Untreated, carious destruction progresses through the enamel and dentin and with bacterial contamination of the pulp ultimately renders the pulp necrotic. The deep pits, fissures, and grooves characteristic of the surfaces of newly erupted teeth are at increased risk for developing carious lesions (Fig. 20-43; and see Fig. 20-5). Sealing these defects with plastic bonding agents may prevent the initiation of caries. Other preventive methods include brushing and flossing on a daily basis (beginning with eruption of the first tooth)

to remove bacteria-containing plaque; implementation of systemic fluoride via the water supply or prescribed supplements; and control of the frequency of intake of fermentable carbohydrates, especially those high in sugar and adhesiveness.

Dental caries is an infectious, communicable disease. Studies have shown that mothers are the main source of *Streptococcus mutans* in their infants, with a greater rate of transmission to female than male infants. Cariogenic microbes can be transmitted vertically or horizontally. Vertical transmission occurs when bacteria, such as *Streptococcus mutans*, pass from caregiver to child through saliva. Horizontal transmission occurs between members of the family or close groups and can also be caused by saliva-sharing activities.

The pregnant mother should be counseled to visit her dentist for routine cleanings and examinations and if necessary should have all carious lesions restored, preferably before pregnancy, but if the decay is active and painful the treatment should be completed during the second trimester and when cleared by her physician. The presence of active dental caries and accompanying levels of *Streptococcus mutans* can lead to vertical transmission of bacteria by the mother to the infant and may increase the risk for the development of carious lesions at a very early age.

Children should be referred to a dentist to establish a dental home within 6 months of the eruption of the first tooth, but no later than 1 year of age. Examining children at a young age can help in preventing dental caries, providing anticipatory guidance, and noting any dental malformations or problems that exist.

Nursing bottle caries (otherwise known as early childhood caries) involve the primary dentition of the child who is habitually put to bed with a bottle containing milk or another cariogenic (sugar-containing) liquid. This form of caries was

Figure 20-37 Hepatic discoloration. Generalized intrinsic discoloration of the primary teeth is seen in this patient with biliary atresia.

Figure 20-39 The reddish-brown tooth discoloration associated with porphyria.

Figure 20-40 Isolated intrinsic discoloration. The central incisor is discolored secondary to trauma. Often, such a change is a manifestation of pulpal necrosis.

Figure 20-41 Radiographic evidence of dystrophic calcification of the pulp and root canal of the upper right primary central incisor.

originally associated with bottle-feeding only; however, an association with frequent and prolonged nocturnal breast-feeding has become apparent. Carious lesions initially develop on the maxillary incisors and later on the molars and canines (see Fig. 20-42, *A* and *B*). The mandibular incisors are spared by the protective position of the tongue during nursing. The particularly deleterious effect of nocturnal nursing is due to the fact that the rates of salivation and swallowing are decreased during sleep. Hence the liquid ingested has more prolonged contact with dental surfaces and oral flora. Brushing before bedtime and after any nocturnal feedings is especially important in prevention. The American Academy of Pediatric Dentistry (AAPD) defines early childhood caries (ECC) as "the presence of one or more decayed (noncavitated or cavitated), missing (due to caries), or filled tooth surfaces in any primary tooth in a child 71 months of age or younger."

The AAPD also specifies that "in children younger than 3 years of age, any sign of smooth-surface caries is indicative of severe early childhood caries (S-ECC)."

The AAPD and the American Academy of Pediatrics (AAP) recommend discontinuation of the nursing bottle by 12 months of age. Frequent bottle-feedings through the night, breast-feeding ad libitum, and extended and repeated use of a training ("sippy") cup are all associated with early childhood caries. Breast milk alone is not implicated in developing early childhood caries, but when given in conjunction with carbohydrates it can be cariogenic.

An especially severe variant of nursing bottle caries, severe early childhood caries, is seen in toddlers whose parents have deferred weaning until well after 1 year of age, continued to provide them with night-time bottles, and failed to ensure regular brushing and to seek dental care for their children. In

Figure 20-42 Caries. **A,** The typical pattern of nursing bottle caries, with the upper incisors being the first involved. **B,** When badly neglected, severe tooth erosion occurs and periapical abscesses may develop. **C** and **D,** This 3-year-old victim of medical and dental neglect represents the extreme end of the spectrum of nursing bottle caries. When placed in foster care, she was still drinking from a bottle and had never had her teeth brushed or seen a dentist. **C,** Marked discoloration, extreme wear, and carious destruction of her entire maxillary dentition are evident. **D,** All of her upper teeth were abscessed, and her mandibular teeth were severely decayed as well.

Figure 20-43 The occlusal surfaces of newly erupted molars exhibit varying degrees of pit and fissure depth. The morphology of these patterns makes these teeth more prone to early decay.

such cases decay is extensive and deep, the teeth show signs of wearing down, and numerous abscesses are found (see Fig. 20-42, *C* and *D*). This constitutes significant dental neglect, and these children often must undergo multiple dental extractions.

Fluoride Use

The frequent and repeated use of fluoride is of critical importance for the control and prevention of dental caries in both children and adults. Optimal fluoride exposure acts as an adjunct in decreasing the incidence of caries, as well as remineralizing enamel. Fluoride is the most effective caries prevention agent and is considered completely safe when properly used. However, the ingestion of high concentrations or incorrect dosages of fluoride can lead to nausea, vomiting, dental fluorosis, or, in extreme cases, death.

Parents should be advised to delay the use of a fluoride dentifrice until the child is older than 24 months and can expectorate. When applying fluoridated toothpaste, a small pea-sized quantity should be placed on the brush. Pediatricians and dentists should take into consideration all sources of fluoride before prescribing supplements, to determine the correct dosage (Table 20-1).

Diet and Nutrition

Between-meal snacking and the frequency of eating and drinking are related to dental caries incidence. When sugary liquids such as watered-down juice, sugar water, flavored milks, and carbonated beverages (such as soda) are given to young children in bottles or training cups, it can greatly increase their caries risk. Frequent intake of these drinks can promote and accelerate caries progression.

According to the guidelines of the AAPD, particular emphasis should be placed on "discontinuation of the nursing bottle by 12 months of age and cessation of at-will breastfeeding after teeth begin to erupt" to decrease the likelihood of early childhood caries.

Dietary screening, assessment, and guidance should be an integral component of the care process for dental clients. A diet high in citrus fruits, snacks containing citric acid, and acidogenic sports drinks can lead to dental erosions. Another cause of dental erosion is excessive regurgitation of gastric contents into the oral cavity, which can be related to gastroesophageal reflux disease (GERD). Sugar-containing carbonated beverages, juices, and sports drinks are also acidic and the combination of acid and sugar may act synergistically to cause the severe caries associated with regular carbonated beverage consumption. It takes repeated cariogenic attacks to produce the mineral loss that presents as dental caries. The frequency and form of cariogenic foods or beverages are more important than the amount of sugar in each food item. Foods such as raisins, starches, and candies that stick to the teeth for an extended period of time will continue to slowly leach and metabolize as sugars and acid. The oral bacteria will use these sugars as food and prolong the decrease in pH in the oral cavity. Similarly, any food or beverage that contains fermentable carbohydrates and is consumed over a prolonged period or with increased frequency will have the same effect. Diet suggestions for healthy teeth and gingiva are listed in Table 20-2.

INFECTIONS

For a summary and description of raised intraoral lesions, see Table 20-3.

Viral Infections

Herpetic Gingivostomatitis

Primary herpetic gingivostomatitis, caused by herpes simplex type 1 virus, is an extremely painful and contagious disease that affects children, especially those between the ages of 6 months and 3 years. The vesicular lesions of the lips, tongue, gingiva, and oral mucosa are preceded by fever, headache, regional lymphadenopathy, and gingival hyperemia and edema. These lesions tend to rupture quickly, leaving shallow ulcerations covered by a gray membrane and surrounded by an erythematous halo (Fig. 20-44; see also Chapter 12). The inflamed gingivae are friable and bleed easily. Lesions heal spontaneously in 1 to 2 weeks without scarring. Because inflammation makes brushing painful, oral hygiene should be maintained with a preparation such as chlorhexidine or glycerin and peroxide (in very young children) to decrease the incidence of secondary infection. A bland diet and rinsing with viscous lidocaine (in children older than 6 or 7 years) or a solution of equal parts Benadryl (diphenhydramine) and

Table 20-1	Dietary Fluoride Supplementation Schedule		
Age	Less Than 0.3 ppm F	0.3-0.6 ppm F	More than 0.6 ppm F
Birth to 6 mo	0	0	0
6 mo to 3 yr	0.25 mg	0	0
3 yr to 6 yr	0.50 mg	0.25 mg	0
6 yr up to at least 16 yr	1.00 mg	0.50 mg	0

From American Academy of Pediatric Dentistry: Guideline on fluoride therapy, *Pediatr Dent* 24:66, 2002 [special issue: reference manual 2002-2003].

Figure 20-44 Herpetic gingivostomatitis. The ulcerations seen on the oral mucosa were preceded by fever, headache, and lymphadenopathy. Note the erythematous halos around the ulcerations.

Table 20-2 Diet Suggestions for Various Oral Conditions

Food Group	Dental Caries	Periodontal Disease	Dentures	Mucositis/Oral Lesions	Oral Impairment and Surgery
General	Limit number of eating times Avoid sticky or retentive foods	Avoid soft, mushy foods	Encourage chewing Begin by chewing on molar area Work up to biting	Avoid hard, sharp, or acid foods Avoid temperature extremes	Aim for soft food, or blenderize foods if needed
Grains/cereals (6-11/d)	Have whole grains Popcorn for snacks Avoid crackers, donuts, potato chips between meals	Avoid popcorn Have whole grains, foods requiring chewing	Begin with softer foods, such as hot cereal, pasta, soft whole-grain bread Work up to bagels, hard rolls	Have soft grains such as warm cereals, pasta, rice, potato Avoid hard crusts	Hot cereals, rice, pasta, soft bread, soups with pasta and rice
Fruits (3-5/d) Fresh, frozen, canned juices	Have fruits for dessert/snacks Avoid dried fruits or fruit roll-ups Don't sip slowly or often on fruit drinks Avoid fruit drinks	Have plenty of fruits high in vitamin C and carotene, such as citrus fruits (oranges, grapefruit), tomatoes, apricots, cantaloupe, fruit nectars, fruit juices	Avoid biting into large raw fruits at first, such as apples Begin with soft or canned fruits, juices Cut whole fresh fruit in small pieces and chew with molars Work up to biting with central incisors	Avoid acidic fruits such as citrus fruits (lemon, lime, orange, grapefruit) Have bland fruits such as banana, apricot, pear Have fruit nectars rather than acid fruit juices	Juices, blenderized fruits, pureed fruits
Vegetables (2-4/d) Fresh, frozen, canned, juices, potatoes	All veggies are fine Watch sweetened salad dressings Have raw veggies for snacks	All veggies are fine but concentrate on fresh and frozen rather than canned mushy vegetables Try vegetable juices	Avoid biting into raw vegetables at first, such as carrots Cut these into pieces and chew with molars Begin with soft or canned vegetables and juices Work up to biting with central incisors	Have bland vegetables, avoid tomatoes and tomato juice	Pureed vegetables, vegetable juices
Protein (2+/d) Meat, fish, poultry, eggs, beans (lentils, etc.), tofu, nuts	All proteins are fine Nuts for snacks	All proteins are fine Avoid nuts that can get stuck in sulcus	Soft meats such as hamburger, ground chicken, or chicken cut in small pieces, eggs, beans Nuts may be difficult to chew	Most protein sources are fine Nuts may be irritating to oral tissues	Eggnogs, liquid breakfast beverages, blenderized meats in broth
Dairy (2-3+/d) Milk, cheese, ice cream, tofu, cottage cheese	Have milk in coffee, soup Cheese in sandwiches, casseroles, etc. Cheese for snacks	Have plenty to maintain oral bone health (see Dental Caries column for other suggestions)	Have plenty to maintain alveolar bone health Cottage cheese, cheese sauces, milk in beverages and soups Ice cream for dessert	All dairy products are fine and bland: see Dental Caries column	Have milk-based beverages with ice cream added, cheese soups, tofu or cottage cheese blended with milk, ice cream in sodas
Sweets/fats Oil, margarine, butter, salad dressing, candy, sweet desserts, soda pop	Avoid slowly dissolving candies Have sweets as dessert only Avoid constant sipping on sweet beverages (soda, sports drinks)	Same as for caries to prevent root caries	Go light on these as they can be filling and take the place of more nutritious foods Avoid hard candies that may crack dentures Avoid sticky sweets, which may be difficult to clean off For partially dentate, see Dental Caries column Have casseroles, lasagna, and other soft combination foods to boost nutrients	Go light on these as they can be filling and take the place of more nutritious foods	As tolerated, have ice cream, sherbet, sorbet for dinner
Other	Have flavored club soda or diet soda Use sugar-free gum	Same as for caries to encourage oral clearance	Have casseroles, lasagna, and other soft combination foods to boost nutrients		Most foods can be pureed and are more palatable than canned liquid supplements Pureed baby foods may work; be careful of psychological implications

From Palmer CA: *Diet and nutrition in oral health,* Upper Saddle River, N.J., 2002, Prentice Hall.

Maalox, in addition to the use of oral analgesics, are indicated to minimize and control pain. In some severe cases, codeine may be required. The use of systemic acyclovir may be indicated in cases with moderate to severe involvement. Topical application of the same drug can be helpful in milder cases.

Recurrent infections caused by reactivation of latent herpes simplex virus are fairly common. Lesions are few in number, and more localized; systemic symptoms are absent unless the host is immunocompromised. Lesions are usually located on the lips, with prodromal symptoms of itching and burning preceding the development of thin-walled vesicles that rupture and become crusty in appearance (see Chapter 12). When intraoral lesions occur, they manifest as small vesicles in a localized group on mucosa that is tightly bound to periosteum. Elective dental treatment should be deferred while the child is infectious.

Table 20-3	Summary of Raised Intraoral Lesions and Intraoral Ulcerations

Lesion/Ulceration	Description
Raised Intraoral Lesions	
Fibroma	Most common tumor of oral mucosa, painless, firm, pedunculated; therapy is excision
Papilloma	Pedunculated with cauliflower surface, caused by HPV; therapy is excision
Abscess	Painful red area with pimple-like appearance; therapy includes antibiotics with root canal or extraction of offending tooth
Pyogenic granuloma	Painless red nodule, pedunculated, with gingival enlargement; therapy is excision
Intraoral Ulcerations	
Herpetic gingivostomatitis	Gingival erythema with multiple oral vesicles, often grouped and more anterior in location; therapy includes pain relief and antivirals for severe cases
Herpangina	Multiple vesicles with erythematous borders on tonsillar pillars, uvula, and soft palate; therapy includes pain relief and palliation
Varicella-zoster	Pruritic vesicles/pustules on skin with ulceration of mucous membranes; therapy includes pain relief and antivirals for severe cases
Aphthous ulcer	Ulceration with erythematous halo, typically on "unbound" mucosa; therapy includes steroids and/or antibiotic rinses
Mucositis	Inflammation and ulceration of oral cavity; therapy includes improved oral hygiene
Trauma	History from parent/patient important to rule out nonaccidental trauma; treatment is palliative
Hand, foot, and mouth disease	Vesicles and ulcerations on hands, arms, feet, and legs, as well as oral mucosa; treat herpangina

HPV, human papillomavirus.

Hand, Foot, and Mouth Disease

Hand, foot, and mouth disease, caused by coxsackievirus A or enterovirus, may present itself with fever, malaise, abdominal pain, cough, and lymphadenopathy. Oral ulcerations (usually 5 to 10 in number) are present, often with vesicles on hands, arms, and feet, for about 10 days. Treatment is palliative. Elective dental treatment should be deferred until oral and skin lesions resolve.

Herpangina

Herpangina, caused by coxsackievirus A, is typically present in summer and fall months. It is spread via the oral–fecal route. Vesicles are present on the soft palate and tonsillar pillars. They often rupture, leaving shallow but painful ulcerations. Malaise, fever, and lymphadenopathy may be present.

Treatment is palliative, and the disease is self-limited. Elective dental treatment should be deferred until oral lesions and other acute symptoms of infection resolve.

Herpes Zoster (Shingles)

Herpes zoster results from reactivation of the varicella-zoster virus and inflammation of a dorsal root or extramedullary cranial nerve ganglion. Although the disease is seen in otherwise healthy children, it is more likely to occur in the severely debilitated or immunosuppressed child. The patient exhibits a prodrome of malaise, fever, headache, and tenderness along the affected dermatome that may last 3 days or more. This is followed by the extraoral formation of painful, grouped vesicular lesions that rupture to form ulcerations. The oral cavity also may be affected with erosions when maxillary and mandibular divisions of the trigeminal nerve are involved (Fig. 20-45).

Recurrent Aphthous Ulcers (Canker Sores)

Aphthous ulcers are similar in appearance to herpetic ulcers. Their specific etiology is unknown, but possible precipitating factors include trauma, stress, sunlight, endocrine disturbances, hematologic disorders, and allergies. Infection with viruses and L-forms; immunologic dysfunction or dysregulation; deficiency of iron, trace elements, vitamin B_{12}, and folate; and genetic factors have all been postulated as causative but have not been proved so by scientific study. The complete pathophysiology is likely due to several factors. Onset is usually during adolescence or young adulthood, and between 5% and 25% of the population is affected at some time during their lives by recurrent ulcers. Unlike herpetic lesions, these ulcerations are not preceded by vesicle formation. They are extremely painful and have a pseudomembrane and an erythematous halo (Fig. 20-46). They can vary in size, number, and distribution. Small aphthae may coalesce into larger lesions. Although any oral mucosal surface may be involved, freely movable mucosa is more frequently involved than tightly bound mucosa. Lesions heal in 1 to 2 weeks without scarring. Recurrences have no regular periodicity and are not accompanied by fever or other systemic symptoms. Absent a recognized etiology, treatment is symptomatic, usually with a topical anesthetic/antiseptic preparation. More recently, use of immunomodulating agents is being studied.

A much less common disorder, seen only in children, in which recurrent aphthous ulcers are a feature is Marshall syndrome (also known as *periodic fever, aphthous stomatitis, pharyngitis,* and *cervical adenitis* [PFAPA]), first described in 1987. Affected patients have onset before 5 years of age and recurring episodes with a distinct periodicity in both duration of symptoms and asymptomatic interval for each given patient. The average duration of episodes is 5 days (range, 3 to 6 days),

Figure 20-45 Herpes zoster. This patient's infection involved the trigeminal nerve including the nasociliary branch. The extraoral (**A**) and intraoral (**B**) lesions stop at the midline.

Figure 20-46   Recurrent aphthous ulcers. The ulceration seen on the labial mucosa is surrounded by a characteristic erythematous halo.

and the average interval is 28 days (range, 2 to 9 weeks). Episodes tend to begin abruptly with a rapid rise in temperature to 39° C or 40° C, accompanied by malaise, chills (not rigors), and often headache with cervical adenitis (seen in 88%) and/or nonexudative pharyngitis (seen in 72%) and/or aphthous ulcers (seen in 70% but thought to be possibly overlooked in some cases). Oral aphthae are three or more in number, shallow, less than 5 mm in diameter, and not described as remarkably painful. Cervical nodes rapidly enlarge bilaterally and, although tender, are not warm, and no overlying erythema, edema, or fluctuance is present. Rhinorrhea, cough arthralgias, and myalgias are not seen. Signs and symptoms tend to clear just as abruptly as they appear, although the aphthous ulcers may take 5 to 10 days to resolve (without scarring). During episodes, affected children look relatively well and between episodes they not only are healthy with normal growth and development but also appear less susceptible to the common cold and other infections their siblings develop. The only associated laboratory abnormalities are mild leukocytosis and an elevated erythrocyte sedimentation rate. Cultures are negative, and antibiotics and antiviral agents have no ameliorative effect. Of note, early administration of one or two doses of prednisone promptly aborts episodes, although its use may shorten the asymptomatic intervals between bouts. Daily administration of cimetidine (used for its immunomodulating properties) for 6 months has stopped episodes in up to 30% of patients; however, they may resume when treatment is discontinued. Tonsillectomy and adenoidectomy have been reported curative in up to 70% of children so treated, and tonsillectomy alone in 50%. Spontaneous resolution has been seen in about 40% after an average of 5 years, but some patients continue to experience recurrences for 15 years or more.

At present, infection with periodic flares and some form of immune dysregulation are considered the major etiologic possibilities. The disorder is distinguished from cyclic neutropenia by finding normal neutrophil counts at 2-week intervals for 6 weeks and by the absence of unusual and serious bacterial infections. In Behçet disease, the periodicity is not so exact; fever is not so prominent; oral aphthous ulcers are large and heal with scarring; and genital ulcers, arthritis, and uveitis are typical features.

Bacterial Infections

Odontogenic infections are caused by both aerobic and anaerobic microorganisms. Streptococci and staphylococci are isolated frequently; however, any oral flora or opportunistic microorganism may be involved. Oral anaerobic organisms, including fusobacteria, anaerobic streptococci, and *Kingella* species are often prominent causes.

Dental Abscesses

Abscesses are most common in children with neglected dental caries as a result of poor dental hygiene and irregular dental care. Once caries extend to the pulp, infection and pulpal necrosis ensue, setting the stage for the formation of a periapical abscess. Children with traumatized teeth may go on to develop abscesses if the resulting pulpal hyperemia is so extreme that it causes pressure necrosis, if the neurovascular bundle is severed, or if the pulp is exposed by a crown fracture.

Periapical abscesses require endodontic therapy or extraction of the offending tooth. The potential for complications makes early diagnosis important, yet frequently this does not occur because often symptoms are insidious in onset and progression and nonspecific in nature. This is in part because the alveolar processes of the mandible and maxilla in young children are fenestrated anteriorly, assisting early decompression of the abscess through the alveolus and gingiva. Patients may complain of headaches as the abscess enlarges and pressure builds up, and then of abdominal pain after decompression as the draining pus is swallowed, causing gastric irritation. Later in childhood, abscessed maxillary teeth may intermittently decompress through the floor of a maxillary sinus, producing recurrent sinus infections. Other symptoms may include anorexia, avoidance of certain foods, halitosis, toothache, a sensitive tooth, or facial swelling. Nonspecific complaints and complaints of referred pain are more common among children than are complaints of a toothache, and some children have no overt symptoms but report feeling better after treatment.

On physical examination the examiner may find localized gingival swelling and/or erythema, a gingival abscess, a fistula, or a granuloma (Figs. 20-47 and 20-48, *A*). On occasion there is increased sensitivity to percussion or palpation. Left untreated, a periapical abscess of a primary tooth may damage the underlying developing tooth bud. Abscesses may also result in formation of an apical granuloma or a radicular cyst,

Figure 20-47   Dental abscesses. **A,** An abscess above the left upper lateral incisor developed after an injury in which the patient had chipped that tooth and his central incisor. **B,** This abscess above the right central incisor has ruptured through the gingiva and begun to drain. The tooth is discolored as a result of pulp necrosis stemming from an injury 2 years earlier.

Figure 20-48   A, A deep, neglected cavity in this mandibular molar predisposed to development of a periapical abscess that, after rupture, resulted in formation of a gingival granuloma. **B,** Left untreated, such abscesses can be responsible for this type of extraoral lesion in which infection has spread by way of a fistulous tract to the skin. Extraction of the offending tooth is necessary for resolution of the extraoral lesion.

or they may rupture and spread through the adjacent soft tissues to create a fistula, which drains through the skin (see Fig. 20-48, *B*). In some instances infection can spread into adjacent facial soft tissues, resulting in facial cellulitis (Fig. 20-49). More ominously, the infection may track through lateral pharyngeal, retropharyngeal, or sublingual spaces, threatening the airway and causing sepsis and/or mediastinitis. Rarely, septic thrombosis of the cavernous sinus or jugular veins may result from badly neglected infections. Necrotizing fasciitis of the facial tissues is extremely rare but a life-threatening complication of these infections.

Ludwig Angina

Ludwig angina is a potentially life-threatening infection of the mandibular floor. It is usually an infection associated with anaerobic streptococci, although any of the anaerobic flora of the mouth may cause this syndrome. Symptoms begin with signs of dental abscess, but progress to a tense swelling of the mandibular floor and then cervical edema resulting in a "bull neck." Pain, fever, and difficulty in swallowing are typical of Ludwig angina, with inability to handle secretions marking late stages of disease with airway impingement. It is extremely important to protect the airway in patients with Ludwig angina, as the disease will progress rapidly even with adequate therapy, and the rapid onset of airway compromise is life-threatening. Treatment includes immediate surgical intervention with stabilization of the airway and removal of infected teeth. Intravenous antibiotics are necessary until the patient stabilizes. There is frequent need for incision and drainage of the infected area, and a multidisciplinary team including dental medicine, anesthesia, and otolaryngology may be needed.

Pericoronitis

Pericoronitis is a bacterial infection of the gingival soft tissue surrounding the crown of a partially erupted tooth. This occurs when food particles and plaque become trapped under the

Figure 20-49 Facial cellulitis associated with an abscessed maxillary tooth. Hospital admission for intravenous antibiotics, incision and drainage, and extraction of the abscessed tooth was necessary.

residual gingiva, stimulating bacterial growth and abscess formation. The third molars are most commonly involved. Symptoms include localized pain and tenderness and occasionally fever and malaise. Erythema and edema are readily apparent on examination (Fig. 20-50, *A*), and an enlarged tender submandibular node is often found. Figure 20-50, *B* demonstrates the presence of both partially impacted and erupted teeth. The maxillary third molars and right mandibular third molar have erupted into a favorable position. The left mandibular third molar is partially erupted; however, it has been unable to erupt into occlusion. Partially erupted mandibular third molars are often associated with pericoronitis and/or periodontal defects distal to the second molar. Treatment options include warm salt water rinses to decrease bacterial counts and dislodge trapped food particles. Antibiotics and possible surgical correction may be necessary.

Acute Necrotizing Ulcerative Gingivitis (Vincent Infection, Trench Mouth)

Acute necrotizing ulcerative gingivitis (ANUG) is a fusospirochetal infection caused by fusiform bacilli and *Borrelia vincentii*, which is seldom seen before the age of 10. Patients experience abrupt onset of fever, malaise, severe mouth pain, and anorexia. The gingiva are reddened, edematous, and friable with necrotic punched-out craters in the interdental papillae. On occasion the palate and tongue are affected as well. Involved areas bleed readily and become covered with a pseudomembrane (Fig. 20-51). The breath is fetid, and cervical and submandibular nodes are enlarged and tender. Treatment generally consists of gentle dental prophylaxis followed by improved oral hygiene measures and topical peroxide applications. In most cases resolution occurs within several days without the use of antibiotics. On occasion, secondary infection or severe involvement may necessitate the use of antibiotics; penicillin is then the antibiotic of choice.

Bacterial Pharyngitis

Pharyngitis is most commonly a bacterial infection of the tonsils and posterior pharynx, caused by *Streptococcus pyogenes* in school-age children and adolescents. It is manifested by erythematous inflammation of the tonsils and posterior pharynx, petechiae of the soft palate, and anterior cervical lymphadenopathy (see Chapter 12). There may be associated headaches, fever, vomiting, or abdominal discomfort. Most symptoms will last for 5 to 7 days, and antibiotic therapy decreases suppurative complications while reducing the risk for rheumatic fever in endemic areas.

Lemierre Syndrome

Lemierre syndrome is a suppurative jugular thrombophlebitis most commonly caused by *Fusobacterium* species, although many anaerobic oral flora can be involved. The most common age group is adolescents. Typically beginning with a local

Figure 20-50   A, Pericoronitis involving a partially erupted third molar. Food particles and bacteria have become trapped under the residual overlying gingiva, resulting in inflammation and abscess formation. This condition can occur with eruption of any molar but is most common with partially erupted third molars (wisdom teeth). **B,** Panoramic radiograph demonstrating the presence of erupted maxillary third molars and mandibular right third molar but only partial eruption of the left mandibular third molar.

pharyngitis, oral anaerobes then progress to parapharyngeal infection and involve the internal jugular vein, invading and causing thrombosis and bacteremia. Embolic disease to the lungs and other tissues as well as septic shock may then be seen. Previously thought to be rare, this syndrome is once again gaining in frequency. Without prompt recognition and aggressive antibiotic therapy, patients may require critical care management for shock and airway compromise. Treatment involves long courses of intravenous therapy and anticoagulation in select cases.

Fungal Infections

Candidiasis (Moniliasis, Thrush)

Oral candidiasis results from infection with the opportunistic pathogen *Candida albicans*. This is seen most commonly as a relatively benign infection in infants (as thrush) and in young children who may be receiving or have recently completed a course of antibiotic treatment. Less frequently, it may be seen in immunocompromised or immunosuppressed children or in those with serious underlying systemic diseases. In the latter the infection is likely to be more extensive and severe. Oral forms can appear to be pseudomembranous or plaquelike. Scraping of the lesion reveals a raw and erythematous base with bleeding from torn capillaries. HIV infection or other immune deficiency must be ruled out when severe or therapy-resistant disease is present in children. Common sites of involvement are the buccal mucosa, tongue, palate, and commissures of the lips (Fig. 20-52). The intraoral lesions of acute infection are soft, elevated, creamy white plaques that do not scrape off easily. Chronic candidiasis, usually

seen in the immunocompromised host, can result in marked hypertrophy and fissuring of the tongue mucosa. Although culturing is difficult and not reliable, diagnosis may be made on the basis of clinical findings or examination of a potassium hydroxide (KOH) preparation. Treatment consists of local application of nystatin (miconazole or other antifungal agents for severe or chronic cases) and control of the underlying causes including sterilization of nipples used for formula feedings.

TRAUMA

Assessment of Patients with Orofacial and Dental Injuries

In evaluating patients with orofacial and dental trauma, key elements of the history include when, where, and how the injury occurred; the child's subsequent behavior; any prior treatment; and general health and tetanus immunization

Figure 20-52   Candidiasis. **A,** Involvement of buccal mucosa with white plaque. **B,** Mucocutaneous infection of the commissures of the lips.

Figure 20-51   Acute necrotizing ulcerative gingivitis. The infected gingiva exhibits localized necrosis and hemorrhage and is covered with pseudomembranes.

status. It is important to note whether there was loss of consciousness, as well as any nausea or vomiting. It is also important to note whether the child has age-appropriate responsiveness, as well as how quickly the child returned to consciousness. In asking about the mechanism of injury, the examiner must determine the forces involved. Did the child trip and fall while walking, or was he or she running; if riding a bike, how fast was he or she going; in the case of falls, from what height, onto what kind of surface? This gives the examiner a better idea of the potential severity of injury and risk of associated injuries. If the mechanism of injury reported is minor and significant injuries are found, if the mechanism does not fit the injuries seen, and/or if a parent tries to prevent an older child from giving a history, the possibility of abuse should be considered.

Physical examination is first directed at determining the adequacy and stability of airway, breathing, and circulation followed by evaluation for associated head and neck injury. When these areas have been cleared and/or stabilized, then the examiner may proceed with the orofacial examination, assessing the extent and nature of injuries. Because the presence of underlying injuries is often indicated by the degree and nature of overlying soft tissue trauma, assessment begins with external inspection of facial structures for swelling, deformity, contusions, abrasions, and lacerations. The presence of associated periorbital ecchymoses or swelling; subconjunctival hemorrhage or edema; diplopia; and nasal bleeding should raise suspicion of frontal skull and midface fractures. Battle sign, bruising of the mastoid process, is an indication of basilar skull fracture and may suggest underlying brain trauma. Meticulous examination of cranial nerve function is essential. This is followed by observation of occlusion and jaw motion on opening and closing, checking for deviation or trismus. Older patients can be asked if it feels normal when they bite down; parents of young children can report if the child's occlusion looks normal. The temporomandibular joint should be palpated while the child's facial expression is observed, assessing for tenderness, snap, or pain on opening and closing.

Next, intraoral soft tissues are inspected for evidence of swelling, hematoma, abrasions, and lacerations. Displacement, loosening, and fractures of teeth are noted. Palpation of facial bones and the labial and lingual surfaces of the dental arches and assessment of abnormal maxillary mobility may be best left until last because resulting pain may reduce cooperation. All internal and external lacerations must be carefully inspected to check for injury to underlying neural and ductal structures.

Recommended radiographs include apical and occlusal views for displacement or loosening of a permanent tooth, panoramic and facial bone radiographs for possible mandibular fractures, and a CT scan for suspected maxillary and midface fractures.

Soft Tissue Injuries

A variety of soft tissue injuries including lacerations, contusions, abrasions, perforations, avulsions, and burns may occur. Although soft tissue injuries may occur in isolation, they are often associated with injuries of teeth and supporting bones. Thus any assessment of a soft tissue injury must include careful attention to the teeth and underlying structures. The injured area should be cleansed of blood clots, debris, and foreign material, and then carefully examined to determine the extent of tissue involvement. Mechanical debridement of any ragged, necrotic, or beveled margins may be necessary. Appropriate tetanus prophylaxis should also be considered. Saline rinses, careful attention to oral hygiene, penicillin prophylaxis, and soft diet are mainstays of management of all intraoral soft tissue injuries.

Abrasions

Superficial abrasions usually heal without complications. Extensive abrasions should be covered with a water-soluble, medicated gauze after irrigation. Extensive deep abrasions may require skin grafting.

Contusions

A contusion, or bruise, usually requires no treatment, and healing proceeds favorably in most instances. However, contusions are often associated with underlying injuries; therefore a careful examination of adjacent structures is indicated.

Perforations

Perforations are small, deep wounds caused by sharp objects and are fairly common in children, especially as a result of falls with such an object in the mouth. Careful examination of the wound and the object is essential. After careful inspection and irrigation, larger wounds should be closed in layers; smaller wounds may not require closure. If doubt exists concerning foreign bodies and/or contamination, a drain should be left in place and proper antibiotics prescribed. The possibility of damage to large vessels should be recognized, especially when the perforation involves the posterolateral palate or a tonsillar pillar (see Chapter 23).

Avulsions (Degloving Injuries)

Avulsions of oral soft tissues are uncommon injuries, yet when they occur they may involve deep and superficial tissues (Fig. 20-53, *A* and *B*). Small avulsions can be treated by undermining and suturing surrounding tissues. Larger avulsions can be treated by reattaching the avulsed tissues or by use of a graft.

Lacerations

Lacerations of facial and oral tissues are common in children. Small intraoral lacerations with well-approximated margins do not require suturing. Bleeding usually subsides spontaneously,

Figure 20-53 Degloving injury, before **(A)** and after **(B)** repair. Such an injury to the oral mucosa requires immediate inspection, irrigation, approximation, and suturing.

Figure 20-54 This laceration of the oral mucosa—deep and not well approximated—requires immediate treatment and surgical closure.

and healing proceeds satisfactorily. Large lacerations, through-and-through lacerations, and those associated with extensive, recurrent, or uncontrolled bleeding require careful assessment and surgical closure (Fig. 20-54). To reduce risk of infection, saline irrigation and antimicrobial prophylaxis are indicated for all intraoral lacerations, regardless of whether sutures are required.

Lip lacerations are often caused by penetration of teeth through the labial soft tissues (Fig. 20-55). Thus the adjacent dentition must be carefully inspected for evidence of chipping and for signs of loosening or displacement. If chipping is found, embedded tooth particles should be suspected. These may be difficult to palpate but are easily detected radiographically. If present, they must be removed to prevent infection.

Because the trauma that results in chin lacerations commonly involves forced occlusion of the dentition with transfer of impact forces to the underlying bone and condyles, these cases warrant assessment of underlying dental and bony structures (see Figs. 20-55, 20-65, and 20-66). Forced occlusion injuries can also produce tongue lacerations. Closure is required for large, gaping wounds with persistent bleeding (Fig. 20-56, *A*), but conservative management is best for smaller lesions (Fig. 20-56, *B*).

Figure 20-56 Tongue lacerations. **A,** A large gaping tongue laceration in a toddler produced by the upper front teeth being forced through the tissue by a fall with the tongue protruded. This type of injury requires suturing. **B,** This small laceration, although gaping slightly, does not require surgical closure.

Soft palate lacerations require a thorough pharyngeal inspection. The possibility of foreign body entrapment, immediate or delayed vascular injury (particularly when the laceration involves posterolateral structures), or formation of pharyngeal abscesses should be seriously considered. Lacerations involving the labial frenulum of infants are common and require only restriction of lip manipulation and a soft diet.

Figure 20-55 **A,** This boy incurred a forced occlusion injury when hit by a car and thrown from his bike. Note the chin laceration and through-and-through lip laceration. **B,** He also had bilateral condylar neck fractures of the mandible. In this radiograph the condyles bend inward at nearly 90 degrees above the fracture lines.

Figure 20-57   This electrical burn was the result of chewing on an extension cord. In this site, delayed hemorrhage after separation of the eschar and deformity with scarring are particular problems.

Burns

Burns involving the oral cavity usually heal rapidly but, when deep, may do so with contracture and scarring. Burns at the angle of the mouth incurred by chewing on an electrical cord (Fig. 20-57) are particularly problematic. After the injury an eschar forms over the necrotic tissue. This tends to separate approximately 10 days later, at which time profuse bleeding from the labial artery may occur. Parents need to be informed of this possibility and instructed on what action to take if it should occur. Splints fabricated from dental materials are important in long-term management to prevent or minimize contracture by maintaining proper anatomic relationships during healing.

Traumatic Ulcers

Painful ulcerations may result from mechanical, chemical, or thermal trauma. Injury may be secondary to irritation by objects, trauma during mastication, toothbrush trauma, or abnormal habits. Large ulcerations involving the buccal mucosa or lower lip may be associated with cheek or lip biting after inferior alveolar nerve block (Fig. 20-58). Topical peroxide application (Gly-Oxide) is useful in cleansing the area. Lesions usually heal without scarring, but secondarily infected lesions may require antibiotic therapy. Identification and elimination of the habit is necessary for resolution of habit-related lesions.

Oral Mucositis

Oral mucositis is an inflammation and ulceration of the oral cavity. It is commonly seen as a complication of cancer treatment. Good oral hygiene is important for patients with oral

Figure 20-58   Traumatic lip ulceration caused by lip biting after administration of local anesthesia.

mucositis. Patients are encouraged to drink plenty of liquids. Patients undergoing chemotherapy are encouraged to brush two or three times per day with a soft bristle toothbrush. If poor oral hygiene is present, chlorhexidine rinses should be encouraged. If a patient develops oral mucositis, chlorhexidine may need to be discontinued as its high alcohol content may dehydrate the tissue. It is also important for patients undergoing chemotherapy to supplement fluoride because of the possibility of xerostomia (dry mouth), which may lead to increased caries risk.

Trauma to the Dentition

As noted earlier, facial injuries in childhood frequently involve the dentition and supporting bones. One prospective study showed that 50% of children had suffered at least one dental injury by age 14. Although falls are the major source in early childhood, bicycle and skateboard accidents, contact sports, fights, and motor vehicle accidents become more prevalent with advancing age. The possibility of child abuse must be considered for all age groups. The risk of facial injuries is relatively high in (1) children with neurologic disorders that impair coordination; (2) children with protruding maxillary anterior teeth; (3) children with a deviant anatomic relationship, such as an anterior open bite or a hypoplastic upper lip; and (4) 2- to 3-year-old children, with immature motor skills and coordination. Preventive measures, such as use of helmets, mouthguards, and seat belts, significantly reduce the incidence and severity of such injuries.

Potential Complications

Pulp hemorrhage and/or vasodilation of the pulp vessels are a common response to concussive injury to a tooth and can lead to development of permanent discoloration within 10 to 14 days. Excessive pulpal vasodilation can actually result in pressure necrosis of the pulp. Injuries that produce loosening or displacement of a tooth disrupt the anchoring periodontal ligament. If disruption is mild, there may be no sequelae, although in some cases it stimulates overactive bony repair, ankylosing the tooth in place. When disruption is more severe, the neurovascular bundle can be torn, resulting in pulpal necrosis, which then may lead to abscess formation. Finally, dental fractures in which dentin and/or pulp are exposed open a pathway for bacteria and may lead to abscess formation. The fracture surface must be sealed emergently.

Several extensive classifications of tooth injuries have been suggested, but for the purpose of this text a more simplified descriptive classification is presented.

Crown Craze or Crack

A significant number of children are discovered during routine physical examination to have "cracks" in the enamel of their teeth. Such cracks are presumably caused by relatively minor trauma or temperature changes. The majority of such teeth are asymptomatic and require no treatment.

Crown Fractures without Pulpal Exposure

Fractures that traverse only the enamel layer often require no treatment other than smoothing down rough edges and ensuring close follow-up (see Fig. 20-47, A). However, any fracture of the crown that results in exposure of the dentin requires emergency treatment to prevent infection and subsequent pulp necrosis (Fig. 20-59) because oral flora enter the dentinal tubules and rapidly migrate to the pulp. The treatment of choice is to seal the exposed dentin with calcium hydroxide and protect it with an acid-etched resin bandage. This procedure should be performed as soon as possible after the injury. As noted earlier, dental fragments are occasionally embedded

Figure 20-59 These crown fractures demonstrate involvement of enamel and dentin, without exposure of the pulp. Immediate dental referral is necessary to prevent contamination of the pulp through the dentinal tubules.

Figure 20-61 A vertical fracture of the upper central incisor extending below the gum line resulted in pulp exposure.

in the soft tissues of the lip or tongue; therefore appropriate examination and palpation of these areas are indicated. The presence of such fragments may be confirmed by radiographic examination.

Crown Fractures with Pulpal Exposure

Fractures that traverse all three tooth layers to expose the pulp usually involve a significant loss of tooth structure. On physical examination, the fracture surface reveals the pink central pulp surrounded by the beige dentinal layer (Fig. 20-60). Severe vertical or diagonal fractures may also result in pulp exposure and can at times extend to involve the root (Fig. 20-61). Such teeth must be treated on an emergency basis by pulp capping, pulpotomy, or root canal therapy, depending on severity.

Root Fractures

Root fractures are less common in the primary dentition, and when they occur they usually require no therapy. If the coronal segment represents an aspiration risk, or the patient has traumatic occlusion, the treatment of choice is extraction of the primary tooth. Root fractures of permanent teeth may occur with or without loss of crown structure and may be asymptomatic (Fig. 20-62). If a seemingly normal tooth is tender or exhibits increased mobility after trauma, root fracture should be suspected and radiographs obtained. In general the prognosis is good, and treatment may include splinting the involved segment, with or without root canal therapy. If the root fracture is in the coronal third of the tooth, splinting is recommended for 2 or 3 months. If the fracture is not in the coronal third, splinting is indicated for 4 weeks.

Displacement Injuries

Displacement injuries result in extrusion, intrusion, or lateral displacement (labially or lingually) and are most commonly seen in the primary dentition, where the combination of a short root length and a "pliable" bony structure seems to permit displacement to occur (Fig. 20-63, *A* and *B*). Displacement injuries are often the cause of significant discomfort, bleeding, and possible interference with mastication and occlusion. All result in some degree of disruption of the periodontal ligament. Further, being the result of moderate to severe mechanisms of injury, fractures of underlying bony structures are common associated findings. Because the primary teeth are most vulnerable to these types of injury, there is always a risk of damage to and interference with normal development of permanent tooth buds; therefore immediate care is advised. Treatment may include observation with or without prophylactic antibiotic coverage, immediate correction when lingual displacement is likely to interfere with mastication, or extraction of the displaced tooth in cases of severe labial or vertical displacement. Most intruded primary teeth re-erupt within 6 to 8 weeks, but may take up to 6 months for spontaneous re-eruption. Sensible oral hygiene and an appropriate diet should be observed after displacement to improve outcomes. In general, displaced permanent teeth should be repositioned and splinted, with close follow-up. It is not uncommon for these teeth to require root canal therapy.

Avulsion and Reimplantation

Avulsion is the complete displacement of a tooth from its socket and is seen mostly in preschool and early school-age children. Reimplantation of primary teeth is not recommended.

Figure 20-60 This crown fracture involves enamel, dentin, and the soft tissue of the pulp as well. Immediate dental referral is mandatory to save the tooth.

Figure 20-62 This radiograph reveals a root fracture in the apical third of an upper primary incisor. This was suspected clinically because of tenderness and increased mobility.

Figure 20-63 Displacement injuries. **A,** This primary lateral incisor was traumatically intruded. Such intrusions usually spontaneously re-erupt. **B,** Lateral displacement. The left upper central incisor is lingually displaced, and its crown appears elongated as a result of partial extrusion. This would require repositioning and splinting.

On the other hand, reimplantation of permanent teeth is an acceptable technique with a relatively good prognosis (Fig. 20-64, *A* and *B*). The major factors in improving prognosis are as follows:

1. A short period between avulsion and reimplantation, preferably less than 15 minutes, or as soon as possible

2. Appropriate storage of the avulsed tooth (the most desirable "medium" is the socket itself, followed in order of preference by ViaSpan, Hanks' balanced salt solution, cold milk, saliva, saline, and water)

3. Appropriate irrigation of the surgical site, replacing the tooth into the socket without pressure, and stabilization with the use of a splint

4. Appropriate removal of the pulp within 2 weeks as a first step in completing root canal treatment, unless the tooth was immature with incomplete root formation

5. Removal of the splint within 2 weeks

Figure 20-65 A panoramic radiograph reveals a nondisplaced mandibular fracture extending through the wall of the third molar tooth bud. An associated hairline fracture exists near the midline on the patient's right.

6. Ensuring that the patient has received complete tetanus immunization. Follow-up care also includes chlorhexidine rinse, appropriate antibiotic, and a soft diet for 2 weeks

Trauma to Supporting Structures

The developing facial bones in the young child are small relative to the calvarium and thus somewhat protected by it. They are compact, spongy, and have greater elasticity, which tends to reduce the risk of fractures. However, the relatively thin outer cortices make alveolar process fractures somewhat more likely with dental displacement injuries, and their growth centers and developing tooth buds serve as weak points and thus are major sites of fractures when they do occur (Fig. 20-65). Finally, their thick periosteum has remarkable osteogenic potential, which speeds healing remarkably. Injuries to these bony supporting structures of the dentition may result from birth trauma (rarely), bicycle accidents, car accidents, various physical and sporting activities, child abuse, and animal bites. Because major forces are required to produce jaw fractures in children, the examiner must carefully search for evidence of associated head and neck injuries (Fig. 20-66) and be vigilant in observing for evidence of expanding hematomas that may later compromise the airway.

Fractures of the Mandible

Excluding nasal fractures, the most common facial fractures in children involve the mandible. The two major mechanisms are forced occlusion and lateral or frontolateral impact. Forced occlusion can produce hemarthrosis of the temporomandibular joint, a compression fracture of the condylar process, or a greenstick condylar fracture (see Fig. 20-55). These injuries can be associated with fractures of the molar crowns. Lateral and frontolateral blows tend to produce fractures of the mandibular body, usually through the wall of a developing tooth

Figure 20-64 **A,** Four permanent incisors have been avulsed. **B,** The teeth have been reimplanted successfully.

Figure 20-66 CT scan reveals intrusion of the mandibular condyle into the middle cranial fossa as a result of an extremely severe forced occlusion injury. Careful "pull back" and splinting is a common treatment for this type of injury.

bud (see Fig. 20-65). Because the mandible is an arch through which the force of the impact is transmitted, these injuries are often associated with a contralateral fracture of the mandibular body or condyle (see Fig. 20-65). Important diagnostic clues may include ecchymosis, facial swelling, deviation on opening or closing (Fig. 20-67), trismus, and malocclusion that may be apparent visibly or only subjectively evident to the patient. Severe bilateral mandibular fractures can result in posterior displacement of the mandible and tongue with secondary airway obstruction. Palpation may reveal localized tenderness and hematoma formation, a step-off, or abnormal mobility with or without gingival tears. Examination of the child with a temporomandibular joint injury may reveal tenderness and decreased motion, clicking, or crepitus when the examiner's fingers are pressed just anterior to the external auditory canal as the child opens and closes the mouth. A panoramic radiograph and a mandibular series should be ordered if there is clinical suspicion of a fracture. If routine views are unrevealing, CT may be called for in certain unusual, difficult, or complex cases.

Management requires careful assessment of the stability and type of erupted dentition, as well as the location of the tooth buds. Nondisplaced fractures with no occlusal abnormalities may require no treatment other than a soft diet. Most displaced fractures can be treated conservatively: first by appropriate reduction, followed by simple intermaxillary fixation or intraoral splints and circumferential wiring (closed reduction). Seldom is open reduction indicated; however, if this technique is used, careful placement of intraosseous holes is essential to avoid damaging the developing tooth buds.

Figure 20-67 A method of measuring deviation of the mandible on opening, showing a shift to the fracture side the width of one lower central incisor.

Fractures of the Maxilla and Midface

Other than minor fractures of the alveolar process seen with dental displacement injuries, fractures of the maxilla and midface are uncommon in infants and young children. This is because the relatively large cranial vault provides protection, with the forehead bearing the brunt of most frontal impacts. The elasticity of the facial bones further reduces the risk of fracture. When such injuries do occur in older children and adolescents, they are generally the result of major impacts and are often associated with injuries to the nose, ethmoid sinuses and orbits, and the frontal portion of the skull. As noted earlier, careful attention must be given to the airway, breathing, and circulation, along with assessment for associated head and neck injuries. Exact diagnosis of the location and extent of maxillary fractures is challenging and necessitates a thorough and detailed examination and specialized imaging techniques. CT scan of the midface in both sagittal and coronal planes is the most reliable diagnostic tool.

The Le Fort classification of midfacial fractures, devised in 1901, divides them into three groups (Fig. 20-68) as follows:

1. Le Fort I, involving primarily the maxilla, separating it from the pterygoid plates and the nasal and zygomatic struts (Fig. 20-69)

2. Le Fort II, in which the maxilla and nasal complex are separated from the orbits and the zygoma (Fig. 20-70)

3. Le Fort III, in which there is complete separation of the midface from the cranial vault at the level of the naso-orbital ethmoid complex and the zygomaticofrontal suture area with extension through the orbits (Fig. 20-71)

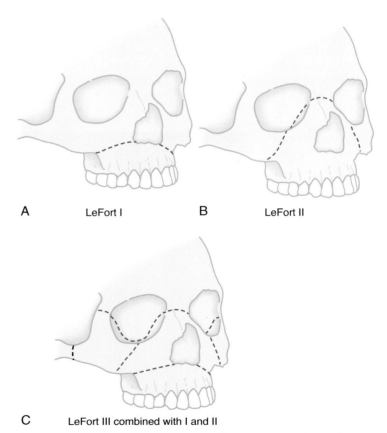

A LeFort I   B LeFort II

C LeFort III combined with I and II

Figure 20-68 Diagrammatic representation of fracture patterns of Le Fort fractures. **A,** Le Fort I: the fracture separates the maxilla from the pterygoid plates and the nasal complex. **B,** Le Fort II: the fracture line separates the maxilla and nasal complex from the orbits and the zygoma. **C,** Le Fort III: the fracture line separates the midface from the cranial vault, traversing the zygomaticofrontal sutures and extending through the orbits and the naso-orbital ethmoid complex. Fracture lines of types I and II are shown as well because they are commonly present with the Le Fort III.

Figure 20-69   CT scan shows a Le Fort I fracture. The maxilla is separated from the midface. The degree is greater on the right.

Often these fractures occur in combination, and the involved maxilla may be further fragmented. It is not unusual to encounter the combination of a Le Fort II on one side and a Le Fort III on the other. Sagittal splitting of the palate, often accompanied by palatal laceration, is seen in about 10% of patients. Associated mandibular fractures are common.

The diagnosis of Le Fort I fracture is often made by finding abnormal mobility of the maxilla when the maxillary dental arch is grasped anteriorly and a vertical "pull–push" maneuver is performed, although on occasion the fracture may be impacted or incomplete and malocclusion without mobility is found. Associated findings may include midfacial swelling or ecchymosis (Fig. 20-72; and see Fig. 20-70), epistaxis, malocclusion, and apparent elongation or shortening of the midface.

Le Fort II fractures should be suspected when both the maxilla and nasal complex are mobile. Physical findings are similar to those noted in Le Fort I fractures, but wrinkling of the skin above the nose may also be seen.

Beyond these findings, patients with Le Fort III fractures tend to have prominent periorbital hematomas and swelling and may have subconjunctival hemorrhage, disconjugate gaze, and limited extraocular motion, any of which should prompt careful assessment for associated orbital rim and frontal bone fractures. Up to 25% of patients with Le Fort II and III fractures have cerebrospinal fluid rhinorrhea and pneumocephaly. Injury to the naso-orbital ethmoid complex can also cause detachment of the medial canthal ligaments, with resultant widening of the intercanthal distance.

Progression of edema and often profuse nasopharyngeal bleeding necessitate frequent reassessment of the patient's airway and circulatory status. The airway may need to be stabilized via orotracheal intubation (or rarely tracheotomy) to protect the patient from aspiration of blood or airway narrowing from edema or an expanding hematoma. Total blood loss must be monitored carefully, the patient typed and crossmatched, and blood replacement initiated when necessary.

Once airway, circulatory status, and head and neck injuries have been stabilized or ruled out, appropriate imaging can be performed and treatment initiated. Primary objectives include control of hemorrhage; reestablishing normal occlusion, vertical dimension, and width of the midface; and immobilization of fractures and restoration of normal fronto-orbital architecture. This often necessitates a team approach. It is preferable to plan and carry out the repair as soon as possible after more serious injuries are stabilized because delays increase infection risk and can make repair more difficult as edema worsens and the bones begin to knit over the first 2 to 3 days postinjury.

CRANIOMANDIBULAR DYSFUNCTION (TEMPOROMANDIBULAR JOINT DISEASE)

The term *craniomandibular dysfunction* (CMD) is used to define a set of signs and symptoms that involve the masticatory musculature, the temporomandibular joint (TMJ), or both. Most clinicians and investigators agree that signs and

Figure 20-70   Le Fort II fracture. This adolescent boy sustained multiple midfacial and naso-orbital injuries in a motor vehicle accident. **A** and **B,** He has a collapsed midface with marked swelling of the upper lip, deviation of the nose, and prominent periorbital swelling and ecchymosis. *(Courtesy Joseph Andrews, MD.)*

Figure 20-71 Le Fort III fracture. This 10-year-old girl was hit by a car while sledding. Clinically, she had bilateral raccoon eyes; severe facial edema with a mobile maxilla; and bleeding from the nose, mouth, and eyes. She had the constellation of fractures that constitutes a Le Fort III fracture and numerous other facial and skull fractures. **A,** CT cut shows multiple fractures involving the anterior, posterior, and medial walls of the maxillary sinuses. **B,** Bilateral zygoma fractures are evident in another cut.

symptoms of CMD may include the following: tenderness or pain of the masticatory muscles, TMJ tenderness, limited or asymmetrical mandibular movements, clicking or crepitation of the joint, and secondary headaches. Reported signs and symptoms are generally mild, fluctuate over time, and exhibit no sex predilection. Their prevalence ranges from 9.8% to 85% of subjects surveyed, with results varying with patient selection, subject age, sample size, and definition of diagnostic criteria. Prevalence has been shown to increase with age. Despite the high frequency of CMD signs and symptoms, it is estimated that only 5% of children and adolescents are in need of treatment. The discrepancy can be attributed to the subclinical nature of many of the signs and symptoms recorded in epidemiologic studies.

The etiology of CMD is multifactorial. Oral parafunctional habits such as bruxism (grinding), bite deviations (malocclusion), trauma to the TMJ or mandible, orthodontic treatments, and history of stress are often cited as etiologic factors. Of these, bruxism and stress (possibly with attendant jaw clenching) are most significantly associated with symptomatic CMD. Trauma, the next most common factor, has been reported to be responsible for TMJ pain in 26% of pediatric patients with CMD. We have also encountered a number of young musicians, especially violinists who practice for long periods daily, who have CMD symptoms. Both cross-sectional and longitudinal studies have failed to show a one-to-one relationship between signs and symptoms of CMD and morphologic and functional malocclusion. Hence malocclusion alone is not a primary etiologic factor. Similarly, orthodontic treatment has not been shown to significantly increase or decrease the frequency of signs and symptoms.

Patients presenting with symptoms of CMD should undergo a comprehensive history and examination. The history should include present illness and time of onset of symptoms, their nature, exacerbating and ameliorating factors, and prior therapy; a complete medical history; and a detailed dental history. The latter should note whether there has been a history of treatment under general anesthesia; trauma to the TMJ or mandible; oral parafunctions such as bruxism, thumb sucking, nail biting, or gum chewing; headaches related to clenching of the teeth; and unusually diligent practice with a musical instrument such as the violin, horn, or reed instrument. In addition, family and social history with emphasis on recent changes and potential sources of emotional stress should be obtained. Clinical examination includes inspection of the head and neck; intraoral examination; palpation of the TMJ and masticatory musculature; auscultation of the TMJ during opening and closing; and observation of mandibular movements in all planes (opening, protrusive, and lateral). Significant deviations from normal mandibular motion, tenderness, clicking or crepitus of the joint, or generalized TMJ pain all suggest the need for further evaluation.

Identification and elimination of etiologic factors is of paramount importance in the treatment of CMD. Studies on children and young adults suggest that conservative or reversible types of treatment are most appropriate. Such modalities may include physical or behavioral modification therapy, bite splints, and judicious use of analgesics. The application of irreversible treatment modalities such as bite adjustment (selective grinding of the teeth), orthognathic surgical intervention, and orthodontics to correct CMD is not supported scientifically.

Figure 20-72 Delineated ecchymosis with hematoma formation on the mucosa of the upper lip is a common sign associated with underlying fractures, in this case a fracture of the anterior nasal spine of the maxilla.

Bibliography

American Academy of Craniomandibular Disorders: Guidelines for evaluation, diagnosis and management. In McNeil C, editor: *Craniomandibular disorders*, Chicago, 1990, Quintessence Publishing.

American Academy of Pediatric Dentistry: Policies and guidelines, *Pediatr Dent* 31, 2009. (Special issue.)

Bhaskar SN: Oral lesions in infants and newborns, *Dent Clin North Am* July:421–435, 1966.

Christensen RE Jr: Soft tissue lesions of the head and neck. In Sanders B, editor: *Pediatric oral and maxillofacial surgery*, St. Louis, 1979, Mosby.

Long SS: Syndrome of periodic fever, aphthous stomatitis, pharyngitis, adenitis (PFAPA)—what it isn't. What is it? *J Pediatr* 135:1–5, 1999.

Martin B, Armanazi Y, Bouquot J, et al: Dental and gingival disorders. In Bluestone CD, Stool SE, editors: *Pediatric otolaryngology*, ed 4, Philadelphia, 2002, WB Saunders.

McDonald R: *Dentistry for the child and adolescent*, ed 8, St. Louis, 2004, Mosby.

Nazif MM, Ruffalo RC: The interaction between dentistry and otolaryngology, *Pediatr Clin North Am* 28:977–1010, 1981.

Nowak A, Casamassimo P: *The handbook of pediatric dentistry*, Chicago, 2007, American Academy of Pediatric Dentistry.

Palmer CA: *Diet and nutrition in oral health*, Upper Saddle River, N.J., 2002, Prentice Hall.

Sanders B, et al: Injuries. In Sanders B, editor: *Pediatric oral and maxillofacial surgery*, St. Louis, 1979, Mosby.

Schuit KE, Johnson JT: Infections of the head and neck, *Pediatr Clin North Am* 28:965–971, 1981.

Sonis A, Zaragoza S: Dental health for the pediatrician, *Curr Opin Pediatr* 13:289–295, 2001.

Vanderas AP: Prevalence of craniomandibular dysfunction in children and adolescents: A review, *Pediatr Dent* 9:312–316, 1987.

Walund K, List T, Dworkin SF: Temporomandibular disorders in children and adolescents: Reliability of a questionnaire, clinical examination, and diagnosis, *J Orofac Pain* 12:42–51, 1998.

ORTHOPEDICS

Vincent F. Deeney | Jennifer Arnold | Morey S. Moreland |
W. Timothy Ward | Holly W. Davis

Children with musculoskeletal injuries and afflictions are brought for care because of pain, deformity, or loss of function. Often the clinical challenge lies not so much in recognizing the impaired or injured part, which in most cases is readily accessible to inspection and examination, but in making an accurate diagnosis in order to plan and initiate appropriate treatment. Because of their rapid physical growth and the special properties of their developing bones, children often pose special problems for the clinician.

Musculoskeletal problems in children fall into several general categories.

1. Trauma (discussed here and in Chapter 6)

2. Congenital problems—malformations resulting from genetic factors and from exposure to teratogens during the first trimester, as well as deformations stemming from insults later in pregnancy, many of which are associated with anomalies of other organ systems (discussed here and in Chapters 1, 2, and 15)

3. Infections (see Chapter 12)

4. Inflammatory processes such as the collagen vascular diseases, the vasculitides, rheumatoid arthritis, and inflammatory bowel disease (see Chapters 7 and 10)

5. Metabolic diseases (see Chapters 9, 10, and 13)

6. Neoplastic disorders (see Chapter 11)

This chapter focuses on primary musculoskeletal problems, and the discussion is divided into eight sections: (1) development of the skeletal system, (2) physical assessment, (3) musculoskeletal trauma, (4) disorders of the neck and spine, (5) disorders of the upper extremity, (6) disorders of the lower extremity, (7) generalized musculoskeletal disorders, and (8) sports medicine.

DEVELOPMENT OF THE SKELETAL SYSTEM

The assessment, diagnosis, and management of pediatric orthopedic problems necessitate a clear understanding of the physiology of the growing musculoskeletal system and especially of the unique properties of growing bone. The process of growth begins in utero and continues until the end of puberty. Linear growth occurs as the result of multiplication of chondrocytes in the epiphyses, which align themselves vertically, forming a transitional zone of endochondral ossification in the metaphyses. The shafts of long bones widen, and flat bones enlarge through the deposition and mineralization of osteoid by the periosteum. Hence genetic and congenital disorders that affect connective tissue (and thus the skeleton) tend to cause abnormal growth. Most commonly this results in dwarfism, with varying degrees of deformity. However, in some conditions such as Marfan syndrome, excessive linear growth occurs, resulting in an abnormally tall stature and unusually long fingers and toes.

The terminal arterial loops and sinusoidal veins that form the vascular bed of growing metaphyses have sluggish blood flow, which increases the risk of thrombosis and of the deposition of bacteria during periods of bacteremia. As a result, there is a greater risk of developing hematogenous osteomyelitis in pediatric patients than in adults. Furthermore, the epiphyseal plates, which are incompletely formed in infancy, are a less effective barrier to extension of infection into adjacent joints, and the relatively thin diaphyseal cortices tend to permit rupture outward under the overlying periosteum. Similarly, penetration of vascular channels through the vertebral end plates into the intervertebral disks makes diskitis more likely than vertebral osteomyelitis in early childhood (see Chapter 12).

A thorough understanding of musculoskeletal development and of the radiographic findings at differing stages is particularly important in the diagnosis and management of orthopedic injuries. At birth only a few epiphyses have begun to ossify; the remainder are cartilaginous and thus are invisible radiographically. With development, other epiphyses begin to ossify, enlarge, and mature in such an orderly fashion that one can estimate a child's age from the number and configuration of ossification centers (Figs. 21-1 and 21-2). The epiphyseal plates (physes), which are sites of cartilaginous proliferation and growth, do not begin to ossify and thereby close until puberty (Fig. 21-3). This process starts and ends earlier in girls than in boys. When skeletal injuries involve sites where ossification has not begun or is incomplete, radiographic findings may appear normal or may not reflect the full extent of the injury. This necessitates greater reliance on clinical findings. Magnetic resonance imaging (MRI) can be of assistance in defining unossified or incompletely ossified structures.

Before closure of the physis during puberty, the growth plate is actually weaker than nearby ligaments. As a result, injuries that occur near joints are more likely to result in physeal disruption than in ligamentous tearing (i.e., sprains and dislocations are seen less commonly in prepubescent children than in adolescents and adults). Similarly, avulsion fractures at sites where strong muscular attachments join secondary ossification centers are unique to children and adolescents. When there is displacement of an epiphyseal fracture and the fragments are not anatomically reduced, growth disturbances may occur. Because the epiphysis may not be ossified, radiographs often fail to reveal the injury, and for this reason children with injuries at or near joints must be examined with meticulous care so that epiphyseal fractures are not missed. Clinically, pain and swelling may be detected over the epiphyseal plate region and, less notably, over the joint itself.

The periosteum of a child is much thicker than that of an adult, strips more easily from the bone, and is rarely disrupted completely when the underlying bone is fractured. Because of

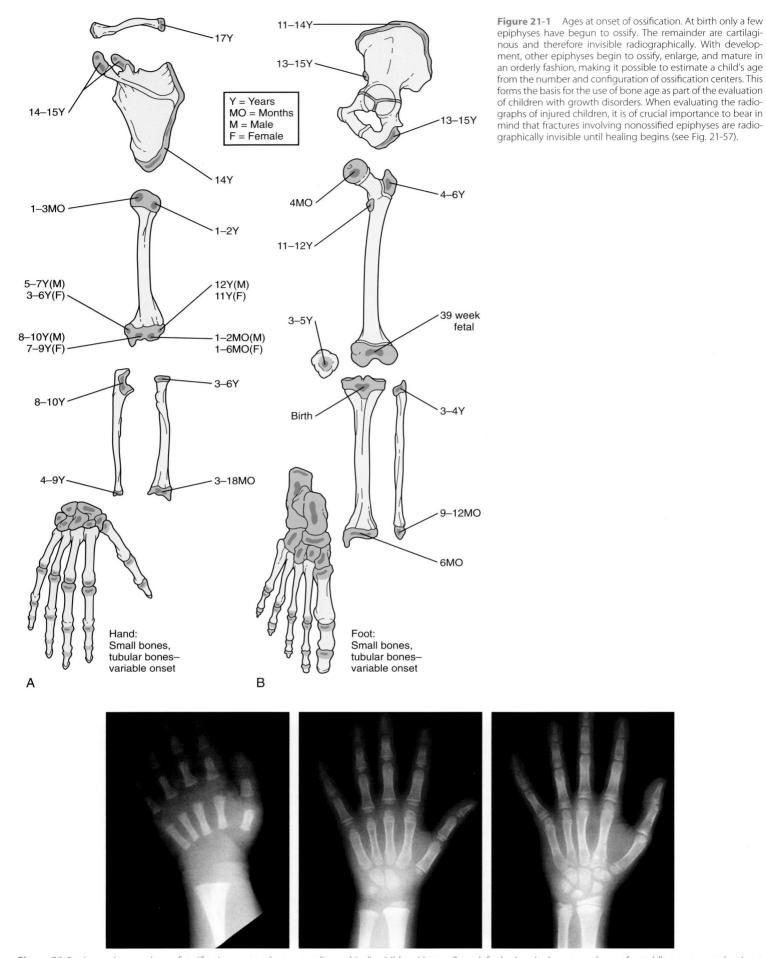

17Y

14–15Y

11–14Y

13–15Y

13–15Y

Y = Years
MO = Months
M = Male
F = Female

14Y

1–3MO

4MO

4–6Y

1–2Y

11–12Y

5–7Y(M)
3–6Y(F)

12Y(M)
11Y(F)

8–10Y(M)
7–9Y(F)

1–2MO(M)
1–6MO(F)

3–5Y

39 week
fetal

8–10Y

3–6Y

Birth

3–4Y

4–9Y

3–18MO

9–12MO

6MO

Hand:
Small bones,
tubular bones–
variable onset

Foot:
Small bones,
tubular bones–
variable onset

A

B

Figure 21-1   Ages at onset of ossification. At birth only a few epiphyses have begun to ossify. The remainder are cartilaginous and therefore invisible radiographically. With development, other epiphyses begin to ossify, enlarge, and mature in an orderly fashion, making it possible to estimate a child's age from the number and configuration of ossification centers. This forms the basis for the use of bone age as part of the evaluation of children with growth disorders. When evaluating the radiographs of injured children, it is of crucial importance to bear in mind that fractures involving nonossified epiphyses are radiographically invisible until healing begins (see Fig. 21-57).

Figure 21-2   Increasing numbers of ossification centers become radiographically visible with age. From left, the hands shown are those of a toddler, a young school-age child, and a young adolescent. Injuries affecting unossified bones or growth centers are invisible radiographically.

Figure 21-3 Ages at physeal closure.

the immature elements in the rapidly growing skeleton of the child, the bone has more viscoelasticity and can sustain plastic deformation more easily than the adult skeleton. Consequently, a given compressive force that would produce a comminuted fracture in an adult tends to be dissipated in a child in part by the bending that occurs in the more flexible bone of the child. Such a force is thus more likely to result in plastic deformation or to produce an incomplete fracture, such as a torus fracture or a greenstick fracture, in a child.

Thus fracture patterns in children often differ from those in adults. Their fractures can be considerably more difficult to detect clinically and radiographically, and because the growing cells in the epiphyseal plate may be injured, growth disturbances may occur. Children do have advantages, however, in that their actively growing bones heal more rapidly and have a remarkable capacity for remodeling.

Finally, numerous genetic, metabolic, endocrine, renal, and inflammatory processes can affect not only growth and ultimate height but also skeletal maturation—in some cases delaying it and in others accelerating it. Comparison of the patient's actual bone age, as determined by the number of radiographically visible ossification centers, with his or her chronologic age can help in the diagnosis of these underlying disorders.

PHYSICAL ASSESSMENT

History

Key historical points in the evaluation of problems not resulting from trauma include the following:

1. Age at onset of symptoms

2. Mode of onset

3. Clinical course, including the manner and rate of progression and associated signs and symptoms

4. Past medical history, with an emphasis on the prenatal and perinatal history in the infant or young child

5. Family history, especially of genetic, metabolic, and musculoskeletal problems

This information helps considerably in narrowing the list of differential diagnostic possibilities.

When the patient's problem is the result of trauma, it is important to obtain the following historical points:

1. The time and place of the accident and whether it was witnessed

2. The mechanism of injury, including the degree of force applied and the direction of force, if known (e.g., if a fall, from what height, onto what surface? Was the child running or walking [momentum]? In what position did the child land? Was there any head injury or loss of consciousness?)

3. The child's behavior since the time of injury (e.g., decreased movement, guarding, refusal to walk or limping, any altered level of consciousness)

4. Complaint of pain (if so, how severe, and can it be localized?)

5. Prior treatment or first aid

6. Past medical history of serious illness and prior injuries

7. Family history of musculoskeletal problems

This information helps localize the site or sites of injury and potential injury severity, points to the risk of possible associated injuries, gives clues to the possible existence of underlying disorders that may predispose to injury, and may occasionally raise a suspicion of abuse.

Physical Examination

The orthopedic examination involves a systematic assessment of posture, stance, and gait; the symmetry or asymmetry of paired musculoskeletal structures and their motion; muscle strength and tone; and neurovascular status. In pediatrics, the patient's developmental level is a major consideration, not only in terms of the interpretation of findings, but also in terms of the manner in which the examination is conducted. Patience and often some degree of creativity are required on the part of the examiner if the patient is very young. Often, much information can be gleaned from an initial period of observation of the child's demeanor and spontaneous activity. This can be assisted by providing age-appropriate toys for him or her to play with while the history is being taken and by engaging the patient in play (if circumstances permit) before starting the more formal physical examination. This also helps to alleviate anxiety and gain the child's trust, enhancing his or her cooperation. As in all examinations of infants and children, taking time to establish the child's trust in the examiner is helpful. After spontaneous activity is observed, the relevant parts of the orthopedic examination are typically done by region.

A complete orthopedic examination that assesses each bone, muscle, joint, tendon, and ligament is lengthy, detailed, and rarely indicated. Even in multiple-trauma victims and patients whose symptoms point toward an underlying systemic disorder, each region is screened and a full assessment done only of those regions where local musculoskeletal abnormalities are found. Similarly, in patients with focal injuries or deformities, the examination can generally be focused on the region involved, with the clinician bearing in mind referral patterns for pain and the maxim that all extremities "begin at

the back." Finally, in performing routine physical examinations on healthy children, after a general screening examination of spontaneous movement, posture, gait, station, and stance, the assessment of the musculoskeletal system is focused on areas at risk for the child's age (e.g., the hip for dislocation in the neonate, the spine for scoliosis in the preadolescent and adolescent).

Regional Musculoskeletal Examination

In the regional examination the area of concern is inspected visually for spontaneous movement, guarding, size, swelling, deformity, and the appearance of overlying skin, and the findings are compared with those for its paired structure. After this, the normal side and then the affected side are gently palpated for warmth, induration, and tenderness. Muscle mass, tone, and reflexes on the affected side are compared with those on the normal side, and the presence or absence of spasm is noted. If asymmetry in muscle mass is detected, the circumference is measured bilaterally at a point equidistant from a fixed bony landmark. The child is then asked to move the extremity or is handed objects to get him or her to do so, and active motion is observed. If this appears limited, passive range of motion is tested first on the normal and then on the affected side, taking care not to cause severe pain. Strength is tested against gravity and then against resistance (Table 21-1), being careful to stay within the limits of pain. Then sensation and vascular status are also evaluated.

Joints are further inspected to determine whether there is erythema, obliteration of landmarks that may indicate the presence of effusion, evidence of deformity, and position of comfort. Further evaluation to detect joint effusion is done by pressing on one side of a visible joint while feeling for the protrusion of fluid on the other. The joints are palpated to check for evidence of heat and tenderness, range of motion is assessed, and evidence of pain on motion is determined.

Assessment of ligamentous stability around joints is discussed under specific sections of the regional examination. However, it is important to remember that in cases of acute trauma, especially when deformity or hemarthrosis is evident on initial assessment, tests of ligamentous stability should be deferred, the extremity splinted, and radiographs obtained to check for possible underlying fracture.

Axial Skeleton and Upper Extremity Examination

Trunk and Neck. With the examiner in front and the patient standing, the sternocleidomastoid muscles, the bony prominences of the clavicles, and the respective heights of the acromioclavicular joints, nipples, and anterior iliac crests and sides of the chest wall are inspected for symmetry. The patient is then turned and viewed from behind, and the shoulder and scapular height, the muscle bulk of the trapezius muscles, and the height of the posterior iliac crests and of the depressions over the sacroiliac joints are checked for symmetry. Trapezius strength is determined by having the patient shrug his or her shoulders, first against gravity and then against resistance, as

Table 21-1	Grading of Muscle Strength
Grade	**Physical Finding**
0/5	No movement seen
1/5	Muscle can move joint with gravity eliminated
2/5	Muscle can move joint against gravity but not against added resistance
3/5	Muscle can move joint against slight resistance
4/5	Muscle can move joint against moderate added resistance
5/5	Normal strength

the examiner presses down on the shoulders. The muscles supplying the scapula are tested by having the patient press his or her outstretched arms against a wall. Winging of the scapula during this maneuver is suggestive of weakness of the serratus anterior muscle. The line of the spinous processes of the vertebrae is observed for straightness, and the position of the head over the trunk is noted. Normally the head is aligned over the midline of the sacrum.

Next, the sternocleidomastoid and paraspinous muscles of the neck are palpated to assess for bulk, tone, tenderness, and spasm, and the spinous processes of the cervical vertebrae are palpated to assess for tenderness and step-off. In the immobilized trauma patient these observations are made largely with the patient supine on a backboard and then log-rolled onto his or her side. Importantly, in checking for neck injury, the cervical spine can be cleared clinically if the patient is awake and alert and has no complaint of neck pain, no evidence of tenderness or paraspinous muscle spasm, and no extremely painful injury elsewhere. If the patient's level of consciousness is not normal or there is a major distracting injury, the cervical spine cannot be cleared, even if radiographic findings are normal, because spinal cord injury can be present in the absence of bony abnormalities.

Range of neck motion is assessed by having the patient move his or her head. A normal child can touch his or her chin to the chest, extend the neck to look directly above, and bend laterally to 45 degrees. He or she is also capable of symmetrical lateral rotation when turning the head from side to side. Strength is tested by applying pressure to the forehead while the patient flexes his or her neck and to the occiput as the patient extends, and by applying resistance to the opposite side of the head as the patient bends and rotates laterally.

Thoracolumbar Spine. Viewed from the side, the normal child has a lordotic curve in the cervical area with a bony prominence at C7, a mild thoracic kyphosis, a lumbar lordosis, and a sacral kyphosis. Each patient is checked for the presence, absence, or accentuation of these curves. The midline of the back is inspected for evidence of abnormal pigmentation and the presence of hemangiomas, nevi, hairy tufts, dimples, masses, or defects, which may be associated with underlying bony or neural anomalies (see Chapter 15).

Flexion, extension, rotation, and lateral bending of the thoracolumbar spine are primarily motions of the thoracolumbar junction and the lumbar area. Most children can bend forward to touch their toes, bend laterally 20 to 30 degrees (with the pelvis held stable by the examiner's hands on the iliac crests), and rotate 20 to 30 degrees in either direction.

Examination of the back for spinal deformity is assisted by the use of the Adams forward bend test (Fig. 21-4). For this, the examiner stands behind the patient, who is then asked to bend forward with arms extended and the palms of the hands

Figure 21-4 Adams forward bend test. **A,** Scoliosis can be difficult to detect on observation of the standing patient. **B,** With the child bending forward and observed from behind, it is much easier to appreciate the asymmetrical trunk rotation seen in scoliosis. **C,** Viewing the patient from the side, one can more easily see even subtle degrees of kyphosis and note lack of reversal of normal lordosis.

together. The surface of the back in the lumbar and thoracic regions is examined for asymmetrical elevation of the paravertebral spinous area, thus indicating a structural rotation of the spine and the possibility of scoliosis (Fig. 21-4, *B*). The examiner should also note any evidence of missing spinous processes (step-off) or their deviation from the midline and palpate the paravertebral muscles for spasm and tenderness. Increased kyphosis, especially in the thoracic region, may be detected when viewing the patient from the side (Fig. 21-4, *C*), as can lack of reversal of the lumbar lordosis, which may indicate muscle spasm or abnormality of the lumbar spine. Leg length inequality may be evaluated during the upright standing portion of this test (see Lower Extremity Examination, later) and, if present, should be corrected with appropriate lifts under the short side in order not to cause a false forward bend test.

Any examination of the spine must include a neurologic assessment of strength, tone, reflexes, and sensation. The straight leg raising test (Fig. 21-5) can be helpful in demonstrating nerve root pathology in patients with slipped disks, spinal or paraspinal masses, or inflammatory processes. The test is performed with the patient lying supine on the examining table. The limb to be tested is grasped behind the ankle and elevated passively into hip flexion with the knee fully extended. This maneuver stretches the sciatic nerve as it passes behind the hip joint, and if one of its several roots has been irritated by a protruded disk, mass, or inflammatory process, pain will be felt with only 15 to 30 degrees of hip flexion. Normally the straight leg can be brought to 90 degrees of hip flexion without difficulty.

Shoulder. When examining the shoulder, first the position of the upper limbs is observed, at the same time noting whether there is any swelling, asymmetry of height, or visible landmarks and looking for any difference in spontaneous movement. Prominent landmarks that are easily palpable include the acromion process lying laterally and subcutaneously, the clavicle, the spine of the scapula, the coracoid process, and the bicipital groove. Any displacement or tenderness of these structures should be noted. Swelling of the glenohumeral joint capsule and atrophy of the shoulder muscles are best appreciated by viewing from above with the patient seated and by comparison with the normal side.

Figure 21-6   Carrying angle. The normal relationship of the extended supinated forearm to the upper arm is not a straight line but involves 5 to 10 degrees of lateral or valgus angulation.

Assessing range of motion is important because many shoulder problems are manifested by a loss of normal motion. The shoulder is a ball-and-socket joint with six components of movement. Abduction, a function of the deltoid muscle, is tested by having the patient raise the extended, supinated arm up so that the hand is directly above the shoulder (180-degree abduction). To test adduction, the patient is asked to flex his or her shoulder to 20 to 30 degrees and then draw the upper arm diagonally across his or her body (75 degrees is normal). Flexion is assessed by having him or her raise the extended pronated arm up and forward until it is parallel to the floor; extension is tested by having him or her return the arm to the neutral position and then lift the arm up and backward (45 to 60 degrees is normal). To check rotation, the upper arm is held to the side with the elbow flexed to 90 degrees and the child is asked to turn the forearm toward the body (medial) and then out to the side (lateral) (60 to 90 degrees is normal).

Elbow. In the normal relationship of the extended, supinated forearm to the upper arm, there is 5 to 10 degrees of lateral (valgus) angulation, termed the *carrying angle* (Fig. 21-6). When this angle is greater than 10 degrees, the deformity is termed *cubitus valgus* and, when less or reversed, *cubitus varus (gunstock deformity)*. The range of motion of the hinge joint of the elbow has four components: extension, a function of the triceps (normally to 0 degrees of flexion); flexion, a function of the biceps (normally to 145 degrees); supination (normally to 90 degrees); and pronation (80 to 90 degrees). The latter two components are tested by having the patient turn the palm up and down respectively, with the elbow flexed.

Because of the proximity of the brachial artery and the median, radial, and ulnar nerves to the elbow joint, injuries of the elbow necessitate a careful neurovascular examination.

Wrist and Hand. During examination of the wrist and hand, one should observe skin color, check capillary refill, and palpate the radial and ulnar pulses to assess circulation. Any swelling or edema should be noted, as well as any abnormal

Figure 21-5   Straight leg raising test. With the patient supine, the limb to be tested is grasped behind the ankle and elevated into hip flexion with the knee in full extension. If pain is produced well before 90 degrees of flexion is achieved, the test is positive, indicating irritation of a sciatic nerve root.

posture or position. The presence of intraarticular fluid in the wrist is manifested by swelling and tenderness, especially evident dorsally, and by restriction of wrist motion. Wrist motion has four components: flexion with the hand held down (normally 70 to 80 degrees); extension with the hand held up (normally 70 degrees); and ulnar and radial deviation (normally 25 degrees and 15 to 20 degrees, respectively).

Examination of hand function can be particularly challenging in young children because of lack of cooperation and developmental limitations. Observation of the position at rest (normally a loose fist with all the fingers pointing in the same direction and with the same degree of flexion) and of use during play is often helpful. Having the parent perform various hand and finger motions while trying to get the child to imitate these can be helpful in some cases. Handing the child a small object such as a key or a thin piece of paper such as a dollar bill may suffice for assessing opposition of thumb to fingers, which in the older child is tested by having him or her touch the tip of the thumb to the tip of the little finger. Normal ranges of motion in the hand are 90 degrees of flexion and 45 degrees of extension for the metacarpophalangeal joints, full extension and 100 degrees of flexion for the proximal interphalangeal (PIP) joints, and full extension and 90 degrees of flexion for the distal interphalangeal joints.

Because the bones of the hand are subcutaneous, displaced fractures and dislocations are readily evident on inspection. Laceration or rupture of the tendons is common because of their superficial location. Those involving flexor tendons result in extensor tendon overpull (Fig. 21-7), with the affected digit lying in greater extension than its neighbors at rest. Conversely, extensor tendon lacerations result in flexor muscle overpull, with the opposite result.

Functional testing of the tendons and intrinsic muscles of the hand is generally possible in older children. They can be asked to extend the fingers at the metacarpophalangeal joints and each interphalangeal joint. Function of the flexor digitorum profundus muscle is tested by holding the PIP joint extended while the patient flexes the tip of the finger. To test the superficialis flexor tendon, adjacent distal interphalangeal

Table 21-2	Signs of Neural Dysfunction with Injury of the Upper Extremity
Nerve	**Sign**
Radial	↓ Strength of wrist and finger extensors ↓ Sensation in web space between thumb and index finger, dorsum of hand to proximal interphalangeal joints, and radial aspect of ring finger
Ulnar	↓ Strength of wrist flexion and adduction ↓ Strength of finger spread ↓ Sensation over ulnar aspect of palm and dorsum of hand, little finger, and ulnar aspect of ring finger
Median	↓ Strength of wrist flexion and abduction ↓ Strength of flexion of proximal interphalangeal joints ↓ Strength of opposition of thumb to base of little finger ↓ Sensation over radial aspect of palm, thumb, index, and long fingers
Anterior interosseous	↓ Strength of flexion of the distal interphalangeal joints of the index finger and thumb

joints are held in extension and the patient is asked to flex the finger being tested at the PIP joint. The intrinsic muscles of the hand are evaluated by having the child adduct and abduct the fingers toward and away from the middle finger. Sensation is best tested using two-point discrimination and pinprick in older children and by touch in very young children.

Muscle strength in the upper extremity is largely tested during assessment of range of motion of the joints, with and without resistance. Signs of neural dysfunction with injury of the upper extremity are listed in Table 21-2.

Lower Extremity Examination

Hip. Examination of the hip begins by assessing gait (see later discussion) and stance, checking the latter to see if the anterior superior and posterior superior iliac spines and the greater trochanters are level. If not, a leg-length discrepancy should be suspected and leg length measured. Total length is measured from the bottom of the anterior superior iliac spine to the medial malleolus of the ankle with the patient supine. If inequality is found, the knees are flexed to 90 degrees with the feet flat on the examination table. If, as the examiner looks from the foot of the examination table, one knee appears higher than the other, the tibias are unequal in length; if one knee is anterior to the other when viewed from the side, the discrepancy involves the femurs. If total leg lengths are equal, the inequality apparent when the patient is standing may be due to pelvic obliquity or flexion contracture of the hip. The latter may also be associated with a compensatory accentuation of lumbar lordosis.

The thighs are checked next for symmetry and signs of atrophy. If atrophy is found, circumference should be measured and compared at a fixed point below the greater trochanters.

Because the hip lies deep and is surrounded by muscles, direct inspection is impossible and palpation is of limited value (although the femoral triangle, greater trochanter, and posterior aspect should be palpated to check for tenderness). As a result, assessment of the position of comfort (abduction and external rotation are seen with effusion, hemarthrosis, and fracture; see Figs. 21-15, *C* and 21-91, *B*), weight bearing, range of motion, and pain on motion are particularly important (for hip examination in the neonate, see Developmental Dislocation of the Hip, later).

Figure 21-7 Extensor tendon overpull. This boy's palm laceration involved the flexor tendons to his index finger. With his hand at rest, his index finger lies in extension, in contrast to his other fingers, which are partially flexed. *(Courtesy Robert Hickey, MD, Children's Hospital of Pittsburgh, Pittsburgh, Pa.)*

Figure 21-8   Thomas test. This test of range of hip extension is performed by flexing both hips, then holding one in flexion while the patient is asked to extend the other leg. **A,** Normally, full extension is achieved. **B,** Inability to fully extend the hip, seen in this boy with Legg-Calvé-Perthes disease, indicates the presence of a flexion contracture of the hip and constitutes a positive Thomas test.

In evaluating range of motion of the hip, care must be taken to distinguish true hip motion from that occurring in combination with pelvic rotation or trunk flexion. The range of hip flexion is normally about 120 degrees. It is tested with the child lying supine. The hip to be tested is passively flexed while the contralateral hip and pelvis are observed or stabilized by one hand. The limit of flexion is reached when movement of the contralateral pelvis is noted. Alternatively, both hips can be flexed simultaneously to stabilize the pelvis and eliminate truncal flexion. The Thomas test is performed by flexing both hips so that the thighs touch the abdomen. Then one is held in place, thereby eliminating lumbar lordosis and movement of the lumbosacral joint, and the patient is asked to extend the hip to be tested. Normally he or she should be able to extend the hip to 0 degrees of flexion (Fig. 21-8, *A*). Failure to do this indicates the presence of a hip flexion contracture, which is a positive result on the Thomas test (Fig. 21-8, *B*). Next, the knee and thigh are held with the hip and knee flexed to 90 degrees and internal and external rotation are tested and recorded in degrees. Abduction and adduction are also checked with the hip flexed to 90 degrees. While the examiner places the thumb and index finger of one hand over the patient's pelvis, attempting to span the distance between the anterior superior iliac spines, the hip to be tested is abducted and then adducted. The limit is determined by the point at which the pelvis begins to move (normally 45 degrees of abduction and 30 degrees of adduction). Extension is tested with the patient prone by having him or her lift the leg up from the table (normal, 20 to 30 degrees). Internal and external rotation are also tested with the patient prone and the hip and leg in extension.

When hip abductor weakness is suspected on the basis of the finding of a gait abnormality, the Trendelenburg test (Fig. 21-9) is performed. This involves having the child stand and asking him or her to lift one leg up. Normally the pelvis should rise slightly on the side of the leg that is lifted. If instead it drops, abductor weakness is present on the opposite side, and the Trendelenburg test is positive.

Knee.   Importantly, knee pain is a common reason for seeking orthopedic care and it is often referred from the hip; thus any patient presenting with knee pain should always be examined for possible limitation of hip motion or pain on motion of the hip.

The knee examination begins with the examiner viewing the joint from the front, side, and back, looking for differences in contour, swelling or masses, and changes in overlying skin. From the front, the knee is inspected for valgus (lower leg points away from the midline) or varus (lower leg deviates toward the midline) deformity and for evidence of effusion, manifested by obliteration of the normal depressions around the patella or by generalized swelling. In viewing the knee from its lateral aspect, the examiner looks for incomplete extension resulting from flexion contracture or excess hyperextension (recurvatum deformity), as well as for symmetry of the tibial tuberosities. From the rear, the popliteal fossae are checked for symmetry and evidence of swelling. The thighs are also observed for comparative size and contour.

The knees are palpated to assess warmth and check for tenderness along the medial and lateral joint lines, the medial and collateral ligaments, the patella and its supporting ligaments, the femoral and tibial condyles, and the tibial tubercles. Palpation is easier with the knee flexed because the skeletal landmarks are more readily seen and felt, and the muscles, tendons, and ligaments are relaxed in this position.

When there is evidence of a marked effusion, landmarks are obscured and the patella is readily ballotable. This is seen with intraarticular hemorrhage, arthritis, and synovitis, and range of motion is usually significantly limited. If landmarks are only mildly obscured (suggestive of a mild joint effusion or fluid collection in the bursae), pressure should be applied over the suprapatellar pouch with the thumb and index finger of one hand, milking down any fluid present while simultaneously pushing the patella up toward the

Figure 21-9   Trendelenburg test. This test is performed to check for weakness of the hip abductors. While lifting his right foot, this patient's left abductor muscles stabilize his pelvis with a slight rise of the pelvis on the right. If left hip abductor weakness were present, the right pelvis would tilt downward when the right leg was lifted.

Figure 21-10   Test for small knee joint effusions. Moderate pressure is applied over the suprapatellar pouch with the thumb and index finger of one hand, milking any fluid present downward. The other hand simultaneously pushes the patella up toward the femur. When an effusion is present, the patella becomes ballotable and a palpable click is felt as the patella strikes the front of the distal femur.

femoral condyles with the other hand (Fig. 21-10). If fluid is present, the patella is ballotable and a palpable click is noted as the patella strikes the front of the femur.

The knee is primarily a hinge joint and is normally capable of 130 to 140 degrees of flexion and 5 degrees of hyperextension. However, it can also rotate approximately 10 degrees internally and externally, and this involves rotation of the tibia on the femur. Flexion is tested with the patient either sitting or lying prone. To test extension, the examiner can have the patient either sit and try to straighten the leg to 0 degrees of flexion or try to lift the straightened leg from the examination table while lying supine. Rotation is assessed by turning the foot medially and then laterally with the knee flexed.

With the knees flexed to 80 to 90 degrees, the patellas should face forward when viewed from the front and be located squarely at the ends of the femurs when seen from the side. The apprehension test (Fig. 21-11) is performed to check for a subluxating or dislocating patella. With the patient sitting, the examiner supports the lower leg and holds the knee flexed to 30 degrees. The patella is then gently pushed laterally. Any abnormal amount of lateral displacement, pain, or apprehension in response to this maneuver indicates a positive test.

Ligamentous stability of the knee should be assessed in the mediolateral and anteroposterior planes. In patients with acute injuries, especially those involving significant pain and swelling, this should be deferred until radiographs have been obtained to check for associated fractures.

The abduction/adduction stress test is used to determine the degree of stability of the medial and lateral collateral ligaments. With the supine patient's thigh moved to the side of the examination table and the knee flexed to 30 degrees, the examiner holds the distal thigh in one hand while grasping the inside of the lower leg with the other. To test the medial collaterals, the examiner applies valgus stress by pressing medially against the distal thigh with the upper hand while gently abducting the lower leg. To check the lateral collaterals, the examiner applies varus stress by pressing laterally on the inside of the distal thigh while gently adducting the lower leg. Normally the joint line should open no more than 1 cm on either side.

Anteroposterior ligamentous stability is provided by the anterior and posterior cruciate ligaments of the knee. They are tested by the anterior and posterior drawer and Lachman tests. The former are performed with the patient supine; the hip and knee flexed to 45 and 90 degrees, respectively; and the foot planted on the examining table, stabilized by the examiner's thigh or buttock. The examiner then grasps the proximal tibia with his or her fingers behind the knee and the thumbs over the anterior joint line and gently pulls and pushes (Fig. 21-12). In a positive anterior drawer test, the tibia moves forward more than 0.5 to 1 cm, indicating instability of the anterior cruciate ligament. Movement backward more than 0.5 to 1 cm indicates instability of the posterior cruciate ligament. In the Lachman test (Fig. 21-13) for anterior cruciate tears, the knee is flexed to 15 degrees. The examiner grasps the distal femur with one hand and the proximal tibia with the other. The thumb of the lower hand is placed on the joint line, and the femur is pushed backward as the tibia is pulled forward. Abnormal anterior displacement of the tibia on the femur can be seen and felt if instability is present. The amount of excursion is estimated in millimeters, and the end point is recorded as soft or firm.

Ankle. Examination of the ankle begins with inspection for evidence of deformity, swelling, change in color of overlying skin, and abnormal position (especially with weight bearing). Palpation is performed to detect warmth and to localize tenderness. In the neutral position the long axis of the foot should be at 90 degrees to the long axis of the tibia. Normally a child

Figure 21-11   Apprehension test for a subluxating or dislocating patella. With the patient sitting and the knee supported in 30 degrees of flexion, the patella is gently pushed laterally. Any abnormal amount of lateral displacement, pain, or apprehension constitutes a positive test.

Figure 21-12   Anterior and posterior drawer tests for cruciate ligament stability. With the patient supine, the hips flexed to 45 degrees, and the knees flexed to 90 degrees, the examiner grasps the proximal tibia with his or her fingers behind the knee and thumbs on the anterior joint line and makes a gentle pull–push motion. Forward movement of more than 0.5 to 1 cm indicates anterior cruciate instability, representing a positive anterior drawer test. Similar posterior motion on pushing indicates posterior cruciate instability, representing a positive posterior drawer test.

Figure 21-13 Lachman test for anterior cruciate ligament tear. With the knee flexed to 15 degrees, the distal femur is grasped with one hand and the proximal tibia with the other, with the thumb on the joint line. The tibia is moved forward while the femur is pushed backward. Any abnormal displacement of the tibia on the femur indicates anterior cruciate instability and represents a positive test.

can dorsiflex 20 degrees and plantar flex 30 to 50 degrees from the neutral position, as well as invert and evert approximately 5 degrees. Dorsiflexion and plantar flexion can be checked by observing passive and active motion (with and without resistance) but are perhaps most easily tested by having the ambulating child walk on his or her heels and toes, respectively. Similarly, inversion is tested by having him or her walk on the outside of the feet and eversion by having him or her walk on the medial sides.

Tests for ligamentous instability can be important after severe ankle sprains. The anterior drawer test is used to assess the stability of the anterior talofibular ligament. With the patient's legs dangling over the side of the examination table and the foot in a few degrees of plantar flexion, the examiner grasps the anterior aspect of the distal tibia with one hand while holding the calcaneus cupped in the palm of the other. The calcaneus is then drawn anteriorly while the tibia is pushed posteriorly. Normally there should be no movement, but with instability of the anterior talofibular ligament, the talus slides anteriorly. Lateral instability is seen only with major tears of the anterior talofibular and calcaneofibular ligaments, occasionally accompanied by tears of the posterior talofibular ligament, and is tested by inverting the calcaneus with one hand while grasping the distal tibia with the other. When instability is present, the talus gaps and rocks in the ankle mortise. Medial instability is exceptionally rare because of the strength of the fan-shaped deltoid ligament. To test for medial instability, the tibia and calcaneus are held in the same manner as they are in testing lateral instability, but the foot is everted instead. Gross gaping of the ankle mortise is felt when there is a major tear.

Gait and Gait Disturbances

Between the onset of walking and 3 years of age, children tend to have a wide-based gait and toddlers often hold their arms out to the side to assist balance. By 3 years of age, children achieve a normal smooth and rhythmic heel-to-toe gait, consisting of two main phases: stance and swing. The stance phase begins when the heel strikes the ground, bears all the weight, and progresses to foot flat, midstance, and push-off as weight is transferred from the heel to the metatarsal heads. The swing phase starts with acceleration after push-off and progresses through midswing to deceleration just before heel strike. During the swing phase, as the leg moves forward, so does the opposite arm. Because stance occupies 60% of the time and weight is borne in this phase, most gait disorders are more evident during the stance phase than during the swing phase. Normally the distance between the two heels

(width of the base) is between 5 and 10 cm, the pelvis and trunk shift laterally about 2.5 cm from stance to stance, the center of gravity rises and falls no more than 5 cm, and the pelvis rotates forward about 40 degrees during swing.

Gait is best observed by having the patient walk back and forth in a hall or in a room with a mirror at one end. As the patient walks, the examiner focuses first on overall movement and then on the motion of the pelvis, hips, thighs, knees, lower legs, ankles, and feet in succession, both coming and going. In doing so, he or she looks for the pattern of heel-to-toe motion, for shortening of the stance phase, for evidence of limitation of joint motion or weakness, and for positional changes of the extremities. Checking the patient's shoes for signs of abnormal wear is also helpful.

Most acute and many chronic disturbances of gait in childhood are caused by pain. Others stem from weakness or spasticity caused by neurologic or muscular disorders, from leg length inequality, or from deformity. Important historical points are the time of onset of the abnormal gait and the circumstances surrounding it; the duration; whether the abnormal gait is constant or intermittent and, if intermittent, the time of day it is most apparent (A.M., juvenile rheumatoid arthritis; P.M., neuromuscular disorders—symptoms becoming more apparent with fatigue); and its relation to activity or exercise including its effect on running or climbing stairs. The examiner should note any associated pain and its location, bearing in mind referral patterns (low back to buttocks and lateral thigh; hip to groin, medial thigh, knee, and sometimes buttock) and attempting to determine whether the pain is constant (suggestive of tumor or infection) or intermittent.

Gait Disturbances Stemming from Pain, Limb Length Inequality, or Stiffness

An antalgic gait is a limp caused by pain on weight bearing that results in shortening of the stance phase on the affected side. It can be due to pain referred from the back or pain anywhere in the lower extremity. Causes include trauma, pathologic fracture, infection, inflammatory disorders and other sources of arthritis, malignancy, tight shoes, foreign body in the shoe, and a lesion on the sole of the foot. Careful physical examination combined with a complete history usually enables localization of the problem.

Patients with leg length inequality manifest depression of the trunk and pelvis during the stance phase on the shorter leg and circumduction of the longer leg during swing. Some children try to compensate for the leg length inequality by toe-walking on the shorter extremity.

Patients with limited hip motion compensate by thrusting the pelvis and trunk forward in the swing phase. When knee flexion is limited, children tend to hike up the pelvis on the involved side during the swing phase and circumduct the leg to clear the foot from the floor. A circumduction gait can also be related to a painful condition involving the ankle or a limitation of ankle motion. By circumducting the leg laterally during swing phase, the patient reduces the need for ankle motion.

Gait Disturbances Resulting from Weakness or Spasticity

Patients with weakness of the hip abductors (gluteus medius muscle) have a Trendelenburg gait. Because they are unable to maintain a level pelvis and linear progression of their center of gravity, their pelvis tilts toward the unsupported side and their shoulder lurches toward the weak side during stance phase to maintain their center of gravity over the foot. Patients with weakness of the gluteus maximus (seen most commonly in children with Duchenne muscular dystrophy) have to hyperextend their trunk and pelvis to maintain their center of gravity posterior to the hip joint (see Chapter 15). Proximal muscle weakness may also be demonstrated by observing a child getting up from the floor unassisted. A Gower sign indicates weak hip extensors and abductors, necessitating that the patient use his arms to assist in standing by placing his hands on his anterior thighs and pushing up, progressively moving his hands upward along the thighs until erect posture is achieved (see Chapter 15). Children with weakness of the quadriceps femoris muscle may have a relatively normal gait on level ground but difficulty climbing stairs. Weakness of the dorsiflexors of the foot results in foot drop and a steppage gait. Because the foot hangs down during the swing phase, the patient must lift the knee higher than usual to help the foot clear the floor and the forefoot tends to slap the floor on impact because smooth deceleration of the foot cannot be controlled. When the plantar flexors are weak, the patient is unable to push off at the end of the stance phase and so the heel and forefoot come off the floor at the same time.

An equine gait, characterized by toe-walking or a toe-to-heel sequence during the stance phase, is seen in children with heel cord contracture and limited dorsiflexion. It is usually indicative of an underlying neurologic problem with spasticity. Patients with spastic cerebral palsy who are able to ambulate often manifest a stiff-legged scissors gait, in which one foot crosses over the other during the swing phase. Vestibular or cerebellar dysfunction or generalized weakness tends to result in a wide-based ataxic gait because of abnormal balance. Absence of the normal arm swing with walking is seen in patients with paresis or cerebellar disease.

Intoeing and Out-toeing. The angular difference between the long axis of the foot and the forward line of progression during walking is called the *foot progression angle*. A minus value is assigned to intoeing, a plus value to out-toeing. The normal range varies from 5 to 10 degrees to 10 to 20 degrees, respectively. The remaining rotational profile of the lower extremities can be examined with the patient in the prone position (Fig. 21-14). The foot axis can be determined by a line marked from the middle of the heel on the plantar surface to the lateral side

Figure 21-14   Evaluation of the rotational profile of the lower extremities. **A,** The foot axis is determined by a line marked from midheel to the lateral aspect of the second toe. Hip excursion is the difference between the angular measure of maximal prone internal rotation **(B)** and maximal prone external rotation **(C).** The tibia–fibula axis is determined by comparing the axis of the plane of motion of the knee with the patient prone and knees flexed **(D)** to the transmalleolar axis **(E).**

of the second toe (Fig. 21-14, *A*). The hip excursion is the difference between the angular measure of the maximal prone internal rotation (Fig. 21-14, *B*) and that for external rotation (Fig. 21-14, *C*), and in the young child is usually negative, representing more internal rotation than external rotation. In the adolescent and adult, usually there is more external rotation, or a positive hip excursion angle. Finally, the axis of the tibia and fibula can be determined by looking down the lower extremity in the prone knee-flexed position and comparing the axis of the plane of motion of the knee (Fig. 21-14, *D*) with the transmalleolar axis (Fig. 21-14, *E*) estimated by palpating the malleoli. The normal axis is 15 to 25 degrees externally rotated.

Femoral anteversion, internal tibial torsion, and metatarsus adductus are common causes of excessive intoeing, or pigeon toe, and femoral eversion and external tibial torsion are common causes of out-toeing, or slew foot (see Disorders of the Lower Extremity, later).

MUSCULOSKELETAL TRAUMA

The normal impulsiveness and inquisitiveness of children combined with their lack of caution and love of energetic activities place them at a relatively high risk for accidental injury. The incidence of trauma is further increased by the prevalence of child abuse (see Chapter 6). In fact, beyond infancy, trauma is the leading cause of death in children and adolescents and is a source of significant morbidity. Musculoskeletal injuries are common, whether seen in isolation or as part of multisystem trauma. Although the management of life-threatening injuries to the airway, circulation, and central nervous system (CNS) must take precedence over treatment of accompanying musculoskeletal injuries in cases of multiple trauma, it must be kept in mind that fractures can result in significant blood loss. This is particularly true of pelvic and femoral fractures. Furthermore, prompt attention must be given to assessment of the status of neurovascular structures distal to obvious fractures because failure to recognize compromise may result in permanent loss of function. Finally, traumatic hip dislocations must be reduced within 6 to 12 hours if the risk of aseptic necrosis and long-term morbidity is to be minimized.

Fractures

Diagnosis

One of the many variables that complicate the diagnosis of the skeletally injured child is that the child, already in pain, is frightened by his or her recent experience and by the strangeness of the hospital or emergency department setting. Many children are too young to give a firsthand history, and the cooperation of toddlers is often limited. The parents are likely to be anxious as well. A calm, empathetic manner is necessary to allay their fears. Taking a thorough history before making any attempt to perform a physical assessment helps the examiner establish rapport with the patient and the family. This should include questions concerning the type and direction of the injuring force, the position of the involved extremity at the time of the accident, and the events immediately following the injury such as measures taken at the scene of the accident. The presence of underlying disorders and the possibility of contamination of an open wound should be determined as well. Physicians also should be alert to signs suggestive of inflicted injury or child abuse. These include a history in which the mechanism of injury does not fit the type and/or severity of the fracture found, an unusual delay in presentation, and/or radiographic evidence of old healing fractures for which no medical attention was ever sought.

In cases of suspected fracture, splinting, elevation, and topical application of ice may help reduce discomfort and local swelling. Splinting is particularly important for displaced and unstable fractures because it prevents further soft tissue injuries and reduces the risk of fat embolization. When pain is moderate to severe and there are no cardiovascular or CNS contraindications, analgesia should be administered promptly. Contrary to the opinion of many physicians, this does not obscure physical findings. Tenderness is not reduced significantly, swelling remains, and patient cooperation during the examination may be considerably greater.

Before beginning the physical examination, it is wise for the examiner to talk with the child to further gain his or her trust. Older infants and toddlers are often more comfortable when allowed to sit on a parent's lap, and use of puppets or toys can reduce fear and help gain their cooperation. Because comparison of paired extremities is an integral part of orthopedic assessment, it is best to begin by examining the uninjured side and it is wise to defer palpation of the most likely site of the injury on the affected side until last. If young children are highly anxious, it can be useful to instruct the parent in how to perform passive range of motion and palpation.

The first step in the physical examination is visual inspection of the injured area. The gross position of the extremity should be noted, and attention given to the presence or absence of deformity, distortion or abnormal angulation, and longitudinal shortening (Fig. 21-15). The overlying skin and soft tissues are examined for evidence of swelling, ecchymoses, abrasions, punctures, and lacerations. Comparison with the opposite extremity and measurement of circumference can be helpful when findings are subtle.

The location of open wounds is important in ascertaining whether an underlying fracture is open or closed and in assessing the risk of joint penetration. Small puncture wounds or lacerations overlying bony structures from which a bloody, fatty exudate is oozing usually reflect communication with the medullary cavity of a fractured bone. Similarly, punctures or tears over joints that weep serous or serosanguineous fluid, especially when drainage is increased on moving the joint, must be assumed to communicate with the joint capsule (Fig. 21-16, *A*). In patients with penetrating joint injuries, radiographs may demonstrate air in the joint, but absence of this does not rule out capsular penetration (Fig. 21-16, *B*). Probing of open wounds that are highly likely to communicate with a fracture or joint is contraindicated. The wound should be cleaned and covered with a sterile dressing until its extent can be determined under sterile conditions in the operating room.

After inspection of the most obviously injured area, palpation and assessment of active and passive motion can be performed. It is crucial to remember that in examining an injured limb the entire extremity must be evaluated in order to detect less obvious associated injuries. Localized swelling and tenderness on palpation are significant findings and should alert the examiner to the high likelihood of an underlying fracture. Pain on motion and limitation of motion signal the need for careful scrutiny as well. Assessment of motion involves observation of spontaneous movement, attempts to get the patient to voluntarily move the involved part through its expected range, and passive movement. Particular attention should be paid to the adjacent proximal and distal joints to avoid missing associated injuries. It can be difficult, however, to determine whether motion is limited because of pain, an associated injury, or fear and lack of cooperation.

Clinical findings vary depending on the nature of the fracture. Undisplaced growth plate fractures typically present with mild, localized swelling and point tenderness at the level of the epiphysis (Fig. 21-17). Because ligamentous injury is relatively uncommon in a child, the finding of point tenderness

Figure 21-15 Visible abnormalities seen on inspection in children with fractures. **A,** Distortion and angulation of the distal forearm in a child with fractures of the radius and ulna. **B,** Swelling and angulation of the proximal thigh resulting from a femur fracture. **C,** Longitudinal shortening of the thigh in a child with a proximal femur fracture. Note the characteristic externally rotated position of the injured leg. The child was struck by a car, sustaining a fracture of the femoral neck.

Figure 21-16 **A,** Penetrating injury of the knee. This child was struck by a stone propelled by the blades of a power lawn mower. Although the laceration appeared to be minor, serosanguineous fluid flowed from it on movement of the knee, suggesting penetration of the joint capsule. This was confirmed on exploration in the operating room. **B,** Air is seen within the knee joint and in the overlying soft tissues in a child who sustained a deep laceration that penetrated the joint capsule. (**A,** *Courtesy Bruce Watson, MD.*)

Figure 21-17 Salter-Harris type I fracture of the distal fibula. **A,** Slight swelling is present over the lateral malleolus. The degree of swelling can be truly appreciated only by comparing the injured ankle with its normal counterpart, shown in **(B).** The patient had point tenderness over the affected malleolus. The findings differ from those seen in an ankle sprain, in which tenderness and swelling are greatest over the ligaments inferior to the malleolus (see Fig. 21-65).

Figure 21-18   Fracture with overlying soft tissue swelling. This child has a displaced supracondylar fracture of the distal humerus with moderate soft tissue swelling. The degree of swelling becomes evident if the size of the elbow area is compared with the size of the patient's wrist.

should suffice to prompt treating the injury as a fracture until proven otherwise. Often initial radiographs appear normal and the fracture is confirmed only on follow-up when repeat radiographs disclose evidence of healing. Swelling is typically mild and occasionally imperceptible in cases of torus or buckle fractures and of undisplaced transverse and spiral fractures. Careful palpation should disclose focal tenderness, however. Usually, the patient also experiences some degree of discomfort on motion in some planes or on weight bearing, but it must be remembered that limitation of movement or function can be minimal in patients with such incomplete fractures. In contrast, fractures that completely disrupt the bone and displaced fractures are accompanied by more prominent swelling; more diffuse tenderness; and severe pain, which is markedly increased on motion (Fig. 21-18; see also Fig. 21-15, *A* and *B*). Crepitus may also be evident on gentle palpation. In examining children with these findings, manipulation must be kept to a minimum to prevent further injury.

Assessment of neurovascular function distal to the injury is essential in evaluating any child with a potential fracture. This includes checking the integrity of pulses and speed of capillary refill, as well as testing sensory and motor function. Strength and sensation should be compared with those of the contralateral extremity. Assessment of two-point discrimination is probably the best test of sensory function. Evidence of neurovascular compromise necessitates urgent, often operative, orthopedic treatment. In addition, this assessment is crucial before and after reduction of displaced fractures to determine whether the procedure itself has impaired function in any way. Persistence of intense pain after fracture reduction should provoke suspicion of ischemia.

Supracondylar fractures of the humerus, fractures of the distal femoral shaft and proximal tibia, fracture–dislocations of the elbow and knee, and severely displaced ankle fractures are particularly likely to be associated with neurovascular injury.

Even relatively minor fractures of the tibia, forearm bones, metatarsals, and femur can result in compartment syndrome, in which bleeding and edema collection within a closed fascial compartment produce increased pressure that causes neurovascular compromise and muscle ischemia. This should be strongly suspected in patients who complain of intense pain that is aggravated by passive stretching of the muscles. On palpation the area is noted to be swollen and tense, at times even hard. The patient may complain of paresthesias and show pallor and decreased pulses. However, it is important also to be aware of the fact that vascular compromise can be

present in a patient who has normal distal pulses and good peripheral perfusion (see Compartment Syndromes, later).

In all cases of suspected extremity fractures the injured part should be properly splinted and elevated, an ice pack applied, and analgesia administered while the patient awaits transport to the radiography suite. However, to obtain high-quality radiographs, obstructing splints must be removed temporarily. This presents no major problem in patients with partial or nondisplaced fractures but can create difficulties in patients with severe displaced fractures. To ensure that manipulation is minimal in these patients, splint removal, positioning for radiographs, and splint reapplication should be supervised by a physician and not done merely at the discretion of the x-ray technician.

At a minimum, two radiographs taken at 90-degree angles are obtained, anteroposterior (AP) and lateral views being the most common. Oblique views are helpful in fully disclosing the nature and extent of many fracture patterns, especially when the injury involves the ankle, elbow, hand, or foot. They can also prove useful in detecting subtle spiral fractures and in cases in which the AP and lateral views are normal, yet a fracture is strongly suspected. Radiographs should include the joints immediately proximal and distal to a fractured long bone, because there may be associated bony or soft tissue injuries in these areas as well. Such associated injuries easily can be missed on clinical examination when assessment of motion is limited by pain or when patient cooperation is limited. It is necessary to obtain comparison views of the opposite side, especially when evaluating patients with suspected physeal injuries who may have very subtle radiographic abnormalities. These views can also prove invaluable in detecting cortical disruptions. In some cases of displaced or angulated fractures, potentially complex intraarticular fractures, and vertebral and pelvic fractures, a computed tomography (CT) scan can be useful. A bone scan may be necessary to detect subtle stress fractures.

Particular care should be taken in interpreting pediatric radiographs because of the high incidence of subtle or even normal findings in patients with fractures. If the clinical picture strongly suggests a fracture, appropriate treatment should be initiated, even if the radiograph appears normal. Reassessment in 1 to 2 weeks can then clarify the exact nature of the injury.

Fracture Patterns

Fractures should be described in terms of anatomic location, direction of the fracture line, type of fracture, and degree of angulation and of displacement. When the growth plate is involved, use of the Salter-Harris classification system is recommended.

Any specific mechanism of injury results in a readily definable pattern of force application, which tends to produce a typical fracture pattern. Because of this, it is often possible to infer the likely mechanism of injury once the fracture pattern is documented radiographically. If the vector of the direct force is perpendicular to the bone, a transverse fracture is most likely to result, whereas direct force applied at any angle to the bone produces an oblique fracture pattern. Examples of situations resulting in transverse and short oblique fractures include falls in which an extremity strikes the edge of a table, counter, or chair; direct blows with an object such as a stick; and karate chops. These fractures are commonly seen as a result of accidents or fights and in the battered child syndrome. Comminuted fractures generally result from high-velocity, direct forces such as those characteristic of vehicular accidents, falls from heights, or gunshot wounds. Impacted fractures are produced by forces oriented in a direction parallel to the long axis of the bone. Application of indirect force

Figure 21-19 Longitudinal fracture. During a motocross competition this teenager missed a jump and was thrown 20 feet in the air, then fell to the pavement below, landing directly on his foot. The force of the impact was transmitted upward through his ankle, resulting in this vertical tibia fracture.

Figure 21-20 Transverse fracture of the midportion of the clavicle. The fracture line is perpendicular to the long axis of the bone.

commonly results in spiral, greenstick, or torus fractures in children.

A common example of a nondisplaced spiral fracture is the toddler's fracture (see Fig. 21-43), which results from a fall with a twist. Typically, the child was either running, turned, and then fell; jumped and fell with a twist; or got his or her foot caught and fell while twisting to extricate himself or herself. If a child's arm or leg is forcibly pulled and twisted, a similar fracture pattern may be seen. Greenstick and torus fractures of the radius or ulna are incurred usually when the child falls on an outstretched arm with the wrist dorsiflexed. Vigorous repetitive shaking while holding a child by the

hands, feet, or chest results in small metaphyseal chip or bucket-handle fractures, a major feature of the shaken-baby syndrome (see Chapter 6). Table 21-3 summarizes the major features of these various fracture patterns, which are illustrated in Figures 21-19 through 21-27.

The anatomic location of the fracture line simply refers to that portion of the bone to which the injury force was applied. Table 21-4 presents types of fractures classified by anatomic location. These fractures are illustrated in Figures 21-28 through 21-36. There is some degree of overlap in this method of categorization, however.

Physeal Fractures

An estimated 15% of all fractures in children involve the physis. Because the adjacent epiphyseal plate is not ossified in the young child and therefore is invisible on a radiograph, the fracture may be mistaken for a minor sprain or missed altogether, only to manifest itself at a later date in the appearance of slowed or failed longitudinal limb growth or in the development of an angular deformity. Even if diagnosed and properly treated, physeal injuries may still result in longitudinal or angular abnormalities. This risk is especially high in children with physeal fractures involving the distal femur,

Table 21-3	Patterns of Fractures	
Fracture Pattern	**Major Feature**	**Radiographic Appearance**
Longitudinal	Fracture line is parallel to the axis of a long bone	Fig. 21-19
Transverse	Fracture line is perpendicular to the axis of a long bone	Fig. 21-20; and see Fig. 21-28
Oblique	Fracture line is at an angle relative to the axis of a bone	Fig. 21-21
Spiral	Fracture line takes a curvilinear course around the axis of a bone	Fig. 21-22; and see Fig. 21-43
Impacted	Bone ends are crushed together, producing an indistinct fracture line	Fig. 21-23
Comminuted	Fracturing forces produce more than two separate fragments	Fig. 21-24
Bowing	Bone bends to the point of plastic deformation without fracturing	Fig. 21-25
Greenstick	Fracture is complete except for a portion of the cortex on the compression side of the fracture, which is only plastically deformed	Fig. 21-26; and see Fig. 21-25, B
Torus	Bone buckles and bends rather than breaks	Fig. 21-27; and see Fig. 21-29

Figure 21-21 Oblique fracture of the midportion of the femur. The fracture line is angled relative to the axis of the bone.

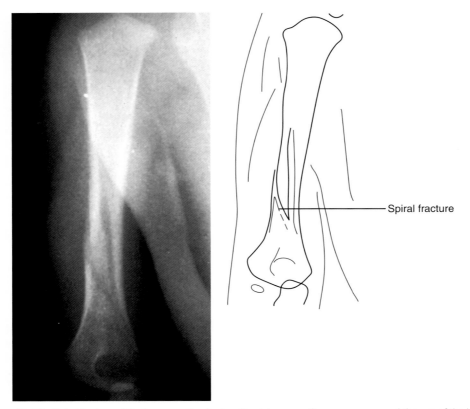

Figure 21-22   Spiral fracture of the humerus. The fracture line takes a curvilinear course around the axis of the bone.

Figure 21-23   Impacted fracture of the base of the proximal phalanx resulting from axial loading. The fracture line is indistinct, and the fragments appear to be crushed together. The fracture does not actually involve the growth plate but is located just distal to it in the proximal metaphysis.

proximal tibia, or radial head and neck. Most physeal disruptions occur through the zone of cartilage cell hypertrophy within the physeal plate and thus do not result in permanent damage to the plate. However, a small proportion of disruptions involve the resting or germinal layer of the physis and may disrupt the cells permanently, resulting in eventual deformity despite adequate reduction of the fracture fragments.

Because of the potential for long-term morbidity in patients with physeal fractures, great attention has been focused on the classification, diagnosis, treatment, and prognosis of physeal fractures. The Salter-Harris classification scheme is the system most commonly used in North America to classify physeal injuries (Fig. 21-37).

Salter-Harris Type I

A Salter-Harris type I injury consists of a fracture running horizontally through the physis itself, resulting in a variable degree of separation of the epiphysis from the metaphysis. The amount of separation depends on the degree of periosteal disruption. Radiographs are often normal; hence the diagnosis frequently must be made clinically on the basis of the findings of point tenderness and mild soft tissue swelling over the site of an epiphysis (Fig. 21-38; see also Fig. 21-17). This injury usually results from a shearing force. Prognosis is usually favorable.

Salter-Harris Type II

Also produced by shearing forces, a Salter-Harris type II injury consists of a fracture line running a variable distance through the physis and exiting through the metaphysis on the side opposite the site of fracture initiation. A fragment consisting of the entire epiphysis with an attached metaphyseal fragment is thus produced (Fig. 21-39). Prognosis is generally favorable with adequate reduction.

Text continued on page 824

Figure 21-24 Comminuted fracture of the femur secondary to a gunshot wound. Notice the numerous small fragments of bone in the adjacent soft tissues.

Myriad bone fragments

Comminuted fracture

Figure 21-25 Plastic deformation. **A,** While playing soccer, this school-age child fell onto his outstretched arm. On impact another player who fell with him landed on the arm, resulting in this bowing deformity of the forearm. **B,** On x-ray plastic deformation of both the ulna and radius are seen, along with a greenstick fracture of the radius. This necessitated manipulation under anesthesia to straighten the arm before casting.

Figure 21-26 Greenstick fracture of the distal radius. **A,** In this anteroposterior view of the distal radius, a fracture line is seen that is complete except for a portion of the cortex on the compression side of the fracture. **B,** The lateral radiograph demonstrates more clearly the disrupted and compressed cortices. This resulted from a fall on the outstretched arm with the wrist in dorsiflexion.

Figure 21-27   Torus fracture of the distal radius resulting from a fall on an outstretched arm. **A,** An anteroposterior radiograph of the wrist shows a minor torus or buckle fracture of the radius. **B,** The lateral radiograph shows the dorsal location of the deformity. This injury can be expected to completely remodel.

Table 21-4	Classification of Fractures by Anatomic Location	
Type	**Site**	**Radiographic Appearance**
Diaphyseal	Fracture involves the central shaft of a long bone	Fig. 21-28; and see Figs. 21-21, 21-22, and 21-25
Metaphyseal	Fracture involves the widened end of a long bone	Fig. 21-29; and see Fig. 21-26 and Chapter 6
Epiphyseal	Fracture involves the chondro-osseous end of a long bone. Such fractures can also be classified as Salter-Harris fractures	Fig. 21-30
Articular	Fracture involves the cartilaginous joint surface	Fig. 21-31; see also Figs. 21-40 and 21-41
Intercondylar	Fracture is located between the condyles of a joint. This is one variant of articular fracture and could also be subclassified as a Salter-Harris fracture	Fig. 21-31, *A*
Physeal	Fracture involves the growth center of long bone. These are subclassified according to the Salter-Harris system	Fig. 21-32
Condylar	Fracture traverses the condyle of a joint	Fig. 21-33
Supracondylar	Fracture line is located just proximal to the condyles of a joint	Fig. 21-34
Epicondylar	Fracture involves an area juxtaposed to the condylar surface of a joint	Fig. 21-35
Subcapital	Fracture is located just below the epiphyseal head of certain bones	Fig. 21-36

Figure 21-28   Diaphyseal fracture. A transverse fracture line crosses the diaphyseal region of the femur. A moderate amount of overlap exists at the fracture site.

Metaphyseal buckle fracture

Figure 21-29   Metaphyseal fracture. This lateral radiograph of the wrist shows a dorsal buckle fracture of the distal radial metaphysis. This fracture resulted from a fall on the outstretched arm with the wrist dorsiflexed and is a common injury in children.

Figure 21-30 Epiphyseal fracture. A fracture involving the medial aspect of the epiphysis of the distal tibia is seen in this anteroposterior radiograph of the ankle in a 4-year-old girl. A slight step-off is present at the articular surface. This could also be classified as a Salter-Harris type III fracture.

Figure 21-31 Articular fractures. **A,** This anteroposterior view of the knee demonstrates intraarticular extension of a fracture line that exits at the junction of the medial and lateral femoral condyles. The condyles are separated by only a few millimeters. This can also be termed an *intercondylar fracture.* **B,** On coming down from a rebound, a 14-year-old basketball player landed with a twist with his knee in extension. The lateral radiograph demonstrates intraarticular extension of a fracture line that starts at the tibial tubercle and exits in the middle of the knee joint. **C,** On computed tomography scan the degree of intraarticular displacement of the fracture is better appreciated.

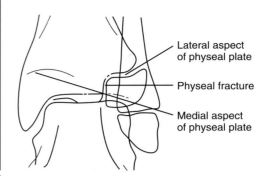

Lateral aspect
of physeal plate

Physeal fracture

Medial aspect
of physeal plate

Figure 21-32 Physeal fractures. **A,** A fracture of the lateral aspect of the tibial epiphysis through the lateral aspect of the physeal plate is seen in this anteroposterior view of the ankle of a 13-year-old boy. Also called a Tillaux fracture, this pattern is seen in adolescents in whom the medial aspect of the distal tibial physis has closed but not the lateral aspect. It can also be classified as a Salter-Harris type III fracture. **B,** A 7-year-old restrained backseat passenger involved in a head-on collision motor vehicle accident suffered a direct impact to the front of his lower leg due to violent displacement of the front seat. This resulted in shearing of the proximal tibial epiphysis from the metaphysis. The lateral view of the knee demonstrates complete separation of the epiphysis from most of the metaphysis. This degree of posterior displacement of the metaphysis can be associated with compression of the popliteal artery. This can also be classified as a Salter-Harris type II fracture because a small metaphyseal fragment remains attached to the epiphysis.

Condylar
fracture

Figure 21-33 Condylar fractures. This anteroposterior radiograph of the elbow shows a fracture of the lateral condyle of the distal humerus. The condyle is displaced proximally and radially. The fragment is always larger than it appears on a radiograph because of the large amount of unossified cartilage present in the distal humerus.

Figure 21-34 Supracondylar humerus fractures. These injuries are typically the result of a fall backward onto an outstretched arm with the elbow in hyperextension. This transmits the force of the impact to the distal humerus, driving the distal fragment posteriorly. Most require surgery to realign, reduce, and stabilize the fracture. **A,** This 8-year-old fell backward off a swing, landing on his hand with his elbow extended. The anteroposterior radiograph shows the fracture line crossing through the olecranon fossa in the supracondylar region of the distal humerus. Although there is marked soft tissue swelling, degree of displacement appears mild. **B,** In the lateral view moderate posterior displacement of the distal fragment is evident. There is also a positive fat pad sign. **C,** In another boy, after a more severe backward fall, the anteroposterior radiograph shows the distal fragment displaced radially, and in the lateral view **(D),** significant posterior displacement is evident. **E** and **F,** In this case an 8-year-old fell backward from a barn window onto his extended arm. This resulted in a severely displaced (type III) supracondylar fracture with associated injury to the brachial artery and vascular insufficiency of the forearm and hand, manifest by a cool hand and absent pulses. The distal fragment is displaced posterolaterally. In such cases the brachial artery may be placed on "stretch" over the proximal fragment or may be entrapped between fragments. This is a true surgical emergency requiring immediate surgery to reduce the fracture and restore distal blood flow. **G,** This boy has cubitus valgus deformity of his left elbow as a result of incorrect healing of a supracondylar fracture. **H,** This was corrected by a distal humerus osteotomy, restoring normal contour to the elbow.

Figure 21-35 Epicondylar fracture. This 10-year-old tripped while playing soccer and fell onto his arm with a valgus strain on the elbow. The anteroposterior radiograph shows a moderately displaced medial epicondylar fracture. These injuries are sometimes associated with dislocation of the elbow, in which case there is marked swelling of the entire elbow.

Salter-Harris Type III

Intraarticular shearing forces can produce a fracture line running from the articular surface through the epiphysis and then exiting through a portion of the physis. This creates a separate epiphyseal fragment with no connection to the metaphysis (Fig. 21-40; see also Figs. 21-30 and 21-32, *A*). Prognosis may be quite poor. Accurate anatomic reduction is required to achieve the best possible outcome.

Salter-Harris Type IV

In this fracture the fracture line starts at the articular surface, runs through the epiphysis across the physis, and exits the metaphysis. A single fragment consisting of both the epiphysis

Figure 21-36 Subcapital fracture. This anteroposterior radiograph of the pelvis shows a displaced subcapital fracture of the left femur. This particular injury may be seen acutely as the result of significant trauma or may develop slowly as a result of gradual slipping at the physeal level.

and attached metaphysis is thus created (Fig. 21-41). Like the Salter-Harris type III fracture, the injury results from the application of a shearing force. Prognosis may be poor despite seemingly good anatomic restoration of the fracture fragments. Open reduction and internal fixation are virtually always necessary. Salter-Harris type III and type IV fractures also can be classified as intraarticular fractures.

Salter-Harris Type V

A Salter-Harris type V fracture is the product of a crushing injury to the physis without physeal fracture or displacement. Radiographic diagnosis is virtually impossible to make at the time of injury; hence this fracture must be diagnosed on clinical grounds. Distinction between Salter-Harris type I and Salter-Harris type V fractures is often possible only when a subsequent growth abnormality has been appreciated. Prognosis is quite poor for normal growth (Fig. 21-42).

Fracture Treatment Principles

The healing and remodeling capacity of the growing bones of a child is considerably greater than that of an adult; the younger the child and the closer the fracture to the epiphysis, the greater is this capacity for regeneration. As a result, healing is rapid, necessitating a shorter period of immobilization; nonunion is rare. Furthermore, in planning fracture

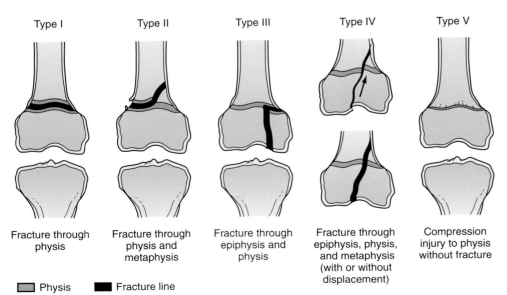

Type I	Type II	Type III	Type IV	Type V
Fracture through physis	Fracture through physis and metaphysis	Fracture through epiphysis and physis	Fracture through epiphysis, physis, and metaphysis (with or without displacement)	Compression injury to physis without fracture

☐ Physis   ■ Fracture line

Figure 21-37 Salter-Harris classification of physeal injuries.

Figure 21-38 Salter-Harris type I injury. Close inspection shows slight widening of the distal humeral epiphysis *(right, arrow)*. Clinically, the patient had pain, tenderness, and decreased range of motion of the elbow. *(Courtesy Jocelyn Ledesma Medina, MD.)*

reductions, the remodeling capability and the likely addition to bone length as a result of overgrowth must be considered. For example, in managing a toddler with a femur fracture that is displaced in the plane of motion of the adjacent joint, the bone ends must overlap to account for overgrowth and a degree of angulation can be accepted because this will ultimately be corrected by remodeling. The amount of angulation and the degree of overlap of fracture fragments that can be accepted are difficult to state in numeric terms. Acceptable position is determined in part by the child's age, the nature and position of the fracture, the bone involved, the appearance and condition of the adjacent soft tissues, and the presence or absence of other systemic injuries. Remodeling has its limitations, however. Rotational deformities and angular deformities that are not in the axis of adjacent joint motion are not effectively remodeled. Thus these must be corrected at the time of initial fracture reduction.

Figure 21-40 Salter-Harris type III injury. Comparison view of both ankles reveals a fracture involving the lateral aspect of the right distal tibial epiphysis. This configuration creates a separate fragment without any connection to the metaphysis.

Nondisplaced fractures are simply casted or splinted. Because of the relative rarity of ligamentous injuries before epiphyseal closure, patients with an appropriate clinical history and point tenderness over an epiphysis are presumed to have a fracture and should be treated accordingly, even if radiographs are normal. Most displaced fractures not involving the physis can be treated by closed reduction and casting. As a general rule, open reduction and internal fixation are usually reserved for the management of Salter-Harris type III and type IV fractures that have any degree of displacement; for certain open fractures; and for fractures associated with continued neurovascular compromise. Depending on the time of presentation, degree of displacement, and severity of soft tissue swelling, reduction or casting may have to be deferred pending application of traction and subsidence of edema.

The importance of adequate analgesia and sedation before the performance of closed-reduction procedures warrants emphasis. Too often reduction is performed without the benefit of appropriate analgesia and justified by the rationale that "it will only hurt for a minute." This reasoning is callous because that excruciating "minute" may seem an eternity to the child. After reduction and/or immobilization in a cast or splint, pain should be markedly alleviated, although some analgesia is likely to be necessary for a day or two. Persistence or recurrence of considerable discomfort signifies a complication and warrants prompt reevaluation.

Care must be taken in describing the nature of the injury and its prognosis and in explaining the rationale for proposed treatment measures to the parents. A simpler explanation in terms geared to his or her developmental level should be given to the child. Written instructions regarding home care measures, necessary parent observations, and worrisome signs that signal the need for prompt reevaluation are invaluable.

Figure 21-39 Salter-Harris type II injury. On this lateral radiograph of the thumb, the fracture is seen to involve the proximal phalanx. The fracture line runs through the physis and exits through the metaphysis on the side opposite the site of fracture initiation. A fragment consisting of the entire epiphysis with the attached metaphyseal fragment is produced.

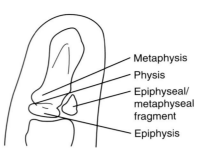

Figure 21-41   Salter-Harris type IV injury. This patient incurred a fracture of the distal phalanx of the index finger. The fracture line starts at the articular surface, runs through the epiphysis across the physis, and exits through the metaphysis. A single fragment consisting of the epiphysis and the attached metaphysis is thus created.

Metaphysis
Physis
Epiphyseal/
metaphyseal
fragment
Epiphysis

Special Cases

Clavicular Fractures

Fractures of the clavicle are common. They are caused by lateral compression forces (as can occur in the process of delivery of the newborn or in falls onto the shoulder), by transmission of forces through the glenohumeral joint in a fall to the side on an outstretched arm, or occasionally by a direct blow or impact on the clavicle itself. Most involve the midshaft or distal clavicle. Greenstick fractures are more common in infants and toddlers, whereas through-and-through fractures are more typical of older children and adolescents (see Fig. 21-20). Severe displacement and angulation are usually prevented by the thick periosteum that envelops the clavicle. Clinically, the child complains of pain in the shoulder, is noted to avoid moving the arm on the involved side, and often splints it by holding the arm close against the chest. Tenderness and mild swelling are evident on palpation of the fracture site. Complications are rare, and treatment consists of the application of a padded figure-of-eight splint for 2 to 3 weeks for purposes of immobilization and to prevent foreshortening of the clavicle on healing. Older children may be more comfortable with the addition of a sling for the first few days.

Slings are not advisable for toddlers because they need to be able to hold both arms out when walking in order to maintain balance. Forewarning parents that a hard bump will appear as the fracture heals and that this is due to callus formation is advisable because the clavicle's superficial location makes the site of callus formation prominent.

Medial clavicular fractures are rare and are caused by high-impact forces and often are associated with injuries of mediastinal structures. Thus, they warrant meticulous evaluation including chest CT and often angiography.

Fractures involving the distal tip of the clavicle in infants (beyond the neonatal period) and toddlers are likely to be the result of abuse (see Chapter 6).

Toddler's Fracture

One of the most common orthopedic injuries seen in children between the ages of 1 and 5 years is the toddler's fracture. The child usually has a sudden onset of refusal to bear weight on one leg or of an antalgic limp. Typically this develops after a fall with a twist, to which the unsteady toddler is unusually prone. The child may have gotten his or her foot caught and fallen while trying to extricate himself or herself, may have

Figure 21-42   Salter-Harris type V injury. This anteroposterior radiograph of the ankle taken several weeks after a crush injury sustained in an automobile accident reveals obliteration of the distal tibial physeal plate. As is often the case, original radiographs taken at the time of injury looked normal. This fracture must be suspected on clinical grounds, and the patient treated and monitored accordingly.

Obliterated
physeal plate

Figure 21-43 Toddler's fracture. This spiral fracture of the distal tibia was the result of a fall with a twist. The fracture was invisible when the child was seen initially but is evident along with subperiosteal new bone formation on this follow-up film taken 2 weeks later.

fallen while running and making a sudden change of direction, or fallen with a twist on jumping. Not uncommonly the actual fall is unwitnessed, and the parents are unsure about the nature of the accident. The injury results in a spiral or short oblique fracture of the distal tibia or the junction of the mid- and distal tibia (Fig. 21-43). Because the thick periosteum tends to be only partially disrupted, soft tissue swelling is often minimal and tenderness may be subtle. Furthermore, many of these fractures are radiographically invisible or so subtle as to be difficult to detect, although some degree of soft tissue swelling may be evident on the film. In some cases an oblique view may be revealing. Without radiographic evidence of a fracture, the physician must rely on the examination findings to make a clinical diagnosis.

It is generally best to allow the child to remain seated in the parent's lap during the examination. This helps calm the child and ensures a more subdued response to palpation of the uninvolved areas. Attention should first be turned to the normal extremity. The ankle, knee, and hip should be placed through their range of motion. Next, the entire foot, tibia, fibula, and femur should be palpated. The child will cry if upset, but nothing about the examination should otherwise exacerbate the child's baseline irritability. Attention is then directed to the involved extremity, and a similar examination is performed. Palpation over the fracture site usually will be revealed either by a withdrawal reaction or, more commonly, by an increase from baseline irritability, usually manifested by a change in the child's facial expression and in the pattern of crying. In suspected cases in which it is difficult to determine whether tenderness is present, a gentle passive twist applied to the tibia may elicit pain. Localized bone tenderness or pain on passive twisting in this setting is clinical proof of a fracture, even if radiographs are normal. In attempting to assess frightened and highly uncooperative toddlers, it is best to give them time to calm down and then either have the parent perform palpation or introduce puppets and palpate using the puppet's hands.

Treatment consists of either long- or short-leg casting for approximately 4 weeks. Infection must be included in the differential diagnosis of the limping child in this 1- to 5-year age group but usually can be ruled out by lack of fever, absence of local erythema, and normal blood values. If there is no clear history of a fall, only a mild limp, no evidence of localized tenderness, and radiographs are normal, it may be best to defer treatment and observe the child closely.

Fractures Involving the Elbow

Supracondylar, condylar, intercondylar, and epicondylar humerus fractures and proximal radius and ulna fractures all involve the elbow, and the major mechanism is a fall onto the arm with the elbow in hyperextension. In a young infant, a fracture through the cartilaginous portion of the distal humerus at the level of the condyles is known as a transcondylar fracture. Because of the lack of ossification, these are difficult to diagnose on routine x-rays. This may necessitate an MRI study or arthrogram to confirm the diagnosis in an infant with a swollen elbow. Given the force necessary to cause these fractures, when they are seen in an infant who is not yet standing and walking, inflicted trauma must be suspected (Fig. 21-44).

Supracondylar fractures account for about 50% of elbow injuries and usually result from a fall backward onto an outstretched hyperextended arm, which typically results in some degree of posterior displacement of the distal humeral fragment (see Fig. 21-34). A grading system, developed by Gartland and useful in describing severity of injury, includes the following: type 1, nondisplaced; type 2, partial displacement with intact posterior cortex; and type 3, displaced with complete disruption of the posterior cortex. When due to abuse, the mechanism is usually a grab and yank into hyperextension (see Chapter 6). More rarely, a direct blow to the posterior aspect of the distal humerus is the cause, in which case the distal fragment is angulated anteriorly. Pain, swelling, and tenderness are most prominent over the posterior aspect of the distal humerus. A significant risk of associated neurovascular injury exists in patients with such fractures.

Lateral condylar fractures are in part interarticular (see Fig. 21-33). Typically they result from a fall onto an extended and abducted arm. Swelling and tenderness are prominent over the lateral aspect of the elbow. These fractures are generally unstable and often require pinning to ensure optimal reduction.

Medial epicondylar fractures stem from falls in which the elbow is hyperextended and abducted from the body, subjecting it to a valgus stress (see Fig. 21-35). They are also commonly seen in association with elbow dislocations. These children have swelling and tenderness centered over the medial aspect of the elbow.

Radial head and neck fractures are usually the result of a fall onto an outstretched, supinated arm (Fig. 21-45). Local swelling and tenderness are centered over the proximal radius, although pain is often referred to the wrist. Because they often are accompanied by other fractures, care should be taken to search for associated injuries.

Radiographic findings in patients with fractures about the elbow can be subtle, and oblique and comparison views may be necessary to reveal them. Key signs suggestive of a fracture in the absence of fracture lines are the posterior fat pad sign and displacement of the anterior humeral line. The fat pad sign consists of the upward and outward displacement of the posterior fat pad of the distal humerus (Fig. 21-46, *A* and *B*; and see Fig. 21-34, *B*), which is normally invisible. The finding of a fat pad indicates the presence of a hemarthrosis, and it can be seen in patients with fractures involving the distal

Figure 21-44 Inflicted elbow fractures. This 10-month-old was brought in with a history of a minor fall and decreased use of his arm. **A,** However, radiographs revealed displaced transverse fractures of both the distal humerus and proximal ulna along with marked soft tissue swelling. These findings were incompatible with the reported mechanism of injury and instead were the result of grabbing the arm and yanking the elbow into hyperextension with severe force. **B,** Follow-up films 1 month later show prolific subperiosteal new bone formation.

humerus, proximal radius, or proximal ulna. The anterior humeral line is a line drawn through the anterior cortex of the humerus and normally intersects the middle third of the capitellum. As just noted, hyperextension injuries of the distal humerus resulting in fractures typically displace the distal humeral fragment posteriorly. As a result, the anterior humeral line intersects the anterior third of the capitellum if displacement is slight or misses it entirely if displacement or angulation is marked (Fig. 21-46, *B*).

Figure 21-45 Radial neck fracture. When this 4-year-old boy fell off his bike, the position of his arm on impact resulted in transmission of a valgus force across the elbow joint, resulting in this impaction fracture of the radial neck. Radial neck fractures may require reduction to restore normal supination and pronation of the forearm.

Hand and Finger Fractures

Although a complete discussion of the examination of the hand and hand injuries is beyond the scope of this chapter, several key points bear emphasis, as appropriate assessment and management are essential if long-term dysfunction is to be prevented (see Figs. 21-87 and 21-88).

Phalangeal Fractures. The most common mechanism of injury producing phalangeal fractures in young children is a crush injury caused by getting their fingers caught in a door or by the weight of a heavy object falling on them. Crush injuries continue to be common in older children and adolescents, but contact sports and fistfights assume an increasing causative role in this age group.

Meticulous attention must be paid to the assessment of neurovascular and tendon function to detect subtle abnormalities that may reflect significant injury with the potential for long-term complications. This can be difficult in young children. However, much information can be gained from observing the position of the hands at rest and during spontaneous movement, as well as by watching motion as the parents hand objects to the child.

Complete phalangeal fractures typically angulate as a result of the action of the intrinsic muscles of the hand. Any fracture associated with shortening, significant angulation (Fig. 21-47), or rotational deformity and any intraarticular fracture must be appropriately reduced. Shortening and rotation are best detected by comparison of the injured hand with its normal opposite. Comparison of the planes of the fingernails of both hands with the forearms supinated and the fingers partially flexed is particularly useful in detecting rotational abnormalities (Fig. 21-48).

Determination of the degree of angulation and identification of intraarticular fractures are best done radiographically. X-ray findings can be subtle, necessitating careful comparison with radiographs of the normal hand. Obtaining oblique, as well as AP and lateral views, is also important.

Chip fractures at the base of the middle or distal phalanges may be associated with avulsion of the flexor or extensor tendons, which may necessitate surgical repair. Clinically, an extensor tendon injury may be manifested by flexor tendon overpull (Fig. 21-49), and conversely, flexor tendon injuries may result in extensor overpull (see Fig. 21-7).

Figure 21-46   **A,** Posterior fat pad sign. Although no clear fracture line is evident in this patient with a supracondylar fracture, the posterior fat pad is readily visible, being displaced upward and outward from the posterior aspect of the distal humerus. The finding indicates the presence of a joint effusion, which after trauma is blood, and in about 70% of cases with no visible fracture line, an occult fracture is present. **B,** Anterior humeral line. A line drawn through the anterior cortex of the humerus in another patient with a positive fat pad intersects the anterior third of the capitellum, indicating posterior displacement of the distal humeral fragment. **C,** Normal elbow for comparison. (**B,** *Courtesy Richard B. Towbin, MD, Children's Hospital of Philadelphia, Philadelphia, Pa.*)

Figure 21-47   Angulated phalanx fracture. Significant angular deformity is seen in this impaction fracture of the proximal phalanx of the thumb. Such fractures require careful reduction to prevent permanent disability.

Figure 21-48   Rotational deformity resulting from a hand injury. With rotational deformity the plane of the nail of the involved finger is seen to deviate from its normal orientation. (*Courtesy Neil Jones, MD, University of California, Los Angeles, Los Angeles, Calif.*)

Figure 21-49   Distal phalanx fracture with extensor tendon injury. **A,** Another player's shoulder landed on this boy's finger. The finger was swollen and painful and maximally tender at the base of the distal phalanx, and the patient was unable to extend the distal interphalangeal joint. **B,** Radiograph revealed separation of the epiphysis at the base of the distal phalanx.

Figure 21-50 Crush injury of the distal phalanx. This child's finger was slammed in a car door. He incurred a crush fracture of the distal phalanx, partial avulsion of the nail, and a nail bed laceration. By definition, this is an open fracture. *(Courtesy Neil Jones, MD, University of California, Los Angeles, Los Angeles, Calif.)*

Crush injuries of the distal phalanges associated with partial or complete nail avulsions often result in open fractures with laceration of the nail bed (Fig. 21-50). These require careful cleansing, debridement, nail bed repair, and antibiotic prophylaxis.

The volar plate is a cartilaginous plate located at the base of the middle phalanx of each finger. Intraarticular fractures involving the PIP joint may fracture or tear this structure as well. The typical mechanism of injury is usually a blow to the end of the finger in hyperextension. Often a chip of bone avulsed from the middle phalanx is seen radiographically. Clinically, pain and swelling are especially marked over the volar aspect of the PIP joint. A hyperextension deformity of the involved PIP joint may be seen when the fingers are extended, or pain or locking may be noted on attempted flexion. Pain is exacerbated on passive hyperextension and reduced on passive flexion. Volar plate injuries may also accompany dislocation of the PIP joint (see Ligamentous Injuries, later).

Metacarpal Fractures. The boxer's fracture, an impacted fracture of the neck of the fifth and often the fourth metacarpal, is among the most common of these injuries (Fig. 21-51). It occurs as a result of direct impact with a partially clenched fist (typically resulting from punching another person or a wall) and is most commonly seen in aggressive adolescents. It can also result from a fall onto a clenched fist. Clinically, depression of the involved knuckle or knuckles may be noted, along with more proximal swelling and discoloration. The involved metacarpals may also appear shortened. An associated rotational deformity, if present, is manifested by rotation of the nails of the corresponding fingers (see Fig. 21-48). If the injury stems from punching another person in the mouth, care must be taken to check for overlying breaks in the skin caused by the opponent's teeth. These are infection-prone wounds and may communicate with metacarpophalangeal joints. Radiographically, volar angulation of the distal segment is typically found. If this exceeds 15 to 20 degrees or a rotational deformity is present, the patient should be referred to an orthopedist or hand surgeon for reduction. Nondisplaced, minimally angulated fractures can be treated with an ulnar gutter splint.

Metatarsal Fractures

Most metatarsal fractures are the result of a heavy object dropping onto the foot and thus are crush injuries. Falls in which the patient twists the forefoot or in which the forefoot is caught in plantar flexion can produce transverse fractures (Fig. 21-52), and injuries of the foot with the ankle inverted and the foot in plantar flexion can avulse the tuberosity from the base of the fifth metatarsal. Mild, localized swelling and point tenderness are noted over the site of a metatarsal fracture; weight bearing is painful, if not impossible. A short-leg cast provides maximal relief. This must be distinguished from the normal finding of a secondary ossification center, termed the *os vesalianum,* at the base of the fifth metatarsal. The edges of the latter are smooth, rounded, and sclerotic (Fig. 21-53).

Adolescents involved in long-distance running or walking may incur stress fractures of the shafts of the second and third metatarsals, which are the site of maximal stress and weight application during the push-off phase of walking and running. Pain often increases insidiously and tends to be poorly localized. Swelling may be imperceptible. These are often microfractures and may be radiographically invisible until healing becomes detectable 3 to 4 weeks after onset. Earlier detection is possible with bone scans.

Lap Belt Fractures

Increased awareness of the importance of using seat belts to prevent serious multiple trauma in auto accidents and adherence to recommendations to place children in the back seat of the car have resulted in an increase in the incidence of lap belt fractures in children. In a head-on collision, the head and torso of a child wearing only a lap belt are thrown forward, resulting in hyperflexion of the lumbar spine over the fulcrum of the lap belt and often causing a flexion/distraction injury. This may produce a compression fracture of a lumbar vertebra or, more likely, a shear fracture through the body of the vertebra, as well as the pedicle and spinous process. This is best seen on a lateral radiograph of the lumbar spine (Fig. 21-54). An AP view of the spine may show lateral displacement of a portion of the involved vertebral body. Because the fulcrum of the injury is anterior where the lap belt contacts the anterior abdominal wall, this injury produces a characteristic rectangular bruise and abrasion over the lower abdomen. Associated intraabdominal injury, especially a ruptured viscus, is common, and the resultant abdominal pain may overshadow that of the

Figure 21-51 Boxer's fracture. This adolescent presented with pain and swelling of the lateral aspect of his right hand after punching a wall in a fit of temper. Radiographically he has typical boxer's fractures of the necks of the fourth and fifth metacarpals with volar displacement of the distal fragments.

Figure 21-52 Transverse metatarsal fractures. **A,** This adolescent fell forward with her forefoot twisted under her. Swelling over the proximal portion of the fifth metatarsal was prominent. **B** and **C,** Anteroposterior and lateral radiographs show a transverse fracture of the proximal fifth metatarsal. **D,** This boy caught his left foot on steps and fell with his forefoot in plantar flexion, thereby incurring a transverse fracture of the distal portion of his second metatarsal.

vertebral injury. Hence whenever a lap belt bruise is seen during the physical examination, great care should be taken in palpating the back for localized tenderness or spasm, and immobilization of the torso and lower back should be maintained until CT scan of the lumbar spine is obtained to confirm the presence or absence of fracture and to determine whether or not a fracture, when present, is stable or unstable. Fortunately, increased use of three-point belts in back seats is reducing the frequency of this injury.

Figure 21-53 Os vesalianum. Many children have a secondary ossification center at the base of the fifth metatarsal. This can be distinguished from a fracture by the fact that its edges are smooth, rounded, and sclerotic. *(Courtesy Jocelyn Ledesma Medina, MD.)*

Pelvic Avulsion Fractures

Pelvic avulsion fractures are a phenomenon unique to adolescents, with a peak occurrence between 13 and 14 years of age in girls and 15 and 17 years of age in boys. This stems from the fact that the secondary centers of ossification in these young people have not yet fused to the pelvis. These fractures are typically seen in adolescents who are in top physical condition and involved in competitive sports, especially track and field (e.g., sprinting and jumping), soccer, and football. The incidence of these fractures is increasing with the rising participation of adolescents in competitive sports. Most result from a sudden, violent muscular contraction while the ipsilateral extremity is held in a static position or when a muscle is suddenly lengthened during isometric contraction. As the muscle power exceeds the strength of the tendinous unit, it is

Figure 21-54 Lap belt fracture. This flexion/distraction injury occurred through the body of the L4 vertebra when the child's body hyperflexed over a lap belt in a head-on automobile collision.

Figure 21-55   Pelvic avulsion fractures. **A,** Ischial tuberosity avulsion fracture. This 14-year-old football player sprinting for a touchdown fell on his stomach and experienced sharp left hip pain. He could not bear weight after the incident and was found to have tenderness over the left buttock and pain with abduction and flexion of the left hip. The avulsed fragment is best seen on this frog-leg view. **B,** Anterior inferior iliac spine avulsion fracture. While running in gym class, this 15-year-old boy experienced the sudden onset of left hip pain and difficulty walking. He had point tenderness over the anterior inferior iliac spine and full range of hip motion but experienced pain on flexion and internal rotation. If compared with the right, the avulsed apophysis is evident. **C,** Another 15-year-old boy, who developed sudden onset of right hip pain and inability to bear weight while kicking a soccer ball, has a large avulsion fracture of the anterior superior iliac spine *(arrows)*. (*A* and *B, Courtesy Janet Kinnane, MD, Children's Hospital of Pittsburgh, Pittsburgh, Pa.)*

torn from the apophysis or secondary ossification center. Avulsion fractures of the ischial tuberosity are the most common. They tend to occur during sprinting and are due to the sudden, powerful contraction of the hamstring muscles when the hip is flexed and the knee extended (Fig. 21-55, *A*). Avulsions of the anterior inferior and anterior superior iliac spines (see Fig. 21-55, *B* and *C*) are caused by strong contractions of the rectus femoris and sartorius muscles, respectively. These, too, tend to happen during running, often during an abrupt directional change. Some cases of anterior inferior/superior iliac spine avulsions occur with kicking. At the time of injury, the patient experiences sudden pain at the site and difficulty walking. On examination, point tenderness and swelling are noted over the involved apophysis and weakness on active hip motion is seen secondary to pain.

In viewing radiographs, it is important to compare the involved side with the normal side to detect displacement of the avulsed fragment and to avoid mistaking a normal apophysis for a fracture.

Treatment is conservative and consists of a few days of bed rest until the pain subsides, followed by 2 to 6 weeks of crutch-walking, with a gradual increase in weight bearing as pain allows. Thereafter, careful reconditioning facilitates a safe return to full activity, usually within 6 to 10 weeks.

Pathologic Fractures

Children with severe osteopenia or osteoporosis, whether stemming from an inherited disorder or disuse secondary to neurologic or neuromuscular disease, are at considerably increased risk of incurring fractures as the result of minor falls or even during routine physical therapy exercises. Localized bone lesions including those caused by osteomyelitis, tumors, or cysts, can cause localized cortical thinning as they expand. Impact on the involved bone can then also result in a pathologic fracture. Examples of some of these conditions and representative fractures are presented in Chapter 6.

Compartment Syndromes

A compartment syndrome arises whenever the interstitial tissue fluid pressure exceeds the capillary perfusion pressure within a muscle compartment. In clinical practice the interstitial pressure elevation must reach approximately 35 to 45 mm Hg for this to occur. Because the enclosed fascial boundary of the involved muscle compartment is unyielding, hemorrhage or edema within it can cause interstitial pressure to rise to such levels, resulting in muscle ischemia and neurovascular compromise. Compartment syndromes are not rare in childhood and can be seen after open or closed fractures, crush injuries, or prolonged pressure on an extremity, which can occur in a comatose child who has been lying on an extremity for several hours. A displaced fracture of the proximal tibial metaphysis is the fracture most likely to be complicated by a compartment syndrome. Other fractures that are well documented to predispose to the development of this problem include supracondylar humerus fractures and displaced forearm fractures.

Prompt and accurate diagnosis of a compartment syndrome is essential because, if definitive treatment is not implemented within 4 to 6 hours of onset, permanent neuromuscular damage will result. The clinical findings in compartment syndrome are quite classic. The involved extremity is swollen and tense to palpation. The patient complains of severe pain that is unrelieved by elevation, immobilization, and routine doses of narcotics. Passive movement of the terminal digits (fingers or toes) exacerbates the pain, and active motion is avoided. In view of the fact that pulses may never be diminished or absent despite a full-blown, florid compartment syndrome, the diagnosis or decision to treat should never be based solely on the presence or absence of the peripheral pulses. Because clinical diagnosis can be difficult, especially in the uncooperative or comatose child, intracompartmental needle pressure readings are recommended.

Emergency surgical decompression of the fascial covering of all involved compartments is necessary to prevent irreversible muscle and nerve damage. After fascial decompression, relief of pain and return of active muscle power are immediate.

Ligamentous Injuries

Dislocations

The ligaments of a child have great elasticity and are relatively strong compared with bony structures, especially the physis (Fig. 21-56). Consequently, joint dislocations and ligamentous disruptions are rather unusual in childhood; when seen, they are usually the result of severe trauma and are commonly associated with fractures. In some instances the dislocation is obvious and the fracture subtle or even invisible radiographically (Fig. 21-57), but often the fracture is the prominent clinical finding and the dislocation less apparent. Hence the emphasis in pediatric orthopedics is on examining the entire extremity and on including the joints proximal and distal to a suspected fracture site in the radiographic examination. Failure to diagnose the full extent of injury can result in permanent morbidity. It must also be remembered that in infants epiphyseal separations before ossification can simulate dislocations. For example, separation of the distal humeral epiphysis in infancy presents a radiographic picture suggestive of posterior displacement of the olecranon. The most frequent sites of dislocation in children are the hip, patellofemoral joint, and interphalangeal joints.

Hip dislocations in the young are usually the result of falls. In children younger than 5 years of age, the softness of the acetabulum and relative ligamentous laxity enable dislocation

Figure 21-57 Fracture–dislocation, right hip. This young infant presented after a serious automobile accident with what appeared to be a traumatic hip dislocation without an associated fracture. **A,** The right femoral head is displaced laterally and superiorly. **B,** The follow-up film taken 2 weeks later reveals vigorous callus formation around the proximal femur and periosteal new bone formation both proximally and distally, thus confirming the existence of associated femoral fractures. *(Courtesy Department of Pediatric Radiology, Children's Hospital of Pittsburgh, Pittsburgh, Pa.)*

Figure 21-56 Epiphyseal separation. Because of the elasticity and relatively greater strength of the ligaments, forces that would have resulted in dislocation in an older adolescent have instead caused epiphyseal separation and displacement of the proximal humeral epiphysis in this prepubescent child. *(Courtesy Department of Pediatric Radiology, Children's Hospital of Pittsburgh, Pittsburgh, Pa.)*

without the application of extreme force, and thus there may be no associated fractures. In older children, violent force is required and dislocation is commonly accompanied by fractures of the femur and acetabulum. In most instances the femoral head dislocates posteriorly. The child presents in severe pain with the involved leg held in adduction, internally rotated and flexed (Fig. 21-58). A position of extension, external rotation, and abduction is adopted by patients with the less common anterior dislocation. When the child also has an impressive femoral fracture, his or her pain may be attributed to that and the positional findings missed, unless the clinician specifically looks for them. Even in patients without an obvious associated fracture, epiphyseal separation or avulsion of an acetabular fragment may have occurred. Prompt reduction is important, both to relieve pain and to reduce the risk of secondary avascular necrosis of the femoral head. Postreduction films are important because these are more likely to disclose the fact that an epiphyseal separation has occurred and tend to show incomplete reduction if a radiolucent intra-articular fragment is present.

In patellofemoral dislocations the patella usually dislocates laterally (Fig. 21-59). This may occur as the result of laterally directed shearing forces or of a hyperextension injury. Patients with ligamentous laxity appear particularly susceptible. In

Figure 21-58 Traumatic posterior hip dislocation. This child suffered an impaction injury in an automobile accident. **A,** In the anteroposterior view the right femoral head appears to be displaced laterally and superiorly. The femur is also adducted and internally rotated. **B,** The frog-leg view discloses the severity of displacement posteriorly.

most instances the patella has relocated by the time the patient is seen. If not, it is seen as a bulge lateral to its usual anterior location and the patient is in severe pain. In such cases x-rays should be deferred, the leg should be extended immediately, and the patella pushed back into place. This maneuver promptly alleviates pain. Other findings on examination include prominent swelling and hemarthrosis, tenderness along the medial patellar border, a positive apprehension test (see Knee and Fig. 21-11), and increased lateral mobility of the patella. Avulsion fractures of the lateral femoral condyle or medial patella are common associated injuries. Application of ice, rest, and use of a knee immobilizer for 3 weeks are recommended. At present there is disagreement on whether surgical intervention should be considered after the first episode or deferred until a recurrence.

True shoulder dislocations are seen only in adolescents after epiphyseal fusion. On examination of the shoulder, a loss of the rounded contours lateral and anterior to the acromion is found. When the humeral head dislocates anteriorly, it is displaced medially beneath the coracoid process, where it can be palpated (Fig. 21-60). These patients usually support the affected arm with the opposite hand, with the shoulder in moderate internal rotation. Patients with posterior shoulder dislocations have evidence of a fullness posterior to the glenoid cavity and are unable to externally rotate the involved upper extremity.

Separation of the proximal humeral epiphysis or major fracture–dislocations are seen in younger children subjected to forces that would cause shoulder dislocation after puberty (see Fig. 21-56).

Elbow dislocations are rare in the absence of an associated fracture. The fracture may be as subtle as a nonossified fragment avulsed from the medial epicondyle or the ulna or as prominent as a displaced fracture of the ulna or radius. An example of the latter is the *Monteggia fracture,* which results from a fall onto the hand with the elbow extended and the forearm rotated radially, producing a varus stress. In this situation a displaced fracture of the proximal ulna is accompanied by dislocation of the radial head. A radial dislocation should be suspected if a line drawn through the long axis of the radius fails to pass through the capitellum on any view (Fig. 21-61). Less frequently, fractures of the radius are associated with dislocation of the radioulnar joint, and fractures of the olecranon may be accompanied by dislocation of the radius. A fall onto an extended or partially flexed arm with the forearm supinated can result in posterior dislocation of both the radius and ulna with tearing of the anterior portion of the joint capsule and of the medial collateral ligaments. This injury may be associated with fracture of the medial epicondyle (see Fig. 21-35), the coronoid process, the olecranon, or the proximal radius. Clinically the forearm is shortened and there is an obvious deformity and marked swelling of the posterior aspect of the elbow. A high risk of neurovascular compromise and compartment syndrome exists in patients with this injury.

Dislocation of an interphalangeal joint results in an obvious deformity and is an intensely painful injury (Fig. 21-62). Avulsion fractures, volar plate fractures, and tendinous or capsular injury may be associated with it and difficult to detect radiographically. These must be suspected if range of motion is incomplete after relocation. In some cases the associated injury makes closed reduction impossible.

Sprains

A sprain is a ligamentous injury in which some degree of tearing occurs, often as a result of excessive stretching or twisting. As noted in the section on fractures, sprains are less common in children with open epiphyses than they are in older adolescents whose epiphyses have fused. When sprains do occur in these younger patients, they tend to be milder and may be associated with Salter-Harris fractures. This stems from the fact that the growth plate, being weaker than the

Figure 21-59 Patellar dislocation. In this flexion view obtained before relocation, the left patella is displaced laterally and there is marked swelling. *(Courtesy Department of Pediatric Radiology, Children's Hospital of Pittsburgh, Pittsburgh, Pa.)*

Figure 21-60 **A,** Anterior dislocation of the right shoulder. The humeral head is not in the glenoid fossa but is displaced anteriorly. **B,** The normal relationship is seen in this comparison view of the left shoulder. The injury occurred when the patient was taking a back swing for a hockey shot. The patient felt a pop with the immediate onset of severe pain. Note that his epiphyses have fused. *(Courtesy Department of Pediatric Radiology, Children's Hospital of Pittsburgh, Pittsburgh, Pa.)*

ligaments, tends to give before significant ligamentous tearing can occur. Thus in children, physeal fractures tend to result from forces that would produce a sprain in older adolescents or adults.

In many other instances a suspected sprain is actually a small avulsion fracture. If the portion avulsed is ossified, the small fragment may be detectable radiographically, but if the fragment is cartilaginous, it will be radiographically invisible. A particular example of this is the gamekeeper's thumb, which is often associated with a small avulsion fracture of the proximal phalanx (Fig. 21-63). In it, an injury causing forceful abduction of the thumb results in rupture of the ulnar collateral ligament at the base of the thumb. Adequate examination necessitates stress testing of the radial and ulnar collateral ligaments by applying varus and valgus stress, respectively, with the thumb in extension. However, this is often impossible until pain has been reduced by a digital nerve block. If more than 20 degrees of instability is found on stressing the ulnar collaterals, the patient should be referred to an orthopedist or

hand surgeon for possible surgical repair. Failure to correct the problem results in a loss of resistance to abduction and a weak pinch.

Before epiphyseal closure, Salter-Harris fractures and avulsion fractures of the distal fibula or tibia should be strongly suspected in children with "sprainlike" injuries of the ankle. Similarly, injuries that rupture the cruciate ligaments of the knee in adults usually avulse the tibial spine in children (Fig. 21-64). These are the result of a blow to the knee, forcing it into hyperextension along with a valgus or varus stress. After physeal closure in adolescence, sprains are seen with some frequency.

Sprains are classified in three grades according to severity (Table 21-5). In contrast to physeal fractures, swelling and tenderness are more likely to be prominent and occur early. They are most evident over the involved ligament or ligaments, not over the epiphysis. Pain on motion is often more marked in patients with sprains than in patients with physeal fractures.

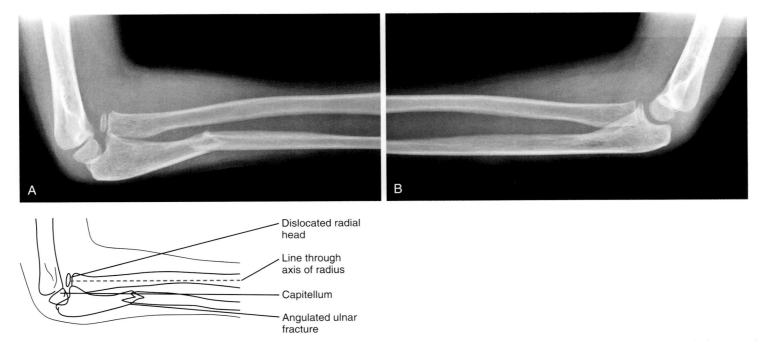

Dislocated radial head

Line through axis of radius

Capitellum

Angulated ulnar fracture

Figure 21-61 Monteggia fracture. **A,** A displaced fracture of the proximal right ulna is accompanied by dislocation of the radial head. A line drawn through the long axis of the radius would intersect the distal humerus above the level of the capitellum. **B,** The comparison view of the left arm shows the normal position of the radial head. *(Courtesy Department of Pediatric Radiology, Children's Hospital of Pittsburgh, Pittsburgh, Pa.)*

Figure 21-62 Interphalangeal joint dislocation. The distal phalanx of the thumb is dislocated dorsally. *(Courtesy Department of Pediatric Radiology, Children's Hospital of Pittsburgh, Pittsburgh, Pa.)*

Figure 21-63 Gamekeeper's thumb. A small avulsion fracture of the epiphysis at the base of the proximal phalanx is associated with rupture of the ulnar collateral ligament. The injury occurred when the patient fell while skiing and the strap of his ski pole forcefully abducted his thumb on impact.

Ankle Sprains

An ankle sprain in an adolescent patient is typically caused by a severe inversion stress injury, and the presenting findings are diffuse pain and tenderness along with swelling centered below the lateral malleolus, although the superior margin of swelling may cover the malleolus (Fig. 21-65). Areas of maximal tenderness may be found over the anterior talofibular ligament alone or over both it and the calcaneofibular ligament. Rarely the posterior talofibular ligament is also torn in patients with particularly severe sprains, and tenderness and swelling are noted over its course as well. Little pain occurs on dorsiflexion or plantar flexion, but marked pain occurs on passive inversion. Tests for ligamentous stability are described earlier (see Ankle).

Knee Sprains

Patients with major knee sprains present with marked pain, refusal to bear weight, and swelling resulting from hemarthrosis. Tears of the medial or lateral collateral ligaments of the knee are seen in adolescents and are usually the result of a direct blow that applies valgus or varus stress, respectively. A football tackle and being hit by a car from the side are common reported mechanisms. Tenderness is prominent over the involved ligaments. Major tears result in ligamentous instability detected by the adduction/abduction stress test (see Knee). Tibial spine avulsion fractures (see Fig. 21-64) and anterior cruciate ligament tears stem from falls in which the knee is hyperflexed, often a fall from a bicycle or a fall while skiing. Tenderness is marked anteriorly, and instability is demonstrated by the anterior drawer and Lachman tests (see Knee, earlier, and Figs. 21-12 and 21-13).

Because of the frequency of associated fractures in children and adolescents, patients with apparent sprains and hemarthroses should not undergo tests of ligamentous stability until radiographs have been obtained and the possibility of an unstable fracture has been ruled out.

Shoulder Separation

A shoulder separation involves a ligamentous tear at the acromioclavicular joint, usually resulting from a fall onto an outstretched, adducted arm. Clinically the lateral aspect of the clavicle appears to ride higher on the injured side than on the normal side, and with application of pressure it may be forced back into its normal position. If it can also be moved forward and backward, the coracoclavicular ligaments have been torn as well.

Evaluation and Management

In evaluating patients with possible sprains, careful attention must be given not only to assessment of swelling, tenderness, and joint stability, but also to evaluation of adjacent bony structures and to musculotendinous function (see Physical Examination, earlier). Complete evaluation may be impossible

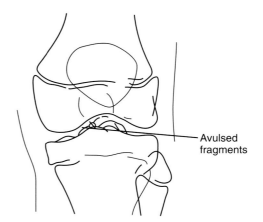

Avulsed fragments

Figure 21-64 Avulsion fracture of the left tibial spine as the result of a soccer injury (anteroposterior view). Also present were a tear in the cruciate ligament and a lipohemarthrosis. *(Courtesy Department of Pediatric Radiology, Children's Hospital of Pittsburgh, Pittsburgh, Pa.)*

Figure 21-65 Ankle sprain. Marked tenderness and swelling were maximal inferior to the malleolus of this 17-year-old youth. The anterior talofibular, calcaneofibular, and posterior talofibular ligaments were all tender. This is in contrast to the findings seen with a Salter-Harris type I fracture of the distal tibia (see Fig. 21-17).

if initial presentation has been delayed for several hours and secondary effusion, soft tissue swelling, and muscle spasm are pronounced. In such instances it may be necessary to immobilize the affected joint with a splint and have the patient return for reevaluation in 24 to 72 hours when the swelling has abated.

Rest, the application of ice, use of analgesic anti-inflammatory agents such as ibuprofen, and perhaps use of an Ace wrap or taping, suffice for grade I sprains. Subjective improvement occurs in a few days. Grade II and grade III sprains require a longer period of immobilization. Splinting or casting for a few to several weeks is generally necessary. Grade III sprains may require surgical intervention.

Subluxation of the Radial Head (Nursemaid's Elbow)

Subluxation of the radial head is the most common elbow injury in childhood and one of the most common ligamentous injuries. The mechanism is one of sudden traction applied to the extended arm. The injury is seen predominantly in children between the ages of 1 and 4 years. The typical history

Figure 21-66 Nursemaid's elbow. **A,** The affected arm is held close to the body with the elbow flexed and the forearm pronated. **B,** The reduction maneuver consists of supinating the forearm while pressing down on the radial head.

is one of a parent's suddenly pulling the child up by the arm to prevent a fall; of the child, in a fit of temper, attempting to pull away from the parent; or of a child being swung by an arm. However, in a number of cases the injury is due to the child's grabbing onto some object in an effort to avoid falling. This type of injury can also occur in an infant who is rolled over with an extended arm trapped beneath his or her trunk. After a brief initial period of crying, the child calms down but is unable to use the affected arm, which is held close to the body with the elbow flexed and forearm pronated (Fig. 21-66, *A*). If old enough to talk, the child may complain of elbow, forearm, or even wrist pain. Physical examination reveals no bony tenderness and no evidence of swelling, but on assessment of passive motion, the child resists any attempt at supination and cries in pain. Mild limitation of elbow flexion and extension may also be noted.

Pathologically, when the radial head is subluxated by the sudden pull on the arm, the annular ligament is torn at the site of its attachment to the radius and the radial head slips through the tear. When the traction is released and the radial head recoils, the proximal portion of the annular ligament

Table 21-5	Classification of Sprains	
Grade of Sprain	**Degree of Tearing**	**Clinical Findings**
I	A small percentage of ligamentous fibers is disrupted	Pain on motion Local tenderness Mild swelling
II	A moderate percentage of fibers is torn	Pain on motion More diffuse tenderness Moderate swelling, may have joint effusion Mild instability
III	The ligament is completely disrupted	Severe pain on motion Marked swelling, usually with joint effusion Marked tenderness Joint instability

Distal humerus

Capitellum

Annular ligament

Ulna

Radius

A   B

Figure 21-67   Nursemaid's elbow. **A,** Sudden traction on the outstretched arm pulls the radius distally, causing it to slip partially through the annular ligament and tearing it in the process. **B,** When traction is released, the radial head recoils, trapping the proximal portion of the ligament between it and the capitellum.

becomes trapped between the radial head and the capitellum (Fig. 21-67). This limits motion and produces the child's pain. Radiographs are normal because the radial head is not truly subluxated. When a patient presents with a typical history, is found to have no evidence of tenderness, and resists supination, x-ray studies are unnecessary. Reduction, as described later, should be attempted.

Treatment consists of supinating the child's forearm with the elbow in a flexed position while applying pressure over the radial head (see Fig. 21-66, *B*). A click can be perceived as the annular ligament is freed from the joint. On occasion this maneuver fails, in which case the forearm should be supinated and extended with traction applied distally while pressing down on the radial head. If this fails as well, pronation with the elbow in extension may be attempted. On reduction, pain relief is immediate and return of function is evident within 10 to 15 minutes. Clinicians often recommend that the child wear a sling for 10 days to reduce use and to allow the annular ligament to heal; compliance is difficult to ensure, however.

If presentation has been delayed for several hours, there may be a longer delay between reduction and resumption of normal use and it may be necessary to administer acetaminophen for 12 to 14 hours to relieve residual aching. Parents should be cautioned to avoid maneuvers that cause excessive traction on the arm because there is a significant risk of recurrence.

Extremity Pain with Ligamentous Laxity

Children with significant and generalized ligamentous laxity have hypermobile joints and are vulnerable to excessive stretching or stress on ligamentous and musculotendinous structures. They are also somewhat more susceptible to joint dislocations. The phenomenon is seen in up to 18% of girls and 6% of boys. After periods of vigorous physical activity, these children often complain of arthralgias, shin or muscular pain, and occasionally have evidence of joint swelling. Episodes tend to occur in the evening or at night; are self-limited, lasting 1 to several hours; and respond to rest and acetaminophen or ibuprofen. Many of these children have been accused of attention-getting behavior and hypochondriasis. Others have been dismissed as having "growing pains," and some have undergone extensive testing for rheumatic disorders. A history of greater than average activity on the preceding day and of recurrent short-lived pain usually without objective swelling, combined with findings of ligamentous laxity on examination (Fig. 21-68), should point to this diagnosis. The rarity of joint swelling and the absence of fever and other systemic symptoms help to rule out rheumatic and collagen vascular disorders.

Once the problem is correctly diagnosed, patients can minimize discomfort by avoiding sudden increases in level of activity, when possible, and by taking a mild analgesic prophylactically before going to bed after a day of unusually vigorous activity. Graduated strengthening exercises may also be helpful. This is particularly true for children who want to participate in gymnastics or competitive sports.

DISORDERS OF THE NECK AND SPINE

Children with disorders of the axial skeleton most commonly present with some type of deformity. Pain or dysfunction of the associated spinal cord and nerve roots may also prompt evaluation. Because these conditions often progress with growth, awareness and early recognition are important to assist early institution of appropriate treatment and to minimize resultant morbidity.

Congenital Torticollis

Congenital torticollis, or "wryneck," is a positional abnormality of the neck produced by fibrosis and shortening of the sternocleidomastoid muscle. It is thought to be secondary to abnormal intrauterine positioning or to birth trauma resulting in the formation of a hematoma within the muscle belly. Usually the condition is recognized at or shortly after birth. A palpable swelling or "tumor" is often noted within the muscle. With subsequent fibrosis, the characteristic deformity of torticollis develops, consisting of head tilt toward the affected side with rotation of the chin to the opposite side (Fig. 21-69). Passive rotation is diminished toward the side of the torticollis, and lateral side bending is limited toward the side away from the torticollis. Although the mass usually disappears in the first several weeks of life, contracture of the muscle persists and, if untreated, may result in craniofacial disfigurement with flattening of the face on the affected side. Gentle passive stretching exercises and positioning the child's crib so that external stimuli will cause him or her to turn the head and

Figure 21-68 Ligamentous laxity. This child shows findings typical of the joint hypermobility seen with ligamentous laxity. **A,** He is able to hyperflex the wrist on the forearm. **B,** He can also hyperextend the distal interphalangeal joint and the metacarpophalangeal joint.

neck away from the side of deformity may be beneficial. If these measures fail, surgical release of the contracted muscle may be indicated.

Considerations in the differential diagnosis include Klippel-Feil syndrome; inflammatory or infectious conditions of the head, neck, or nasopharynx; posterior fossa or brainstem neoplasm; traumatic cervical spine injury; and atlantoaxial rotary subluxation. However, with the exception of the Klippel-Feil anomaly, the other conditions tend to occur considerably later in childhood. In addition, a hip examination should be performed and an AP pelvis radiograph obtained for each infant with torticollis because hip instability or dysplasia is present in approximately 20% of these children.

Klippel-Feil Syndrome

Patients with Klippel-Feil syndrome have a congenital malformation of the neck that results from a failure of segmentation in the developing cervical spine. The condition varies greatly in severity, depending on the number of vertebrae that are

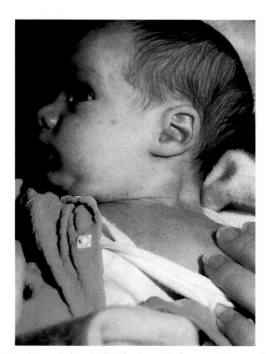

Figure 21-69 Congenital torticollis. The "tumor" of congenital torticollis is seen as a swelling in the midportion of the sternocleidomastoid muscle. It is firm on palpation, and the muscle itself is shortened. The head tilts toward the affected side, and the chin rotates in the opposite direction. *(Courtesy James Reilly, MD, Nemours/Alfred I. duPont Hospital for Children, Wilmington, Del.)*

fused (Fig. 21-70, *A* and *B*). More severely affected individuals exhibit a short, broad neck with the appearance of "webbing," a low hairline, and gross restriction of motion (Fig. 21-70, *C* and *D*). The condition may be associated with other congenital malformations such as a Sprengel deformity (see Fig. 21-81); rib deformities; scoliosis; CNS defects; and cardiac, pulmonary, and renal anomalies. Secondary neurologic problems are rare, but accelerated degenerative changes may occur at mobile spinal segments adjacent to the involved vertebrae.

On occasion, range-of-motion exercises or bracing may be tried to improve mobility or correct the deformity. Surgery, except for cosmesis or the treatment of neurologic dysfunction, is rarely indicated. Mild forms of the malformation may be diagnosed only as a result of radiographs taken for other reasons.

Scoliosis

Scoliosis is a condition in which there is curvature of the spine occurring in the lateral plane. It occurs in structural forms, characterized by a fixed curve, and "functional" forms, characterized by a flexible or correctable curve. By anatomic necessity, this lateral deviation is associated with vertebral rotation, such that when this deformity occurs in the thoracic spine, a chest wall deformity, or "rib hump," develops (Fig. 21-71). When it occurs in the lumbar spine, a prominence of the flank may be noted (Fig. 21-72). Often there is a primary structural curve with an adjacent secondary compensatory curve. Most cases of structural scoliosis are idiopathic and have their onset in early adolescence. A familial predisposition has been documented, but inheritance appears to be multifactorial. Females are affected more often than males, and their curvature is more likely to worsen. Infantile (0 to 3 years) and juvenile (3 to 10 years) forms of idiopathic scoliosis are seen, although much less commonly. Those with onset in infancy rapidly develop plagiocephaly with flattening of the head on the concave side of the curve and a corresponding prominence on the opposite side of the head. Affected infants also have an increased incidence of associated hip dysplasia, congenital heart disease, inguinal hernia, and mental retardation. Structural scoliosis can also occur in conjunction with neuromuscular conditions such as cerebral palsy (Fig. 21-73), myelomeningocele, spinocerebellar degeneration, polio, and spinal cord tumors; myopathic disorders including arthrogryposis and muscular dystrophy; congenital spinal anomalies (Fig. 21-74, *A* and *B*) such as hemivertebrae, trapezoidal vertebrae, and unsegmented vertebrae; neurofibromatosis (Fig. 21-75) and mesenchymal disorders; and a variety of other conditions (Table 21-6). These neuromuscular and congenital forms of scoliosis tend to

Figure 21-70 Klippel-Feil syndrome. **A,** This radiograph shows mild osseous involvement with fusion of the upper cervical segments. **B,** In this radiograph another patient has severe osseous involvement in which C3-C7 are fused and hypoplastic. **C,** Clinically the neck appears short and broad in the anterior view of this young child. **D,** In this posterior view the hairline is low and an associated Sprengel deformity is present, the left scapula being hypoplastic and high riding. As a result, the patient is unable to fully raise his left arm. Typical webbing of the neck is not appreciable in this child.

Figure 21-71 Moderate idiopathic thoracic scoliosis in an adolescent. **A,** Scapular asymmetry is easily discernible in the upright position. This results from rotation of the spine and attached rib cage. **B,** Forward flexion reveals a rib hump deformity.

Figure 21-72 Lumbar scoliosis. Pelvic obliquity is present, with prominence of the left flank.

Figure 21-73 Neuromuscular scoliosis. This 12-year-old boy has cerebral palsy and scoliosis. Note that his sitting balance is affected by the curve of his spine, which extends from the upper thorax to his pelvis, resulting in pelvic obliquity and inability to sit independently. This is typical of spinal deformity in patients with neuromuscular disorders.

Figure 21-74 Congenital scoliosis. **A,** This 7-year-old was born with fusion of ribs 5 to 10 on her right side. She also has congenital failure of segmentation of several vertebrae. Both of these anomalies contributed to her progressive scoliotic deformity. **B,** She was treated with an opening thoracostomy (separation of the ribs) and insertion of a vertical expandable prosthetic titanium rib (VEPTR; Synthes, Solothurn, Switzerland). This device allows for spinal growth and expansion of the chest cavity by repeated surgical expansions at 6-month intervals.

have more rapid progression of curvature than is true of idiopathic scoliosis, and infants with congenital spinal anomalies have a high incidence of associated genitourinary anomalies.

Apparent nonstructural, flexible, or "functional" scoliosis may be seen in association with poor posture; limb length inequality; or flexion contracture of a hip or knee, in which case the curve disappears when the child is seated. It can also be seen with paraspinous muscle spasm after a back injury; as the result of splinting because of pain in cases of pyelonephritis, appendicitis, or pneumonia; or in patients with a herniated intervertebral disk and secondary nerve root pain (see Fig. 21-80, *A*; see also Table 21-6). These forms resolve with treatment of the primary disorder.

Except in curvatures resulting from inflammatory or neoplastic processes and from herniation of an intervertebral disk, pain is rarely a complaint in children and adolescents with scoliosis. In fact, patients with pain, signs of nerve root compression, or evidence of new-onset peripheral neurologic deficits should undergo thorough evaluation for a treatable underlying cause.

The clinical signs found during examination in a patient with scoliosis can be separated into true pathognomonic findings and associated stigmata, which may also occur in otherwise normal, nonscoliotic children. The only true pathognomonic sign of scoliosis is the presence of a curve noted on forward bending, which constitutes a positive Adams forward bend test (see Thoracolumbar Spine, earlier). An associated convex posterior chest wall prominence (termed *rib hump*) or paralumbar prominence may also be noted on forward bending (see Fig. 21-71, *B*). The rib hump and paralumbar prominence are manifestations of the vertebral rotational deformity seen in scoliosis.

Table 21-6	Causes of Scoliosis
Structural Scoliosis	• Metabolic disorders
Idiopathic	• Trauma, surgery, irradiation, burns
Congenital	
Neuromuscular	***Functional Scoliosis***
Other conditions that may result in scoliosis:	Herniated lumbar disks
	Postural derangements
• Myopathic disorders	Limb length inequality
• Neurofibromatosis	Irritative or inflammatory disorders
• Mesenchymal disorders	Hysteria
• Osteochondrodystrophies	

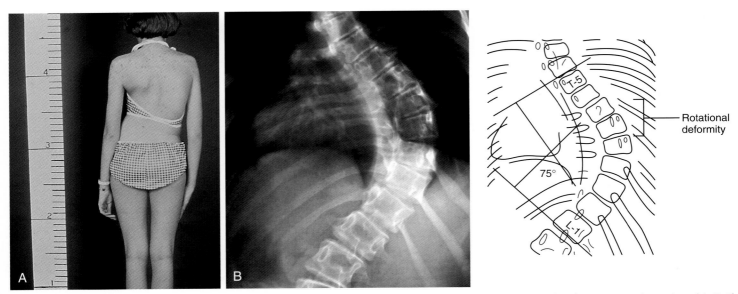

Figure 21-75   Severe thoracic scoliosis secondary to neurofibromatosis. **A,** Note the chest wall deformity and that the patient's head is not centered over the pelvis. **B,** The severe curvature is more apparent on this radiograph. The angle of measurement (here, 75 degrees) is determined by the intersection of lines drawn perpendicular to the vertebrae at the ends of the curve (Cobb method).

Frequently a diagnosis of scoliosis is based not on a positive forward bend test, but rather on the presence of so-called stigmata signs. These signs include shoulder asymmetry, unilateral scapular prominence, waist asymmetry, and small chest or paralumbar humps (see Figs. 21-71, *A*; 21-72; and 21-75, *A*). Any or all of these stigmata signs may be present in a child with true scoliosis, but the mere presence of these stigmata does not always imply the presence of scoliosis. Body asymmetry is a frequent occurrence in the normal nonscoliotic child. A carefully performed Adams forward bend test always determines whether the stigmata signs are associated with true scoliosis or simply evidence of body asymmetry.

Because screening studies have shown that up to 5% of school-age children and adolescents have lateral curvatures, routine screening by primary care physicians is important. Hence the forward bend test should be part of all examinations in children from age 6 to 7 years until the end of puberty (see Thoracolumbar Spine, earlier). When true clinical scoliosis is found, the patient should be referred for orthopedic evaluation no matter how small the curve is believed to be. It is probably safer and more cost-effective for the primary care physician to make the referral without obtaining prior radiographs, because typical office radiographs done for scoliosis screening are usually not of high quality. Standing, full-torso x-rays taken on 36-inch-long (90 cm) cassette films with special grids are much more helpful and more readily available in the orthopedic clinic or office. Once a diagnosis of scoliosis has been made, follow-up x-rays are routinely obtained no more frequently than at 6- to 9-month intervals. The goal of close follow-up is to detect progression of curvature early and to implement treatment to prevent or reduce it when needed. Idiopathic curves of 25 to 30 degrees or more and lesser curves showing rapid progression are treated by spinal bracing and an exercise program. Children with curves exceeding 45 to 50 degrees or those with curves that progress rapidly despite bracing require operative intervention.

Patients with untreated curvatures exceeding 75 to 80 degrees inevitably suffer significant secondary cardiopulmonary problems including decreased vital capacity, shunting, decreased oxygen saturation, and cor pulmonale.

Newborns and infants should be screened for congenital and infantile forms of scoliosis. This is often best done by holding the infant prone on the examiner's hand and can be done while assessing for parachute reflex.

Kyphosis

Kyphosis is a condition in which there is curvature of the spine in the sagittal plane. The thoracic spine normally has a kyphotic curvature of 25 to 50 degrees, with a similar amount of lordosis in the lumbar spine in the sagittal plane. Excessive kyphosis may be purely postural in nature or may be associated with a number of pathologic conditions. The latter include congenital vertebral anomalies, a spinal growth disturbance known as Scheuermann disease (Fig. 21-76), neuromuscular afflictions, skeletal dysplasias, and metabolic diseases (Fig. 21-77). Kyphosis can also develop after spinal trauma or surgery. Patients with a structural deformity may complain of backache aggravated by motion. The deformity is best viewed from the lateral position on forward bending. Evaluation of the effects of posture and of application of pressure over the apex of the curve assists diagnosis and decisions regarding treatment.

Postural kyphosis is usually seen in preadolescents and consists of a flexible thoracic kyphosis that is correctable on hyperextension. Most affected children have a compensatory increase in lumbar lordosis. Radiographic findings are normal. Treatment consists of an exercise program designed to strengthen trunk and abdominal muscles, which are usually weak in these patients.

Scheuermann disease, a disorder of unknown etiology, is the most common cause of fixed kyphotic deformity. It can be distinguished clinically from postural kyphosis by its inherent stiffness and the greater magnitude of the deformity. The deformity fails to correct or is only partially correctable on hyperextension or on the application of pressure over the apex of the curve. Lateral radiographs reveal anterior wedging of three or more consecutive vertebral bodies that are located at the apex of the curve. Radiographic evidence of end-plate erosion of the involved vertebrae often exists, and Schmorl nodules are a common associated finding (see Fig. 21-76).

Exercises and bracing are quite effective in treating mild structural kyphosis in the growing spine. However, when the deformity is severe and fixed, surgical correction and stabilization may be indicated.

Figure 21-76 Moderate thoracic kyphosis secondary to Scheuermann disease. **A,** The patient is attempting to correct the deformity, but because of its fixed nature, he cannot do so and must compensate for this with an increased lumbar lordosis. **B,** This tomographic cut shows anterior wedging of three consecutive vertebral bodies and clearly demonstrates the associated erosion of the vertebral end plates and Schmorl nodules.

Wedging of vertebra

Irregular end-plate

Figure 21-77 **A,** Severe kyphosis of the thoracic spine secondary to vertebral wedging in a patient with glycogen storage disease. To stand upright, the patient must increase his lumbar lordosis and thrust his head forward to center it above the pelvis. **B,** The kyphotic deformity is accentuated on forward bending. **C,** Radiographically, the vertebral wedging that underlies the kyphotic deformity is evident.

Spondylolisthesis

Spondylolisthesis is a condition characterized by the translation or forward displacement of one vertebral body over another and is seen most commonly at the lumbosacral articulation. The problem may develop as a result of insufficiency or fatigue fractures of the pars interarticularis (isthmic), congenital dysplasia of the posterior spinal elements (dysplastic), or degenerative changes in the disk and facets (degenerative), or it may occur secondary to pathologic lesions within the vertebra and its elements (pathologic). Isthmic spondylolisthesis (spondylolysis) is by far the most common type (Fig. 21-78). Patients with a congenital predisposition may show alarming degrees of slippage. The condition is often associated with low back pain that increases with strenuous activities and abates with rest. Some patients have symptoms of nerve root irritation. This necessitates differentiation from inflammatory and neoplastic processes and from disk herniation.

Examination often reveals loss of normal lumbar lordosis, tenderness of the involved posterior elements, paravertebral muscle spasm, and secondary tightness of the hamstring muscles. A step-off deformity may be evident on palpation of the spinous processes. Range of motion is often limited in extension because of pain. Nerve root signs may be present. In its most severe form, spondyloptosis, the L5 vertebral body may completely translate off the sacrum, and the patient characteristically exhibits a waddling gait, a transverse abdominal crease, flattened buttocks, and flexion deformities of the hips and knees, as well as foreshortening of the torso (Fig. 21-79, A and B). Characterization and grading of the process are accomplished with radiographs. The oblique view may reveal a spondylolysis and the lateral view the degree of spondylolisthesis (Fig. 21-79, C; see also Fig. 21-78).

In mild to moderate cases, treatment consists of appropriate exercises and bracing. Patients with progressive slippage require surgical fusion, and those with neural involvement may also require nerve root decompression. In cases of severe spondylolisthesis with cosmetic deformity, functional impairment, and neurologic dysfunction, surgical reduction of the deformity may be attempted but is not easy, nor is it without risk to the adjacent neural structures.

Herniated Intervertebral Disk

Although relatively common in adults, herniated disks occur only rarely in children and infrequently in adolescents. They are almost always limited to the lower two segments of the lumbar spine. A history of antecedent trauma is not uncommon. Lower extremity radicular symptoms predominate. Patients often describe a peculiar "pulling" sensation in a lower extremity or liken their pain to a "toothache" in the distribution of the L5 or S1 nerve roots (see Chapter 15). They also may complain of numbness or weakness in the involved limb. Forward flexion, sitting, coughing, and straining aggravate the neurologic symptoms.

On examination, an antalgic scoliosis of the lumbar spine may be apparent, which the patient is unable to reduce (Fig. 21-80, A). Inability to reverse the normal lumbar lordosis is noted, and symptoms may be aggravated by attempts at flexion. The straight leg raising test is often positive (radicular symptoms being reproduced when the limb is raised by the examiner; see Thoracolumbar Spine, earlier; and Fig. 21-5), and neurologic abnormalities may be found on sensory, motor, and reflex testing, although these may be subtle. Plain radiographs usually show no abnormality, other than a possible diskogenic scoliosis, but the diagnosis may be verified by myelography, CT, or MRI (Fig. 21-80, B). The differential diagnosis may include hematogenous disk space infection or vertebral osteomyelitis, spinal cord or neural element tumor, and spondylolisthesis with nerve root irritation.

Nonsurgical treatment consisting of rest and anti-inflammatory agents may be successful, but if a profound neurologic deficit is present or if incapacitating symptoms persist, surgical disk excision may be indicated. Intradiskal chemonucleolysis, as employed for adults, is contraindicated for children, and conservative treatment of radiographically proven disk herniation is not as effective in adolescents as it is in adults.

DISORDERS OF THE UPPER EXTREMITY

Because of the importance of prehensile function, disorders affecting any area of the upper limb can result in significant impairment of motor development during childhood.

Defect in pars interarticularis

Slippage of L-5 forward on S-1

Figure 21-78 Radiograph of a moderate isthmic spondylolisthesis in a 14-year-old boy. The forward slippage of L5 on the sacrum was the result of a fatigue fracture of the pars interarticularis.

Figure 21-79 Spondyloptosis in a 16-year-old girl. **A,** A cosmetic deformity is common with this magnitude of spondylolisthesis. The torso is foreshortened, and a transverse abdominal crease is present. **B,** In the lateral view the torso is thrust forward, the buttocks are flattened, and there are flexion deformities of the hips and knees. **C,** The L5 vertebra has completely translocated off the sacrum as the result of a congenital insufficiency of the posterior elements; the lumbar spine has essentially migrated anteriorly and into the pelvis.

No visible continuity between anterior and posterior elements of spine

Severe slippage of L-5 off of S-1

Vertical orientation of sacrum

L-5

S-1

Knowledge of the normal anatomy and actions of the shoulder, arm, elbow, forearm, wrist, and hand is vital for assessment of abnormalities and institution of appropriate treatment.

Sprengel Deformity

A Sprengel deformity is a congenital malformation characterized by an abnormally small, high-riding scapula. In most cases it is unilateral. The etiology is unknown, but there appears to be a familial predisposition and the condition may be associated with a variety of other congenital anomalies including Klippel-Feil syndrome (see Fig. 21-70) and rib and vertebral malformations. Scoliosis and torticollis may be associated abnormalities. Cosmetic deformity and limited shoulder motion on the affected side are the usual complaints.

On examination, the scapula is noted to be hypoplastic and high riding in association with asymmetry of the base of the neck and shoulders (Fig. 21-81, *A*). Shoulder motion is usually severely limited, particularly in abduction (Fig. 21-81, *B*). This is due to limited scapular motion because the scapula is often

Figure 21-80 Herniated intervertebral disk. **A,** Diskogenic scoliosis is evident in a 16-year-old girl with a herniated disk at L4-L5. The trunk is shifted away from the affected side. The normal lumbar lordosis is absent, and spinal motion is severely limited. **B,** On sagittal magnetic resonance imaging, the L4-L5 disk bulges posteriorly, compressing the cauda equina. (**B,** *Courtesy Department of Pediatric Radiology, Children's Hospital of Pittsburgh, Pittsburgh, Pa.*)

Figure 21-81   Sprengel deformity. **A,** The left scapula is high riding and hypoplastic, and its vertebral border is prominent. **B,** Shoulder motion is severely limited, particularly in abduction. *(Courtesy Dana Mears, MD.)*

tethered to the cervical spine by a fibrous omovertebral band, which is frequently ossified. Radiography confirms the abnormal size and position of the scapula.

Nonsurgical treatment consisting of stretching and range-of-motion exercises may be instituted but is rarely successful. Surgery may be undertaken on occasion for cosmetic and functional reasons and may consist of excision of the prominent superior aspect of the scapula or of release and reduction of the scapula accomplished by positioning it inferiorly on the chest wall. Although care must be taken during the procedure to prevent brachial plexus injury, surgery performed before adolescence usually improves appearance and restores some function.

Congenital Pseudarthrosis of the Clavicle

Congenital pseudarthrosis of the clavicle is a rare congenital disorder usually manifested by a painless, nontender bulbous deformity in the region of the midclavicle. It is thought to result from a failure of maturation of the ossification center of the clavicle. It generally involves the right side and on occasion may be associated with other congenital anomalies and can be seen in patients with neurofibromatosis 1. In cleidocranial dysostosis the entire clavicle may be absent or may have an appearance similar to that of congenital pseudarthrosis.

On examination, the clavicle appears foreshortened with a prominence evident in its midportion (Fig. 21-82; see Chapter 6 for radiographic appearance). Palpation reveals hypermobility of the two ends of the clavicle and crepitance. In general, range of motion of the shoulder is normal. This condition characteristically involves no functional impairment and requires no treatment. Although clavicular fracture as a result of birth trauma may present a similar appearance, it is easily distinguished because of tenderness over the region of deformity.

Radial Club Hand

Radial club hand is the result of congenital absence or hypoplasia of the radial structures of the forearm and hand. Associated muscular structures and the radial nerve are hypoplastic or absent. The anomaly is rare and affects more male than female subjects. Its characteristic clinical presentation is one of a small, short, bowed forearm and aplasia or hypoplasia of the thumb, and the residual hand is deviated radially (Fig. 21-83, *A* and *B*). Radiographs show absence of bones in the affected area (Fig. 21-83, *C*).

Treatment is best instituted early with passive stretching exercises and corrective casting. Surgical treatment consists of centralization of the hand on the "one-bone forearm" to maximize function.

Ganglion of the Wrist

A ganglion is a benign cystic mass consisting of an accumulation of synovial fluid or gelatin in an outpouching of a tendon sheath or joint capsule. The exact etiology is unknown, but it is thought to be related to a herniation of synovial tissue with a ball–valve effect. Antecedent trauma may be reported. These masses may be present over the dorsal or volar aspects of the wrist and are generally located toward the radial side (Fig. 21-84). On occasion they are seen on the dorsum of the foot or adjacent to one of the malleoli of the ankle (see Fig. 21-108). Their size may fluctuate with time and activity. On examination they may be either firm or fluctuant, and they can be transilluminated. Although most are asymptomatic, an occasional patient may complain of pain and tenderness.

Treatment is generally unnecessary for patients who are asymptomatic, and surgery is not routinely advised because the recurrence rate may be as high as 20%. On occasion, patients desire removal for cosmetic or psychological reasons.

Figure 21-82   Congenital pseudarthrosis of the clavicle. There is a bulbous, nontender swelling in the region of the midclavicle. The medial aspect of the clavicle is prominent. This patient has associated anomalies. Radiographic appearance is shown in Chapter 6.

Figure 21-83 Radial club hand. **A,** The forearm is shortened with radial deviation of the hand and wrist on the ulna. **B,** A flexion deformity of the hand and wrist on the forearm and a hypoplastic thumb are present. **C,** Radiograph shows absence of the radius, dislocation of the carpus, and a rudimentary thumb, all characteristic of radial club hand. *(Clinical photographs courtesy Joseph Imbriglia, MD, Allegheny General Hospital, Pittsburgh, Pittsburgh, Pa.)*

Aspiration, injection, or rupture of these cysts does not eradicate them. Surgical excision with obliteration of the base of the ganglion is the most successful treatment for the occasional patient in whom treatment is indicated.

Syndactyly

Syndactyly is a relatively common congenital anomaly involving failure of the digits of the hands or feet to separate. It is both more common and more disabling in the upper extremity. Bilateral involvement is usual, and a positive family history is not uncommon. It may be associated with other congenital anomalies, particularly Apert syndrome and Streeter dysplasia. Great variation in the degree of fusion exists. In mild cases, only the skin is joined, making reconstructive surgery simple (Fig. 21-85). In more severe cases the nails, deeper structures, and bones may be conjoined, contributing to deformity and growth abnormalities and making reconstructive treatment more difficult.

Figure 21-84 Ganglion of the wrist. This cystic mass overlying the wrist joint and flexor tendons was asymptomatic and nontender.

Figure 21-85 Syndactyly. This child has mild syndactyly involving soft tissues of the middle and ring fingers without bony involvement. *(Courtesy Joseph Imbriglia, MD, Allegheny General Hospital, Pittsburgh, Pa.)*

Figure 21-86 Congenital trigger thumb. There is a fixed flexion deformity at the interphalangeal joint of the thumb resulting from tightness of the tendon sheath of the flexor pollicis longus. The remainder of the hand appears normal.

Congenital Trigger Thumb

A congenital trigger thumb is characterized by a fixed or intermittent flexion deformity of the interphalangeal joint of the thumb that may be present at birth or may develop shortly thereafter (Fig. 21-86). It is thought to result from tightness of the tendon sheath of the flexor pollicis longus in the region of the metacarpophalangeal joint. The flexion deformity generally cannot be reduced, although in milder cases it may be passively correctable, with a snapping sensation felt as the tendon passes through the stenosed pulley mechanism. If passively correctable, splinting in extension occasionally results in correction; otherwise, surgery is required.

Boutonnière (Buttonhole) Deformity

A boutonnière deformity of a finger is the end result of a traumatic avulsion of the central portion of the extensor tendon at its insertion on the middle phalanx that went unrecognized at the time of initial injury. The mechanism of injury is usually a blow to the tip of the finger that drives it into forced flexion against resistance, although a laceration over the dorsum of the finger involving the extensor tendon may produce a similar deformity if tendon involvement is not recognized and repaired at the time. Initially, there may be local tenderness over the dorsal aspect of the PIP joint without deformity. With time, however, the lateral bands of the extensor mechanism migrate volarly, producing a flexion deformity of the PIP joint with a secondary extension deformity of the distal joint (Fig. 21-87). If the injury is recognized early, healing may occur with splinting of the PIP joint in extension. Later, open surgical repair may be necessary to improve function.

Mallet Finger/Swan-Neck Deformity

A mallet finger is the result of avulsion of the extensor tendon from its insertion at the base of the distal phalanx of a finger. It occurs as a result of a blow to the extended finger against resistance. The tendon alone, or a portion of the distal phalanx into which it inserts, may be involved. The clinical appearance

Figure 21-87 Boutonnière deformity of the finger. A fixed flexion contracture of the proximal interphalangeal joint exists, along with hyperextension of the distal joint secondary to volar migration of the lateral bands of the extensor mechanism. This is the result of an unrecognized or inadequately treated injury to the extensor tendon at its insertion on the middle phalanx.

is that of a "dropped finger" or flexion deformity of the distal interphalangeal joint with inability to actively extend the joint (see Fig. 21-49). If not recognized and treated at the time of the initial injury, the condition becomes chronic and contracture of the extensor mechanism may occur, with a secondary hyperextension deformity of the PIP joint producing a swan-neck deformity (Fig. 21-88). Treatment consists of splinting the distal joint in an extended position, open reduction if a large fragment of bone is involved, or surgical repair in chronic cases.

DISORDERS OF THE LOWER EXTREMITY

Normally developed and functional lower extremities permit locomotion with ease and a minimal amount of energy expenditure. A disability resulting from a deformed, shortened, or painful lower limb can be considerable (see Gait and Gait Disturbances, earlier).

Many problems of the lower extremities occurring in childhood are congenital and, if they remain unrecognized or are unsuccessfully treated, can result in lifelong disability. Knowledge of the normal anatomy and function of the hip, knee, ankle, and foot is necessary to accurately recognize and treat abnormalities in this region (see Lower Extremity Examination, earlier).

Developmental Dislocation of the Hip

Developmental dislocation of the hip, formerly referred to as *congenital dislocation of the hip,* consists of displacement of the femoral head from its normal relationship with the

Figure 21-88 Mallet finger with secondary swan-neck deformity. This is the result of avulsion of the extensor tendon from its insertion at the base of the distal phalanx, which was not recognized at the time of injury. The patient shows a flexion deformity of the distal interphalangeal joint and secondary hyperextension of the proximal interphalangeal joint.

acetabulum. It is a relatively frequent problem, with an incidence of 1 to 2 per 1000 births. It is generally detectable at birth or shortly thereafter. Female infants are affected significantly more frequently than male infants, and unilateral dislocation is twice as frequent as bilateral. Developmental dislocation may be divided into idiopathic and teratogenic types. Idiopathic dislocation is more frequent, and patients often have a positive family history for the defect. Its severity varies from subluxated, to dislocated and reducible, to dislocated and irreducible. This type of developmental dislocation may be related to abnormal intrauterine positioning or restriction of fetal movement in utero, which impedes adequate development and stability of the hip joint complex. The relaxing effect of hormones on soft tissue during pregnancy may also contribute, with affected infants perhaps being more sensitive to the pelvic relaxation effects of maternal estrogen. A history of breech presentation is not uncommon, and these patients often exhibit generalized ligamentous laxity. Teratogenic dislocations of the hip represent a more severe form of the disorder and are probably the result of a germ plasm defect. They occur early in fetal development and result in malformation of both the femoral head and the acetabular socket. Associated congenital anomalies are common in infants whose dislocations are teratogenic, including clubfoot deformity, congenital torticollis, metatarsus adductus, and infantile scoliosis.

The importance of careful hip evaluation in the newborn and at early infant visits cannot be overemphasized. Early diagnosis enables prompt institution of treatment and results in a better outcome. A knowledge of the clinical signs and skill in techniques of examination are necessary.

Typically, the infant with a dislocated hip has no noticeable difference in the position in which the leg is held, although some affected infants may hold the leg in a position of adduction and external rotation. If the dislocation is unilateral, the skin folds of the thighs and buttocks are often asymmetrical and the involved lower extremity appears shorter than the opposite side (Fig. 21-89, A). This foreshortening is accentuated by holding the hips and knees in 90 degrees of flexion (Galeazzi sign). In patients with bilateral dislocations, this asymmetry is not present. In a truly dislocated hip, the most consistent physical finding is that of limited abduction (see Fig. 21-89, B). Additional diagnostic maneuvers may assist in establishing the diagnosis. In patients with reducible dislocations, the Ortolani sign is positive when a palpable clunk is felt on abduction and internal rotation (relocation) of the hip. The Barlow test is positive if, with the knees flexed and hips flexed to 90 degrees, the hips are gently adducted with pressure applied on the lesser trochanter by the thumb. A palpable clunk indicating posterior dislocation is appreciated if the hip is unstable or dislocated. When the hip is dislocated and irreducible, only limitation of abduction is apparent.

The radiographic findings of a developmental hip dislocation are characteristic. The femoral head is generally located lateral and superior to its normal position, and the acetabulum may be shallow, with lateral deficiency and a characteristic high acetabular index or slope (Fig. 21-89, C and D). Reduction of the dislocated hip is apparent if, on abduction of the hip to 45 degrees, a line drawn through the axis of the metaphysis of the neck crosses the triradiate cartilage (Fig. 21-89, diagram). Because ossification is not evident radiographically until 3 to 6 months of age, ultrasound evaluation of the hip is often helpful in determining the acetabular–femoral head relationships. Furthermore, in developmental dislocation, ossification may be delayed even longer, because normal articulation forces are absent.

In teratogenic hip dislocation, there may be hypoplasia of both the acetabular and femoral sides with noncongruent development of one or both of these structures. The early radiographic findings, however, are similar to those already mentioned.

Successful correction of congenital hip dislocation depends on early diagnosis and institution of appropriate treatment. In the first 6 months of life, use of a Pavlik harness, which permits gentle motion of the hip in a flexed and abducted position, may achieve and maintain a satisfactory reduction. Between 6 and 18 months of age, gentle closed reduction and immobilization in a spica cast with or without surgical release of the contracted iliopsoas and adductor muscles is indicated. After the age of 18 months, reduction by manipulative measures is difficult owing to contractures of the associated soft tissues. In such instances open reduction is usually indicated. In cases of teratogenic dislocation, underlying maldevelopment makes the outcome less satisfactory, even with optimal management.

With early recognition and appropriate treatment, a relatively normal hip with satisfactory function can be anticipated in cases of idiopathic hip dislocation. Failure of concentric reduction or complications such as avascular necrosis of the femoral head, resulting from overzealous attempts at closed reduction in long-standing cases, may result in a lifelong disability characterized by pain and stiffness in the hip; an antalgic, lurching gait; and shortening of the involved limb.

Legg-Calvé-Perthes Disease

In Legg-Calvé-Perthes disease (coxa plana), impairment of the blood supply to the developing femoral head results in avascular necrosis. The etiology is unknown. Current theories implicate traumatic disruption of the blood supply and recurrent episodes of synovitis, during which increased intra-articular pressure compromises blood flow to the developing ossific nucleus, as causative. The disorder generally becomes manifest between the ages of 4 and 11 years, with a higher incidence in boys. Affected children often exhibit delayed skeletal maturation and are small for their age. Unilateral involvement is the rule, and if a bilateral case is suspected, some form of epiphyseal dysplasia must be ruled out. The severity of the disease varies greatly, depending on the extent to which the femoral head is affected. Younger children generally have milder involvement, as a larger portion of the femoral head is still cartilaginous and less dependent on vascular supply.

Typically onset is insidious. The child may present with symptoms characteristic of toxic synovitis without radiographic findings. Many children present with a painless limp, and others complain of thigh or knee pain, fatigue on walking, or hip stiffness. In general, the patient bears less weight on the involved leg when standing and there is a flexion contracture of the involved hip (Fig. 21-90, A; see also Fig. 21-8, B), with the lower extremity held in a slightly externally rotated position. Pain and limitation of motion are encountered on attempts at internal rotation and abduction. The Trendelenburg sign (failure to maintain a level pelvis when standing on the involved limb) is positive.

Early radiographic findings may include failure of progressive development of the femoral ossific nucleus, a subchondral radiolucent fracture line (Caffey sign), and evidence of slight subluxation. However, in early cases, radiographs may be completely normal, although a nuclear bone scan may be useful in verification of impairment of the blood supply to this region. Later, fragmentation of the femoral ossification center may be evident with flattening of the femoral head, extrusion, and frank subluxation (Fig. 21-90, B).

The disease is self-limited, typically lasting for 1 to 2 years. Although revascularization and reconstitution of the femoral

Figure 21-89   Developmental dislocation of the hip. **A,** In cases of unilateral dislocation, the involved extremity is foreshortened and the thigh and groin creases are asymmetric. **B,** Limited abduction of the involved hip is seen. This is a consistent finding in infants with a dislocated and irreducible hip. **C,** In this anteroposterior radiograph obtained in a 3-month-old child, the proximal left femur is displaced upward and laterally, and the acetabulum is shallow. The femoral head is not visible on the radiograph because of the delayed ossification associated with developmental hip dislocation. **D,** In the frog-leg view, the long axis of the affected left femur is directed toward a point superior and lateral to the triradiate cartilage, in contrast with that of the right, which points directly toward this structure.

head always occur, loss of mechanical integrity of the head with flattening and fragmentation of its surface may result in an irreversible predisposition to degenerative change. Most treatments are based on the principle of "containment" and the maintenance of a normal relationship of the femoral head within the acetabulum so as to minimize permanent joint incongruity. In young children with minimal symptoms and radiographic findings, decreased activity and close observation may be all that is necessary. Antiinflammatory agents and traction are used during episodes of synovitis. In more severe cases, abduction casting, bracing, or surgical treatment with femoral or acetabular osteotomy to reposition the femoral head deeper within the acetabulum may be employed. In patients whose disease is recognized late or who fail to respond to

appropriate measures, permanent degenerative change is common and salvage-type surgery may be necessary.

Slipped Capital Femoral Epiphysis

Slipped capital femoral epiphysis, a disorder seen early in puberty, involves displacement of the femoral head from the femoral neck through the epiphyseal plate. It is seen more frequently in males and occurs bilaterally in approximately 25% of cases. Most commonly, it occurs at the onset of puberty in obese children with delayed sexual maturation. Although the etiology is unclear, it is generally thought that hormonal changes at the time of puberty may result in loss of mechanical integrity of the growth

Figure 21-90 Legg-Calvé-Perthes disease. **A,** This 7-year-old boy is small for his chronologic age. He is bearing less weight on the involved right leg (note the slightly flexed right knee). On examination a hip flexion contracture, detected by a positive Thomas test (see Fig. 21-8, *B*), and an abductor lurch gait were found. **B,** In this anteroposterior radiograph, the right femoral epiphysis is flattened and fragmented. The proximal femur is also displaced inferiorly and laterally.

plate, and that if the epiphysis is then subjected to excessive shear stress, slippage through this area may occur. This condition differs from traumatic epiphyseal fractures because the translational displacement occurs through a different portion of the growth plate. In some cases an underlying connective tissue disorder such as Marfan syndrome or an endocrinologic problem such as hypothyroidism can be identified.

The clinical presentation is quite characteristic, although the duration of symptoms varies. The patient presents with a painful limp and may or may not have a history of recent trauma, which is usually minor, or pain may have developed after jumping. This injury may have precipitated a slip in the previously weakened epiphysis or may have increased the degree of displacement of a slip that was already in progress. The pain may be perceived as being in the hip or in the thigh or knee. The lower extremity is held in an externally rotated position secondary to deformity at the site of physeal displacement (Fig. 21-91, *A* and *B*). An antalgic and abductor lurch gait is usually apparent. A flexion contracture may be noted, and range of hip motion tends to be diminished in all planes, particularly internal rotation. Slight shortening of the involved lower extremity is observed in some patients.

Radiographic findings vary from a widened and radiolucent physis (preslip) to a frank deformity with displacement of the femoral head on the proximal femur posteriorly and inferiorly in relation to its normal counterpart (Fig. 21-91, *C* and *D*). The degree of slippage and deformity correlates with the extent of incongruity of the hip joint and the later development of degenerative change and painful symptoms. Prompt intervention to prevent further displacement is an important factor in preventing lifelong problems, and awareness of the condition, a high index of suspicion, and early recognition are key factors in improving prognosis.

In patients with minimally or moderately displaced slips, stabilization of the slip by in situ pin fixation is indicated. In severe slips, especially those that have slipped acutely, pinning

may be the treatment of choice initially, but development of avascular changes secondary to disruption of the blood supply to the femoral head may occur and complicate the outcome. When the disease is recognized late and deformity is severe, proximal femoral osteotomy may be necessary. Children with unilateral slipped epiphyses must be monitored closely for signs of involvement of the opposite limb.

Femoral Anteversion

Femoral anteversion may be viewed as a normal variation of lower extremity positioning in the developing child. In utero and at birth, the femoral neck sits in an anteverted position relative to that of the adult. During childhood it remodels to a position of slight anteversion and normal alignment of the lower extremities. In certain children, however, delayed rotational correction may result in persistent intoeing. An unsightly gait, kicking of the heels, and tripping on walking or running are frequent related complaints. There may be a history of sitting on the floor with knees bent and the lower legs turned outward in a reversed tailor position. In general, the condition is bilateral and is not associated with other musculoskeletal problems.

On examination, the child is noted to stand with the thighs, knees, and feet all turned inward. An increase in internal rotation over external rotation is apparent on assessment of range of motion of the hip (Fig. 21-92). Radiographic findings are normal. No treatment is indicated, other than reassurance that the condition will correct with growth and instructions to avoid sitting in the predisposing position.

Genu Varum (Physiologic Bowleg)

Genu varum, or bowleg, is usually a normal variation of lower extremity configuration, seen in the 1- to 3-year-old age group. It is generally recognized shortly after ambulation begins and may be associated with laxity of other joints and internal tibial

Figure 21-91   Slipped capital femoral epiphysis. **A,** This obese boy presented with a painful limp during early puberty. Note his reluctance to bear weight on the involved right leg. **B,** When he lies supine, the affected leg is positioned in external rotation because this minimizes discomfort. Attempts at motion produce pain in the acutely slipped epiphysis. **C,** In the anteroposterior radiograph the right femoral head is displaced medially in relation to the femoral neck as a result of epiphyseal separation. **D,** In the lateral view the femoral head is seen to be displaced posteriorly in relation to the femoral neck. A line drawn along the axis of the femoral neck should normally touch the head.

torsion. Examination reveals diffuse bowing of the lower extremities with an increased distance between the knees that is accentuated on standing (Fig. 21-93). Varus positioning of the heel with pronation of the feet may be noted on weight bearing. The child may walk with a waddling gait and kick the heels on running to clear the feet from the ground and avoid hitting the contralateral limb. Laxity of joint capsular structures may be noted with application of a reduction force.

Radiographs of children with physiologic bowing show normal osseous and physeal development and may reveal a gentle symmetrical bowing of the femur and tibia. Although there may be slight beaking of the medial metaphyses of the femur and tibia adjacent to the knee joint, there is no fragmentation of the epiphyses or irregularity of the growth plate, as is seen in *Blount disease* (see Fig. 21-96).

Treatment is rarely indicated, as this condition resolves with growth; in fact, a valgus deformity of the knees may be noted later, at approximately 4 to 5 years of age. Casting, bracing, and corrective shoes are unnecessary, and there is no indication for surgery.

Less commonly, genu varum is of pathologic origin. Conditions such as rickets (see Chapter 6) or other metabolic

Figure 21-92   Femoral anteversion. **A,** The condition occurs bilaterally, and in the standing view, both legs appear to turn inward from the hip down. **B,** On assessment of range of motion, the degree of internal rotation of the hips is found to be greater than normal. *(Courtesy Michael Sherlock, MD, Lutherville, Md.)*

abnormalities, epiphyseal dysplasia, various forms of dwarfism, and pathologic growth disturbances such as Blount disease may be causative and can be diagnosed on the basis of radiographic findings if the diagnosis is not obvious clinically. Unilateral bowing is not a result of intrauterine positioning and should prompt investigation for an underlying disorder (Fig. 21-94).

Genu Valgum (Physiologic Knock-Knee)

Genu valgum, or knock-knee, is a normal variation of lower extremity configuration, generally noted in children between 3 and 5 years of age. The phenomenon is part of the normal process of remodeling of the lower extremities during growth and development. It is more frequently seen in females and may be associated with ligamentous laxity. While standing, the child is noted to have an increased distance between the feet when the medial aspects of the knees touch one another (Fig. 21-95). Not uncommonly, the child will place one knee behind the other in an attempt to get the feet together. In some cases, valgus alignment of the feet and a pes planus deformity may be noted. Radiographs reveal no osseous or physeal abnormalities, but accentuation of the angular deformity of the knee secondary to ligamentous laxity is seen on weight-bearing views. One must rule out the possibility of an underlying metabolic condition such as rickets or renal disease. Treatment is generally not indicated, as the condition gradually corrects with time.

Blount Disease

Blount disease is an isolated growth disturbance of the medial tibial epiphysis manifested as an angular varus deformity of the proximal tibia with apparent progressive genu varum.

Figure 21-93   *Physiologic genu varum.* **A,** The mild symmetrical bowing seen in this 1-year-old boy represents a normal variation of lower extremity configuration that occurs in toddlers; correction occurs with growth and remodeling. The bowing is diffuse and involves the upper and lower portions of the legs. **B,** This child has more severe physiologic bowing, which resulted in frequent tripping and a waddling gait. He also had associated ligamentous laxity and intoeing on the left.

Figure 21-94 Pathologic genu varum. **A,** This 11-month-old child has a unilateral, right-sided bowleg deformity. When unilateral, genu varum is not a result of intrauterine positioning and necessitates radiographs to determine the cause of the deformity. **B,** In this case the bowing was caused by a congenital pseudarthrosis of the tibia, a condition frequently associated with neurofibromatosis 1 (see Chapter 15).

Unilateral and bilateral involvement are seen with nearly equal frequency. The etiology of this condition is unknown, although it appears to be more common in African Americans. It may represent a compression injury to the medial growth plate of the proximal tibia.

On careful examination, a localized angular deformity of the proximal tibia is apparent (Fig. 21-96, *A* and *B*), in contrast to the diffuse bowing of the lower extremities seen in patients with physiologic bowleg. In general, there is no evidence of the ligamentous laxity commonly associated with physiologic bowing. Radiographs reveal fragmentation of the medial epiphysis of the tibia associated with beaking and loss of

height in this region, as well as the characteristic angular deformity (Fig. 21-96, *C*). A satisfactory response to treatment depends on accurate diagnosis and early recognition, as bracing or surgical osteotomy with realignment of the leg may prevent further progression.

Osgood-Schlatter Disease

Osgood-Schlatter disease is a traction apophysitis of the tibial tubercle that tends to develop during the adolescent growth spurt. It occurs somewhat more frequently in males than in females. It is thought that differential rates of growth in the osseous and soft tissue structures and stress on the apophyses produced by vigorous physical activity are contributing factors. Bilateral involvement is usual. Patients have a history of gradually increasing pain and swelling in the region of the tibial tubercle. Discomfort is accentuated by vigorous physical activity, kneeling, or crawling and is relieved by rest.

On examination, a localized tender swelling is noted in the region of the tibial tubercle and patellar tendon (Fig. 21-97, *A*). The knee joint is otherwise normal on examination, with the exception that some patients show limitation of knee flexion with reproduction of their pain. Radiographs may reveal only soft tissue swelling in the region of the proximal tibial apophysis or irregularity of ossification of this structure (Fig. 21-97, *B*). In long-standing cases, frank fragmentation of the apophysis may be seen.

The problem, although self-limited, typically persists for 6 to 24 months. If the condition is only occasionally bothersome and does not limit activities, treatment is unnecessary. Use of ibuprofen, as needed, for relieving pain and curtailing activities that produce pain are sufficient treatment for most patients. If severe pain and a limp are present, a short period of immobilization in a splint or cast may be beneficial. Steroid injection is contraindicated because this may cause deterioration of the tendon and provides little in the way of long-term relief.

Figure 21-95 Genu valgum. This 3½-year-old girl shows moderate knock-knee. Ligamentous laxity and mild pes planus are associated problems.

Collapsed medial
epiphysis

Normal position
of proximal tibia

Figure 21-96 Blount disease. **A,** This patient has a unilateral angular deformity of the proximal left tibia that gives the appearance of genu varum. **B,** Both proximal tibias are bowed in another patient as a result of fragmentation and loss of height of the medial epiphyses. In contrast with physiologic bowing, the thighs are straight. **C,** This radiograph shows the typical fragmentation, loss of height, and angular deformity or beaking of the medial portion of the proximal tibia.

Popliteal (Baker) Cyst

Popliteal cysts occurring in childhood are encountered most commonly in children between 5 and 10 years of age and occur significantly more frequently in boys than in girls. They are located in the posteromedial aspect of the knee joint in the region of the semimembranosus tendon and medial gastrocnemius muscle belly. Pathologically, a fibrous tissue or synovial cyst filled with synovia-like fluid is seen. In contrast to those seen in adults, popliteal cysts in childhood generally do not communicate with the joint capsule but originate instead beneath the semimembranosus tendon, presumably as a result of chronic irritation. On occasion vague pain is noted, but evaluation is usually sought because of a recently noted painless mass.

On examination, a soft, nontender, cystic mass is found in the described location (Fig. 21-98, *A*). Range of motion of the joint is normal unless the cyst is particularly large, limiting flexion. The knee is otherwise normal, and radiographs show no osseous abnormality. An MRI clearly delineates the cyst and its position in relation to nearby structures (Fig. 21-98, *B*

Figure 21-97 Osgood-Schlatter disease. **A,** Localized swelling is evident in the region of the tibial tubercle. This is generally tender on palpation. The knee is otherwise normal on examination, with the possible exception of mild limitation of flexion. **B,** Irregularity and fragmentation of the tibial tubercle are seen in this radiograph. In less severe cases of shorter duration, soft tissue swelling or irregularity of ossification may be the only finding.

Figure 21-98 Popliteal (Baker) cyst. **A,** A localized swelling appears in the region of the semimembranosus tendon. This may arise from the synovial lining of the semimembranosus bursa. **B,** Sagittal plane magnetic resonance imaging (MRI) from another child with a Baker cyst shows the posterior location. **C,** A transverse plane MRI demonstrates the posterior and medial position of cyst and its close relation to the gastrocnemius muscle.

and *C*). Popliteal cysts are benign and may resolve over time, although surgical excision is reasonable if desired.

Anterior Patellar Disorders

Pain located in or around the patella is a frequent complaint, especially in the adolescent. Once thought to involve irregular changes in the articular cartilage of the patella and termed *chondromalacia*, the true sources of pain in this region are still not completely understood. Two primary causes for this group of symptoms have been identified, however. One is mechanical malalignment of the patellofemoral mechanism, either congenital or acquired. In such cases the patella does not track congruously in the femoral groove, and subsequent alignment problems or quadriceps atrophy can lead to increased stress on the tissues, producing pain. The second cause may relate to overuse of the patellofemoral joint, leading to chronic fatigue of the tissues, intrasubstance failure, and a painful inflammatory response.

Onset of symptoms may be insidious or may abruptly follow trauma. The patient complains of diffuse aching behind the patella that is exacerbated by climbing stairs, pedaling a bicycle, or prolonged sitting. On examination the patella is found to be tender, and application of pressure over the patella with the knee slightly flexed elicits pain. In the case of mechanical malalignment, tenderness may be greatest on palpation of the lateral or medial edge of the patella near the facets. In overuse problems, tenderness may be noted either at the quadriceps attachment proximally or at the inferior pole where the infrapatellar tendon attaches. In either case, when the examiner holds a hand over the patella as the patient flexes and extends the knee, a grating sensation may be felt.

Treatment is aimed at the underlying cause. If malalignment is the primary source of the problem, quadriceps strengthening exercises and avoidance of high mechanical loads such as deep knee bends and weight lifting may suffice. On occasion, surgical release of the retinaculum on the lateral side may be necessary. When overuse is causative, a reduction of activities to assist initiation of healing and oral administration of antiinflammatory agents followed by a stepwise return to normal activities is effective. Evaluation of training schedule and techniques and modifications where indicated may prevent recurrence.

Internal Tibial Torsion

Internal tibial torsion is a nonpathologic variation in the normal development of the lower leg in children younger than the age of 5 years. It is a rotational deformity that is thought to result from internal molding of the foot and leg in utero. The child is usually brought for evaluation because of concern about prominent intoeing on walking and frequent tripping.

On examination, the hips and knees are found to be normally aligned, with the patellas facing anteriorly, but the lower legs and feet are rotated inward. The lateral malleolus, which is normally positioned slightly posterior to the medial malleolus, may be in alignment with it or even anteriorly displaced, thus causing the ankle mortise to shift to a medially directed orientation, resulting in intoeing (Fig. 21-99). The rotational deformity can be detected by having the patient lie prone on the examining table with the knees flexed (see Fig. 21-14, *E*). Radiographs reveal no osseous abnormalities. Treatment is seldom indicated; remodeling gradually corrects the condition as the child grows and develops. Children who have a habit of sitting on their feet on the floor may inhibit the normal remodeling process and should be discouraged from doing so. Bracing and special shoes have little effect and are not recommended.

Congenital Clubfoot

Congenital clubfoot (talipes equinovarus) is a teratogenic deformity of the foot that is readily apparent at birth. It is seen more frequently in male infants than female infants and has an incidence of 1 in 1000 live births. Etiology is probably multifactorial. Findings from familial incidence studies point toward an underlying genetic predisposition. Abnormal intrauterine positioning and pressure at a critical point in development may contribute as well. Neural, muscular, and osseous abnormalities are other proposed predisposing conditions. A near equal frequency of unilateral and bilateral involvement exists. The deformity is characterized by three primary components: (1) the entire foot is positioned in plantar flexion (equinus); (2) the hindfoot is maintained in a position of fixed inversion (varus); and (3) the forefoot exhibits an adductus deformity, often combined with supination (Fig. 21-100, *A-C*). In the newborn period the deformity may be passively

Figure 21-99 Internal tibial torsion. **A,** On weight bearing the hip, thigh, and knee are normally oriented and the patella faces anteriorly, but the lower leg and foot turn inward. The deformity results in prominent intoeing on walking, which may cause the child to trip frequently. **B,** In this view of the child while sitting, it is easy to appreciate that the lateral malleolus is positioned anteriorly to the medial malleolus. This shifts the ankle mortise and foot to a medially oriented position.

correctable to some extent. With time, however, deformities become more fixed as a result of contracture of soft tissue structures.

The primary pathologic finding is that of a rotational deformity of the subtalar joint with the os calcis internally rotated beneath the talus, producing the characteristic varus deformity of the heel and mechanically creating a block to dorsiflexion of the foot. The navicular bone is in a medially displaced position on the head or neck of the talus, producing the characteristic adductus deformity of the forefoot (Fig. 21-100, *D* and *E*). Contractures of the Achilles and posterior tibial tendons and of the medial ankle and subtalar joint capsules appear to be secondary factors that contribute to the difficulty in obtaining anatomic reduction. Congenital absence of certain tendinous structures may be found in rare instances. A small atrophic-appearing calf is frequently noted without pathologic change in its osseous or soft tissue structures. The typical congenital clubfoot deformity must be differentiated from similar foot deformities secondary to neurologic imbalance resulting from myelodysplasia, spinal cord tethering, or degenerative neurologic conditions. On occasion, tibial hemimelia with deficiency of this bone may present a similar clinical picture. The condition should not be confused with the nonteratogenic occurrence of isolated metatarsus adductus. Its association with arthrogryposis and congenital dislocation of the hips should also be kept in mind.

The roentgenographic difference between a clubfoot and a normal foot can be appreciated by comparing Figure 21-100, *D* and *E* with Figure 21-101, *A* and *B*.

Early treatment consists of attempts at manipulation and serial casting or cast wedging with progressive correction. When the child is seen late or closed treatment is unsuccessful, open reduction and surgical release of the contracted soft tissues is indicated. In general, these measures should be undertaken before the age at which walking is expected in order to prevent the deformity from impeding the child's motor and social development.

Metatarsus Adductus

Metatarsus adductus (metatarsus varus) is a deformity of the forefoot in which the metatarsals are deviated medially. The condition is probably the result of intrauterine molding and is

usually bilateral. Other than the deviation, there are no pathologic changes in the structures of the foot. There is a wide spectrum of severity and resultant intoeing, but otherwise patients are asymptomatic. Clinically it should be distinguished from the more severe and complex deformity of congenital clubfoot, as it carries a more benign prognosis.

Examination is best performed with the foot braced against a flat surface or with the patient standing. With the hindfoot and midfoot positioned straight, the affected forefoot assumes a medially deviated or varus position (Fig. 21-102, *A* and *B*). A skin crease may be located over the medial aspect of the longitudinal arch. When mild, the deviation may be passively correctable by the physician or actively correctable by the patient. Active correction may be demonstrated by gentle stroking of the foot, stimulating the peroneal muscles to contract. In more severe cases, the deviation may be only partially corrected by these maneuvers. Some patients have an associated internal tibial torsion deformity, but their calf muscle is normal in size. Radiographs demonstrate the abnormal deviation of the metatarsals medially without other osseous abnormalities (Fig. 21-102, *C*).

Treatment depends on the severity of the condition. In mild cases, passive manipulation of the deformity by the mother several times a day may suffice. In moderate cases, a combination of manipulative stretching and reverse or straight-last shoes may be indicated. More severe cases, which are not passively correctable and which exhibit a prominent deformity and skin crease, necessitate serial manipulation and casting for 6 to 8 weeks. If the deformity persists despite these measures, surgical intervention may be required. Treatment should be undertaken before anticipated ambulation so as to prevent impairment of the patient's motor and social development.

Metatarsus Primus Varus (Adductus)

Metatarsus primus varus is a congenital and often hereditary foot deformity characterized by a broad forefoot with medial deviation of the first metatarsal. It is significantly more frequent in females than in males. Examination reveals a wide forefoot with medial deviation of the first metatarsal and normal orientation of the second through fifth metatarsals. Often an associated varus deviation of the great toe exists (Fig. 21-103, *A*). Over time, a secondary hallux valgus deformity and

Figure 21-100 Clubfoot. This deformity has three primary components. **A,** The foot is positioned in plantar flexion (equinus). Note the pathologic skin creases over the heel and arch. **B,** The heels or hindfeet are fixed in inversion (varus). **C,** The forefeet are fixed in an adducted and supinated position. **D,** In the anteroposterior radiograph, the talus overlies the os calcis (stacking) and the forefoot is adducted. A line drawn through the longitudinal axis of the talus normally aligns with the first metatarsal, and one drawn through the axis of the os calcis normally aligns with the fifth metatarsal. **E,** This lateral radiograph shows that the foot is in equinus and the axes of the talus and os calcis are nearly parallel. They normally intersect at an approximately 45-degree angle. (Compare with normal shown in Fig. 21-101.)

Figure 21-101   Normal foot. Anteroposterior **(A)** and lateral **(B)** views of the foot of a slightly older child show the normal orientation of the tarsal bones, as compared with the findings in congenital clubfoot (shown in Fig. 21-100, *D* and *E*).

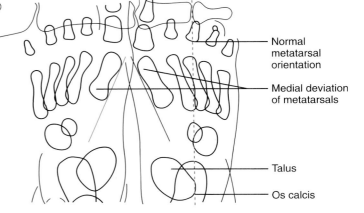

Normal metatarsal orientation

Medial deviation of metatarsals

Talus

Os calcis

Figure 21-102   Metatarsus adductus. **A,** In this view from above, the forefeet are seen to be deviated medially, but otherwise the feet are normal. **B,** When the feet are viewed from the plantar aspect, rounding of the lateral border can be appreciated, along with a crease on the medial side. **C,** In the anteroposterior radiograph, all five metatarsals can be seen to be deviated medially with respect to the remainder of the foot; otherwise, the bony structures are normal. The relationship of the talus and os calcis is normal, unlike the relationship in clubfoot.

Figure 21-103   Metatarsus primus varus. **A,** The first metatarsal and great toe are deviated medially, and the forefoot is broad. The other metatarsals are normally oriented. **B,** Bilateral metatarsus primus varus with hallux valgus. The forefeet are broad, and the great toes deviate laterally. (**A,** *Courtesy Michael Sherlock, MD, Lutherville, Md.*)

bunion may be produced by the abnormal forces exerted on the great toe with weight bearing and ambulation (see Fig. 21-103, *B*). The heel may seem narrow, but this is more apparent than real. Pronation of the forefoot may be present as well. Radiographs confirm the diagnosis by revealing an increased space between the first and second metatarsals and a large first intermetatarsal angle. The first ray through the tarsometatarsal joint may be medially oriented, forming the basis for the deformity.

In mild cases no treatment may be necessary. In moderate or severe cases, foot strain symptoms, bunion pain, and shoe-fitting problems may necessitate treatment. Surgical osteotomy of the medial cuneiform or first metatarsal in conjunction with bunion correction can satisfactorily eliminate the deformity.

Congenital Vertical Talus

Congenital vertical talus is a teratogenic anomaly of the foot noted at birth and characterized by a severe flatfoot deformity. The underlying pathology is a malorientation of the talus, which assumes a more vertical position than normal. The adjacent navicular is dorsally displaced, articulating with the superior aspect of the neck of the talus and causing the forefoot to assume a dorsiflexed and valgus orientation. In effect, these deformities are the opposite of those seen in congenital clubfoot. The etiology of this condition is unknown, although it may be associated with other musculoskeletal or organ system anomalies. Pathologic analysis reveals normal development of the bones but an abnormal relationship. As in clubfoot, associated soft tissue contractures may occur, particularly of the Achilles tendon, toe extensors, and anterior tibial tendon.

Clinically the deformity is recognizable as a calcaneovalgus foot with loss of the arch or, on some occasions, a rocker bottom–type foot with a prominent heel (Fig. 21-104, *A* and *B*). The head of the talus is often palpable on the medial plantar aspect of the midfoot. The deformity is usually fixed, but passive correction may be obtainable in some instances, particularly if the talus is oriented in a less severe oblique position. Radiographs mirror the clinical appearance, showing a vertical orientation of the talus, a calcaneus deformity of the os calcis, and valgus orientation of the forefoot (Fig. 21-104, *C*; see also Fig. 21-101, *B* for a normal comparison).

Initially, attempts at manipulation and serial casting are indicated. However, if this is unsuccessful, as is often the case, surgery may be necessary.

Calcaneovalgus Foot Deformity

Physiologic calcaneovalgus is another deformity of the foot thought to result from intrauterine molding. It is normally a supple deformity that is passively correctable, in contrast with the rigid foot characteristic of congenital vertical talus. The condition is evident at birth and at times is associated with a contralateral metatarsus adductus. No underlying pathologic changes occur in the foot, and no osseous deformities other than the positional one exist. On examination, the foot is noted to be held in a dorsiflexed and everted position with some loss of the normal longitudinal arch (Fig. 21-105). Tightness of the anterior tibial tendon and laxity of the Achilles tendon may be noted in association with the positional deformity. Radiographs reveal no pathologic bony changes. Nonoperative treatment is usually successful and consists of serial casting to eliminate the deformity. Later, wearing shoes with inner heel wedges and longitudinal arch supports may help prevent recurrence and improve ambulation.

Pes Planus (Flatfoot)

Pes planus, or physiologic flatfoot, is an extremely common condition to which there is a familial predisposition. It is characterized by laxity of the soft tissues of the foot resulting in loss of the normal longitudinal arch, with pronation or eversion of the forefoot and valgus or lateral orientation of the heel (Fig. 21-106). Secondary tightness of the Achilles tendon may exist. In general, the condition is asymptomatic in children, and evaluation is sought primarily because of parental concern about the appearance of the foot and the possibility of future problems. On occasion, affected patients report discomfort after long walks or running.

On examination the characteristic appearance is easy to recognize, and laxity of other joints, particularly the thumb, elbow, and knee, may be noted. Weight-bearing radiographs reveal loss of the normal longitudinal arch without osseous abnormality. Treatment is unnecessary if the condition is asymptomatic. Corrective shoes with arch supports are of no use unless symptoms of foot strain are present.

Accessory Tarsal Navicular

An accessory tarsal navicular results from formation of a separate ossification center on the medial aspect of the developing tarsal navicular at the insertion site of the posterior tibial

Figure 21-104 Congenital vertical talus. **A,** The normal longitudinal arch of the foot is absent; a rocker bottom–type deformity is present; and the forefoot is fixed in dorsiflexion, which is even more evident in **(B). C,** On this radiograph the talus is oriented vertically, and its position does not change with flexion or extension of the ankle. The calcaneus is also fixed in equinus position, resulting in a rigid flatfoot deformity (see Fig. 21-101, *B* for comparison).

tendon. The condition is not uncommon and is usually associated with a pes planus deformity. Clinically, patients exhibit a bony prominence on the medial aspect of the foot that tends to rub on the shoe, thus producing a painful bursa (Fig. 21-107, *A*). Radiographs reveal either a separate ossification center or bone medial to the parent navicular, or a medial projection of the navicular when fusion has occurred (Fig. 21-107, *B* and *C*). Cast immobilization may be helpful in acutely painful cases. Long-term improvement can be obtained by wearing soft, supportive shoes with longitudinal arches and a medial heel wedge. Recalcitrant symptoms warrant surgical intervention.

Ganglion of the Foot

A ganglion, or synovial cyst, may develop on the foot. These benign masses are similar to those more commonly seen on the wrist. They originate from outpouchings of a joint capsule or tendon sheath. Trauma may be a predisposing factor in their formation. They are most commonly found on the dorsal or medial aspect of the foot. The mass is soft and nontender and transilluminates. It does not produce symptoms, other than difficulty in fitting shoes (Fig. 21-108). If this occurs, surgical excision may be indicated.

Cavus Feet and Claw Toes

Cavus feet and claw toes are deformities produced by a muscular imbalance within the foot. Although they may occur for unknown reasons, often they are manifestations of an underlying neurologic disorder such as Charcot-Marie-Tooth disease, Friedreich ataxia, or spinal cord tethering (see Chapter 15). These conditions should be considered in evaluating each patient presenting with these deformities, particularly if the problem is unilateral. Cavus feet exhibit a high arch with a varus or inversion deformity of the heel. Usually the metatarsal heads appear prominent on the plantar aspect of the foot (Fig. 21-109). This phenomenon is accentuated by overlying callosities that develop as a result of abnormal weight bearing. With claw toes, the metatarsophalangeal joints are held in

Figure 21-105 Calcaneovalgus foot deformity. The right foot is held in a position of eversion and dorsiflexion. This deformity is supple and thus is passively correctable. The contralateral foot exhibits a metatarsus adductus deformity, giving the feet a "windswept" appearance.

Figure 21-106   Pes planus (flatfoot). **A,** Laxity of the soft tissue structures of the foot results in a loss of the normal longitudinal arch and pronation or eversion of the forefoot. **B,** Viewed from behind, the characteristic eversion of the heels is appreciated more readily.

extension with the PIP joints in flexion and the distal joint in the neutral or slightly flexed position (Fig. 21-110). Calluses tend to develop over the PIP joints as the result of rubbing against shoes. Neurologic examination may reveal motor weakness, most often involving the anterior tibial, toe extensor, and peroneal muscles.

Logical treatment necessitates identifying and treating the underlying pathologic condition when possible. Nonsurgical measures for managing the deformities and ameliorating the symptoms consist of the wearing of customized shoes and use of a metatarsal bar to relieve pressure on the metatarsal heads and to correct the extension deformities at the base of the toes. However, surgical correction is often necessary.

GENERALIZED MUSCULOSKELETAL DISORDERS

Numerous systemic disorders have significant musculoskeletal manifestations. Those relating to genetic, endocrine, collagen vascular, neurologic, and hematologic problems are discussed in their respective chapters. Five conditions with major musculoskeletal manifestations—skeletal dysplasias, cerebral palsy, spina bifida, osteogenesis imperfecta, and arthrogryposis—are discussed in this section.

Skeletal Dysplasias

Overview

Skeletal dysplasias are a heterogeneous group of disorders characterized by abnormalities of bone and cartilage growth, development, and differentiation that often result in short stature (dwarfism), as well as orthopedic and medical complications. Despite the more than 300 types of identified skeletal dysplasias, many individuals with a presumed skeletal dysplasia remain unclassified. Whereas some dysplasias may be lethal at birth (e.g., type IIA osteogenesis imperfecta, thanatophoric dysplasia, and a number of short-rib syndromes), many are not and even some patients with rare, presumed lethal dysplasias may survive into adulthood. Although skeletal dysplasias comprise a heterogeneous group of disorders, two major categories exist: osteochondrodysplasia and dysostosis. The osteochondrodysplasias result from abnormal growth and development of bone and/or cartilage. These are progressive and generalized disorders and are the

Figure 21-107   Accessory tarsal navicular. **A,** A bony prominence produced by the formation of a separate ossification center of the tarsal navicular is present over the medial aspect of the midfoot. It is covered by a painful bursa, produced by chronic rubbing of the prominence against the medial side of the patient's shoe. Patients with this problem usually have a pes planus deformity as well. **B** and **C,** Anteroposterior and lateral radiographs of the foot demonstrate the accessory navicular. The posterior tibialis tendon attaches to the small accessory bone and may contribute to continued irritability and tenderness in this area. Similar extra ossicles are often present asymptomatically on the opposite foot.

Figure 21-108 Ganglion of the foot. A prominent soft tissue mass is present over the medial aspect of the midfoot. This represents a ganglion of the posterior tibial tendon sheath.

Figure 21-110 Unilateral claw toes. This child with a tethered spinal cord has unilateral claw toe deformities. The metatarsophalangeal joints are held in extension while the proximal interphalangeal joints are fixed in flexion.

focus of this section. Dysostosis is a disorder of an individual bone, either singly or in combination (e.g., skull and fingers). Examples include poly/syndactyly and craniosynostoses. There are 33 groups of osteochondrodysplasia and 3 categories of dysostosis in the current classification system. Table 21-7 shows a list of common skeletal dysplasias, osteochondrodysplasias, and common lethal skeletal dysplasias that may be encountered. Although individual skeletal dysplasias are rare, as a group they are relatively common. The incidence of all

Figure 21-109 Bilateral cavus feet. **A,** The feet are inverted and have high arches. The deformity is often a feature of neuromuscular disorders, as in this case where it is the result of Charcot-Marie-Tooth disease. **B,** In addition to the high arches and varus (inverted) heels seen in the view of the plantar surface, the prominence of the metatarsal head region is apparent. Callosities have developed over the lateral borders of the feet as a result of abnormal weight bearing.

skeletal dysplasia is approximately 1 case per 4000 to 5000 births. A Danish study found that skeletal dysplasias represented 9% of the Danish population and that the incidence of congenital generalized skeletal dysplasias at birth was found to be 75.7 per 100,000 births. Because a proportion of skeletal dysplasias are lethal, the prevalence in the general population in that study was found to be much lower (33 per 100,000 population). Thanatophoric dysplasia (Fig. 21-111) and achondrogenesis account for 62% of all lethal skeletal dysplasias. Achondroplasia is usually regarded as the most common nonlethal skeletal dysplasia worldwide.

Diagnosis

Accurate diagnosis can be important for genetic counseling regarding future pregnancies and is helpful in predicting the clinical course as well as in aiding in treatment strategies for complications. Diagnosis of specific skeletal dysplasias can be challenging because of limited availability of genetic testing. Often diagnoses are made on the basis of distinctive radiographic and physical findings. In addition, when growth halts after puberty, it is difficult to distinguish radiographically between the types of skeletal dysplasias, making it important to make a diagnosis as early as possible. Because diagnosis often relies on radiographic findings, it is important to obtain a skeletal survey of any infant or child in whom a dysplasia is suspected.

Prenatal detection of a skeletal dysplasia is important as it determines the obstetric and perinatal management of an affected fetus. Because up to 30% of skeletal dysplasias can

Table 21-7	Skeletal Dysplasias
Nonlethal Skeletal Dysplasias	**Lethal Skeletal Dysplasias**
Achondroplasia—most common	Thanatophoric syndrome—most common
Hypochondroplasia	
Pseudoachondroplasia	Achondrogenesis
Diastrophic dysplasia	Homozygous achondroplasia
Spondyloepiphyseal dysplasia	Chondrodysplasia punctata (recessive form)
Ellis–van Creveld syndrome	
Cartilage hair hypoplasia	Camptomelic dysplasia (sometimes)
Metatropic dysplasia	Congenital lethal hypophosphatasia
Multiple epiphyseal dysplasia	Perinatal lethal type of osteogenesis imperfecta
Kniest dysplasia	
Acromesomelic dysplasia	Short-rib polydactyly syndromes
Larson syndrome	
Jarcho-Levin syndrome	

Figure 21-111   Thanatophoric dysplasia. **A,** Chest and abdomen radiograph showing newborn with lethal thanatophoric dysplasia. Note the severe pulmonary hypoplasia and spinal abnormalities. **B,** Postmortem photo of a newborn who died of asphyxia due to lethal pulmonary hypoplasia, in turn due to thanatophoric dysplasia.

be lethal, accurate diagnosis is imperative for decision-making regarding possible termination. Unfortunately, prenatal diagnosis of specific skeletal dysplasias can be even more challenging than postnatal diagnosis. Factors that lead to difficulty in diagnosis include the large number of skeletal dysplasias, their phenotypic variability and overlapping features, the lack of precise genetic diagnoses for many disorders, the inability of prenatal ultrasonography to provide a detailed view, and variability in the time at which findings manifest for some skeletal dysplasias. Prenatal ultrasound of a suspected skeletal dysplasia involves systematic imaging of the long bones, thorax, hands and feet, skull, spine, and pelvis. Evaluation of thoracic dimensions revealing a hypoplastic thorax is suggestive of severe or lethal skeletal dysplasias. This leads to pulmonary hypoplasia and is a frequent cause of death in patients within the first year of life. The mainstay of prenatal diagnosis remains two-dimensional ultrasound, but it has a sensitivity of only 60%. Assessment of the fetus by three-dimensional ultrasonography improves diagnostic accuracy, because additional phenotypic features may be identified. The precise diagnosis of a specific dysplasia is often difficult prenatally even with accurate imaging, because of variable phenotypic presentations; the variability in the time at which they manifest; and, often, the lack of precise molecular diagnosis. Although the radiologist plays a major role in making an accurate diagnosis, specialists in other disciplines, such as medical genetics, obstetrics, and neonatology, may make valuable contributions to the diagnosis and clinical management.

After birth, a skeletal survey is imperative in the evaluation of a child with a skeletal dysplasia. Certain characteristics that are critical for diagnosis are present only in children, because of their skeletal immaturity. The epiphyseal characteristics of affected children can be pathognomonic of specific disorders, such as the anterior tongue–like protrusion of the spine in pseudoachondroplasia. However, many of these characteristics will disappear with skeletal maturity.

Although specific skeletal abnormalities can be identified radiographically, most skeletal dysplasias are diagnosed by careful physical examination. Clues in the physical examination, such as abnormalities in limbs, spine, trunk, and facial features, help to differentiate types on the basis of phenotypic

features. Findings include abnormalities of the limbs, spine, and trunk. Abnormalities of the limbs include rhizomelic shortening (short proximal segments such as humerus or femur), mesomelic shortening (short middle segments such as radius, ulna, tibia, fibula), acromelic shortening (short distal segments such as metacarpals or phalanges), acromesomelic shortening (short middle and distal segments such as forearms and hands), and micromelia (shortening of extremities involving entire limb). Examples of some of the skeletal dysplasias correlated with specific physical examination findings are listed in Table 21-8. Although the molecular basis is known for some dysplasias, a working diagnosis based on clinical and radiographic findings may better guide the use of existing molecular testing.

Genetics

There has been a recent explosion of knowledge regarding the genetic basis of many skeletal dysplasias. The need for specific genetic tests arises from the complex phenotypes and individual variations that occur according to age, treatment, and

Table 21-8	Limb Abnormalities Seen in the Skeletal Dysplasias
Limb Abnormality	**Examples**
Rhizomelia (shortening of proximal limb)	Achondroplasia, hypochondroplasia, chondrodysplasia punctata, metaphyseal dysplasia, spondyloepiphyseal dysplasia (SED) congenita, thanatophoric dysplasia, atelosteogenesis, and diastrophic dysplasia
Mesomelia (shortening of middle limb segments)	Langer and Nievergelt types of mesomelic dysplasias, Robinow syndrome, and Reinhardt syndrome
Acromelia (shortening of distal limb segments)	Acrodysostosis and peripheral dysostosis
Acromesomelia (shortening of middle and distal limb segments)	Acromesomelic dysplasia
Micromelia (shortening of entire limb)	Achondrogenesis, fibrochondrogenesis, Kniest dysplasia, dyssegmental dysplasia, and Roberts syndrome

Table 21-9	Common Genes Associated with the Skeletal Dysplasias

Skeletal Dysplasia	Gene Mutation
Achondroplasia, thanatophoric dysplasia	Fibroblast growth factor receptor gene-3 (FGFR3)
Pseudoachondroplasia	Cartilage oligomeric protein gene (COMP)
Diastrophic dysplasia	Diastrophic dysplasia sulfate transporter gene (DTDST)
Spondyloepiphyseal dysplasia congenita	Collagen 2A (COL2A1)
Camptomelic dysplasia	SRY (sex-determining region Y)-box 9 protein (SOX9)

environment. The genes responsible for skeletal dysplasia have been identified in more than 150 diseases (Table 21-9 lists some common skeletal dysplasias with their respective genes). Almost all of the skeletal dysplasias are the result of single gene mutations. Up to 80% of skeletal dysplasias are the result of spontaneous mutations with no prior family history. However, almost all are subsequently inheritable in an autosomal dominant manner with few exceptions.

Specific Skeletal Dysplasias

Achondroplasia

Achondroplasia is the most common of all the skeletal dysplasias, with an estimated incidence of 1 per 10,000 live births. It is caused by a mutation in the fibroblast growth factor receptor-3 gene *(FGFR3)*, found on the short arm of chromosome 4 (4p16.3). FGFR3 is one of many fibroblast growth factors involved in skeletal development. Although achondroplasia is an autosomal dominant disorder, 75% of new diagnoses are due to de novo spontaneous mutations. Physical examination findings in persons with achondroplasia include disproportionate short stature with rhizomelia (Figure 21-112). Typical facial features include a flattened nasal bridge, upturned nose, protruding jaw, deep-set eyes, frontal bossing, and midface hypoplasia. Most children with achondroplasia have macrocephaly. Because infants and children are also at risk of hydrocephalus, occipital–frontal circumference should be monitored, using American Academy of Pediatrics growth charts. Children with achondroplasia have normal intelligence and development with the exception of delayed motor milestones. They are at risk for complications including otitis media, obstructive sleep apnea, hydrocephalus due to foramen magnum stenosis, thoracolumbar kyphosis, and bowing of the lower limbs that may necessitate surgical repair.

Diastrophic Dysplasia

Diastrophic dysplasia is one of the few skeletal dysplasias inherited in an autosomal recessive manner. It results from a mutation in the diastrophic dysplasia sulfate transporter gene *(DTDST)* located on chromosome 5. The mutation results in deficient uptake of sulfur by chondrocytes, resulting in abnormal cartilage. It is characterized by short limb dwarfism, severe joint deformities, kyphoscoliosis, clubbed feet, an abducted "hitchhiker's" thumb, and characteristic malformed

Figure 21-112 Achondroplasia. **A,** Radiograph of the femur in an infant with achondroplasia. The proximal ends of the femurs are relatively clublike with metaphyseal flaring and rhizomelic shortening of the lower extremities. **B,** Radiograph of the hand, showing shortened metacarpals and phalanges. **C,** Radiograph of the spine, showing thoracic lumbar kyphoscoliosis. **D,** A 4-month-old female with distinctive facial features: upturned nose, flat nasal bridge, and large forehead.

Figure 21-113   Diastrophic dysplasia. **A,** A 6-month-old female with diastrophic dysplasia showing characteristic facial features of a long, full face; broad forehead; and prominent cheeks and perioral fullness. **B,** Hand showing characteristic, abnormally positioned or "hitchhiker's" thumb. **C,** Lower extremities showing bilateral clubfeet. **D,** Ear showing malformed pinna; this is called a "cauliflower ear" because of the blister-like sacs filled with fluid on the upper part of the ear. These swollen sacs will drain naturally, but most often leave a misshapen upper ear.

pinnae of the ears (Fig. 21-113). Persons with diastrophic dysplasia have normal intelligence, but orthopedic complications due to joint contractures and dislocations can lead to severe osteoarthritis and disability.

Pseudoachondroplasia

Pseudoachondroplasia is a skeletal dysplasia inherited in an autosomal dominant manner. It results from mutations in the gene encoding cartilage oligomeric matrix protein (COMP). Pseudoachondroplasia is often not discovered until a child begins to walk; difficulties with walking or a waddling gait lead to the diagnosis. Because short stature is often not detected until 2 to 3 years after birth (because initial growth velocity is within normal limits), it should be included as a potential diagnosis in the workup of the short-statured child. Children usually exhibit marked short stature and deformity of the legs, short fingers, loose joints, and significant ligamentous laxity.

Spondyloepiphyseal Dysplasia Congenita

Spondyloepiphyseal dysplasia congenita (SEDc) is one of a spectrum of skeletal disorders caused by mutations in the COL2A1 gene, which is responsible for making a protein that forms type II collagen, found in cartilage and in the vitreous humor. Persons born with SEDc have short stature from birth, with a very short trunk and neck and shortened limbs; and they sometimes have cleft palate and clubfeet. Severe orthopedic complications are common throughout childhood, including cervical spine instability necessitating surgical fusion, scoliosis, hip dysplasia, knock-knee deformity, and osteoarthritis as early as the teenage years. SEDc may also be associated with vision problems (myopia and retinal detachment) and hearing loss (sensorineural).

Complications

Each dysplasia has unique characteristics, making generalizations about medical and surgical complications difficult. Treatments for individuals with skeletal dysplasia should be directed at preventing neurologic and orthopedic complications due to spinal cord compression, joint instability, joint degenerative disease, and long bone deformity. The following sections list general types of medical and surgical complications that are experienced by children with skeletal dysplasias.

Neurologic Complications

Hydrocephalus is a common complication in infants and children with achondroplasia. This results from poor cerebrospinal fluid drainage, due primarily to foramen magnum stenosis.

Screening should include careful neurologic examinations at every well-child visit, regular occipital–frontal circumference measurements based on achondroplasia growth charts, head ultrasound at birth and bimonthly until 6 months, and head CT or MRI for evaluation between 6 months and 1 year. Because an enlarged head is normal in achondroplastic children, pediatricians can use a special head circumference growth chart to distinguish between normal growth and possible hydrocephalus. Treatment for hydrocephalus is surgical, including decompression surgery and placement of a ventriculoperitoneal shunt. Clinical symptoms of hydrocephalus and foramen magnum stenosis include brisk reflexes, numbness, weakness, difficulty walking, loss of bowel and bladder control, and central sleep apnea. This complication can be a cause of sudden death in the first year of life.

In the neonatal period it is important to monitor the cervical spine for C1-C2 instability due to odontoid hypoplasia and ligamentous laxity. Although common in many skeletal dysplasias such as spondyloepiphyseal dysplasia congenita and pseudoachondroplasia, it is not found in achondroplasia. All children at risk for having a skeletal dysplasia should have cervical spine x-rays and/or undergo cervical spine MRI. Screening should be performed within the first 6 months of life and then yearly as indicated. Treatment involves surgical fusion of C1-C2 to prevent slippage of vertebrae and subsequent death or paralysis.

Lumbar–sacral stenosis can be a common complication for adults with achondroplasia. Progressive narrowing of the spinal canal in the lumbar and sacral regions can lead to pain, difficulty in walking, loss of bowel and bladder control, and ultimately paralysis. The risk of lumbar–sacral stenosis can be lessened by providing adequate support to infants in the first year of life who exhibit significant kyphosis. Recent evidence suggests that counseling families on selective bracing and prohibiting unsupported sitting in the first 18 months of life can prevent fixed lumbar lordosis and reduce to zero the risk for severe lumbar–sacral stenosis requiring surgery later in adulthood. This finding demonstrates the positive impact of anticipatory guidance and monitoring early in life for these patients.

Orthopedic Complications

There are a variety of orthopedic complications seen with skeletal dysplasias. One of the more common and more troublesome adult sequelae is premature and severe osteoarthritis that can develop as early as adolescence. Patients with dysplasias with epiphyseal involvement (e.g., spondyloepiphyseal dysplasia congenita) are especially at risk for osteoarthritis and should avoid long distance running, obesity, and high-impact activities. Another complication is scoliosis in childhood. Progression is more rapid than scoliosis in patients without skeletal dysplasia, and may result in mechanical, neurologic, and heart/lung complications that necessitate bracing or early surgical repair. Valgus and varus deformities are also common in many of the skeletal dysplasias, due to irregular bone growth. Surgical treatment may be indicated to preserve function and ameliorate pain.

Other Complications

Obstructive sleep apnea is common in many skeletal dysplasias, but especially achondroplasia. The condition arises from small bony air passages of the midface or a crowded hypopharynx, resulting from a tiny jaw or thickened soft tissues. Symptoms include snoring, apnea, and sweating during sleep; failure to thrive; and developmental delay. Treatment includes tonsillectomy and adenoidectomy, continuous positive airway pressure, supplemental oxygen, or a tracheostomy in severe cases. Severe cases may require oral/maxillofacial reconstructive surgery. Eustachian tube dysfunction due to abnormal craniofacial shape, midface hypoplasia, and shortened eustachian tubes is common in many forms of dwarfism, but most often achondroplasia, resulting in recurrent otitis media. Children should have ear examinations with every upper respiratory infection to prevent chronic otitis media, hearing loss, and speech delay. Treatment may include tympanostomy tube placement, tonsillectomy and adenoidectomy, and repair of cleft palate when present.

Development for Children with Skeletal Dysplasias

Growth should be monitored using specialized growth charts for height, weight, and head circumference. Special growth charts now exist for achondroplasia, spondyloepiphyseal dysplasia, diastrophic dysplasia, and pseudoachondroplasia. Children with skeletal dysplasias frequently have delayed motor milestones, but typically have normal cognitive, social, and language development.

Cerebral Palsy

Cerebral palsy refers to a group of fixed, nonprogressive neurologic syndromes resulting from static lesions of the developing CNS. Depending on the timing of injury, signs may be present at birth or they may become evident in infancy or early childhood. The primary cerebral insult may be intrauterine or perinatal infection; a prenatal or perinatal vascular accident; anoxia due to placental insufficiency, difficult delivery, or neonatal pulmonary disease; hyperbilirubinemia resulting in kernicterus; or neonatal hypoglycemia. After the newborn period, CNS infections, trauma, and vascular accidents may, when severe, produce the disorder. Abnormal motor function is the most obvious result and may take the form of a spastic neuromuscular disorder (65% of cases), athetosis (25%), or rigidity and/or ataxic neuromuscular dysfunction (10%). Sensory deficits and intellectual impairment are common, and there is a significant incidence of associated seizure disorders.

Because of the number and variety of possible insulting factors, each of which has its own spectrum of severity, there is a broad range in the location and extent of neural damage, and thus in the degree of functional impairment. Patients with severe afflictions generally have early evidence of gross neuromuscular dysfunction. Those with milder involvement may have subtler abnormalities and may be diagnosed only after they fail to achieve normal developmental and motor milestones. Patterns of the affliction include involvement of one or two limbs (monoplegia or hemiplegia), of both lower extremities (diplegia), of all four extremities (quadriplegia) (Fig. 21-114), or of all limbs with poor trunk and head control (pentaplegia). Those patients with a spastic disorder exhibit flexion contractures of the involved limbs, hyperreflexia, and spasticity; those with athetosis exhibit the characteristic movement disorder. Mixed involvement is apparent in some patients. Neurologic examination often reveals the persistence of primitive reflexes. Patients with severe involvement that inhibits sitting and ambulation suffer disuse atrophy of involved muscles and skeletal demineralization that increases their risk of pathologic fractures (see Chapter 6).

Although cerebral palsy is by definition a nonprogressive neurologic condition, the orthopedic manifestations of the condition are frequently progressive. The progression of orthopedic problems is related to the severity and distribution of spasticity in the child. Increased spasticity in certain muscle groups leads to shortening and contractures in muscles and tendons, imbalance of mechanical forces across a joint or extremity, and eventual bone and joint deformity secondary to the Hueter-Volkmann principle. This principle states that

Figure 21-114   Cerebral palsy. Typical patient with spastic quadriplegia. Note the secondary muscle atrophy especially evident in the lower extremities. He requires crutches to ambulate, seizure medication, and a specialized educational program. His neuromuscular abnormalities are the result of a one-time central nervous system insult and are not progressive.

nonambulatory may be significant because the spasticity of their muscles generates forces across the hip joints that are equivalent to those of ambulatory children.

Treatment goals in cerebral palsy are to prevent musculoskeletal deformity, to improve function and reduce pain, and to attempt to "balance" the muscle forces across the bones and joints in those children with severe spasticity. Administration of medications that reduce muscle spasm, and carefully timed and selected surgical procedures, are helpful. Oral baclofen can also be helpful in reducing spasticity, ameliorating the pain due to associated muscle spasm, and preventing contractures and bone and joint deformity. In cases in which the maximal oral dosage is not sufficient to control spasticity or produces unwanted side effects, consideration should be given to intrathecal baclofen administration via a baclofen pump, as delivery of the drug directly to the spinal cord/CNS does not produce the systemic effects seen with the oral route. Botulinum toxin injections into spastic muscles can also be used to reduce spasm, and these injections can be given in an outpatient clinic. The effect on the muscle can last for up to 3 months.

In evaluating patients with apparent cerebral palsy, one must be careful to rule out a progressive neurologic disorder such as intracranial or spinal cord neoplasia, degenerative neurologic conditions, and tethering of the spinal cord. Spasticity of the extremities can be a physical finding indicative of upper motor neuron pathology from numerous etiologies.

Optimal treatment of cerebral palsy necessitates a team approach. In addition to general pediatric, neurologic/neurosurgical, and orthopedic care, these patients often require the services of a urologist and physical, occupational, and speech therapists, and they may need to be enrolled in individualized educational programs. Family counseling is a necessity. From an orthopedic standpoint, emphasis is placed on optimizing neuromuscular function by attempting to assist the achievement of progressive motor milestones including the ability to sit, stand, walk, and perform activities of daily living. Exercises, bracing, and surgical procedures all have a role, and the institution of specific measures must be timed to fit the pace of growth and development of the individual child. Encouragement and cautious optimism are important.

Surgical treatment usually takes the form of soft tissue release to relieve flexion deformities, tendon transfer to optimize functional use of the extremities, osteotomy to correct deformities, and occasionally selective neurectomy to inhibit

the growth of any bone or joint can be altered by uneven, nonphysiologic mechanical forces across the bone or joint, leading to permanent deformity. One example of this biologic response to muscle imbalance in the growing child, frequently seen in children with severe spasticity, especially with quadriplegia, is hip dislocation (Fig. 21-115). Hip deformity, dislocation, and associated arthritic changes are the result of significant and prolonged imbalance of muscle pull about the hip. It is estimated that in 50% of children with untreated hip dislocation, pain may become significant and problematic, necessitating hip resection or replacement in adolescent or adult life. The development of pain in these children who are

Figure 21-115   Hip dislocation in cerebral palsy (CP). **A,** This 9-year-old with quadriplegic CP has a dislocated left hip as a result of spasticity and unbalanced muscle pull. This is a source of significant pain in about 50% of cases whether or not the child is ambulatory, and surgical treatment is indicated. Note the baclofen pump on the right. **B,** This is the proximal femur removed from another child with severe spasticity and a painful dislocated hip. Note the erosion of the articular cartilage. This and disuse osteoporosis make it easy for a metal probe to perforate the femoral head.

Figure 21-116 Pre- and postoperative spinal radiographs of a 15-year-old female with cerebral palsy and scoliosis. **A,** Preoperative radiograph indicating pelvic obliquity (tilt), which makes sitting in a chair difficult. The patient is nonambulatory. **B,** Postoperative radiograph. Note improved symmetry of chest and leveling of pelvis, which made sitting easier and more comfortable.

overactive muscle units. The most common orthopedic surgical procedures are directed at achieving a plantigrade foot (heel cord lengthening, split posterior tibial tendon transfer), correcting a crouch gait at the knee (hamstring lengthening), and keeping the hips in place (soft tissue release, femoral and pelvic osteotomy).

The spine is one of the major areas of concern in children with significant spasticity and who are wheelchair dependent. Scoliosis develops frequently and contributes to pelvic tilt (pelvic obliquity), which impairs sitting balance (Fig. 21-116, A and B). Bracing is used for children with flexible curves to help them sit better in their chairs, but bracing does not alter the natural history of the scoliosis. The curves will progress in spite of the brace even into adult life. The decision to surgically correct the spine should be discussed with the family when the child's curvature becomes significant enough to interfere with sitting, if there is significant back pain, or if the quality of the child's life is adversely affected because of the magnitude of the curve. The risks of complications are higher in spinal surgery for children with cerebral palsy than in adolescent idiopathic scoliosis because of greater overall health issues and because the spinal fusion is more extensive, usually extending from the upper thoracic spine to the pelvis. The complications include excessive blood loss, increased risk of infection, pulmonary problems, failure of fusion and breakage of instrumentation, neurologic injury, and a risk of perioperative death. However, in spite of the increased risk of complications, most children do very well and although their functional limit remains, their quality of life can be significantly improved (Fig. 21-116, B). Successful surgical outcome requires a team approach in the pre- and postoperative evaluation and treatment of the child that includes general pediatrics, pulmonology, neurology, anesthesia, critical care, and on occasion hematology for assessment of coagulopathies. The final decision on spine surgery is made by the family after a thorough discussion with the surgeon concerning risks and benefits.

Spina Bifida Cystica (Myelomeningocele)

The myelodysplasias are a group of congenital deformities that result from defective closure of the caudal portion of the neural tube during embryonic development. When the failure of closure involves only the posterior vertebral elements, it is termed a *meningocele;* when it involves neural and vertebral elements, it is called a *myelomeningocele.* In patients with myelomeningocele, the loss of neurologic function that results from abnormal cord and spinal root development has dire consequences for the developing musculoskeletal system. Affected children often require neurosurgical closure of the defect at birth to allow healing and prevent infection, and most need a ventriculoperitoneal shunt to prevent or control hydrocephalus. Because of lack of bladder innervation and control, careful urologic follow-up is necessary as well.

The skeletal manifestations seen in spina bifida are the result of imbalances in muscle function of the trunk and extremities. The neurologic loss roughly corresponds to the level of the spine at which the defect lies. In those patients with thoracic myelomeningocele, complete lack of sensation and motor function is seen in the lower extremities, and ambulating and functional capacity are limited. On the other hand, in those individuals whose defect is at a low lumbar or sacral level, the weakness and subsequent deformity may be limited to the foot, or hip extensors and abductors, and to bladder dysfunction.

As with cerebral palsy, treatment by a multidisciplinary team of physicians, nurses, and therapists is helpful in reducing complications and maximizing function. Physical therapy (PT) is important in helping to maintain motion and maximize strength of those muscles that are working. Bracing, in addition to PT, helps prevent secondary joint contractures, which can significantly impair function. Surgical intervention may be necessary to help rebalance unequal muscle forces and to release contractures if they occur. A kyphotic deformity

Figure 21-117 Spina bifida. **A,** This child with thoracic-level spina bifida has an obvious kyphotic deformity. The scars on her back are from surgical closure of her myelomeningocele. **B** and **C,** Anteroposterior and lateral radiographs of the spine demonstrate that kyphosis is secondary to incomplete posterior osseous support.

(Fig. 21-117) of the spine can make bracing, sitting, and lying uncomfortable and may necessitate surgical correction with spinal rods and fusion.

Osteogenesis Imperfecta

Osteogenesis imperfecta (OI) is a family of inherited disorders characterized most notably by brittle bones. Nearly 90% of cases have been determined to be the result of mutations in either the *COL1A1* or *COL1A2* gene. These genes encode production of the pro-α1 and pro-α2 polypeptide chains, which are then assembled into a triple helix composed of two pro-α1 chains and one pro-α2 to form type I collagen—the major structural protein of bone and other connective tissues. Thus far, hundreds of different mutations of these genes have been identified as causative of varying phenotypes of OI. Nearly all are autosomal dominant. Some of these mutations are characterized by production of structurally abnormal collagen. In other cases, the mutant allele is not expressed, resulting in secretion of about 50% of expected levels of structurally normal type I collagen (see also Chapter 1). Histologically, bone mass is decreased and trabeculae are reduced in both number and thickness. Ossification is decreased, and when structurally abnormal collagen is produced, osteoid is poorly organized. The end result is a significant increase in susceptibility to fractures.

The most widely accepted system of classification of these disorders, developed by Sillence and colleagues (1979), uses a combination of clinical features and course, radiographic findings, and genetic factors to divide cases into four main types. In type I, nearly all cases are characterized by reduced production of structurally normal collagen, whereas in types II to IV some proportion of the type I collagen produced is structurally abnormal. Phenotypically, patients with types I and IV have mild to moderate (less often moderately severe) fragility, and those with types II and III have severe disease. Patients with the two milder forms typically experience a distinct decrease in fracture frequency with the onset of

puberty, which then reverses in the fifth or sixth decade, or after menopause in women.

Considerable phenotypic variation exists between and within types, due predominantly to the large number of possible sites for mutations to occur on the *COL1* genes. Some cases of intrafamilial variability are the result of genetic mosaicism within a parent.

Although the causative mutations affect all connective tissues in the body, their primary clinical manifestations involve the skeleton because of the greater structural demands placed on bones. Estimates of incidence of cases of type I range from 1 in 15,000 to 30,000 live births, and for type II from 1 in 20,000 to 60,000. Type III occurs in approximately 1 in 70,000 live births. Cases of type IV are thought to be much less common, but the exact incidence of type IV is unknown because it is likely that many patients with milder disease are never diagnosed, and there is evidence that a number of other cases have been misclassified as type I in the past. The same is probably true of patients with milder forms of type I whose sclerae are not noticeably blue.

Osteogenesis Imperfecta Type I

OI type I is the most common form and is usually the mildest clinically. Two subtypes exist: A (the great majority), in which teeth are normal, and B (unusual), in which dentinogenesis imperfecta is a feature (see Chapter 20). All those with OI type I have blue or grayish-blue sclerae at birth (Fig. 21-118), although the degree varies and tends to lessen with age.

Bony fragility ranges from mild to moderate (up to 10% have no fractures). Although an occasional patient incurs a fracture during delivery, most experience their first after they begin to cruise or walk. The most common sites are the long bones of the arms and legs. Healing is normal with good callus formation and occurs without deformity.

Radiographically, bones appear normal in infancy, save for the presence of wormian bones within the sutures of the calvarium (Fig. 21-118, *B*; and see Chapter 15); however, over time, some degree of osteopenia becomes evident along with

Figure 21-118   Osteogenesis imperfecta (OI) type I. **A,** Blue sclera. **B,** Wormian bones. Multiple wormy, irregular lucencies are seen over the occipitoparietal area. This finding is characteristic of all children with OI types I, II, and III and is seen in more than 50% of patients with OI type IV. **C,** Cortical thinning is evident, especially distal to the oblique fracture of the tibia in this child with OI type I who incurred his fractures while jumping off a chair. (*A* and *C, Courtesy Thomas Daley, MD, St. Joseph's Hospital, Paterson, N.J.*)

thinning of the cortices (Fig. 21-118, *C*). In some patients vertebral flattening is noted in later childhood and adolescence.

Growth is normal, with ultimate stature within the expected range or at its lower limits. Kyphoscoliosis is seen only occasionally. Other common clinical features include mild femoral bowing at birth and generalized ligamentous laxity with joint hypermobility. Easy bruisability and slight thinning of the skin are present in some patients. Approximately 50% of individuals with OI type I develop progressive hearing loss beginning in the late teens or twenties. The loss has both sensorineural and conductive components, the latter stemming from fractures and/or fusion of the ossicles of the middle ear.

Osteogenesis Imperfecta Type II

OI type II is the severest form and is usually lethal in the perinatal period. Most cases are the result of new mutations, although parental germ line mosaicism is occasionally causative. Intrauterine growth is severely retarded, and affected infants are born prematurely with innumerable poorly healed fractures and prominent deformities due to extreme bony fragility. The sclerae are a dark blue-black; the facies is triangular with micrognathia and a small beaked nose; and the calvarium is large in relation to the face and remarkably soft. Other clinical features include marked shortening of the extremities and severe bowing of the legs with hips flexed and thighs fixed in abduction and external rotation (Fig. 21-119). The combination of a short trunk (due to vertebral flattening) and a small chest cage predisposes to severe/progressive pulmonary insufficiency and congestive heart failure.

Radiographs reveal extreme undermineralization of the entire skeleton; prominent vertebral flattening; very thin hypoplastic beaded ribs; and long bones (especially the femurs) that are broad and telescoped, resembling a concertina in appearance.

Death usually supervenes within a few days to weeks of delivery, due to cardiopulmonary complications.

Osteogenesis Imperfecta Type III

Like OI type II, OI type III is usually the result of new mutations, less commonly of parental germ line mosaicism. The majority are born with multiple fractures and deformities due to fractures in utero. Those who are not incur multiple fractures within the first 1 to 2 years. Birth weights are usually low, and length is short. The extremities are foreshortened, and tibial bowing is prominent (Fig. 21-120, *A*). Sclerae are blue to pale blue and gradually lighten with age. The calvarium is

Figure 21-119   Osteogenesis imperfecta type II. This infant was born with multiple fractures and limb deformities. The thighs are fixed in abduction and external rotation. His sclerae are a dark bluish-gray. He died of respiratory insufficiency in the first month of life as the result of his small thorax.

Figure 21-120   Osteogenesis imperfecta type III. **A,** Note the extremely small stature of this 5-year-old child and the deformities of the rib cage and lower extremities. A recent fracture has been splinted. **B,** In this close-up, the characteristic craniofacial features are seen, consisting of a triangular facies, a broad nose, and frontal and temporal bossing. The sclerae may be normal in color, as in this child, or light blue or gray. **C,** Radiograph of an affected infant shows dwarfed, deformed femurs with a new fracture in the midshaft of the right femur. Note also the thin, peculiarly shaped ribs.

relatively large in comparison with the face, which is triangular with a small chin and frontotemporal bossing (Fig. 21-120, *B*). Dentinogenesis imperfecta is seen in more than half of cases. Bony fragility is moderately severe to severe, and fractures occur with minimal trauma. Healing is impaired and often associated with hyperplastic callus and angulation. Repeated fractures of long bones over time result in progressive limb shortening and deformity.

Radiographically severe diffuse osteopenia and thin cortices are evident, and this tends to worsen with age (Fig. 21-120, *C*). The calvarium is markedly undermineralized, with wormian bones seen within sutures (see Fig. 21-118). The ribs are thin and hypodense. In some patients cystic changes develop in the metaphyses of long bones between 2 and 5 years of age. These are a manifestation of severe disorganization of growth plate structure, which significantly impairs linear growth, and combined with vertebral flattening results in markedly reduced stature. Rapidly progressive kyphoscoliosis is a feature in many older patients and predisposes to cardiopulmonary complications. Other clinical features include ligamentous laxity (seen in 50%) and early-onset hearing loss. About 25% experience easy bruisability, and a number of affected children also report heat intolerance and excessive sweating.

Osteogenesis Imperfecta Type IV

OI type IV, generally considered the least common of the four major types of OI, is divided into two major subsets: A (a minority) with normal dentition and B (the majority) with dentinogenesis imperfecta (see Chapter 20). Sclerae are normal in color or slightly gray. The degree of bony fragility ranges widely from mild to moderately severe. Birth weight and length are normal, and mild femoral bowing is seen in most affected newborns. On occasion fractures occur in utero or at

delivery, but most do not experience their first break until after the perinatal period, usually after they begin to walk. Although most fractures heal without deformity, in some instances mild angulation and long bone shortening may occur.

Radiographically, bones may appear normal early on, but with age cortical thinning and osteopenia become increasingly evident. Linear growth tends to be mildly impaired, and by age 2 to 3 years most affected children are at or below the third percentile. Generalized ligamentous laxity with joint hypermobility and bowing of the lower extremities and/or valgus knees are not uncommon. Up to one third develop scoliosis in late childhood/early adolescence. Hearing loss is unusual.

Other Types of Osteogenesis Imperfecta

Since the Sillence classification was formulated in the 1970s, major advances in testing for defects in type I collagen have enabled more accurate classification of cases into the four major types of OI. In addition, three other clinical types have been identified more recently (types V through VII), none of which has any detectable deficit in type I collagen. Types V and VI are autosomal dominant, and type VII is autosomal recessive. All are rare.

Osteogenesis Imperfecta Type V

Affected children have normal sclerae and teeth but moderate to severe fragility of long bones and vertebrae, as well as ligamentous laxity. Callus produced in the course of fracture healing is distinctly hyperplastic. Radiographically, a radiodense band is seen in the metaphyses of long bones near the epiphyses in all affected patients who are still growing. Another feature unique to this type is calcification of the interosseous membrane between the ulna and radius, which limits supination and pronation of the forearm.

Osteogenesis Imperfecta Type VI

Patients with OI type VI have normal to slightly blue sclerae and normal teeth. Mild to moderate osseous fragility is seen (often to a greater degree than in type IV), with onset of fractures occurring in the first 6 to 18 months. Vertebral compression fractures are especially common. Histologically there is evidence of defective mineralization of the bony matrix with accumulation of osteoid.

Osteogenesis Imperfecta Type VII

In children with OI type VII, sclerae are blue but teeth are apparently normal. Osteopenia is significant, and bony fragility is moderate to severe. Fractures are often present at the time of delivery and those involving long bones of the lower extremities often result in deformity. Both coxa vara, a downward curvature of the femoral neck causing adduction of the thigh, and rhizomelia (shortening of the proximal extremities) have been described.

Diagnosis

With close attention to clinical findings and course, as well as radiographic features and family history, the diagnosis of OI types II and III is relatively obvious and that of types I and IV is usually straightforward. The major exception involves the very small minority of patients with OI type IVA—with normal teeth and sclerae—and of patients with OI type IA, whose sclerae are not noticeably blue. Routine laboratory studies that reflect bone and mineral metabolism are normal and thus unhelpful. Thus far determination of standards for the normal range of bone density in growing children is in its infancy. Further, although measurements in children with mild forms of OI reveal that densities are usually somewhat low, many are still within what is currently considered the normal range.

When a clinical diagnosis cannot be made with any degree of assurance and when an exact diagnosis is necessary, analysis of collagen synthesis by fibroblasts obtained via skin biopsy can be performed. However, the process takes 3 to 4 months. It must also be remembered that the results will be normal in children with OI type VI or VII.

Prenatal diagnosis, for families who have had a child with OI type II or III (the genetic defect of which has been identified), involves analyzing fetal DNA obtained by chorionic villus sampling. Ultrasound is also of use in detecting these types of OI between 15 and 18 weeks of gestation. Routine specific genetic testing is as yet infeasible.

Differential Diagnosis

In general there is no confusion in the diagnosis of type III OI. The same is true of most type II cases, although occasionally they must be distinguished from thanatophoric dysplasia, achondrogenesis, and autosomal recessive hypophosphatasia.

The major differential diagnostic considerations in cases of types I and IV are child abuse and idiopathic juvenile osteoporosis.

Distinction from abuse (see Chapter 6) is usually possible clinically because infants and children with previously undiagnosed mild OI and an acute fracture are brought in for care promptly, by parents who are appropriately concerned and give a history of a mechanism of injury that fits the fracture pattern found, although the amount of force reported is somewhat less than is usually required to cause a fracture. Further, most of these fractures involve the diaphyses of the long bones of the extremities. The metaphyseal fractures seen commonly in abuse victims are exceptionally rare in children with OI, and typically one does not find multiple fractures of varying ages for which no prior care has been sought. Finally, skull fractures are rare in OI and retinal hemorrhages, subdural hematomas, and visceral injuries are not seen, with the rare exception of the infant or child with OI who is also a victim of abuse.

The major source of potential confusion is the infant with mild OI and normal sclerae who has incurred one or more nondisplaced fractures in utero or during delivery that were not diagnosed in the newborn period. If he or she then presents with a first symptomatic fracture within the ensuing few months, old healing fractures will be found. Again, timing of presentation, parental demeanor, consistency with mechanism, and family history and psychosocial history should all be scrutinized carefully in making the distinction. Consultation with a specialist in abuse and neglect can be very helpful.

Idiopathic juvenile osteoporosis is an exceptionally rare disorder of unknown etiology. In affected children osteopenia and fractures are most evident in the vertebrae, less so in the long bones, and measurements of bone density are well below normal. This condition improves dramatically in adolescence. Family history is negative for unusually frequent fractures.

Treatment

Patients with OI types I and IV usually require only routine orthopedic care for their fractures and counseling regarding accident prevention and safety. Palliative supportive care and minimal handling are the only measures available for infants with OI type II. Treatment of infants and children with OI type III is geared toward minimizing the frequency of fractures and preventing deformities. In infancy this may mean limited handling of the child and use of a padded carrying device. Later, bracing and surgical treatment in the form of osteotomies and internal stabilization of long bones with intermedullary rod fixation may be necessary. Maintenance of activity and the avoidance of repeated prolonged periods of immobilization help prevent disuse atrophy.

Early investigational trials of intravenous pamidronate in patients with severe fragility have shown some promise in reducing fracture frequency. However, only preliminary results on small numbers of patients are available, and data on long-term side effects do not exist. Growth hormone, which stimulates bone and collagen metabolism, has shown some promise in children with more severe forms of OI type I. It is, however, contraindicated in patients with kyphoscoliosis because it increases the rate of progression of deformity, and also in children with OI types II to IV because its stimulant effect on collagen metabolism only serves to increase secretion of abnormal collagen.

Arthrogryposis

Arthrogryposis is a nonprogressive muscular disorder of unknown etiology that appears to be related to either failure of development of or degeneration of muscular structures. Neural factors have been implicated in its pathogenesis because in some instances the spinal cord has been found to be reduced in size, with a decreased number of anterior horn cells. In general, all limbs are involved. On occasion the disease may be confined to one or a few limbs only. Primary manifestations consist of joint contractures with secondary deformities and limited motion. Deformities include clubfoot; dislocated hips; and contractures of the knees, elbows, wrists, and hands (Fig. 21-121). Motion of the involved joints is severely limited, but patients can generally compensate for this functional limitation. Radiographs show relatively normal-appearing bones and joints, but fat density is noted in the areas where muscles are normally seen. On pathologic

Figure 21-121   Arthrogryposis. **A,** Two sisters with the generalized form of the disorder. Note the stiff posture and tubular appearance of the limbs. Motion of all joints is limited as a result of failure in the development, or the degeneration, of muscular structures. Their stature is short. **B,** The lateral view highlights the flexion contractures of the elbows.

analysis, there is a striking absence of muscle tissue with strands of fat permeating the area.

Orthopedic treatment is aimed at providing optimal motor function. Range-of-motion exercises may maintain what motion is present but rarely result in an increase. Surgery rarely results in improved range of motion but is indicated to restore functional position in those patients with clubfoot and/or hip dislocation. Gradual recurrence of the deformity after surgery is not uncommon, however.

SPORTS MEDICINE

The benefits of physical activity and sports have been touted not only by the health care professions but also by school officials, sports enthusiasts, the media, and insurers. They include improved physical fitness and flexibility; an increased sense of physical well-being; and reduction of stress, tension, and anxiety at all ages. Further, a well-selected activity can be a source of considerable physical pleasure and enjoyment. In childhood and adolescence, physical activity and sports can increase self-confidence and self-esteem, especially when the child is able to achieve mastery of skills and, thereby, a sense of competence and accomplishment. Participation in team sports can also assist development of interactive social skills including cooperation, conflict resolution, and discipline and

give a child a sense of "fitting in." Furthermore, when physical activity is and remains a source of fun and enjoyment from an early age, it can set the stage for a lifelong pattern or habit of being active with the attendant long-term benefits of cardiovascular health, good weight control, optimal bone density, and reduction of risk of developing type 2 diabetes.

In the first half of the 20th century, sports in childhood consisted primarily of free play and "pick-up games" in yards, on streets, in alleys, and on empty lots with little or no adult supervision. Spontaneity, flexibility, and in many cases greater inclusiveness (kids of differing ages and skill levels) were typical, and although competition was a feature, it tended to be less prominent than is true of organized sports. In contrast, today greater danger in many urban neighborhoods; limited numbers of children in others; lack of access to playgrounds or other sports facilities; and competing demands of television, computers, and homework have reduced the opportunity for unstructured free play. Furthermore, with many children entering day care at an early age and progressing through preschool to elementary school and beyond, constant adult supervision of play is often the norm. These factors have contributed to the strong trend over the past few decades toward increasing organization of sports. As a result, participation of children in either formally or informally organized sports activities is nearly universal and has become part of normal childhood experience. Physical education may begin as early as age 4 and extend through adolescence and is now nearly equal for boys and girls.

This trend toward increasing organization has had its pluses and minuses. It can be positive when there is good coaching and supervision that takes developmental levels and readiness into consideration, has reasonable goals for participation, and good methods for achieving them. Elements of such programs include emphasis on learning basic skills while gradually increasing level and intensity of activity; on developing the social skills necessary for good teamwork; on good sportsmanship and having fun more than winning; and use of praise, encouragement, and enthusiasm to motivate progress. Other good practices include fair processes in team selection; matching competitors by size and skill level; teaching the rules and the reasons for them; placing emphasis on safety and setting strict limits on dangerous practices; and teaching safe practice techniques with reasonable time limits on practices and games to reduce risk of overuse and other injuries. An added benefit has been a trend toward construction of better facilities and development and use of improved equipment. Conversely, when coaches and parents place unrealistic demands and expectations on children that exceed their developmental abilities and readiness to participate, when competitiveness and winning become the goals and only the best players get praise and the opportunity to play, and when criticism and demeaning remarks are used as "motivators," then spontaneity and enjoyment are lost and sports become a source of stress. In such situations, many children lose interest and motivation and come away with a sense of frustration and failure. In fact, greater emphasis on competition from peers, coaches, and parents and higher expectations for increased performance in ever-younger children now account for a significant rise in the incidence of adult-type injuries appearing in children. This is in addition to the injury patterns that are unique to childhood. It also may be partially responsible for a significant drop-off in sports participation during the middle school teen years.

Development of Athletic Skills

Having a basic understanding of child development is integral to optimal parental encouragement of physical activity and to safe and effective coaching of sports programs. Acquisition

Table 21-10	Average Age at Acquisition of Mature Patterns of Sports-related Motor Skills	
Skill	**Boys (Years)**	**Girls (Years)**
Throwing	6	8
Kicking	7	8
Hopping and catching	7-8	7-8
Hitting balls and shooting baskets	10-14	10-14

of motor milestones during infancy and childhood follows a relatively orderly and predictable course, albeit with a wide range of normal variation in rate. This development in concert with advances in cognitive and social ability is dependent on physical growth and on myelination and neural maturation with corresponding increases in sensory/motor integration, as well as on each child's own curiosity and desire to master new movements and activities. Although it has been demonstrated that having freedom and encouragement to explore and experiment at their own pace (without undue restriction or criticism) fosters developmental advances, there is no evidence that participation in early training programs either hastens this process or improves later performance in sports.

In the early school years, further maturation assists acquisition of additional basic motor skills, development of mature patterns of sport-related skills (Table 21-10), and then the trying out of these skills in varying combinations (transitional skills). There is evidence that instruction and practice can help refine motor skills in children in this age range. Cognitively and socially, young school-age children do not have the wherewithal to make true teamwork or team play realistic, however. During later childhood and early puberty, ongoing maturation enhances the ability to further refine skills and enables understanding of strategy and practice of true teamwork. Throughout the elementary and middle school years, there is a gradual increase in cardiopulmonary endurance in

both sexes, and this, coupled with the fact that strength is relatively comparable in boys and girls, makes coed participation and competition feasible and safe.

With puberty, the growth spurt results in major increases in muscle mass and strength, as well as in exercise capacity or cardiopulmonary endurance. Girls tend to mature earlier and more gradually, while boys often enter puberty somewhat later but at a more rapid rate, ultimately ending up much larger and stronger than most of their female counterparts. This makes coed participation, especially in contact sports, less safe for girls. During the pubertal growth spurt, bones grow relatively faster than surrounding soft tissues, resulting in a temporary period of decreased flexibility or tightness, especially of the hamstring muscles and ankle dorsiflexors. This phenomenon can predispose to injury, and preparticipation stretching exercises are advisable as a preventive measure (see Fig. 21-124). Throughout childhood and well into puberty, the open epiphyses of growing bones are vulnerable to injury when subjected to shearing stresses and heavy weight loads. This necessitates care in strength training and avoidance of weight lifting and related sports until skeletal maturity is achieved.

The wide range of normal variation of onset and pace of puberty results in significant differences in size and maturation of individuals of the same age and sex. This has led to the practice of matching children and teams by weight or size to reduce risk to smaller children in contact sports. Use of maturation indexing, matching by Tanner stage or maturity level, is gaining interest, and although there are no hard data yet regarding effectiveness, it does have an inherent logic and may be preferable, given the fact that a pubertal child of the same size as a prepubertal child is likely to be much stronger. To date, however, this practice has not gained wide acceptance.

Table 21-11 presents in summary form the developmental progression of motor and cognitive development along with corresponding recommendations for athletic education and training. Importantly, no data currently exist regarding optimal age for beginning participation in the various organized sports.

Table 21-11	Developmental Skills for Sports and Sports Recommendations during Childhood	
Early Childhood (2 to 5 Years)	**Middle Childhood (6 to 9 Years)**	**Late Childhood (10 to 12 Years)**
Motor skills • Limited fundamental skills • Limited balance skills Learning • Extremely short attention span • Poor selective attention • Egocentric learning—trial and error • Visual and auditory cues are important Vision • Not fully mature before ages 6 to 7 (farsighted) • Difficulty tracking and judging velocity of moving objects Sports recommendations • Emphasize fundamental skills with minimal variation and limited instruction • Emphasize fun, playfulness, exploration, and experimentation rather than competition • *Activities:* Running, swimming, tumbling, throwing, catching	Motor skills • Continued improvement in fundamental skills • Posture and balance become more automatic • Improved reaction times • Beginning transitional skills Learning • Short attention span • Limited development of memory and rapid decision-making Vision • Improved tracking • Limited directionality Sports recommendations • Emphasize fundamental skills and beginning transitional skills • Flexible rules of sports • Allow free time in practices • Short instruction time • Minimal competition • *Activities:* Entry-level soccer and baseball	Motor skills • Improved transitional skills • Ability to master complex motor skills • Temporary decline in balance control at puberty Learning • Selective attention • Able to use memory strategies for sports such as football and basketball Vision • Adult patterns Sports recommendations • Emphasis on skill development • Increasing emphasis on tactics and strategy • Emphasize factors promoting continued participation • *Activities:* Entry level for complex skill sports (football, basketball)

Modified from Nelson MA: Developmental skills and children's sports, *Phys Sportsmed* 19:67-79, 1991.

The Preparticipation Sports Physical Examination

Recognition of the rise in injury incidence and of new types of injury in children, especially when participating in programs that do not adequately factor in neuromuscular and cognitive development, has led to increased interest in more formal medical monitoring of child and adolescent athletes.

In an effort to foster safer participation, a task force was formed, composed of representatives from the American Academy of Family Physicians, the American Academy of Pediatrics, the American Medical Society for Sports Medicine, the American Orthopaedic Society for Sports Medicine, and the American Osteopathic Association for Sports Medicine. Their charge was to develop recommendations and standards for the format of the preparticipation evaluation (PPE) of youngsters before entry into competitive sports programs. Initial recommendations were published in 1992 and were subsequently refined and updated in 1997.

The primary goals of the PPE are as follows:

1. Detection of underlying medical problems or conditions that are characterized by the following:
   - May predispose to injury (e.g., patellofemoral malalignment)
   - Are potentially disabling (e.g., prior injury)
   - Are potentially life-threatening (e.g., hypertrophic cardiomyopathy)

Such conditions may warrant further evaluation and testing, a rehabilitation or preconditioning program, or selection of an alternative sport.

2. Assessment of the following:
   - General health
   - Physical maturation
   - Fitness level and proficiency for a particular sport (including strength, flexibility, and joint stability)

This helps in determining whether a preconditioning program may be indicated or whether selection of an alternative sport may be advisable.

3. Compliance with insurance and legal requirements

4. Counseling regarding health-related issues
   - Nutrition and healthy diet
   - Avoidance of high-risk or unhealthy behaviors (e.g., drugs, alcohol, fighting, promiscuity)
   - Importance of safe training and play techniques and safety equipment
   - What sports are safe for the individual

5. Ideally, assessment of cognitive and social readiness; interest level, goals, and motivation; psychosocial supports at home and at school; and current life stresses

The person performing the examination may be the primary care physician or, in some instances, a sports medicine physician or a physician with a specific interest in this area. It is generally recommended that an examination be done at least every 2 years, more frequently if there is a change in the physical condition of the child or a change in the sports level. However, most states and school systems require yearly examinations. The assessment is best performed at least 6 to 8 weeks before beginning participation to allow for time to correct any deficiencies that may need rehabilitation or warrant a preconditioning program.

Three major formats/sites of examination may be used.

- Locker room examination: Students line up and are seen one at a time by a team physician who usually has an interest in or expertise in sports medicine.
- Station method: The examination is divided into components, each with a station that may be staffed by a nurse, physician, trainer, or coach. Stations include weight/height, vision, vital signs, and general examination. Dental and nutrition stations are optional.
- Office method: The child is examined by his own primary care physician.

Both the locker room and station methods tend to be performed in a noisy milieu (making auscultation difficult). They afford limited privacy and have the disadvantage of the physician's not knowing or having an established relationship with the child or adolescent. They do, however, have the advantage of having physicians who tend to be more well versed in sports medicine, are reputed to be more efficient, and are less costly. The office method affords privacy, a quiet environment, and greater opportunity for individual attention and counseling. When there has been long-standing continuity of care, the physician knows the child's past medical, surgical, injury, growth, developmental, family, and psychosocial histories. Furthermore, the established physician–patient relationship assists assessment of maturity, readiness, motivation, and psychosocial stressors that may affect performance, and it can enhance efficacy of counseling and compliance with recommendations. It may have the disadvantage of the physician's having limited knowledge of the sport and its requirements.

The forms designed by the PPE task force for the history, physical examination, and clearance to participate are well crafted for meeting the goals of the PPE. They are regarded by experts as the best available, and we encourage their use (especially the history form), although states and school systems often have their own, less inclusive forms.

Ideally, the history form is given to the prospective athlete in advance of the examination date, with instructions to complete it together with his or her parents. (Requiring a parental signature may be advisable to ensure that the parent's input is included.) Athletes may need to be reassured that the primary goal of the PPE is to identify potential problems that can be remedied, whenever possible, not to exclude them from play. This form is then reviewed with the athlete at the time of the examination. Questions are designed to screen for conditions most likely to result in problems or to be associated with significant risk for injury, reinjury, disability, or sudden death. Positive responses also help to highlight areas that need special attention in performing the physical examination. Particular areas of emphasis include exercise- or postexercise-related cardiopulmonary, neurologic, and musculoskeletal symptoms; family history of early and sudden cardiac deaths; past medical, surgical, injury, and heat illness histories; and identification of chronic or recent illnesses (especially the possibility of myocarditis and mononucleosis) that may be sources of increased risk or necessitate limits on participation.

The cardiovascular, pulmonary, and musculoskeletal portions of the physical examination have the highest yield in identifying potential problems. Attention is also paid to identifying visual problems that warrant protective eyewear (i.e., being functionally one-eyed), the abdominal examination for detection of visceromegaly, and genital examination (when having a single testicle warrants extra protection during contact sports).

In addition to screening for hypertension, the cardiac examination should focus on findings that may suggest a previously undetected disorder that may place the athlete at risk when playing sports of high aerobic intensity. These include hypertrophic cardiomyopathy, aortic stenosis, coarctation, other cardiomyopathies, myocarditis, and certain arrhythmias. Attention is paid to pulse quality and regularity; amplitude of pulses in upper and lower extremities; precordial activity; and auscultation in supine, as well as squatting and standing, positions because in some (although not all) cases of hypertrophic cardiomyopathy and other sources of left ventricular outlet obstruction, a systolic murmur that increases on rising from squatting is noted. This is in contrast to the flow murmur heard in well-conditioned athletes that decreases on standing.

Murmurs that increase on standing from a squat position, diastolic murmurs and those that are grade III or greater, pulse irregularities other than physiologic changes with respiration, unequal pulses in upper and lower extremities, and decreased pulse amplitude all warrant further evaluation by a cardiologist, as do any positive responses to cardiovascular questions on history.

Exercise-induced asthma, the most common pulmonary problem affected by exercise, can often be identified by history of cough, shortness of breath, or chest tightness with exercise. Nevertheless, in many cases the condition remains unrecognized. Although peak flow readings before and after exercise challenge done in the office (running up and down stairs or jumping rope for 3 to 5 minutes) may detect additional cases, research suggests that the best method is field testing of pulmonary function before and after a 1-mile run. Unfortunately, the latter is often impractical.

The contours, symmetry, range of motion, and stability of the neck, back, shoulders, elbows, wrists, hands, hips, knees, ankles, and feet can be assessed quickly and efficiently using the 2-minute musculoskeletal screening examination (Fig. 21-122). When this is combined with additional attention to areas highlighted by the history, the vast majority of

1. Inspection, athlete standing, facing toward examiner (symmetry of trunk, upper extremities).
2. Forward flexion, extension, rotation, lateral flexion of neck (range of motion, cervical spine).
3. Resisted shoulder shrug (strength, trapezius).
4. Resisted shoulder abduction (strength, deltoid).
5. Internal and external rotation of shoulder (range of motion, glenohumeral joint).
6. Extension and flexion of elbow (range of motion, elbow).
7. Pronation and supination of elbow (range of motion, elbow and wrist).
8. Clench fist, then spread fingers (range of motion, hand and fingers).
9. "Duck walk" four steps (motion of hip, knee, and ankle; strength; balance).
10. Inspection, athlete facing away from examiner (symmetry of trunk, upper extremities).
11. Back extension, knees straight (spondylolysis/spondylolisthesis).
12. Back flexion with knees straight, facing toward and away from examiner (range of motion, thoracic and lumbosacral spine; spine curvature; hamstring flexibility).
13. Inspection of lower extremities, contraction of quadriceps muscles (alignment, symmetry).
14. Standing on toes, then on heels (symmetry, calf; strength; balance).

Figure 21-122   Two-minute musculoskeletal screening examination. *(From Smith DM, editor:* Preparticipation physical evaluation monograph, *ed 2, Minneapolis, 1997, American Academy of Family Physicians in association with the American Academy of Pediatrics, American Medical Society for Sports Medicine, American Orthopaedic Society for Sports Medicine, and American Osteopathic Association for Sports Medicine, pp. 1-49.)*

musculoskeletal abnormalities that may benefit from preconditioning programs or rehabilitation are identified, with concomitant reduction of risk of injury and disability.

Use of routine laboratory tests has been found unnecessary. Furthermore, studies of mass electrocardiographic and echocardiographic screenings have proved to have high cost and low yield in detecting potentially life-threatening cardiac abnormalities (probably because of their low incidence). Hence these studies should be reserved for cases in which results of history and physical examination indicate the need for further cardiac assessment. Although the rare case of an asymptomatic child with no findings on examination may escape detection, use of a thorough screening assessment as just described will identify the vast majority of children at risk.

As noted earlier, although maturation indexing has generated interest it has not gained wide acceptance. Nevertheless, Tanner staging may have a role in selecting lower-risk activities and providing advice with regard to intensity of training. For example, a girl at Tanner stage 2 is entering a period of maximal growth velocity, during which female athletes may have limited joint flexibility and may be particularly predisposed to overuse syndromes.

Strength and endurance may be other factors that are potentially helpful in the preparticipation evaluation. These include body composition (skin folds); endurance (12-minute or 1.5-mile run); flexibility (stretch, reach); agility (Illinois agility test); power (vertical jump); and balance (single-leg stance), although exact standards for many of these have yet to be defined.

In addition, participation clearance for a particular level of sport must be matched with the safety of the sport. The American Academy of Pediatrics has classified sports into risk categories (Tables 21-12 and 21-13) on the basis of contact/collision risk, degree of aerobic intensity required, and static and dynamic demands placed on the body during play. Although the categorizations are quite helpful, it is important to recognize that they do not factor in the competitiveness of a given sports program or its intensity of training, and they do not include factors that predispose to overuse injuries.

Clearance for participation in organized youth sports is generally divided into three categories: (1) full, unrestricted participation is allowed; (2) approval of coach, trainer, or team physician is required, and the athlete may have defined limits on participation or require rehabilitation; and (3) clearance is deferred because of underlying disease process or the need to evaluate further for such a process before giving clearance.

Risk of Injury

In early and middle childhood, risk of sports-related injury is relatively low. Being smaller and having less muscle strength than adolescents, children achieve less velocity and thus encounter less force in falls and collisions. In this age range, injuries are more likely to be incurred during recreational play and in the process of learning a new sport. With puberty, gains in size, strength, and speed combine with increased competitiveness and intensity of play to substantially increase both the incidence and severity of injuries. Even so, the majority of injuries incurred during organized sport are minor in nature; less than 10% are serious; and catastrophic spinal and head injuries and sudden cardiac, pulmonary, and heat-related deaths are rare events. Injuries are more likely to occur during practice sessions because practices outnumber formal competitions or games, although incidence of injuries per unit of time played is greater during the latter.

The incidence of overuse injuries, in particular, has risen in parallel with the trend toward increasing organization of

Table 21-12	Classification of Sports by Contact/Collision Risk	
Contact or Collision	**Limited Contact**	**Noncontact**
Basketball	Baseball	Archery
Boxing*	Bicycling	Badminton
Diving	Cheerleading	Body building
Field hockey	Canoeing or kayaking	Bowling
Football (tackle)	(white water)	Canoeing or kayaking
Ice hockey†	Fencing	(flat water)
Lacrosse	Field events	Crew or rowing
Martial arts	High jump	Curling
Rodeo	Pole vault	Dancing‡
Rugby	Floor hockey	Ballet
Ski jumping	Football (flag)	Modern
Soccer	Gymnastics	Jazz
Team handball	Handball	Field events
Water polo	Horseback riding	Discus
Wrestling	Racquetball	Javelin
	Skating	Shot put
	Ice	Golf
	In-line	Orienteering§
	Roller	Power lifting
	Skiing	Race walking
	Cross-country	Riflery
	Downhill	Rope jumping
	Water	Running
	Skateboarding	Sailing
	Snowboarding‖	Scuba diving
	Softball	Swimming
	Squash	Table tennis
	Ultimate Frisbee	Tennis
	Volleyball	Track
	Windsurfing or surfing	Weight lifting

*Participation not recommended by the American Academy of Pediatrics.
†The American Academy of Pediatrics recommends limiting the body checking allowed for hockey players 15 years and younger to reduce injuries.
‡Dancing has been further classified into ballet, modern, and jazz since previous statement was published.
§A race (contest) in which competitors use a map and compass to find their way through unfamiliar territory.
‖Snowboarding has been added since previous statement was published.
From American Academy of Pediatrics, Committee on Sports Medicine and Fitness 2000-2001: Medical conditions affecting sports participation, *Pediatrics* 107:1205-1209, 2001.

sports. Children are especially prone to overuse injuries during periods of rapid growth, when the rate of bone growth exceeds that of surrounding soft tissues, resulting in decreased flexibility. Intensive training for a particular sport, especially when initiated at a low level of fitness; abrupt increases in level of activity; lack of preconditioning; and participation in multiple sports during the course of a year are other predisposing factors, as are training practices that fail to teach children proper athletic techniques and to monitor and limit repetitive motions.

Youths with ligamentous laxity (up to 7% of school-age children) and joint malalignment (such as patellofemoral tracking disorder) may be injury prone without special preconditioning. Children and adolescents who resume competitive participation after a musculoskeletal injury, without full rehabilitation (return of normal strength, flexibility, and range of motion), have a significant risk for reinjury.

In female athletes, especially gymnasts, dancers, and long-distance runners, undue calorie restrictions to maintain "ideal weight," in combination with intensive training regimens, result in amenorrhea; decreased estrogen levels; and loss of bone density, which has been demonstrated to predispose to early hip and vertebral fractures.

Environmental factors can also be sources of significant risk. These include weather conditions such as high heat and

| Table 21-13 | Classification of Sport by Level of Aerobic Intensity and by Degree of Static and Dynamic Demands |

HIGH TO MODERATE INTENSITY

High to Moderate Dynamic and Static Demands	High to Moderate Dynamic and Low Static Demands	Low Dynamic and High to Moderate Static Demands
Boxing*	Badminton	Archery
Crew or rowing	Baseball	Auto racing
Cross-country skiing	Basketball	Diving
Cycling	Field hockey	Horseback riding
Downhill skiing	Lacrosse	(jumping)
Fencing	Orienteering	Field events (throwing)
Football	Race walking	Gymnastics
Ice hockey	Racquetball	Karate or judo
Rugby	Soccer	Motorcycling
Running (sprint)	Squash	Rodeo
Speed skating	Swimming	Sailing
Water polo	Table tennis	Ski jumping
Wrestling	Tennis	Water skiing
	Volleyball	Weight lifting

LOW INTENSITY

Low Dynamic and Low Static Demands
Bowling
Cricket
Curling
Golf
Riflery

*Participation not recommended by the American Academy of Pediatrics.
From American Academy of Pediatrics, Committee on Sports Medicine and Fitness, 2000-2001: Medical conditions affecting sports participation, *Pediatrics* 107:1205-1209, 2001.

humidity (with attendant risk of dehydration and heat illness) and extreme cold or swimming in cold water (frostbite, hypothermia). Children are particularly prone to hyperthermia and hypothermia because of their larger surface area–to-volume ratio. They also have a decreased rate and delay in onset of sweating, compared with adults, making it more difficult for them to dissipate heat. Finally, they have to be encouraged to drink adequate fluids, as their own thirst levels tend not to be adequate to ensure replacement of losses. Finally, uneven or unsafe field conditions or playing surfaces; improper, poorly designed, or ill-fitting equipment (including shoes); and lack of or failure to use appropriate safety gear are other significant factors.

Participation in some types of organized sports carries an inherently greater risk and thus higher rates and degrees of severity of injury. This is by virtue of their requiring higher levels of aerobic intensity, their placing high static and/or dynamic stresses on the body, or because high-velocity contacts or collisions are part of the activity. Among these, competitive wrestling, football, and gymnastics are the top three, followed by cross-country skiing, soccer, basketball, track, volleyball, softball, and baseball in approximate order of frequency (see classification system of sport activities based on contact/collision risk [Table 21-12], as well as on aerobic intensity required and on static and dynamic demands encountered [Table 21-13]). Such sports may present especially high risks to children with underlying chronic health conditions (see Sport Selection and Participation for Children with Underlying Problems or Chronic Conditions, later).

Two areas of sport are specifically not recommended by the American Academy of Pediatrics: boxing because of high risk of eye and head injury; and weight lifting, power lifting, maximal lifts, and body building because of concerns regarding epiphyseal injuries (especially of the wrist) and apophyseal separations of the vertebrae in children and adolescents who have not reached skeletal maturity.

Nonorganized recreational sports are not without their own hazards, in part because of less supervision and inconsistent compliance with recommended safety measures. Those in which high-speed or angular momentum is attained carry particularly high risks for significant trauma. These include bike riding, skateboarding, in-line skating, trampoline jumping, and riding motor bikes and all-terrain vehicles.

Risk Reduction and Injury Prevention

One of the first steps in prevention is identification of children at potential risk for injury, using the PPE and referral for further evaluation, if indicated, to a preconditioning exercise program to increase strength, aerobic fitness and/or flexibility, or for preseason sport-specific training, as indicated. When children are found to have conditions that make certain activities potentially harmful, counseling by physicians and coaches regarding safe and enjoyable alternative sports that are of interest to the child can be most helpful.

Coaches who are well trained in teaching and coaching their sport, as well as in health and safety issues, and who place their players' interests first are crucial figures in promoting safety. Best practices include the following:

1. Meeting with prospective players before the preseason to do the following:
   - Emphasize the importance and purpose of the PPE and of honesty in completing the history form.
   - Outline expected skill and fitness levels for preseason tryouts.
   - Suggest or oversee safe, well-supervised preparticipation conditioning or sport-specific training programs.

2. During the preseason and season
   - Implementing graduated training regimens in which youths can improve skills at a reasonable pace. Such regimens also emphasize the following:
   - Warm-up and cool-down periods
   - Learning proper skill techniques (e.g., throwing, kicking)
   - Limiting the number of repetitions of a single activity (such as throws for a pitcher)
   - Placing appropriate limits on practice duration and time in play
   - Having flexibility to modify the regimens to meet individual athletic needs
   - Familiarizing athletes with the rules of the game and their basis in consideration for safety, along with promotion of strict officiating
   - Promoting, even insisting on, safe playing facilities and conditions
   - Ensuring appropriate use of proper equipment of good design and good fit
   - Insisting on use of recommended safety gear (Table 21-14)
   - Fostering gradual acclimatization to hot/humid weather conditions, ensuring frequent rest periods, encouraging drinking fluids, and limiting time for practice
   - Insisting on prompt evaluation of injuries or worrisome symptoms, as well as complete rehabilitation before return to play

In Table 21-15 common injuries seen in athletes participating in a number of specific sports are enumerated along with

Table 21-14	Safety Gear and Field Safety Modifications
Recommended/Required Devices	**Specific Sport(s)**
Helmets	Bike riding, skating, baseball (batting), football, hockey
Elbow/wrist/knee guards	Skating, skateboarding
Shin guards	Soccer
Chest protectors	Baseball catcher
Mouthguards	Contact sports
Protective eyewear*	Racquet sports, water sports, contact sports (unless incorporated into helmet)
Groin cups	Football, hockey
Field Modifications	**Sport**
Breakaway bases	Baseball
Stationary goal cages	Soccer

*Mandatory for all functionally one-eyed individuals and those who have had eye surgery or prior eye trauma per American Academy of Pediatrics, Committee on Sports Medicine and Fitness.
From American Academy of Pediatrics, Committee on Sports Medicine and Fitness, 1995-96: Protective eyewear for young athletes, *Pediatrics* 98:311-313, 1996.

prevention strategies recommended by the American Academy of Orthopaedic Surgeons and the American Academy of Pediatrics.

Conditioning and Training

The rise in participation of youth in sports activities and the ever-increasing desire to improve performance have led to new concern for understanding the physiologic responses of the growing child to regular and increasingly demanding exercise regimens. The most general of these measures is the maximal oxygen uptake (VO$_2$max). Studies of VO$_2$max, which includes cardiovascular, pulmonary, and musculoskeletal function, have shown that there is relatively little difference between children and adults, and only slightly less function in girls versus boys. It is of note, however, that training does not improve VO$_2$max in children. The biggest increase seems to occur with the pubertal growth spurt. In contrast to aerobic function, children do not do as well anaerobically (as measured by the anaerobic threshold), apparently because they cannot utilize glycogen as efficiently as adults. These factors are important in considerations of the two major types of sports training programs: endurance and strength training.

Endurance training consists of a long-term specific exercise program designed to increase exercise capability during prolonged sports participation; in many instances its purpose is to increase the athlete's fatigue resistance. This is done by specifically increasing the amounts of "overload" on a graduated basis and may be sport specific, for example, running. Basic to endurance training is aerobic conditioning, which requires sustained rhythmic movement of large muscle groups at a level of intensity that results in increases in heart rate and respiratory rate. The recommended frequency is three to five times per week for approximately 15 minutes. In monitoring the training program of the pediatric athlete, it is essential to avoid overload situations that can cause tissue damage and lower performance. All programs need to take into account duration, frequency, and intensity. In young children, conditioning is often best approached through play activities that are more attractive to them with their shorter attention spans. Importantly, those devising training programs should take into consideration that children are not miniature adults.

Strength training involves the use of progressive resistance exercises to increase the ability to exert force or resist force.

It is designed to enhance ability to perform a sport and to assist in injury prevention by increasing strength. This is to be distinguished from weight lifting, which is considered a sport, is not a conditioning program, and is not recommended for the immature skeleton. Experts generally agree that a carefully controlled and closely supervised progressive program in the prepubescent athlete may be effective in increasing strength, although it does not increase muscle mass before puberty. Rather, it appears to increase firing of motor neurons and synchronization of motor units. Close supervision by a knowledgeable adult, who monitors technique and the intensity and duration of sessions, is essential to ensure optimal benefit and prevent injury. Training begins with no added load until the child has developed consistently good technique. Then low weight or resistance can be added. When the child is comfortably able to do between 8 and 15 repetitions, then weight or resistance can be added in small increments. The American Orthopaedic Society for Sports Medicine (AOSSM) Workshop on Strength Training recommends two or three sessions per week of 20 to 30 minutes each, including a warm-up and cool-down period. When improved general fitness is also a goal, strength training should be combined with a tailored aerobic conditioning program. Specific strengthening exercises and their target muscle groups are presented in Table 21-16, and exercises designed to strengthen the muscles of the shoulder girdle are shown as an example in Figure 21-123.

Strength training can be especially beneficial in preconditioning athletes with ligamentous laxity and in those with patellofemoral malalignment. By strengthening muscles around the involved joints, most commonly the shoulder and knee, joint stability may be improved and the risk of glenohumeral and patellar subluxations and of other injuries may be reduced. Finally, carefully supervised and graduated strength training is an important part of postinjury rehabilitation.

Stretching exercises can prove valuable as part of a preconditioning program, in warm-ups before sport participation, and in rehabilitation. They are designed to enhance flexibility or ease of movement of a joint through its normal range of motion. A stretching program is particularly important for children and adolescents during growth spurts, when bone growth outstrips that of the soft tissues surrounding adjacent joints, thereby decreasing flexibility. Examples of stretching exercises are presented in Figure 21-124. Children should be supervised closely, at least initially, to ensure that their movements are slow and smooth, progressing to the point at which resistance is felt, whereupon they should hold still without bouncing for a count of 10.

Sport Selection and Participation for Children with Underlying Problems or Chronic Conditions

The prevalence of children and adolescents with chronic health problems has significantly increased over the past few decades, largely due to advances in medical and surgical treatment modalities that have substantially increased life span and quality of life. With improved general health has come greater interest in participation in sports on the part of these children. This has been bolstered by increased recognition of the importance of avoiding the natural tendency to overprotect "vulnerable" children by concerned parents and subspecialists and by programs like the Special Olympics. The latter has greatly expanded opportunities for handicapped children in sports and clearly demonstrated the benefits of sport and the enjoyment that can be derived. Indeed, research and experience have shown that the majority of children with chronic health conditions can reap many of the same benefits as those

Table 21-15	Sport-Specific Injury Prevention Strategies*

Common Injuries	Prevention Strategies
Ballet/Dance	
Repetitive hyperextension of the spine	Initiate a program of strengthening and stabilization exercises for the trunk
Sprains, tendinitis, stress fractures of the lower extremity	Initiate a stretching and strengthening program for tight hip flexors and weak abductors/external rotators; work the hip within available range of motion
Talar impingement	Treat precursor conditions (shin splints, metatarsalgia)
Snapping hip (iliopsoas tendinitis, trochanteric bursitis)	Initiate a program of strengthening and proprioception exercises for the ankle and calf; encourage low-impact training (Pilates method, pool workouts)
	Avoid pointe work until strength and skill permit; ensure that pointe shoes are fitted professionally
	Limit pointe work and pliés if the ankle is swollen or if there is any restricted joint motion
	Ensure calcium intake is adequate
Baseball/Softball	
Throat injuries (to catchers)	Use proper protective equipment (helmets, throat guards for catchers, breakaway bases)
Head and eye injuries	
Rotator cuff impingement/tendinitis	Limit the number of throws and teach proper throwing technique
Medial epicondylitis	Initiate a program of strengthening for the shoulder and a graduated preseason training program
Ankle injuries	
Basketball	
Patellar tendinitis	Initiate a program of stretching, strengthening, and overall conditioning exercises
Ankle injuries	Use braces and taping for ankles
Field Hockey	
Ankle sprains	Use proper protective equipment (lace-up ankle braces and/or tape)
Knee sprains	Initiate a program of strengthening exercises for the quadriceps and hamstrings
Back pain (often discogenic or vertebral end plate)	Initiate a program of exercises to maintain overall flexibility and neutral spine posture
Football	
Concussions	Teach proper tackling techniques
Neck injuries	Use proper protective equipment (helmets, face masks, mouthguards)
Stingers and burners	
Low back stress fractures	
Pelvic contusions	
Dehydration	Ensure frequent water breaks are scheduled in high-temperature/high-humidity conditions
Heat-related illnesses	Remove helmet frequently
	Ensure proper hydration during practice and competition
Gymnastics	
Repetitive flexion, hyperextension, and compression stresses at the thoracolumbar junction and on the lumbar vertebrae	Initiate a program of strengthening exercises for the abdomen and trunk and exercises to maintain the spine in a neutral position
Capsulitis and dorsal impingement at the wrist	Use tape or braces to protect the wrist
Radial epiphysitis	Limit weight bearing and impact on the upper extremities to protect the elbow and wrist
Osteochondritis dissecans at the elbow	
Ulnar collateral sprains of the elbow	
Shoulder instability	Limit extreme or repetitive abduction and external rotation of the shoulder
Tendinitis of the biceps and supraspinatus muscles	Initiate a program of strengthening exercises for the rotator cuff and scapular stabilizers
Ice Hockey	
Concussions	Use proper protective equipment (mouthguard, well-padded full-cage helmet with good strap *around* the chin) (*Note:* Many helmets are equipped with only a strap that goes under the chin)
Lacerations about the head and face	
Acromioclavicular sprains	Initiate a program of strengthening exercises for the upper body, especially the rotator cuff and scapular stabilizers, and the quadriceps and hamstrings
Glenohumeral subluxations/dislocations	
Ligament sprains in the knee	Ensure that the net can slide out of the holes in the ice when athletes strike the pipes
Contusions of the quadriceps	Increase padding in the thigh guard by using football thigh pads because these are larger and thicker
Soccer	
Concussion	Teach proper "heading" techniques and avoid excessive heading
Contusions about the head	Avoid heading a water-soaked ball
Tibial shaft fractures	Use shin guards
Swimming	
Rotator cuff impingement/tendinitis	Initiate program of strengthening, stretching, and flexibility exercises for the shoulder, rotator cuff, upper back, and scapular stabilizers
Medial patellofemoral pain (from breaststroke)	Limit use of hand paddles or devices that create added resistance in the water
Spondylolysis	Use fins to provide greater leg drive and reduce demands on the shoulder
Tennis	
Rotator cuff impingement/tendinitis	Initiate a program of strengthening and flexibility exercises for the back, shoulder, and abdominal muscles, especially strengthening the rotator cuff and scapular stabilizers and improving flexibility in the hamstrings and hip flexors
Medial epicondylitis	Use proper mechanics and equipment to prevent elbow injuries
Lateral epicondylitis	
Spondylolysis	

Continued

Table 21-15	Sport-Specific Injury Prevention Strategies—cont'd
Common Injuries	**Prevention Strategies**
Track and Field	
Stress fractures of the lower extremity	Ensure proper diet and conditioning, gradually increasing speed and intensity
Sesamoiditis	Initiate a cross-training program
Shin splints	Ensure good shoe fit
Iliotibial band syndrome	Avoid downhill running and sudden stops
Wrestling	
Glenohumeral subluxation/dislocation	Initiate a preseason program of strengthening exercises for the rotator cuff, scapular stabilizers, quadriceps mechanism, and hamstrings
Acromioclavicular and sternoclavicular sprains	
Meniscal tears	Avoid quick stops in dangerous positions during practice and competition
Skin infections (herpesvirus, bacteria [impetigo], tinea corporis)	Ensure that mats are cleaned daily with commercial antiseptic solution
	Teach athletes to seek medical attention for rapid treatment of any questionable skin lesions to prevent spread of infection
	Conduct skin checks before tournaments
Auricular hematomas (with resultant cartilage deformity [cauliflower ear])	Use proper protective equipment (snug-fitting head gear with ear protectors)
	Drain any blood in the auricle promptly to prevent cartilage deformity

*Injuries and prevention strategies are not listed in any particular sequence. Both lists provide general examples and are not intended to represent each injury or prevention strategy.

From Barfield WR, Gross RH: Injury prevention. In Sullivan JA, Anderson SJ, editors: *Care of the young athlete,* Elk Grove Village, Ill., 2000, American Academy of Orthopaedic Surgeons, American Academy of Pediatrics.

Position: Standing with elbow straight and thumb pointing toward floor; arm adducted 30° toward the midline.
Action: Slowly raise arm to eye level and hold for a count of 2 seconds; slowly lower arm.
Amount: Three sets of 10 repetitions.
Options: A ½-pound to 3-pound weight may be added as child gets stronger.

A

B

Position: Prone on table with arm hanging straight toward floor.
Action: Raise arm (with thumb toward ceiling) out to the side to eye level; hold for a count of 2 seconds and slowly lower.
Amount: Repeat 10 times.

Position: Prone on table with shoulder abducted 90° and upper arm supported on table with elbow bent.
Action: Keeping shoulder and elbow fixed, raise externally rotated arm 90°; hold for 2 seconds and slowly lower.
Amount: Repeat 10 times.

C

Position: Lie on opposite side with involved arm at side and elbow bent 90°.
Action: Keeping elbow fixed to side, raise arm into external rotation; hold for 2 seconds and slowly lower.
Amount: Repeat 10 times.
Options: A ½-pound to 3-pound weight may be added as child gets stronger.

D

E

Position: Prone with arms outstretched and palms flat on table.
Action: With head remaining down, raise arms as high as possible overhead; hold for a count of 3.
Amount: Repeat 10 times.

Figure 21-123   Shoulder-strengthening exercises. **A,** Empty can. **B,** Prone horizontal abduction. **C,** 90-degree/90-degree external rotation. **D,** Side-lying external rotation. **E,** Superman. *(From Goldberg B, Pappas AM, Cummings NM: Consideration for sports selection and preparatory training. In Goldberg B, editor:* Sports and exercise for children with chronic health conditions: Guidelines for participation from leading pediatric authorities. *Champaign, Ill., 1995, Human Kinetics Publishers.)*

Table 21-16	Preconditioning Strengthening Exercises
Exercise	**Target Muscle(s)**
The empty can	Supraspinatus
Prone horizontal abduction	Deltoid, infraspinatus, teres minor
90-degree/90-degree external rotation	Teres minor
Side-lying external rotation	Infraspinatus, teres minor
Superman	Lower trapezius
Abdominal curls	Rectus abdominis
Quad set	Quadriceps
Straight leg raise	Quadriceps: May perform progressive resistance exercises with more weight on ankle
Knee curls	Hamstrings: Progressive resistance exercises with more weight on ankle
Toe raises/toe-walking	Gastrocnemius/soleus
Heel walking	Anterior tibialis

Modified from Goldberg B, Pappas AM, Cummings NM: Considerations for sports selection and preparatory training. In Goldberg B, editor: *Sports and exercise for children with chronic health conditions: Guidelines for participation by leading pediatric authorities,* Champaign, Ill., 1995, Human Kinetics Publishers.

Table 21-17	Disease-Specific Benefits of Exercise
Disease	**Benefits**
Cardiac disorders	Improved cardiac function and aerobic capacity
Asthma	Possible reduced severity of EIB
Cystic fibrosis	Improved respiratory muscle endurance
	Improved clearance of airway mucus
Insulin-dependent diabetes mellitus	Increased insulin sensitivity
	Increased glucose utilization
	Prevention of obesity
	Reduction in associated CAD risk factors
Muscular dystrophy	Maintain muscle strength and endurance
	Prevention of disuse atrophy
	Maintain ambulation
Cerebral palsy	Prevent joint contractures
	Improve ambulation and other motor function
	Improved aerobic capacity
Arthritis	Preserve range of motion
	Decreased joint stiffness
	Prevent disuse muscle atrophy and osteopenia
	Possible decreased rate of progression of joint disease
Renal disease	Improved blood pressure
	Improved lipoprotein profiles
	Improved glucose tolerance

CAD, coronary artery disease; EIB, exercise-induced bronchospasm.

From Nelson MA, Harris SS: The benefits and risks of sports and exercise for children with chronic health conditions. In Goldberg B, editor: *Sports and exercise for children with chronic health conditions: Guidelines for participation by leading pediatric authorities,* Champaign, Ill., 1995, Human Kinetics Publishers.

noted in normal children and that the benefits well outweigh the risks when careful attention is given to safe sport selection and preconditioning. Furthermore, many such children are actually able to significantly improve their physical health and reduce risk for obesity as a result (Table 21-17). Psychosocial benefits may be even greater in terms of reducing the sense of isolation many such children feel, increasing their level of enjoyment in life and even helping them to forget their disease, for at least a time.

The preparticipation evaluation of these youngsters, although similar to that for children in good general health, must focus additional attention on the following:

1. The exact nature of and current status of the child's disease

2. The effect of the disorder on stamina and skill acquisition

3. The child's current fitness and skill levels

4. Whether specific sports pose undue risk for injury or complications

5. Whether special considerations are necessary in terms of the following:
   - Therapeutic intervention
   - Preconditioning and training
   - Special protective devices
   - Modifications in training techniques, rules, duration of play periods, rest periods, etc.

Children with PPE findings suggestive of high-risk cardiac abnormalities and children with moderate to severe pulmonary disease need referral to a subspecialist for complete evaluation including exercise stress testing.

After the PPE and any necessary subspecialty or physical therapy assessment, level of clearance for participation can be determined, and the child and his or her parents can be informed of necessary limits. Suggestions can be made regarding activities that are not only safe but also at which the child has a realistic chance of success.

To facilitate decision-making, the American Academy of Pediatrics, through the Committee on Sports Medicine, has recommended specific participation levels for competitive sports for children and adolescents with either chronic disease or underlying physical defects on the basis of risk (Table 21-18). This classification system has a number of "Qualified yes" recommendations that indicate the need for consultation with relevant subspecialists regarding the individual child's needs. This is necessitated by the fact that there are often significant differences in level of severity of a disorder and degree of disability, and therefore in ability to participate.

Specific examples of clearance decisions might include the following:

1. No restrictions: Small ventricular septal defect or atrial septal defect

2. Clearance with recommendations
   - Child with exercise-induced asthma—cleared but must take bronchodilator 15 to 20 minutes before exercise; must be allowed to stop and rest if becoming short of breath or otherwise symptomatic
   - Girl with patellofemoral malalignment—cleared after preparticipation strengthening program

3. Qualified clearance
   - Down syndrome child who wants to participate in contact sport—cleared pending cervical spine x-rays to rule out atlantoaxial instability

4. Not cleared
   - For swimming—child with poorly controlled seizure disorder
   - For contact sport—child with osteogenesis imperfecta, cardiac pacemaker, hemophilia

5. No competitive sports
   - Child with hypertrophic cardiomyopathy
   - Child who has undergone open heart surgery within past 6 months
   - Symptomatic mitral valve prolapse

The classification and clearance process is often further defined by specific organizations for the disability. For example, the National Association of Sports for Cerebral Palsy, the

National Wheelchair Athletic Association, and the International Sports Organization for the Disabled are responsible for deciding which disabled athletes will compete in the Special Olympics, as well as in what category. The need for adaptive equipment is controlled and classified by the organizing agencies and can include such devices as wheelchairs, custom seating devices for boats, and outrigger ski poles.

In helping these children with sport selection, the physician must try to achieve a balance between necessary limits and encouraging activity. This is aided by clear knowledge of the nature of the child's problem and of the demands and risks

of specific sports, as well as information on the level of competitiveness and training demands of the proposed sports program. Although children with chronic conditions may not be able to participate in some sports, there is still a wide array of safe alternative sports available to them (see Tables 21-12 and 21-13; and Goldberg, 1995). In conferring with the child and family, it is generally possible to find one or more activities that are of interest to the child, that are safe for him or her, and at which the athlete has a reasonable chance to improve and succeed. Teaching the child to recognize when to stop and rest (e.g., starting to get short of breath or to tire)

A
Position: Sitting on a stool with hips extended and externally rotated.
Action: Gradually bend forward toward floor until a gentle stretch is felt in the lower back; hold for 10 seconds.
Amount: Repeat 10 times.

B
Position: Sitting with back against a wall and soles of feet together.
Action: Gently push down on the inside of thighs; hold for count of 30 and then relax.
Amount: Repeat 10 times.

C

Position: Supine on table.
Action: Bring one knee toward chest while keeping opposite leg straight; gently pull on knee and hold for a count of 30.
Amount: Repeat 10 times each side.

D
Position: Either standing with ipsilateral arm against wall for support or in prone position.
Action: Grab right foot with left hand and gently pull foot toward buttock. Hold for a count of 10.
Amount: Repeat 20 times, alternating legs.

E
Position: Supine with one leg bent to chest and hands locked behind knee.
Action: Slowly straighten knee until gentle stretch is felt; hold for count of 10.
Amount: Three sets of 10 repetitions on each side.

Figure 21-124 Stretching exercises to enhance flexibility. **A,** Lumbar stretch. **B,** Hip adductor stretch. **C,** Hip flexor stretch. **D,** Quadriceps stretch. **E,** Hamstring stretch. *Note:* Stretching slowly until resistance is felt and then holding still in that position for 10 seconds are important. *(From Goldberg B, Pappas AM, Cummings NM: Consideration for sports selection and preparatory training. In Goldberg B, editor:* Sports and exercise for children with chronic health conditions: Guidelines for participation from leading pediatric authorities. *Champaign, Ill., 1995, Human Kinetics Publishers.)*

F

Position: Stand a little distance from wall, resting forearms and forehead against wall.
Action: Bend one knee while keeping opposite leg straight and foot flat on the floor until a gentle stretch is felt in calf of straight leg. Hold for a count of 10.
Amount: Three sets of 10 repetitions on each side.

G₁

Position: Sitting with elbows bent 90°.
Action: Raise (abduct) arm to shoulder level; pinch shoulder blades together; rotate arms toward ceiling, hold for a count of 5, then slowly reverse movements.
Amount: 25 sets of 5 repetitions.

G₂

Position: Supine on table; assistant must stabilize scapula on the thoracic wall.
Action: Slowly push arm across chest; hold for a count of 5.
Amount: Repeat 10 times.

G₃

Position: Supine with assistant stabilizing scapula on thoracic wall and arm in neutral rotation.
Action: Slowly bring arm up overhead toward table; hold for a count of 5.
Amount: Repeat 10 times.

Figure 21-124, cont'd   F, Gastrocnemius/soleus stretch. **G,** Shoulder stretches: G₁, standing abduction/external rotation; G₂, glenohumeral adduction stretch; G₃, glenohumeral forward elevation stretch. *Note:* Stretching slowly until resistance is felt and then holding still in that position for 10 seconds are important. *(From Goldberg B, Pappas AM, Cummings NM: Consideration for sports selection and preparatory training. In Goldberg B, editor: Sports and exercise for children with chronic health conditions: Guidelines for participation from leading pediatric authorities. Champaign, Ill., 1995, Human Kinetics Publishers.)*

Table 21-18	Sport Participation Recommendations for Children with Underlying and Chronic Health Conditions*	
Condition		**May Participate**
Atlantoaxial Instability (instability of the joint between cervical vertebrae 1 and 2)		Qualified yes
Explanation: Athlete needs evaluation to assess risk of spinal cord injury during sports participation		
Bleeding Disorder		Qualified yes
Explanation: Athlete needs evaluation		
Cardiovascular Disease		
Carditis (inflammation of the heart)		No
Explanation: Carditis may result in sudden death with exertion		
Hypertension (high blood pressure)		Qualified yes
Explanation: Those with significant essential (unexplained) hypertension should avoid weight and power lifting, body building, and strength training. Those with secondary hypertension (hypertension caused by a previously identified disease) or severe essential hypertension need evaluation. The National High Blood Pressure Education Working Group defined significant and severe hypertension		
Congenital heart disease (structural heart defects present at birth)		Qualified yes
Explanation: Those with mild forms may participate fully; those with moderate or severe forms or who have undergone surgery need evaluation. The 26th Bethesda Conference defined mild, moderate, and severe disease for common cardiac lesions		
Dysrhythmia (irregular heart rhythm)		Qualified yes
Explanation: Those with symptoms (chest pain, syncope, dizziness, shortness of breath, or other symptoms of possible dysrhythmia) or evidence of mitral regurgitation (leaking) on physical examination need evaluation		
All others may participate fully		
Heart murmur		Qualified yes
Explanation: If the murmur is innocent (does not indicate heart disease), full participation is permitted. Otherwise, the athlete needs evaluation (see congenital heart disease and mitral valve prolapse)		
Cerebral Palsy		Qualified yes
Explanation: Athlete needs evaluation		
Diabetes Mellitus		Yes
Explanation: All sports can be played with proper attention to diet, blood glucose concentration, hydration, and insulin therapy. Blood glucose concentration should be monitored every 30 minutes during continuous exercise and 15 minutes after completion of exercise		
Diarrhea		Qualified no
Explanation: Unless disease is mild, no participation is permitted because diarrhea may increase the risk of dehydration and heat illness. See Fever		
Eating Disorders		Qualified yes
Anorexia nervosa		
Bulimia nervosa		
Explanation: Patients with these disorders need medical and psychiatric assessment before participation		
Eyes		Qualified yes
Functionally one-eyed athlete		
Loss of an eye		
Detached retina		
Previous eye surgery or serious eye injury		
Explanation: A functionally one-eyed athlete has a best-corrected visual acuity of less than 20/40 in the eye with worse acuity. These athletes would suffer significant disability if the better eye were seriously injured, as would those with loss of an eye. Some athletes who previously have undergone eye surgery or had a serious eye injury may have an increased risk of injury because of weakened eye tissue. Availability of eye guards approved by the American Society for Testing and Materials and other protective equipment may allow participation in most sports, but this must be judged on an individual basis		
Fever		No
Explanation: Fever can increase cardiopulmonary effort, reduce maximal exercise capacity, make heat illness more likely, and increase orthostatic hypertension during exercise. Fever may rarely accompany myocarditis or other infections that may make exercise dangerous		
Heat Illness History		Qualified yes
Explanation: Because of the increased likelihood of recurrence, the athlete needs individual assessment to determine the presence of predisposing conditions and to arrange a prevention strategy		
Hepatitis		Yes
Explanation: Because of the apparent minimal risk to others, all sports may be played that the athlete's state of health allows. In all athletes, skin lesions should be covered properly, and athletic personnel should use universal precautions when handling blood or body fluids with visible blood		
Human Immunodeficiency Virus Infection		Yes
Explanation: Because of the apparent minimal risk to others, all sports may be played that the athlete's state of health allows. All athletes should cover their skin lesions properly, and athletic personnel should use universal health precautions when handling blood or body fluids with visible blood		
Kidney, Absence of One		Qualified yes
Explanation: Athlete needs individual assessment for contact, collision, and limited-contact sports		
Liver, Enlarged		Qualified yes
Explanation: If the liver is acutely enlarged, participation should be avoided because of risk of rupture. If the liver is chronically enlarged, individual assessment is necessary before collision, contact, or limited-contact sports are played		
Malignant Neoplasm		Qualified yes
Explanation: Athlete needs individual assessment		
Musculoskeletal Disorders		Qualified yes
Explanation: Athlete needs individual assessment		

Table 21-18 Sport Participation Recommendations for Children with Underlying and Chronic Health Conditions—cont'd	
Condition	**May Participate**
Neurologic Disorders	
History of serious head or spine trauma, severe or repeated concussions, or craniotomy	Qualified yes
Explanation: Athlete needs individual assessment for collision, contact, or limited-contact sports and also for noncontact sports if deficits in judgment or cognition are present. Research supports a conservative approach to management of concussion	
Seizure disorder, well-controlled	Yes
Explanation: Risk of seizure during participation is minimal	
Seizure disorder, poorly controlled	Qualified yes
Explanation: Athlete needs individual assessment for collision, contact, or limited-contact sports. The following noncontact sports should be avoided: archery, riflery, swimming, weight or power lifting, strength training, and sports involving heights. In these sports, occurrence of a seizure may pose a risk to self or others	
Obesity	Qualified yes
Explanation: Because of the risk of heat illness, obese persons need careful acclimatization and hydration	
Organ Transplant Recipient	Qualified yes
Explanation: Athlete needs individual assessment	
Ovary, Absence of One	Yes
Explanation: Risk of severe injury to the remaining ovary is minimal	
Respiratory Conditions	
Pulmonary compromise including cystic fibrosis	Qualified yes
Explanation: Athlete needs individual assessment, but generally, all sports may be played if oxygenation remains satisfactory during a graded exercise test. Patients with cystic fibrosis need acclimatization and good hydration to reduce the risk of heat illness	
Asthma	Yes
Explanation: With proper medication and education, only athletes with the most severe asthma will need to modify their participation	
Acute upper respiratory infection	Qualified yes
Explanation: Upper respiratory obstruction may affect pulmonary function. Athlete needs individual assessment for all but mild disease. See Fever	
Sickle Cell Disease	Qualified yes
Explanation: Athlete needs individual assessment. In general, if status of the illness permits, all but high exertion, collision, and contact sports may be played. Overheating, dehydration, and chilling must be avoided	
Sickle Cell Trait	Yes
Explanation: It is unlikely that persons with sickle cell trait have an increased risk of sudden death or other medical problems during athletic participation, except under the most extreme conditions of heat, humidity, and possibly increased altitude. These persons, like all athletes, should be carefully conditioned, acclimatized, and hydrated to reduce any possible risk	
Skin Disorders (boils, herpes simplex, impetigo, scabies, molluscum contagiosum)	Qualified yes
Explanation: While the patient is contagious, participation in gymnastics with mats, martial arts, wrestling, or other collision, contact, or limited-contact sports is not allowed	
Spleen, Enlarged	Qualified yes
Explanation: A patient with an acutely enlarged spleen should avoid all sports because of risk of rupture. A patient with a chronically enlarged spleen needs individual assessment before playing collision, contact, or limited-contact sports	
Testicle, Undescended or Absence of One	Yes
Explanation: Certain sports may require a protective cup	

*Table 21-18 is designed for use by medical and nonmedical personnel. "Needs evaluation" means that a physician with appropriate knowledge and experience should assess the safety of a given sport for an athlete with the listed medical condition. Unless otherwise noted, this is because of variability of the severity of the disease, the risk of injury for the specific sport, or both.

From American Academy of Pediatrics, Committee on Sports Medicine and Fitness, 2000-2001: Medical conditions affecting sports participation, *Pediatrics* 107:1205-1209, 2001.

is also important. For further details on evaluation of risks, clearance considerations, and sport selection for individual disorders, see Goldberg (1995).

Having helped with sport selection, the physician can also encourage and help assist in devising an individualized and graduated preparticipation conditioning or training program, which can often incorporate rehabilitative physical therapy. He or she can also help to identify sport programs that allow participation with flexibility and modifications. Monitoring the child's progress over time is also advisable.

Rehabilitation and Return to Play

Rehabilitation of the pediatric athlete after injury involves restoring the individual to normal activity so that he or she may return to sports as quickly as possible. Decisions regarding timing of return to play must be made with the athlete's best interest and safety foremost. This necessitates monitoring of progress, assessment of readiness, and determination (in consultation with coaches) of the usefulness of additional protective equipment and/or of the need for changes in skill technique or training regimen (especially important for children with overuse injuries).

Return to Play after Musculoskeletal Injury

Rehabilitation of musculoskeletal injury encompasses the reparative and healing process and assists return to prior level of activity through the use of physical modalities and therapeutic exercises. Inflammation and repair are important phases that have different interventions. In the inflammatory stages of an acute injury, tissue swelling and the inflammatory response require rest or splinting to prevent further injury and protect the injured part during the early phase of the healing process, along with application of ice packs or ice massage and judicious use of oral antiinflammatory agents. Once the acute phase of injury has passed, then protected mobility and the use of heat to mobilize the repair process are appropriate. Use of ultrasound, a high-energy source that when applied to the body can produce deep heat and is selectively absorbed by muscle and connective tissue (because of their high water content), can be quite helpful.

Therapeutic exercises are effective after initial healing is well under way, although well-moderated early exercises may be used on occasion. These are applied in a graduated manner to bring back strength and flexibility. They fall into the categories of passive, active-assisted, active, active-resistive, isometric, and strengthening exercises. These therapeutic exercises may be viewed as a transition between the acute injury and conditioning exercises. Programs must be specific to the area of injury, goal oriented, appropriately paced, and well supervised by physical therapists or knowledgeable trainers. *Return to play is safe when the athlete is symptom free with normal strength, flexibility, and range of motion.*

Return to Play after Concussion

The issue of timing of return to play of the athlete who has incurred a concussion is one of particular importance, the reason being that suffering a second concussion while the athlete is still symptomatic from a first can result in the catastrophic phenomenon known as *second impact syndrome*. This is characterized by relentless cerebrovascular congestion and edema with loss of autoregulation of cerebral blood flow, usually culminating in herniation and death.

Concussion is defined as a condition characterized by temporary impairment of neurologic function after a head injury. Important to remember is that loss of consciousness and amnesia, although common, are not always seen. Other acute symptoms may include dizziness, headache, drowsiness, confusion, disorientation, delayed response times, difficulty concentrating, emotional lability or inappropriateness, visual changes, and impaired coordination. These may be seen singly or in any combination.

In the acute situation, obviously any athlete with prolonged loss of consciousness, abnormal neurologic findings, persistently altered mental status, or progression of acute symptoms merits prompt transfer to the hospital for further evaluation and imaging. In milder cases of head injury, a sideline assessment of mental status (orientation, ability to concentrate, and short-term memory) and of neurologic status (strength, sensation, coordination) is indicated to determine whether any signs and symptoms of concussion are present. If these are negative, provocative exertional tests that increase intracranial pressure (push-ups, sit-ups, sprints, or Valsalva maneuver) are performed. If any concussive symptoms are present on mental status or neurologic screening or are provoked by exertional tests, further participation is contraindicated. If symptoms are mild and duration is brief (<15 minutes), some authorities believe the youth may return to play, whereas others advocate deferring return for a day or so. When symptoms persist, it is generally agreed that the athlete should not compete until he or she has been asymptomatic both at rest and on exertion for at least 1 week. Most recommend neurosurgical evaluation and/or neuroimaging when symptoms persist beyond 1 week. Athletes who have a prior history of concussion may warrant a longer period of inaction (2 to 4 weeks or more).

Return to Play after Exacerbation of Underlying Disorder

For recommendations regarding return to play of athletes who incur other injuries or exacerbation of symptoms of chronic diseases, see Goldberg (1995), Sullivan and Anderson (2000), and Garrett and coworkers (2001) in the Bibliography.

Bibliography

Ablin DS, Greenspan A, Reinhart M, et al: Differentiation of child abuse from osteogenesis imperfecta, *Am J Radiol* 154:1035–1046, 1990.

Aegerter E, Kirkpatrick JA Jr: *Orthopedic diseases: Physiology, pathology, radiology*, ed 4, Philadelphia, 1975, WB Saunders.

American Academy of Neurology, Quality Standards Subcommittee: Practice parameter: The management of concussion in sports (summary statement), *Neurology* 48:581–585, 1997.

American Academy of Pediatrics, Committee on Sports Medicine: Participation in competitive sports, *Pediatrics* 81:737–739, 1988.

American Academy of Pediatrics, Committee on Sports Medicine and Fitness: Strength training by children and adolescents, *Pediatrics* 107:1470–1472, 2001.

American Academy of Pediatrics, Committee on Sports Medicine and Fitness and Committee on School Health: Organized sports for children and pre-adolescents, *Pediatrics* 107:1459–1461, 2001.

American Orthopaedic Association: *Manual of orthopaedic surgery*, ed 6, Philadelphia, 1985, The Association.

American Society for Surgery of the Hand: *The hand: Examination and diagnosis*, Edinburgh, 1983, Churchill Livingstone.

American Society for Surgery of the Hand: *The hand: Primary care of common problems*, Aurora, Colo., 1985, Churchill Livingstone.

Bachman D, Santora S: Orthopedic trauma. In Fleisher GR, Ludwig S, editors: *Textbook of pediatric emergency medicine*, ed 4, Philadelphia, 2000, Lippincott Williams & Wilkins.

Canale GT: *Campbell's operative orthopaedics*, ed 9, St. Louis, 1999, Mosby.

Chang FM: The disabled athlete. In Stanitski CL, DeLee JC, Drez D, editors: Pediatric and adolescent sports medicine, vol 3, Philadelphia, 1994, WB Saunders.

Ferguson AB Jr: *Orthopedic surgery in infancy and childhood*, ed 5, Baltimore, 1981, Williams & Wilkins.

Garrett WE, Kirkendall DT, Squire DL, editors: *Principles and practice of primary care sports medicine*, Philadelphia, 2001, Lippincott Williams & Wilkins.

Garrick JG: Sports medicine, *Pediatr Clin North Am* 24:737–747, 1977.

Goldberg B, editor: *Sports and exercise for children with chronic health conditions: Guidelines for participation from leading pediatric authorities*, Champaign, Ill., 1995, Human Kinetics Publishers.

Herring JA: *Tachdjian's pediatric orthopedics*, ed 3, Philadelphia, 2002, WB Saunders.

Hoppenfeld S: *Physical examination of the spine and extremities*, New York, 1976, Appleton-Century-Crofts.

Kelly JP, Rosenberg JH: Diagnosis and management of concussion in sports, *Neurology* 48:575–580, 1997.

Lombardo JA: Preparticipation physical evaluation, *Primary Care* 11:3–21, 1982.

Lonstein JE: *Moe's textbook of scoliosis and other spinal deformities*, ed 3, Philadelphia, 1995, WB Saunders.

Lovell WW, Winter RB: *Pediatric orthopedics*, ed 4, Philadelphia, 1996, JB Lippincott.

Ogden JA: *Skeletal injury in the child*, ed 3, New York, 2000, Springer.

Rang M: *Children's fractures*, ed 2, Philadelphia, 1983, JB Lippincott.

Rockwood CA Jr, Wilkins KE, King RE: *Fractures in children*, vol 3, ed 3, Philadelphia, 1991, JB Lippincott.

Salter RB: *Textbook of disorders and injuries of the musculoskeletal system*, ed 3, Baltimore, 1999, Williams & Wilkins.

Scoles PV: *Pediatric orthopedics in clinical practice*, ed 2, Chicago, 1988, Year Book.

Sillence DO, Senn A, Danks DM: Genetic heterogeneity in osteogenesis imperfecta, *J Med Genet* 16:101–116, 1979.

Simon RR, Koenigsknecht SJ: *Orthopedics in emergency medicine: The extremities*, New York, 1982, Appleton.

Smith DM, editor: *Preparticipation physical evaluation monograph*, ed 2, Minneapolis, 1997, American Academy of Family Physicians in association with the American Academy of Pediatrics, American Medical Society for Sports Medicine, American Orthopaedic Society for Sports Medicine, and American Osteopathic Association for Sports Medicine, pp. 1–49.

Staheli LT: *Fundamentals of pediatric orthopedics*, ed 2, Wickford, R.I., 1998, Lippincott-Raven.

Stanitski CL, DeLee JC, Drez D, editors: Pediatric and adolescent sports medicine, vol 3, Philadelphia, 1994, WB Saunders.

Sullivan JA, Anderson SJ, editors: *Care of the young athlete*, Elk Grove Village, Ill., 2000, American Academy of Orthopaedic Surgeons, American Academy of Pediatrics.

Sullivan JA, Grana WA, editors: *The pediatric athlete*, Parkridge, Ill., 1989, American Academy of Orthopaedic Surgery.

PEDIATRIC PLASTIC SURGERY

Alexander Y. Lin | Joseph E. Losee

The word "plastic" is derived from the Greek word for "shape," and therefore plastic surgery is "shape surgery" that improves form and function. Form is often related to appearance, which is why aesthetics usually plays an important role in plastic surgery. Although all surgeons repair function to some degree, plastic surgery has an emphasis on functions that improve quality of life, rather than vital life functions. The prime example is in craniofacial anomalies, as one of the main functions of the face is to appear normal, so that an individual is not outcast. Similarly, although speech is not vital, in a patient with a cleft palate speech can sound hypernasal and abnormal, which is stigmatizing and jeopardizes normal social interactions.

Given that plastic surgery involves visible deformities, pediatric plastic surgery problems can be especially distressing to the parents and the patient. The newborn's anomalies are immediately apparent, causing emotions that range from guilt to fear. The face is so central to human uniqueness and recognition that craniofacial abnormalities can affect integration and socialization from infancy onward. As children learn to recognize self and non-self, apparent differences can lead to teasing and suffering that can stymie normal psychological development. Defects that are cosmetic in adults can be devastating in children.

Many of these anomalies can be associated with genetic syndromes, making visual recognition pivotal in arriving at a diagnosis and predicting the ultimate welfare of the child. In addition to congenital abnormalities, similar plastic surgery principles apply to acquired defects from trauma or tumor extirpation. Complex, uniquely human structures include the face and the hands, where both skeletal and soft tissue reconstruction is required. For the trunk and lower extremities, the primary reconstructive concern is typically soft tissue coverage.

This chapter familiarizes the pediatrician or neonatologist with the more common pathologies of form and function that the pediatric plastic surgeon can treat. It is important to educate parents that although improvements are likely, severity of the defect, variability in wound healing, and the growth of the patient make the final result difficult to predict. In addition, all surgical incisions will leave scars, which is a normal physiologic process that cannot be eliminated, and postoperative swelling and remodeling may take months to years to resolve.

CRANIOFACIAL ANOMALIES

There is no more human quality than the familiar external form of the head and face, which is the domain of the plastic surgeon specializing in craniofacial surgery. Likewise, human speech is complex and shared by no other creature, and thus palate and speech surgery are also within the same field. On the other hand, all animals share the common *internal* structures and functions involved with hearing and ear drainage, nasal drainage, airway, sight, and mastication—these are treated by non–plastic surgery subspecialists. The *external* shapes of the ear, nose, or lips are clearly the realm of the plastic surgeon.

This section divides the craniofacial arena didactically into upper third, middle third, and lower third. The upper third deals with abnormalities of the skull and forehead, including deformational plagiocephaly, and both nonsyndromic and syndromic craniosynostoses. The middle third covers the maxilla, orbits, and the external ear and nose. The lower third includes the mandible and tongue. Cleft lips, noses, and palates are discussed separately because they are so common.

Craniofacial Embryology

Congenital anomalies are best understood from an embryologic perspective. Craniofacial development occurs 4 to 7 weeks after conception. At 4 weeks, the fetus has a clear cephalic–caudal axis and differentiated endoderm, mesoderm, and ectoderm. On either side of the neural tube, the paraxial mesoderm divides into segmented tissue blocks called *somitomeres* cephalically and somites from the occiput caudally, which ultimately form the bones of the neurocranium, or protective vault of the brain. Simultaneously, mesenchymal differentiation of neural crest cells participates in the formation of the viscerocranium, or the facial skeleton.

The neurocranium consists of plates that ultimately become the adult frontal, occipital, sphenoid, ethmoid, paired temporal, and paired parietal bones (Fig. 22-1). They are separated by sutures and fontanelles that serve two main purposes: to allow molding of the head as it passes through the birth canal in parturition, and to allow rapid increase of brain volume, which doubles in the first 6 months of life and again by 2 years of age.

The longitudinal suture between the paired parietal bones is the sagittal suture. Anteriorly, the sagittal suture becomes anterior fontanelle where it intersects the transverse coronal sutures that separate the frontal bones from the parietal bones. Posteriorly, the sagittal suture becomes the posterior fontanelle where it meets the oblique L-shaped lambdoid sutures. Finally, the metopic suture runs longitudinally between the two paired frontal bones (Fig. 22-2). Closure of the posterior fontanelle occurs within the first 6 months of life, whereas the anterior fontanelle closes between 12 and 18 months of age. The metopic suture closes at about 7 months of age, and completely fuses such that the adult frontal bone has no

Figure 22-1   Bones of the human skull in lateral **(A)**, anteroposterior **(B)**, and oblique **(C)** presentation. A, frontal; B, parietal; C, occipital; D, temporal; E, ethmoid.

evidence of a former metopic suture. The sagittal and coronal sutures are next to fuse, in a posterior-to-anterolateral direction. Prenatal or postnatal premature fusion is called *craniosynostosis*, which causes abnormal skull shape by restricting growth in the direction of the fusion, which can sometimes lead to pressure on the growing brain.

The facial skeleton, or viscerocranium, is supported on a scaffold of 14 bones: the vomer; the mandible; and the paired nasal, maxilla, lacrimal, zygoma, palatal, and inferior nasal concha. By the end of the fourth gestational week, the neural crest–derived mesenchyme differentiates to form three facial prominences: the maxillary, mandibular, and frontonasal. Over the course of the next 2 weeks, migration and fusion result in the sculpture of the facial features supported by the underlying bony face. The frontal–nasal prominence gives rise to the forehead, bridge of the nose, and medial and lateral nasal prominences that further define the lower nose. The maxillary prominence evolves into the cheeks, palate, and lateral aspect of the upper lip, and the mandibular prominence develops into the lower lip. Abnormal migration, fusion, or disruption of established events during this cascade results in anomalies.

Cleft Lip, Nose, and Palate

Cleft lip, nose, and palate are the most frequent presentations of orofacial clefts, which are the most common congenital birth defects in the United States, estimated to be 1 in 590 live births annually (Basseri, 2011; Centers for Disease Control and Prevention, 2006; Parker, 2010) (Table 22-1). Approximately 1 in 700 individuals in the United States is affected, or about 15,000 live births per year. Although the cleft may be a component of an identifiable syndrome, it more commonly occurs as a solitary nonsyndromic defect. The clefting of the lip always affects the shape of the nose as well. Facial clefting is frequently categorized into cleft lip with or without cleft palate (CLP) and the isolated cleft palate (CP). Epidemiologically, a distinction is notable between the two with respect to incidence, race, and sex. Approximately 1 in 700 live births is affected with a CLP, occurring twice as often in males. Asians constitute the largest population of affected infants, followed by the white population, and then African Americans. CP has a lower incidence of approximately 1 in 1000 live births, with slightly more females affected, but no ethnic predilection.

Embryologically, at the end of the fifth week the maxillary prominences grow medially, and the medial nasal prominences are displaced toward the midline, where they fuse and ultimately form the premaxilla, which contains the philtrum of the upper lip, the portion of the upper jaw carrying the incisors, and the triangular primary (anterior) palate. Simultaneously, maxillary prominences develop outgrowths called the *palatine shelves*, which fuse in the midline, forming the secondary (posterior) palate. The primary and secondary palates join at the incisive foramen to separate the nasal and oral cavities. Failure of fusion of the palatine shelves results in secondary palatal clefting, whereas partial or complete lack of fusion of the maxillary prominence with the medial nasal prominence on one or both sides results in lip clefting with or without clefting of the primary and secondary palates (Fig. 22-3). This developmental cascade is complete by the 12th week of gestation. During this vulnerable period anatomic interference (malposition of the tongue due to mandibular hypoplasia, as in Pierre Robin sequence), miscues in cell differentiation and migration, or teratogens (phenytoin, retinoids, steroids, lithium, and maternal smoking) may lead to clefting in the developing fetus.

Initial difficulties develop from the inability of the infant to create an airtight seal to suckle effectively, which is related to the size of the clefts. Nasal regurgitation is frequent. Upright positioning and adaptive nipples can assist with preventing regurgitation and achieving effective closure around the nipple to obtain a seal. Breast-feeding is possible for infants with clefting; in fact, because the breast is more compliant, the infant may fare better in creating a seal around the breast. As with any newborn, infant weight and growth should be monitored closely; however, in this patient population it is not unusual for poor weight gain to be noted in the first 2 to 3 months of life. Thereafter, infants typically progress well and are able to make up weight.

Cleft palates have disruption of the muscular levator veli palatini sling, which often disrupts eustachian tube ventilation, leading to frequent bouts of otitis media. Persistent effusions may result in conductive hearing loss with subsequent delays in speech and language development. Careful monitoring of middle ear effusions often leads to the placement of tympanostomy tubes by the pediatric otolaryngologist to allow adequate drainage. In addition, hearing loss may be identified

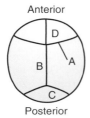

Figure 22-2   Cranial sutures as viewed from the vertex of the skull. A, coronal; B, sagittal; C, lambdoidal; D, metopic.

Table 22-1	Clefting Characteristics	
	Cleft Lip/Nose ± Cleft Palate	**Isolated Cleft Palate**
Incidence	1 in 700	1 in 1500
Sex	M > F (2:1)	F > M (3:2)
Race	Asian > Caucasian > African (4:2:1)	No difference
Syndromic association	15%	50%

Figure 22-3 The spectrum of lip clefting. **A,** Left-sided unilateral cleft lip with minimal soft tissue involvement or "forme fruste." **B,** Incomplete bilateral cleft lip. **C,** Complete left-sided unilateral cleft lip. Note the associated nasal deformity. **D,** Complete bilateral cleft lip with associated palatal clefting.

in up to one third of children with palatal clefting, under-scoring the importance of continued audiology surveillance through adulthood.

Plastic surgery reconstruction of facial clefts is a multistep endeavor, depending on the type and degree of deformity. The goals are aesthetic improvement, maintenance of normal maxillofacial growth, and restoration of palatal function in an effort to assist normal phonation. Reparative strategies continue to evolve, and controversy exists as to optimal timing and optimal procedure. Typically the cleft lip–nose deformity repair is scheduled at 3 to 6 months of age. For wide unilateral and bilateral clefts, most centers will preoperatively narrow the cleft to obtain better results. Some centers perform a lip adhesion, or simpler approximation of the defect, when the infant is less than 3 months of age; others preoperatively narrow the cleft defect by presurgical orthopedics (PSO), or customized intraoral mouth-nosepieces adjusted by pediatric orthodontists.

In some centers palate repair may be combined with the initial lip repair, but in most the palate repair is performed several months later, closer to 12 months of age. Optimal hearing and speech acquisition evolve when palatal integrity is restored before the second birthday. As such, palate closure is typically performed before 2 years of age despite concerns that early surgical interventions involving the midface may

have a negative impact on maxillofacial growth and result in midface retrusion. Studies continue to try to define intervals when palatal procedures can be performed with a minimum of untoward effects.

Unique errors of speech articulation are common to patients with cleft palate and are more likely to develop in children who undergo delayed palatal repair. Hypernasal speech, also called *velopharyngeal insufficiency,* may occur in patients in whom the soft palate is foreshortened and allows air to escape into the posterior nasal vestibule. For these patients a pharyngeal flap procedure may be performed whereby a peninsula of the posterior pharynx is attached to the soft palate. This recruited tissue serves to lengthen the palate and substantially alleviates hypernasal speech.

As the child develops an awareness of self, the lip scar resulting from earlier repair often becomes an issue and revisions can be performed to improve the upper lip's appearance. Between ages 7 and 10, during the time of mixed dentition, an alveolar bone graft is usually indicated to permit normal eruption of the canine on the affected side(s), as well as to restore the maxillary arch, provide nasal support, and close the alveolar cleft.

The end of adolescence marks the completion of the child's facial skeletal growth. At this time residual nasal deformities, which usually involve a broad and inferiorly displaced nasal ala, may be targeted by a formal rhinoplasty. Malalignment of the upper and lower jaws may additionally exist because of deficient maxillary growth. Once mandibular growth is complete, surgical advancement of the midface can be performed to restore normal occlusion.

As this brief discussion outlines, the family of a newborn with a facial cleft can anticipate numerous procedures spanning the entire childhood of their infant before reaching the end of the restorative journey. The impact of these interventions on the child is certainly profound.

Deformational Plagiocephaly

The general term *plagiocephaly*, derived from the Greek word *plagio* meaning "oblique," describes an asymmetric cranium. Etiologies can be intrinsic, such as genetic factors causing premature suture synostosis, or extrinsic, such as mechanical factors in utero or postnatally.

Deformational plagiocephaly refers to perinatal occipital flattening due to mechanical forces, with resulting changes in the malleable infant craniofacial skeleton. About 10% of cases are congenital, from pressure causes such as multiple gestations or reduced maternal pelvic volume. Postnatally, occipital flattening is acquired from persistent supine sleep positions. The high incidence (5% to 48% of healthy newborns) is because newborns cannot lift and midline their heads until 3 months of life, when neuromotor control has matured. In addition, supine positioning has become even more popular since the 1990s, when the American Academy of Pediatrics recommended supine sleeping to reduce the incidence of sudden infant death syndrome. In fact, compliance rates with the "Back to Sleep" campaign correlate with the incidence of deformational plagiocephaly, with the white population affected the most, followed by African Americans and Hispanics. Other associated factors are male gender, multiparity, and torticollis, of which the latter is associated with up to 20% of infants with deformational plagiocephaly.

Right-sided deformational plagiocephaly is more common, possibly due to right-handed mothers holding infants in a right-side-down position to nurse, causing pressure and flattening of the right occiput. Regardless of the side, once a preferential supine position develops, it becomes habitual and difficult to correct. History usually confirms a normal head at birth and acquired asymmetry that worsens with time. As the occiput becomes flatter, up to 80% of infants will have anterior displacement of the ipsilateral forehead, with concomitant increase in the height of the ipsilateral palpebral fissure, anterior displacement of the ipsilateral ear, and anterior displacement of the ipsilateral cheek, which can be seen from the anterior view (Fig. 22-4). These changes are shaped like a parallelogram on vertex view (Fig. 22-5). Posteriorly, the mastoid skull bases should be symmetric, otherwise there would be suspicion for a true unilateral lambdoid synostosis, described in The Skull, later.

Torticollis is often associated with deformational plagiocephaly, with patients typically having contralateral sternocleidomastoid (SCM) muscle "stiffness" rather than true muscle atrophy or fibrosis. For a given SCM, muscle contraction twists the head contralaterally but tilts the head ipsilaterally. In typical deformational plagiocephaly, the contralateral SCM is foreshortened and resists full extension, yielding a contralateral head tilt and ipsilateral head twist that makes the mandibular midline appear to be deviated ipsilaterally to the side of the occipital flattening. Physical examination can reveal tenderness of this contralateral SCM or resistance and agitation on contralateral head twist.

Treatment is by careful monitoring and prevention. Whenever not sleeping, infants should be placed prone ("tummy

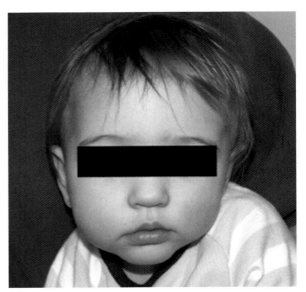

Figure 22-4   Infant with right-sided deformational plagiocephaly demonstrating anterior craniofacial changes: an advanced forehead, ear, and cheek.

time") to decrease preferential supine positioning and to increase shoulder girdle strength. Parents should alternate infant supine positions during feeding and sleeping. During feeding, pressure should be avoided on the side of the flattened occiput. Changing the position of stimuli in the crib may also influence the infant to turn to a different side, and a rolled-up towel or foam pinned to the clothes on one side will prevent the infant from sleeping on that side. If there is torticollis, at each diaper change neck exercises should be performed so that the chin can touch each shoulder for at least 10 seconds. These infants are monitored monthly until 6 months of age.

For infants older than 6 months or with more severe craniofacial deformities that are not improved with positioning, external cranioplasty with an orthotic device is a more intense treatment method. Before 10 months of age, an orthotic helmet worn 23 or more hours per day allows the malleable infant skull to grow into the shape of the symmetric helmet. Infants are typically monitored every 2 to 3 months for contour and neurologic development. After 10 months of age, helmet therapy has minimal effect.

The Skull

Craniosynostosis is defined as premature closing of the sutures between the cranial bones during development, resulting in deformities of the skull. *Primary* craniosynostosis originates from pathology at the involved suture level, whereas *secondary* craniosynostosis results from dysgenesis of the underlying brain that then misdirects cranial expansion. The latter usually does not require plastic surgical skull reconstruction as the defect is in the brain itself.

The growth of bone can be visualized as occurring at the sutures in a direction perpendicular to the suture's axis. Therefore when a suture is fused and normal growth is interrupted, resulting compensatory growth is in the direction parallel to the suture, resulting in characteristic skull shapes with their own Greek descriptive terms. So a sagittal craniosynostosis results in abnormal growth parallel to the fused sagittal suture leading to anteroposterior elongation and temporal narrowing, resulting in a *scaphocephaly*, or "boat-shaped head." *Simple* craniosynostosis refers to single suture fusion, whereas *complex* craniosynostosis is multiple suture fusion (Table 22-2).

Table 22-2	Skull Shape Nomenclature	
Name	**Suture(s) Involved**	**Shape**
Acrocephaly	Bilateral coronal	Skull height greater anteriorly, slanting downward posteriorly
Brachycephaly	Bilateral coronal	Wide, taller skull shortened in anteroposterior dimension
Oxycephaly	Bilateral coronal	Taller skull, shortened width and anteroposterior dimension
Turricephaly	Bilateral coronal	Tall skull
Plagiocephaly	Unilateral coronal or unilateral lambdoidal	Asymmetrical skull
Scaphocephaly	Sagittal	Anteroposterior elongation with bitemporal narrowing
Trigonocephaly	Metopic	Narrow, triangular, ridged forehead
Kleeblattschädel	Bilateral coronal, lambdoidal, and metopic	Cloverleaf deformity

The incidence of craniosynostosis is approximately 1 in 2500 live births across ethnic populations, but varies between genders depending on the sutures involved. In simple craniosynostosis, genetics and fetal environment may both play roles, as twins and infants delivered from breech position have a higher incidence. The genes involved in many of the *syndromic* craniosynostoses are known and are described later.

On physical examination, normal patent sutures (which may overlap slightly) move when palpated by the examiner's thumbs. Prematurely fused sutures can have a palpable ridge. To confirm, a computed tomography (CT) scan of the face and skull with fine cuts and three-dimensional reconstructions will reveal the skeletal pathoanatomy.

Increased intracranial pressure is the main concern of craniosynostosis, although its clinical significance and risk are likely low in simple craniosynostosis, and high in complex and syndromic craniosynostoses. Intracranial hypertension (ICH) could potentially lead to retardation and blindness. Therefore, along with routine neurologic and developmental examinations, at least yearly pediatric ophthalmology funduscopic examinations are mandatory, and more frequently if symptoms of ICH occur. In the syndromic craniosynostosis with midface hypoplasia, patients should also be routinely evaluated for retruded midface causing airway obstruction and obstructive sleep apnea.

Treatment usually occurs before 12 months of age, while the skull is relatively malleable and the dura can stimulate osteogenesis. Surgery consists of a bicoronal scalp incision to expose the calvarium; the plastic surgeon then draws the outlines of the bony pieces to make, and the neurosurgeon then elevates the pieces off the brain. When the deformity extends to the supraorbital rim, the elevation of the fronto-orbital bar for reconstruction adds considerable length to the operation as both the brain and globes must be protected. The plastic surgeon then reassembles the skull pieces with absorbable plates, screws, and sutures to reshape the head. Many centers also offer limited-incision, endoscopically assisted suturectomy, in which the fused suture is simply cut open and then the patient's head placed postoperatively into a molding orthotic helmet to allow growth into a normal shape; but this must be done before 6 months of age. Regardless of treatment, patients need to be monitored postoperatively at least yearly, for neurologic, ophthalmologic, and developmental changes, and for recurrence of craniofacial deformities.

Nonsyndromic, Simple Craniosynostoses

Up to 70% of simple, isolated craniosynostoses occur sporadically. Autosomal dominant and recessive familial patterns have been identified in 8% of cases. If one parent and child are affected, subsequent pregnancies are quoted to have a 50% incidence risk. Simple sagittal synostosis is the most commonly encountered simple craniosynostosis, representing 57% of cases. Coronal synostosis can be unicoronal or bicoronal, and is less common. Metopic synostosis is still less frequent, and true lambdoid synostosis is extremely rare.

Sagittal Synostosis

Sagittal synostosis, the premature fusion of the sagittal suture, leads to increased anteroposterior length and biparietal narrowing, known as *scaphocephaly* (Fig. 22-6). Isolated nonsyndromic sagittal synostosis is the most common form of craniosynostosis. It is almost always sporadic, with only 2%

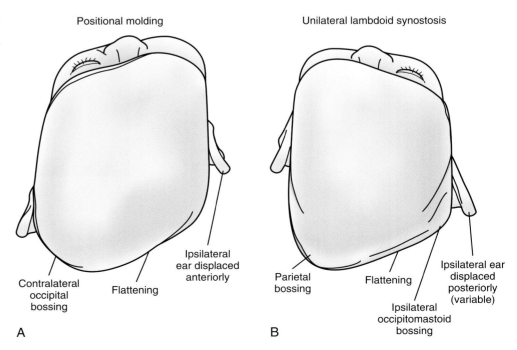

Figure 22-5 Vertex views. **A,** Right-sided deformational plagiocephaly exhibiting a parallelogram head shape. **B,** Right-sided lambdoid craniosynostosis exhibiting a trapezoid-like head shape.

Positional molding

Contralateral occipital bossing

Flattening

Ipsilateral ear displaced anteriorly

A

Unilateral lambdoid synostosis

Parietal bossing

Flattening

Ipsilateral ear displaced posteriorly (variable)

Ipsilateral occipitomastoid bossing

B

Figure 22-6 Sagittal synostosis. Lateral **(A)** and vertex **(B)** views of a child with sagittal synostosis. Anterior **(C)**, lateral **(D)**, and vertex **(E)** views of the craniofacial skeleton of a child with sagittal synostosis.

of patients having a genetic etiology. A 4 : 1 male predominance is recognized, with no race predilection. There is low risk for ICH and abnormal brain development, as the remaining cranial sutures allow compensatory expansion of the neurocranium.

Sagittal suture synostosis can range from predominantly anterior fusion, to predominantly posterior fusion, to complete fusion, causing slightly different skull shapes. Isolated anterior sagittal suture fusion will manifest frontal bossing, whereas

posterior sagittal suture fusion will exhibit occipital bossing. Bossing of both the frontal and occipital domains with associated biparietal narrowing results from complete fusion of the suture.

A ridged sagittal suture may be palpable as discussed previously, but intracranial and ophthalmic risks are low. The goals of repair are therefore appearance-related, to reduce the anterior and posterior prominences while widening the biparietal dimension. Anterior and posterior vault remodeling can be

Figure 22-7   Metopic synostosis. Anterior **(A)** and vertex **(B)** views of a child with metopic synostosis. Anterior **(C)** and vertex **(D)** views of the craniofacial skeleton of a child with metopic synostosis.

staged or simultaneous. Endoscopic strip suturectomy is also frequently successful.

Metopic Synostosis

The metopic suture is the first cranial suture to fuse, typically at about 7 months of age. It is the only suture that disappears and is indiscernible in the adult skull. Significantly premature fusion leads to a "keel"-shaped, trigonocephalic head (Fig. 22-7). Metopic synostosis has an incidence of between 1:2500 and 1:15,000 births, accounting for 10% to 20% of isolated craniosynostoses. Males are affected more often than females at about 3:1. Physical examination shows the keel-shaped forehead with hypotelorism, upward slanting of the eyelids laterally, and a triangular shape to the forehead and

supraorbital ridge. Although typically isolated, 8% to 15% of children affected with trigonocephaly will have associated anomalies involving the extremities or the central nervous, cardiac, or genitourinary system.

A ridged metopic suture may be palpable. These patients may have higher risk of astigmatism and strabismus. Although its incidence in this population is less than 4%, the presence of intracranial hypertension must be excluded. Some literature suggests cognitive delay in these patients not attributable to the sequelae of ICH, but the data are conflicting.

The severity of the deformity indicates the need for surgery. For instance, in some families the infant has slightly premature metopic fusion at 5 or 6 months of age, resulting in a prominent forehead without significant keel-shape or hypotelorism,

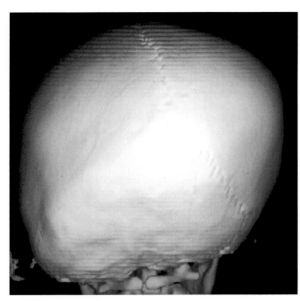

Figure 22-8   Lambdoid synostosis. Posterior view of the craniofacial skeleton of a child with left-sided lambdoid synostosis.

and no surgery is indicated. Severe shape changes can be corrected by anterior cranial vault remodeling with reshaping of the triangular fronto-orbital rim.

Lambdoid Synostosis

Lambdoid synostosis may involve one or both of the lambdoid sutures and is the rarest of the craniosynostoses. When it occurs, it is usually unilateral and causes a synostotic posterior plagiocephaly. A raised ridge may be palpable over the involved suture, and there is often a mastoid bulge of the affected side of the occiput with contralateral parietal bossing (Fig. 22-8). From the vertex view (see Fig. 22-5), a trapezoid head shape is seen, with contralateral frontal bossing, posterior displacement of the ipsilateral ear, and ipsilateral

occipitomastoid bossing. This view best distinguishes rare true lambdoid suture synostosis from common deformational plagiocephaly. True lambdoid craniosynostosis requires cranial vault remodeling, whereas deformational plagiocephaly is treated by positioning or helmet therapy.

Coronal Synostosis

The coronal sutures may be affected either unilaterally or more infrequently bilaterally, resulting in synostotic anterior plagiocephaly or anterior brachycephaly ("short skull" in the anteroposterior dimension that is wider and taller), respectively. Bicoronal synostosis is more often associated with a syndrome. Nonsyndromic unilateral coronal synostosis has an estimated incidence of 1 in 2500 live births and accounts for 15% to 30% of cases of craniosynostosis. Its etiology is unknown, but proposed causes include fetal head constraint, thyrotoxicosis, and certain vitamin deficiencies.

Synostosis of a single coronal suture results in a widened ipsilateral palpebral fissure, an elevated and anteriorly positioned ipsilateral ear, nasal root deviation toward the affected suture, chin deviation away from the affected suture, and a superiorly and posteriorly displaced supraorbital rim and eyebrow known as the "harlequin eye" deformity (Fig. 22-9). Bilateral craniosynostosis restricts anteroposterior growth and causes retrusion of the fronto-orbital region, leading to compensatory widening and raised height of the anterior cranium; the result is described as brachycephaly, acrocephaly, oxycephaly, or turricephaly (Table 22-2). In bilateral craniosynostosis, there is increased incidence of ICH.

Treatment of coronal synostosis includes anterior cranial expansion with vault remodeling and fronto-orbital advancement. Some centers perform suture craniectomy with helmet therapy, especially for the unicoronal coronal synostosis, where symmetry is difficult to achieve.

Multiple Suture Synostoses

The most severe skull dysmorphology and ICH result from multiple suture fusion. When the coronal and lambdoid sutures fuse bilaterally with fusion of the anterior metopic

Figure 22-9   Unilateral coronal synostosis. **A,** Photograph of a child with left-sided unilateral coronal synostosis. **B,** Anterior view of the craniofacial skeleton of a child with right-sided unilateral coronal synostosis.

Table 22-3	Gene Mutations Associated with Craniofacial Syndromes	
Gene/Protein	**Syndrome**	**Chromosome**
FGFR1	Pfeiffer	8
FGFR2	Apert	10
	Crouzon	10
	Pfeiffer	10
	Jackson-Weiss	10
	Beare-Stevenson	10
FGFR3	Muenke	4
	Crouzon with AN	4
TWIST	Saethre-Chotzen	7
Treacle	Treacher Collins	5

AN, acanthosis nigricans; FGFR, fibroblast growth factor receptor.

suture, compensatory bulging at the remaining open sagittal suture leads to a trifoliate appearance described as the cloverleaf deformity, or *kleeblattschädel*. Although multiple suture synostoses can be sporadic, they are much more likely to be associated with syndromes.

Syndromic, Complex Craniosynostoses (Table 22-3)

Craniosynostoses involving more than one suture are much rarer, tend to be syndromic, and are usually caused by sporadic mutations, although if transmitted tend to be autosomal dominant. The most characterized are the acrocephalosyndactyly syndromes, which share the features of bicoronal craniosynostosis, midface hypoplasia, abnormal facies, and limb abnormalities. The genetic defect usually inactivates fibroblast growth factor receptor *(FGFR)* genes that are involved in restraining bone growth, leading to hypermorphic bone development. *FGFR1*, *-2*, and *-3* are differentially involved in these phenotypic syndromes. The key craniofacial issues are that all of these patients have bicoronal craniosynostoses with retruded supraorbital rims, and midface hypoplasia with weak infraorbital support, resulting in shallow orbits and high risk of exorbitism and exposure keratitis that can lead to blindness, and other ophthalmologic problems. Craniofacial anomalies such as cleft palate, mandibular growth problems, stylohyoid calcification, and other cranial suture involvement are common. There is variability in neurosurgical conditions such as ICH; hydrocephalus; neurocognitive development; and cranial base, cervical spine, and other vertebral abnormalities. Inner ear problems such as otitis media requiring myringotomy tubes; and inner nose and airway issues such as choanal, tracheal, and laryngeal abnormalities require consultation with an otolaryngologist. Cardiac, renal, and other visceral anomalies are also common.

Apert Syndrome

Apert syndrome is autosomal dominant with incomplete penetrance and a birth prevalence of 5.5 to 16 per 1 million live births. The majority of cases are sporadic; more than 98% of patients with Apert syndrome have identifiable mutations in the *FGFR2* gene, resulting in multiple anomalies in all systems (Fig. 22-10). Two distinguishing features include symmetric complex syndactylies of the hands and feet, and cognitive defects.

Their bicoronal synostosis results in brachycephaly with a high cranium that is described as turricephalic. They have delayed closure of their metopic and sagittal sutures between 2 and 4 years of age, resulting in hypertelorism. Their abnormal facies have more severe features, including ptosis and downward-slanting palpebral fissures. Their midface deficiency is often associated with hypoplastic or stenotic choanae, leading to airway obstruction requiring tracheostomy. A sleep study can diagnose obstructive sleep apnea requiring treatment with a continuous positive airway pressure device.

Their shallow orbits can result in proptosis, but patients with Apert syndrome also commonly have strabismus with a V-shaped pattern: exotropic upward gaze divergence with esotropic downward gaze, as well as other ophthalmic problems.

Although significant hydrocephalus is not common, the risk of neurosurgical abnormality is high and therefore baseline magnetic resonance imaging (MRI) is recommended along with the usual CT scan to evaluate the bone on a regular basis.

Seventy-two percent of children with Apert syndrome are noted to have brain anomalies, leading to developmental delays and cognitive deficits. Infants operated on before their first birthday but after 3 months of age are more likely to have intelligence quotients (IQs) greater than 80. Unfortunately, children who underwent similar procedures before 3 months of age trended toward lower IQs and required additional operations.

A hallmark of Apert syndrome is complex symmetric syndactyly of the hands and feet, especially of the middle three digits, leaving the first and fifth digits separate; this results in a "mitten hand" appearance (Fig. 22-10, *B*). Plastic surgeons can separate the digits to produce a more functional hand.

Finally, the skin of patients with Apert syndrome may display excessive sweating. Patients have been shown to have an increased number of sweat glands and prominent sebaceous glands. During adolescence the skin becomes oily, and in 70% of patients acne erupts on the face, chest, and back.

Crouzon Syndrome

Crouzon syndrome is another autosomal dominant acrocephalosyndactyly with incomplete penetrance that presents as a sporadic new mutation 60% of the time. The birth prevalence is 15 to 16 per 1 million live births and is also associated with mutations in *FGFR2*. Its distinguishing features include normal extremities.

The heads of patients with Crouzon syndrome are overall brachycephalic from the bicoronal synostosis although other sutures can be involved, leading to other skull shapes (Fig. 22-11). Their midface hypoplasia similarly leads to proptosis, and also an illusion of mandibular prognathism with a severe underbite called *class III malocclusion*.

Intracranially they may have anomalous venous drainage, and are more likely to have hydrocephalus than are patients with Apert syndrome. They are also more likely to have Chiari I malformations, likely due to their tendency to have early closure of the lambdoid sutures; because of this an early MRI scan is recommended. Some may also develop suture fusion postnatally, and thus early CT scans may show relatively patent coronal sutures.

Some variants of Crouzon syndrome are associated with acanthosis nigricans, a verrucous hyperplasia and hypertrophy of the skin with associated hyperpigmentation and accentuated skin markings. It is distributed in the axillae, neck, chest, abdomen, breasts, perioral and periorbital regions, and nasolabial folds. Multiple melanocytic nevi are also frequently noted over the face, trunk, and extremities.

Pfeiffer Syndrome

Pfeiffer syndrome, a type of acrocephalosyndactyly, has the distinguishing characteristic of broadened thumbs and toes. Mutations in the *FGFR1* and *FGFR2* genes have been implicated. Most patients have bicoronal synostosis with brachycephaly and midface hypoplasia with associated ocular findings. The distinguishing feature is broad, symmetric thumbs that deviate radially, and great toes that deviate medially, often with phalangeal malformations and simple soft tissue syndactyly (Fig. 22-12).

Apert Syndrome: Features and Findings

Craniofacial
Brachycephaly due to coronal suture synostosis
Hypertelorism
Proptosis
V-pattern exotropia
Midface hypoplasia
Choanal stenosis
Cleft palate
Stylohyoid calcification
Conductive hearing deficits
Extracranial Skeletal
Symmetrical syndactyly of the hands
Cervical spine fusion
Shortened humeri

Other
Cardiovascular anomalies
Hydronephrosis
Cryptorchidism
Tracheal anomalies
Obstructive sleep apnea
Diffuse acne

Figure 22-10   Apert syndrome. **A,** Lateral view of a child with Apert syndrome. **B,** Syndactyly of the hand. Anterior **(C)** and lateral **(D)** views of the craniofacial skeleton of a child with Apert syndrome. Note the expansive anterior fontanelle in the anteroposterior view.

There are some subtypes with more severe symptoms, including *kleeblattschädel* deformity (cloverleaf skull) with hydrocephalus, and more severe midface hypoplasia with ICH, mental retardation, and a poorer prognosis.

Jackson-Weiss Syndrome

Jackson-Weiss syndrome is an autosomal dominant acrocephalosyndactyly that is associated with mutations in *FGFR2*. Patients usually have coronal synostosis with a broad or towering forehead, hearing deficits, and foot anomalies such as short metatarsals. Their hands are usually normal.

Saethre-Chotzen Syndrome

Saethre-Chotzen syndrome has similar characteristics to the Jackson-Weiss syndrome but does not involve the *FGFR3* gene family. The etiology involves a mutation in the *TWIST* gene with a pattern of autosomal dominant inheritance. Patients frequently have coronal craniosynostosis with

Crouzon Syndrome: Features and Findings

Craniofacial
Brachycephaly due to coronal suture synostosis
Hydrocephaly with Chiari I malformation
Hypertelorism
Proptosis
Midface hypoplasia
"Beaked" nose

Cleft palate
Stylohyoid calcification
Conduction and/or neurosensory hearing deficit
Extracranial Skeletal
Cervical spine fusion
Other
Acanthosis nigricans

Figure 22-11   Crouzon syndrome. **(A)** Frontal view; **(B)** anterior skeletal view; **(C)** lateral skeletal view

Pfeiffer Syndrome: Features and Findings

	Type I	Type II	Type III
Craniofacial	+		+
Acrocephaly, or turribrachycephaly (oxycephaly), due to coronal suture synostosis			
Kleeblattschädel sutural deformity		+	
Hydrocephaly		+	
Midface hypoplasia	+	++	++
"Beaked" nose	+	+	+
Hypertelorism	+	+	+
Proptosis	+	++	+
Blindness		+	
Choanal atresia		+	+
Mental retardation		+	+
Extracranial Skeletal			
Broad, radially deviated thumbs	+	+	+
Broad, medially deviated great toes	+	+	+
Soft tissue syndactyly	+	+	+
Elbow ankylosis		+	+

Figure 22-12   Pfeiffer syndrome. **(A)** Lateral view; **(B)** anterior skeletal view; **(C)** great toe anomalies.

brachycephaly. Their facies include abnormally downward-sloped palpebral fissures with ptosis, low forehead hairline, and ear abnormalities. They often have incomplete syndactyly of their hands.

The Midface

Midface craniofacial syndromes can be quite complex because they affect many facial structures including the eyes, ears, soft tissues, and skeleton of the midface. Accordingly, the defects are among the most challenging to reconstruct, with patients requiring multiple procedures and interventions. These syndromes are often also associated with mandibular hypoplasia, which can lead to upper airway obstruction. In general, securing the airway and feeding will be priorities in the neonatal period and may necessitate a tracheostomy and gastrostomy tube placement. Early intervention with an otologist to optimize hearing is important. Although pediatric plastic surgery reconstruction of the midface and mandible is usually performed as late as possible to avoid interrupting normal skeletal growth, exposure of sclerae from midface hypoplasia or airway obstructive symptoms (such as sleep apnea) could warrant earlier augmentation of the maxilla or mandible. External ear reconstruction is usually performed at about 6 to 7 years of age, when there is enough rib cartilage for the procedure and the patient is mature enough to tolerate the three- or four-stage procedure, each stage separated by several months.

Mandibulofacial Dysostosis (Treacher Collins Syndrome)

Treacher Collins syndrome (TCS) affects mainly the midface and mandible, and is suspected to have an incidence of approximately 1 in 50,000 live births (Fig. 22-13). Inheritance is autosomal dominant with variable expression, but probably about half the cases are sporadic new mutations. The genetic defect is in the gene that encodes the protein Treacle, which is thought to affect the development of the first branchial arch (mandible), second branchial arch (maxilla), and nasal placode in the developing fetus.

The facial dysmorphology tends to be bilateral with involvement of the mandible, malar region (cheek), eyes, and ears. There is both bony and soft tissue hypoplasia of the malar region or zygoma, resulting in a lateral facial cleft. This extends to the lateral orbit walls, leading to temporal concavity, reduced bitemporal distance, and reduced cephalic length. Thus the neurocranium may appear misshapen, although there is no craniosynostosis. Intelligence is usually average to above average.

Overlying these deficient orbitozygomatic regions are, frequently, abnormalities in eyelid structure, preauricular cheek skin, temporal fossa, and external ears. The palpebral fissures are downwardly slanted and the lower eyelids can have colobomas, lack of eyelashes, or hypoplasia. External ears are often symmetrically malformed or malpositioned, with stenosis or atresia and parallel middle ear abnormalities. The latter causes a conductive hearing loss that can usually be improved by hearing aids (see Chapter 23).

The mandible is usually hypoplastic, resulting in retrognathia, malocclusion, temporomandibular joint (TMJ) dysfunction, and misformed muscles of mastication, resulting in an open bite. A *type I mandible* refers to a retrognathic mandible with minor anterior open bite and mild glenoid fossa hypoplasia, whereas the worse grade, type III, is a free-floating severely retrognathic mandible without any articulation to the cranial base (lack of TMJ), usually requiring a postnatal tracheostomy. In between are type IIA with moderate hypoplasia but intact TMJ, and type IIB with greater hypoplasticity and a nonfunctioning TMJ.

Mandibulofacial Dysostosis (Treacher Collins Syndrome): Features and Findings

Craniofacial (Usually Bilateral Findings)	Preauricular hair
Bilateral zygoma hypoplasia	Bilateral external ear deformities
Bony deficiency of lateral orbits	Bilateral external auditory canal stenosis or atresia
Maxillary hypoplasia	Auditory ossicle hypoplasia or ankylosis
Choanal stenosis	Conductive hearing deficits
Cleft palate with or without cleft lip	Retrognathia due to mandibular hypoplasia
Downward-slanting palpebral fissures	
Colobomas	Bite malocclusion
Lower eyelid hypoplasia	Temporomandibular joint dysfunction
Absent lower eyelashes	

Figure 22-13 Mandibulofacial dysostosis. **A,** Photograph of a child with mandibulofacial dysostosis. **B,** Anterior view of the craniofacial skeleton of a child with mandibulofacial dysostosis.

Given the midface anomalies and mandibular hypoplasia, a CT scan of the head and face is usually recommended. Mandibular hypoplasia leads to glossoptosis and airway compromise, compounded by midface hypoplasia with some degree of choanal stenosis or atresia. Other early issues concern feeding and corneal exposure. Non–plastic surgery specialists can assist in tracheostomies, placement of gastrostomy tubes, ophthalmic assessment, and hearing aids. Pediatric plastic surgeons are involved in cleft palate repair if indicated, and reconstruction of the hard and soft external structures of the face.

A cleft palate should be treated as described previously, timed around the time of developing speech. Unless corneal exposure is threatened, most reconstruction is delayed as long as possible, to avoid inevitable recurrence as the face ages. In symptomatic retrognathia where glenoid fossae are present (types I, IIA, IIB), the mandible can be lengthened by distraction osteogenesis, in which mandibular osteotomies are subsequently serially lengthened by hardware. This is usually performed at early skeletal maturity (females, ages 13 to 15; males, ages 15 to 16). Type III deformities first need TMJ reconstruction at about age 6 to 10 years, before the mandible lengthens. A rhinoplasty can improve mid-dorsal humps and wide nasal bridges, but should usually be postponed until after jaw surgery, as the latter moves the base of the nose. Eyelid defects can be repaired with skin or muscle flaps. Ear reconstruction, described below, requires an autologous rib cartilage graft and multiple surgical stages. The hollow temporal fossa and lateral cleft can be augmented, but there is a high resorption rate.

In summary, TCS yields significant multiple perimaxillary and mandibular anomalies with a range of severities, and usually leads to tracheostomies and multiple reconstructive efforts. The underlying genetic anomalies make it impossible to regain a normal appearance, but improvements can usually be made.

Acrofacial Dysostosis (Nager Syndrome)

In 1948 Nager and de Reynier characterized a series of infants with branchial arch deformities similar to TCS but with, in addition, upper extremity anomalies (Fig. 22-14). It is, similarly, autosomal dominant and usually presents sporadically, with prevalence twice as frequent among males as females. It presents similar craniofacial abnormalities, and its distinguishing feature is the presence of preaxial (radial) abnormalities, including radioulnar synostosis (proximal fusion) and hypoplasia or aplasia of the thumbs. Other findings include toe abnormalities and visceral involvement. Patients progress developmentally, provided hearing deficits are addressed by otolaryngologists.

Oculo-Auriculo-Vertebral Spectrum (Goldenhar Syndrome and Craniofacial or Hemifacial Microsomia)

The oculo-auriculo-vertebral syndrome, or spectrum, is a collection of facial anomalies that are believed by many experts to represent a spectrum of phenotypes exhibited secondary to a heterogeneous developmental field defect (Fig. 22-15). It includes several named entities including Goldenhar syndrome, craniofacial microsomia, and hemifacial microsomia. Classically, hemifacial microsomia defined a condition that affected primarily ear, oral, and mandibular development; Goldenhar syndrome additionally included vertebral anomalies and epibulbar dermoids. They are likely variants of a common underlying developmental aberration.

The findings witnessed in Goldenhar syndrome and hemifacial microsomia are referred to as the oculo-auriculo-vertebral spectrum, the incidence of which varies from 1 in 3500 to 19,500 live births. A male-to-female ratio of 3:2 is observed, with a similar ratio of lateralization favoring the right side of the body. Up to one third may have bilateral involvement, but still be asymmetric. Most cases are sporadic, although familial patterns have been identified.

Findings may be divided into those affecting the craniofacial domain, the central nervous system, the skeleton, the cardiovascular system, and other systemic findings. The majority of cases have some degree of facial asymmetry that may become apparent only as the child grows. The acronym

Acrofacial Dysostosis (Nager Syndrome): Features and Findings

Craniofacial (Usually Bilateral Findings)	Bilateral external auditory canal stenosis or atresia
Bilateral zygoma hypoplasia	Auditory ossicle hypoplasia or ankylosis
Bony deficiency of lateral orbits	Conductive hearing deficits
Maxillary hypoplasia	Severe mandibular hypoplasia
Choanal stenosis	Bite malocclusion
Cleft palate with or without cleft lip	Temporomandibular joint dysfunction
Downward-slanting palpebral fissures	***Extracranial Skeletal***
Colobomas	Radioulnar synostosis
Lower eyelid hypoplasia	Thumb hypoplasia or aplasia
Absent lower eyelashes	
Preauricular hair	
Bilateral external ear deformities	

Figure 22-14 Acrofacial dysostosis. **A** and **B,** Photographs of children with acrofacial dysostosis.

OMENS describes the major findings of hypoplasia of the orbit, mandible, external ear, nerve (facial), and soft tissue, usually asymmetrically. The maxillary, temporal, and malar bones are hypoplastic and flattened on the affected side. The mandible may be either aplastic or hypoplastic. Smooth epibulbar dermoids, often with fine hairs, are common unilateral findings inferotemporally at the limbus of the eye. Unilateral colobomas of the upper eyelids and oculomotor disorders including esotropia and exotropia are other ocular findings. The region of the ear is always involved to some degree and may exhibit preauricular appendages, pretragal blind-ended fistulae, and hypoplastic or malpositioned pinnae. The external auditory canal may be atretic or stenotic, leading to conductive hearing impairment, which is far more common than neurosensory losses. Involvement of nearly all cranial nerves has been reported, with lower facial weakness a frequent observation. There can be a lateral facial cleft at the oral commissure, also known as macrostomia. The palatal and tongue muscles may be hypoplastic and paralyzed, affecting feeding success. Furthermore, a unilateral or bilateral cleft lip and/or palate occurs in up to 15% of infants.

Neurosurgical issues such as brain anomalies, spine deformities, or congenital heart disease may also be present, and thus these patients often need a complete tertiary workup.

The Mandible

Isolated mandibular malformations are rarer, with the exception of Pierre Robin sequence (PRS). PRS is not a syndrome; rather, it is an original gestational event that likely leads to

Oculo-Auriculo-Vertebral Spectrum: Features and Findings

Craniofacial
Facial asymmetry
Unilateral maxillary, temporal, and
    zygomatic hypoplasia
Epibulbar dermoids with fine hairs
Unilateral colobomas of upper eyelids
Esotropia or exotropia
Preauricular appendages
Pretragal fistula
External ear deformities
External auditory canal stenosis or atresia
Conductive hearing deficits
Macrostomia due to mandibular
    dysgenesis
Lateral facial cleft
Cleft lip with or without cleft palate

Central Nervous System
Seventh cranial nerve palsy
Microcephaly
Hydrocephaly
Encephaloceles

Extracranial Skeletal
Cervical vertebral fusion
Spina bifida
Hemivertebrae
Butterfly, fused, or hypoplastic vertebrae
Scoliosis
Rib anomalies

Cardiovascular
Ventricular septal defect
Tetralogy of Fallot
Transposition of the great vessels
Coarctation of the aorta
Pulmonic stenosis
Dextrocardia

Other
Pulmonary dysplasia
Tracheoesophageal fistula
Renal anomalies
Imperforate anus

Figure 22-15   Oculo-auriculo-vertebral (OAV) spectrum. **A** and **B,** Photographs of a child with oculo-auriculo-vertebral spectrum. **C,** Anterior view of the craniofacial skeleton of a child with right-sided OAV spectrum anomalies (hemifacial microsomia).

sequential developmental sequelae. It may appear as an entity alone or in association with other syndromes.

Pierre Robin Sequence

PRS describes symptomatic microretrognathia (small mandible) that leads to glossoptosis (tongue falling posteriorly) resulting in airway obstruction (Fig. 22-16). The glossoptotic tongue in the developing fetus often interrupts palatal shelve fusion, typically resulting in a U-shaped cleft palate. Symptomatic airway obstruction demands close observation (pulse oximetry, blood gases, sleep studies) and possible intervention.

Figure 22-16   Pierre Robin sequence. **A,** Lateral view of a child with Pierre Robin sequence, characterized by severe micrognathia and cleft palate. **B,** Lateral view of the craniofacial skeleton of a child with Pierre Robin sequence. Note the small, retruded mandible. (**A,** Courtesy Wolfgang Losken, MD.)

PRS may occur as frequently as once in 2000 live births, with reported mortalities ranging from 19% to 65%, the result of airway issues. The mandibular hypoplasia may be due to the intrauterine environment, but coexisting malformation syndromes, such as Stickler syndrome, can play a role as well. PRS is associated with a syndrome in 25% to 40% of cases.

Glossoptotic airway obstruction leads to substernal breathing, stridor, and distress. The prone position or a nasopharyngeal airway can temporize the airway obstruction. Because of respiratory insufficiency, up to 55% of infants with PRS may experience feeding difficulties, including reflux. Antireflux medication is almost always necessary, and those with significant hypoxemia during feedings or inadequate caloric intake or weight gain require gavage feeding. A swallow evaluation may reveal aspiration or worse, with the tongue likely contributing. If airway obstruction occurs at rest or with feeding, exploration under anesthesia by otolaryngology is necessary to rule out primary tracheolaryngeal pathology.

Because a tracheostomy is a great social burden to caregivers and nursing resources, pediatric plastic surgeons are involved with manipulating the soft and hard tissues to restore more normal anatomy. Often mandibular growth will catch up during the temporizing stage.

Tongue–lip adhesion (TLA), or glossopexy, involves layered suturing of the tongue to the lower lip to reduce glossoptosis. Earlier versions of the surgery resulted in a high dehiscence rate; at present the plastic surgeon will often include muscular sutures, bolster with "buttons" over sutures, and allow prolonged intubation to improve healing. TLA can allow transition from nasogastric tube feeding to oral feeding and hence avoid a tracheostomy. At the time of the cleft palate repair, usually at about 9 to 12 months of age, the adhesion is taken down. This coincides nicely with the amount of time necessary for infant mandibular growth to overcome its contribution to airway compromise. Should a TLA fail to alleviate airway obstruction, either distraction of the mandible or a tracheostomy is indicated. As described previously, mandibular osteotomies followed by distraction osteogenesis can lengthen the mandible. As a last resort, tracheostomy bypasses the obstructed nasopharynx.

Outcomes for children with PRS vary. Advances in monitoring have led to improved outcomes, and generally children do well. Strategies for initial and long-term management continue to evolve, however. As such, care plans that foster optimal outcomes for these children should be individually developed.

External Structures of the Face

Whereas other subspecialists take care of the eye (globe), the inner ear (eardrum, ossicles, cochlea), the nasal sinuses and choanae, the laryngotracheal system, and the dentition, pediatric plastic surgeons are usually consulted to repair and reconstruct the external structures of the face: eyelids, outer ears (pinnae), nose and septum, lips and tongue, nerves, and muscles. Among their other functions, these structures constitute our unique human appearance. Skeletal diagnosis and treatment are described in Craniomaxillofacial Trauma (later). As for soft tissue, we briefly discussed cheiloplasty of the lips and rhinoplasty of the nose in the previous section Cleft Lip, Nose, and Palate, but similar principles are applicable in treating acquired defects of the lips and nose, such as from trauma or lesion removal. Tongue manipulation, described previously in the section The Mandible, also includes shaping the tongue such as in macroglossia (e.g., Beckwith-Wiedemann syndrome). Although there are many specific external facial problems with well-described solutions, there are such a large variety of unique potential

defects, especially given the random nature of trauma, that basic principles of soft tissue reconstruction (described later in this chapter) may need to be creatively put together for a customized solution.

Because of space limitations, we highlight the external ear as an example of an external face defect with a well-described reconstruction. Abnormalities of the ear appear in many of the craniofacial syndromes described previously, including craniofacial microsomia and Goldenhar syndrome. Other isolated forms of microtia exist, and although there are usually lobule-like vestiges, microtia can range from hypoplastic ears to full anotia (Fig. 22-17, A). There are usually three or four stages of surgery, each separated by at least several months, to accomplish the reconstruction. The first stage is the harvest of autologous rib cartilage, which is then carved, constructed, and placed as a graft under very thin auricular skin (Fig. 22-17, B). The rest of the stages include a skin graft to elevate the construct and soft tissue rearrangements to create an earlobe and tragus to finish the details of the ear (Fig. 22-17, C and D).

Other ear abnormalities include prominent ears and constricted ears. Prominent ears are usually due to a loss of the antihelical fold (Fig. 22-18, A) and an excessive conchoscaphal angle (Fig. 22-18, B), and reconstructive efforts are directed toward correcting these issues (Fig. 22-18, C and D). Constricted ears refer to the variety of helical abnormalities referred to as lop ear, cup ear, hidden ear, and others. These repairs are based on soft tissue rearrangements but may need cartilage grafts. Extremely constricted ears may also be treated as microtia, with staged reconstruction as described previously.

Craniofacial Summary

Clefting and craniofacial syndromes represent a number of interesting and at times challenging medical and surgical entities that fortunately afflict a relatively small number of newborns. Medical science has only recently begun to delineate why these developmental anomalies occur and, unfortunately, may have little to offer in the way of intervention owing to the early occurrence of the developmental miscues. The impact on those affected and their families can be devastating. It is encouraging, however, that early thorough evaluations and appropriate interventions can significantly benefit the lives of these children. Many health care providers are pivotal to the success of these endeavors. Indeed, multidisciplinary teams consisting of plastic surgeons, nurse care coordinators, speech therapists, otologists and audiologists, orthodontists, occupational therapists, psychologists, and social workers convincingly optimize the outcomes for these children and should be enlisted where available.

CRANIOMAXILLOFACIAL TRAUMA

Management of craniofacial trauma in children differs from that for adults in that the pediatric craniofacial skeleton is still developing and growing. Relative to adults, there is more cartilage, cancellous bone, and malleable growth centers, resulting in more absorption of energy and less likelihood of fracturing. Even when there are fractures, they are more likely to be partial (greenstick) than complete. Other major differences include the higher skull-to-face ratio, lack of pneumatized sinuses, and presence of adult tooth buds in the maxilla and mandible. Finally, children heal faster, so the decision to repair fractures needs to be made sooner, and the posttreatment immobilization period made shorter.

The facial skeleton develops more slowly than the cranial skeleton, such that facial dimensions at 5 years of age are approximately 80% of an adult's face. The growth then

Figure 22-17 Ear reconstruction. **A,** Microtia; **B,** constructed costal cartilage framework beneath scalp skin flap; **C,** ear lobe transposition stage; **D,** completed ear reconstruction.

plateaus until the pubertal growth spurt, which lasts until about age 17, when another plateau is reached that eventually halts. Overall, the upper third grows fastest because of the development of the brain and orbits, the middle third is next, and the lower third, or mandible, is the last to finish growing after puberty. Modern methods of open reduction internal fixation with titanium plates and screws could restrict growth. In addition, pediatric maxillae and mandibles contain both pediatric and adult teeth, making it imperative to avoid hardware that could injure unerupted permanent teeth. Therefore, wires and absorbable plates are preferred whenever possible. Because of the potential growth disturbance, pediatric patients

with craniofacial fractures are monitored on a yearly basis until skeletal maturity.

The evaluation of any trauma patient must still progress according to Advanced Trauma Life Support (ATLS) guidelines, including securing the airway and circulation before proceeding to the focused craniofacial examination. Brain trauma and cervical spine injury must be ruled out, as there is a high incidence of concomitant injury that may require neurosurgical consultation. Orbital examination including visual assessment and extraocular movement must be undertaken, which could lead to an ophthalmologic consultation. The nasal septum should be inspected visually to rule out a

Figure 22-18 Prominent ear. **A,** Prominent ear with absence of antihelical fold. **B,** Prominent ear with excessive conchoscaphal angle. **C,** Frontal view of repaired prominent ear. **D,** Lateral view of repaired prominent ear: note the newly formed antihelical fold.

septal hematoma that could lead to cartilage necrosis; the dental occlusion should be examined as well, and the patient asked about symptoms of malocclusion. Although requiring more cooperation than some children can muster, facial animation should be checked for symmetry, and facial sensation can be tested in the trigeminal nerve distribution (V_1, forehead; V_2, cheeks; V_3, chin). Palpating the facial skeleton for tenderness or bony step-offs needs to include the forehead, periorbital borders, cheeks, nasal bones, and jaws. Suspicion for fractures warrants a fine-cut noncontrast CT scan of the head and face for definitive diagnosis. Finally, preinjury photos should always be obtained if possible for comparison, as facial asymmetries and dental problems are common.

Although craniofacial trauma deals with both bony and soft tissue injuries, in this section we discuss skeletal injuries only, as soft tissue principles are discussed elsewhere in this chapter. However, the facial nerve (cranial nerve VII) and parotid duct are specialized structures that must be examined if in the zone of injury. In addition, the pediatric skeleton also contains growth centers that drive the growth of the craniofacial region, with the overlying soft tissue following that growth.

Skull and Forehead Fractures

The ratio of cranium to face is greater in younger patients, and thus skull fractures are more common than facial fractures at younger ages. The frontal sinus does not form until about 5 or 6 years of age, and then pneumatization continues until well past puberty. This lack of a frontal sinus allows fractures to the forehead and skull to directly transmit their forces to the skull base, orbit, and zygoma, resulting in an extended skull fracture or an "oblique craniofacial fracture." When minimally displaced, skull fractures can be treated conservatively, but otherwise these fractures require neurosurgical repair of the dura and plastic surgical reconstruction of the bone.

Another unique pediatric injury is a growing skull fracture: the "growth" likely originates from a clinically insignificant dural tear at the time of injury that stretches and allows brain herniation between the fracture edges, resulting in nonunion and expansion. If the growing skull fracture contains the supraorbital ridge, this can lead to changes in the orbit, including pulsatile exophthalmos and vertical dystopia, shifting the position of the globe.

As in an adult, the goals of forehead reconstruction in the pediatric patient are to isolate the intracranial contents (to prevent cerebrospinal fluid leaks and communication with the nasal sinuses), restore facial contour, and avoid posttraumatic sequelae (such as mucoceles and pyoceles from an inadequately drained frontal sinus). If the patient is old enough to have a pneumatized frontal sinus, then the frontonasal ducts must be adequately draining or the mucosal lining of the sinus must be stripped away. The remaining dead space within the demucosalized frontal sinus must then be obliterated with bone graft or cranialized, that is, the posterior table (wall of the sinus) removed so that the brain can expand into the frontal sinus, with a muscle flap protecting the brain from potential communication with the frontonasal duct.

Orbital Fractures

Pediatric orbital fractures differ from their adult counterparts in several ways. The lack of a frontal sinus means that impact in this area can often translate into an isolated orbital roof fracture. Blowout fractures through the orbital floor (which is anatomically the ceiling of the maxillary sinus) are less likely because the maxillary sinuses are well buttressed by being small (without a big hollow into which to collapse) and filled with tooth buds. However, when they do occur, children are much more likely than adults to have a true trapdoor-type fracture, in which the inferior eye muscles have become trapped under the fractured floor segment (Fig. 22-19, A and B). This is a surgical urgency, as the muscle becomes ischemic if not released. There will be restriction of extraocular movement (usually the affected globe is tethered inferiorly by the entrapped muscle and the patient cannot look up; Fig. 22-19, C) and often disproportionate pain and nausea on upward gaze against the tethered muscle. It is thought that true trapdoor orbital floor fractures are more common in children because their periosteum and other supporting structures are more

elastic and snap the fractured bone back into place, entrapping the muscle.

On examination, orbital fractures frequently have periorbital and subconjunctival hematomas. The clinical indications for repairing an orbital floor fracture are vertical dystopia (globe appears to be at a different height) (Fig. 22-19, D), extraocular muscle dysfunction (especially entrapment), increased orbital volume causing enophthalmos (globe looks posteriorly seated with pseudoptosis of the lids), and symptomatic diplopia. Without these abnormal findings, nonsurgical management can usually be offered to pediatric patients, regardless of the size of the fracture, as the elastic supporting structures seem to allow normal orbital support and restoration of volume. However, these findings can be difficult to assess in the immediate postinjury period because of swelling, which can mask any bony defects and cause temporary diplopia.

If surgery is needed, multiple approaches (e.g., the transconjunctival, subciliary, or mid-lid approach) can be used. Regardless of exposure, the goal is to place an autologous bone graft or small implant into the floor without injuring orbital muscles, the infraorbital nerve, or the optic nerve, and to reconstruct the orbital volume so that there is almost symmetry in globe position with the contralateral, uninjured eye.

Zygomaticomaxillary Complex Fractures

The zygoma, or cheek bone, articulates at five points: with the lateral maxilla along the lateral zygomaticomaxillary buttress, with the superior maxilla along the infraorbital rim, with the temporal bone forming the zygomatic arch, at the lateral orbital *rim* at the zygomaticofrontal suture, and along the lateral orbital *wall* at the zygomaticosphenoid suture. Because of underdevelopment of the maxillary sinus and resiliency of the immature bone, isolated zygomatic fractures are relatively uncommon in children, who present more often with orbital fractures.

Figure 22-19 Orbital floor trapdoor fracture with entrapped muscle. **A,** Coronal CT view of left inferior rectus muscle entrapped. **B,** Sagittal CT view of left inferior rectus muscle entrapped. **C,** Left-sided limited upward gaze. **D,** Left-sided enophthalmos and vertical ocular dystopia.

Like orbital fractures, the functional deformities are related to changes in orbital volume that could lead to vertical globe dystopia or enophthalmos that could have an appearance deformity or lead to diplopia, which would require operative reduction. Minimally displaced fractures can be treated conservatively. If displaced enough, the cheek is usually rotated in the direction of the injury with malar flattening or blunting (although it may be difficult to clinically discern in the initial period because of swelling) and will need to be reduced and then fixed at two or three articulating points for stability.

Maxillary and Midface Fractures

Isolated midface fractures in children are rare given the prominence of their cranium and mandible, which absorb the majority of forces. Therefore, a true pediatric midface fracture is highly likely to be associated with other injuries. Given the underdeveloped maxilla that is relatively solid and not pneumatized, classic pure Le Fort fracture patterns are rare (see Chapter 20, Fig. 20-68). Classic Le Fort fractures are diagnosed by grabbing the maxilla and palate and pulling anteriorly: Le Fort I fractures have a mobile maxilla; Le Fort II fractures have a mobile maxilla that pulls the nasal pyramid with it; and Le Fort III fractures present a complete craniofacial dysjunction, in which the entire midface pulls anteriorly. Transverse maxillary, or Le Fort I, fractures are extremely uncommon in children. The Le Fort II fracture presents as a naso-orbital ethmoid (NOE) fracture combined with a Le Fort I maxillary fracture. Le Fort III fractures are also rare in children, and are more likely to present as combined NOE and zygomaticomaxillary complex (ZMC) fractures.

When maxillary fractures are greenstick or minimally displaced, a conservative approach with a liquid or very soft diet should be attempted, as children undergo rapid remodeling. Significant displacement may require maxillomandibular fixation with open reduction internal fixation, but injury to unerupted adult tooth buds must be avoided.

Nasal Fractures

Nasal fractures are one of the most common facial fractures in children, and can include the nasal bones, cartilages, and septum. They are diagnosed by history of trauma to the nose and epistaxis that self-resolves. Often the workup will include a fine-cut face CT to rule out other injuries, although it is not absolutely necessary if clinically confident that the nasal fractures are isolated. Examination must include an intranasal examination with a speculum to rule out septal hematoma. In children, there is only a loose attachment of the upper lateral cartilages to the nasal bones, so it is possible to develop hematomas in this area as well. Untreated hematomas cause pressure necrosis to the septal cartilage, leading to a saddle-nose deformity. Therefore it is recommended that cartilaginous nasal hematomas be drained urgently.

The indication for surgical treatment of the fracture is clinical. Regardless of the actual fracture pattern, it is the appearance of the nose and the septum that determine the need for surgery. Like adults, closed reductions of nasal fractures have a fairly high subsequent revision rate. Most plastic surgeons will perform a closed reduction on a pediatric nasal fracture, and if a revision septorhinoplasty is needed later, will delay until closer to skeletal maturity.

Mandibular Fractures

The prominent mandible is the most common site of pediatric facial fractures, and likely represents 20% to 40% of pediatric facial fractures. Before the age of 6, mandibular fractures are less common and concomitant injuries should be sought. The incidence of mandibular fractures increases from 6 years to about 15 years of age. The mandible is a symmetric ring with a central symphysis, and paired on either side the parasymphysis, body, angle where the body transitions to ramus, ascending ramus giving off anteriorly the coronoid process where the temporalis muscle inserts, and posteriorly the condyle that articulates with the glenoid fossa forming the temporomandibular joint (TMJ). Condylar fractures are common before age 6, but decrease from then onward. In children older than 15 years, angle and body fractures have the highest proportion.

Clinically, these present with pain and malocclusion, as well as pain on opening (trismus), drooling, and decreased maximal incisal opening. Intraoral examination can show a dental step-off at the fracture site. Whereas bilateral condylar fractures often present as an anterior open bite, unilateral condylar fractures present as contralateral posterior open bites. In condylar neck fractures, the condylar head is often displaced medially out of its glenoid fossa by the strong pull of the pterygoid muscles medially.

In addition to symptomatic malocclusion, the examiner can assess the TMJ by placing fingers in the external auditory canals while the patient opens and closes his or her mouth. Palpating along the edge of the entire mandible for tenderness can sometimes indicate the location of the fractures. The mandible has some ringlike structure properties, and can often break in two places. Placing the heel of the examiner's hand against the child's symphysis and asking the patient to protrude the chin against the hand may yield pain, indicating a mandibular fracture.

The key to treatment is to restore normal occlusion. Given the remodeling ability of the pediatric mandible, minor occlusal discrepancies will improve on their own or with orthodontic manipulation later. For significant malocclusion, surgical reduction is attempted, and a stable reduction can be treated by maxillomandibular fixation (MMF) with guiding elastics (rubber-banding rather than wiring the jaws shut). Unstable or irreducible fractures need MMF, possibly with open reduction internal fixation (ORIF), but standard MMF arch bar placement can be difficult because of the shape of pediatric teeth. Primary dentition appears from 6 months to 6 years of age, and then mixed dentition is present from 6 to 12 years of age.

Condylar and subcondylar fractures are difficult to approach surgically; there is also the risk of damaging the facial nerve, resulting in ipsilateral weakness or loss of facial animation. These fractures are also at risk for TMJ ankylosis, and early range-of-motion therapy is important. The infrequent indications for an open repair include displacement of the condyle into the middle cranial fossa or auditory canal, or bilateral fractures without the ability to establish occlusion and mandibular height. The side of the fracture usually results in a shorter ramus height with the teeth meeting earlier, causing a contralateral open bite or crossbite. Operative closed reduction by MMF, with contralateral elastics, can correct this defect and allow remodeling with a soft diet.

In general, more seriously displaced mandibular fractures will be obvious on physical examination, with malocclusion or even gross instability of the mandible. ORIF should be performed by the most minimal fixation techniques possible to avoid damaging the tooth buds and to prevent impingement on dental growth; this can be accomplished by using only the cortex on the inferior border of the mandible. Intraoral incisions are preferred, and absorbable plates and wires are preferred over metal plates. If metal plates are used, it is preferable to remove them once bony healing is complete to reduce the risk of affecting growth.

Panfacial Trauma

Patients who have experienced trauma severe enough to cause craniofacial fractures of the upper, middle, and lower thirds of the face often have multiorgan injuries complicating their management. Physical examination usually reveals a flattened face appearance, as loss of the multiple skeletal buttresses reduces the anterior projection. There are many approaches to these reconstructions, with the overall goals of re-establishing occlusion, maintaining anterior projection, and maintaining height. Along with pediatric ophthalmology, an otolaryngologist may be consulted for securing the airway with a temporary tracheostomy, neurosurgery may be needed for intracranial access, and an anesthesia team needs to be prepared for patients requiring significant lengths of time to treat. One approach is to use the cranial base as a guide and reduce the NOE to the nasion, the mandible to the glenoid fossas, the maxilla to the occlusal surface of the mandible, the ZMC to the sphenoid and maxilla, and then adjust orbital volumes, followed by soft tissue repairs.

RECONSTRUCTIVE PEDIATRIC PLASTIC SURGERY

As reviewed previously, plastic surgeons can improve congenital and acquired defects such as trauma by reshaping the tissue, based on the principles of wound healing and blood supply. These principles also apply to problems regarding soft tissue deformities and coverage of wounds. This places plastic surgeons in close contact with all of the other surgical specialties when they cannot induce a surgical wound to close, such as after debridement of devitalized tissue or tumor extirpation.

Every piece of tissue in the human body is alive because the blood supplies oxygen and nutrition and carries away waste products such as carbon dioxide. Not only does the cardiovascular system need to deliver oxygenated blood and immune factors to every cell in the body, but also the capillary bed, where oxygen exchange takes place, averages a modest perfusion pressure of 20 to 30 mm Hg. This surprisingly low pressure plays an important role in pathophysiologic states such as compartment syndromes and pressure ulcers.

Therefore, plastic surgeons are limited, because every incision made removes more blood supply. Chronic and complex wounds often are in areas that have decreased blood supply, such as the dependent areas of sitting and standing, which leads to infection, increased oxygen consumption, and relative ischemia, in turn leading to a downward spiral of more infection or oxygen demand and ischemia.

The main tools by which a plastic surgeon moves tissue around the body to restore form and function are grafts, flaps, and molding of the tissue. A *graft* is tissue that is completely removed from one part of the body and placed in a new recipient site in hopes that a new blood supply will grow into it to keep the graft alive. A *flap* is a vascularized block of tissue that is transferred to another location with its own blood supply. *Molding of tissue* refers to new and developing technologies to shape tissues: two common techniques involve the use of tissue expanders and negative-pressure wound therapy devices.

The main difference between a graft and a flap is that a graft has no blood supply and must gain a new blood supply at its recipient site. It takes about 48 hours before the first stages of revascularization, and therefore the graft must find other mechanisms to survive in the early period. It is thought that it survives by diffusion of nutrients and wastes across an osmotic gradient, and therefore it must be in close contact with a moist, nonepithelialized, vascular bed such as muscle. For example, in a skin graft, if fluid gets in between the graft and its recipient bed, as with a seroma, hematoma, or pus, or if the graft shears and does not keep close contact with its vascular bed, then those areas of the skin graft will not survive or "take." This is one of the reasons that skin grafts are often meshed, so that extra fluid can egress and improve take. Another example is autologous fat grafting that can be used to augment soft tissue. Because of their mechanism of revascularization, grafts tend to have a certain percentage take, and the rest may resorb.

There are many types of grafts, including skin, fat, cartilage, bone, nerve, and composite grafts containing more than one type of tissue. Skin grafts come in split-thickness and full-thickness versions. Split-thickness grafts are thin enough that the donor site will heal on its own, and their thinness also implies that they survive more easily. However, thin skin grafts have worse cosmetic outcomes and can contract as they heal. Full-thickness skin grafts look much better and are much more pliable, but they have more difficulty surviving and create a donor site defect that needs to be repaired. The key issue to recognize is that skin grafts cannot cover nonvascularized tissue such as bone without periosteum, cartilage without perichondrium, tendon without paratenon, or exposed hardware. To cover such nonvascularized structures, a vascularized flap must be used.

Flaps are thicker blocks of tissue that have a blood supply. They usually contain a mix of the following tissue types: skin, subcutaneous fat, fascia, muscle. They can be based on presumed vascular plexuses (known as *random pattern flaps*) or on known blood vessels by knowledge, visualization, or Doppler (known as *pedicled flaps*); or completely detached with a known pedicle and brought to a distant location to revascularize via microvascular anastomosis to recipient vessels (known as *free flaps*). Free flaps may be thought of as autologous tissue transplantation, as they can survive only on the basis of technically performed vascular anastomoses (called *microsurgery* because of the requirement for an operating microscope) with concomitant risks of thrombosis and flap failure that could necessitate an emergency return to the operating room to explore or re-do the anastomoses. Because a flap leaves a donor site defect when it is moved to cover another tissue, the donor site may sometimes need a skin graft to cover it if it cannot be closed primarily (Fig. 22-20, *A-E*).

Molding describes the direct manipulation of tissue and can refer to numerous techniques that plastic surgeons have innovated to directly shape tissue. Naso-alveolar molding for the cleft lip–nose, implants, and hyaluronidase and collagen fillers are among the many technologies available. Two of the most commonly used techniques in pediatric plastic surgery are tissue expansion and negative-pressure wound therapy.

Tissue expansion can potentially solve the problems of tissue mismatch of grafts and the limited availability of local flaps. It involves the placement of inflatable silicone elastomer balloons under skin, fascia, or muscle with a port to inject saline. After months of weekly saline injections into the tissue expanders, the soft tissue has grown to accommodate the expanders, and the expanders can be removed to advance these expanded local flaps. Studies have shown there is actual growth of tissue rather than mere stretching. This solution works well to produce enough specialized neighboring tissue, such as hair-bearing scalp in scalp reconstruction. The main drawbacks are related to the implantable hardware: infection, bleeding, extrusion, skin necrosis, pain, and neurapraxia.

Negative-pressure wound therapy (NPWT) involves shrinking an open wound to a smaller size to allow treatment with

Figure 22-20   Soft tissue defect of the ankle with exposed bone. **A,** Ankle defect with flap designed; **B,** elevated flap; **C,** rotated flap; **D,** flap donor site skin grafted; **E,** well-healed ankle.

a smaller, safer, simpler reconstruction such as a skin graft, rather than a larger one, such as a free flap. An air-filled substance such as a sponge or gauze is placed in the wound, covered by airtight elastic, and then connected to a vacuum suction device to create negative pressure. The force draws the wound edges toward each other, reduces edema, stimulates cell mitosis, and may also increase healing and granulation by increasing blood flow and the availability of wound-healing factors. Basic steps of wound healing, such as debridement of devitalized tissue, need to be performed to optimize the wound before sealing it shut by NPWT. The NPWT dressing is usually changed about twice per week (depending on the type of wound), and as it is a form of wound dressing, can be changed by nursing staff on an inpatient or outpatient basis.

Pressure Sores

Pressure sores demonstrate the tenets of wound healing. Capillary perfusion pressure is a mere 20 to 30 mm Hg, which is easily exceeded when tissue is compressed between two unyielding surfaces: a bony prominence and a chair or bed. Although any bony surface could potentially cause a pressure sore depending on the patient's positioning, the bony surfaces most commonly involved are the sacrum, calcaneus, ischium,

and greater trochanter. In fact, these areas are naturally subject to pressure greater than 30 mm Hg when we are sitting or lying down, but our autonomic nervous system prompts us to shift our weight frequently to avoid chronic pressure. Therefore, patients who develop pressure sores either are obtunded and hence too unaware to move or have decreased sensation, as in the case of spina bifida or spinal cord injury.

As little as 1 to 2 hours of chronic pressure exceeding capillary perfusion pressure leads to compromised oxygenation, ischemia, and eventually tissue necrosis. Therefore, patients with risk factors, and their caregivers, must be taught strict pressure precautions, such as shifting the patient's weight every 1 to 2 hours while in bed or in a wheelchair. The management goals in treating pressure sores are to identify the intrinsic and extrinsic etiologic factors in order to reduce them, and to perform wound care and debridement to prevent chronic infection from becoming acute infection. Because a postsurgical wound would break down easily if subject to pressure sore–inducing forces, and surgical wounds take at least 6 weeks to heal, patients need to demonstrate nonworsening of their pressure sores for at least 6 to 8 weeks before becoming candidates for surgical coverage of their wounds.

Sacral pressure sores are the result of lying down too long in a supine position. Ischial pressure sores result from the sitting position. Greater trochanter pressure sores are caused by lying on the side. Extrinsic factors such as moisture and incontinence in these areas, and shearing forces from patient repositioning, add to the difficulty in treating these wounds. Intrinsic factors such as malnutrition are common and further impede wound healing. These factors can be elucidated from a detailed history and physical examination.

Pressure sores are typically staged according to the National Pressure Ulcer Advisory Panel consensus development conference scale developed in 1989, which stages pressure sores according to four main layers of tissue: does not pass skin; does not pass fat; does not pass muscle; involves bone. A stage I pressure sore therefore has intact skin, but the skin stays reddened for more than 1 hour even after pressure is removed. In a stage II pressure sore there is a break in the dermis with or without infection, and subcutaneous fat may be exposed. In stage III there is subcutaneous destruction extending into the muscle layer. Stage IV pressure sores involve bone. There are also two designations for suspected deep wounds: a *suspected deep tissue injury* has intact skin with the purple or discolored hue suggestive of deep tissue injury, and *unstageable* implies full-thickness loss with eschar that hides how much deep involvement there is. It is important to note that when bone is exposed, the most superficial aspect of bone is desiccated and thus relatively devascularized and superficially colonized by bacteria. This is osteitis, or inflammation of bone, rather than osteomyelitis, or deep bone infection. If the deep bone has good blood supply, a healthy patient can tolerate osteitis for protracted periods as long as there is good wound care and pressure precautions that prevent the wound from worsening.

After a pressure sore is cleaned, there are three keys to treatment: reduction of pressure and other extrinsic factors via patient education and mechanical low-pressure devices such as air mattresses and mapped wheelchair cushions (consider physiatrist consult), good wound care (consider wound care nurse consult), and adequate nutrition (consider nutrition or feeding consult). Only when these factors are optimized can there be healing of the wound, potentially enough either to avoid surgery or to become a candidate for surgery. Because in pressure sores undergoing surgical treatment there is usually bone exposure, a vascularized flap is used to cover the wound rather than a skin graft.

Soft Tissue Lesions

Plastic surgeons deal with many soft tissue lesions, including congenital melanocytic nevi (CMNs), vascular anomalies, neurofibromas, and others. Some of these lesions are described in Chapter 8. Many physicians are comfortable treating small lesions that can be removed with local anesthetic and closed by simple primary closure, but pediatric plastic surgeons are often consulted for larger lesions, as they require general anesthesia and multiple reconstructive techniques. Some large lesions can be covered by local flaps or skin grafts, but one particularly challenging category concerns large CMNs. Large or giant CMNs have an approximately 4% to 8% risk of malignant transformation to melanoma, and thus they need to be monitored closely or excised. Given their size, local flaps often do not suffice, and skin grafts cannot match the tissue type (e.g., hair-bearing scalp would be replaced by a hairless skin graft), and thus tissue expansion is often the best type of reconstruction (Fig. 22-21, *A-F*). When large CMNs are near complex areas of the body such as the eyelids, a customized combination of skin grafts, flaps, and tissue expansion may be necessary.

Vascular anomalies are broadly categorized into hemangiomas and vascular malformations. Hemangiomas are endothelial tumors that usually appear within the first year of life

Figure 22-21 Giant congenital melanocytic nevus. **A,** Nevus; **B,** serial excision; **C,** scalp tissue expansion; **D,** scalp tissue expansion with planned nevus excision and flap coverage; **E,** after nevus excision and expanded flap coverage; **F,** well-healed flap.

(infantile hemangiomas) and go through a proliferative phase (with growth in size), followed by an involution phase that usually leaves residual fibrofatty tissue. Some hemangiomas are present at birth *(congenital hemangiomas);* these may involute rapidly or not involute. Vascular malformations, the result of an error in development, are present at birth and grow proportionately with the child. They can be arterial, venous, capillary, lymphatic, or distinct combinations of these, and each has its own characteristics and natural history. Vascular anomalies can cause increased growth of underlying soft and bony tissues, or directly extend into or exist separately in other tissues, such as leptomeninges, viscera, and muscle.

Indications for treating vascular anomalies include current or predictable future symptoms of abnormal appearance, pain, ulceration, bleeding, infection, growth, or psychosocial dysfunction. Rapid intervention must be sought for interference with airway, vision development, conductive hearing, or other organ function, with appropriate consultation with a pediatric otolaryngologist, ophthalmologist, or other subspecialists. Although the pediatric plastic surgeon can perform excisions or laser treatments, a multidisciplinary team approach is usually offered, including the dermatologist, pediatrician, and interventional radiologist, as therapies range from observation to systemic therapies (such as steroids or propranolol) to embolization.

Hand and Upper Extremity

Like the face, the hand is a complex organ that is unique to humans. Its function is unsurpassed, allowing humans the gift of creation, and thus reconstructive efforts focus on its functionality. Like most aspects of plastic surgery, the function is very much based on form: the structures of the bones, tendons, and muscles, and the neurovascular conduits connecting them, act together to orchestrate hand function. In addition, the socialization aspect of the hand should not be neglected, as it plays a key role in the patient's interaction with parents and others. Given the wide variety of potential defects, the timing of surgery must be customized: the patient needs to be old enough to observe how the abnormal hand is being used and what the functional deficits are, but also young enough that postoperative neurologic retraining will be effective. Function is usually more important than aesthetics in these cases, and sometimes surgery is not indicated at all. The overall goals are to optimize function before the patient is 4 years of age, but preferably earlier, at about 1 year of age, when the three-digit pinch is being mastered. Parents should understand that although a normal hand cannot be restored, improving function is still beneficial in the developing child.

Upper limb buds emerge at 4 weeks of gestation and, via at least three distinct signaling gradients, develop along all three dimensions: the apical ectodermal ridge signals proximal-to-distal mesenchymal differentiation, the dorsal ectoderm delineates dorsal (extensor) to palmar or volar (flexor) surfaces, and the zone of polarizing activity creates a gradient in an anterior (preaxial, or toward the radius and thumb)-to-posterior (postaxial, or toward the ulna and small finger) direction. By 6 to 7 weeks, digits have fully segregated via apoptosis of the mesenchyme between the digits, and further growth and ossification of cartilage proceed.

These three axes of development lead to a wide variety of congenital defects, and they are classified as (1) failure of formation, (2) failure of differentiation, (3) duplication, (4) overgrowth, (5) undergrowth, (6) congenital constriction band syndrome, and (7) generalized skeletal abnormalities. Some of these conditions may be associated with genetic syndromes. These can range from unusual conditions such as cleft hands to the more common syndactylies and polydactylies. Syndactyly (fusion of digits), which occurs in about 1 in 2000 births, can be simple (not involving bone) or complex (involving bone). Polydactylies, or extra digits, are most common on the radial aspect as thumb duplication, or on the ulnar aspect as a small finger accessory. Separation of digits requires flaps and grafts, and excision of digits requires attention to excise the redundant nerve to avoid neuromas, and to reconstruct tendons or ligaments. For more complex anomalies, web space reconstruction can increase the size of an object that can be held, pollicization may be needed to move a digit into the position of the absent or nonfunctioning thumb, or toe-to-hand microvascular transfer can use one or more toes to simulate the thumb or other digits.

Trunk and Lower Extremities

Given that there is typically excess tissue at the trunk, local flaps can usually provide reconstructive coverage, such as for breast reconstruction, gynecomastia treatment, or abdominal reconstruction. On the other hand, the lower extremity has thin soft tissue relative to the bone, and overall a paucity of soft tissue, so local flaps are often not an option. Negative-pressure wound therapy can improve wounds on both the trunk and lower extremity, as it can shrink the wounds and encourage granulation tissue, sometimes converting a large wound into a smaller one that can be covered in a simpler manner, such as with a skin graft.

Similar principles therefore apply: if coverage can be delayed, a large wound can often receive NPWT to reduce its dimensions and possibly avoid surgery altogether. If there is no bone exposure, a skin graft may suffice. Otherwise a local flap or free flap is needed. For the lower extremity, the distal third of the calf near the ankle typically has the least amount of local tissue, and therefore a free flap is often needed.

CONCLUSION

Plastic surgery solves problems of form and function that are exclusive to humans, such as appearance and speech, to improve quality of life. These deformities can prevent normal functional and psychological development in infants and children, given that unique human features play such an important role in socialization with caregivers and peers. Congenital and acquired deformities can be treated by similar principles of hard and soft tissue reconstruction. Parents should be educated that although pediatric plastic surgeons can often improve outcomes, they are limited by the patient's innate wound healing and scarring, by the severity of the defect, and by changes that occur as the child grows.

Bibliography

Ades LC, Mulley JC, Senga LP, et al: Jackson-Weiss syndrome: Clinical and radiographical findings in a large kindred and exclusion of the gene from 7p21 and 5qter, *Am J Med Genet* 51:121–130, 1994.

Aleck K: Craniosynostosis syndromes in the genomic era, *Semin Pediatr Neurol* 11:256–261, 2004.

Basseri B, Kianmahd BD, Roostaeian J, et al: Current national incidence, trends, and health care resource utilization of cleft lip–cleft palate, *Plast Reconstr Surg* 127(3):1255–1262, 2011.

Centers for Disease Control and Prevention: *Birth defects 2006.* Available at http://www.cdc.gov/ncbddd/birthdefects/data.html.

Cohen MM, Kreiborg S: An updated pediatric perspective on the Apert syndrome, *Am J Dis Child* 147:989–993, 1993.

Cohen MM Jr, Rollnick BR, Kaye CI: Oculoauriculovertebral spectrum: An updated critique, *Cleft Palate J* 26:276–286, 1989.

Danziger I, Brodsky L, Perry R, et al: Nager's acrofacial dysostosis: Case report and review of the literature, *Int J Pediatr Otorhinolaryngol* 20:225–240, 1990.

Gorlin RJ: Fibroblast growth factors, their receptors and receptor disorders, *J Cranio-Maxillofac Surg* 25:69–79, 1997.

Keating RF: Craniosynostosis: Diagnosis and management in the new millennium, *Pediatr Ann* 26:600–620, 1997.

Losee JE, Mason AC: Deformational plagiocephaly: Diagnosis, prevention, and treatment, *Clin Plastic Surg* 32:53–64, 2005.

National Pressure Ulcer Advisory Panel: Pressure ulcer prevalence, cost and risk assessment: Consensus development conference statement, *Decubitus* 2:24–28, 1989.

Ocampo RV, Persing JA: Sagittal synostosis, *Clin Plastic Surg* 21:563–574, 1994.

Parker SE, Mai CT, Canfield MA, et al: Updated National Birth Prevalence estimates for selected birth defects in the United States, 2004-2006. *Birth Defects Res A Clin Mol Teratol* 88(12):1008–1016, 2010.

Posnick JC: Unilateral coronal synostosis (anterior plagiocephaly): Current clinical perspectives, *Ann Plast Surg* 36:430–447, 1996.

Posnick JC: Treacher Collins syndrome: Perspectives in evaluation and treatment, *J Oral Maxillofac Surg* 55:1120–1133, 1997.

Prevel CD, Eppley BL, McCarty M: Acrocephalosyndactyly syndromes: A review, *J Craniofac Surg* 8:279–285, 1997.

Singer L, Sidoti EJ: Pediatric management of Robin sequence, *Cleft Palate Craniofac J* 29:220–223, 1992.

Wilkie AO, Wall SA: Craniosynostosis: Novel insights into pathogenesis and treatment, *Curr Opin Neurol* 9:146–152, 1996.

Facial Fractures

Losee JE, Afifi A, Jiang S, et al: Pediatric orbital fractures: Classification, management, and early follow-up, *Plast Reconstr Surg* 122:886–897, 2008.

Losee JE, Jiang S, Deleyiannis FWB: Craniofacial fractures. In Bentz ML, Bauer BS, Zuker RM, editors: *Principles and practice of pediatric plastic surgery*, ed 2, vol 2, St. Louis, 2008, Quality Medical Publishing, Chapter 38, pp 1047–1072.

Reconstructive Pediatric Plastic Surgery

Arneja JS, Gosain AK: Vascular malformations, *Plast Reconstr Surg* 121:195e–206e, 2008.

Arneja JS, Gosain AK: Giant congenital melanocytic nevi, *Plast Reconstr Surg* 124(1 Suppl):1e–13e, 2009.

Beck DO, Gosain AK: The presentation and management of hemangiomas, *Plast Reconstr Surg* 123:181e–191e, 2009.

Lin AY, McGrath MH: Pressure sores in the elderly. In Rosenthal RA, Zenilman ME, Katlic MR, editors: *Principles and practice of geriatric surgery*, ed 2, New York, 2011, Springer, Chapter 93, p 1257.

Riddle RD, Tabin C: How limbs develop, *Sci Am* 280:74–79, 1999.

Swanson AB. A classification for congenital limb malformations, *J Hand Surg* 1:8–22, 1976.

OTOLARYNGOLOGY

Robert F. Yellon | David H. Chi

The importance of pediatricians and family physicians having an understanding of and experience with otolaryngologic problems and being skilled in techniques of examination of the head and neck region cannot be overemphasized. One study revealed that more than one third of all visits to pediatricians' offices were prompted by ear symptoms. When nasal and oral symptoms are included, ear, nose, and throat pathology accounts for more than 50% of all visits. With patience and proper equipment, pediatricians can complete a thorough examination on almost all children. If a disorder fails to respond to therapy or becomes chronic or recurrent, or if an unusual problem is encountered, then consultation with a pediatric otolaryngologist should be sought.

Successful examination of the ears, nose, and oropharynx of a young child can present some challenges, especially with older infants and toddlers, who fail to appreciate the need for (and thus often vigorously resist) examination. This can be a particular problem in children who have had previous bad experiences. Patience, warmth, humor, and careful explanation on the part of the examiner help reduce fear and enhance cooperation.

Whenever possible, the child should be allowed to sit on the parent's lap. Pacifiers, puppets and other toys, and tongue blades with faces drawn on them can all serve to reduce anxiety, enlist the child's trust, and distract attention. Gradual introduction of the equipment can also be helpful, especially if done in a playful way. The child can be asked to blow out the otoscope light while the examiner turns it off, urged to catch the light spot as the examiner moves it around, and even allowed to look in the parent's or examiner's ears (Fig. 23-1, A-D). Parents can also help demonstrate maneuvers for opening the mouth, panting to depress the tongue, and holding the head back. Although this may take a little additional time at the outset, it often saves considerable time in the long run and makes future follow-up examinations far easier.

EAR DISORDERS

Ear pain (otalgia), discharge from the ear (otorrhea), and suspected hearing loss are three of the more common and specific otic symptoms for which parents seek medical attention for their children. Less specific symptoms such as pulling or tugging at the ears, fussiness, and fever are also frequently encountered, particularly in children younger than 2 years of age.

History should center on the nature and duration of symptoms, character of the clinical course, and possible antecedent treatment. Because many infections of the ear are recurrent and/or chronic, the parent should be asked about previous

medical or surgical therapy (e.g., antibiotics, myringotomy, tube insertion).

A brief review of the anatomy of the ear is helpful in developing a logical approach to any clinical abnormalities that may be encountered. The ear is conveniently divided into the following three regions (Fig. 23-2):

1. The *external ear* includes the pinna, or auricle, and the external auditory canal, up to and including the tympanic membrane.

2. The *middle ear* is made up of the middle ear space, the inner surface of the eardrum, the ossicles, and the mastoid.

3. The *inner ear* comprises the cochlea (hearing), the labyrinth and semicircular canals (balance), and the main nerve trunks of the seventh and eighth cranial nerves.

The examination should include inspection of the auricle, periauricular tissues, and external auditory canal and visualization of the entire tympanic membrane, including assessment of its mobility in response to positive and negative pressure with pneumatic otoscopy. This necessitates clearing the canal of cerumen or discharge by using a curette, cotton wick, lavage, or suction, and presumes that the tympanic membrane is intact (Fig. 23-3, A and B). Use of a surgical otoscope head or an examining microscope assists visualization during the cleaning process. These procedures should be performed carefully and gently and attempted only after the child has been carefully immobilized to avoid trauma (Fig. 23-4). It is extraordinarily easy to injure the canal during the process of cleaning the external ear. Hence great care must be taken; otherwise bleeding from the ensuing trauma obscures the examination and upsets the patient and parent. Steadying of the examiner's hands on the child's head while using the otoscope and instruments is an essential skill to avoid ear trauma. Both the patient and parent should be given a clear explanation of the procedure beforehand. Allowing older children to handle and look through the equipment before cleaning the ear reduces anxiety and enhances cooperation (see Fig. 23-3, C).

Because the external auditory canal is often angulated in infants and young children, gentle lateral traction on the pinna is frequently necessary to assist visualization of the eardrum itself (Fig. 23-5). In infants the tympanic membrane tends to be oriented at a greater angle (Fig. 23-6, A and B); the landmarks are less prominent; and the skin that lines the canal, being loosely attached, moves readily on insufflation of air, simulating a normally mobile eardrum. To avoid confusion, the canal should be inspected as the speculum is inserted to

Figure 23-1 Techniques to assist examination of a child's ears, nose, and oropharynx. **A,** Young infants often can be examined on their mother's lap, with gentle immobilization provided by the parent and the examiner's hand. **B,** Having a toddler or preschooler sit on the mother's lap and using puppets, other toys, and tongue blades with faces drawn on them while gradually introducing the examining instruments reduces anxiety and enlists cooperation. **C** and **D,** Making a game of blowing out the otoscope light and allowing the patient to check the examiner first convey that otoscopy does not have to hurt.

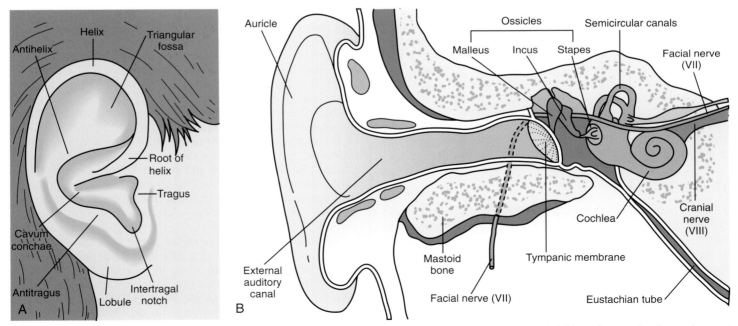

Figure 23-2 Anatomy of the ear. **A,** A normal external ear (auricle or pinna) is shown, with its various landmarks labeled. It is helpful to refer to such a diagram in assessing congenital anomalies. **B,** This coronal section shows the various structures of the hearing and vestibular apparatus. The three main regions are the external ear, middle ear, and inner ear. The eustachian tube connects the middle ear and the nasopharynx and serves to drain and ventilate the middle ear.

Figure 23-3   A, Equipment for cleaning the external auditory canal. The curette *(1)* is the implement most commonly used to remove cerumen. Use of a surgical otoscope head *(2)* makes the process considerably easier. Additional implements include cotton wicks *(3)* and a suction tip *(4)* for removal of discharge or moist wax, alligator forceps *(5)* for removing foreign bodies, and an ear syringe *(6)* and motorized irrigation apparatus *(7)* for removing firm objects or impacted cerumen. Lavage is contraindicated when there is a possible perforation of the tympanic membrane. If the motorized apparatus is used for irrigation, it must be kept on the lowest power setting to avoid traumatizing the eardrum. **B,** Use of suction is often necessary when there is copious exudate. **C,** Allowing the child to look through the examining microscope may help him or her cooperate with the examination.

ensure that the transition between canal wall and tympanic membrane is visualized.

The pneumatic otoscope is the most valuable diagnostic tool when signs or symptoms of otitis media are present. Pediatricians, family practitioners, and otolaryngologists who treat children should be skilled in its use. Practical advice on the use of this instrument is as follows:

1. Use adequate light. A bright halogen lamp is better than an ordinary light bulb. Replace bulbs routinely every 4 to 6 months, and provide for routine battery charging.

2. Choose a speculum of sufficient diameter and length to allow adequate penetration (10 to 15 mm) into the external canal for good eardrum visualization and a good seal for pneumatic otoscopy.

3. Restrain the patient (on the parent's lap or on the examining table).

4. Brace the hand holding the otoscope on the child's head to avoid ear canal trauma.

When otoscopic findings are unclear or when it is difficult to obtain a good air seal for pneumatic otoscopy, tympanometry can be highly useful in evaluating patients older than 8 months of age (Fig. 23-7). The procedure is not of value in young infants because the abundance of loose connective tissue lining the ear canal and the laxity of the cartilage at the entrance increase canal wall compliance and invalidate the results.

Because otitis media can be a reflection of both immunologic and anatomic abnormalities, the practitioner should be suspicious of possible underlying immune or temporal bone defects when seeing patients with chronic or frequently recurrent otitis media. The temporal bone is the bony housing for the auditory and vestibular systems. In addition, it provides bony protection for the facial nerve as it crosses from the brainstem to the facial muscles. The growth and development of this bone are affected in syndromes such as Treacher Collins that are characterized by altered midface growth (Fig. 23-8). The soft tissues attached to the temporal bone, such as the muscles controlling eustachian tube function, can be abnormal in children with cleft palates (see Palatal Disorders, later). As a result, children with these disorders tend to have an increased incidence of otitis media.

Children with chronic effusions who complain of hearing loss, those whose parents complain that they do not listen, those with speech delays, or those with suspected congenital malformations must have their hearing evaluated by audiometry, evoked otoacoustic emissions, or brainstem evoked potentials. Patients with vertigo and/or problems of balance and those with facial weakness or asymmetry warrant testing of hearing, facial nerve, *and* vestibular function. These children, and those suffering from malformations, may require computed tomography (CT), magnetic resonance imaging

Figure 23-4   Method of immobilization for cleaning. An assistant holds the child's arms and simultaneously immobilizes the child's head with the thumbs. The parent firmly holds the hips and thighs. This critical immobilization prevents dangerous motion by the child during cleaning of the ear canal and is also useful for otoscopy in young children.

Figure 23-5   Because the external auditory canal usually is angulated in children, lateral traction on the pinna is often required to straighten the canal and improve visualization of the tympanic membrane.

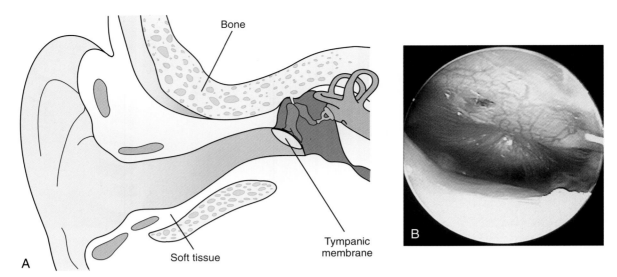

Figure 23-6   Angulation of the tympanic membrane in infancy. **A,** The relationship between the ear canal and eardrum is different in the infant, with the drum being tilted at an angle of 130 degrees. **B,** Greater care is required in examining an infant's eardrum because of this angulation and because the landmarks are less prominent.

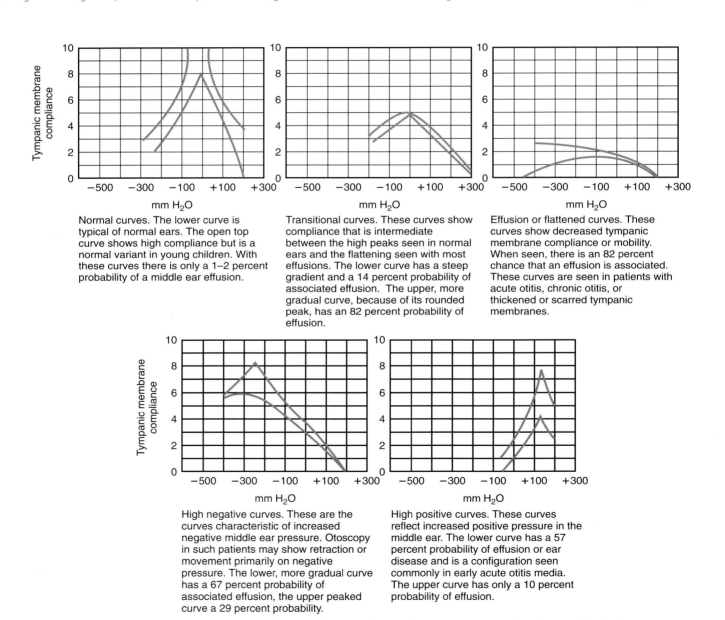

Normal curves. The lower curve is typical of normal ears. The open top curve shows high compliance but is a normal variant in young children. With these curves there is only a 1–2 percent probability of a middle ear effusion.

Transitional curves. These curves show compliance that is intermediate between the high peaks seen in normal ears and the flattening seen with most effusions. The lower curve has a steep gradient and a 14 percent probability of associated effusion. The upper, more gradual curve, because of its rounded peak, has an 82 percent probability of effusion.

Effusion or flattened curves. These curves show decreased tympanic membrane compliance or mobility. When seen, there is an 82 percent chance that an effusion is associated. These curves are seen in patients with acute otitis, chronic otitis, or thickened or scarred tympanic membranes.

High negative curves. These are the curves characteristic of increased negative middle ear pressure. Otoscopy in such patients may show retraction or movement primarily on negative pressure. The lower, more gradual curve has a 67 percent probability of associated effusion, the upper peaked curve a 29 percent probability.

High positive curves. These curves reflect increased positive pressure in the middle ear. The lower curve has a 57 percent probability of effusion or ear disease and is a configuration seen commonly in early acute otitis media. The upper curve has only a 10 percent probability of effusion.

Figure 23-7   Tympanometric patterns of various conditions of the middle ear. *(Courtesy Mrs. Ruth Bachman, Pittsburgh, Pa.)*

Figure 23-8 Syndromes affecting the growth of the temporal bone and midface that predispose patients to recurrent or chronic otitis media and chronic recurrent sinus infections. **A** and **B,** Treacher Collins syndrome. Note the maxillary hypoplasia, micrognathia, and auricular deformity. **C,** Apert syndrome. **D** and **E,** Crouzon syndrome. Both Apert and Crouzon syndromes are characterized by severe maxillary and midfacial hypoplasia. **F,** Hemifacial microsomia with unilateral hypoplasia. (**B-F,** *Courtesy Wolfgang Loskin, MD, University of North Carolina, Chapel Hill, N.C.*)

(MRI), or genetic studies in select cases to clarify the nature of the problem.

DISORDERS OF THE EXTERNAL EAR

The "Four D's"

Examination of each child's ear begins with inspection of the auricle and periauricular tissues for four important signs—discharge, displacement, discoloration, and deformity (the "four D's"). The canal is normally smooth and angulated slightly in an anterior direction. Cerumen is often present; it varies in color from yellowish-white to tan to dark brown. It is secreted from glands interspersed among the hair follicles at the entrance to the ear canal, and it may have some bacteriostatic activity. When cerumen obstructs the view, it must be removed to allow adequate visualization of the canal and tympanic membrane. When soft and moist, cerumen is easily removed with a curette. Removal may be more difficult if the cerumen is dry and flaky and may require removal with otologic forceps or, at times, instillation of drops. In some children, cerumen solidifies or has been packed in with cotton-tipped applicators, forming a firm plug that impedes sound conduction and requires softening for removal. Irrigation is contraindicated if there is any possibility that the eardrum may not be intact, as infection may be driven into the ear by blind irrigation.

Discharge

Discharge is a common complaint with a number of possible causes. When there is thick, white discharge and erythema of the canal wall, the physician should gently pull on the pinna. If this maneuver elicits pain and the canal wall is edematous, primary otitis externa is the likely diagnosis (Fig. 23-9), although prolonged drainage from untreated otitis media with perforation may present a similar picture (see Disorders of the

Figure 23-9 External otitis. Acute bacterial external otitis is characterized by intense pain that is worsened by traction on the pinna, along with purulent exudate and intense canal wall inflammation with normal tympanic membrane mobility on pneumatic otoscopy.

Middle Ear, later). When the middle ear is the source of otic discharge, the tympanic membrane is abnormal and should show evidence of perforation (see Fig. 23-26). The major predisposing condition to primary otitis externa is prolonged excessive moisture in the ear canal, which promotes bacterial or fungal overgrowth. Thus this is a common problem in swimmers. Another major source is the presence of a foreign body in the ear canal (see Fig. 23-19), which stimulates an intense inflammatory response and production of a foul-smelling purulent discharge. Thus when otic drainage is encountered, the discharge must be gently removed under appropriate magnification to assess the condition of the tympanic membrane and to rule out the presence of perforation and foreign objects. This can be accomplished either by gentle siphoning and wiping with cotton wicks or by careful suctioning (see Fig. 23-3).

If the history indicates that the drainage is persistent or recurrent despite therapy, a culture should be obtained to determine both the causative organism and its sensitivity to antimicrobial agents. Treatment consists primarily of topical otic antimicrobial/steroid preparations. Systemic antibiotics should be given when pain is severe; when there is evidence of otitis media; or when, despite attempts at cleaning, there is still uncertainty about an infection of the middle ear. Parenteral antibiotics may be required when the process has extended, producing cellulitis of the periauricular soft tissues or frank mastoiditis.

Displacement

Displacement of the pinna away from the skull is a worrisome sign. The most severe condition causing displacement is mastoiditis, resulting from extension of a middle ear infection through the mastoid air cells and out to the periosteum of the skull. In addition to displacement, important clinical signs of mastoiditis include erythema and edema and possibly fluctuance of the skin overlying the mastoid, exquisite tenderness on palpation of the mastoid process, a sagging ear canal, purulent otorrhea, fever, and usually toxicity (Fig. 23-10). This condition is now considered unusual and is seen mainly in patients with long-standing, untreated, or inadequately treated otitis media. Recognition, prompt institution of parenteral antibiotic therapy, and myringotomy with culture and sensitivity testing are crucial because there is significant risk of central nervous system (CNS) extension. The use of a CT scan will delineate the extent of involvement and assist the surgical approach (Fig. 23-11). Mastoidectomy is indicated in cases complicated by bone erosion, or CNS extension, and in those in whom intravenous (IV) antibiotics and myringotomy fail to produce complete resolution.

Other conditions characterized by displacement of the pinna away from the head include parotitis, primary cellulitis

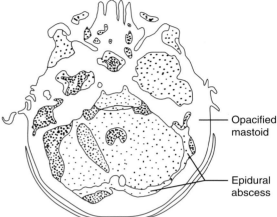

Opacified
mastoid

Epidural
abscess

Figure 23-11   Mastoiditis. The CT image shows acute left-sided mastoiditis with the complication of an associated epidural abscess delineated in the diagram.

of the periauricular tissues, and edema secondary to insect bites or contact dermatitis. Parotitis is differentiated by finding prominent induration and enlargement of the parotid gland anterior and inferior to the external ear, together with blunting of the angle of the mandible on palpation (see Chapter 12). Primary cellulitis is characterized by erythema and tenderness but can often be distinguished clinically from mastoiditis by the presence of associated skin lesions that antecede the inflammation (Fig. 23-12). In cases secondary to untreated external otitis or otitis media with perforation, the picture may be clinically similar. Localized contact dermatitis and angioedema may be erythematous, but they are also pruritic and nontender. The former condition is characterized by microvesicular skin changes (Fig. 23-13), whereas in the latter condition, a precipitating insect bite can often be identified on inspection (Fig. 23-14).

Figure 23-10   Mastoiditis. **A,** This frontal photograph clearly shows the left auricle displaced anteriorly and inferiorly. **B,** In another patient, viewed from the side, erythema can be appreciated over the mastoid process. **C,** On otoscopy, erythema and edema of the canal wall are evident and the posterosuperior portion of the canal wall sags inferiorly. (**C,** Courtesy Michael Hawke, MD.)

Figure 23-14 Angioedema. This youngster had pruritic, nonpainful, nontender erythema and swelling of his ear and infraorbital region. Close examination of the latter revealed the punctum of an insect bite. Another punctum on his ear was obscured by crusting following scratching. *(Courtesy Michael Sherlock, MD, Lutherville, Md.)*

Figure 23-12 Periauricular and auricular cellulitis. This infant had mild postauricular seborrhea and developed varicella. The vesicular varicella lesions that clustered at sites of prior skin irritation became secondarily infected with group A β-streptococci, resulting in cellulitis with intense erythema, edema, and tenderness of the auricle and periauricular tissues. In this case the external canal was normal. *(Courtesy Ronald Chludzinski, MD.)*

Discoloration

Discoloration is another important sign and is commonly a feature of conditions producing displacement. Erythema of the pinna is common when there is inflammation, with or without infection (see Fig. 23-10, *B* and Figs. 23-12 to 23-14). Ecchymotic discoloration may be encountered with trauma. When this overlies the mastoid tip, the area immediately posterior to the pinna, it is termed a *Battle sign* (Fig. 23-15, *A*) and usually reflects a basilar skull fracture. In such cases the canal wall should be checked for tears and the tympanic membrane for perforation or a hemotympanum (blood behind the tympanic membrane; Fig. 23-15, *B*). These findings are generally more helpful in making the diagnosis than routine skull x-rays, which are often inconclusive. CT can usually confirm the diagnosis of a basilar skull fracture. Recognition that bruising

Figure 23-15 Basilar skull fracture. **A,** The presence of a basilar skull fracture involving the temporal bone is often signaled by postauricular ecchymotic discoloration, termed the *Battle sign.* **B,** The force of the blow may also cause tearing of the ear canal or, as shown here, middle ear hemorrhage with hemotympanum. Depending on the timing of examination, this may appear red or blue. *(B, Courtesy Michael Hawke, MD.)*

Figure 23-13 This young girl became sensitive to the nickel posts of her earrings and developed periauricular contact dermatitis. The auricle and periauricular skin are erythematous and covered by a weeping, pruritic microvesicular eruption. *(Courtesy Michael Sherlock, MD, Lutherville, Md.)*

Figure 23-16   **A,** Grade 3 microtia and congenital aural atresia of the right external ear. In this otherwise normal child, the pinna failed to develop properly and the external canal was atretic. Audiometric testing revealed a 60-dB hearing loss. **B,** Grade 2 microtia. Note deficiency of superior portion of auricle. Such isolated deformities stem from abnormal development of the first and second branchial arches.

of the pinna and/or postauricular area can be a manifestation of child abuse is most important (see Chapter 6).

Deformity

When the external ear is grossly misshapen or microtic, associated anomalies of middle ear structures are common and hearing loss may be significant (Fig. 23-16, *A* and *B*). Severe deformities stem from developmental anomalies of the branchial arches, which contribute to both external ear and middle ear structures. Such abnormalities warrant a thorough evaluation in infancy to ensure early recognition and treatment of hearing loss. Deformity of the pinna can be the result of hereditary factors or exposure to teratogens, but at times it is simply produced by unusual intrauterine positioning. Most deformities are minor and represent isolated malformations of mostly cosmetic significance (Fig. 23-17, *D*). In some instances they may be part of a picture of multiple congenital anomalies (Fig. 23-17, *A-C*; see also Fig. 23-8 and Chapter 1).

Figure 23-17   Minor congenital auricular deformities. **A,** In this infant the superior portion of the helix is folded over, obscuring the triangular fossa; the antihelix is sharply angulated; and there are three preauricular skin tags. **B,** This neonate with orofaciodigital and Turner syndromes has a simple helix and a redundant folded lobule. The ear is low set and posteriorly rotated, and the antitragus is anteriorly displaced. **C,** This infant with Rubinstein-Taybi syndrome has an exaggerated elongated intertragal notch. **D,** Prominent ear in an otherwise normal child. The auricular cartilage is abnormally contoured, making the ear protrude forward. (**C,** *Courtesy Michael Sherlock, MD, Lutherville, Md.*)

Figure 23-18 Preauricular sinuses. **A,** These congenital remnants are located anterior to the pinna and have an overlying surface dimple. **B,** In this child the sinus has become infected, forming an abscess. (**A,** Courtesy Michael Hawke, MD.)

Trauma to the pinna may result in a hematoma between the skin and cartilage, the recognition of which requires otolaryngologic consultation. An unrecognized hematoma may result in a permanent deformity if left undrained, or if superinfection of the hematoma results. Either complication can result in permanent cosmetic damage to the pinna.

Preauricular sinuses and cysts constitute two of the more common congenital abnormalities. These are congenital remnants located anterior to the pinna with an overlying surface dimple (Fig. 23-18, A). These cysts are vulnerable to infection and abscess formation (Fig. 23-18, B), which necessitate needle aspiration or incision and drainage in conjunction with antistaphylococcal antibiotics. Once infection has occurred, recurrence is common unless the entire sinus is completely excised. This procedure should be undertaken once inflammation has subsided. A preauricular sinus may also result from branchio-oto-renal syndrome (also known as Melnick-Fraser syndrome), an autosomal dominant disorder characterized by bilateral preauricular sinuses, ear anomalies, branchial cleft anomalies in the neck, and renal problems.

Foreign Objects and Secondary Trauma

It is not unusual for children to put paper, beads, and other foreign objects into their ear canals (Fig. 23-19, A). Small insects also on occasion may become trapped in the external ear (Fig. 23-19, B). In some cases small objects may be embedded in cerumen and missed on inspection. As noted earlier, if present for more than a few days, the foreign material stimulates an inflammatory response and production of a purulent discharge that is often foul-smelling and may obscure the presence of the inciting foreign body. Removal of some objects can be accomplished by use of otologic alligator forceps or by irrigation of the ear canal; others—particularly spherical objects—require use of a Day (right angle) hook or suction (Fig. 23-19, C; see also Fig. 23-3). Foreign objects may also be the cause of painful abrasions or lacerations of the external auditory canal or even perforation of the tympanic membrane. Insertion of pencils or sticks into the ear canal by the child and parental attempts to clean the canal with a cotton swab are the most common modes of such injury.

Exposure to concussive forces such as a direct blow (which may be accidental or inflicted) or an explosion can also result in perforation (Fig. 23-20, A and B). Patients with traumatic perforations must be carefully assessed for signs of injury to deeper structures. If tympanic membrane perforation occurs as a result of penetration by a foreign object or of concussive forces, the physician must be particularly aware of the possibility of middle ear or inner ear damage. Evidence of hearing loss, vertigo, nystagmus, facial nerve injury, or cerebrospinal fluid leak should prompt urgent otolaryngologic consultation because an emergency surgical exploration may be indicated.

DISORDERS OF THE MIDDLE EAR

The normal tympanic membrane is thin, translucent, neutrally positioned, and mobile. The ossicles, particularly the malleus, are generally visible through the membrane (Fig. 23-21). Adequate assessment of the tympanic membrane requires that the examiner note four major characteristics: (1) thickness, (2) degree of translucence, (3) position relative to neutral, and (4) mobility. Application of gentle positive and negative pressure, using a properly sealed pneumatic otoscope (Fig. 23-22), produces brisk movement of the eardrum when the ear is free of disease and abnormal movement when fluid is present, when

Figure 23-19 Otic foreign bodies. **A,** This child inserted a bead into her ear. The object must be removed carefully to prevent further trauma. **B,** This patient experienced a period of intense buzzing, pain, and itching in the ear that abated after a few hours. If the tympanic membrane is intact, olive or mineral oil may be used to drown the insect. **C,** A blunt-tipped, right-angled Day hook, small wire loop curette, Hartmann forceps, and an alligator forceps (and see Fig. 23-3, A) are useful instruments for removing foreign bodies from the external auditory canal.

Figure 23-20 Traumatic perforations of the tympanic membrane. **A,** This 8-year-old boy's tympanic membrane was perforated by a forceful slap on the ear. **B,** Even more severe damage with thickening and hemorrhage is seen in this victim of a blast injury caused by an explosion. (**A,** *Courtesy Michael Hawke, MD.*)

the drum is thickened or scarred, or when there is an increase in either positive or negative pressure (Fig. 23-23). An abnormality in any one of the four major characteristics suggests middle ear pathology.

Acute Otitis Media

Acute otitis media is the term used to describe acute infection and inflammation of the middle ear. Associated inflammation and edema of the eustachian tube mucosa appear to play key roles in the pathogenesis by impeding drainage of the middle ear fluid. In some children, anatomic or chronic physiologic abnormalities of the eustachian tube predispose to infection. The problem is commonly seen in conjunction with an acute upper respiratory tract infection, and its onset is often heralded by a secondary temperature spike one to several days after the onset of respiratory symptoms. The major offending organisms are bacterial respiratory pathogens. The most commonly isolated organisms and their relative frequency, shown in Table 23-1, demonstrate the rise of penicillin-resistant *Streptococcus pneumoniae.* A small proportion of cases constitute an exception to these percentages, that is, those in which otitis is accompanied by conjunctivitis. Nontypable *Haemophilus influenzae* is found to be causative in 70% to 75% of these cases. Increasing rates of β-lactamase positivity in these organisms, as well as the rising incidence of penicillin-resistant *S. pneumoniae,* has necessitated the use of high-dose amoxicillin and/or greater use of β-lactamase–resistant antibiotic regimens whenever this scenario is seen. Sulfa drugs may also be useful for therapy of community-acquired methicillin-resistant

Staphylococcus aureus, which is becoming increasingly common.

In acute otitis media the classic findings on inspection of the tympanic membrane are erythema and injection; bulging that obscures the malleus; thickening, often with a grayish-white or yellow hue, reflecting a purulent effusion; and reduced mobility (Fig. 23-24, *A*). However, crying produces erythema of the eardrum, and thus tympanic erythema in a crying child is of little diagnostic value. The patient is usually febrile and, if old enough, typically complains of otalgia. However, in many cases this "textbook picture" is not seen. This is probably due in part to time of presentation, the virulence of the particular pathogen, and host factors.

Accuracy in diagnosis necessitates meticulous inspection during otoscopy and knowledge of the various modes of presentation. Children may have fever of a few hours' duration and otalgia (or if very young, fever and irritability) yet have no abnormality on otoscopy. If re-examined the next day,

Table 23-1	Acute Otitis Media: Most Commonly Isolated Bacterial Pathogens and Their Relative Frequency		
Bacterial Pathogen		**Number of Isolates (% of Total)**	**Number Resistant (%)**
Streptococcus pneumoniae		49 (44)	18 (37)
Haemophilus influenzae		46 (41)	21 (46)
Moraxella catarrhalis		16 (14)	16 (100)
Staphylococcus aureus		0 (0)	0 (0)
Total		111 (100)	55 (50)

Figure 23-21 A normal tympanic membrane. The drum is thin and translucent, and the ossicles are readily visualized. It is neutrally positioned with no evidence of bulging or retraction. *(Courtesy Sylvan Stool, MD.)*

Figure 23-22 Pneumatic otoscopy. This procedure requires proper equipment including a pneumatic otoscope head and an appropriately sized speculum to achieve a good air seal. When a seal is difficult to obtain despite proper speculum size, the head and tubing should be checked for air leaks. If none is found, application of a piece of rubber tubing to the end of the speculum (shown attached to the otoscope) or use of a soft speculum *(1)* may solve the problem.

Figure 23-23 Technique and findings in pneumatic otoscopy. **A,** The speculum is inserted into the ear canal to form a tight seal. The bulb is then gently and slowly pressed and released while the mobility of the drum is assessed. Pressing on the bulb applies positive pressure; letting up applies negative pressure. **B,** A normal drum moves inward and then back. **C,** In cases of acute otitis media, in which the middle ear is filled with purulent material, the drum bulges toward the examiner and moves minimally. **D,** In cases of acute otitis media with an air–fluid level, mobility may be nearly normal. In some patients, however, the drum may be retracted, indicating increased negative pressure. If this is the case, mobility on positive pressure may be reduced whereas movement on negative pressure is nearly normal or only mildly decreased. **E,** This is the same pattern as that seen commonly in children with chronic serous otitis. **F,** In cases of high negative pressure and no effusion, application of positive pressure produces little or no movement, but on negative pressure the drum billows back toward the examiner.

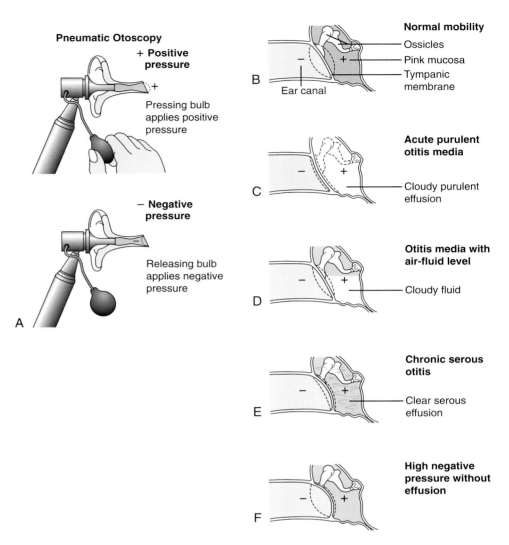

many of these patients have clear evidence of acute otitis media. Some have erythema and bubbles or air–fluid or air–pus levels (a result of venting by the eustachian tube) without bulging and with nearly normal mobility of the eardrum (Fig. 23-24, B). In still other cases the drum may be full and poorly mobile with cloudy fluid behind it but with minimal erythema (Fig. 23-24, C). In some patients the drum is retracted, moves primarily or only in response to negative pressure, and shows signs of inflammation and/or a cloudy effusion.

On occasion the signs and symptoms of otitis media may be accompanied by formation of a bullous lesion on the surface of the tympanic membrane, a condition termed *bullous myringitis* (Fig. 23-25). These children usually complain of intense pain. Whereas this phenomenon is most commonly associated with *Mycoplasma* infection in adults, any of the usual pediatric pathogens (see Table 23-1) can be causative in children. Finally, acute otitis media may, by virtue of increasing middle ear pressure, result in acute perforation of the tympanic membrane. On presentation the canal may be filled with purulent material; however, tugging on the pinna usually does not elicit pain, and erythema and edema of the canal wall are minimal or absent. Cleansing with a cotton wick or

Figure 23-24 Acute otitis media. **A,** This is the textbook picture: an erythematous, opaque, bulging tympanic membrane. The light reflex is reduced, and the landmarks are partially obscured. Mobility is markedly reduced. **B,** In this acutely febrile child who complained of otalgia, the presence of both air and fluid formed bubbles separated by grayish-yellow menisci. Even though the drum was not injected, this finding, combined with fever and otalgia, is consistent with acute infection. **C,** In this child the tympanic membrane was injected at the periphery, and a yellow purulent effusion caused the inferior portion to bulge outward. Mobility was markedly reduced. (**A,** *Courtesy Michael Hawke, MD.*)

Figure 23-25   Acute otitis media with bullous myringitis. This patient was febrile and extremely uncomfortable. On otoscopy an erythematous bullous lesion is seen obscuring much of the tympanic membrane. This phenomenon, called *bullous myringitis*, is caused by the usual pathogens of otitis media in childhood. The bullous lesion often ruptures and drains spontaneously, providing immediate relief of pain.

Figure 23-27   Serous otitis media. This patient has a chronic serous middle ear effusion. The tympanic membrane is retracted, thickened, and shiny. Behind it is a clear yellow effusion. Mobility was decreased and primarily evident on negative pressure. The child was not acutely ill but did have decreased hearing. *(Courtesy Sylvan Stool, MD.)*

suction usually reveals an inflamed drum with a barely visible perforation (Fig. 23-26).

Just as clinical findings of acute otitis media vary, so do symptoms. Although some patients have severe otalgia, others may complain of sore throat, mild ear discomfort, ear popping, or decreased hearing yet have floridly inflamed eardrums. Fever may be absent. As a guideline, the American Academy of Pediatrics and the American Academy of Family Physicians recommend that the diagnosis of acute otitis media be made with (1) a history of acute onset of signs and symptoms, (2) the presence of middle ear effusion, and (3) signs and symptoms of middle-ear inflammation.

Radiographic studies are generally of little value in the diagnosis of acute otitis media. When a temporal bone CT scan is obtained in a patient with acute otitis media and fluid in the middle ear, fluid is often present in the mastoid cavity. This will be interpreted by a radiologist as opacification of the mastoid because it may be difficult to distinguish between the CT findings of acute otitis media and those of acute mastoiditis. In such instances it is important that the physician look at the patient's clinical signs rather than rely on radiographic findings to make the diagnosis.

Treatment for acute otitis media may include the option of observation without use of antibiotics based on diagnostic certainty, age, illness severity, and assurance of follow-up. In addition to treating patients with an appropriate antimicrobial agent and analgesics when necessary, follow-up examination is important. This is best done 2 to 3 weeks after diagnosis,

when complete resolution can be expected in more than 50% of children. The purpose of reevaluation is to identify those patients who have persistent serous effusions and require ongoing surveillance. Selected older patients with mild, uncomplicated acute otitis media may be observed without antimicrobial therapy, but follow-up examination is still necessary.

Otitis Media with Effusion (Serous Otitis Media)

Serous effusion in the middle ear may result from an upper respiratory tract infection, or it may be the residual of treated acute otitis. In many instances this effusion is not spontaneously cleared but instead remains in the middle ear for weeks or months, resulting in a persistent clear gray or yellow effusion behind the eardrum (Fig. 23-27). Persistence appears to result in part from eustachian tube dysfunction with poor drainage and ventilation. Pneumatic otoscopy often reveals poor mobility of the tympanic membrane, and mobility is noted primarily on negative pressure. The latter is thought to develop as a result of absorption of middle ear gases by mucosal cells, creating a vacuum that persists with the fluid because of failure of ventilation by the eustachian tube. Such long-standing effusions impair hearing. Persistence of bilateral serous effusions for more than 3 to 4 months with hearing loss is an indication for myringotomy and insertion of tubes (see Fig. 23-29, *A* and *B*) to improve hearing.

Chronic–Recurrent Otitis Media

Chronic or chronic–recurrent otitis media with effusion (COME) is common in young children. Patients subject to this condition appear to have significant and prolonged eustachian tube dysfunction. This "otitis-prone" state may be a seemingly isolated phenomenon, or it can be a feature of a number of syndromes characterized by palatal dysfunction or malformation or by facial hypoplasia or deformity. These conditions include cleft palate, Crouzon syndrome, Down syndrome, and the mucopolysaccharidoses and mucolipidoses (see Fig. 23-8; and see Palatal Disorders, later). Chronic obstructive adenoidal hypertrophy may also be a predisposing condition. Less commonly, immunodeficiency and immotile cilia syndrome are identified as underlying etiologic conditions.

Chronic otitis media is associated with significant morbidity in terms of intermittent or chronic hearing impairment, intermittent discomfort, and the sequelae of recurrent infection.

Figure 23-26   Acute otitis media with perforation. In this child, increased middle ear pressure with acute otitis resulted in perforation of the tympanic membrane. The drum is thickened, and the perforation is seen at the 9 o'clock position.

Figure 23-28 Sequelae of chronic otitis media. **A,** Much of this child's tympanic membrane is scarred and thickened, and a thinned dimeric area balloons out of the inferior central portion. **B,** The eardrum is markedly thickened, scarred in an arc from 12 to 5 o'clock, and has a large chronic perforation. **C,** Severe retraction of the tympanic membrane is seen in this patient. The membrane adheres to the malleus. (**A** and **B,** Courtesy Sylvan Stool, MD; **C,** courtesy Alejandro Hoberman, MD, Children's Hospital of Pittsburgh, Pittsburgh, Pa.)

Over months or years, the process produces permanent myringosclerotic changes in which the tympanic membrane becomes whitened, thickened, and scarred (Fig. 23-28, A). Chronic perforations are common (Fig. 23-28, B). Patients with persistent middle ear infections despite medical therapy, those with frequent recurrences, and children with chronic severe tympanic membrane retraction (Fig. 23-28, C) appear to benefit from surgical drainage and insertion of tympanostomy tubes that vent the middle ear (Fig. 23-29). Persistence of a serous effusion for longer than 3 to 4 months with significant hearing loss is also an indication for myringotomy and insertion of tubes. Once placed, tubes should be checked at intervals for presence and patency. Spontaneous extrusion generally occurs

Figure 23-29 **A,** Tympanic membrane of patient with a history of chronic otitis media, with tympanostomy tube in place. The tube serves to vent the middle ear, improve hearing, and reduce the frequency of infection. **B,** The tympanic membrane is slightly smaller than the size of a dime. A typical tube takes up approximately 15% of the tympanic membrane's surface area. There are many different types in a variety of shapes, materials, sizes, and colors. Selection is based on specific pathology and surgeon preference. (**A,** Courtesy Sylvan Stool, MD.)

6 to 24 months after insertion. When tubes have been inserted, it is wise to prevent contamination of the middle ear with water. The need for earplugs in children with tubes or a perforation is the subject of some controversy, but in general their use is still recommended.

Protection of the Exposed Middle Ear with Earplugs

Earplugs come in all shapes and sizes. They vary in cost from inexpensive, premolded earplugs to expensive, custom-molded devices. The general purpose of an earplug is to prevent water from entering the external ear canal and contaminating the middle ear space. "Wax" earplugs act like a putty that can be molded into the particular shape that comfortably blocks the individual's ear canals. A preformed earplug is held in place by the conchal bowl and provides reasonable protection for children. Although custom-made earplugs are not of critical importance, they do provide a better fit and are more comfortable, and compliance with their use tends to be greater. Children have a propensity to lose or misplace these devices, and it is best to focus on obtaining functional earplugs that are easily replaceable at minimal cost.

Other Middle Ear Disorders

Although considerably less common than otitis media and serous otitis media, a number of other disorders involving the tympanic membrane are important because of potential severity.

Mass Lesions Involving the Tympanic Membrane

The most common and one of the most serious mass lesions of the eardrum is a *cholesteatoma*. It can present as a defect in the tympanic membrane through which persistent drainage occurs, or it can appear as a white cystic mass behind or involving the eardrum. It consists of trapped epithelial tissue that grows beneath the surface of the membrane (Fig. 23-30). Although a few are congenital with an intact tympanic membrane, the majority are sequelae of untreated or chronic–recurrent otitis media with a tympanic membrane defect. If a cholesteatoma is not removed surgically, it continues to enlarge; becomes locally destructive; and can erode the mastoid bone, destroy the ossicles, and even invade the inner ear structures or cranium. Progressive hearing impairment is usually a feature of this condition. Congenital cholesteatoma

Figure 23-30 Cholesteatomas. **A,** Congenital cholesteatoma noted in a young child with spontaneous ear drainage. No previous history of ear infections existed. **B** and **C,** Acquired cholesteatomas, which generally present after a long history of chronic middle ear disease.

is rare. It is seen under an intact tympanic membrane in the anterior superior quadrant of the middle ear.

Granulomas or *polyps* of the tympanic membrane (Fig. 23-31) can also develop in children with chronic middle ear infections. The most common cause of aural polyps in children is an old, retained tympanostomy tube. Cholesteatoma is another predisposing condition. These tissues often bleed easily, which can frighten the patient, the parent, and the physician. Left untreated, polyps can enlarge to fill the canal and by expansion can progressively damage the drum and the ossicles. Therefore prompt surgical removal is indicated if therapy with topical and oral antimicrobials is unsuccessful.

Distortions of the Tympanic Membrane

Thin, dimeric portions of the eardrum may be observed in patients with chronic middle ear disease, or they may develop after extrusion of a tympanostomy tube (Fig. 23-32; see also Fig. 23-28, *A*). These thinned areas are the result of abnormal healing of perforations and are hypermobile on pneumatic otoscopy. The important points to note on examination are whether the full depth of the pocket is visible or partly hidden, its location with respect to the ossicles, and whether or not it is dry. If the ear canal and drum are not dry, an active infection and/or cholesteatoma is present. In cases of severe deformity, aggressive therapy including ventilation of the middle ear and surgical excision of the pocket may be necessary.

NASAL DISORDERS

A child's nose is examined most commonly for disturbances in external appearance, excessive drainage, or blockage of airflow and interference with breathing. Epistaxis is also frequently encountered.

Figure 23-32 Dimerism of the tympanic membrane. Otoscopy demonstrates a severely retracted atrophic segment of the eardrum that also has multiple white scars (tympanosclerosis). The thinned portions are the result of abnormal healing of perforations and tend to be hypermobile on otoscopy. *(Courtesy Sylvan Stool, MD.)*

Nasal Examination

The nasal examination can be difficult in younger children. It is best done with the child sitting on a parent's lap or in a chair. The child's head is held in a neutral position, not tilted up.

An otoscope with a wide speculum (≥4 mm) is the most practical instrument. The examiner should gently brace his or her free hand on the child's upper lip to prevent sudden head movement from pushing the speculum tip into the nose, which could lead to nasal trauma, and should try to look toward the back of the nose rather than up into the nose. If the child is old enough to comply, he or she is asked to

Figure 23-31 Granulomas and polyps of the tympanic membrane. **A,** Growth of this polypoid granuloma was stimulated by the inflammatory process of chronic middle ear infection. **B,** These polyps, which protrude through a tympanic membrane perforation, have enlarged to entirely fill the external ear canal. Because of the possible attachment of the polyp to the facial nerve or the ossicles of the middle ear, removal of polyps requires extreme caution. *(**A,** Courtesy Sylvan Stool, MD.)*

Figure 23-33 Nasal endoscopic examination. **A,** A child holding and feeling the endoscope. **B,** When he shines the light on himself, the endoscope shows his face on the monitor. **C,** By holding it at the entrance to his nose, he sees that the instrument is neither hot nor painful.

breathe through his or her mouth so as not to fog up the lens on the otoscope. If a nasal spreader-type speculum is used, a headlight is desirable. The septum, the anterior edges of the middle and inferior turbinates, and the nasal floor are inspected, and the quality of nasal secretions is noted. With practice and when there is minimal congestion, adenoidal size can be assessed.

A more thorough examination is possible with a nasal endoscope; this enables full visualization of internal nasal structures. Before starting, the nose is sprayed with a decongestant to shrink the nasal mucosa and with a topical anesthetic. With patience, older children can be coaxed through the insertion and examination. Allowing them to hold and inspect the device, test the light, look at themselves on the monitor, and even insert the tip into their nose assists cooperation (Fig. 23-33, A-C). Most children younger than 5 years of age require immobilization, either on a papoose board or with parental and nursing assistance. The nasal endoscope is a useful tool, and this type of examination can be done readily in the otolaryngologist's office.

Nasal Congestion and Obstruction

Upper Respiratory Infections in Early Infancy

In infancy and early childhood the nasal passages are small and easily obstructed by processes that produce mucosal edema and coryza, whether infectious, "allergic," or traumatic. In the first 1 to 3 months, infants are obligate nose breathers and therefore can have significant respiratory distress from nasal congestion alone. Young infants with upper respiratory tract infections may, in addition to nasal discharge, have tachypnea and mild retractions and often have to interrupt feeding to breathe, which can result in the swallowing of significant amounts of air, leading to a secondary increase in spitting up after feeding and to intestinal gas pain. These secondary problems can be minimized by instructing parents to hold these infants up on their shoulders and burp them for 10 to 15 minutes after feedings. Instillation of saline nose drops to loosen secretions, followed by nasal suctioning before meals and naps, also provides a measure of relief. Oral decongestants are ineffective and often produce marked irritability when given to infants in the first year of life; they are no longer approved for pediatric use because of serious adverse events including deaths in children under 2 years of age. Fortunately, upper respiratory tract infections are generally brief and clear within a few days.

On occasion, infants with upper respiratory tract infection go on to have persistent, purulent, or serosanguineous nasal discharge. Culture of discharges persisting longer than 10 to 14 days may disclose heavy growth of a single pathogen. Preliminary studies of empirical antimicrobial therapy in such infants suggest that this produces rapid and effective resolution of symptoms when compared with a placebo. Thus this picture of prolonged nasal discharge probably represents a *bacterial ethmoiditis,* the infant equivalent of sinusitis.

Nasopharyngitis Secondary to Gastroesophageal Reflux (Reflux Rhinitis)

Infants with gastroesophageal reflux disease (GERD) may develop persistent nasal congestion and rhinorrhea with varying degrees of mucosal inflammation and edema in response to exposure to gastric contents. Snoring and/or coughing during sleep are common associated symptoms. Although vomiting or frequent spitting, sometimes with passage of regurgitated material through the nose, may be reported, often such symptoms are absent. The section Otolaryngologic Manifestations of Gastroesophageal Reflux Disease near the end of this chapter details the spectrum of signs and symptoms that may assist in diagnosis of GERD-related nasal disorders.

Congenital Causes of Nasal Obstruction

Congenital causes of nasal obstruction include choanal atresia, choanal stenosis, and mass lesions such as tumors, cysts, and polyps.

Choanal Atresia and Stenosis

Choanal atresia may be bony (90%) or membranous (10%), bilateral or unilateral. Newborns with bilateral choanal atresia manifest severe respiratory distress at delivery, with cyanosis that is relieved by crying and returns with rest (paradoxic cyanosis). The true nature of the problem can elude detection if the physician relies solely on passing soft feeding catheters through the nose to determine patency, because these can buckle or curl within the nose. The correct diagnosis is best made with a van Buren urethral sound or a firm plastic suction catheter (both no. 8 French). This is passed gently along the floor of the nose, close to the septum. If bony resistance is encountered, the diagnosis of choanal atresia is suspected (Fig. 23-34, *A*) and can be confirmed by endoscopy or by obtaining a CT scan of the nose and nasopharynx with fine overlapping cuts (Fig. 23-34, *B*).

Immediate relief of neonatal respiratory distress from bilateral choanal atresia may be accomplished by insertion of an oral airway (or a firm nipple from which the tip has been cut away) into the mouth. Definitive studies can then be performed to aid in planning surgical correction. Infants

Figure 23-34 Choanal atresia. **A,** This infant manifested severe respiratory distress at delivery, with paradoxic cyanosis. Attempts to pass a urethral sound suggested bony obstruction of the choanae bilaterally. **B,** A CT scan done after instillation of radiopaque dye reveals pooling of the dye within the nose anterior to the choanae, confirming complete obstruction.

with unilateral choanal atresia (Fig. 23-35) are usually asymptomatic at birth; however, with time they develop a persistent unilateral nasal discharge.

Choanal stenosis or anterior nasal (piriform aperture) stenosis is also generally asymptomatic in the newborn period,

Figure 23-35 Unilateral choanal atresia. Viewed through the nasopharyngoscope, the left choana is clearly patent, whereas the right is atretic. The child had a history of unilateral nasal discharge.

but acquisition of an upper respiratory tract infection can result in significant respiratory compromise. When either lesion is suspected, nasal endoscopy or probing with a urethral sound is indicated. If the sound meets resistance, further evaluation is required. In most cases symptomatic therapy using saline nose drops and nasal suctioning is sufficient to help the infant through the upper respiratory tract infection. With growth, the problem usually abates, but in some cases surgery may be required.

Congenital Mass Lesions

Congenital mass lesions are another source of nasal obstruction. These are particularly likely to become apparent during the first 2 years of life. The modes of presentation vary; some lesions are manifest primarily by symptoms of obstruction and are detected by diagnostic radiography; others become visually evident within a nostril or as a subcutaneous mass located near the root of the nose. On occasion, these patients have recurrent nasal infections and/or epistaxis. All such masses merit thorough clinical and radiographic evaluation because many have intracranial connections.

An *encephalocele* is an outpouching of brain tissue through a congenital bony defect in the midline of the skull. Some patients have craniofacial deformities and a rounded subcutaneous swelling between the eyes or adjacent to the nose. In other instances the neural tissue prolapses into the nasal cavity or nasopharynx, resulting in signs and symptoms of nasal obstruction without obvious external anomalies (Fig. 23-36, *A*). On occasion, a grapelike mass may be seen within the nares or protruding into the back of the mouth. The mass is usually identified by diagnostic radiography. CT (Fig. 23-36, *B*) is particularly helpful in delineating the extent of the mass and the underlying bony defect. Repair requires a collaborative effort by specialists in otolaryngology, neurosurgery, and in some cases plastic surgery.

Nasal dermoids are embryonic cysts containing ectodermal and mesodermal tissue. They present as round, firm subcutaneous masses located on the dorsum of the nose, close to the midline (Fig. 23-37, *A*). Examination of the overlying skin frequently reveals a small dimple, at times with extruding hair. Some of these cysts have deep extensions down to the nasal septum or through the cribriform plate into the cranium. Thorough evaluation by axial and coronal CT scans (Fig. 23-37, *B*) and MRI is necessary to determine extent and to plan repair. If such cysts are not removed, secondary infection is common and often results in fistula formation.

Papillomas (Fig. 23-38) are similar growths that occur on the distal nasal mucosa near the mucocutaneous junction. These growths should be excised to improve appearance and confirm diagnosis; they do not cause obstruction.

Acquired Forms of Nasal Obstruction

Adenoidal and Tonsillar Hypertrophy

The lymphoid tissue that constitutes the tonsils and adenoids is relatively small in infancy, gradually enlarges until 8 to 10 years of age, and then usually begins to shrink in size. In most instances this normal process of hypertrophy results in mild to moderate enlargement of these structures and does not constitute a problem. A small percentage of children, however, develop marked adenoidal and tonsillar hypertrophy, with attendant symptoms of nasal obstruction and rhinorrhea. A few even have difficulty swallowing solid foods. Recurrent infection appears to be the most common inciting factor, although atopy may play a role in some cases. On occasion, mononucleosis is the initiating event, resulting in rapid enlargement of adenoidal and tonsillar tissues that is then slow to resolve (see Tonsillitis/Pharyngitis, later; and

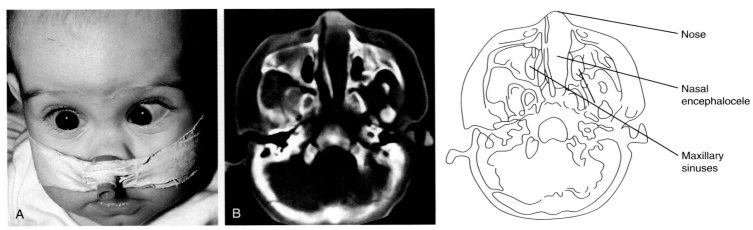

Figure 23-36   Nasal encephalocele. **A,** This normal-appearing infant had signs of severe nasal obstruction, necessitating insertion of a nasopharyngeal airway to relieve distress. **B,** A CT scan shows a large nasal mass lesion that fills one nostril and pushes the nasal septum into the other. This lesion proved to be an encephalocele extruding through a bony defect in the skull base (extrusion seen on another CT cut).

see Chapter 12). In most children, progressive adenoidal enlargement appears to be the cumulative result of a series of upper respiratory tract infections. The consequent obstruction to normal flow of secretions then starts a vicious circle, making the child more vulnerable to recurrent infections of the ears, sinuses, and nasopharynx, which in turn further exacerbate the adenoidal and tonsillar hypertrophy.

Regardless of the mode of origin, when adenoidal hypertrophy is marked, blockage of the nasal airway becomes severe and results in mouth breathing, chronic rhinorrhea, inability to blow the nose, and snoring during sleep (Fig. 23-39, *A*). Speech becomes hyponasal and muffled. The child holds his or her mouth open and has little or no airflow through the nares, and his or her tonsils may also meet at the midline (Fig. 23-39, *B*). A lateral neck x-ray examination reveals a large adenoidal shadow impinging on the nasal airway (Fig. 23-39, *C*). For many patients these features are noted primarily in the course of acute illness; however, a number of children have symptoms even when free of acute infection. When obstruction is severe, sleep disturbance may result. This is characterized by restlessness and retractions when recumbent, snoring, and frequent waking. Some patients begin to sleep sitting up, and many manifest daytime fatigue, irritability, and short attention span. Symptoms are worse during sleep because relaxation of the pharyngeal muscles further increases the degree of upper airway obstruction. In severe cases this results

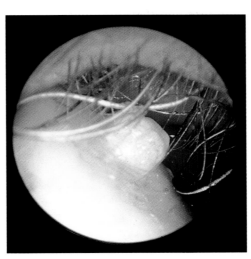

Figure 23-38   Nasal papillomas present as warty growths at the mucocutaneous junction of the nares. *(Courtesy Michael Hawke, MD.)*

in periods of hypoxia and hypercarbia. Because a patient may look relatively healthy when awake (with the exception of having to breathe through the mouth), it is important to observe for retractions and to assess the pattern of breathing after the child has been recumbent for a period of time or,

Figure 23-37   Nasal dermoid. **A,** A firm, round mass with a central dimple is seen over the bridge of this infant's nose. **B,** CT scan demonstrates a bony dehiscence of the nasal bridge with a nasal dermoid extending into the anterior cranial vault in the area of the foramen cecum.

Figure 23-39 Adenoidal and tonsillar hypertrophy. **A,** External appearance of a child with marked enlargement of tonsils and adenoids. He must keep his mouth open to breathe and shows signs of fatigue as a result of sleep disturbance caused by his upper airway obstruction. **B,** On examination of the pharynx, his tonsils are seen meeting in the midline. **C,** A lateral neck radiograph shows a large adenoid shadow impinging on the nasopharyngeal airway. **D,** If obstruction is prolonged, as was the case in this patient, cor pulmonale, abnormal facial elongation, and widening of the nasal root may result. **E,** When the palate is retracted before adenoidectomy, the extent of overgrowth of adenoidal tissue is readily appreciated.

better still, during a nap. Use of polysomnography or continuous pulse oximetry may help confirm or establish the diagnosis and determine the severity of sleep apnea. Polysomnography may be useful to assess the severity of the sleep-disordered breathing. If severe obstruction persists for a prolonged period of time, cor pulmonale (with signs of right ventricular hypertrophy on electrocardiogram and chest radiograph) and abnormal facial growth may result (Fig. 23-39, *D*).

Management of patients with adenoidal hypertrophy depends in part on the severity and the duration of the obstruction. In milder cases of short duration or in patients with intermittent symptoms, careful monitoring; treatment of atopy with intranasal steroids, when present; or institution of a 2- to 4-week course of antimicrobial therapy with a β-lactam–stable agent may result in significant shrinkage of hypertrophied tonsillar and adenoidal tissues. Children with persistent symptoms despite therapy and those with sleep disturbance or cor pulmonale should undergo adenoidectomy, during which the extent of adenoidal overgrowth can be fully appreciated (Fig. 23-39, *E*). Children with major orthodontic abnormalities and nasal obstruction also should be considered for adenoidectomy before orthodontic correction.

Nasal Foreign Bodies

As with the external ear, it is not unusual for small children to put beads, paper, pieces of sponge, plastic toys, or other foreign material into their noses. Such foreign objects are irritating to the nasal mucosa and soon incite an intense inflammatory reaction with production of a thick, purulent, foul-smelling discharge that helps to hide their presence. Intermittent epistaxis may accompany the discharge. Because most children younger than 5 years of age are unable to blow their noses and are afraid or unable to tell their parents what they have done, the object is not expelled and the problem often goes unrecognized until symptoms develop and medical attention is sought. A unilateral nasal discharge and/or a foul smell are the typical chief complaints and should lead the clinician to suspect a foreign body immediately (Fig. 23-40, *A*).

Speculum examination may readily disclose the object (Fig. 23-40, *B* and *C*), but often the purulent discharge obscures the view, necessitating removal with an absorbent swab or via gentle suction. Even when visualization is accomplished, removal can be difficult because children are easily frightened at the prospect of instrumentation, and their struggling can result in mucosal injury during attempts at removal. To minimize problems, topical anesthetic spray and a topical vasoconstrictor can be applied, and the child can be restrained with a papoose board. Older patients or calm young children may do well sitting in a parent's lap, if the examiner is patient, reassuring, and willing to explain each step carefully. The discharge may then be removed by swab or suction. If the object is anterior to the turbinates, removal can be attempted using suction; a small wire loop curette; a right-angled Day hook for spherical objects; or otologic forceps for material that can be grasped (Fig. 23-40, *C*). Consultation with an otolaryngologist should be sought for removal of objects located more posteriorly or those not readily removed on initial attempts. A major concern is that in the attempted removal, a deeply situated foreign body may be dislodged into the nasopharynx, leading to aspiration or, worse, laryngeal obstruction. In such cases the best course of action is to remove the object after the airway has been secured with an endotracheal tube in the operating room, with the patient under general anesthesia. Significant bleeding may occur during attempted removal of an intranasal foreign body, and this is another reason to strongly consider general anesthesia with an endotracheal tube to secure the airway. Small batteries such as watch batteries in the nose can cause a great deal of tissue injury from the electric current. Therefore, all batteries should be removed as quickly as possible (Fig. 23-40, *D* and *E*).

Nasal Polyps

Polyps are thought to be the end result of recurrent infection and/or inflammation, although in a portion of cases, atopy may play a contributing role. Polyps originate in the ethmoid or, less commonly, the maxillary sinuses and protrude through the sinus ostia into the nasal cavity. The phenomenon is unusual in children younger than 10 years of age, with the exception of patients with cystic fibrosis, 25% of whom develop polyps, some as early as infancy. Symptoms consist of those of progressive nasal obstruction, frequently with associated discharge. Recurrent sinusitis is a common complication as a result of impaired sinus drainage. In some cases chronic sinusitis may be the cause of polyp formation. Affected patients with acute infections may also have intermittent epistaxis. Involvement may be unilateral or bilateral. On examination, moist, glistening pedunculated growths that may have a smooth or a grapelike appearance are seen (Fig. 23-41).

Figure 23-40 Nasal foreign body. **A,** This child had a unilateral, foul-smelling nasal discharge. **B,** Aspiration of the discharge in this patient revealed a red bead that was removed with a Day hook. **C,** Hartmann forceps, a small wire loop curette, and a right-angle Day hook are the instruments used most commonly for removal of nasal foreign bodies. Nasal spreaders assist visualization and create a wider space for inserting the desired instrument. Note that bleeding or aspiration of the nasal foreign body may occur, especially with uncooperative toddlers. Thus consideration should be given for removal of nasal foreign bodies in the operating room with general anesthesia and a controlled airway. **D,** Severe intranasal damage resulting from a nasal foreign body: a tiny watch battery. **E,** The watch battery removed. (**A,** *Courtesy Michael Hawke, MD.*)

Figure 23-41   Nasal polyp. This 2-year-old girl with cystic fibrosis was referred because of nasal obstruction and nocturnal snoring of a few months' duration. A large grayish polyp was found in the left nostril. Any child presenting with a nasal polyp should be tested for cystic fibrosis.

Figure 23-42   Sequelae of chronic nasal polyps. This 7-year-old girl with cystic fibrosis and recurrent nasal polyps shows secondary alteration in facial growth consisting of a broadened nasal root and prominence of the malar areas. This occurred despite several resections.

Bilateral opacification of the ethmoid and maxillary sinuses is commonly found on radiography. Polyps must be distinguished from a nasal glioma or encephalocele, which may have a similar appearance and can produce identical symptoms. These neural mass lesions are more common in infancy but may present in older children. Therefore, before biopsy or removal a CT scan of the sinuses and skull base should be considered for children with polypoid nasal lesions who do not have cystic fibrosis.

Surgical removal of the polyps is indicated to relieve nasal obstruction, reduce the risk of secondary sinusitis, and diminish the possibility of altered facial growth. Another problem seen in children with chronic polyps (most frequently those with cystic fibrosis) consists of widening of the nasal root and prominence of the malar areas of the face (Fig. 23-42).

Nasal Trauma

Blunt nasal trauma is frequently encountered in pediatrics. In the majority of instances it results only in minor swelling and mild epistaxis, which is readily controlled by application of pressure over the nares (see Chapter 2 for nasal trauma

incurred during delivery). However, more severe injuries do occur and have a significant potential for long-term morbidity and deformity if not identified and treated appropriately. These injuries include displaced nasal fractures (Fig. 23-43, *A* and *B*), which, if not reduced, result in permanent deformity; septal deviation or dislocation, with or without an associated fracture (Fig. 23-44), which produces unilateral impairment of airflow; and septal hematomas (Fig. 23-45, *A*), which, if not drained promptly, may lead to abscesses (see Chapter 6) and cause destruction of nasal cartilage, resulting in a saddle-nose deformity (Fig. 23-45, *B*). Finally, profuse bleeding that is difficult to stop or that recurs readily suggests trauma to deeper structures of the face or frontal bones and warrants prompt stabilization and meticulous clinical and radiographic assessment (see Chapter 20).

In evaluating patients with nasal trauma, the nasal bridge should be inspected for swelling or deformity (the latter may not be apparent if swelling is marked) and the septum palpated for tenderness, crepitus, or excessive mobility. The nares should be cleared of clots, and the septum assessed for position and presence of swelling, which would suggest a hematoma. A hematoma is soft on palpation of the septum with a

Frontal bone

Displaced fracture

Figure 23-43   Displaced nasal fracture. **A,** This teenager was hit on the nose while playing football. On external inspection there is obvious deformity, and there are ecchymoses under both eyes. Crepitus was evident on palpation. **B,** A lateral radiograph of another patient shows a displaced fracture of the proximal portion of the nasal bone, delineated on the diagram.

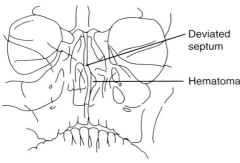

Figure 23-44 Deviated nasal septum. This patient was punched in the nose, resulting in a leftward deviation of the cartilaginous portion of the nasal septum, which is clearly visible in the radiograph and is delineated in the diagram. The small arc of mucosal swelling along the septum proved to be a small septal hematoma that necessitated drainage. No visible fracture occurred. Septal deviation requires correction to prevent deformity and to relieve secondary nasal obstruction.

Figure 23-45 Septal hematoma. This patient incurred facial trauma **(A)** resulting in multiple fractures of the nasal and orbital bones and submucosal bleeding along the nasal septum. Such septal hematomas must be drained promptly to reduce the risk of abscess formation and to prevent cartilage necrosis, which ultimately results in a saddle-nose deformity **(B)**. (*A, Courtesy Robert Hickey, MD, Children's Hospital of Pittsburgh, Pittsburgh, Pa.*)

cotton-tipped applicator. Examination of the oropharynx is also helpful in determining whether blood is flowing posteriorly. When marked swelling, severe tenderness, deformity, crepitus, or septal deviation is found, radiologic evaluation may be considered. However, radiographs should be interpreted with caution because a large portion of the nasal skeleton in children is composed of cartilage rather than bone and serious nasal injuries can be present despite a seemingly normal x-ray film. Septal hematomas, displaced fractures, and bleeding that fails to cease readily with direct pressure necessitate prompt consultation with an otolaryngologist.

Epistaxis

Although often due to direct trauma, nasal bleeding in childhood has a number of other causes including infection, mucosal irritation, bleeding disorders, vascular anomalies, and hypertension. Patients with these conditions may have apparently spontaneous bleeding or epistaxis triggered by minor external trauma or by forceful sneezing and blowing. Profuse bleeding that is difficult to stop is most characteristic of acute thrombocytopenia, vascular anomalies, and severe hypertension. Mild bleeding that is readily controlled by application of pressure suggests mucosal infection or irritation that promotes bleeding from small superficial veins located on the anterior nasal septum (Fig. 23-46). In all cases the problem should be taken seriously and investigated carefully to correctly diagnose and appropriately treat the primary source of the problem.

In approaching patients with epistaxis, the following historical points should be addressed:

1. Is the problem acute or recurrent?

2. Was external or intranasal trauma, sneezing, or blowing a triggering event?

3. What is the duration of the current bleed and the approximate volume of blood loss (handkerchiefs soaked, hemodynamic status, etc.)?

4. Is the bleeding unilateral or bilateral?

5. Are there any unilateral nasal obstructive symptoms?

Figure 23-46 Dilated septal vessels of Kiesselbach plexus, which tend to bleed in response to mucosal drying, cracking, infection, or irritation. (*From Becker W: Atlas of ear, nose, and throat diseases, ed 2, Stuttgart, 1983, Thieme.*)

6. Has the patient been having symptoms suggestive of an upper respiratory tract infection or nasal allergy?

7. Has the child manifested other signs and symptoms of an underlying coagulopathy or of hypertension?

8. Has the patient been taking medication, especially aspirin, ibuprofen, intranasal steroid sprays, or other nonsteroidal antiinflammatory or anticoagulant agents?

Physical assessment must address the patient's general well-being in addition to careful examination of the nose. Hemodynamic status is of particular importance when hemorrhage has been profuse.

After observation of the external appearance of the nares, the nose is cleared of clots and discharge, if present. The septum and mucosa are then inspected for possible points of hemorrhage, signs of obstruction, mass lesions, and foreign objects. The oropharynx should also be examined for posterior flow of blood, especially when no point of bleeding is evident on inspection of the nasal mucosa. Otolaryngologic consultation should be sought in cases involving profuse bleeding that does not readily cease on application of pressure and may require nasal cautery or packing or other surgical treatment.

Epistaxis Caused by Infection and Mucosal Irritation

In many patients with nontraumatic epistaxis, examination reveals unilateral or bilateral septal erythema and friability or excoriation (Fig. 23-47). The history given is one of intermittent bleeding, especially with sneezing, blowing the nose, or during sleep (the child's pillow is found spotted with blood). The phenomenon is commonly attributed to digital manipulation of the nose in response to itching. However, in view of the sensitivity of the mucosa to painful stimuli, picking to the point of excoriation is rather unlikely. In many instances erythematous friable areas are impetiginous or represent the combined effects of inflammation (the result of nasopharyngitis, sinusitis, or allergic rhinitis) and trauma caused by forceful sneezing and blowing. When infection is suspected, culturing of the friable area for a predominant bacterial pathogen (especially group A β-hemolytic streptococci or coagulase-positive staphylococci) may prove rewarding. In patients with no history of or no findings consistent with upper respiratory tract infection, mucosal drying may be responsible. This occurs most commonly in winter as a result of drying of the air by central heating systems. Although application of topical antibiotic ointment, water-based lubricants, humidification, and antihistamines (for atopic patients) may provide some relief, when bacterial pathogens are found, oral antimicrobial therapy is more likely to be successful.

Patients with nasal polyps who have an intercurrent infection and children with nasal foreign bodies with secondary infection and inflammation are also highly prone to intermittent epistaxis and blood-tinged nasal discharge.

Epistaxis Caused by Bleeding Disorders

Despite application of pressure, epistaxis in patients with coagulopathies is more likely to be prolonged and carries a greater risk of significant blood loss. Although many such patients have known bleeding disorders, a few may present with prolonged or recurrent nosebleeds as one of the initial manifestations of their problem. This is most typical of idiopathic thrombocytopenia, aplastic anemia, and acute leukemia. When epistaxis arises in the context of a bleeding disorder, the personal history, family history, and/or other physical findings should point to the diagnosis (see Chapter 11), which can then be confirmed by hematologic studies (complete blood count and differential, platelet count, prothrombin time and partial thromboplastin time, and coagulation profile).

Acute management depends in part on the source of the coagulopathy (e.g., factor replacement or platelet transfusion) and in part on the severity of bleeding. Topical application of a vasoconstrictor such as epinephrine and insertion of absorbable synthetic material that aids coagulation (Gelfoam or Surgicel) can be helpful in patients with thrombocytopenia and an anterior point of bleeding. The risks of secondary infection with packing must be given careful consideration in patients undergoing immunosuppressive therapy. Prophylactic antimicrobials should be administered to patients requiring packing to avoid secondary infections.

Epistaxis Caused by Vascular Abnormalities

In a minority of children with recurrent epistaxis, the history reveals significant bleeding that typically drains from one side of the nose. This suggests a localized vascular abnormality. The most commonly encountered problem is that of a dilated septal vessel or plexus, which may be a sequela of prior inflammation (see Fig. 23-46). This may be visible anteriorly but also can be located high on the septum, requiring nasal endoscopy for identification. Cauterization is generally curative. In children older than 7 years of age, anterior septal lesions can be cauterized in the office with silver nitrate after application of a topical anesthetic and vasoconstrictor. Younger children and many patients with posterior lesions may need general anesthesia for cauterization.

Two relatively rare vascular anomalies also may be the source of recurrent nasal bleeding: telangiectasias and angiofibromas. Patients with *hereditary hemorrhagic telangiectasia* (Osler-Weber-Rendu disease) have an autosomal dominant disorder characterized by formation of cutaneous and mucosal telangiectatic lesions that begin to develop in childhood and gradually increase in number with age. These lesions appear as bright red, slightly raised, star-shaped plexuses of dilated small vessels that blanch on pressure (Fig. 23-48). Mucosal telangiectasias may bleed spontaneously or in response to minor trauma. Recurrent epistaxis is a common mode of presentation in childhood. Multiple telangiectasias are evident on close examination. Hematuria and/or gastrointestinal bleeding may be seen separately or in combination with epistaxis.

Juvenile nasopharyngeal angiofibroma is a rare vascular tumor seen predominantly in adolescent boys. Although benign, it is locally invasive and destructive and may involve the maxillary sinuses, palate, sphenoid sinus, and portions of

Figure 23-47 Excoriated nasal septum. This child presented with an upper respiratory tract infection and a history of intermittent epistaxis with nasal blowing and nocturnal epistaxis, with blood noted on his pillow in the mornings. He had a purulent nasal discharge *(lower right)* and a diffusely excoriated erythematous septum. Cultures of nose and throat specimens grew group A β-streptococci.

Figure 23-48 Hereditary hemorrhagic telangiectasia. Numerous telangiectasias dot the lips and the nasal and palatal mucosa of this boy who had problems with recurrent epistaxis. *(Courtesy Bernard Cohen, MD, Johns Hopkins Hospital, Baltimore, Md.)*

the skull base. The most common mode of presentation is one of profuse, often recurrent epistaxis. Some patients also have symptoms of unilateral nasal obstruction with secondary rhinorrhea, and a small percentage may have visual, auditory, or other cranial nerve disturbances. On examination, a purplish soft tissue mass may be seen through the nares or on nasal endoscopy. In addition to standard radiographs, CT, MRI, and angiography may be necessary to assess the extent of the tumor (Fig. 23-49). Carefully planned excision is then the treatment of choice.

Epistaxis Caused by Hypertension

In contrast to the adult population, hypertension is an unusual source of epistaxis in childhood. However, it should be considered, especially in patients with antecedent headache and spontaneous, profuse bleeding that is difficult to stop. Patients with such a history may have previously undiagnosed coarctation of the aorta or chronic renal disease with severe secondary hypertension, and they should be examined with these possibilities in mind. It must be remembered that after significant blood loss, blood pressure may drop to normal levels.

DISORDERS OF THE PARANASAL SINUSES AND ADJACENT STRUCTURES

The paranasal sinuses are air-filled, bony cavities that lie within the facial bones of the skull, adjacent to the nasal passages. They develop through a gradual enlargement of

pneumatized cells that evaginate from the nasal cavity. This process occurs over the course of childhood and adolescence; there is a wide normal range in the duration of this process and in the ultimate size of the sinuses and their ostia (Fig. 23-50). In infancy the ethmoid and maxillary sinuses are partially pneumatized, but they are small and not readily demonstrable on radiographs (although they can be readily seen on a CT scan). Therefore radiographs are of little diagnostic value until after the first 2 years of life. The sphenoid sinus is not evident until about 5 to 6 years, and the frontal sinuses are not well developed until after 7 to 8 years of age (Fig. 23-51).

The sinuses are lined by ciliated respiratory epithelium, which produces and transports mucous secretions. They drain into the nasal cavity through various small openings, which are located under the middle turbinate. Several points of clinical importance warrant emphasis. First, the ostia of the sinuses are small and thus easily obstructed by mucosal edema. Further, there are many important structures adjacent to the sinuses that are vulnerable to involvement if a disease process spreads beyond a sinus. These include the orbit, the brain, and the cavernous sinus. The roots of the maxillary teeth lie in the floor of the maxillary sinuses. Therefore dental infections may drain into the maxillary sinuses, resulting in recurrent or chronic sinusitis. Hence the dentition should be thoroughly inspected in evaluating any child with suspected sinus infection (see Chapter 20).

Sinusitis

During the first several years of life, infection of the maxillary and/or ethmoid sinuses is more common than is generally appreciated. Frontal sinusitis becomes important after about 10 years of age. The probable pathogenesis is mucosal swelling (whether the result of upper respiratory tract infection, allergic rhinitis, or chemical irritation), resulting in obstruction of the sinus ostia. This impedes drainage of secretions; promotes mucous plugging; and, if prolonged, sets the stage for proliferation of bacterial pathogens with resultant infection. Both bacterial and viral pathogens have been isolated from pediatric patients. The most commonly identified bacteria are *S. pneumoniae,* nontypable *H. influenzae,* and *Moraxella catarrhalis.* The viral agents include adenoviruses and parainfluenza viruses. As in adults, no good correlation exists between results of nasopharyngeal and sinus aspirate cultures. There is, however, an approximately 80% correlation between middle meatus and sinus cultures. The middle meatus is the space between the middle and inferior turbinates where the frontal, maxillary, and ethmoid sinuses all drain. A culture of the middle meatus may be obtained by means of an otoscope and a small culture swab.

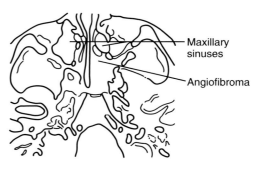

Maxillary sinuses

Angiofibroma

Figure 23-49 Juvenile nasopharyngeal angiofibroma. A CT scan is helpful in assessing the extent of this locally invasive vascular tumor. In this cut, an enhancing mass (an angiofibroma, as delineated in the diagram) is seen occupying the posterior portion of the left nostril, deviating the septum and compressing the ipsilateral maxillary sinus.

THE PARANASAL SINUSES

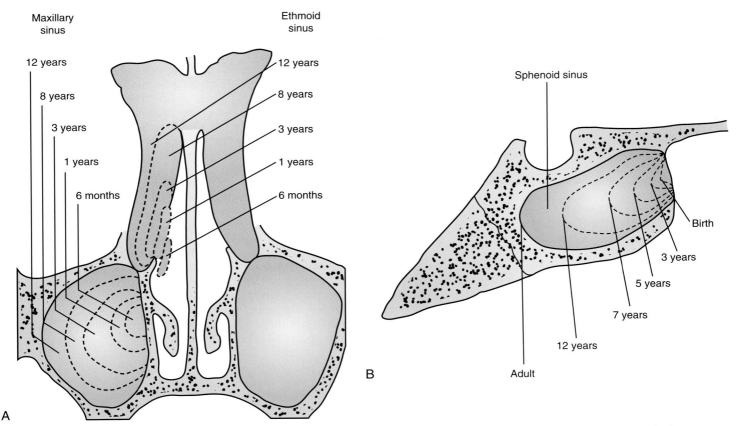

Figure 23-50   Development of the paranasal sinuses. **A,** This schematic diagram shows the development of the maxillary and ethmoid sinuses. Note that development occurs throughout childhood and may not be complete until 12 years of age. **B,** The sphenoid sinus, which sits under the pituitary fossa, develops slowly and may not even be well aerated for the first 5 to 6 years of life.

As with otitis media, a number of conditions predispose children to sinus infections by virtue of alterations in anatomy and/or physiology. These conditions include midfacial anomalies or deformities, particularly when maxillary hypoplasia is part of the picture (see Fig. 23-8); cleft palate (see Palatal Disorders, later); nasal deformity and/or septal deviation, whether congenital or acquired; mass lesions including hypertrophied adenoids, nasal foreign bodies, polyps, and tumors; abnormalities of mucus production and/or ciliary action such as cystic fibrosis and ciliary dyskinesia; immunodeficiency; atopy; dental infection; and barotrauma.

Clinical Presentations

In young children, sinusitis is primarily a disorder of the ethmoid and maxillary sinuses, and the clinical picture differs considerably from that seen in adolescents and adults. The most common picture is one of a prolonged upper respiratory tract infection that has shown no sign of amelioration after 7 to 10 days. Cough and/or persistent nasal discharge (of any character—thin, thick; clear, cloudy; white, yellow, or green) are the major complaints. The cough is usually loose or wet; it is prominent during the day but may be worse on waking in the morning and/or on first going to bed at night. Patients tend to clear their throats and sniff or snort frequently, especially after sleep. Halitosis or "fetor oris" is commonly noted by parents. In a minority of children, periorbital swelling, most noticeable on awakening, may be reported (Fig. 23-52). A small percentage of patients have a low-grade fever, and a few may complain of headache, facial discomfort, sore throat, or abdominal pain (thought to be due to gastric irritation from swallowing the infected postnasal discharge).

Often, physical examination alone is of little help in distinguishing sinusitis from an upper respiratory tract infection. Findings may include purulent nasal and postnasal discharge with erythema of the nasal mucosa and pharynx, but, as noted previously, this is not uniformly seen. Halitosis may be pronounced and strongly suggests sinusitis in the absence of evidence of dental infection, severe pharyngitis, or nasal foreign body. Sinusitis is also probable when features of the aforementioned picture are accompanied by signs of a maxillary dental abscess (see Chapter 20). Tenderness to percussion over the sinuses suggests sinusitis but is not seen in the majority of patients with the "prolonged upper respiratory tract infection" picture. The clinical spectrum is wide; any combination of the aforementioned symptoms and signs may be present, and sinusitis should be suspected, even if the course is relatively brief, whenever clinical findings are strongly suggestive.

A less frequent mode of presentation in young children is that of an acute upper respiratory tract infection that is unusually severe, which is characterized by high fever and copious purulent nasal discharge. Facial discomfort and periorbital swelling (nontender, nonindurated, and most marked on waking) are common with this picture. The edematous area may be normal in color or mildly erythematous (Fig. 23-53) and is thought to result from impairment of venous blood flow caused by increased pressure within the infected sinuses. Some of these patients also have conjunctival erythema and discharge. If periorbital erythema is intense or the area is indurated or tender, periorbital cellulitis should be suspected. On occasion a child with sinusitis has the typical findings of sympathetic edema but without high fever or the prolonged upper respiratory tract infection picture.

Figure 23-51   Normal radiography of the sinuses. Radiography is currently the most helpful noninvasive tool for evaluating the paranasal sinuses. Interpretation requires appreciation of the normal pattern of development and the findings in health and with disease. **A,** Anteroposterior, or Caldwell, view shows clear ethmoid sinuses in an 18-month-old child. The bony margins are sharp, and the sinus cavities are dark. **B,** The Waters view of the same child shows normal maxillary sinuses with sharply defined bony margins. The cavities appear black. **C,** After age 6 or 7, the Caldwell view is taken posteroanteriorly. In this 8-year-old boy, the bony margins of both the ethmoid and frontal sinuses are sharply defined. Because the calvarium is superimposed, it can be difficult to appreciate frontal sinus clouding on this view alone, particularly with bilateral disease. Therefore evaluation of the frontal sinuses requires close scrutiny of both Caldwell and lateral views. **D,** Lateral view of an 8-year-old child shows pneumatization of the frontal and sphenoid sinuses. Bony margins are sharply defined. The frontal sinuses appear black, but the sphenoid is somewhat gray because there are more overlying structures. Note that the roots of the maxillary teeth are embedded in the floor of the maxillary sinus. Note that plain sinus radiographs are quite inaccurate when compared with sinus CT for the diagnosis of sinusitis.

Figure 23-52   Sympathetic periorbital swelling with sinusitis. This 2-year-old boy was seen late in the afternoon with fever, wet cough, decreased activity, and mild infraorbital puffiness. The swelling was neither red, indurated, nor tender and reportedly had been more marked on awakening in the morning. He also had a scant cloudy nasal discharge. His chest radiograph was normal, but sinus films showed opacification of the maxillary sinuses.

Older children and adolescents with acute maxillary and/or ethmoid sinusitis may have either of the previously described symptom pictures but are more likely to complain specifically of headache and/or facial pain. The headache may be perceived as frontal, temporal, or even retroauricular. Facial discomfort can be described as malar pain or a sense of pressure or fullness. On occasion, patients complain that their teeth hurt (in the absence of dental pathology). When the frontal sinuses are involved, frontal or supraorbital headache is prominent, often perceived as dull or pulsating. The sphenoid sinus is rarely a site of isolated sinus infection, but it is often involved in pansinusitis, in which case occipital or vertex pain may be reported in addition to discomfort in other sites. Frequently the headache is intermittent. When constant, it varies in severity. This variability appears to be related to degree of drainage. Patients reporting copious "postnasal drip" tend to have less pain. Discomfort and congestion are often most marked on waking, probably as a result of recumbency and lack of gravity-promoted drainage. Some patients also report

Figure 23-53   This child with sinusitis had prominent erythematous periorbital edema and signs of purulent conjunctivitis. The redness raised concerns of periorbital cellulitis, but the area was nontender and not indurated. Presence of periorbital swelling is a helpful clue in diagnosing sinusitis in children with other suggestive signs and symptoms. *(Courtesy Ellen Wald, MD, Children's Hospital of Pittsburgh, Pittsburgh, Pa.)*

aggravation of pain with head movement, particularly on bending down and then straightening up. Swallowed discharge may produce significant abdominal discomfort as well. Coughing is often a feature but tends to be less prominent than in younger children. Physical findings include purulent (often blood-streaked) nasal and postnasal discharge, erythema of the nasal mucosa, and halitosis. Tenderness on sinus percussion is common. As with younger children, the clinical spectrum is wide and highly variable.

Ancillary Diagnostic Methods

When patients have most of the signs and symptoms of sinusitis, the diagnosis can be made on clinical grounds and treatment started empirically. This is particularly true for the younger child with the prolonged upper respiratory tract infection picture. Amoxicillin remains the drug of first choice for patients who are not allergic to penicillin. If there is no clear clinical improvement in 3 to 4 days, switching to amoxicillin/clavulanate or a comparable antimicrobial is indicated. If this also fails to produce clinical improvement in 3 to 4 days, resistant pneumococci may be the likely culprits, and high-dose amoxicillin/clavulanate, clindamycin, or an agent to which the organism is likely to be sensitive is indicated. Sulfa drugs or clindamycin often cover community-acquired methicillin-resistant *Staphylococcus aureus*. In less clear-cut cases, ancillary tools and tests are often necessary. The usefulness of the various diagnostic methods in evaluating suspected sinusitis is still under study. Radiography appears to be the most helpful noninvasive tool in children older than 2 years of age. Radiographs are most useful in patients in whom the clinical picture is not distinct enough to distinguish between sinusitis and allergic rhinitis and in patients who fail to respond to antimicrobial therapy as noted earlier. Findings of complete opacification, mucosal thickening greater than 4 mm, or an air–fluid level on standard radiography (Fig. 23-54) are strongly associated with positive findings on sinus aspiration. However, the wide range of variability in development and configuration of the sinuses can make interpretation difficult. Plain radiographs of the sinuses have been shown to both overestimate and underestimate the degree of sinusitis when compared with CT of the sinuses. The CT scan (Fig. 23-55) is the most sensitive modality for diagnosis and is considered the gold standard, but it can be falsely positive in patients with viral upper respiratory tract infections, is expensive, and may require sedation of the younger patient for an adequate examination. Thus it should be reserved for patients with possible complications of sinusitis, underlying anatomic abnormalities, or suspected chronic sinusitis who fail to respond to a prolonged course of antimicrobial therapy. Needle aspiration of the sinuses is conclusive but invasive and not without risk. It is, however, justified in patients with severe symptoms, patients with CNS or orbital extension, those not responding to treatment, and those who are immunocompromised or immunosuppressed. Middle meatus culture is also useful to detect the bacterial pathogen in sinusitis. Middle meatus cultures correlate with sinus cultures about 80% of the time.

At minimum, therapy consists of a 10- to 14-day course (or until the patient is symptom free for 7 days) of an antimicrobial agent suitable to the likely spectrum of organisms (see preceding paragraph). It is not unusual for a 3- to 4-week course of therapy with a β-lactam–stable agent to be required. Analgesia is given as needed for discomfort and perhaps an oral antihistamine or topical intranasal steroid spray in patients known to have allergic rhinitis. Some children with intense headaches or facial pain experience symptomatic relief by using topical nasal vasoconstrictors and warm compresses during the first 1 or 2 days of therapy. Patients with sinusitis

Figure 23-54 Radiographic findings in sinusitis. **A,** In this Caldwell view, the right ethmoid is clouded and the bony margins are less distinct than on the left. **B,** In this Waters view, complete opacification of both maxillary sinuses is evident. The bony margins are visible but faint. **C,** This child has significant mucosal thickening of the maxillary sinuses. Thickening greater than 4 mm has a strong association with positive culture on sinus aspirate. **D** and **E,** In another patient an air–fluid level can be seen in the left maxillary sinus on both Waters and lateral views. **F,** Differential opacification of the right frontal sinus is evident in this child who had fever and headache. (**D** and **E,** Courtesy J. Ledesma-Medina, MD; **F,** courtesy C.D. Bluestone, MD, Children's Hospital of Pittsburgh, Pittsburgh, Pa.)

Figure 23-55 CT findings in acute sinusitis. **A,** In the topographic view the examiner can identify the position of each slice and also has an excellent view of the adenoid bed. **B,** The coronal view shows the maxillary–ethmoidal relationship in conjunction with the orbit. Note that the ethmoids are clear but the right maxillary sinus is completely opacified, and the left maxillary sinus is nearly so with only a small air pocket visible. **C,** This axial view shows patchy ethmoidal clouding. **D,** Marked mucosal thickening of both maxillary sinuses is shown in this axial view.

should be instructed to avoid swimming underwater or diving until completion of therapy because the resultant barotrauma aggravates symptoms and may promote intracranial spread of infection.

Complications of Sinusitis

Infectious sinusitis is important not only because of the discomfort it causes, but also because there is a significant risk of extension of infection and secondary complications. This risk stems from several anatomic factors. First, the sinuses surround the orbits superiorly, medially, and inferiorly. The bony plates that make up the sinus walls are thin and porous, and their suture lines are open in childhood. This is especially

true of the lamina papyracea, which separates the ethmoid air cells from the orbits (Fig. 23-56). Increased sinus pressure occurring as a result of ostial blockage and fluid collection can cause separation of portions of these bony structures and extension of the sinus infection into the orbit. Facial vascular anatomy also contributes to the spread of infection. The veins of the face, nose, and sinuses drain in part into the orbit and then into the ophthalmic venous system, which is in direct continuity with the cavernous sinus. The ophthalmic veins have no valves and thus may provide less defense against spread of infection. The orbit is also devoid of lymphatics, which helps explain the ease of periorbital edema formation when there is increased sinus pressure. The relative looseness

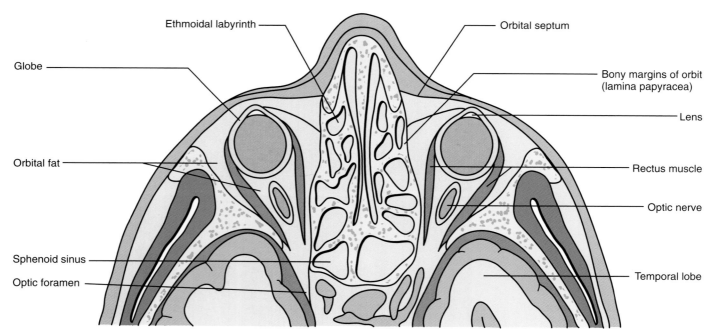

Figure 23-56 The anatomy of the orbit. **A,** Sagittal section shows the relationship of the orbit to the maxillary and frontal sinuses and the position of the orbital septum within the eyelid. The latter structure appears to serve as an anatomic barrier, helping to prevent the spread of infection from periorbital tissues into the orbit. **B,** In this horizontal section the close relationship of the orbit to the ethmoid sinuses is apparent.

Figure 23-57   Pott puffy tumor. **A** and **B,** This patient had fever, headache, and an erythematous swelling over the forehead that was exquisitely tender and had a doughy consistency. **C,** A lateral radiograph shows frontal sinus clouding, irregularity of the frontal bone, and marked soft tissue swelling that is highlighted by a wire placed over the forehead and scalp. (**C,** *Courtesy Kenneth Grundfast, MD, Boston Medical Center, Boston, Mass.*)

of the subcutaneous tissues of the face also assists edema collection and may aid in spread of infection. As a result of these factors, direct extension of infection can occur (1) into the periorbital soft tissues, producing periorbital cellulitis; (2) through the bony walls into the orbits, resulting in orbital cellulitis or a subperiosteal abscess within the bony orbit; (3) via erosion outward through the frontal bone, producing a Pott puffy tumor; or (4) via erosion inward through the frontal bone, resulting in an epidural abscess. On rare occasions, hematogenous seeding of bacteria may occur.

Fortunately, improved recognition of sinus infection and early use of antimicrobial therapy, whether before or early in the course of recognized extension, have reduced the frequency, severity, and morbidity of these disorders.

Pott puffy tumor and epidural abscess, being direct complications of frontal sinusitis, are discussed next. Periorbital and orbital cellulitis, stemming at times from sinusitis and at times from other predisposing conditions, are covered in the subsequent section.

Pott Puffy Tumor

Frontal sinusitis assumes importance after 8 to 10 years of age (once the frontal sinuses have begun to form) and has the potential for serious complications, particularly when neglected or inadequately treated. Erosion occurring anteriorly through the frontal bone results in formation of a subperiosteal abscess, classically known as a *Pott puffy tumor*. This is seen as an erythematous frontal swelling with a doughy consistency and exquisite tenderness (Fig. 23-57). Affected patients tend to be toxic, febrile, and extremely uncomfortable. Prompt surgical drainage is of utmost importance. A CT scan should be obtained before surgical drainage to evaluate the extent of the abscess and to identify other sites of spread. Osteomyelitis of the frontal bone is present, and long-term IV antimicrobials are required for Pott puffy tumor.

Epidural Abscess

Another potential complication of frontal sinusitis is the formation of an epidural abscess as the result of erosion through the posterior wall of the frontal bone. This should be suspected in patients with frontal sinusitis who have unusually high temperature, unusually severe headache, signs of toxicity, or altered sensorium. Diagnosis is best confirmed by CT scan (Fig. 23-58) and MRI. Although IV antimicrobial therapy and careful monitoring may suffice in the management of

small lesions, larger abscesses necessitate neurosurgical consultation and surgical intervention. Further extension of these infections may result in brain abscess (see Chapter 15).

Periorbital and Orbital Infections

Periorbital Cellulitis Caused by Spread from Adjacent Sinusitis

Periorbital cellulitis is the mildest of the complications of infectious sinusitis. The cellulitis is confined to tissues outside the orbit, with spread blocked in part by the orbital septum (see Fig. 23-56). When sinusitis is the underlying condition, the ethmoid or maxillary sinuses are the structures primarily affected. Typically, patients are younger than 4 or 5 years of age and have an antecedent history of upper respiratory tract infection with or without conjunctivitis, otitis, or sinusitis. This is superseded by the sudden appearance of lid and periorbital swelling. In contrast to the uncomplicated sympathetic edema seen in some patients with sinusitis, the swelling in

Figure 23-58   Epidural abscess. This patient had lethargy, high fever, left eye pain, and periorbital swelling after 1 week of severe nasal congestion. A CT scan, obtained to rule out orbital involvement, revealed a small epidural abscess behind the left frontal bone. Note the small central air pocket.

Figure 23-59 Periorbital cellulitis. Intense erythema and edema of the lids are evident. The swollen tissues were indurated and tender on palpation. Ocular motion was normal. Underlying ethmoid sinusitis was confirmed by CT scan.

children with periorbital cellulitis is usually unilateral and is erythematous, indurated, and tender (Fig. 23-59). Conjunctival injection and discharge may also be seen. In many patients a secondary increase in temperature accompanies the onset of swelling, but although most patients appear uncomfortable, toxicity is unusual. The course of periorbital cellulitis resulting from extension of sinus infection is milder and characterized by much slower progression than is true of cases resulting from hematogenous spread.

Periorbital Cellulitis Caused by Hematogenous Spread

When periorbital cellulitis is the result of hematogenous seeding, the organisms tend to be more virulent, the onset more explosive, and the course more fulminant. Typically the patient experiences sudden onset of high fever (often after a mild upper respiratory tract infection) accompanied by the appearance of erythematous, indurated, and tender periorbital swelling, which progresses rapidly and is accompanied by signs of systemic toxicity. The majority of these patients are younger than 1 year of age or only slightly older, and bacteremia with *S. pneumoniae* or *H. influenzae* type B is usual. Widespread use of the *H. influenzae* type B vaccine has dramatically reduced the incidence of *H. influenzae* B–induced cellulitis.

Periorbital Cellulitis Caused by Spread from Adjacent Facial Infection

More than 50% of children with periorbital cellulitis have neither sinusitis nor bacteremia as a predisposing condition. Rather, the patients appear to suffer from extension of nearby facial infection to periorbital tissues. They may have a history of antecedent trauma to the orbit or nearby facial structures, often with a break in the skin (Fig. 23-60) or one of a primary skin infection (impetigo, a pustule, a chalazion, infected dermatitis, or insect bite). They subsequently experience a temperature spike and evolution of periorbital and eyelid edema. This group tends to be somewhat older, generally older than 5 years of age. *Staphylococcus aureus* and group A β-hemolytic streptococci are the predominant offending organisms.

Diagnostic Studies

A number of cultures are often obtained in an attempt to isolate the causative pathogen in cases of periorbital cellulitis. Needle aspiration of the leading edge of the cellulitis has perhaps the highest yield but requires caution. It is perhaps best avoided when the inflamed area does not extend well beyond the orbital rim because of the risk of eye injury if the patient moves suddenly, despite efforts to immobilize his or her head.

Cultures of adjacent skin wounds, when present, are also commonly positive. Nasopharyngeal and conjunctival drainage reveals the offending organism in about one half to two thirds of cases, respectively. Blood cultures are positive in about one third of patients overall, with the highest incidence found in cases caused by hematogenous spread. Sinus radiographs show opacification in more than two thirds of patients without antecedent trauma or skin lesions and in about 40% to 50% of patients with such a history. Ethmoid opacification is the predominant finding. Middle meatus culture, but not nasal culture, may be useful for detection of the sinus pathogen. Radiographic interpretation can be difficult, however, because overlying edema may give a false impression of clouding. In addition, standard radiographs are relatively useless in most cases of hematogenous origin because the patients are typically younger than 1 year of age. CT, however, is an excellent tool for assessing the extent of infection and the presence or absence of sinus opacification, as well as for detecting evidence of early orbital involvement.

Because of the severity and the potential for further extension and hematogenous spread, aggressive IV antimicrobial therapy is urgently required. This necessitates empirical selection of agents to cover likely pathogens, pending culture results. Patients also require close monitoring for signs of complications.

Orbital Cellulitis

In orbital cellulitis, infection extends into the orbit itself. It may take the form of undifferentiated cellulitis, or it may later evolve into a subperiosteal or orbital abscess. Patients tend to have a history similar to that of patients with periorbital cellulitis but are generally more ill, toxic, and lethargic. The most common source of spread is from an adjacent infected ethmoid sinus, although extension from nearby frontal sinusitis or a facial or dental infection occasionally occurs. Causative organisms are the same as those in periorbital cellulitis. Patients old enough to be articulate describe intense, deep retro-orbital pain aggravated by ocular movement. Edema and erythema of the lid and periorbital tissues are often so marked that it is impossible to open the eye without the use of lid retractors (Fig. 23-61, *A* and *B*). Tenderness is exquisite. If the lid can be retracted, the clinician may find proptosis, conjunctival inflammation with chemosis and purulent discharge, decreased extraocular motion, and some loss of visual acuity. Ophthalmologic consultation is required.

Aggressive IV antimicrobial therapy and close monitoring for evolution and CNS complications are vital in the

Figure 23-60 Periorbital cellulitis caused by spread of an adjacent facial infection. This child developed fever and erythematous, tender periorbital swelling a few days after incurring an abrasion as a result of a fall.

Figure 23-61   Orbital subperiosteal abscess. **A** and **B,** This child had a fever, severe toxicity, and marked lethargy. He experienced intense orbital and retro-orbital pain and showed a limited range of ocular motion with associated exacerbation of pain. **C,** This CT scan shows preseptal swelling, proptosis, and lateral displacement of the globe and orbital contents by a subperiosteal abscess.

management of orbital cellulitis. CT is exceptionally useful for determining the presence or absence of abscesses (Fig. 23-61, *C*). When a subperiosteal abscess is present or the clinical ocular examination shows deterioration, surgical drainage combined with an ethmoidectomy are indicated. It is now possible to perform the ethmoidectomy and abscess drainage endoscopically in most patients. Optimal management necessitates a team approach involving pediatrics, otolaryngology, ophthalmology, and at times neurosurgery.

Local complications of orbital cellulitis include abscess formation, optic neuritis, retinal vein thrombosis, and panophthalmitis. CNS complications may result from direct extension or spread of septic thrombophlebitis. Meningitis, epidural and subdural abscesses, and cavernous sinus thrombosis have been described. All are characterized by marked toxicity and alteration in level of consciousness. Cavernous sinus thrombosis is heralded by sudden, bilateral, pulsating proptosis and chemosis in association with increased toxicity and obtundation.

Atopic Disorders

Allergic Rhinitis with Postnasal Discharge

Patients with allergic rhinitis appear to be more susceptible to infectious sinusitis than nonatopic individuals, probably as a result of mucosal swelling in response to allergen exposure and alterations in ciliary action. They can also have symptoms mimicking sinusitis in the absence of infection, and this can be a source of confusion. Two major clinical pictures are seen. In the first, nasal congestion, nighttime cough, and morning throat clearing are prominent. Some patients may complain of morning nausea, and a few may have morning emesis with vomitus containing large amounts of clear mucus. Fever is absent, and in contrast to infectious sinusitis, nasal discharge is never purulent, there is no halitosis, and daytime cough is not prominent. Patients may complain of itching of the nose and eyes, and some have frequent sneezing. On examination, the nasal mucosa is edematous but does not appear erythematous. Discharge, if present, is clear. Patients also tend to have the typical allergic facies (see Chapter 4) with Dennie lines, allergic shiners, and cobblestoning of the conjunctivae. Environmental control and antihistamines provide symptomatic relief for most of these children.

Vacuum Headache

The second potentially confusing clinical picture is that of the allergic sinus headache, or vacuum headache. In this condition, older atopic individuals complain of intense facial or frontal headache, without fever or other evidence of infection. This occurs during periods in which patients are having

exacerbation of allergic symptoms, after swimming in chlorinated pools, or while flying on an airplane. The phenomenon appears to be caused by acute blockage of sinus ostia by mucosal edema, with subsequent creation of a vacuum within the sinus as a result of resorption of sinus gases by mucosa. The resultant negative pressure pulls the mucosa away from the walls of the sinus, producing the pain. In these patients the nasal mucosa tends to be pale and swollen but without discharge. Sinuses may be tender to percussion but are clear radiographically. Symptoms respond promptly to application of a topical vasoconstrictor and warm compresses over the face. Improvement is maintained by antihistamines and decongestants.

OROPHARYNGEAL DISORDERS

Oropharyngeal Examination

Adequate examination of the pharynx is important in pediatrics because of the frequency of pharyngeal infections. However, the procedure can be challenging at times. The small size of the mouth and difficulty in depressing the tongue in infancy; lack of cooperativeness in toddlers; and the fear of causing older children to gag when using tongue blades can impede efforts. These problems can be minimized by a few simple techniques. Infants and young children, when placed supine with the head hyperextended on the neck, tend to open their mouths spontaneously, enabling visualization of the anterior oral cavity and assisting insertion of a tongue blade to depress the tongue and inspect the posterior palate and pharynx. When examining older children, asking them to open their mouths as wide as possible and pant "like a puppy dog" or say "ha ha" usually results in lowering of the posterior portion of the tongue, revealing the posterior palatal and pharyngeal structures. Because conditions involving the lips, mucosa, and dentition are presented in Chapter 20, this section concentrates on palatal and pharyngeal disorders.

Palatal Disorders

Palatal malformations range widely in severity and can significantly affect feeding, swallowing, and speech. In addition, by altering normal nasal and oropharyngeal physiology, they place affected patients at increased risk for chronic recurrent ear and sinus infections.

Cleft Palate

Palatal clefts are among the most severe abnormalities encountered. They stem from a failure of fusion during the second month of gestation and have an incidence of about 1 in every

Figure 23-63 Cleft palate. This child has a midline cleft of the soft palate. The hard palate, alveolar ridge, and lip are spared. *(Courtesy Ms. Barbara Elster, Cleft Palate Center, Pittsburgh, Pa.)*

Figure 23-62 Pierre Robin sequence, characterized by severe retromicrognathia and cleft palate. In this infant the micrognathia produced posterior displacement of the tongue, resulting in airway obstruction that necessitated a tracheotomy. *(Courtesy Wolfgang Loskin, MD, University of North Carolina, Chapel Hill, N.C.)*

2000 to 2500 births. They are usually but not always associated with a cleft lip. The defect is often isolated in an otherwise normal child. In many cases there is a positive family history for the anomaly. A number of teratogens have also been linked to the malformation. In a small percentage of cases the cleft palate is one of multiple congenital anomalies in the context of a major genetic syndrome such as the Pierre Robin sequence (Fig. 23-62) and trisomies 13 and 18 (see Chapter 1).

The extent of the cleft varies: Some involve only the soft palate (Fig. 23-63); others extend through the hard palate but spare the alveolar ridge (Fig. 23-64, *A*). Still others are complete (Fig. 23-64, *B* and *C*). The defect may be unilateral or bilateral. The four major types of congenital cleft palate are as follows:

Type I: Soft palate only (see Fig. 23-63)

Type II: Unilateral cleft of soft and hard palate (see Fig. 23-64, *A*)

Type III: Unilateral cleft of soft and hard palate, extending through the alveolar ridge (see Fig. 23-64, *B*)

Type IV: Bilateral cleft of soft and hard palate, extending through the alveolar ridge (see Fig. 23-64, *C*)

These anomalies create a number of problems beyond the obvious cosmetic deformity. In infancy, a cleft palate prevents the child from creating an effective seal when nursing and hampers feeding. In addition, formula tends to reflux into the nasopharynx with resultant choking. This necessitates patience during feeding, use of palatal obturators or specially designed nipples or feeding devices, and careful training of parents in feeding techniques that facilitate nursing and prevent failure to thrive. Eustachian tube function is uniformly abnormal, and before palate repair, all patients have chronic middle ear effusions that are frequently infected. Even after repair, recurrent middle ear disease (characterized by negative pressure and effusions, and possibly cholesteatomas) remains a problem. Hearing loss, with its potential for hampering language acquisition, ultimately occurs in more than 50% of patients. Despite corrective surgery, palatal function is never totally normal, and many patients continue to have hypernasal speech and difficulties in articulation, necessitating long-term speech therapy. Secondary dental and orthodontic problems are routine as well.

The multitude of problems and the need for frequent medical visits and multiple operations, in combination with the often-associated cosmetic deformity, can have a significant psychological impact on the child and family. Optimal management necessitates a multidisciplinary team, preferably coordinated by a primary care physician who is aware of the patient's individual needs and those of his or her family.

Figure 23-64 Cleft palate. **A,** Cleft of the hard and soft palate, sparing the alveolar ridge. Complete clefts of the palate, alveolar ridge, and lip may be unilateral (**B**) or bilateral (**C**). (**A** and **C**, *Courtesy William Garrett, MD;* **B**, *courtesy Michael Sherlock, MD, Lutherville, Md.)*

Figure 23-65   Submucous cleft of the palate. **A,** This girl shows failure of normal midline fusion of the palatal muscles, resulting in midline thinning of the soft palate. Palpation confirms the area of weakness. A U-shaped notch can also be felt in the midline at the junction of the hard and soft palate. She also has a bifid uvula. **B,** This child was found to have a notched uvula on pharyngeal examination. This may serve as a clue to the presence of a submucous palatal cleft, or it may be an isolated anomaly.

Timing of corrective surgery remains somewhat controversial. Cleft lips are repaired at about 3 months, but scheduling of palatal repair must be individualized depending on the size and extent of the cleft. Defects of the soft palate are generally repaired at about 8 months, and the hard palate is closed either surgically or by use of a prosthetic plate. Most patients also require early myringotomy with insertion of tubes at the time of lip repair to help manage the chronic middle ear disease. Adenoidectomy is contraindicated because of adverse effects on palatal function, unless airway obstruction is severe and resistant to antimicrobial therapy. Upper (partial) adenoidectomy may be required in selected patients with severe airway obstruction.

Another disorder of clinical importance, *submucous cleft of the palate,* is often overlooked in infancy. The condition is characterized by a bony U-shaped notch, palpable in the midline, at the juncture of the hard and soft portions of the palate (Fig. 23-65, *A*). There also may be palpable midline thinning of the soft palate. The anomaly results from a failure of the tensor veli palatini muscle to insert properly in the midline. Some children have an associated double or notched (bifid) uvula that, when present, serves as a clue to the existence of the palatal abnormality (Fig. 23-65, *A* and *B*). The bifid uvula may be an isolated asymptomatic anomaly, however. Although not subject to the feeding difficulties seen in children with overt clefts, children with submucous clefts have similar problems with eustachian tube dysfunction and chronic middle ear disease. Speech is often mildly hypernasal, because the soft palate is of inadequate length or cannot elevate sufficiently to separate the nasopharynx from the oropharynx. Problems therefore occur with the sounds of "f," "b," and "p." Recognition is particularly important when considering tonsillectomy and adenoidectomy for recurrent tonsillitis and otitis because surgical removal of the adenoids in these children can result in severe speech and swallowing dysfunction; hence these procedures may be contraindicated. In selected cases of severe adenoidal hypertrophy or severe adenotonsillitis, upper (partial) adenoidectomy may be an option.

High-arched Palate

High-arched palate, a minor anomaly, is a common clinical finding (Fig. 23-66). Although usually an isolated variant of palatal configuration, it occasionally occurs in association with congenital syndromes. Long-term orotracheal intubation of premature infants creates an iatrogenic form of the problem. Although generally clinically insignificant, the high arch can be associated with increased frequency of ear and sinus infections and hyponasal speech in severe cases.

Tonsillar and Peritonsillar Disorders

Tonsillitis/Pharyngitis

As noted earlier, the tonsils and adenoids are quite small in infancy, gradually enlarge over the first 8 to 10 years of life, and then start to regress in size. When evaluating the tonsils, particularly during the course of an acute infection, or when monitoring patients for chronic enlargement, it is helpful to use a standardized size-grading system, as shown in Figure 23-67. Inspection of the palate is also important in assessing patients with tonsillopharyngitis because lesions characteristic of particular pathogens are often present on the soft palate and tonsillar pillars (see Chapter 12).

The tonsils appear to serve as a first line of immunologic defense against respiratory pathogens and are frequently infected by viral and bacterial agents. The most commonly identified organisms are group A β-hemolytic streptococci, adenoviruses, coxsackieviruses, and the Epstein-Barr (EB) virus. There is a wide range of severity in symptoms and signs, regardless of the pathogenic organism. Sore throat is the major symptom, and it may be mild, moderate, or severe. When severe, it is typically associated with dysphagia. Erythema is the most common physical finding and varies from slightly to intensely red (Fig. 23-68). Additional findings may include acute tonsillar enlargement, formation of exudates over the tonsillar surfaces, and cervical adenopathy. In a small percentage of cases the findings suggest a given pathogen. Patients with fever, headache, bright red and enlarged tonsils (with or without exudate), palatal petechiae (Fig. 23-68, *B*), tender and

Figure 23-66   High-arched palate. This is a common minor anomaly, usually isolated, but occasionally associated with genetic syndromes.

1+ 2+

3+ 4+

Figure 23-67 Grading of tonsillar size for children with acute tonsillopharyngitis and those with chronic tonsillar enlargement. This grading system is particularly useful in serial examinations of a given patient. *(Modified from Feinstein AR, Levitt M: Role of tonsils, N Engl J Med 282:285-291, 1970. Copyright © 1970 Massachusetts Medical Society. All rights reserved.)*

enlarged anterior cervical nodes, and perhaps abdominal pain are likely to have streptococcal infection. Patients with marked malaise, fever, exudative tonsillitis, generalized adenopathy, and splenomegaly are probably suffering from Epstein-Barr virus mononucleosis (Fig. 23-68, *C*; and see Chapter 12). Those with conjunctivitis, nonexudative tonsillar inflammation, and cervical adenopathy may have adenovirus. Yellow ulcerations with red halos on the tonsillar pillars strongly suggest coxsackievirus infection, whether or not other oral, palmar, or plantar lesions are present (see Chapter 12). Unfortunately, the majority of patients with tonsillopharyngitis do not have such clear-cut clinical syndromes. Patients with streptococcal infection may have only minimal erythema; in its early stages, mononucleosis may consist of fever, malaise, and nonexudative pharyngitis without other signs; and although streptococci and EB virus are the most common sources of exudative tonsillitis and palatal petechiae, other pathogens produce these findings as well.

Because of the variability in the clinical picture and the importance of identifying and treating group A β-hemolytic

streptococcal infection to prevent both pyogenic (e.g., cervical adenitis, peritonsillar, retropharyngeal, and parapharyngeal abscesses) and nonpyogenic (e.g., rheumatic fever) complications, a screening throat culture is advisable for patients with even mild signs or symptoms of tonsillopharyngitis. In obtaining this culture, the clinician swabs both tonsils and the posterior pharyngeal wall to maximize the chance of obtaining the organism. In the first 3 years of life, when streptococcal infection is suspected (because of history of exposure, signs of pharyngitis, or scarlatiniform rash), it is helpful to obtain a nasopharyngeal culture as well. For reasons as yet unclear, the nasopharyngeal culture is often positive when the throat culture is negative in this age group.

Treatment is symptomatic for all forms of tonsillopharyngitis except that caused by group A β-hemolytic streptococci, which requires a 10-day course of penicillin, amoxicillin, or erythromycin. As the secondary attack rate of group A β-hemolytic streptococci within families is 50%, parents should be instructed to notify the physician if other family members develop symptoms of upper respiratory or pharyngeal infection within the ensuing few weeks. If so, they can then be examined and specimens obtained for culture, or they can be treated empirically. Follow-up is also important. As noted earlier, the tonsillitis of mononucleosis may appear mild early in the course of the illness, yet tonsillar inflammation and enlargement may progress over a few to several days to produce severe dysphagia and even airway obstruction. Thus parents should be instructed to notify the physician if such signs develop. Follow-up is also important in monitoring for other complications and for frequent recurrences.

Recurrent Tonsillitis

Frequent recurrences of tonsillitis, despite antibiotic therapy when indicated, must be handled on an individual basis. In some cases frequent recurrences of streptococcal infection can be traced to other family members. When they are treated along with the patient, the cycle of recurrences often ends. In other instances frequent recurrent tonsillar infections have no traceable source within the family, and they are significantly debilitating. In children with six or more episodes in any one year, five episodes per year for two consecutive years, or three episodes per year for three consecutive years, tonsillectomy has a favorable outcome in reducing both frequency and severity of sore throats. Tonsillar hypertrophy with obstructive sleep apnea is also an indication for tonsillectomy.

Uvulitis

Uvulitis is characterized by inflammation and edema of the uvula. In addition to throat pain and dysphagia, affected patients commonly complain of a sense of having "something in their throat" or a gagging sensation. The phenomenon has

A B C

Figure 23-68 Tonsillopharyngitis. This common entity has a number of causative pathogens and a wide spectrum of severity. **A,** The diffuse tonsillar and pharyngeal erythema seen here is a nonspecific finding that can be produced by a variety of pathogens. **B,** This intense erythema, seen in association with acute tonsillar enlargement and palatal petechiae, is highly suggestive of group A β-streptococcal infection, although other pathogens can produce these findings. **C,** This picture of exudative tonsillitis is most commonly seen with either group A streptococcal or Epstein-Barr virus infection. *(**B,** Courtesy Michael Sherlock, MD, Lutherville, Md.)*

Figure 23-69   Uvulitis. **A,** The uvula appears markedly erythematous and edematous, with pinpoint hemorrhages, in this case caused by β-streptococci. **B,** In this child with mononucleosis the tonsils are enlarged and covered with a gray membrane, and the uvula is edematous and erythematous. The patient had respiratory compromise because of the severity of his tonsillar and adenoidal hypertrophy. **C,** The vesicular lesions on the swollen, painful uvula of this patient suggest a viral etiology, probably involving an enterovirus.

been reported in association with pharyngitis caused by group A β-hemolytic streptococci, in which cases the uvula is bright red and often hemorrhagic (Fig. 23-69, *A*). The condition has also been noted in association with mononucleosis, both in the presence and the absence of exudative tonsillitis (Fig. 23-69, *B*), and with other viral agents as well (Fig. 23-69, *C*). Uvulitis has also been reported in a patient with concurrent epiglottitis. In this case the child was anxious, toxic, febrile, and drooling, with a more severe clinical picture than that seen with streptococcal or EB virus infection. Culture of the uvular surface grew *H. influenzae* type B.

Peritonsillar Abscess or Cellulitis

A peritonsillar abscess is one that forms between the tonsil and constrictor muscle and extends into the soft palate. Patients are usually school age or older, and they typically have a history of having developed an antecedent sore throat a week or two earlier, which was not cultured or treated, or for which the child was given an incomplete course of antimicrobial therapy. The patient may experience initial improvement but then has a sudden onset of high fever and severe throat pain, which is worse on one side. The pain usually radiates to the ipsilateral ear and is associated with marked dysphagia, such that the patient spits out saliva to avoid swallowing. On examination, the child often appears toxic and has obvious enlargement of the ipsilateral tonsillar lymph node, which is exquisitely tender. Many patients have torticollis, tilting the head toward the involved side to minimize pressure of the sternocleidomastoid muscle on the adjacent tonsillar lymph node (Fig. 23-70*A*). Speech is thick and muffled because

of splinting of the tongue and pharyngeal muscles. Trismus, or limitation of mouth opening, is often noted as a result of inflammation of the internal pterygoid muscles (Fig. 23-70, *B*). If visualization of the pharynx is possible (despite the trismus), a bright red, smooth bulge is seen in the supratonsillar area projecting forward and medially, obscuring the tonsil, and deviating the uvula to the opposite side (Fig. 23-70, *C*). Group A β-hemolytic streptococci and *S. aureus* are the most common pathogens. Mixed infections with gram-positive and gram-negative aerobic, as well as anaerobic, pathogens are common. Patients with mononucleosis, concurrently infected with group A streptococci and treated with steroids, are reportedly at risk for developing a rapidly evolving peritonsillar abscess and complications.

On the basis of the age and level of cooperation from the child, the otolaryngologist may drain peritonsillar abscesses transorally in the office. If examination and cooperation are limited, the abscess may require incision and drainage in the operating room.

Tonsillar Lymphoma

The majority of children, whether well or acutely ill with tonsillitis, have tonsils that are symmetrical in size. When a child has an asymmetrically enlarged tonsil without evidence of infection, the possibility of a lymphoma should be considered (Fig. 23-71). Thorough history of recent health status and meticulous regional and general examination are in order. Particular attention should be paid to cervical and other nodes and to the size and consistency of abdominal viscera. Hematologic studies may also be helpful. In the absence of other

Figure 23-70   Peritonsillar abscess. **A,** This patient demonstrates the torticollis often seen with a peritonsillar abscess in an effort to minimize pressure on the adjacent inflamed tonsillar node. **B,** Sympathetic inflammation of the pterygoid muscles causes trismus, limiting the patient's ability to open the mouth. **C,** This photograph, taken in the operating room, shows an intensely inflamed soft palatal mass that obscures the tonsil and bulges forward and toward the midline, deviating the uvula.

Figure 23-71   Tonsillar lymphoma. This adolescent had painless dysphagia. Examination revealed marked unilateral tonsillar enlargement. The asymmetry and degree of enlargement prompted tonsillectomy. Pathologic examination confirmed a tonsillar lymphoma.

evidence, a brief period of observation may be justified. If other findings are suggestive or enlargement continues during observation, excisional biopsy is indicated.

Penetrating Oropharyngeal Trauma

Penetrating oral injuries are fairly common in childhood and are usually the result of falling with a stick, pencil, straw, or lollipop in the mouth. Gunshot wounds and external stab wounds are unusual occurrences in the pediatric population, but their incidence begins to increase in adolescents. Prophylactic antimicrobial therapy is indicated for all penetrating injuries because of the high risk of secondary infection.

The majority of intraoral injuries involve the palate and consist of simple lacerations. Many of these injuries heal spontaneously and require no repair. Large lacerations producing excessive bleeding or mucosal flaps must be sutured (Fig. 23-72).

Penetration of the posterior pharyngeal wall may result in a number of complications. These patients merit careful clinical evaluation of the oropharynx and neck; neck radiographs

Figure 23-73   Retropharyngeal air dissection. This lateral neck radiograph of a child with a puncture wound of the posterior pharyngeal wall reveals extensive air dissection through the retropharyngeal soft tissues. Subcutaneous air has tracked anteriorly as well.

should also be obtained. Whenever an object penetrates the pharyngeal wall, it introduces oral flora into the retropharyngeal soft tissues, setting the stage for development of infection and abscess formation (see Retropharyngeal Abscess, later; and Fig. 23-75). This complication is seen predominantly in patients who fail to seek care immediately after the injury. However, it can develop even in treated patients. Symptoms generally begin a few to several days after the initial trauma. Fever, pain, dysphagia, and signs of airway compromise predominate.

In a number of patients with posterior pharyngeal tears, penetration results in dissection of air through the retropharyngeal soft tissues (Fig. 23-73). Such children may complain of throat and neck pain. Subcutaneous emphysema may be noted clinically. On occasion, signs of airway compromise develop with this complication. Therefore hospitalization for observation is advisable when this sequela is encountered. Serial plain radiographs should document resolution of subcutaneous emphysema before discharge.

When penetration involves posterolateral structures (e.g., the tear is located near the tonsil or tonsillar pillar), the possibility of vascular injury must be considered. Deep penetration in this area can puncture or nick the internal carotid artery or nearby vessels, resulting in hemorrhage or, more commonly, gradual hematoma formation. Clues to vascular injury are lateral pharyngeal or peritonsillar swelling and fullness or tenderness on palpation of the neck on the side of the wound. Radiographs should confirm soft tissue swelling. Patients with peritonsillar tears should be admitted for observation even in the absence of these signs. Findings that suggest vascular involvement warrant magnetic resonance or CT angiography or, more rarely, formal angiography. Thrombosis and embolic stroke are possible.

Figure 23-72   Palatal laceration. This large, complex laceration occurred when this boy fell with a piece of metal tubing in his mouth. A flap of palatal tissue has retracted away from the tear, warranting surgical approximation.

UPPER AIRWAY OBSTRUCTION

Acute Upper Airway Obstruction

Few conditions in pediatrics are as urgent and potentially life-threatening as those causing acute upper airway obstruction. In these conditions, expeditious assessment and appropriate stabilization are often life-saving. In contrast, underestimation of the severity of distress, overzealous attempts at examination or invasive procedures, and efforts by the unskilled to intervene may have catastrophic results.

The major causes are severe tonsillitis with adenoidal enlargement (see Tonsillar and Peritonsillar Disorders, earlier; and Fig. 23-69, *B*), retropharyngeal abscess, epiglottitis, croup or laryngotracheobronchitis, foreign body aspiration, and angioedema (see Chapter 4). All are characterized by stridor, retractions that are primarily suprasternal and subcostal (unless distress becomes severe and retractions generalize), and mild to moderate increases in heart and respiratory rates. For purposes of assessment, it is helpful to classify the disorders into two categories—supraglottic and subglottic—on the basis of major signs and symptoms listed in Table 23-2.

The key to appropriate management is a brief history detailing the course and associated symptoms, followed by rapid assessment of clinical signs to determine the approximate level of airway involvement and the degree of respiratory distress (Table 23-3). This can be done for the most part through visual inspection, without ever touching the patient. It is particularly important to avoid upsetting a child with upper airway obstruction who shows signs of fatigue or cyanosis or meets any of the other criteria for severe respiratory distress. Such disturbances can serve only to worsen distress and may precipitate complete obstruction. Therefore when a child has signs of moderately severe or severe obstruction, his or her parents should be allowed to remain with him or her; any positional preference (if manifested) should be honored; and oral examination, venipuncture, IV line placement, and radiographs should be deferred until the airway is secure. Once the initial assessment is done, the most skilled personnel available are assembled to stabilize the airway. This procedure is best accomplished under controlled conditions in the operating room, or if necessary in the emergency department.

Supraglottic Disorders

See also "Tonsillar and Peritonsillar Disorders," earlier.

Table 23-2	Clinical Features of Acute Upper Airway Disorders	
Clinical Finding	**Supraglottic Disorders**	**Subglottic Disorders**
Stridor	Quiet and wet	Loud
Voice alteration	Muffled	Hoarse
Dysphagia	+	−
Postural preference*	+	−
Barky cough	−	+ Especially with croup
Fever	+	+ Usually with croup
Toxicity	+	−
Trismus	+ Usually with peritonsillar abscess	−
Facial edema	−	+ Usually with angioedema

Epiglottitis—patient characteristically sits bolt upright, with neck extended and head held forward; *retropharyngeal abscess*—child often adopts opisthotonic posture; *peritonsillar abscess*—patient may tilt head toward affected side.
From Davis HW, Gartner JC, Galvis AG, et al: Acute upper airway obstruction: Croup and epiglottitis, *Pediatr Clin North Am* 28:859-880, 1981.

Table 23-3	Estimation of Severity of Respiratory Distress		
Clinical Finding	**Mild**	**Moderate**	**Severe**
Color	Normal	Normal	Pale, dusky, or cyanotic
Retractions	Absent to mild	Moderate	Severe and generalized with use of accessory muscles
Air entry	↓ (mild)	↓ (moderate)	↓ (severe)
Level of consciousness	Normal or restless when disturbed	Anxious, restless when undisturbed	Lethargic, depressed

↓, decreased.
From Davis HW, Gartner JC, Galvis AG, et al: Acute upper airway obstruction: Croup and epiglottitis, *Pediatr Clin North Am* 28:859-880, 1981.

Retropharyngeal Abscess

A retropharyngeal abscess usually involves one of the retropharyngeal lymph nodes that run in chains through the retropharyngeal tissues on either side of the midline. Because these nodes tend to atrophy after 4 years of age, the disorder is seen primarily in children younger than 3 or 4 years old. The major causative organisms are group A β-hemolytic streptococci, although *S. aureus* is found in some cases. Mixed infections with gram-positive and gram-negative aerobes, as well as anaerobes, are common as well.

The child with a retropharyngeal abscess generally has a history of an acute, febrile upper respiratory tract infection or pharyngitis beginning several days earlier, which may have improved transiently. Suddenly, the child's condition worsens with development of a high spiking fever, toxicity, anorexia, drooling, and dyspnea. On examination, the patient is irritable and tends to lie with the head in a neutral position, as neck movement exacerbates neck tenderness. Quiet gurgling and stertor are often heard. If respiratory distress is not severe, the pharynx can be examined, and asymmetrical swelling of the posterior pharyngeal wall may be observed pushing the uvula and ipsilateral tonsil forward (Fig. 23-74, *A*). Even with direct examination, this swelling can be difficult to appreciate at times. A portable lateral neck radiograph taken on inspiration and with the neck in extension (with a physician in attendance) shows marked widening of the prevertebral soft tissues (Fig. 23-74, *B*), which are normally no wider than a vertebral body.

It should be noted that false-positive radiographic findings of prevertebral soft tissue swelling, in the absence of retropharyngeal pathologic findings, are common when lateral neck radiographs are not taken on inspiration and with the neck extended. When a retropharyngeal abscess is diagnosed, prompt otolaryngologic consultation should be sought to determine whether the mass is fluctuant, necessitating surgical drainage, or if it is in an early cellulitic phase, requiring serial re-examination. A CT scan can be helpful in this regard (Fig. 23-74, *C*). High-dose parenteral antimicrobial therapy is necessary whether or not drainage is required.

As noted earlier, a retropharyngeal abscess may occasionally form in an older child after a puncture wound of the posterior pharyngeal wall (Fig. 23-75). Signs of infection develop acutely a few days later. In these cases oral flora are found on culture.

Parapharyngeal Abscess

Lateral neck space abscesses can also occur in infants and young children. Most patients are toxic with high spiking fevers. The history and clinical picture are nearly identical to those of children with retropharyngeal abscess. However,

Figure 23-74   Retropharyngeal abscess. A young child presented with high fever, drooling, quiet stridor, and an opisthotonic postural preference. **A,** Pharyngeal examination in the operating room revealed an intensely erythematous, unilateral swelling of the posterior pharyngeal wall. **B,** A lateral neck radiograph shows prominent prevertebral soft tissue swelling that displaces the trachea forward. **C,** On CT scan, a thick-walled abscess cavity is evident in the retropharyngeal space. The highly vascular wall enhanced with contrast injection.

Figure 23-75   Retropharyngeal abscess after a puncture wound. This child tried to swallow a tack that punctured and became lodged in the posterior pharyngeal wall. The incident was unwitnessed, and he came to medical attention only when he developed fever and began drooling. *(Courtesy Robert Gochman, MD, Schneider Children's Hospital, Long Island Jewish Medical Center, New Hyde Park, N.Y.)*

these patients have torticollis, bending toward the affected side, and examination of the neck reveals diffuse anterolateral swelling that is exquisitely tender (Fig. 23-76, *A*). Oral inspection may reveal medial displacement of the tonsil or lateral pharyngeal wall. A CT scan is essential to confirm the diagnosis (Fig. 23-76, *B*). Parapharyngeal cellulitis is treated with IV antimicrobials. Abscesses are treated by prompt drainage to prevent rupture with aspiration of purulent material, erosion into vascular structures, and extension to adjacent sites or into the mediastinum.

Epiglottitis (Supraglottitis)

Epiglottitis, a now uncommon but life-threatening form of acute upper airway obstruction, is an infection caused most often by *H. influenzae* type B. Its incidence has dropped precipitously since introduction of the *H. influenzae* B vaccine. Hence many younger practitioners have never seen a case, increasing the risk of delayed diagnosis. Epiglottitis is characterized by marked inflammation and edema of the pharynx, epiglottis, aryepiglottic folds, and ventricular bands. The peak age range is 1 to 7 years, but infants and older children may be affected. Onset is sudden and progression rapid; most patients are brought to medical attention within 12 hours of the first appearance of symptoms. In general, the child is entirely well until several hours before presentation, when he or she abruptly spikes a high fever. This is rapidly followed by progressive quiet stridor, severe throat pain with dysphagia and drooling, and soon thereafter by dyspnea and anxiety.

On examination, the child is usually toxic, anxious, and remarkably still, sitting bolt upright with neck extended and head held forward (unless obstruction is mild or fatigue has supervened) (Fig. 23-77, *A-C*). Quiet gurgling, stridor, and

Figure 23-76 Parapharyngeal abscess. **A,** This infant had high fever, toxicity, and marked, exquisitely tender anterolateral neck swelling with overlying erythema. These manifestations followed a week of upper respiratory tract symptoms and decreased feeding. **B,** His CT scan reveals an encapsulated abscess in the right parapharyngeal area.

drooling are evident, along with dyspnea and retractions. If the child will talk, which is unusual, the voice is muffled. This clinical picture is so typical that, when seen, the best course of action after initial assessment is prompt airway stabilization, usually intubation under controlled conditions by experienced personnel in the operating room. At this time the epiglottis/supraglottis is found to be markedly swollen and erythematous (Fig. 23-77, *D* and *E*). After airway stabilization, cultures can be obtained and parenteral antimicrobial therapy initiated. Obtaining a radiograph or repeating oral physical examinations before transfer to the operating room is contraindicated; it adds nothing and may precipitate total airway obstruction.

On occasion, children present with a similar history but milder symptoms and signs. In these cases, presentation is early or the child is older than average. Respiratory distress is minimal, and visualization of the pharynx can be attempted (without use of a tongue blade) if the child will voluntarily open his or her mouth. In some instances a swollen epiglottis is seen projecting above the tongue. When the history suggests epiglottitis/supraglottitis but clinical findings are mild and the diagnosis is not confirmed by attempted noninvasive visualization, a portable lateral neck x-ray examination (done in the emergency department with a physician in attendance) can be useful. It may reveal mild epiglottic enlargement ("thumbprint sign"; Fig. 23-78) or merely swelling of the aryepiglottic folds

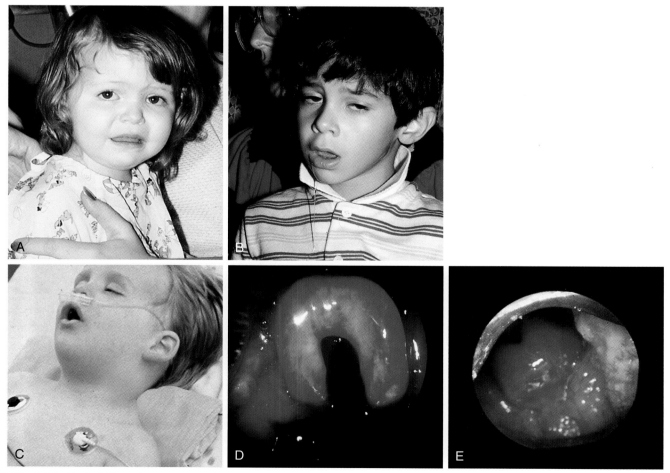

Figure 23-77 Epiglottitis. **A-C,** These three patients with acute epiglottitis demonstrate the varying degrees of distress that may be seen, depending on age and time of presentation. **A,** This 3-year-old seen a few hours after onset of symptoms was anxious and still but had no positional preference or drooling. **B,** This 5-year-old, who had been symptomatic for several hours, holds his neck extended with head held forward, is mouth breathing and drooling, and shows signs of tiring. **C,** This 2-year-old was in severe distress and was too exhausted to hold his head up. **D** and **E,** In the operating room the epiglottis can be visualized and appears intensely red and swollen. It may retain its omega shape or resemble a cherry.

Figure 23-78 Mild epiglottitis or supraglottitis. This lateral neck radiograph demonstrates mild epiglottic swelling and thickening of the aryepiglottic folds.

and ventricular bands. If either is found, the diagnosis is confirmed. Hypopharyngeal dilatation may also be seen. Intubation is generally advisable in the former instance despite mild symptoms, but close observation in the intensive care unit on intravenous antibiotic therapy (covering for *H. influenzae* type B) may suffice when mild supraglottitis is the only finding.

Subglottic Disorders

Croup or Laryngotracheobronchitis

Croup, an acute respiratory illness, is characterized by inflammation and edema of the pharynx and upper airways, with maximal narrowing in the immediate subglottic region. There is probably a component of laryngospasm as well. The majority of cases are caused by viral pathogens, with parainfluenza, respiratory syncytial virus, adenoviruses, influenza viruses, and echoviruses being the agents most commonly identified. The peak season is between October and April in the northern hemisphere. The disorder primarily affects children between the ages of 6 months and 3 years. This is probably because their airways are narrower, and the mucosa is both more vascular and more loosely attached than in older children, enabling greater ease of edema collection. Older children can be affected, however.

Typically the child has had symptoms of a mild upper respiratory tract infection with rhinorrhea, cough, low-grade fever, and perhaps a sore throat for 1 to 5 days before developing symptoms of croup. The change is generally sudden and usually occurs at night or during a nap. The child awakens with fever, loud inspiratory stridor, a loud "barky" or "seal-like" cough, and hoarseness. The severity of symptoms and the course vary widely and are highly unpredictable. Duration averages 3 days but can be as brief as 1 day or as long as 1 week. Most patients have a waxing and waning course, with symptoms more severe at night, but it is impossible to predict which night will be the worst. Some patients remain relatively mildly affected throughout the course, whereas others progress either slowly or rapidly to severe distress. Airway drying, probably in part as a result of mouth breathing necessitated by nasal congestion (especially while sleeping), appears to aggravate the cough and possibly the element of laryngospasm.

Physical findings are highly variable, depending on degree of distress at the time of presentation. Most affected children are moderately febrile but not toxic and have a loud barky cough and loud inspiratory stridor, with suprasternal and subcostal retractions (Fig. 23-79) and a mild decrease in air entry. A small percentage of patients with more extensive airway inflammation may have wheezing on auscultation. Distinguishing the stridor of croup from the wheezing of asthma is most important. Many patients improve substantially as a result of exposure to cool night air during the trip to the emergency department. Some have restlessness or agitation reflecting hypoxia, and a few have severe distress. In these more severely affected patients, stridor may be both inspiratory and expiratory, with generalized retractions. If impairment of airflow is extreme, fatigue supervenes, stridor abates, and retractions diminish. *This must not be mistaken for clinical improvement.* A clinical scoring system that helps in grading severity of distress is presented in Table 23-4. In mild to moderate cases the pharynx can be visualized and reveals only mild erythema. *Oral examination should be deferred in severe cases until the airway is secure.* Radiography can be helpful in demonstrating subglottic narrowing—the "steeple sign" (Fig. 23-80, *A*). However, this is not necessary for patients with mild disease, and it is contraindicated for those with severe distress. Gastroesophageal reflux disease is commonly associated with recurrent croup. Thus, management with medication; a low-fat, low-acid, low-spice diet; and avoidance of overeating and excessive drinking can be helpful.

Management depends largely on severity of distress when the child is seen and on clinical response to mist therapy. Most patients have mild disease, improve considerably on mist alone, and can be managed at home with humidification. Parents must, however, be instructed to watch for signs of increasing distress, which would warrant return to the hospital. Aerosolized racemic epinephrine is effective in reducing airway obstruction caused by croup. It is particularly useful for children with moderate obstruction who do not show marked improvement on mist alone, and it can provide significant relief for children with severe distress. This agent, although effective, is short-acting, and rebound airway edema tends to occur. Thus patients requiring racemic epinephrine should generally be admitted for further observation.

Figure 23-79 Croup. This toddler with moderate upper airway obstruction caused by croup had suprasternal and subcostal retractions. Her anxious expression was the result of mild hypoxia confirmed by pulse oximetry.

Table 23-4	Croup Scoring System			
Clinical Finding	**0**	**1**	**2**	**3**
Stridor	None	Mild	Moderate inspiratory at rest	Severe, on inspiration and expiration, or none with markedly decreased air entry
Retractions	None	Mild	Moderate	Severe, marked use of accessory muscles
Air entry	Normal	Mild decrease	Moderate decrease	Marked decrease
Color	Normal	Normal (0 score)	Normal (0 score)	Dusky or cyanotic
Level of consciousness	Normal	Restless when disturbed	Anxious, agitated when undisturbed	Lethargic, depressed

Modified from Taussig LM, Castro O, Beaudry PH, et al: Treatment of laryngotracheobronchitis (croup): Use of intermittent positive-pressure breathing and racemic epinephrine, *Am J Dis Child* 129:790-793, 1975.

Administration of intramuscular dexamethasone (sometimes followed by a 2- to 3-day course of oral prednisone) appears to reduce the severity of symptoms and thus the need for hospitalization.

Patients in severe distress who do not improve dramatically after treatment with racemic epinephrine, as well as those who steadily worsen in the hospital despite mist and aerosol treatments, merit airway endoscopy and stabilization, via intubation or tracheotomy under controlled conditions in the operating room. The choice of procedure remains controversial and is perhaps best made in accordance with the skills of the personnel and facilities available at the individual institution. In some instances, subglottic narrowing is so severe as to necessitate tracheotomy (Fig. 23-80, *B*). Attempts at emergency tracheotomy in the emergency department are fraught with hazard and should be avoided at all costs.

Bacterial Tracheitis

In a small percentage of cases, children with a crouplike picture are atypically toxic, markedly febrile, and have rapidly progressive airway obstruction necessitating urgent intubation and occasionally tracheotomy. Bronchoscopy before airway stabilization reveals severe inflammation; edema; and a copious, purulent subglottic exudate that contains large numbers of bacteria. Most of these patients appear to have a history of viral croup with sudden worsening. It is thus thought that the disorder may represent secondary bacterial infection, and staphylococci including methicillin-resistant strains are often isolated.

Foreign Body Aspiration

Foreign body aspiration is seen for the most part in older infants and toddlers. The story is usually one of a sudden choking episode while the child was eating material that the immature dentition is ill equipped to chew. Such foods include nuts, seeds, popcorn, raw vegetables such as carrots and celery, and hot dogs. On occasion, the episode occurs when the child is chewing on a small object, a toy, or a detachable portion of a toy. If the object lodges in the larynx, asphyxiation results unless the Heimlich maneuver or back blows are performed promptly. In the majority of cases the foreign material clears the larynx and lodges in the trachea or a bronchus (more commonly, the right mainstem because of its more vertical orientation). After the choking spell, there is a silent period usually lasting up to several hours (occasionally days or weeks), after which the child develops cough, stridor (if

Figure 23-80 Croup. **A,** This radiograph reveals a long area of narrowing extending well below the normally narrowed area at the level of the vocal cords. The finding is often termed the *steeple sign.* **B,** In this patient, direct visualization revealed subglottic narrowing so severe that only tracheotomy would enable establishment of an adequate airway. (**A,** *Courtesy Sylvan Stool, MD.*)

Steeple sign

Subglottic narrowing

Figure 23-81   Foreign body aspiration. Radiopaque objects and those well outlined by air are readily visualized on radiographs. **A,** A piece of eggshell is seen in the subglottic portion of the trachea, clearly outlined by the air column. **B,** An earring lies in the entrance of the right mainstem bronchus. **C,** A screw is seen lodged in the right mainstem bronchus and projecting into the trachea. (**A,** *Courtesy Mananda Bhende, MD, Children's Hospital of Pittsburgh, Pittsburgh, Pa.;* **B** *and* **C,** *courtesy Robert Gochman, MD, Schneider Children's Hospital, Long Island Jewish Medical Center, New Hyde Park, N.Y.*)

the object is lodged in the trachea) or wheezing (if it is lodged in a bronchus), and respiratory distress. In this acute phase, when the object is situated in a bronchus, wheezing may be unilateral and associated with decreased breath sounds. Later, diffuse wheezing may be heard, simulating asthma or bronchiolitis.

Lateral neck and chest radiographs may reveal aspirated objects that are radiopaque or outlined by the air column (Fig. 23-81, *A-C*), enabling localization before endoscopy. However, most cases involve materials not visible on radiographs, although other radiographic clues may be present. Partial obstruction of a bronchus creates a ball-valve effect, allowing air in during inspiration but preventing its egress on expiration. This produces hyperinflation of one or more lobes of the lung on the same side as the foreign body (Fig. 23-82), which may be evident on the plain chest film. In subtler cases, chest fluoroscopy may highlight the differential inflation and

Figure 23-82   Foreign body aspiration with ipsilateral hyperinflation. This 18-month-old child was eating popcorn when he suddenly began choking. Within a few hours, he developed significant respiratory distress and his chest radiograph revealed massive hyperinflation of the right lung caused by the ball-valve effect of a piece of popcorn lodged in the right mainstem bronchus. (*Courtesy Department of Radiology, Uniontown Hospital, Uniontown, Pa.*)

deflation, showing mediastinal shift away from the side of the foreign body on exhalation (Fig. 23-83). These findings are particularly likely if the patient is seen fairly soon after the aspiration episode.

When there is a delay in seeking medical attention (usually because the aspiration episode was unwitnessed and onset of symptoms insidious), the patient may have cough and fever. In these instances, atelectasis and a mediastinal shift toward the side of the foreign body may be found on the chest radiograph (Fig. 23-84). This finding also may be seen acutely when the bronchus is totally obstructed. Many patients presenting acutely have no detectable radiographic abnormality after foreign body aspiration. Hence when clinical suspicion is high, given the history and physical findings, rigid endoscopic examination (with forceps for foreign body removal available) is indicated despite normal plain films. Conversely, when physical findings and x-ray films are normal and the history is questionable, a period of close observation may be indicated.

Unfortunately, in up to 50% of cases, the aspiration episode is not reported because the parent does not relate it to the child's symptoms or did not witness the choking spell. For this reason, this diagnosis should be considered and specific questions asked regarding possible aspiration whenever a young child has acute onset of cough and stridor, develops asymmetric breath sounds, or experiences a first episode of wheezing. Persistent cough or wheezing after a choking episode warrants endoscopic evaluation for possible foreign body removal. A missed retained foreign body may lead to total airway obstruction if the foreign body lodges in the larynx, or it may chronically obstruct a bronchus leading to lung abscess and the need for lobectomy.

Chronic Upper Airway Obstruction

Laryngeal Examination

In children with a subacute or chronic airway disorder, a laryngeal examination is necessary to arrive at a definitive diagnosis. If a child is in distress or has acutely decompensated, this examination should be done in an operating room where rigid

Figure 23-83 Foreign body aspiration, inspiratory and expiratory radiographs. **A,** This inspiratory film taken during fluoroscopy suggests hyperinflation of the right lower and middle lobes. **B,** This becomes much more evident on exhalation, when the hyperinflation persists and the mediastinum shifts to the opposite side. *(Courtesy Robert Gochman, MD, Schneider Children's Hospital, Long Island Jewish Medical Center, New Hyde Park, N.Y.)*

ventilating bronchoscopes and an anesthesiologist are available as backup. When the child is not in significant distress and the airway has been stable, laryngoscopy can be performed by an otolaryngologist in the office or emergency department, using a flexible fiberoptic nasopharyngolaryngoscope (Fig. 23-85, *A*). These are now available in a range of diameters suitable for pediatric patients. Letting the older child handle the scope (with close supervision) and look through the lens assists cooperation. The child is then prepared by spraying the nasal mucosa with a decongestant and topical lidocaine. With careful preparation, most patients can be examined in the parent's lap or an examination chair, but the toddler usually requires immobilization on a papoose board. The fiberoptic tube is then gently inserted into the nose and guided through past the palate (Fig. 23-85, *B*). If the child is exclusively mouth breathing, the soft palate may be apposed to the posterior pharyngeal wall. Asking the child to try to breathe through the nose a few times moves the palate forward, assisting passage. Anatomic abnormalities and dynamic motion of the supraglottic and glottic structures are easily seen with this device. Asking the child to phonate by saying the letter *e* enables observation of cord movement. In infants, cord movement is generally observed with crying. Although less well seen, the subglottic space can generally be viewed as well.

Subglottic Stenosis

Subglottic stenosis is a disorder in which the subglottic region of the trachea is unusually narrow in the absence of infection. In some instances the stenosis is the result of abnormal cricoid development and is therefore congenital. In other cases narrowing is the long-term result of injury and scarring from prior intubation. Regardless of the source, these children tend to develop stridor and respiratory distress with each upper respiratory tract infection. A few are identified by virtue of having an atypically prolonged episode of croup. Some also have stridor with crying, even when well. Neck x-rays may present a similar appearance to that seen with croup (steeple sign; see Fig. 23-80, *A*).

The problem generally improves with growth, but up to 40% of these children develop such severe distress with colds that tracheotomy and reconstruction are required. Figure 23-86, *A* shows laryngeal findings resulting from endotracheal tube trauma with formation of obstructing granulation tissue that later developed into severe glottic and subglottic stenosis requiring tracheotomy (Fig. 23-86, *B*). Figure 23-87 shows the endoscopic view of a child with a laryngeal laceration and fracture due to blunt neck trauma who required tracheotomy and later developed subglottic stenosis.

Figure 23-84 Foreign body aspiration—delayed presentation. **A,** With delay in presentation of partial obstruction or with complete obstruction of a bronchus, radiographic findings consist of atelectasis and a mediastinal shift *toward* the side of the foreign body. **B,** In this case a peanut was found completely obstructing the bronchus. *(Courtesy Robert Gochman, MD, Schneider Children's Hospital, Long Island Jewish Medical Center, New Hyde Park, N.Y.)*

Figure 23-85 Fiberoptic laryngoscopy. **A,** The flexible fiberoptic laryngoscope. **B,** With careful preparation the patient can tolerate insertion of the flexible fiberoptic scope and the examination.

Laryngomalacia

Laryngomalacia, a congenital condition, accounts for greater than 70% of cases of persistent inspiratory stridor in infants. The problem is the result of unusual flaccidity of the laryngeal structures, especially the epiglottis and the arytenoid cartilages. The etiology is uncertain, but it is thought to be caused by lack of neural coordination of the laryngeal muscles, with the result that supraglottic structures hang over the airway entrance like a set of loose sails over a sailboat (Fig. 23-88).

Because the stridor is inspiratory, it does not represent true wheezing and bronchodilators should not be used.

Clinically these infants tend to have mild inspiratory stridor that is worse when they are lying supine and tends to improve when they are placed in the prone position or when their necks are slightly hyperextended. The condition is usually benign and rarely interferes with feeding or respiration. The diagnosis can be confirmed only by visualization of the larynx during active respiration. This is important in that it is necessary to document that the stridor is not the result of a more dangerous condition. Once the examination has been completed, the parents can be reassured that the condition is usually benign and that with growth the stridor typically abates by the end of the first year and a half of life. Management consists of observation, with particularly close monitoring during upper respiratory tract infections. GERD often occurs concomitantly with laryngomalacia, and empirical treatment of GERD often results in reduction of stridor. The occasional infant with unusually severe obstruction must be managed surgically with supraglottoplasty.

Even though a child has the classic presentation of laryngomalacia, other significant airway problems may mimic this disorder, and thus endoscopy in the office or operating room to confirm the diagnosis is always required. For example, Figure 23-89, *A* shows an endoscopic view of a vallecular cyst that displaced the epiglottis in a posterior direction, creating airway obstruction that mimicked laryngomalacia. Cyst excision was curative (Fig. 23-89, *B*).

Vocal Cord Paralysis

Paralysis of the vocal cords may be present at birth, or it may develop in the first 2 months of life. It may be bilateral or unilateral. The underlying problem is generally located somewhere along the vagus nerve and may be found in the central nervous system or in the periphery. Even though many cases are idiopathic, a thorough evaluation must be done in an effort to locate the lesion and identify its source. Ten percent of chronic stridor cases in neonates are thought to be due to this condition.

Infants with unilateral cord paralysis have stridor, hoarseness, and a weakened voice or cry. The airway diameter is generally adequate for respiration, and unless a secondary lesion is present, it is rarely necessary to perform a tracheotomy. This problem is most often caused by a cardiac abnormality or cardiovascular surgery because the recurrent

Figure 23-86 **A,** Glottic granulation tissue from prolonged intubation. **B,** Severe posterior glottic and subglottic stenosis. The granulation tissue and mucosal injury in **(B)** are organized into a severe scar with a pinhole airway necessitating chronic tracheotomy.

Figure 23-87 Laryngeal trauma. This child sustained a fracture of the thyroid cartilage from blunt neck trauma. This is the endoscopic view of the laceration to the right side of the right true vocal cord. This child required open repair and tracheotomy for airway stabilization.

laryngeal nerve is looped around these structures as it passes through the chest.

In contrast, bilateral vocal cord paralysis is a life-threatening condition that presents with stridor and cyanosis because the vocal cords are unable to abduct on inspiration with consequent severe narrowing of the aperture between the cords (Fig. 23-90). As the problem is usually associated with a depressed laryngeal cough reflex, aspiration is common. A tracheotomy may be essential to secure the airway. Hydrocephalus or an Arnold-Chiari malformation is often the underlying problem because each causes compression of the vagus nerves as they leave the brainstem. Neurosurgical intervention may correct the problem and allow eventual decannulation.

Juvenile Laryngeal Papillomatosis

Juvenile laryngeal papillomatosis is a condition in which multiple benign papillomas develop and grow on the vocal cords and supraglottic structures. In a few patients they may extend to involve the pharyngeal walls or tracheal mucosa. They are of viral (human papillomavirus) origin, and there is some evidence of transmission during delivery to children born to mothers with condylomata acuminata. The main symptom is hoarseness, but stridor may develop in children with large lesions or tracheal extension. Radiographs are usually normal. The diagnosis should be considered in patients with chronic hoarseness and in those with atypically prolonged croup. On laryngoscopy, irregular warty masses are seen (Fig. 23-91). Biopsy is required to confirm the diagnosis. Excision can be performed with forceps, a laser, or a powered microdebrider, but it is often followed by regrowth. Tracheotomy should be avoided if at all possible because this may promote seeding farther down the tracheobronchial tree.

Vascular Compression of the Trachea

Persistent expiratory wheezing or stridor that is unresponsive to bronchodilators may result from vascular compression of the trachea (Fig. 23-92) or tracheobronchomalacia. Symptoms are exacerbated by infections with increased respiratory requirements and increased secretions. Importantly, vascular compression of the trachea and tracheomalacia produce *expiratory* stridor. This is in sharp contrast to laryngomalacia, which produces *inspiratory* stridor.

Figure 23-88 Laryngomalacia. **A,** Note the omega shape of the epiglottis and the elongation of the arytenoid cartilages. **B,** This is the larynx during inspiration. Note that the forces of the inspired air lead to collapse of the laryngeal inlet. Infolding of the epiglottic surfaces and the arytenoid cartilages causes partial airway obstruction.

Figure 23-89 **A,** Vallecular cyst. Large mucous retention cyst in the vallecula, displacing the epiglottis in a posterior direction and leading to severe airway obstruction and stridor that mimicked laryngomalacia. **B,** Endoscopic excision of the superior cyst wall was curative.

Figure 23-90 Bilateral vocal cord paralysis. **A,** The marked narrowing of the aperture between the cords stems from loss of ability to abduct on inspiration. The voice may be normal in some cases because the vocal cords can adduct. This is in contrast to normal opening and closing on inspiration and expiration as seen in **(B)** and **(C).**

ESOPHAGEAL FOREIGN BODIES

Ingestion of foreign objects is relatively common in older infants and toddlers, who are prone to putting almost anything they can pick up into their mouths. Coins, small toys, and pieces of toys are the objects most frequently found. Most traverse the esophagus, stomach, and intestines without incident and are of little concern. A small percentage of swallowed foreign bodies, being too large to pass through to the stomach, become lodged in the esophagus (usually at the level of the cricopharyngeus [C6] and less commonly at the level of the aorta [T4] or the diaphragmatic inlet [T11 to T12]). With mild obstruction, the child may refuse solid foods (although 17% of patients are asymptomatic); with moderate obstruction, liquids often are refused as well, or the child may appear to choke with drinking. When obstruction is nearly complete, the child may begin drooling. If the object is particularly large or produces an inflammatory mass over time, it may compress the trachea as well, producing signs of airway obstruction. Older patients may complain of neck or substernal pain or discomfort, especially with swallowing.

Patients who have significant symptoms of esophageal or respiratory obstruction and those who have ingested sharp, potentially toxic, or caustic objects should undergo prompt endoscopic removal. Those who have ingested smooth objects and have mild symptoms can be observed for 12 hours and then have a repeat x-ray examination. If the object has passed into the stomach, endoscopy can be avoided. Otherwise, endoscopic removal is indicated.

Although in many cases there is a clear history of ingestion, in a significant percentage the ingestion was not witnessed. A high level of suspicion is often required to make the diagnosis, and the possibility of an esophageal foreign body should be considered in evaluating any young child for a sudden change in eating pattern. Plain radiographs detect metallic and other radiopaque objects (Fig. 23-93). Most ingested objects are plastic, however, and require barium swallow or in some cases endoscopy for detection. Delays in diagnosis can result in stricture formation or, more rarely, esophageal perforation with secondary pneumomediastinum, mediastinitis, pneumonia (Fig. 23-94), and/or large vessel hemorrhage.

Similar to the concerns for button battery foreign bodies in the nose, special comment is necessary for button battery esophageal foreign bodies. When a button battery is suspected on the basis of history or radiographic imaging, prompt removal is warranted. The button battery is extremely destructive and may lead to esophageal perforation or tracheoesophageal fistula if it is not removed immediately.

OTOLARYNGOLOGIC MANIFESTATIONS OF GASTROESOPHAGEAL REFLUX DISEASE

Over the past two decades, increased recognition and study of gastroesophageal reflux disease (GERD) have led to greater understanding of the disorder and its protean manifestations. As noted earlier, infants with GERD may develop nasopharyngeal congestion with varying degrees of mucosal inflammation, edema, and rhinorrhea. This is the result of exposure of

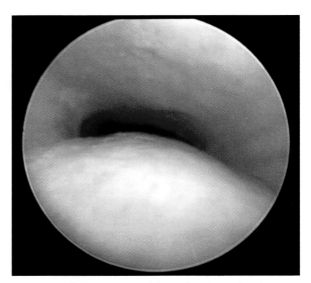

Figure 23-92 Vascular compression of the trachea. Anomalous innominate artery compression of the distal anterior tracheal wall. The presentation of this child was that of intractable wheezing during expiration that did not respond to bronchodilators. The child improved after thoracotomy for lifting (*pexy*) of the innominate artery off the trachea by sewing it to the inner surface of the sternum.

Figure 23-91 Laryngeal papillomas. Multiple smooth, warty growths are seen nearly occluding the larynx in this child who had a history of chronic hoarseness.

Figure 23-93 Esophageal foreign bodies. **A,** This youngster accidentally swallowed a coin. He complained of throat pain and refused oral intake. When initially seen, the coin was lodged high in the esophagus. **B,** After observation overnight, repeat radiography revealed that the coin had moved down but was still lodged in the esophagus. The patient underwent endoscopic removal. Note that asymmetrical objects in the esophagus are oriented in the coronal plane, whereas in the larynx, they lie in the sagittal plane (see Fig. 23-81, *A*). *(Courtesy Robert Gochman, MD, Schneider Children's Hospital, Long Island Jewish Medical Center, New Hyde Park, N.Y.)*

Figure 23-94 Esophageal foreign body. An unwitnessed ingestion of this safety pin led to a period of anorexia followed by fever and respiratory distress. The point of the pin had perforated the esophageal wall and pleura, causing a secondary right upper lobe pneumonia. *(Courtesy Robert Gochman, MD, Schneider Children's Hospital, Long Island Jewish Medical Center, New Hyde Park, N.Y.)*

mucosal surfaces to gastric juices. Affected infants who are still obligate nose breathers may have respiratory distress with feeding (sucking) and are often reported to snore during sleep. Some, but by no means all, have a history of vomiting and/or frequent spitting up, and parents may report that at times some of the regurgitated material comes out the nose.

Reflux has also been associated with cough and wheezing, especially during sleep. In most cases this reflects a reflex bronchospastic response to esophageal mucosal irritation, whereas in others, more severe reflux into the posterior pharynx with aspiration may be causative. In the latter, severe bouts of coughing and bronchospasm with patchy infiltrates on chest radiograph may be seen. Infants who aspirate repeatedly may be noted on bronchoscopy to have cobblestoning of the posterior tracheal mucosa (Fig. 23-95, *A*) and may also have prominent edema and inflammation of glottic structures (Fig. 23-95, *B*). Chronic or intermittent hoarseness can be an associated feature. GERD has also been found to be causative in cases of recurrent croup and contributes to laryngeal edema in laryngomalacia. In still other infants, reflux of even a minute amount of gastric contents onto the vocal cords can precipitate intense laryngospasm with attendant apnea. This tends to occur when the baby is laid down shortly after a feeding. If the apnea is unwitnessed and laryngospasm is prolonged, this can prove fatal. As noted earlier, subclinical GERD is common in infants with laryngomalacia and it is also present in the majority of infants with acquired subglottic stenosis.

In addition to vomiting or spitting up, infants with GERD may have a range of symptoms of esophagitis. These may include crying after every few swallows with feeding (as reflux is induced by swallowing); refusal to feed; and arching and writhing movements of the neck and back, which constitute Sandifer syndrome. It is important to recognize that Sandifer movements; other symptoms of esophagitis; and snoring,

Figure 23-95 Airway manifestations of gastroesophageal reflux. **A,** This cobblestoned appearance of the posterior tracheal mucosa is the result of chronic inflammation in an infant with severe gastroesophageal reflux and recurrent aspiration. **B,** In this infant there is so much edema of the arytenoid mucosa that the arytenoids obscure the view of the posterior portion of the vocal cords. (**A,** *Courtesy Anil Gungor, MD, Anadolu Foundation Healthcare System, Cayirova Mevkii, Gebze, Turkey.)*

cough, and bronchospasm that are worse during sleep can all occur in isolation or in any combination, and that they are often seen in the absence of overt vomiting and spitting. Hence when infants have these symptoms persistently, evaluation for GERD and/or empirical therapy should be instituted.

NECK DISORDERS

Neck disorders including adenitis, congenital cysts, and vascular and lymphatic masses and tumors are commonly managed by otolaryngologists. Limitations of space have required us to be selective in presenting disorders in this chapter. The reader is referred to Chapter 12 for a discussion of cervical adenitis and to Chapter 17 for a description of mass lesions.

ACKNOWLEDGMENTS

The authors acknowledge and thank Children's Hospital of Pittsburgh, Department of Radiology, and University of Pittsburgh School of Medicine, Department of Neuroradiology, for providing many of the radiographs and CT scans in this chapter.

Bibliography

American Academy of Pediatrics, Subcommittee on Management of Acute Otitis Media: Diagnosis and management of acute otitis media, *Pediatrics* 113:1451–1465, 2004.

Bluestone CD, Stool SE, editors: *Pediatric otolaryngology*, ed 4, Philadelphia, 2002, WB Saunders.

Bluestone CD, Wald ER, Shapiro GC: The diagnosis and management of sinusitis in children: Proceedings of a closed conference, *Pediatr Infect Dis J* 4:549–555, 1985.

Bowen AD, Ledesma-Medina J, Fujioka M, et al: Radiologic imaging in otorhinolaryngology, *Pediatr Clin North Am* 28:905–939, 1981.

Casey J, Adlowitz D, Pichichero M: New patterns in the otopathogens causing acute otitis media six to eight years after introduction of pneumococcal conjugate vaccine, *Pediatr Infect Dis J* 29:304–309, 2010.

Davis HW, Gartner JC, Galvis AG, et al: Acute upper airway obstruction: Croup and epiglottitis, *Pediatr Clin North Am* 28:859–880, 1981.

Gellady AM, Shulman ST, Ayoub EM: Periorbital and orbital cellulitis in children, *Pediatrics* 61:272–277, 1978.

Gwaltney JM Jr, Phillips CD, Miller RD, et al: Computed tomographic study of the common cold, *N Engl J Med* 330:25–30, 1994.

McAlister WH, Lusk R, Muntz HR: Comparison of plain radiographs and coronal CT scans in infants and children with recurrent sinusitis, *Am J Roentgenol* 153:1259–1264, 1989.

Melnick M, Bixler D, Nance WE, et al: Familial branchio-oto-renal dysplasia: A new addition to the branchial arch syndromes, *Clin Genet* 9:25, 1976.

Orobello P, Park R, Belcher L, et al: Microbiology of chronic rhinosinusitis in children, *Arch Otolaryngol Head Neck Surg* 117:980–983, 1991.

Rosenfeld R, Bluestone CD, editors: *Evidence-based otitis media*, Hamilton, ON, Canada, 1999, BC Decker.

Rowland PS, Smith TL, Schwartz SR, et al: Clinical practice guideline: Cerumen impaction, *Otolaryngol Head Neck Surg* 139(3 Suppl 2):S1–S21, 2008.

Ungkanont K, Yellon R, Weissman J, et al: Head and neck space infections in infants and children, *Otolaryngol Head Neck Surg* 112:375–382, 1995.

Wald ER: Acute sinusitis in children, *Pediatr Infect Dis J* 2:61–68, 1983.

Wald ER, Milmoe GJ, Bowen A, et al: Acute maxillary sinusitis in children, *N Engl J Med* 304:749–754, 1981.

Zhang L, Mendosa-Sassi R, Cesar J, et al: Intranasal corticosteroids for nasal airway obstruction in children with moderate to severe adenoidal hypertrophy, *Otolaryngol Head Neck Surg* 140:451–454, 2009.

FUNDAMENTALS OF PEDIATRIC RADIOLOGY

Sameh Tadros | Vera Sperling | Sunhee Kim

The last three decades have produced an enormous era of technical advance, data acquisition, and data transfer especially pertaining to imaging. This has resulted in significant changes in protocols for imaging of various symptom complexes. New imaging modalities such as computed tomography (CT), magnetic resonance (MR), and positron emission tomography (PET) have expanded our ability to diagnose previously hidden conditions and also our knowledge of these conditions.

The goal of this chapter is to highlight pediatric imaging and to review the imaging issues faced in routine pediatric practice. This chapter is not meant to be a comprehensive review of the subject because many well-selected radiology images and related discussions have been included in the other chapters. The first section includes an introduction to pediatric radiology and radiation safety, and conveys concise, up-to-date information on imaging modalities as they are applied to each body part. The second section describes the various CT and MR applications in neuroimaging. The last section covers key concepts on how and why nuclear medicine and PET procedures are performed.

INTRODUCTION

Children have special needs and different disease processes, and thus the diagnostic imaging approaches are also different. Pediatric imaging should be problem oriented. Communication between the referring physician and the pediatric radiologist is encouraged (e-Table 24-1). The essential components of a pediatric imaging facility are listed in Table 24-1.

Imaging Modalities

Pediatric diagnostic imaging can be achieved by various modalities (Table 24-2). X-rays are used in conventional radiography, computed radiography (CR), fluoroscopy, angiography, and computed tomography (CT). Gamma rays are used in nuclear scintigraphy and positron emission tomography (PET). Ultrasonography uses inaudible sound waves ranging in frequency from 1 to 20 MHz to produce images, whereas magnetic resonance (MR) images are generated with a strong magnetic field and radiofrequency (RF) pulse. The digital age has provided us with picture archiving and communication systems (PACS). A PACS eliminates the use of films, permits rapid retrieval of images and remote viewing, and compacts storage.

Child-friendly Atmosphere

A few simple techniques can help create a positive hospital experience for the child. Distraction in the waiting room may be beneficial for children of all ages, and can be achieved with posters, pictures, and toys. Effective distraction for toddlers includes interactive toys, pinwheels, blowing bubbles, and singing. School-age children enjoy blowing bubbles, TV/video games, books, counting, and deep breathing. Teenagers may prefer deep breathing, stress balls, TV/video games, books, and music.

The well-trained imaging staff can relieve the patient's apprehension and decrease time and effort to obtain the optimal examination. Technologists should have a gentle demeanor and wear child-friendly, cheerful uniforms.

Child life specialists are specially trained to help children prepare for health care experiences and enable them to cope with imaging or invasive procedures. If aspects of a procedure are painful or uncomfortable, any child older than age 2 is prepared in advance with truthful information, using words that can be understood. The child life specialist is especially useful in some situations, such as (1) a child whose injuries have resulted from suspected child abuse; (2) a child admitted with accidental injuries (e.g., a motor vehicle accident); (3) a child newly diagnosed with chronic illness; (4) a child who recently experienced traumatic loss or has a chronic illness (developmental delay); (5) a child who exhibits oppositional behavior; (6) a child having difficulty coping with a necessary procedure, that is, crying, fighting or hiding; and (7) a child who needs preparation for an invasive procedure.

Environment

The imaging room's environment is modified to reduce a child's anxiety. Smaller equipment can be hidden or concealed with covers and images. Large equipment such as CT scanners can be decorated to give a sense of adventure (Fig. 24-1), and allow study acquisition without sedation. Other distraction techniques include lamps placed in the line of vision of the patient and displaying entertaining images on the ceiling (Fig. 24-2), or the release of piquant aromas in the imaging room (e.g., coconut). Movie goggles allow the child to watch a favorite movie while undergoing magnetic resonance imaging (MRI) or a nuclear medicine scan.

Positioning

The technologist usually allows parents to be present in the examining rooms and even to assist with some studies. This decreases the repeat rate and so decreases the radiation dose to the child. When a child lies supine, he or she may feel vulnerable. Comfort positions can give children a sense of control and help them feel more relaxed, that is, sitting on a chair or in a parent's lap, hand-holding with a parent, or hugging. The child is encouraged to participate in producing the best possible examination by being permitted to make individual choices (e.g., placement of a toy or blanket, the position of a parent, the flavor of oral contrast material, or the selection of a bandage).

Figure 24-1 PET/CT suite known as "Camp Cozy."

Figure 24-2 Child-friendly light display that shines on the walls and ceiling of the ultrasound examination room.

Language

The radiology team should always remember to use simple language for child-friendly explanations. For children of any age, the wrong choice of words can have a negative impact and potentially long-lasting effects. Avoid saying "dye/contrast"; say instead, "a drink/sticky water that helps the doctor see the inside of your belly clearer in your pictures." Also, describe the imaging room environment in ways that can be related to the child's home, for example, the noise of a CT scanner can be described to be like that of a "washing machine," or a urinary catheter can be described as a "tiny straw that takes out pee-pee and puts in the x-ray water." Young children have little sense of time; the radiology team should always prepare them to know when they will be done with their examination. For example, if a child is undergoing a voiding cystourethrogram (VCUG), avoid saying, "this will only take 15 minutes"; instead, say "you'll be all finished and get up after you potty on the table for us."

Table 24-1	Essential Components of Pediatric Imaging

- Communication and consultation between practitioners and radiologists
- Patient and parent preparation
- Child-friendly atmosphere
- Safe patient immobilization and sedation
- Radiation protection
- Age-appropriate imaging techniques

From Osborn LM, DeWitt TG, First LR, et al, editors: *Pediatrics,* Philadelphia, 2005, Mosby Elsevier.

Table 24-2	Advantages and Disadvantages of Imaging Modalities	
Modality	**Advantages**	**Disadvantages**
X-ray film	Fast; relatively inexpensive; available	Uses radiation; poor soft tissue contrast; two-dimensional imaging only
Fluoroscopy	Real-time imaging; relatively inexpensive; available; useful in operating room; can be portable	Uses radiation; no cross-sectional imaging
CT	Readily available; excellent delineation of bones, soft tissues, and calcification; multiplanar and 3D reconstruction; minimally invasive (CT angiography); assists in interventions	Intermediate to high radiation dose; relatively expensive; IV contrast side effects (nephrotoxicity and anaphylaxis); weight limit
MRI	Excellent soft tissue characterization; no ionizing radiation; multiplanar imaging; minimally invasive (MR angiography); functional imaging; assists in interventions	Less readily available; expensive; claustrophobia often a problem; lengthy exams; limited use in unstable patients; may need sedation/GA; metal artifact; contraindicated with cardiac pacemakers and some devices; gadolinium-induced nephrogenic systemic fibrosis (NSF) in patients with renal impairment; weight limit
Ultrasound	Portable; inexpensive machine; real time; least expensive cross-sectional imaging modality; no radiation; differentiates cystic vs. solid masses; multiplanar imaging; Doppler evaluation of blood flow; assists in interventional procedures	Difficult with obese and immobile patients; highly operator dependent; bone and gas obscure anatomy
Nuclear medicine	Readily available; functional/molecular imaging	Intermediate to high radiation dose; weak anatomic analysis; may need sedation; radioactive urine and body fluids; expensive

3D, three-dimensional; CT, computed tomography; GA, general anesthetic; IV, intravenous; MRI, magnetic resonance imaging.

Table 24-3	Estimated Medical Radiation Doses for a 5-Year-Old Child	
Imaging Area	**Effective Dose (mSv)**	**Equivalent No. of CXRs**
Three-view ankle	0.0015	1/14th
Two-view chest	0.02	1
Anteroposterior and lateral abdomen	0.05	2½
Tc-99 m radionuclide cystogram	0.18	9
Tc-99 m radionuclide bone scan	6.2	310
FDG PET scan	15.3	765
Fluoroscopic cystogram	0.33	16
Head CT	4	200
Chest CT	3	150
Abdomen CT	5	250

CT, computed tomography; CXRs, chest x-rays; FDG PET, fluorodeoxyglucose positron emission tomography; Tc-99 m, technetium-99 m.

Data provided by R. Reiman, MD (Occupational and Environmental Safety Office, Radiation Safety Division [www.safety.duke.edu/RadSafety], written communication, 2006). From Brody AS, Frush DP, Huda W, et al: Radiation risk to children from computed tomography, *Pediatrics* 120:677-682, 2007.

Effective Radiation Dose

Effective dose is expressed as an SI unit, the millisievert (mSv) (Table 24-3). A major benefit of the effective dose is that it permits all radiologic examinations that use ionizing radiation to be directly compared, using a simple common scale. Note that the effective radiation dose of one adult chest radiograph (0.1 mSv) is comparable to natural background radiation for 10 days (background radiation is 3 mSv/year in the United States; people living in Colorado or New Mexico receive about 1.5 mSv more per year than those living near sea level, that is, 4 to 5 mSv/year).

Radiation Safety

The radiologist as "consultant" can triage imaging examinations to eliminate inappropriate referrals or to use procedures with less or no ionizing radiation. Imaging protocols must be as evidence-based as possible and the American College of Radiology (ACR) and the Society of Pediatric Radiology (SPR) guidelines should be implemented.

Americans were exposed to more than seven times as much ionizing radiation from diagnostic medical procedures in 2006 than they were in the early 1980s. The increase over the past quarter century puts the cumulative national medical exposures on a level with natural background radiation exposure (Fig. 24-3). The estimated cumulative individual dose from all sources in the early 1980s was 3.6 mSv and in 2006 was 6.2 mSv, almost double the previously reported value. The increase in medical exposure was the only significant change in the two estimates. The largest part of the increase in medical exposure was from CT scans, amounting to almost one half of the imaging exposure, and nuclear cardiac scans, amounting to one fourth of the current total (Fig. 24-4). In 2006 alone, more than 63 million CT scans were performed in the United States. Approximately 7 million CT scans were obtained in children in 2007. Children are at increased risk from radiation because of their greater sensitivity to radiation and a longer lifetime to manifest those changes. To be safe, we should act as if low doses of radiation cause harm using the ALARA (as low as reasonably achievable) principle routinely.

The exact radiation risk in CT examinations, and even whether a risk absolutely exists, are controversial topics. However, most scientific and medical organizations support the concept of the linear, no-threshold model for ionizing radiation risk of cancer induction, and believe that radiation even at low levels (doses below 100 mSv) may have a harmful effect. This assumption, however, overlooks cellular repair mechanisms. Some researchers estimate the increased risk that a young child might develop cancer related to an abdominal CT scan is in the magnitude of 1:4000. This is based on the most widely used estimate of risk of cancer from ionizing radiation at 5% per sievert (Sv), and the diagnostic imaging doses are in the millisievert (mSv) range (5 mSv for abdominal CT). One should also note that the background lifetime risk of fatal cancer is 20% to 25% (1 in 4 or 5). The benefits of CT are real and known, and the risks are tiny and unknown.

Conservative estimations of potential risk (i.e., any required assumptions are made toward the direction of overestimating risk rather than underestimating it) show that the potential risk of dying from undergoing a CT examination is less than that of drowning or of a pedestrian dying from being struck by any form of ground transportation, both of which most Americans consider to be extremely unlikely events (e-Table 24-2); this provides a comparison of the statistical odds of dying from an abdominopelvic CT examination relative to other causes of death. It can be seen that the lifetime risk of a fatal cancer from all causes is 22.8%, and the lifetime potential risk of a fatal cancer from the radiation associated with a body CT examination is approximately 0.05%.

The ordering physician needs to ensure that a CT scan is justified, and the radiologist needs to optimize the scan. Because children are smaller than adults and need less radiation to create the same signal-to-noise ratios, the tube current (milliamperes, or mA) can be greatly reduced when imaging a small child. Other techniques include reducing the peak kilovoltage (kVp); using in-plane shielding for areas such as the eye, thyroid, and breasts; increasing beam pitch; and picking a CT manufacturer that has put effort into dose-reducing technology (e.g., adaptive statistical iterative reconstruction, or ASIR) (Fig. 24-5).

The "Image Gently" Campaign

The Alliance for Radiation Safety in Pediatric Imaging has created resources to address the relative risk of CT for children, including parent information pamphlets and a convenient medical imaging record card, similar to the familiar immunization card, for parents to track their child's imaging history. This card may be distributed by pediatricians or downloaded by parents from the Image Gently website (e-Fig. 24-1). This card alerts families and their doctors to the frequency of patient imaging examinations. With relocation of families and the use of different hospital centers in the same community, this card may help decrease the number of repeat examinations performed.

RADIOGRAPHY

Introduction

Advantages of Radiography in Pediatric Imaging

The advantages of radiography in pediatric imaging include the following:

1. Fast
2. Relatively inexpensive
3. Available

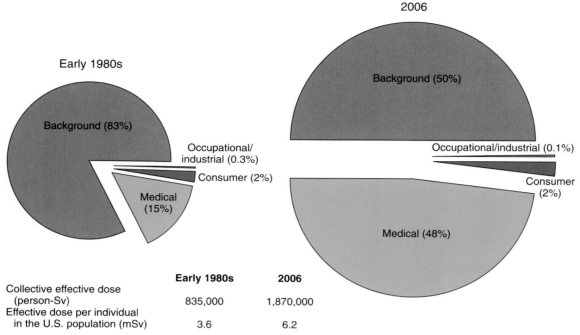

	Early 1980s	**2006**
Collective effective dose (person-Sv)	835,000	1,870,000
Effective dose per individual in the U.S. population (mSv)	3.6	6.2

Figure 24-3 Exposure of the population of the United States to ionizing radiation in the early 1980s and in 2006, according to National Council on Radiation Protection and Measurements (NCRP) report no. 160 (*Ionizing radiation exposure of the population of the United States*). (*From Schauer DA, Linton OW: National Council on Radiation Protection and Measurements report shows substantial medical exposure increase*, Radiology 253:293-296, 2009.)

4. No need for sedation

5. Portable

6. Plain films of the chest and skeletal system are important (about 50% of all pediatric imaging consists of chest radiographs)

Disadvantages

The disadvantages of radiography in pediatric imaging include the following:

1. Uses ionizing radiation

2. Poor soft tissue contrast

3. Two-dimensional imaging only

Physics

X-rays are a form of short electromagnetic radiation produced by energy conversion when fast-moving electrons from the cathode filament of the x-ray tube interact with the tungsten anode (target) (Fig. 24-6). The amplitude of the tube current

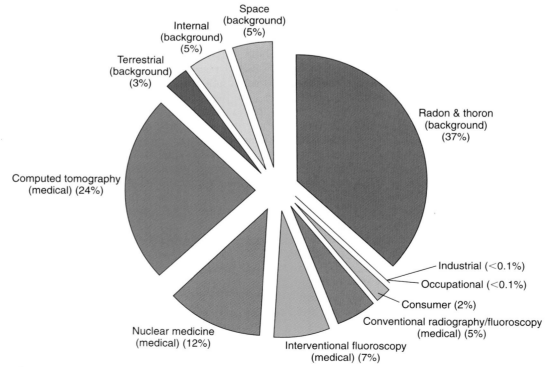

Figure 24-4 Collective effective dose as a percentage for all exposure categories in 2006, according to National Council on Radiation Protection and Measurements (NCRP) report no. 160 (*Ionizing radiation exposure of the population of the United States*). (*From Schauer DA, Linton OW: National Council on Radiation Protection and Measurements report shows substantial medical exposure increase*, Radiology 253:293-296, 2009.)

Figure 24-5 Targeted low-dose CT of the upper chest of a 12-year-old for follow-up of left upper lobe cavity *(arrow)*; effective dose, 0.5 mSv. **A,** Axial image; **B,** coronal reformatted image.

(expressed as milliamperes, or mA) depends on the emission rate of electrons from the cathode, which is determined by the cathode temperature. The speed of the electrons as they are propelled from the cathode to the anode is determined by the x-ray tube potential (kilovoltage peak, or kVp). When an x-ray beam is directed toward the examined part of the body, an image is formed. The resultant image is a recording of internal body structures in which the black areas represent the least dense body structures that have allowed the x-rays to pass through (i.e., lungs) and the more dense structures (i.e., bone), which have absorbed the x-rays, appear white (e-Fig. 24-2).

Computed radiography (CR) has replaced conventional film-based radiography. The acquired image is displayed instantly on the high-resolution monitor of the PACS. e-Table 24-3 lists common indications for plain radiography.

Radiography of the Airway

The anteroposterior (AP) and lateral views of the neck are useful in assessing the trachea, pharynx, retropharynx, epiglottis, tonsils, adenoids, and bony skeleton. Stridor is one of the most common indications for imaging the neck. Other indications include snoring, hoarseness, abnormal cry, neck mass, suspected foreign body, epistaxis, trauma, and caustic ingestion.

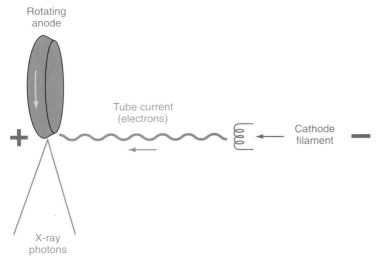

Figure 24-6 X-ray production.

Lateral Soft Tissues of the Neck

The retropharyngeal soft tissues extend from the adenoids, which are visible by 3 to 6 months of age, to the origin of the esophagus at the level of C4 to C5. A useful ratio is the width of the retropharyngeal soft tissue to that of the C2 vertebral body. The ratio varies in inspiration from almost 1.0 before 1 year of age to 0.5 by 6 years of age. The soft tissue width should not exceed 50% of the accompanying vertebral body to C4 (Fig. 24-7). Expiratory tracheal buckling can create buckling of the trachea anteriorly, causing an apparent increase in retropharyngeal soft tissues and creating a "pseudo-retropharyngeal abscess" (Fig. 24-8). Pseudo-retropharyngeal abscess can be differentiated from a true abscess when the appropriate inspiratory film demonstrates supraglottic airway and hypopharyngeal distention with air (Fig. 24-9). Appropriate patient positioning is critical. The examination of the lateral view of the soft tissues of the neck must be performed in slight extension and during inspiration (Fig. 24-10). The most common cause of a pseudo-retropharyngeal abscess is a film taken during expiration or swallowing, or with an improperly positioned child.

The lateral view of the neck is optimal for evaluating the supraglottic airway (see Fig. 24-7). The lower border of the nasopharynx is the hard palate, soft palate, and uvula. The oropharynx (below the hard and soft palate) leads to the air spaces at the base of the tongue, which are the valleculae. Immediately behind the valleculae is the epiglottis. The hyoid bone is inferior and anterior to the valleculae. The oropharynx also merges posteriorly with the nasopharynx to form the hypopharynx. The tonsils are seen in the lateral walls of the hypopharynx. Anteriorly, the hypopharynx leads to the larynx and becomes the esophagus. The pyriform sinuses are the most lateral and inferior margins and provide a landmark for the level of the vocal cords.

The lateral film is important in the assessment of (1) the encroachment of adenoidal tissue on the nasopharyngeal airway; (2) retropharyngeal swelling/abscess (air in the retropharyngeal space); (3) the degree of hypopharyngeal airway distention as a measure for airway encroachment (croup); and (4) identification of a radiopaque foreign body. Calcification in respiratory cartilage, although very rare in children, is pathologic; it is seen in chondrodysplasia punctata and relapsing polychondritis. The hyoid bone may be ossified at birth.

Anteroposterior Film of the Neck

The frontal radiograph is best for evaluation of tracheal position. Normally, the trachea is slightly deviated to the right by the aortic arch (deviation to the left is always abnormal). A normal thymus will not affect the trachea. Expiration causes

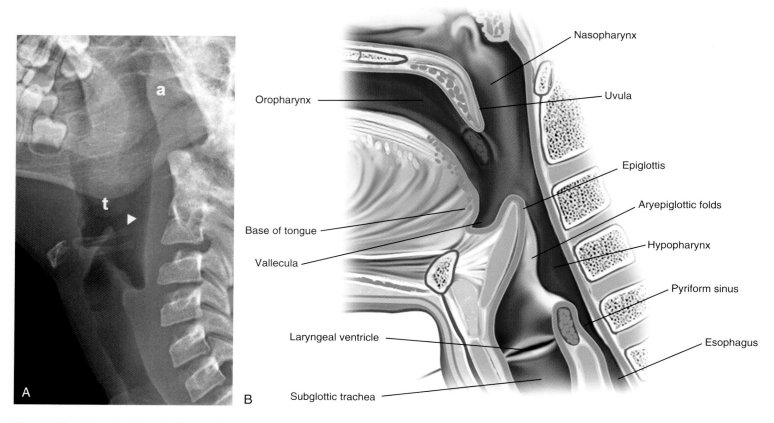

Figure 24-7 **A,** Lateral radiograph of a normal airway. The cornua of the hyoid *(arrowhead)* point to the epiglottis. a, adenoids; t, tonsil. **B,** Diagrammatic representation of the normal anatomy of the upper airway. (**B,** *From Blickman JG, Parker BR, Barnes PD: Pediatric radiology: The requisites, ed 3, Philadelphia, 2009, Mosby Elsevier.)*

buckling of the trachea to the right (see Fig. 24-8). Note that the airway is a dynamic system and changes in caliber and position so that an isolated, single film may be quite misleading. Nonetheless, an abnormal configuration of the airway should be pursued in light of the clinical history.

Chest Radiograph

Interpretation of the Chest Film:
1. The Radiologist's Circle

A systematic approach to the radiographic evaluation is crucial for anyone dealing with children. Comparison with previous imaging studies is mandatory and is facilitated by the use of a PACS. A chest film is always examined for information about the heart and lungs, but radiologists look first at the nonpulmonary areas, that is, the abdomen, bones, soft tissues, and airway, to be sure that they do not miss any abnormality. Only then should one progress to the mediastinum. A good habit to develop is to imagine a circle on the film so as to dispense with all the noncardiopulmonary areas. Begin at the corners, where the patient information is. Check the name, date, and especially the left and right markers. An easy way to complete the circle is to progress from the name tag to the markers to the ABCS of the film: A, abdomen; B, bones; C, chest (airway, mediastinum, lungs, and diaphragm); and S, soft tissues. Carefully observe the easily missed areas: under the

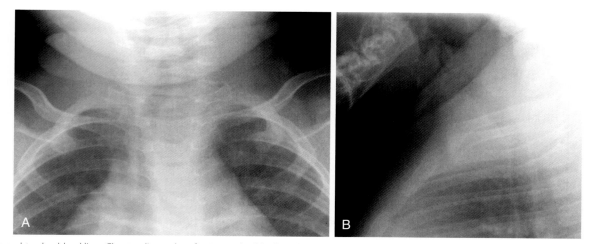

Figure 24-8 Normal tracheal buckling. Chest radiographs of a 4-month-old infant demonstrate tracheal buckling, a normal occurrence when the film is exposed during flexion and/or expiration. **A,** In the frontal projection, normal tracheal buckling occurs rightward, away from the aortic arch. **B,** Anterior buckling is evident on the lateral projection. This normal anterior tracheal displacement frequently causes confusion because it simulates a retropharyngeal mass. Note that the airway should be visible on all normal chest films.

Figure 24-9 Effect of phase of respiration on the prevertebral soft tissue space. *Arrow* in **A** demonstrates the prevertebral soft tissue widening on expiration that disappears on inspiration **(B).** *(From Blickman JG, Parker BR, Barnes PD:* Pediatric radiology: The requisites, *ed 3, Philadelphia, 2009, Mosby Elsevier.)*

diaphragm, through the heart, paraspinal lines, lung apices, shoulders, and soft tissues of the neck.

On every chest film, read the abdominal portion as you would read an abdominal film. Evaluate the abdomen (regardless of how little of it can be seen) on every chest film, and note whether the stomach bubble is on the left and the liver on the right. Is it an erect film? If so, examine it specifically for calcifications, gallstones, or pancreatic calcification.

Determine the presence of bowel distention, air–fluid levels, and free intraperitoneal air. The heart and liver are transparent organs; one can see opacities or bronchial markings projecting over their shadows. Then look at bones and soft tissues; one can often see portions of the arms, shoulders, ribs, sternum, and mandible, as well as cervical, thoracic, and lumbar vertebrae. Be alert for fractures (Fig. 24-11), congenital abnormalities (e.g., absent clavicles), bone destruction, or other signs of disease. Examine the soft tissues of the neck, thorax, and abdomen to detect any swelling, foreign body, calcifications, and so on. The soft tissues may reveal multiple artifacts, such as hair braids, buttons, bandages, electrocardiogram (ECG) electrodes, or redundant skin folds. Soft tissue swelling or subcutaneous calcifications can be clues to systemic disease.

Figure 24-10 False-positive identification of a retropharyngeal mass. **A,** An examination with poor head extension suggests a retropharyngeal mass. **B,** A repeat examination with better head extension and pressure applied to the anterior neck with a lead-gloved finger; the retropharyngeal soft tissues are normal. Intervention with a gloved finger is seldom necessary if the film is repeated in full extension and inspiration. *(From Hilton SvW, Edwards DK III:* Practical pediatric radiology, *ed 3, Philadelphia, 2006, Saunders Elsevier.)*

Figure 24-11   Supine chest radiograph of a 3-day-old newborn with surfactant deficiency. A radiologist interpreting this chest film systematically, that is, by examining the ABCS (A, abdomen; B, bones; C, chest [airway, mediastinum, lungs, and diaphragm]; and S, soft tissues), shouldn't miss the fracture involving the right humerus at the edge of the image. Note that the patient is rotated to the left with the heart appearing prominent, likely due to rotation.

Interpretation of the Chest Film: 2. Technical Factors

Degree of Inspiration: Lung Volumes

On an adequate film obtained during deep inspiration, nine posterior ribs and five anterior ribs should be seen above the diaphragm. If the child is too young to cooperate, expose on full inspiration, during normal respiration. Babies' and toddlers' breathing is abdominal: watch for an expanded abdomen in the AP position. The child/baby must not be crying during exposure. If so, inspiration will be too deep, and the overinflated lungs may create a misleading appearance that can be mistaken for pathology. The differences in appearance on inspiration and expiration are more marked than in adults. With a good inspiratory effort on the frontal view, less than one third of the heart projects below the dome of the diaphragm; the domes of the diaphragm are rounded (if very domed, the film is expiratory). If the child has taken a shallow breath, the heart may appear enlarged; the vessels may coalesce to give a false impression of an opacity, especially in the region of the bases and hila. On the lateral view, obliquely oriented hemidiaphragms are seen in good or possibly increased lung volume (if horizontally oriented, the film is expiratory). The vertebral bodies become blacker as we progress from superior to inferior on the lateral view.

Position of the Patient

Conventional radiographs of the chest are frequently produced with a portable machine and with the younger patient (less than 2 years of age) placed supine. Upright films can be obtained after age 2; until 3 or 4 years old the patient is usually sitting for an AP projection. Children aged 5 years and over can stand for a posteroanterior (PA) projection. Proper immobilization and positioning are mandatory. For radiation protection purposes, the primary beam must be collimated within the area of the cassette, and pediatric lead rubber aprons, obtainable in several sizes, should be used for gonadal protection. Frontal views are often the only ones necessary, but lateral views can be obtained as indicated.

When the x-ray passes through the patient from back to front (a PA projection), the heart is closer to the film and is less magnified. Conversely, if the x-ray beam enters the front of the patient's chest, passes through the back and onto the film (an AP projection), the magnified heart and great vessels may give the impression of cardiomegaly. This is a common problem with portable chest films, which are taken in the AP projection. Also, the closer the tube to the film, the more the

magnification. Routinely, portable films are exposed 40 inches (1 m) from the tube, adding to the magnification. This is compared to 6 feet (1.8 m) used in the erect patient, which causes less magnification.

When the patient is supine, the vascular supply to the upper and lower lobes of the lungs is equal because gravity has no effect. When sitting or standing, gravity plays a significant role, and the upper lobe vessels are less distended than the lower lobe vessels and consequently smaller (one third to two thirds size). One can determine that a film was produced with the patient in the erect position by looking at the air–fluid level in the stomach and by comparing the relative sizes of the upper and lower pulmonary vasculature.

Determining Rotation

If the patient is well centered on the frontal view: (1) the medial aspects of the clavicles are symmetrical in relation to the midline; (2) the anterior ribs are equidistant from ipsilateral pedicles; (3) the position of the carina approximates the right pedicles; and (4) the two lungs are symmetrical in density. The signs of rotation include asymmetrical clavicles, a difference in lung aeration, heart projected over one hemithorax and not the other, and asymmetrical ribs when relating the anterior rib to the pedicles (see Fig. 24-11). On the lateral view, the ribs are not seen posteriorly in the straight (unrotated) patient. If the patient is slightly rotated, the ribs are shown on each side posterior to the spine.

Adequacy of Exposure

Adequacy of exposure can be assessed on the frontal film by examining the vertebral column behind the heart. The exposure is correct when we can see (1) the detailed spine and pedicles behind the heart, and (2) the pulmonary vessels in the peripheral lung. If we can see only the spine but not the pulmonary vessels, the film is too dark (overexposed).

Mediastinum

The mediastinum is composed of the thymus, trachea, heart, great vessels, esophagus, lymph nodes, and neural elements. The mediastinum is divided on the lateral radiograph into (1) the anterior portion, including the space in front of the heart and great vessels; (2) the middle portion, that is, the space between the anterior and posterior mediastinal components, including the heart, airway, esophagus, and lymph nodes; and (3) the posterior portion, including everything behind a line connecting the mid-portion aspects of the vertebrae, including the vertebrae, neural elements, and paraspinal lymph tissue. In some classifications the posterior mediastinum begins with the anterior aspect of the vertebral body.

Thymus

The thymus may make interpreting pediatric chest radiographs difficult. It can simulate cardiac enlargement, lobar collapse, pulmonary infiltrates, and mediastinal masses. The thymus constitutes the major portion of the mediastinal silhouette in a normal newborn. It may extend from the lung apex to the diaphragmatic surfaces; be insinuated into the minor fissure on the right, giving a "sail sign" (see e-Fig. 24-2); and may be bilaterally symmetrical or predominantly one-sided (Fig. 24-12). The normal thymus is a "soft" organ situated in the anterior mediastinum and never "pushes" on the airway or any other intrathoracic structure. The thymus appears smaller as the child becomes older, but the thymus weighs most in adolescents. It is prominent in some children until 4 to 5 years of age, and may persist beyond 5 years, confounding interpretation. Thymic remnants can remain in adults and will be gradually replaced by fat. In an unwell child the thymus can decrease in size and is often not seen. The contour of the

Figure 24-12 Coronal MRI of the chest (short tau inversion recovery [STIR] sequence) demonstrates a left-sided normal thymus in a 7-month-old infant. An anterior cut shows the "wavy thymus sign" *(arrows)* as the thymus insinuates itself between the anterior ribs (r).

Figure 24-13 Chest radiograph of a 1-day-old newborn shows the wavy thymus contour.

thymus is "wavy" because it insinuates itself between the anterior ribs (Fig. 24-13; and see Fig. 24-12).

Effect of Age on the Normal Appearance of the Heart

The shape of the heart on plain radiographs changes with the patient's age. The heart in younger individuals appears more globular in shape, making analysis of specific chamber abnormality difficult. The newborn right heart chambers are larger than the left, and before closure of the patent ductus arteriosus, right-sided cardiac output is greater than left-sided output. This makes identification of the aortic arch difficult or impossible. The right atrial contour in the frontal view and the right ventricular contour in the lateral view will appear abnormally enlarged in these patients. Furthermore, the transverse diameter of the heart is increased, thus increasing the normal cardiothoracic ratio. The thymic shadow regresses by the end of the first year of life, and the heart appears to rotate and descend into the chest. The typical "normal" appearance of the heart does not begin to become apparent until 6 to 8 years of life. However, through adolescence, the apparent size of the main pulmonary artery segment remains increased. Through the teens and early twenties, the size of the main pulmonary artery and base of heart continue to decrease, and the size of the aortic arch increases in caliber, so that by the mid-twenties, the appearance of a "normal" heart may be characterized (Fig. 24-14).

Neonatal Chest Radiograph

Manipulating preterm infants for radiographs must be done with care. Attention must be directed to maintaining oxygen levels, preventing cardiorespiratory complications, preventing heat loss, warming cassettes, and paying attention to good hand washing. Gonad/thyroid shielding is placed on top of

Figure 24-14 **A,** Posteroanterior radiograph of a 30-year-old woman is shown. The lateral border of the left-sided aortic arch (Ao) and proximal descending aorta *(short arrows)* are clearly seen. The main (MP) and proximal left (L) pulmonary artery are seen cephalad to the left bronchus *(long arrow)*. The left atrial appendage section *(small arrowhead)* is inferior to the crossing of the left bronchus and cephalad to the left ventricular contour *(curved arrows)* of the left heart border. The superior vena cava is not seen on this examination. However, the ascending aorta *(small open arrow)* is seen barely over the hilar right pulmonary artery (R). The right atrial contour *(large arrowheads)* extends just to the right of the spine. **B,** Spin-echo MRI obtained from a different 30-year-old woman is shown. The left heart border–forming structures are the aortic arch (Ao), which is to the left of the trachea (T), the distal main pulmonary artery (PA), left atrial appendage (aa), and anterolateral portion of the left ventricle (LV). The transverse right pulmonary artery (RP) passes over the left atrium (LA). Notice that the Ao and PA are equal in caliber. The mitral valve *(small arrows)* and coronary sinus *(large arrow)* are shown. *(From Boxt LM: Plain-film examination of the normal heart, Semin Roentgenol 34:169-180, 1999.)*

the incubator rather than inside it. The cross-table lateral film is used when there is a possibility of free air (pneumothorax or pneumomediastinum). Because the infant is supine, and air rises to the most nondependent location, air can be seen under the sternum.

The airway should be visible on all chest films. The trachea is not a midline structure (the carina projects adjacent to the right pedicles). Buckling of the trachea is normal. The airway is a dynamic structure that changes in caliber; however, if on all views the airway is persistently small, further investigation is necessary. It is normal for neonates and young infants to occasionally have some air in the esophagus (not so in older children). The ideal position of the endotracheal tube is at the level of the inferior margins of the clavicles, or about 1.5 vertebral bodies above the carina.

The aortic arch frequently cannot be seen in a neonate, and its position must be inferred from the position of the carina. If the carina overlies the right pedicles, the aortic arch is left-sided. A right-sided aortic arch may be inferred if the position of the carina is at the midline or to the left. A right aortic arch should alert the physician to the possibility of congenital heart disease and/or a vascular ring. In neonates and infants the cardiothoracic ratio can be up to 60% (the adult dimension is 50%). Measuring the heart size on an AP film is accurate in this age group as there is minimal magnification of the heart (unlike in adult AP chest radiographs). If the heart is large, it should appear so in both frontal and lateral views. On the lateral radiograph, the retrocardiac air space should be seen in a normal-sized heart, and the carinal line (a perpendicular line drawn from the carina to the diaphragm) should not intersect the heart. A second method to evaluate heart size on the lateral film is the anterior tracheal line (a line parallel to the anterior wall of the trachea that extends inferiorly to the diaphragm). This line should not intersect the heart, nor should the line be pushed back to "hit" the spine above the diaphragm. Both methods work best on nonrotated lateral films. If a frontal film shows questionable cardiac enlargement, look at the lateral film. If the lateral film is normal, the heart size is normal.

In infants and older children, pulmonary vascular changes may help in detecting a left-to-right shunt circulation. In the newborn, however, the pulmonary vessels can be seen at the hila and only in the medial third of the lungs. When there is vascular congestion secondary to congestive heart failure or overcirculation from a left-to-right shunt, the vascularity becomes much easier to see in the lateral two thirds of the lung. It is much more difficult to detect decreased pulmonary vascularity (as found in severe pulmonary stenosis or atresia).

Categorization of Congenital Heart Disease on the Basis of Pulmonary Blood Flow

Cyanotic Heart Disease

Cyanotic heart disease may involve the following:
- Increased pulmonary blood flow: Truncus arteriosus and total anomalous pulmonary venous return
- Decreased pulmonary blood flow: Tetralogy of Fallot, Ebstein anomaly, and pulmonary atresia with intact ventricular septum
- Variable flow: D-transposition of the great arteries and tricuspid atresia

Acyanotic Heart Disease

Acyanotic heart disease may involve the following:
- Normal pulmonary blood flow (obstructive lesions): Coarctation of the aorta, aortic stenosis, and pulmonary artery stenosis
- Increased pulmonary blood flow (left-to-right shunt): Ventricular septal defect, atrial septal defect, atrioventricular septal defect, and patent ductus arteriosus

Congestive Heart Failure of the Newborn (Increased Pulmonary Venous Flow)

Left-sided Anatomic Obstruction

Left-sided anatomic obstruction may involve the following:
- Coarctation of the aorta
- Aortic stenosis

Left Ventricular Dysfunction

Left ventricular dysfunction may involve the following:
- Abnormal origin of the left coronary artery
- Myocarditis
- Shock
- Birth asphyxia
- Hypoplastic left heart
- Pulmonary venous atresia/stenosis

General Systemic Illness

General systemic illness may involve the following:
- Anemia
- Polycythemia
- Hypoglycemia
- Sepsis
- Atrioventricular malformations such as hemangioendothelioma of the liver and vein of Galen malformation (e-Fig. 24-3, *A* and *B*).

Diffuse Pulmonary Disease in the Newborn

The differential diagnosis of the various diffuse pulmonary conditions is described in Table 24-4. Premature infants are prone to complications related to therapy, such as:
- Air leak secondary to barotrauma: pulmonary interstitial emphysema, pneumomediastinum, pneumopericardium, pneumothorax, pneumoperitoneum, and air embolism
- Misplaced or perforated tubes: If the infant who is intubated is having unexplained respiratory distress, two views (frontal and lateral) may help define tube position
- Stone formation: gallstones (secondary to hyperalimentation), and renal stones (secondary to diuretic therapy, e.g., furosemide)
- Central nervous system hemorrhage
- Oxygen toxicity (retinopathy of prematurity)
- Line infection and vascular thrombosis

Focal Lung Lesions in Neonates on Chest Radiography

Lucent Lesions

Lucent lesions may involve the following:
- Congenital lobar emphysema
- Congenital cystic adenomatoid malformation
- Persistent pulmonary interstitial emphysema
- Congenital diaphragmatic hernia

Solid Lesions

Solid lesions may involve the following:
- Sequestration
- Bronchogenic cyst
- Congenital cystic adenomatoid malformation

Mediastinal Masses

The following outline is a useful summary of the etiology of mediastinal masses:

Table 24-4	Neonatal Chest Vignettes			
	Hyaline Membrane Disease	**Transient Tachypnea of the Newborn**	**Meconium Aspiration**	**Neonatal Pneumonia**
Typical patient	Premature	Term Cesarean section	Post-term meconium-stained fluid below the vocal cords	Premature rupture of membranes
Time course	Within hours	24-48 h	12-24 h	Onset < 6 h
Lung volume	Decreased	Increased	Increased	Increased
Radiographic characteristics	Ground-glass granular	Interstitial edema	Coarse, nodular, asymmetrical	Perihilar "streaking"
Effusions	No	Yes	No	Maybe
Complications and possible therapy	Pulmonary interstitial emphysema or pneumothorax, respiratory distress syndrome, patent ductus arteriosus	None	Persistent fetal circulation, extracorporeal membrane oxygenation (ECMO)	Sepsis, ECMO

From Blickman JG, Parker BR, Barnes PD: *Pediatric radiology: the requisites,* ed 3, Philadelphia, 2009, Mosby Elsevier.

- Anterior mediastinum (the four T's and a C)
  - Thyroid (ectopic thyroid)
  - "Terrible" lymph node enlargement by either infection or malignancy
  - Teratoma
  - Thymoma
  - Cystic hygroma (lymphatic malformation)
- Middle mediastinum (an abnormality for each organ)
  - Esophagus: Duplication cysts
  - Great vessels: Aneurysmal dilatation
  - Hila: Enlarged lymph nodes (leukemia, lymphoma, tuberculosis, etc.)
  - Trachea: Bronchogenic cysts
  - Pericardium: Cyst
- Posterior mediastinum
  - Tuberculosis (Pott disease) or any spinal infection
  - Extramedullary hematopoiesis (almost always in adults)
  - Neural tumors: Neuroblastoma, ganglioneuroma, neurofibroma, neurenteric cyst

Tips when viewing mediastinal masses include the following: (1) middle mediastinal masses silhouette the heart border and aorta; and (2) posterior mediastinal masses may spread the ribs or cause vertebral changes.

Abdominal Radiograph

The abdominal x-ray is the initial examination in the workup of abdominal and pelvic symptoms, and may provide useful information for tailoring the examination to the individual patient's problem. Supine and upright radiographs are obtained, although left lateral decubitus views are used in newborns and in ill or uncooperative patients. Single supine examinations may be obtained when the clinical suspicion is constipation or foreign body ingestion or if the examination is being performed for tube or catheter localization. On a cross-table lateral view it may be difficult to differentiate intraluminal air from extraluminal air, and decubitus or upright views are more useful in that context.

Abdominal Radiograph: Child versus Adult

The liver takes up a relatively larger space in the peritoneal cavity of a child. The spleen may not be visible and usually does not displace the gastric contour in a child. Likewise, retroperitoneal fat "stripes" (psoas shadows) are frequently not seen on a child's radiograph because of the relative paucity of fat in the infant's and small child's retroperitoneum. The lack of fat in the capsules of the solid organs makes evaluation of their size nearly impossible on radiographs. In contrast, properitoneal fat stripes are visible from infancy. A soft tissue pseudomass in the abdomen may be the urinary bladder, the fluid-filled stomach or intestine, or an umbilical hernia. Children up to the toddler age group typically have air throughout the entire gastrointestinal (GI) tract.

Bowel Gas after Birth

Newborns should have air in the stomach at birth, consisting mainly of swallowed air. The small bowel should be filled with air by 6 hours at the latest; the colon by 12 hours; and by 24 hours of life air should appear in the rectum, although rectal air is typically present much earlier (by 12 hours). A prone film is frequently helpful because air rises into the rectum when obstruction is not present. The normal newborn abdomen demonstrates monotonous polygons of gas. In neonates and infants it is often impossible to reliably differentiate small from large bowel except for stomach and rectum, especially if the bowel becomes dilated.

Absence of air in the stomach at 1 hour of life should raise the possibility of esophageal obstruction: esophageal atresia (EA) without tracheoesophageal fistula, or EA with fistula between proximal esophagus and trachea. A gasless abdomen in an infant for more than 12 hours indicates a serious disease. The most common cause of a lack of intestinal air in the newborn is depression of crying and swallowing in ill babies, especially those with newborn lung disease. Other causes of a gasless abdomen are vomiting, medication that decreases peristalsis, obstruction of a fluid-filled bowel, peritonitis, ascites, and congenital diaphragmatic hernia (a chest radiograph is diagnostic). Other causes of disturbed swallowing and/or diminished peristalsis include septicemia, metabolic disorders, and fatigue. The neonate in whom an orogastric or nasogastric tube has been placed may have a relatively gasless abdomen without other underlying pathology. Absence of meconium passage by 24 hours is abnormal, and abdominal distention or marked dilatation of any viscus in the first day of life should lead to further imaging evaluation.

Umbilical Venous and Arterial Lines

The ideal location for the tip of the umbilical venous line is in the right atrium. The umbilical arterial line tip may be at L4 to L5 (bifurcation of the aorta) or at T8 above the diaphragm (Fig. 24-15, *C*). The course of the umbilical venous line is as follows: umbilical vein → umbilical recess → left portal vein → ductus venosus → inferior vena cava → right atrium (Fig. 24-15, *A*). The umbilical arterial line dips inferiorly in the umbilical artery to join the internal iliac artery (creating a deep loop in the pelvis) and then rises posteriorly in the abdominal aorta (Fig. 24-15, *B*). The lateral view (not

Cranial portion of the inferior vena cava

Right hepatic vein

Inferior vena cava

Right portal vein

Portal vein

Ductus venosus

Left portal vein

Umbilical recess

Umbilical vein

A

Ascending aorta

Right coronary artery

Thoracic aorta (T9 level)

Splenic artery

Inferior phrenic artery

Proper hepatic artery

Celiac trunk

Gastroduodenal artery

Superior mesenteric artery

Inferior mesenteric artery

Level of aortic bifurcation

Common iliac arteries

Umbilical arteries   External iliac arteries   Internal iliac arteries

B

C

Figure 24-15   A, Postmortem demonstration of the umbilical recess with its junction to the ductus venosus and the left portal vein. Twin premature, 27 weeks of gestation, deceased on the first day of life. **B,** Male term newborn. Postmortem normal angiography. The angle between the umbilical arteries and the internal iliac arteries may make catheterization via the umbilical artery more difficult. **C,** Supine radiograph of the abdomen of a 3-day-old newborn shows the umbilical venous line *(blue arrow)* with the tip in the right atrium, and the umbilical arterial line *(red arrow)* with the tip in the aorta at T8. *Arrowhead,* nasogastric tube. (*A and* **B,** *From Hilton SvW, Edwards DK III: Practical pediatric radiology, ed 3, Philadelphia, 2006, Elsevier Saunders.*)

shown) confirms which catheter is arterial (equivalent to posterior) and which is venous (equivalent to anterior).

Adynamic Ileus

Ileus should be suggested only when loops of intestine are dilated. The presence of air in normal-caliber large and small bowel is a common and normal finding in newborns and infants. In adynamic (without peristalsis) ileus (distention), the small bowel is less distended than the colon, and there is gas in the rectum. In infants and older children, adynamic ileus occurs (1) after surgery, (2) with sepsis, (3) with gastroenteritis, (4) subsequent to electrolyte disturbances such as dehydration and hypokalemia, and (5) after administration of drugs such as opiates and anticholinergics.

Dynamic (Mechanical) Ileus

A more uniform, generalized increase in all or parts of the small or large bowel along with multiple air–fluid levels and no air in the rectum denotes mechanical bowel obstruction. The prone film is helpful in directing gas to the rectum for assessment of its caliber when bowel obstruction is a concern; a prone horizontal-beam (cross-table lateral) film of the rectum is helpful in these cases. The most common causes of mechanical obstruction in the neonate are as follows: (1) duodenal atresia or stenosis, (2) malrotation with midgut volvulus, and (3) obstructing peritoneal bands (Ladd bands). Beyond the neonatal period, the most common causes in descending order of frequency consist of (1) appendicitis, (2) intussusception, (3) inguinal hernia, (4) postoperative adhesions, (5) post–necrotizing enterocolitis strictures, and (6) midgut volvulus. In older children, valvulae conniventes and haustral markings may distinguish dilated small bowel and large bowel, respectively, and the distended colon is more peripheral in location than the more centrally located distended small bowel. These findings may not be applicable in the neonate or the child with malrotation and midgut volvulus.

Pneumoperitoneum

Free air in the peritoneal cavity most commonly results from perforation of a hollow viscus. Large amounts of free air are readily identifiable on supine abdominal radiographs, which may show the presence of the Rigler sign (where both sides of the bowel wall can be visualized), the football sign (where the liver is blacker than the adjacent soft tissues), and visualization of the falciform ligament. Small amounts of free air typically require a lateral decubitus or upright view. A cross-table lateral supine view may show a long colonic collection of air mimicking pneumoperitoneum. Perforation of a hollow viscus typically leads to intraperitoneal air–fluid levels as intraluminal fluid as well as air leaks into the peritoneal cavity. Other causes of pneumoperitoneum include (1) postoperative air and (2) tracking of air from pneumomediastinum, usually in children undergoing pressure ventilation and in asthmatic patients. The latter condition results when mediastinal air extends into the retroperitoneum and then along the course of the mesenteric vessels, resulting in subserosal air, which can rupture into the peritoneal cavity. It can be differentiated from visceral perforation by the lack of intraperitoneal air–fluid levels on horizontal-beam radiographs.

Calcifications

The abdominal radiograph can be used to assess calcifications, which may be present in meconium peritonitis; abdominal masses such as hepatoblastoma; and stones in the gallbladder, urinary tract, pancreas, or appendix. A phlebolith in an infant is definitely abnormal; it occurs far more often in adults.

Musculoskeletal System

Radiography remains the primary method of detecting and analyzing skeletal abnormalities. Most fractures and congenital deformities are sufficiently imaged by radiography without the need for additional imaging. The spatial resolution of radiography is superior to that of all other modalities. Radiography is cost-effective and radiation exposure to the patient is minimal. Radiographs often guide the selection of additional imaging modalities. Adequate radiography must include imaging in at least two perpendicular directions.

The skeletal survey remains an important component in the evaluation of many patients with a skeletal dysplasia or syndrome and in suspected victims of child abuse. However, these surveys have largely been replaced by technetium-99m methylene diphosphonate (MDP) nuclear scintigraphy for the detection of metastatic disease to the skeleton. Positron emission tomography (PET) and/or whole body MRI may soon supplant scintigraphy for this function. Surveys for malignant disease are particularly useful in Langerhans cell histiocytosis when the isotope scan may be unremarkable.

Radiographs are less relevant to the study of soft tissues because of their narrow contrast range, but plain films can depict calcifications, fat, gas, or foreign material within a soft tissue lesion, and can show the effect of the lesion on the adjacent bone.

Anatomy

Bone develops by intramembranous (flat bones) and endochondral (long bones) ossification. The long bone of a child is made up of four parts: the physis, or growth plate, and the epiphysis, metaphysis, and diaphysis. Each long bone (humerus, tibia) has a physis, and thus metaphyses and epiphyses, on either end. A secondary ossification center appears in the epiphysis after birth. Some long bones (e.g., the femur) have a nonarticulating apophysis, which is similar to the epiphysis but does not contribute to the length of the bone (e.g., the greater trochanter of the femur).

In the growing child's skeleton, blood supply is primarily to the metaphysis, and many of the disease processes and imaging findings are seen in this region. For example, hematogenous osteomyelitis is visible most often in the metaphysis; similarly, metastases travel hematogenously to the metaphysis.

The child's bones are still growing, developing, and modeling; therefore, many ossification centers are constantly appearing and fusing with the main skeleton. For example, the mnemonic "CRITOE" refers to the approximate age of ossification of secondary centers in the elbow: *c*apitellum (1 year), *r*adial head (4 years), *i*nner (medial) epicondyle (7 years), *t*rochlea (10 years), *o*lecranon (10 years), and *e*xternal (lateral) epicondyle (11 years).

In children the periosteum is less firmly attached to the diaphysis (or shaft) of the long bone and is more likely to tear and thus be elevated by trauma or hematoma formation. The periosteum reacts by laying down a thick layer of new bone. In contrast, the periosteum at the ends of the long bones is not loosely attached but rather firmly adherent to the metaphyseal regions. Shaking injuries here cause avulsion of a piece of bone from the metaphysis. This type of "bucket-handle" injury or avulsion "corner fracture" is commonly found in cases of child abuse (see Chapter 6).

Trauma

The commonest indication for radiography is the assessment of trauma. As a general rule, two orthogonal views are obtained to assess for fracture. When imaging a long bone, both the proximal and distal joints must be included so that the entirety of the bone is imaged.

Contralateral comparison views are not routinely obtained, but frequently aid in differentiating normal developmental variation from pathology. Comparison views are most helpful in areas of complex anatomy, such as the elbow with its six ossification centers. Normal variants are common and may mimic a fracture.

The child's bones are more plastic and less brittle than adults and so pediatric fractures differ from adult fractures. The greenstick fracture is characterized by a bowed long bone with a break on the convex surface but apparent cortical continuity on the concave surface. In the torus fracture there is buckling on one side of the cortex.

Some fractures are more prevalent in different age groups. For example, infants previously able to walk may suddenly limp because of a subtle spiral fracture of the tibia (a *toddler's fracture*). This fracture can be difficult to see on initial films. If there is suspicion that a fracture has occurred but none is definitely identified, repeat films in 7 to 10 days, or a bone scan may help. Periosteal reaction around a fracture indicates healing, and means that the injury is certainly more than several days old.

Periosteal reaction, with the exception of so-called physiologic appositional new bone found symmetrically in infants 2 to 6 months of age, should be regarded as abnormal. The normal physiologic periosteal bone deposition is bilaterally symmetrical and found in the humeri, femora, and tibias and extends to the metaphysis but no further. The periosteum is normally not seen.

Causes of periosteal reaction include (1) infection; (2) trauma; (3) metabolic origin (rickets, scurvy); (4) tumors (osteosarcoma, Ewing sarcoma, histiocytosis); (5) idiopathic origin (Caffey disease); and (6) iatrogenic/toxic origin (prostaglandin, hypervitaminosis A).

If a fracture involves a joint then a joint effusion (particularly in the knee or elbow) is a useful sign indicating that a fracture may have occurred. At the elbow a joint effusion most likely indicates that a supracondylar fracture (younger child) or radial neck fracture (older child) has occurred.

Fractures involving the growth plate are called Salter-Harris fractures and carry a prognostic rating according to the severity of the growth plate injury (types I to V, with type V being the worst; see Chapter 21, Fig. 21-37). Severe length discrepancies and other growth disturbances can occur from fractures in these regions.

The skeleton of children is unique in that it has a low incidence of dislocations of otherwise normal joints as compared with the adult skeleton. Because children's capsular and ligamentous structures are two to five times stronger than the weakest part of the growth plate, the growth plate fractures first, and dislocation occurs less frequently. The zone of calcifying cartilage is the weakest portion of the growth plate.

Nonaccidental Trauma (Child Abuse)

If the imaging findings are suspicious, it is the radiologist's legal obligation to report these findings as compatible with child abuse. Usually, reporting the findings to the referring (pediatric) clinician, either in the report or via telephone (preferable), is sufficient. See Chapter 6 for an in-depth discussion of nonaccidental trauma.

Skeletal Dysplasia

With the short stature of the pediatric age group, it is crucial to clinically determine whether the skeletal dysplasia involves proportionate or disproportionate short stature. The differential diagnosis of proportionate short stature consists of constitutional delay, familial short stature, a small group of endocrinopathies, and some dysmorphology syndromes. A left hand-and-wrist radiograph for bone age determination is required. For the bone age to be considered normal, it should lie within 2 standard deviations of the patient's chronologic age. Most of the bone dysplasias result in clinically disproportionate short stature. The skeletal survey for dysplasia need only include the limbs on one side of the body. See Chapter 21 for an in-depth discussion of skeletal dysplasias.

Bone Tumors

Clear radiographic signs of a benign lesion include sharp demarcation between the lesion and the normal bone, a sclerotic margin around the lesion, and a nonaggressive pattern of growth. The characteristics most often associated with a malignancy include an accompanying soft tissue mass; periosteal reaction; an indistinct zone of demarcation between the normal and abnormal bone; and permeative, destructive changes in the bone. Plain film radiography is usually adequate to diagnose most benign tumors. MRI is the modality of choice to define the extent of the abnormality once a malignant bone lesion has been suggested.

Bone Infection

The clinical symptoms of osteomyelitis precede the radiographic findings by 7 to 14 days. For this reason a radioisotope study or MRI is frequently more helpful in the early diagnosis of acute osteomyelitis.

The radiographic findings of acute osteomyelitis (0 to 2 weeks) include (1) soft tissue swelling initially; (2) loss of cortical margin; (3) focal demineralization of bone; and (4) faint periosteal new bone formation (7 to 14 days after onset).

The radiographic findings of the healing phase (>4 weeks) include (1) destroyed bone with irregular areas of sclerosis and lysis; (2) sequestrum, that is, a dense devascularized bone fragment within an area of pus and granulation tissue; and (3) involucrum, that is, a peripheral shell of supporting bone laid down by the periosteum around the old disease.

Chronic osteomyelitis (either unusual localized osteomyelitis or improperly treated) appears as (1) diffuse bone production with little or no destruction, and (2) an occasional draining sinus or lucent area in the midst of the sclerotic bone.

FLUOROSCOPY

Introduction

Indications, Contraindications, Advantages, and Disadvantages of Fluoroscopy in Pediatric Imaging

For a summary of the indications, contraindications, advantages, and disadvantages of fluoroscopy in pediatric imaging, see Table 24-5.

Fluoroscopic Contrast Agents

For a summary of fluoroscopic contrast agents, see e-Table 24-4.

Clinical Applications

Diaphragm Paralysis

In diaphragm paralysis, fluoroscopy is reserved for patients in whom ultrasound (US) has been unsuccessful or has given results contrary to the clinical impression, such as when the

Table 24-5 Indications, Contraindications, and Advantages/Disadvantages of Fluoroscopy

Organ System	Common Indications	Contraindications/Precautions	Advantages	Disadvantages
Airway/chest (noncontrast)	Laryngomalacia Tracheomalacia Vocal cord paralysis Diaphragm paralysis	None Widely available Dynamic Requires no contrast or sedation	Noninvasive	Radiation exposure Requires brief immobilization of uncooperative children
Gastrointestinal Tract (Contrast-Enhanced)				
Upper gastrointestinal (UGI) series	Vascular ring or pulmonary sling Tracheoesophageal fistula Esophageal stricture Hiatal hernia Gastroesophageal reflux Gastritis Peptic ulcer disease Gastric outlet obstruction (sonography favored for hypertrophic pyloric stenosis) Duodenal stenosis or atresia Malrotation/midgut volvulus	Hyperosmolar water-soluble contrast is contraindicated in patients with reflux or tracheoesophageal fistula Barium is contraindicated in patients with perforation or leak	Noninvasive (or minimally invasive if feeding tube required) Widely available Dynamic Requires no sedation	Radiation exposure Requires ingestion of contrast or tube feeding Requires brief immobilization of uncooperative children
Oropharyngeal motility examination	Swallowing dysfunction	Examination should be terminated if severe aspiration occurs Because of a high risk of aspiration in population studied, barium is the contrast agent of choice Hyperosmolar water-soluble contrast is contraindicated	Allows dynamic assessment of oropharyngeal motility (not included in standard UGI series) Noninvasive Requires no sedation	Requires radiation exposure (often more than for UGI series) Requires contrast/food ingestion and patient cooperation Must be scheduled in advance to ensure simultaneous radiologist and speech pathologist availability
Small bowel series	Small bowel obstruction, pseudo-obstruction, or atresia Malabsorption or immune deficiency Inflammatory bowel disease Mass Short-gut syndrome	Same as for UGI series	Allows assessment of small bowel distal to duodenal-jejunal junction (not included in UGI series) Noninvasive (or minimally if feeding required)	Requires radiation exposure (more than for UGI series alone) Requires ingestion of contrast or tube feeding Requires brief immobilization of uncooperative children May take several hours to complete
Contrast enema* (single contrast)	Distal small bowel obstruction Colonic atresia Microcolon Meconium plug Meconium ileus or equivalent Hirschsprung disease Assessment of postoperative anatomy	To avoid perforation, contrast enemas are relatively contraindicated in patients with necrotic bowel, toxic megacolon, pneumatosis intestinalis, or peritonitis In patients with known bowel perforation or recent surgery, water-soluble contrast is preferred over barium In neonates and infants at risk for dehydration, iso-osmolar water-soluble contrast or barium is preferred over hyperosmolar water-soluble contrast	Requires no sedation Minimally invasive Requires no sedation	Requires radiation exposure Requires rectal tube Requires brief immobilization of uncooperative children
Air-contrast enema	Inflammatory bowel disease Polyposis or colonic mass			
Air enema	Intussusception	Bowel perforation	Advantage over contrast enema: Smaller tears and reduced fecal spillage when bowel perforation occurs	Disadvantage over contrast enema: Slightly higher rate of bowel perforation
Contrast Urography				
Intravenous urography	Urinary calculi	Contrast allergy Renal insufficiency or failure	Minimally invasive	Results in radiation exposure Requires intravenous contrast Less sensitive than CT for calculi
Voiding cystourethrography	Urinary tract infection Hydronephrosis or hydroureter Vesicoureteral reflux Enuresis Cloacal and/or anorectal malformations Ambiguous genitalia Neurogenic bladder Posterior urethral valve Other urethral anomalies (i.e., stricture, polyp)	Acute UTI Prophylactic antibiotics warranted in patients with congenital heart disease Latex avoidance in patients at risk for latex allergy	Minimally invasive More sensitive to grade 1 vesicoureteral reflux than nuclear cystography Provides better anatomic resolution than nuclear cystography	Results in more radiation exposure than nuclear cystography

CT, computed tomography; UTI, urinary tract infection.

*Precaution: A manometer and pop-off valve must be used to keep intraluminal pressure below 120 mm Hg; intravenous access and surgical back-up must be secured before the procedure is begun.

From Osborn LM, DeWitt TG, First LR, et al, editors: Diagnostic imaging (CD-ROM, T 272-1: Indications, contraindications, advantages and disadvantages of fluoroscopy). In *Pediatrics*, Philadelphia, 2005, Mosby Elsevier.

US results are normal but the patient cannot be weaned from the ventilator.

The movement of the hemidiaphragm is complex. The left hemidiaphragm may occasionally be higher than the right, and inequality of movement is common. The anterior part (dome) is the only part of the hemidiaphragm routinely visualized on frontal fluoroscopy. Lateral or oblique fluoroscopy is often useful but occasionally may be difficult to interpret and can be hazardous to a sick child.

Tracheomalacia/Laryngomalacia

In the right lateral position the airway is observed for backward bowing of the epiglottis or fluttering of the aryepiglottic folds (laryngomalacia) and tracheal caliber change (tracheomalacia) or deviation. Laryngomalacia is noisier on quiet breathing, whereas tracheomalacia is noisier with crying.

Upper Gastrointestinal Series and Esophagography

For an upper gastrointestinal (UGI) series or esophagography, the patient should have nothing by mouth for 3 to 4 hours (infants) or 6 to 8 hours (older children). Observe swallowing while the child is in the right lateral position. Note sucking, swallowing coordination, nasopharyngeal reflux, vocal cord penetration, or tracheal aspiration. Examine the esophagus for stricture, indentation, fistula, and peristalsis. The aortic arch

and left atrium are often seen as normal indentations. Anterior indentation of the esophagus with soft tissue structure interposed between esophagus and trachea represents a pulmonary artery sling (Fig. 24-16). Posterior vascular indentation represents an aberrant subclavian artery (see Fig. 24-16).

With the child in the right lateral position, the partially filled stomach should be observed until it empties into the duodenum. Gastric size, shape, and emptying should be noted. Duration of gastric emptying is variable in normal infants and children. Elongation of the pylorus combined with the "string sign" indicates pyloric stenosis. Identify the duodeno–jejunal junction (DJJ) position to exclude or confirm malrotation. The normal position of the DJJ is to the left of the spine and at the level of the bulb/pylorus (Fig. 24-17, A). On the lateral view, both the descending (D2) and ascending (D4) segments of the duodenum are retroperitoneal structures (i.e., close to the spine) (Fig. 24-17, B). The DJJ is also posterior in location on the lateral view. Evaluate for gastroesophageal reflux (GER). The UGI series has an overall lower sensitivity for reflux (38%, compared with 88% with a radionuclide study).

Proximal neonatal bowel obstruction (occurring proximal to the mid-jejunum) includes midgut volvulus (Fig. 24-18), duodenal atresia, duodenal stenosis, duodenal web, annular pancreas, and proximal jejunal atresia. Patients usually present with vomiting. Abdominal radiographs demonstrate a few dilated small bowel loops.

Trachea Esophagus

A

B

Figure 24-16   Four patterns of vascular compression anomalies on the trachea and esophagus. Lateral projections are shown. **A,** Double aortic arch or right aortic arch with aberrant left subclavian artery. **B,** Innominate artery compression. **C,** Left aortic arch with aberrant right subclavian artery. **D,** Pulmonary sling. (*Modified from Berdon WE, Baker DH: Vascular anomalies and the infant lung: Rings, slings, and other things, Semin Roentgenol 7:39-64, 1972.*)

C

D

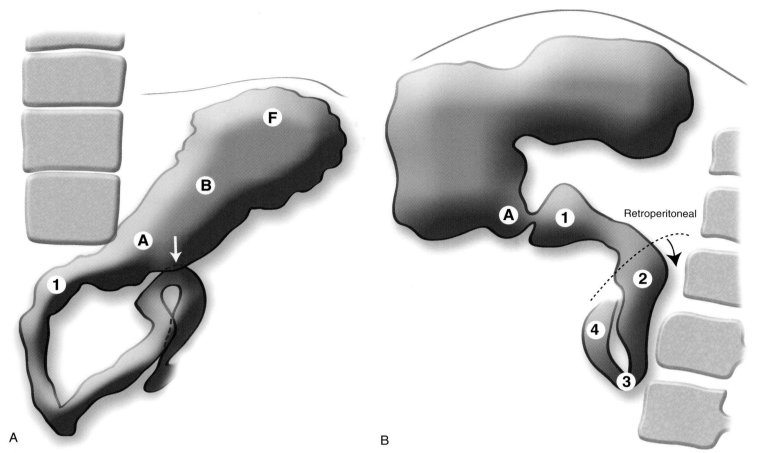

A   B

Figure 24-17   Upper gastrointestinal (UGI) study demonstrating normal duodenal course in a 3-year-old. **A,** Anteroposterior projection: the duodeno–jejunal junction *(arrow)* is at the level of the duodenal bulb and to the left of the left spinal pedicle. 1, duodenal bulb; A, antrum; B, body; F, fundus. **B,** Lateral projection: Note the four portions of the duodenum (1, 2, 3, 4). The second, third, and fourth portions of the duodenum are posterior, within the retroperitoneum. Slight obliquity allows visualization of both the descending (2) and ascending (4) duodenum. A, antrum.

Diagnostic Contrast Enema

Diagnostic contrast enema is performed to identify causes of lower GI bleeding (i.e., polyps), small bowel obstruction (i.e., intussusception or distal bowel atresia), and complications of inflammatory disease (i.e., post–necrotizing enteroco-

Figure 24-18   Upper gastrointestinal (UGI) study in a 6-day-old showing malrotation with midgut volvulus. The duodenal sweep fails to cross the midline and assumes a corkscrew appearance *(arrow)* projecting on the right side of the spine.

litis strictures), and to evaluate functional abnormality (i.e., Hirschsprung disease) or colonic anomaly (i.e., imperforate anus before complete repair). A UGI study is preferred for evaluation for malrotation because contrast enema will miss the diagnosis in 20% of cases (because the cecum is malpositioned in 80% of patients with malrotation and is normally located in the right lower quadrant in the remainder of patients). Low neonatal bowel obstruction (involving the distal jejunum, ileum, or colon) includes meconium ileus, ileal atresia, Hirschsprung disease, and meconium plug syndrome (Fig. 24-19). Patients present with abdominal distention and failure to pass meconium.

Barium or water-soluble contrast (osmolality, 600 mOsm/kg; diluted 1:1 in water) is used. Mucosal detail depicted with barium is better than that shown by water-soluble contrast. In the setting of Hirschsprung disease, barium can harden and remain in the colon as a barium ball. Barium can cause scarring when extravasated into the peritoneal cavity; therefore it is contraindicated in potential GI leak and after recent GI surgery. Water-soluble contrast material can soften meconium plugs and can be used to treat meconium ileus. Administration of barium into the GI tract can interfere with subsequent CT scans of the abdomen or with nuclear studies of the genitourinary (GU) or GI system, such as a Meckel scan. If an abdominal CT scan is contemplated, a barium swallow or UGI series should follow the CT scan, rather than vice versa.

The caliber of the rectum should be compared with that of the sigmoid colon. Normally, the rectum is larger than the sigmoid colon, for a rectosigmoid ratio greater than 1

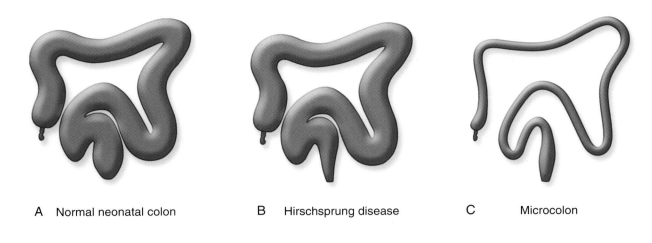

A Normal neonatal colon   B Hirschsprung disease   C Microcolon

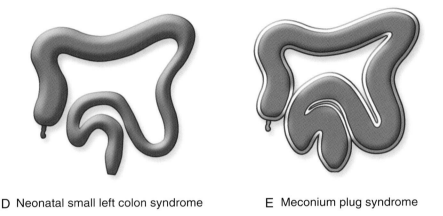

D Neonatal small left colon syndrome   E Meconium plug syndrome

Figure 24-19   **A-E,** Schematic representation of mechanical and functional obstruction in the neonatal period. *(From Hilton SvW, Edwards DK III: Practical pediatric radiology, ed 3, Philadelphia, 2006, Elsevier Saunders.)*

(in Hirschsprung disease, the rectum typically is smaller than the sigmoid).

Reduction of Intussusception

Fluoroscopy-guided air or water-soluble contrast reduction of intussusception is the treatment of choice after sonographic confirmation (see Ultrasound, later). Contraindications to reduction include peritonitis, pneumoperitoneum, shock, and sepsis. The choice of enema medium depends on the radiologist's preference. At present, an air enema is considered superior at reduction, cleaner (based on the appearance of the peritoneal cavity at surgery when perforation occurs), faster, with less radiation when compared with a liquid enema. A water-soluble enema is recommended for infants less than 6 months of age. Barium is no longer the liquid contrast medium of choice for intussusception reduction because of the risk of barium peritonitis, infection, and adhesions if perforation occurs during the enema. Radiologists should strive for enema reduction rates of 80%, but it will depend on their patient population. Neither sedation nor medications increase the enema success rate. Predictors of failure of pneumatic reduction include ileoileocolic intussusception (27%), long duration of symptoms (>2 days), and performance following failed hydrostatic reduction. The perforation rate is about 0.8% and will require immediate surgical intervention. Reduction should not be attempted without surgical back-up, and all children should have surgical consultation before enema. Some reports estimate that the rate of spontaneous reduction based on sonographic and/or enema diagnosis before surgery is 10%.

Insufflated air rapidly fills the colon and outlines the head of the intussusception. Air pressure should be kept below 120 mm Hg to avoid the risk of perforation.

Reduction is defined as complete elimination of the intussusceptum through the ileocecal valve and free reflux of air into the distal small bowel (Fig. 24-20). Perforation complicating air enema may cause tension pneumoperitoneum; some centers advise having an 18-gauge needle readily available in the fluoroscopy room for emergency decompression.

The recurrence rate is 10% postreduction. There is no contraindication to again reducing the intussusception by an enema procedure. Many centers refer patients to surgery after more than three recurrences in order to evaluate for underlying pathologic lead points (PLPs). Approximately 5% to 6% of intussusceptions in children are caused by PLPs, which are due to either focal masses or diffuse bowel wall abnormality. The most common focal PLPs are (in decreasing order of incidence) Meckel diverticulum, duplication cyst, polyp, and lymphoma. Diffuse PLPs are most commonly associated with cystic fibrosis or Henoch-Schönlein purpura. The rate of detection of PLPs by US, liquid enema, and air enema is 66%, 40% and 11%, respectively.

Contrast Enema Reduction of Meconium Ileus Uncomplicated by Bowel Atresia, Perforation, or Volvulus

Contrast enemas may be used for reduction of uncomplicated meconium ileus (see Fig. 24-19, *C*). The study should be performed in conjunction with a pediatric surgeon.

Figure 24-20 Ileocolic intussusception in the proximal transverse colon of a 2-year-old. **A,** Ultrasound shows the characteristic "target sign" on transverse section (hypoechoic ring with an echogenic center). **B-D,** Air enema reduction: **B,** Intussusception (*) is initially located in the right upper quadrant; **C,** intussusception (*) has moved retrograde and is now in the region of the ileocecal valve; **D,** successful reduction with resolution of the soft tissue mass and reflux of air into the terminal ileum.

Contrast Enema for Hirschsprung Disease

No preparation of the colon is necessary when performing contrast enema for Hirschsprung disease. Recent manipulation including rectal examination or rectal thermometry shortly before contrast enema can make diagnosis more difficult by decompressing the distended colon. Normally, the rectum is larger than the sigmoid colon (in Hirschsprung disease, the rectum typically is smaller than the sigmoid). Identify a transition zone between the narrowed distal aganglionic segment and the dilated proximal, normal colon. Although contrast enema remains a useful test, suction biopsy provides definitive diagnosis.

Voiding Cystourethrography

Wash the external genitalia with antiseptic solution. For male patients, squirt lidocaine (Xylocaine viscous 2%) into the penile meatus to locally anesthetize the urethra and make catheterization less painful. Catheterize the urethra with an appropriately sized catheter (5-French feeding tube for newborns and young infants or girls less than 2 to 4 years of age, 8-French feeding tube for older children, 10- to 12-French rubber catheter for teenagers). Under fluoroscopic guidance, the bladder is filled with iodinated contrast. The size, shape, and capacity of the bladder are noted, and the dome of the bladder is examined for irregularities, the presence of filling defects (mass or ureterocele), or sinus tract (urachal remnant). While on the fluoroscopy table, the patient is asked to void (Fig. 24-21). As the child voids, the caliber of the urethra and dilatation of the posterior urethra are noted (Fig. 24-22), as well as caliber change and completeness of voiding. The predicted bladder capacity (in milliliters) for children younger than 1 year is the child's weight in kilograms multiplied by 7. In children older than 1 year, the predicted capacity is the child's age in years plus 2, multiplied by 30.

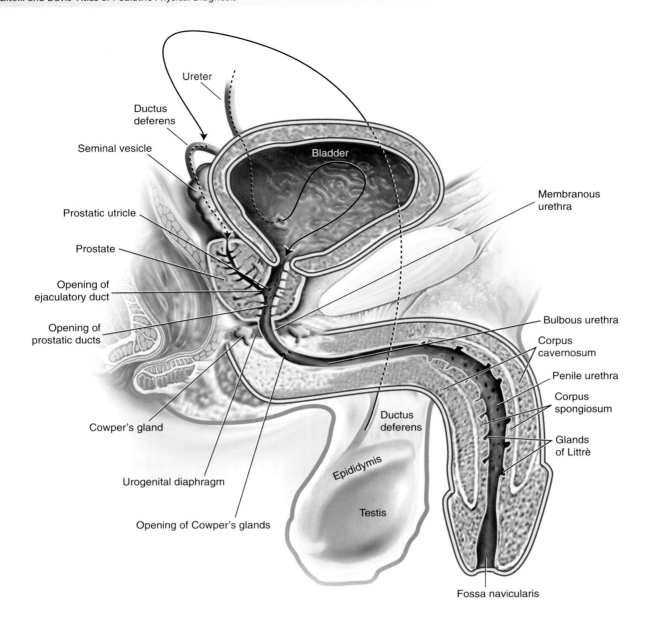

Figure 24-21 Normal anatomy of the male urethra. A schematic drawing demonstrates the anatomy of the male urethra and its relationship with periurethral structures. *(From Kim B, Kawashima A, LeRoy AJ: Imaging of the male urethra, Semin Ultrasound CT MR 28:258-273, 2007.)*

Figure 24-22 Voiding cystourethrogram (VCUG) in a 1-day-old boy. Lateral view during voiding after catheter removal demonstrates the posterior urethral valve as a lucent line *(arrow)* separating the dilated posterior urethra (P) from the distal urethra. Note the trabeculated thick-walled bladder (B).

In patients with neurogenic bladder and myelomeningocele, voiding is usually impossible, and detecting reflux is the most important part of the study. In these cases, the bladder is filled to a volume appropriate for age or corresponding to typical volumes obtained during catheterization, with images obtained over the kidneys and ureters to evaluate for reflux. The bladder is then emptied through the catheter.

ULTRASOUND

Introduction

Advantages of Ultrasound in Pediatric Imaging

Ultrasound presents the following advantages in pediatric imaging:

1. No ionizing radiation is used

2. Real-time image acquisition is possible, allowing a study to be performed in uncooperative or crying patients without the need for sedation

3. Small patient size results in improved image quality

Figure 24-23 Ultrasound image orientation of the right kidney of a 2-day-old male in the supine position. **A,** Sagittal plane. **B,** Transverse plane. D, diaphragm; L, liver; RA, right adrenal; RK, right kidney; S, spine; T, transducer. Note the normal undulating contour of the right kidney secondary to fetal lobulation and the corticomedullary differentiation with hypoechoic renal pyramids. The right adrenal gland is Y-shaped with a bright (echogenic) center and dark (hypoechoic) cortex. The diaphragm appears as a curvilinear echogenic structure.

4. Imaging can be performed in any plane

5. The equipment is portable, allowing the study to be performed at the bedside or in the operating room

6. It is relatively inexpensive compared with CT and MRI and therefore can be used in screening and in multiple follow-up studies

Disadvantages

Ultrasound presents the following disadvantages in pediatric imaging:

1. Ultrasound is operator dependent and therefore should be performed by a well-trained technologist (sonographer) and reviewed by a radiologist (sonologist) before the study is terminated

2. Deep structures are poorly visualized in obese patients

3. Sound penetrates poorly in air-filled viscera and bones

Image Orientation

By convention, when images are acquired in the supine position, the US transducer (or probe) should be held such that the right or cranial portion of the body is viewed on the left side of the image (Fig. 24-23).

Physics

Ultrasound is sound above the audible range, that is, greater than 20 kilohertz (kHz). Diagnostic US frequency ranges between 1 and 20 megahertz (MHz). The speed of sound in soft tissue is 1540 m/second. Various frequency probes are available: the higher the frequency of the probe the better the resolution, but the less the depth of tissue that can be imaged. Depth indicates the distance from the transducer surface to the body part of interest.

The transmitted sound wave is reflected at interfaces of different acoustic impedance. The reflected sound creates a structure and contrast between different tissues and allows a two-dimensional image to be formed. Three-dimensional US is available and is useful in echocardiography and fetal imaging.

Dense structures such as bone, calcifications, and surgical clips/vascular coils within organs will not allow sound to pass through them (absorb sound totally) and appear bright (hyperechoic) with an acoustic shadow behind them (Fig. 24-24, *A*). Cystic structures are dark with no internal echoes (anechoic); very little sound is absorbed, leading to the opposite effect with increased through-transmission of the sound waves, that is, increased signal behind them (Fig. 24-24, *B*). Solid structures produce internal echoes of variable intensity (ranging from hypoechoic to echogenic). An interface between soft tissue and air will cause total reflection of sound so that the deeper structures cannot be imaged, resulting in an acoustic shadow (Fig. 24-24, *C*). Good transducer–skin contact, using a US coupling gel, is necessary to generate an image.

Doppler imaging: The Doppler technique relies on frequency data. Sound reflected from a moving target (e.g., red cells in a blood vessel) undergoes a change in frequency. The difference between the transmitted and the received frequencies is the Doppler shift. If the US beam strikes a reflector moving toward it, the reflected sound will have a higher frequency and shorter wavelength than the original beam. If the US beam strikes a reflector moving away from it, the reflected sound will have a lower frequency and longer wavelength than the original beam.

Duplex Doppler ultrasonography uses the gray-scale image as a road map; Doppler interrogation of a blood vessel in the image can then be performed by positioning a cursor within the vessel. The Doppler waveform depicts the relationship between velocity and time and is unique to the flow pattern within the vessel. Color flow Doppler assigns red and blue colors to vessels according to their flow toward or away from the transducer, respectively (Fig. 24-25).

Arterial flow indexes: The resistive index (RI; or Pourcelot index) is a popular parameter that is altered by vascular resistance and vascular compliance. The pulsatility index (PI) is a measure of the variability of blood velocity in a vessel (e-Fig. 24-4).

Figure 24-24   Ultrasound image characterization. **A,** Gallstone (s) in the neck of the gallbladder (GB) with "acoustic shadowing" posterior to it *(arrows).* **B,** Liver cyst (C) reveals "increased through-transmission" of the sound waves as a bright band posterior to the cyst *(arrows).* **C,** Bowel gas (BG) in a right upper quadrant bowel loop causing "dirty" acoustic shadowing *(arrows);* this explains why excessive bowel gas can limit the quality of the study by obscuring the deep structures. L, liver.

Figure 24-25   Direction of blood flow in the left kidney as indicated by color Doppler imaging. Flow in the main renal artery (A) is directed toward the transducer (T) and is thus red. Color flow is blue in the main renal vein (V), as it is directed away from the transducer. AO, abdominal aorta; IVC, inferior vena cava.

Figure 24-26 Acute bacterial pyelonephritis. **A,** Ultrasound (US) scan shows a wedge-shaped hyperechoic focus *(arrowhead)* in the upper pole of the right kidney related to acute bacterial pyelonephritis. **B,** Color flow US image demonstrates diminished flow through the involved area. *(From Craig WD, Wagner BJ, Travis MD: Pyelonephritis: Radiologic–pathologic review,* Radiographics *28:255-276, 2008.)*

Power Doppler: The power Doppler technique measures the density rather than the velocity of the red blood cells in the sample area. The amplitude of the signal depends on the blood within the sample volume. Large-amplitude signals appear as a bright color and weak signals as a dim color. The technique is also called US angiography, as it gives a detailed road map to blood flow in an organ. The technique is three times more sensitive than conventional Doppler and shows smaller blood vessels at deeper depths. It also provides better edge enhancement of blood vessels. The main disadvantage is the inability to provide functional information such as direction of flow and flow velocity measurements. In acute bacterial pyelonephritis, a positive power Doppler US finding (area of hypoperfusion) can obviate the need for further imaging, that is, ^{99m}Tc-dimercaptosuccinic acid (DMSA) scintigraphy (Fig. 24-26).

Selected topics of pediatric US are described later (e-Table 24-5).

Chest Ultrasound

Thymus

Ultrasound is useful to confirm that a widened mediastinum is due to a normal thymus, particularly when the child presents with stridor thought to be due to airway obstruction. The thymus has a homogeneous fine granular echo texture that is slightly more echogenic than the liver, and less echogenic than the thyroid. It passes from right to left across the anterior mediastinum in front of the great vessels, which are not compressed.

Neck and Superior Mediastinal Masses

Ultrasound can assess the consistency of neck and superior mediastinal masses, whether cystic or solid.

Pleural Effusion

Ultrasound is useful in the assessment of the radiopaque hemithorax. A peripheral pneumonia may appear as a hypoechoic area in the air-filled lung. A parapneumonic effusion appears as anechoic fluid in the costophrenic recess (e-Fig. 24-5). A complicated effusion and/or empyema shows pleural thickening, septations, fibrin strands, and hyperechoic debris.

Diaphragmatic Motion

In unilateral diaphragmatic elevation, US can differentiate between a subphrenic mass or fluid collection, subpulmonary pleural effusion, or impaired diaphragmatic excursion. Diaphragmatic paralysis may be due to damage to the phrenic nerve during a difficult delivery or after a surgical procedure. US can assess paradoxic or asymmetrical diaphragmatic movement with respiration. This is best evaluated in the transverse plane, which allows simultaneous visualization of both hemidiaphragms.

Neck Vessels

Venous duplex US is performed to assess vascular access before major surgeries. It can also detect venous clots, particularly in the presence of central lines.

Echocardiography

Cardiac US is performed in the pediatric cardiology echocardiography laboratory and is useful in the assessment of cardiac morphology and function in congenital and acquired heart disease. It is the first-line modality before cardiac catheterization, CT, or MRI.

Abdominal and Retroperitoneal Ultrasound

Abdominal Mass

Ultrasound will characterize an abdominal mass whether it is cystic or solid. US has high sensitivity for the detection of a primary abdominal mass in patients with neuroblastoma, given the large mean diameter of the tumor (6 to 8 cm). US cannot reliably identify local tumor extent; it has limited value in demonstrating the extent of vessel encasement, involvement of the retroperitoneal and retrocrural nodes, and intraspinal tumor extension compared with CT and MRI.

Ultrasound is the initial imaging modality in the evaluation of suspected Wilms tumor; US confirms the renal origin of the mass (mean diameter, 5 to 10 cm) and evaluates patency of the renal vessels and inferior vena cava. CT is the next imaging study of choice, as it can also demonstrate small lesions in the opposite kidney and liver metastases that may be missed by US as well as pulmonary metastases.

Ultrasound is the initial examination of choice in confirming the presence and character of a suspected hepatic mass. This is followed by CT or MRI to further characterize the lesion and determine its extent and resectability.

Ascites

Ultrasound of the four quadrants of the abdomen and pelvis is sensitive for localizing peritoneal fluid. Uncomplicated ascites is anechoic. Internal echoes can indicate the presence of blood, exudates, chyle, or neoplastic cells.

Figure 24-27 Hypertrophic pyloric stenosis. Longitudinal image shows the thickened pyloric muscle measuring 5.7 mm *(yellow arrows)* and the elongated pyloric channel measuring 22 mm *(red arrows)*. The redundant pyloric mucosa *(blue arrow)* protrudes into the gastric antrum (A), forming the antral nipple sign. The *arrowheads* show the double-track sign.

Abscess

In experienced hands and using meticulous technique, US can localize an intraabdominal abscess. There are both more false negatives (due to overlying bowel gas) and more false positives (fluid-filled bowel loops) with US, and it requires more time and experience than contrast-enhanced CT.

Hypertrophic Pyloric Stenosis

Ultrasound is the diagnostic study of choice to confirm the diagnosis of hypertrophic pyloric stenosis (HPS). Images are acquired in the right posterior oblique position, which allows fluid in the gastric fundus to flow into the antropyloric area, distending this region. The stomach should not be emptied before the examination, because this makes identification of the antropyloric region difficult. If the antrum does not contain adequate fluid, a glucose solution or water can be given orally or via a nasogastric tube. The sonographic hallmark of HPS is the thickened pyloric muscle, defined as wall thickness equal to or greater than 3 mm, and an elongated pyloric channel, defined as a length equal to or greater than 17 mm as measured on the longitudinal images (Fig. 24-27).

Intussusception

Intussusception is an invagination of proximal bowel into its distal lumen. The invaginating portion is termed the *intussusceptum*, and the recipient bowel is called the *intussuscipiens*. Approximately 90% of intussusceptions are ileocolic, with the remaining 10% being ileoileal and colocolic (Fig. 24-28). The diagnostic approach should include (1) abdominal radiographs if concern for other diagnoses or for perforation; (2) sonography for diagnosis or exclusion of intussusception. US shows the intussusception as a "donut," "target," or "pseudo-kidney" sign, and has high accuracy,

approaching 100% in experienced hands. If positive, a surgical consult should be obtained before the air enema reduction. Risk factors for reduction include free intraperitoneal fluid, bowel obstruction, loss of Doppler flow in the intussusception, and fluid trapped within the colon due to incarceration. US can also assess the presence of a pathologic lead point (PLP) mass and intussusception limited to the small bowel, and can be used to diagnose or exclude residual intussusception after enema.

Appendicitis

Obstruction of the appendiceal lumen results in distention of the appendix, superimposed infection, ischemia, and eventually perforation. There is much debate about appropriate imaging algorithms for suspected appendicitis. Some investigators have advocated primary use of US, with CT being performed in equivocal cases. US is much more useful in girls and in patients of thin body habitus than in boys and patients who are obese. In girls, in whom ovarian causes of right lower quadrant pain such as hemorrhagic cyst or torsion are not uncommon, US may be the first test of choice. CT is favored when perforated appendicitis is highly suspected, in evaluation for abscess, in postoperative evaluation, and in obese patients.

Technically adequate examinations are achieved in about 95% of patients. Technical failures are caused by the presence of severe pain, marked ascites, or obesity. In the longitudinal plane, the inflamed appendix is a fluid-filled, noncompressible, blind-ending tubular structure with a diameter of 6 mm or more. Other findings include the presence of a shadowing echogenic appendicolith; pericecal or periappendiceal fluid (Fig. 24-29); enlarged mesenteric nodes; increased periappendiceal echogenicity representing inflamed fat (termed "phlegmon"); abscess; and wall thickening of the cecum or terminal ileum. In the axial plane, the inflamed appendix has a target appearance.

Perforation occurs in 20% to 30% of children with appendicitis. The appendix may disintegrate and hence not be identifiable on US. In general, the appendix is visible in 40% to 60% of children with perforation. Peritonitis is characterized by dilated bowel loops with thick echogenic walls and ascites, and increased blood flow in the bowel wall as demonstrated by color Doppler imaging.

Midgut Malrotation

The upper gastrointestinal examination is the imaging study of choice to diagnose malrotation. US is not needed for the diagnosis, but the findings need to be recognized because they may be encountered on examinations performed for other clinical indications. The sonographic diagnosis of midgut malrotation is predicated on identifying the relative positions of the superior mesenteric artery (SMA) and superior mesenteric vein (SMV) (anterior and to the right of the artery). Reversal of this relationship, with the SMV positioned to the left of the SMA, suggests midgut malrotation. However, some patients with malrotation have a normal position of the artery and vein, and some patients with reversal of the vessels do not have malrotation. Approximately 15% to 28% of patients with midgut malrotation will have a ventral position of the SMV relative to the SMA (described as an indeterminate pattern).

Gastrointestinal Duplication Cysts

Duplication cysts are uncommon congenital anomalies resulting from abnormal canalization of the GI tract. The most common locations are the terminal ileum, where they lie along the mesenteric border, and the distal esophagus. They are usually round and attached to the GI tract, and the majority of the cysts do not communicate with the GI lumen. They

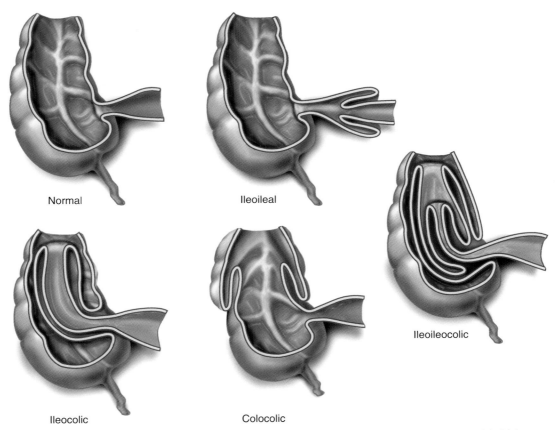

Normal   Ileoileal

Ileoileocolic

Ileocolic   Colocolic

Figure 24-28   Diagrammatic representation of intussusception. *(From Hilton SvW, Edwards DK III: Practical pediatric radiology, ed 3, Philadelphia, 2006, Elsevier Saunders.)*

have a mucosal lining and about 43% contain ectopic gastric mucosa. A duplication cyst may act as a lead point of an intussusception. US will demonstrate a cystic mass with the typical "bowel wall signature." It will have an inner echogenic mucosal layer and an outer hypoechoic muscular layer. This is contrasted with the mesenteric cyst wall, which consists of a single layer.

Hepatic Vascular Assessment

Color Doppler ultrasound is useful in the assessment of liver cirrhosis, portal hypertension, and liver transplantation for intraoperative ultrasound guidance and postoperative

Figure 24-29   Acute appendicitis. A small fluid collection *(arrow)* is surrounding the tip of the inflamed appendix (asterisk), consistent with perforation.

follow-up. US will assess vascular patency and the direction of flow in the hepatic artery, portal vein, hepatic veins, and inferior vena cava. The normal portal venous flow is hepatopetal (i.e., toward the liver) on Doppler US, whereas hepatofugal flow (i.e., away from the liver or reversed flow) is suggestive of portal hypertension.

Gallbladder Disease

The patient should fast for 6 hours before US examination to allow adequate demonstration of the bile-filled gallbladder. The sensitivity of US for detecting gallstones is greater than 95%. The demonstration of posterior acoustic shadowing correlated with cholelithiasis in virtually all patients (see Fig. 24-24, *A*), whereas nonshadowing echogenic foci may represent stone disease, polyps, or other masses. US has a sensitivity greater than 90% for the diagnosis of acute cholecystitis. The most common sonographic findings of acute calculus cholecystitis include cholelithiasis, an enlarged gallbladder, a thickened gallbladder wall (thickness > 3 mm), localized tenderness (sonographic Murphy sign), sludge, and pericholecystic fluid. The most sensitive criteria for diagnosing acute cholecystitis are gallbladder tenderness in association with stones.

Biliary Tree

Because of their small size, normal intrahepatic bile ducts and the cystic duct are not routinely seen at sonography. The intrahepatic ducts are considered dilated if their diameter exceeds 2 mm or is more than 40% of the diameter of the adjacent portal vein. The use of Doppler techniques allows a more confident diagnosis of intrahepatic ductal dilatation.

The main right and left hepatic ducts join to form the common hepatic duct. The common bile duct extends from the junction of the cystic duct and common hepatic duct to the level of the ampulla of Vater, where it joins the main pancreatic duct in 60% to 70% of individuals. In the remainder of individuals, the ducts enter the duodenum separately.

The upper limits of the common duct should not exceed 1 mm in neonates, 2 mm in infants up to 1 year of age, 4 mm in children 1 to 10 years of age, and 6 mm in adolescents and young adults. The distal portion of the common duct is usually larger than the proximal portion. Ductal size may increase by 1 mm or more during deep inspiration and the Valsalva maneuver. An increase in ductal diameter also occurs after cholecystectomy.

About 70% to 80% of cases of neonatal jaundice result from biliary atresia, neonatal hepatitis syndrome, and choledochal cyst. Other biliary abnormalities include bile duct paucity (Alagille syndrome), inspissated bile syndrome, and spontaneous perforation of the extrahepatic bile duct. In older children jaundice is most often due to hepatocellular disease, such as hepatitis and cirrhosis, and less often due to biliary tract inflammation (cholangitis) or obstruction. The causes of obstructive jaundice include choledochal cyst; neoplasms, particularly rhabdomyosarcoma, lymphoma, or neuroblastoma; cholelithiasis; and, rarely, stricture.

Pancreatitis and Pseudocysts

In most patients with mild pancreatitis, the pancreas appears normal on sonography. With more severe disease, a focally or diffusely enlarged pancreas with irregular margins and hypoechoic parenchyma is seen. Pancreatic and common bile duct dilatation are other signs of acute pancreatitis. Pancreatic ducts greater than 1.5 mm in diameter in children between 1 and 6 years of age, greater than 1.9 mm in children aged 7 to 12 years, or greater than 2.2 mm in children aged 13 to 18 years are often associated with acute pancreatitis. Approximately 50% of children with acute pancreatitis have extrapancreatic fluid collections.

Pseudocyst formation is the most common complication of acute pancreatitis, requiring 4 to 6 weeks to develop. Cysts are surrounded by thick-walled capsules of fibrous and granulation tissues and lack epithelial lining (hence, they are called *pseudocysts* rather than true cysts). Unlike acute fluid collections, which resolve spontaneously, resolution of a pseudocyst is less likely. At sonography, pseudocysts are usually well-circumscribed, anechoic or hypoechoic masses with through-transmission. The fluid often contains septations or internal echoes due to debris or hemorrhage.

Blunt Trauma

Both US and CT are useful in assessing abdominal trauma. The "FAST" (*f*ocused *a*ssessment with *s*onography for *t*rauma) technique determines the presence of free intraperitoneal or pericardial fluid in the setting of trauma. The following regions are scanned: (1) the right and left upper quadrants; (2) the right and left paracolic gutters; (3) the pelvis; and (4) the pericardium, using the subxiphoid window.

Congenital Hydronephrosis

When intrauterine hydronephrosis is diagnosed, postpartum US is indicated to confirm the diagnosis. It is recommended that sonography not be performed until 4 to 5 days after delivery. A sonogram performed earlier may be falsely negative or may underestimate the severity of hydronephrosis, because of a relative state of dehydration and decreased glomerular filtration rate (GFR) immediately after delivery. After rehydration in the first few days of life, the GFR increases, thereby increasing urine flow. Pelvicaliceal dilatation secondary to an obstructing lesion then becomes more apparent. If the postnatal sonogram shows moderate to severe hydronephrosis, a VCUG and diuretic scintigraphy are performed. A VCUG assesses the presence of reflux and diuretic scintigraphy assesses differential renal function. When the initial postnatal US is normal or shows mild dilatation, it is generally repeated

at 6 weeks of age. If follow-up sonography shows mild hydronephrosis, a VCUG is performed.

Ureteral Duplication

Complete ureteropelvic duplication has two separate pelvicaliceal systems and two ureters. The upper pole ureter often has an ectopic insertion and is prone to obstruction. It typically inserts medial and inferior to the trigone (Weigert-Meyer rule). The lower pole moiety ureter is orthotopic and inserts into the trigone. It lies lateral and superior to the upper moiety ureter and often has a perpendicular course entering the bladder (rather than the normal oblique course), predisposing it to reflux. The termination of the ureter from the upper pole can end as an ectopic ureter or ectopic ureterocele (Fig. 24-30; e-Fig. 24-6, *A* and *B*).

Urinary Tract Calcifications

Nephrocalcinosis refers to a pathologic deposition of calcium in the renal parenchyma. Calcification is more common in the medulla than in the cortex. *Urolithiasis* refers to the presence of stones in the renal collecting system or in the ureter. Nephrocalcinosis and urolithiasis appear as areas of increased echogenicity. Acoustic shadowing can usually be seen if the stone is 5 mm or greater in size. Nonopaque stones, such as uric acid calculi, can produce as much acoustic shadowing as opaque or calcium-containing renal calculi.

Renal Artery Stenosis

Peak systolic velocity (PSV) is measured in the aorta at the level of the origins of the renal arteries and is also measured in the main renal artery at the origin, mid-hilum, and hilum, and at any area of focal color aliasing. Waveforms from the interlobar or segmental intraparenchymal renal arteries at the upper and lower poles should be obtained to measure the acceleration index (AI), acceleration time (AT), and resistive index (RI). Optimally, three Doppler waveforms of the intraparenchymal renal arteries should be obtained at each pole. The AI is derived by calculating the slope of the line from the onset of systole to the early systolic peak complex, and the AT is the length of time from the onset of systole to the early systolic peak complex. A schematic demonstrating how to measure the AI and AT is presented in e-Figure 24-7.

On pulse Doppler examination, the renal arteries normally have a low resistance waveform with continuous forward diastolic flow and a sharp systolic upstroke (e-Fig. 24-8). PSV typically is less than 100 cm/second in the main renal artery and decreases as the arterial tree is traced distally. The RI should be less than 0.7 in the intraparenchymal renal arteries, and the AT is normally less than 70 milliseconds.

Diagnostic Criteria for Renal Artery Stenosis

Anatomic evaluation of the main renal arteries on the basis of gray-scale images will identify areas of stenosis. Post–stenotic dilatation may also be observed. On color Doppler interrogation, focal color aliasing or a "soft-tissue color bruit" (color artifact in the surrounding soft tissues) suggests an underlying stenosis with increased PSV. Asymmetry of renal length (>1.5 cm) and asymmetry of cortical thickness or echogenicity are also suggestive of underlying renal vascular pathology.

Acute Scrotal Ultrasound

See Table 24-6 for a summary of color Doppler ultrasound findings in acute scrotal conditions.

Acute Epididymitis/Orchitis

Sonographic findings of acute epididymitis include a focally or diffusely enlarged epididymis, with the epididymal head being

Anatomic

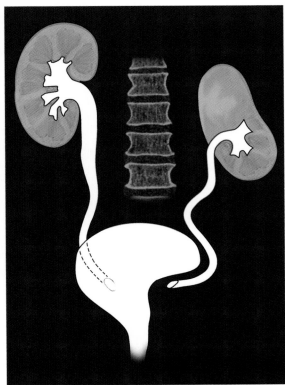

Urographic

Figure 24-30 Ectopic ureterocele. Diagrammatic representation of the anatomic and urographic appearances of an ectopic ureterocele of the left kidney upper moiety without function. Diagnosis of this entity on a urogram depends on recognition of indirect signs: 1, increased distance from the top of the visualized collecting system to the upper border of the nephrogram; 2, abnormal axis of the collecting system; 3, impression on the upper border of the renal pelvis; 4, decreased number of calices compared with the contralateral kidney; 5, lateral displacement of the kidney and ureter; 6, lateral course of the visualized ureter; and 7, filling defect in the bladder. *(From Adam A, Dixon AK: Grainger & Allison's diagnostic radiology, ed 5, Philadelphia, 2008, Elsevier Churchill Livingstone.)*

most commonly involved. Adjacent scrotal skin thickening and a reactive hydrocele are also seen. Spread of inflammation occurs in 20% to 40% of postpubertal males with acute epididymitis, producing epididymo-orchitis. Conversely, 85% of boys with orchitis have signs of epididymitis as well. Color Doppler shows increased blood flow in the inflamed epididymis and/or testis compared with the asymptomatic side.

Testicular Torsion

Torsion of the testis results when the testis and spermatic cord twist one or more times, obstructing blood flow. With testicular torsion the testis usually is enlarged and loses its normal echotexture. On color flow Doppler there will be absence of blood flow to the center of the testicle (Fig. 24-31, *A* and *B*). With torsion and detorsion, one can be led astray by the fact that after detorsion blood returns to the testicle. In these cases the clinical history is exceptionally important because there will be an abrupt cessation of pain with detorsion.

Table 24-6	Color Doppler Ultrasound Findings in Acute Scrotal Conditions	
Diagnosis	**Intratesticular Flow**	**Peritesticular Flow**
Acute torsion	Absent	Normal
Missed torsion	Absent	Increased
Spontaneous detorsion	Normal or increased	Increased
Orchitis	Increased	Normal
Epididymitis	Normal	Increased

From Feld R, Middleton WD: Recent advances in sonography of the testis and scrotum, *Radiol Clin North Am* 30:1033-1051, 1992.

Nonetheless, even with this history, the patient should be surgically explored and the problem corrected.

Hip Ultrasound

Hip Effusion

Ultrasound is useful for delineating fluid in the hip joint (Fig. 24-32, *A* and *B*). At this site the two conditions most commonly encountered are transient synovitis and septic arthritis.

Developmental Dysplasia of the Hip

Breech presentation at birth increases the risk for developmental dysplasia of the hip (DDH) by a factor of 5.5, with the frank breech (hips held in adduction and knees extended) representing the greatest risk. DDH is almost nonexistent in African children as the mothers tend to hold their children against their waist, which holds the hips in flexion and abduction, a position leading to proper acetabular–femoral development. Sonography is well suited to evaluation of the infant hip (Fig. 24-33). The patient must be quiet and relaxed for successful US examination. Ossification of the femoral head interferes with US examination beyond 4 to 6 months of age. Thus, radiography may be useful after about 3 months of age. Manipulation of the hip for dynamic examination may be impossible in the older, stronger infant.

Neonatal Spine Ultrasound

Tethered Cord

Tethered cord, or low-lying conus medullaris, may occur as a primary problem or in association with other components of

Figure 24-31   Testicular torsion. **A,** The left testis (T) is enlarged and hypoechoic. **B,** Color flow Doppler fails to demonstrate flow to the center of the testis. Exuberant flow is present around the testis *(arrows)* and the epididymis (E).

spinal dysraphism, such as lipomyelomeningocele, hemangioma, or a dermoid tract. The filum terminale may be short and abnormally thick (>2 mm). Sonographically, tethered cord is diagnosed in neonates by the presence of low-lying conus (below the L2-L3 disk space). The conus and nerve roots do not move freely in the cerebrospinal fluid (CSF) space and may be positioned posteriorly (Fig. 24-34).

Neonatal Head Ultrasound

Germinal Matrix Hemorrhage

The germinal matrix develops deep to the ependyma and consists of proliferating cells that give rise to neurons and glia

Figure 24-32   Left hip fluid; ultrasound detection. **A,** Plain film demonstrates widening of the left hip joint *(arrow)*. **B,** Ultrasound study of the left hip (LT) in the sagittal plane demonstrates fluid in the bursal extension *(arrows)* over the femoral neck. Also note that the overlying capsule is slightly thickened. Normal side (RT) is shown for comparison. Note that there is no fluid and that the potential bursal joint space over the femoral neck is collapsed *(arrow)*.

of the cerebral cortex and basal ganglia. The germinal matrix vascular bed consists of immature fine capillaries and extremely thin-walled veins. By 24 weeks of gestation the germinal matrix persists only in the caudothalamic groove and is not visualized on US; it is the anatomic site where hemorrhage occurs in premature infants (Fig. 24-35, *A* and *B*). By 40 weeks the germinal matrix has disappeared completely. On US, germinal matrix hemorrhage is seen as an ovoid echogenic mass within the caudothalamic groove. The normal choroid plexus, which is also echogenic, does not extend anterior to the caudothalamic groove into the frontal horn or into the occipital horn. Echogenic material in these segments of the lateral ventricle is consistent with blood.

There are four grades of intraventricular hemorrhage (IVH): grade 1, hemorrhage confined to the germinal matrix (Fig. 24-35, *B*); grade 2, germinal matrix and IVH without ventricular dilatation; grade 3, germinal matrix and IVH with ventricular dilatation; and grade 4, germinal matrix, IVH with or without ventricular dilatation, and intraparenchymal hemorrhage.

COMPUTED TOMOGRAPHY

Introduction

In 1917 Austrian mathematician Johann Radon presented an algorithm for creating an image from a set of measured data. After further theoretical work by Allan Cormack between 1950 and 1970, the British engineer Sir Godfrey Hounsfield built the first CT scanner in 1972 while working for the Electric and Musical Industries (EMI) group, the Beatles' record company, with funding from the Beatles' string of massive successes in the 1960s. Hounsfield and Cormack were awarded the 1979 Nobel Prize in Medicine for their work. Indeed, CT imaging, along with magnetic resonance imaging, was rated the first of 30 major medical innovations in the last three decades of the twentieth century by leading internists.

CT relies on measuring and displaying the varying x-ray attenuations (absorption) of the tissues in a section of the body during the simultaneous rotation of the x-ray tube and detectors around the patient while passing x-rays through this section from different angles (Fig. 24-36). It then uses reconstruction algorithms to display the differing densities in a

transducer

Figure 24-33 The coronal flexion sonogram of the normal left hip **(A)** is oriented vertically to match the anteroposterior radiograph **(B).** The femoral head (FH) is well seated within a nicely rounded acetabulum. The triradiate (T) cartilage, also known as the Y cartilage, is clearly seen between the iliac (IL), pubic (P), and ischial (IS) bones. The *arrow* on the sonogram points to the fibrous tip of the cartilaginous labrum. G1 refers to the gluteus minimus muscle, G2 to the gluteus medius muscle, and G3 to the gluteus maximus muscle. *(Modified from Smergel E, Losik SB, Rosenberg HK: Sonography of hip dysplasia,* Ultrasound Q *20:201-216, 2004.)*

gray-scale image. It is the contrast resolution of CT that distinguishes the modality: CT has, by far, the best contrast resolution of any clinical x-ray modality, allowing small differences in x-ray attenuation values to be visualized. CT can detect lesions that differ approximately 0.5% from the surrounding tissues, whereas conventional (screen-film) radiography requires the lesion to differ by about 5% for detection (i.e., the range of densities recorded is increased 10-fold by CT). To improve lesion conspicuity on CT scans, contrast material may be injected intravenously.

In conventional (serial) CT scanning, the x-ray tube/detector array rotates 360 degrees around the patient to acquire a slice with the patient stationary (see Fig. 24-36). Typically an examination consists of several successive slices of the patient's volume of interest, and the table is incremented and the process repeated for each slice. In helical CT, developed by Willi Kalender in 1989, the x-ray tube/detector array rotates continuously about the patient, and the patient is moved at a constant speed. The x-ray tube focal spot locus defines a spiral or helix (Fig. 24-37). The four Cs of spiral CT consist of (1) Continuously rotating tube/detector system, (2) Continuous radiation, (3) Continuous data acquisition, and (4) Continuous table feed (i.e., each acquisition provides a complete volumetric data set). This single-row detector helical CT scanner (SDCT) is generally much faster than a serial scanner. In the second half of 1998, the major CT manufacturers launched

the multiple-row detector helical CT (MDCT) scanner, capable of acquiring four CT slices in one x-ray tube rotation. In 2004, the 64-slice CT scanner became available. More detectors (currently 64 or more) means that fewer x-ray tube rotations are required to cover the same volume of the patient and therefore data can be acquired more quickly. A short scan time in the pediatric age group may allow more examinations to be performed without sedation. The reduced scanning time significantly decreases the respiratory artifact, affecting the lungs in particular. High-speed imaging also allows high-quality CT angiography and cardiac imaging. On MDCT scanners, thin (submillimeter) slices can be obtained, allowing reconstruction in multiple planes and generation of three-dimensional (3D) images (Fig. 24-38).

CT dose reduction in pediatric imaging requires a combination of different approaches to achieve the goals of ALARA and Image Gently. These include the optimization of scanning protocols for children according to weight-based adjustments, the limitation of unnecessary multiphase contrast studies, replacement of nonessential CT examinations by ultrasonography or magnetic resonance imaging, and development of automatic exposure control devices and dose reduction software by CT manufacturers.

Applications for Pediatric MDCT

CT is useful in imaging many disorders of the brain and spine (see Imaging of the Central Nervous System, later). Common nonneurologic indications for CT are listed in Table 24-7.

Noncontrast CT studies are useful for detecting calcification (e.g., renal stone). Nonionic intravenous contrast is universally used and has significantly reduced the incidence of contrast reactions. In the setting of trauma, intravenous contrast is indicated for CT of the neck, chest, abdomen, and pelvis but not for the head, face, spine, or extremities. For CT of the abdomen and pelvis, enteric contrast medium may be given by mouth or rectum in conjunction with intravenous contrast. The intraluminal gastrointestinal opacification helps to differentiate normal bowel from abnormal bowel, abscesses, and masses. Administration of oral contrast is contraindicated when a patient lacks a gag reflex or might require general anesthesia. Oral contrast should be drunk in small proportions over a period of about 60 minutes before the CT examination starts so that the entire gastrointestinal tract is completely opacified. The patient should therefore arrive at least 1 hour before an abdominal CT examination.

Figure 24-34 Tethered cord. Longitudinal sonogram shows low-lying conus *(arrow)* at the L5 vertebra. Note that the cord and nerve roots are positioned posteriorly.

Figure 24-35 **A,** Normal germinal matrix–caudothalamic groove. A paramedian sagittal plane shows the caudate nucleus (C), thalamus (T), caudothalamic groove (CTG), and choroid plexus (CP). FL, frontal lobe; PL, parietal lobe. **B,** Acute subependymal hemorrhage (grade 1 intraventricular hemorrhage). Left parasagittal image shows increased echogenicity in the caudothalamic groove *(arrow)*.

Chest

Regions and structures evaluated include the lung parenchyma, airway, mediastinum, cardiovascular structures, and chest wall.

Lung Parenchyma

CT is useful to evaluate infection and can differentiate between pulmonary consolidation, abscess formation, and empyema.

Contrast enhancement will outline the vascular pleura, leaving the contents of an empyema unopacified.

CT is invaluable in pulmonary metastatic disease detection and surveillance.

Multiplanar and 3D depictions of parenchymal abnormalities can improve the display of bronchopulmonary foregut malformations for surgical intervention (e-Fig. 24-9). CT has advantages over MR imaging for evaluation of sequestration,

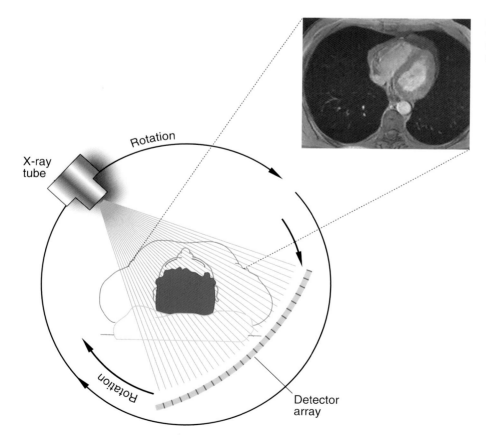

Figure 24-36 Diagram of a modern third-generation computed tomography (CT) scanner, which acquires data by rotating both the x-ray tube with wide fan beam geometry and the detector array around the patient.

3rd generation CT scanner

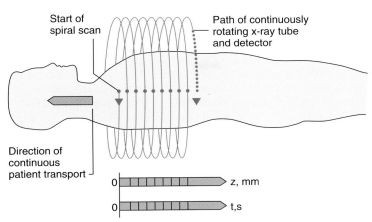

Figure 24-37 Sketch of the scanning geometry in spiral volumetric CT. t, s, time in seconds; z, mm, section position in millimeters. *(Modified from Kalender WA, Seissler W, Klotz E, et al: Spiral volumetric CT with single-breath-hold technique, continuous transport, and continuous scanner rotation,* Radiology *176:181-183, 1990.)*

Table 24-7	Nonneurologic Indications for Computed Tomography
Organ	**Indications**
Chest	Trauma
	Mass
	Metastatic disease
	Infection
	Acute or chronic lung disease
	Pleural disease
	Congenital anomalies, including vascular ring, pulmonary sling, cystic lesions of lung or mediastinum, and sequestration
	Pulmonary embolus
Abdomen/pelvis	Pulmonary embolus
	Trauma
	Mass
	Infection/abscess
	Unexplained pain
	Inflammatory bowel disease
	Portal hypertension
	Pancreatitis
	Urinary calculi (CT preferred over intravenous urography)
	Congenital anomalies
Extremities	Soft tissue or bone mass
	Osteoid osteoma
	Developmental or acquired dysplasia of the hip
	Femoral anteversion
	Leg length discrepancy
	Tarsal coalition
	Fracture

CT, computed tomography.
Modified from Osborn LM, DeWitt TG, First LR, et al, editors: *Pediatrics,* Philadelphia, 2005, Mosby Elsevier.

including a superior depiction of lung parenchyma and improved spatial resolution (e-Fig. 24-10). CT demonstrates primary pulmonary diseases such as cystic fibrosis, bronchiectasis (Fig. 24-39), and interstitial lung disease. In suspected air trapping, sections on inspiration and expiration are evaluated.

Airway

Airway evaluation includes assessment of congenital abnormalities, endobronchial or extrinsic processes with airway effects (Fig. 24-40), postoperative stenosis, and trauma. Virtual CT bronchoscopy can be obtained in children to evaluate endoluminal lesions.

Mediastinum

Most mediastinal masses are initially identified on chest radiography and then further evaluated by CT, which confirms the presence of a mediastinal mass, evaluates its relation to the contrast-enhanced adjacent structures, demonstrates potentially characteristic enhancement of the lesion, and evaluates for potential complications. Depiction of these abnormalities in multiplanar and 3D reconstructions is useful.

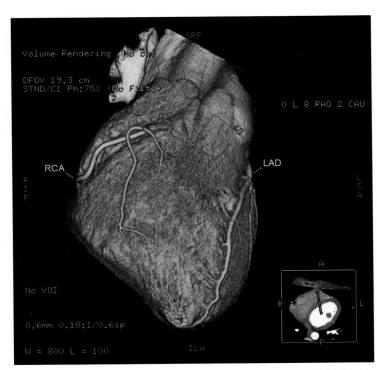

Figure 24-38 Three-dimensional volume-rendering reconstruction of the heart in a pediatric patient, showing normal coronary arteries as demonstrated with a 64-slice multidetector spiral CT scanner. A, Anterior; I, inferior; L, left; LAD, left anterior descending artery; P, posterior; R, right; RCA, right coronary artery; S, superior.

Figure 24-39 Coronal reformatted image of the chest (lung window) demonstrates cystic bronchiectasis.

Figure 24-40   Axial image produced by enhanced 64-slice multiple-row detector helical CT (MDCT) reveals separate right and left aortic arches with right dominance. The trachea and esophagus are surrounded by a vascular ring made by the double aortic arches and are moderately compressed.

Cardiovascular Structures

Cardiovascular evaluation by MDCT has been an important advancement. Assessment of cardiovascular structures includes evaluation of the aorta (e.g., for aneurysm, dissection, vascular rings, and postoperative changes); pulmonary arteries (e.g., for congenital or postoperative stenosis and pulmonary embolism) and veins; congenital anomalies of the coronary arteries (Fig. 24-41); and complex cardiovascular assessment that may not be rendered sufficiently by echocardiography.

Chest Wall

Metastatic involvement of the chest wall by neuroblastoma, lymphoma, or leukemia is more common than are primary tumors (e.g., Ewing sarcoma). MDCT is valuable in the proper depiction of the involved structures and surgical planning. One of the most common abnormalities in chest wall configuration is pectus excavatum. Before surgical repair by the Nuss procedure, a CT examination using low tube current is obtained through the level of the greatest degree of pectus deformity.

Figure 24-41   Axial maximal intensity projection image of a gated cardiac CT reveals a malignant course of the right coronary artery, taking origin from the left coronary artery and coursing between the aorta and pulmonary trunk.

Abdomen and Pelvis

MDCT is a valuable modality for evaluation of the abdomen and pelvis in children. In contrast to the chest, however, there are multiple imaging modalities that are suitable options for evaluation of multiple processes of the abdomen. This includes ultrasound and MR imaging. For many disease processes, there is marked debate concerning which imaging modalities are the primary choice for imaging in the diagnostic workup. Imaging algorithms vary from nation to nation and from institution to institution.

CT is the imaging study of choice for pediatric trauma, evaluation of suspected pediatric tumors, anatomic evaluation of solid abdominal parenchymal organ masses, and evaluation of suspected abscess or inflammatory disorders. The increased use of CT over the past several years in the evaluation of children with abdominal pain, suspected appendicitis, or suspected urolithiasis is related mostly to CT being considered more routine, the increased speed of MDCT, and changes in the patient population. As obesity becomes an increasing pediatric problem, other imaging modalities, such as ultrasound, are less well suited to evaluate pediatric patients for certain abdominal problems, such as appendicitis. The specific areas in which MDCT has been used with increased frequency to evaluate abdominal disorders include appendicitis and abdominal pain, urolithiasis, and inflammatory bowel disease.

Appendicitis and Abdominal Pain

Appendicitis is one of the more common surgical disorders of the abdomen. Between 7% and 9% of the general population develops appendicitis at some time during their life. Clinical examination is somewhat insensitive to appendicitis. Approximately one fourth to half of children with appendicitis are missed at initial clinical examination. This number is even greater for those children less than 2 years of age, of whom nearly 100% are missed at initial clinical examination. In addition, other clinical evaluators, such as the white blood count, are nonspecific and may be normal in cases of appendicitis and elevated in association with many nonsurgical causes of abdominal pain. Because of these reasons, imaging plays a critical role in the evaluation of children with appendicitis.

The reported sensitivity of CT for appendicitis ranges from 95% to 100%. The specificity ranges from 93% to 100%. Direct signs of acute appendicitis include enlarged appendix (greater than 7 mm in transverse diameter); a nonopacified appendiceal lumen; enhancement of the appendiceal wall; or an appendicolith within the appendix (Fig. 24-42). Secondary signs include stranding of the fat surrounding the appendix, associated free fluid, or thickening of the cecal wall and terminal ileum. Small bowel obstruction or abscess may be associated. In one study, the frequency of appendicitis in a population of patients evaluated by CT for abdominal pain was 38%. Sagittal and coronal reconstructed images may be helpful in identifying the appendix.

Identification of alternative diagnoses is another important role of CT in the evaluation of patients with abdominal pain and possible appendicitis. Alternative diagnoses revealed by CT scan in patients with suspected appendicitis included those involving the peribowel (46%); ovaries (16%); bowel (13%); urinary tract (8%); and other (17%). "Peribowel" refers to the mesentery and tissues associated with the bowel.

Urolithiasis

MDCT has gained acceptance as a primary modality for the evaluation of children with abdominal pain and hematuria in the search for urolithiasis. No oral or intravenous contrast is

Figure 24-42 Coronal reformatted CT image produced after the administration of oral, rectal, and intravenous contrast shows dilated appendix *(arrows)* with a thickened enhancing wall and stranding of the surrounding fat. Note the round calcified appendicolith located near the orifice of the appendix.

administered. In one reported series, approximately 40% of patients evaluated with CT for suspected stones demonstrated urolithiasis. In addition, alternative diagnoses were suggested in 17% of patients. CT findings in urolithiasis include visualization of the radiodense stone, dilatation of the ureter or collecting system, asymmetrical enlargement of the kidneys, and perinephric stranding.

Inflammatory Bowel Disease

MDCT is being used in the evaluation of children in adolescence with inflammatory bowel disease, such as Crohn disease or ulcerative colitis. The technique, termed "CT enterography," uses neutral oral contrast and intravenous contrast and is useful in the evaluation of patients with suspected active inflammatory processes, abdominal abscesses, or a fistula. CT enterography is becoming increasingly used, in contrast to various fluoroscopic studies such as small bowel followthrough. CT is superior to fluoroscopy in the demonstration of inflammatory changes within the bowel, and in particular extraluminal manifestations, such as peribowel inflammatory change or abscess. At present, MR enterography is being used at increased frequency, with images comparable to those of CT enterography without exposing patients to ionizing radiation.

Skeletal System

MDCT is indicated to better delineate the extent of a bony lesion (e.g., stress or comminuted fractures, metastatic and primary bone lesions) and in preoperative and postoperative imaging. The role of CT in tumor staging has been largely replaced by MR imaging. The reformatting and 3D reconstruction capabilities (Fig. 24-43) and the superior visualization of trauma, the casted skeleton, and complex osseous structures are the most useful features of CT imaging. CT measurement of leg lengths and femoral anteversion can be performed by a low-dose technique.

MAGNETIC RESONANCE IMAGING

Introduction

Magnetic resonance imaging is based on the electromagnetic activity of atomic nuclei. Nuclei are made up of protons and neutrons, both of which spin about their own axes. The direction of spin is random so that some particles spin clockwise, and others counterclockwise. When a nucleus has an even mass number the spins cancel each other out, and therefore the nucleus has no net spin. When a nucleus has an odd mass number, the spins do not cancel each other out and the nucleus spins. As protons have a charge, a nucleus with an odd mass number has a net charge as well as net spin. Owing to the laws of electromagnetic induction, a moving unbalanced charge induces a magnetic field around itself. The direction and size of the magnetic field are denoted by a magnetic moment or arrow (Fig. 24-44, *A*). Nuclei with an odd number of protons are said to be MR active. They act like tiny bar magnets. The hydrogen nucleus is the MR active nucleus used in clinical MRI. This nucleus consists of a single proton (atomic number 1; ^{1}H). It is used for MR imaging because it is abundant in the human body (e.g., in fat and water), and its solitary proton gives it a large magnetic moment. Each cubic millimeter of tissue contains about 1018 protons (^{1}H).

When the hydrogen nuclei (^{1}H) are exposed to an external magnetic field (B_0), they produce a secondary spin or spin wobble. This wobble is called *precession* and causes the magnetic moments of the hydrogen nuclei to describe a circular path around B_0. The speed at which the magnetic moments wobble about the external magnetic field is called the *precessional* or *resonance frequency*. The precessional frequency becomes higher when the magnetic field strength increases. The precessional frequency corresponds to the range of frequencies in the electromagnetic spectrum of radiowaves. The precessional frequency of ^{1}H at 1.5 tesla (T) is 63 megahertz (MHz).

Until the ^{1}H nuclei are exposed to B_0 magnetization, their axes are randomly aligned. However, when B_0 magnetization is applied, the magnetic axes of the nuclei align with the

Figure 24-43 Three-dimensional volume-rendering reconstruction of a displaced comminuted fracture involving the distal humerus.

Figure 24-44   Basic physics of the magnetic resonance (MR) signal. **A,** As ^{1}H nuclei spin, they induce their own magnetic field (tan), the direction (magnetic axis) of which is depicted by an *arrow* (orange). The ^{1}H nuclei initially spin at various angles, but when they are exposed to an external magnetic field (B_0), they precess with a wobble and align with it. The sum of all magnetic moments is called the net magnetization vector (NMV). **B,** When a radiofrequency (RF) pulse is applied, the net magnetization vector is flipped at an angle (α), which produces two magnetization components: longitudinal magnetization (M_z) and transverse magnetization (M_{xy}). As the transverse magnetization precesses around a receiver coil, it induces a current (i). When the RF generator is turned off, T_1 recovery and T_2 decay occur. *(Modified from Bitar R, Leung G, Perng R, et al: MR pulse sequences: What every radiologist wants to know but is afraid to ask,* Radiographics 26:513-537, 2006.)

magnetic axis of B_0, some in parallel and others in opposition to it (Fig. 24-44, *A*). The cumulative effect of all the magnetic moments of the nuclei is the net magnetization vector (NMV). When a radiofrequency (RF) pulse at an appropriate frequency (resonant frequency) is applied, the absorbed RF energy causes the net magnetization vector to momentarily flip by a certain angle to a higher energy state, and this produces two magnetization vector components: longitudinal magnetization and transverse magnetization. As the transverse magnetization precesses around an RF receiver coil, a current is captured in accordance with the Faraday law of induction. This current becomes the MR signal.

When the RF energy source is turned off, the net magnetization vector realigns with the axis of B_0 through the process of T_1 recovery, during which the longitudinal magnetization increases in magnitude. At the same time, the transverse magnetization decreases (decays) through a mechanism known as T_2 decay. Different tissues have different T_1 and T_2 values. Fat has a shorter T_1 (i.e., recovers faster) and a shorter T_2 (i.e., decays faster) than water, which has a relatively long T_1 (i.e., dark) and long T_2 (i.e., bright) (Fig. 24-44, *B*).

MRI has superior soft tissue contrast resolution compared with other imaging modalities. T_1-weighted images best depict the anatomy, and, if contrast material is used, they also may show pathologic entities; however, T_2-weighted images provide the best depiction of disease, because most tissues that are involved in a pathologic process have higher water content than is normal, and the fluid causes the affected areas to appear bright on T_2-weighted images. The levels of signal intensity that characterize various tissues on T_1- and T_2-weighted images are shown in Figure 24-45. Air is black because of its extremely low concentration of hydrogen, and cortical bone is black because of its lack of mobile protons. Flowing blood is black on spin-echo images because of the flow of protons away from the area before the signal can be received.

An MRI scanner consists of a large circular magnet. The magnetic resonance signal from the body is detected from fixed receiver coil arrays that are built into the patient table and from flexible arrays that can be placed on top of the patient. MRI scanners use magnetic fields that are about 30,000 to 60,000 times stronger than the earth's magnetic field. Magnetic fields are measured in teslas (T); 1 T = 10,000 gauss (G). The earth's magnetic field is weak (50 µT or

0.5 G). No adverse biologic effects from diagnostic MRI have been demonstrated. The strong magnetic field, however, means that it is at present contraindicated in patients with cardiac pacemakers, internal ferromagnetic objects such as surgical aneurysm clips, and intraocular metal shards. Electronic monitoring equipment cannot be used while the patient is scanned. Thus, for most traumas, CT is preferred.

One advantage of MRI over CT is that it can acquire images in any plane and without the need of ionizing radiation. However, acquisition of the highest quality images by MRI requires tens of minutes, whereas a CT scan of most body parts requires only a few seconds. Thus, for patients in whose motion cannot be controlled (i.e., uncooperative, disoriented or claustrophobic patients, and infants/young children), CT is often used or MRI can be performed under sedation. Unavoidable movements from breathing, cardiac pulsation, and peristalsis often degrade the image. Fast image acquisition techniques using special coils, and motion-limiting techniques using gating devices, have made it possible to produce imaging of the motion-prone thorax and abdomen.

Gadolinium-based paramagnetic contrast agents increase the signal intensity of tissues on T_1-weighted images with fat saturation. Pathologic processes such as tumors and inflammation tend to show greater enhancement than normal tissues. Accumulated experience has shown that gadolinium is very safe for administration in children. Contrast-enhanced magnetic resonance angiography (CE-MRA) provides high-resolution imaging of the vasculature and may eventually replace conventional angiography (Fig. 24-46).

Nephrogenic Systemic Fibrosis in Children

Nephrogenic systemic fibrosis (NSF, or nephrogenic fibrosing dermopathy) is a recently defined disease with a potentially deleterious outcome and not yet completely clarified etiology. A common factor in many patients is underlying kidney disease (with renal insufficiency, often requiring dialysis). Another commonly observed factor is repeated gadolinium administration, although there are patients with NSF without previous known gadolinium exposure. Additional independent risk factors are metabolic acidosis and inflammatory and postoperative conditions. Although only a few reports have described a partial linkage between children with NSF and

T1WI

Dark — Air, mineral-rich tissue (cortical bone, stones), fast-flowing blood

Low — Collagenous tissue (ligaments, tendons, scars), high free water tissue (kidneys, gonads, edema, fluids [urine, bile], simple cysts, bladder, gallbladder, spleen, CSF), high bound water tissues (liver, pancreas, adrenals, hyaline cartilage, muscle)

Intermediate — Proteinaceous tissue (abscess, complex cysts, synovial fluid)

Bright — Fat, fatty bone marrow, blood products (methemoglobin [metHB]), slow-flowing blood, radiation change, paramagnetic contrast agents

T2WI

Dark — Air, mineral-rich tissue (cortical bone, stones), fast-flowing blood

Collagenous tissue (ligaments, tendons, scars), bone islands

Low — High bound water tissue (liver, pancreas, adrenals, hyaline cartilage, muscle)

Fat, fatty bone marrow

Intermediate

Bright — High free water tissue (kidneys, gonads, edema, fluids [urine, bile], simple cysts, bladder, gallbladder, spleen, CSF), proteinaceous tissue, blood products (oxyhemoglobin, extracellular metHb)

Figure 24-45 Diagram showing the signal intensity of various tissues at T_1- and T_2-weighted imaging. However, note that the signal characteristics of proteinaceous tissues vary according to the amount of protein content: Tissues with high concentrations of protein may have high signal intensity on T_1-weighted images (T1WI) and low signal intensity on T_2-weighted images (T2WI). CSF = cerebrospinal fluid. *(Modified from Bitar R, Leung G, Perng R, et al: MR pulse sequences: What every radiologist wants to know but is afraid to ask, Radiographics 26:513-537, 2006.)*

gadolinium exposure, the pediatric radiology community is urged to consider NSF when performing MRI (e-Table 24-6).

Applications for Pediatric MRI

MRI is the imaging modality of choice for many disorders of the brain and spine (see Imaging of the Central Nervous System, later).

Figure 24-46 Contrast-enhanced magnetic resonance angiography. Time-resolved imaging of contrast kinetics (TRICKS) MR angiogram in a 7-month-old.

Chest

Regions and structures evaluated include airway, mediastinum, cardiovascular structures, and chest wall. MRI has become an important modality for the evaluation of mediastinal lesions. MRI is ideal for characterizing posterior mediastinal masses such as neuroblastoma because it better defines their intraspinal extension. MRI is useful in characterizing the tissue nature of mediastinal masses. Fat-containing masses in children usually are teratomas. Lymphatic malformations and other cystic lesions usually present as water signal. MRI is useful in the diagnosis of congenital anomalies such as vascular ring and pulmonary sling, and MR angiography may show the systemic vascular supply to the bronchopulmonary malformation and its relationship to the solid or solid component of the lung lesion. Pulmonary metastases can be reliably diagnosed from 5 mm in size, using MRI (Fig. 24-47); however, because of the clinical relevance of early identification of pulmonary metastases, CT is the established gold standard for initial diagnosis. Therefore, MRI of the lung in children has so far been performed solely to monitor the regression of known pulmonary metastases under therapy. Calcifications are readily seen on CT but cast no signals on MR.

Cardiac Magnetic Resonance

Echocardiography is the first-line modality of cardiac imaging. It is portable, noninvasive, and provides immediate high-resolution anatomic and physiologic information. But echocardiography does have several limitations. The quality of images can be compromised in those who are noncooperative or if there are poor acoustic windows. Echocardiography is also limited in providing the position and course of extracardiac vascular structures (e.g., vascular rings, collateral vessels). Cardiac magnetic resonance (CMR) is gaining increasing importance in the management of pediatric congenital heart disease (CHD). It is a powerful tool, giving anatomic and hemodynamic information that echocardiography and

Figure 24-47   Eleven-year-old with metastatic rhabdomyosarcoma. **A,** Coronal CT image of the chest (lung window) demonstrates a 5.2-mm right upper lobe metastatic nodule *(arrow)*. **B,** The same nodule *(arrow)* is hyperintense on a coronal short tau inversion recovery (STIR) image obtained 3 weeks later.

catheterization alone do not provide. Extracardiac anatomy can be delineated with high spatial resolution, intracardiac anatomy can be imaged in multiple planes, and functional assessment can be made accurately and with high reproducibility. CMR is the gold standard for the quantification of ventricular volume, mass, and ejection fraction. Finally, CMR surpasses both catheterization and echocardiography in its ability to create high-resolution 3D reconstructions of complex CHD, without the use of ionizing radiation.

Common Indications for the Use of CMR

1. Shunts (atrial septal defect, ventricular septal defect, and partial anomalous pulmonary venous drainage [PAPVD] and associated sinus venosus defects): CMR can accurately identify the location of the shunt and characterizes its hemodynamics by measuring flow through the pulmonary artery and ascending aorta (Qp:Qs), using through-plane phase-contrast flow sequences.

2. Quantification of valve regurgitation: Through-plane phase-contrast flow sequences give forward and reverse flow volumes through a vessel, allowing the regurgitant fraction to be calculated (RF% = reverse flow/forward flow × 100). Examples of regurgitant valves that require accurate serial imaging to guide management include bicuspid aortic valves and pulmonary regurgitation in patients after tetralogy of Fallot (TOF) repair (Fig. 24-48).

3. Determination of the extracardiac anatomy in patients with complex CHD such as relationship of great vessels, major aortopulmonary collateral arteries (MAPCAs), airway branching pattern, and abdominal situs.

4. Aortic root/arch abnormalities: Assessment of the extent and severity of aortic coarctation (Fig. 24-49). CMR is useful in patients who have undergone coarctation repair in whom echocardiography does not sensitively demonstrate aneurysmal formation or restenosis. Patients with suspected vascular rings benefit from 3D evaluation. CMR is performed in patients with a dilated aortic root, such as a bicuspid aortic valve and Marfan syndrome, to assess morphology and competency/patency of the aortic valve.

5. Evaluation of size and patency of pulmonary arteries: CMR provides detailed anatomy of the branch pulmonary arteries and the main pulmonary trunk in postoperative patients who have had pulmonary arteries mobilized and/or reconstructed (e.g., arterial switch operation, after repair of TOF). Patients with inherently abnormal pulmonary arteries due to syndromes such as Noonan and Alagille may also require CMR.

6. Evaluation of pulmonary venous anatomy/stenosis and systemic veins.

7. Assessment of anomalous coronary arteries, coronary aneurysms in Kawasaki disease, and coronary anatomy after arterial switch operation.

8. T_2^* (pronounced "T_2 star") CMR is an accurate, noninvasive method for the diagnosis and monitoring of patients at risk for iron deposition cardiomyopathy.

9. Evaluation of arrhythmogenic right ventricular dysplasia, hypertrophic cardiomyopathy, and myocarditis.

10. Assessment of intracardiac masses/thrombi and pericardial masses.

11. Takayasu arteritis: MRI can detect arterial wall thickening, edema, and late gadolinium enhancement (LGE) consistent with active disease; and can also assess complications such as vascular narrowing and/or dilation.

12. CMR tissue tagging: This noninvasive tool quantifies 3D intramural myocardial function and provides detailed data on contraction/relaxation of the heart.

Role of CT Imaging

CT imaging is useful for patients who are unable to cooperate with CMR, have contraindications to MRI, or who are too clinically unstable. In addition, when CMR provides inadequate images for clinical decision-making (e.g., small

Figure 24-48   Assessment of pulmonary regurgitation in a 20-year-old with repaired tetralogy of Fallot. **A,** Localizer sagittal spin-echo MR image indicates the imaging plane of the flow images *(white line)* perpendicular to the main pulmonary artery (PA). RV, right ventricle. **B,** Phase-velocity image obtained during systole reveals low signal intensity within the pulmonary artery (PA), indicating antegrade flow. **C,** Phase-velocity image obtained during diastole demonstrates high signal intensity within the pulmonary artery (PA), indicating retrograde flow. **D,** Graph depicts the flow profile in the main pulmonary artery. A pulmonary regurgitant fraction of 55% was calculated (RF% = reverse flow/forward flow × 100).

Figure 24-49   Coarctation of the aorta in an 18-year-old. Sagittal maximal intensity projection **(A)** and volume-rendering **(B)** reconstruction images from magnetic resonance angiography show a three-vessel aortic arch with severe narrowing of the aorta just distal to the origin of the left subclavian artery. There are prominent collateral vessels feeding the proximal descending aorta just beyond the coarctation.

Figure 24-50 Undifferentiated (embryonal) sarcoma in a 14-year-old. **A,** Axial T₂-weighted image shows a well-circumscribed hyperintense mass, in the right lobe of the liver, containing hypointense septa. **B,** Magnetic resonance cholangiopancreatography image demonstrates obstruction of the intrahepatic bile ducts caused by the tumor.

structures such as coronary arteries), ECG-gated CT angiography is the modality of choice.

Abdomen

Abdominal Masses

MRI is increasingly advocated for initial diagnosis of various abdominal masses as well as for preoperative imaging, assessment of complications, and follow-up.

Abdominal masses in the pediatric population are predominantly retroperitoneal in location, with the kidney being the source in more than half of the cases. In neonates, most abdominal masses are benign; beyond the neonatal period, the percentage of malignant neoplasms increases. Retroperitoneal tumors encompass the neonatal mesoblastic nephroma, neuroblastoma, ganglioneuroma, ganglioneuroblastoma, Wilms tumor, rhabdoid renal tumor, renal cell carcinoma (in older children), and pheochromocytoma.

Liver tumors in the pediatric population frequently include hemangioma and hemangiomatosis, hepatoblastoma, embryonal hepatocellular sarcoma (Fig. 24-50), rhabdomyosarcoma, and hepatocellular carcinoma (in cirrhotic liver diseases). Particularly in patients after chemotherapy, liver adenoma and focal nodular hyperplasia may be seen and—in early stages—can be challenging to differentiate from metastasis or recurrent disease. Choledochal cyst is the most common mass arising in the biliary tree. Rhabdomyosarcoma of the biliary tract is rare, but it is the most common malignancy of the biliary tract in children.

Focal pancreatic lesions in children are usually exocrine neoplasms or cystic lesions. Pancreatoblastoma is the most common exocrine pancreatic neoplasm in young children. Cystic pancreatic lesions are usually associated with inherited disorders such as cystic fibrosis, von Hippel-Lindau disease, and autosomal dominant polycystic disease.

Focal splenic lesions in children include abscesses, neoplasms (most commonly lymphoma), vascular malformations (lymphatic malformation and hemangioma), and cysts.

Mesenteric masses include lymphatic malformation, mesenteric cyst, and teratoma. Lymphoma is the most common malignant neoplasm of the bowel and mesentery.

Genital tumors may be encountered; the most common are ovarian teratoma and various ovarian and testicular stromal tumors. Congenital uterine malformations are easily assessed by MRI.

Magnetic Resonance Cholangiopancreatography

Magnetic resonance cholangiopancreatography with heavily T₂-weighted sequences has been shown to be safe and accurate in depicting pancreatobiliary anatomy and can be applied to evaluate pancreatitis, choledochal cysts, choledocholithiasis, primary sclerosing cholangitis, masses, and trauma. It is also useful for evaluation before and after liver transplantation.

Magnetic Resonance Enterography

Magnetic resonance enterography is reliable to assess the degree of disease activity, the severity and extent of bowel involvement, and the presence of extraintestinal complications, including abscesses, fistulas, and sinus tracts (Fig. 24-51).

Figure 24-51 Magnetic resonance enterography. Coronal T₂ single-shot fast spin echo image in a 14-year-old with Crohn disease shows two segments of small bowel wall thickening and luminal narrowing consistent with strictures *(arrows)*. Note the dilation of the ileal loops proximal to the strictures.

Magnetic Resonance Urography

Pediatric magnetic resonance urography has gained importance for assessment of complex GU tract anomalies and severely hydronephrotic kidneys; to a large extent (if available) it has replaced intravenous urography.

Quantification of Iron Accumulation in the Liver

MR imaging does not image iron directly but instead detects the effect of iron on water protons in the tissue of interest. The distribution of iron overload is usually diffuse and homogeneous, but it may be heterogeneous. In patients with cirrhosis, the accumulation also may be focal, reflecting selective accumulation of iron in siderotic nodules.

The pattern of organ involvement reflects the etiology. In patients with hereditary hemochromatosis, there is preferential involvement of the liver, pancreas, and heart, with sparing of extrahepatic reticuloendothelial (RE) organs (spleen, bone marrow, lymph nodes). By comparison, in thalassemia and other transfusion-dependent anemias, preferential involvement of the RE system (liver, spleen, bone marrow, lymph nodes) is characteristic. Involvement of the pancreas and heart suggests the storage capacity of the RE system has been exceeded. In sickle cell disease (SCD), the renal cortex may show iron accumulation related to intravascular hemolysis. The liver in SCD is usually spared in the absence of transfusion therapy; involvement of the liver in nontransfused patients with SCD suggests a coexisting cause for hepatic iron overload such as hereditary hemochromatosis.

Musculoskeletal System

MRI has had a major impact on musculoskeletal imaging because of its ability to produce high-contrast images of structures that are invisible or that are poorly visualized by x-ray–based modalities. This feature is especially important in children, because the immature skeleton contains a high proportion of radiolucent cartilage. Radiographs obtained before MRI guide the selection of the proper MRI protocol (imaging planes and pulse sequences) to fully delineate and characterize anatomy and pathology; and can improve the diagnostic specificity of soft tissue lesions by depicting calcifications, fat, gas, or foreign material within the lesion.

Imaging protocols should include T_1-weighted, T_2-weighted, proton density (PD) sequences (with at least one of these combined with fat saturation); a short tau inversion recovery (STIR) sequence; and, when indicated, T_1-weighted images with fat saturation after intravenous application of gadolinium in two planes. T_2-weighted images with fat saturation and STIR images are used to diminish signal from fat and to increase the conspicuity of pathologic processes. Proton density and gradient echo sequences with fat saturation are useful for displaying cartilage, which appears intense on these images.

On MRI, bone and other dense tissues, including intact ligaments and tendons, show a lack of signal. This characteristic absence of signal provides negative contrast in comparison with muscle, which is of intermediate intensity, and yellow marrow, which is hyperintense on T_1-weighted images. Accumulations of fluid within joints and bursae are hyperintense on T_2-weighted images, as are fluid-containing lesions such as abscesses and cysts. Intravenous gadolinium is useful for the delineation of areas of inflammation, ischemia, and revascularization in patients with avascular necrosis and in patients with tumors. Gadolinium enhancement helps to demonstrate acute inflammatory changes in the joints, especially in the hypertrophied synovium in children with arthritis, and is also helpful in distinguishing the various types of vascular malformations. MR arthrography with dilute gadolinium is now commonly used in the diagnosis of some joint disorders, most notably labral abnormalities in the shoulder and hip.

Bone marrow edema, indicated by alterations in marrow signal (dark on T_1-weighted images, bright on T_2-weighted images with fat suppression and on STIR images), may indicate the presence of subtle or radiographically undetectable microfractures. MRI has proved sensitive to injuries and malformations involving the physis and epiphysis. This permits diagnosis of radiographically occult fractures and allows for early detection of posttraumatic bony physeal bridges. Osteochondritis dissecans involves most often the epiphyseal cartilage of the femoral condyles, talus, and the capitellum. A T_2-weighted sequence is able to demonstrate the grade and stability of the lesions, and visualize the cartilage, thus contributing to treatment planning. MRI is also useful during the course of inflammatory conditions such as juvenile rheumatoid arthritis, hemarthroses associated with blood coagulation disorders, and internal articular derangements from trauma or sports injury. MRI is the method of choice to detect meniscal injuries, ligamentous tears, patellar dislocation, cartilaginous injury, and avulsion fractures. Congenital abnormalities, such as discoid meniscus and tarsal coalition, are also easily recognizable on MRI.

MRI is of extreme value in the imaging of osteomyelitis. Acute inflammation manifests as signal loss on T_1-weighted images and elevated signal on T_2-weighted fat-saturated and STIR images, as early as 24 to 48 hours after the onset of symptoms, allowing early diagnosis. Adjacent soft tissue changes demonstrate similar signal intensity changes. Abscess formation is characterized by a central hypointensity and peripheral enhancement on T_1-weighted images after gadolinium administration (Fig. 24-52).

MRI is the modality of choice in the initial staging of primary malignant bone tumors. First, the entire affected bone and neighboring joint should be scanned in order to determine the exact tumor extension, skip lesions, and joint involvement. Then, high-resolution images of the tumor itself should be obtained. MRI plays a major role in demonstrating the intra- and extramedullary tumor components, and involvement of the growth plate, surrounding muscle components, neurovascular structures, and joints. MRI alone cannot reliably distinguish between benign and malignant tumors, and even

Figure 24-52 Acute hematogenous osteomyelitis in an 8-month-old. Coronal T_1-weighted fat-saturated image with contrast demonstrates bone marrow infection with cortical breakthrough and associated subperiosteal abscess *(arrow)* in the proximal right tibial metaphysis.

associated bone marrow and soft tissue edema or enhancement gadolinium administration are not reliable criteria of malignancy; in many instances only biopsy can establish the definite diagnosis.

MRI remains the only modality that permits direct visualization of normal bone marrow. The amount and distribution of red (hematopoietic) and yellow (fatty) marrow change with age. At birth, nearly the entire skeleton is composed of red marrow. Normal conversion from red to yellow marrow occurs in a predictable manner and is completed by the time an individual has reached the mid-20s (e-Fig. 24-11). Conversion from red to yellow marrow proceeds from the extremities to the axial skeleton, occurring in the distal bones of the extremities (feet and hands) first, and progressing finally to the proximal bones (humeri and femora). Whole body MRI (WBMRI) is a novel technique that is targeted for maximal coverage of the body within the shortest possible time, using the minimal number of sequences. The common scan plane is coronal with additional planes being added depending on the indication. Evaluation of the bone marrow has been the primary indication and thus a STIR sequence is typically used, with the T_1-weighted sequence being added variably. For correct evaluation of the bone marrow in the pediatric age group, understanding the normal pattern of marrow transformation is essential. The primary role of WBMRI has been in oncology for the detection of tumor spread and also for follow-up and the evaluation of complications. The initial comparative studies of WBMRI with scintigraphy and PET in children have shown the high diagnostic potential of WBMRI. Emerging potential applications of WBMRI include evaluation for osteonecrosis, chronic multifocal recurrent osteomyelitis, myopathies, and generalized vascular malformations.

IMAGING OF THE CENTRAL NERVOUS SYSTEM

Introduction

Advances in CT and MRI have vastly improved the delineation of central nervous system (CNS) anatomy and the diagnosis and extent of CNS pathology.

In CT imaging, the development of multidetector CT (MDCT) scanners has resulted in greater resolution, faster imaging and reconstruction times, and reduction of the radiation dose due to focused collimation. All the images acquired can be displayed according to various algorithms and the scout views obtained for each examination may also provide additional information, not unlike that of a plain radiograph. The incredible speed of multidetector CT has also minimized the need for sedation.

Safety issues with CT pertain primarily to the radiation exposure. The American College of Radiology (ACR) is committed to radiation safety and has implemented practice guidelines, technical standards and accreditation programs, as well as Appropriateness Criteria (e-Table 24-7).

MRI is noninvasive and does not involve ionizing radiation. MRI defines CNS anatomy in exquisite detail. Physiology and function can also now be evaluated and assessed by MRI. New sequences such as DWI/DTI (diffusion-weighted imaging and diffusion tensor imaging), MRS (MR spectroscopy), PMRI (perfusion MRI), and fMRI (functional MRI) provide information complementary to that obtained by anatomic imaging and provide additional characterization of disease pathophysiology, response to therapy, and/or disease progression. Faster sequences and MR-compatible goggles (which permit the patient to watch videos/movies and listen to music) have reduced the need for sedation although it remains a significant factor in pediatric MRI examinations (e-Table 24-8).

CURRENT ROLE OF CT IN CNS IMAGING

CT of the brain, head and neck, and spine is often used as a first-line screening modality because of its availability. CT is the modality of choice in the setting of trauma. It may also suffice as the expedient or screening examination in patients with uncomplicated headaches, macrocephaly, or hydrocephalus, particularly in younger patients who may require sedation for an MRI examination. In the elective setting, balancing the availability of CT and concern about the ionizing radiation involved versus the risks of possible sedation are often the determining factors. In acute situations, such as acute mental status change, signs of increased intracranial pressure or acute onset of neurologic symptoms, or in the unstable patient, CT is often the primary imaging modality, again because of its availability and ability to rapidly exclude or provide information related to life-threatening intracranial hemorrhage, edema, hydrocephalus, mass, or mass effect (Table 24-8).

CT still provides the most sensitive detection of subarachnoid hemorrhage and calcifications. The latter may provide added diagnostic specificity for CNS tumors, the sequelae of congenital infections/TORCH, and in the diagnosis of certain phakomatoses such as Sturge-Weber syndrome and tuberous sclerosis. Osseous lesions or lesions with a chondroid matrix are also exquisitely detailed by CT.

The CT density characteristics of many entities can be characterized by their Hounsfield unit (HU) values. The scale defines the density of water as 0 HU, and the density of air as −1000 HU. A change of 1 HU represents a change of 0.1% in density related to the attenuation coefficient of water. The scale defines the calibration for CT scanners (Table 24-9).

Unenhanced CT of the Brain

Indications for various CT imaging modalities depend on the clinical scenario. Use of unenhanced CT of the brain is useful in acute stroke if MRI is not available and excluding hemorrhage and/or large territorial infarction, which may preclude thrombolytic therapy (Fig. 24-53). In patients with acute mental status changes, unenhanced CT scan can evaluate for

Figure 24-53 Unenhanced axial CT image of a patient with a stroke at the level of the basal ganglia delineates hypodense right caudate and putamen *(arrow)*. The left caudate and putamen are hyperdense, as are the thalami; the central and peripheral gray matter appear normal. Right basal ganglia show ischemic changes and infarction.

Table 24-8	Table of Clinical Symptoms and Suggested Diagnostic Modalities: A Guideline			
	Symptom(s)	**Clinical Presentation**	**U/E**	**Modality**
Brain	Headache	No ND or signs of ↑ICP	E	MRI
		ND and/or signs of ↑ICP	U	MRI ± MRA/MRV; if unavailable, CT to exclude mass effect, hemorrhage, or hydrocephalus
	Macrocephaly Hydrocephalus	Without ND, HA, irritability, seizures, or signs of ↑ICP	E	CT or MRI: Balance concern for radiation versus possible need for sedation
		With ND, HA, irritability, seizures, signs of ↑ICP	U	MRI; if unavailable, CT to exclude hydrocephalus, hemorrhage, or mass effect
	Microcephaly	Regardless of presentation	E	MRI (and CT if congenital infection is suspected, to detect calcifications)
	Seizures	Without persistent ND, fever, or signs of ↑ICP	E	MRI ± contrast
		Fever, AMS, ND, or signs of ↑ICP	U	MRI, MRA, MRV, ± MRS; if not available, CT ± contrast
	Stroke	ND, HA, seizures	U	MRI, MRA, MRV, ± MRS and PMRI; if not available, CT
	Perinatal HIE, seizures, ↑bilirubin		U	MRI/MRA/MRV/MRS; if not available, CT
	Congenital anomalies		E	MRI
	Trauma		U	CT for initial evaluation; and MRI in severe trauma to assess full extent of brain injury
Spine	Pain	Without ND or systemic signs	U/E	Plain films and MRI
		With radiculopathy	U/E	Plain films and MRI
		Malignancy, fever, systemic signs	U/E	Plain films and MRI with contrast
	Scoliosis	Without ND or pain	E	Plain films ± MRI
		With ND and/or pain	E	Plain films ± MRI
	Congenital anomalies	Lesion on back, ND	E	MRI and plain films, and/or CT if complex spinal dysraphism is present
	Trauma		U	Plain films ± CT
				MRI in severe trauma for assessment of cord and ligamentous injury and possible intraspinal hematoma
Neck	Mass	Without fever, erythema, dysphagia, or airway compromise	E	CT or MRI with contrast; balance consideration of ionizing radiation with possible need for sedation with MRI
		With fever, erythema, dysphagia, and/or airway compromise	U	CT with contrast
	Pain/infection	With fever, swelling, dysphagia, and/or airway compromise	U	CT with contrast
	Metastases		E	CT or MRI with contrast; if perineural spread of concern, MRI
Orbits, head, and skull base	Skin lesion	No pain or erythema	E	MRI with contrast
	Hemangioma		E	MRI with contrast
	Infection	Pain, fever, swelling, or cranial nerve deficit	U	CT with contrast; MRI if perineural spread or intracranial extension is suspected
	Cranial nerve deficit	Without pain or fever	U	MRI; MRI if perineural spread or intracranial extension is suspected
	Trauma		U	CT
	Anomalies		E	High-resolution CT with 3D reconstruction
	Leukocoria		U/E	MRI (and CT to assess for calcifications)
	Strabismus		E	MRI

AMS, altered mental status; CT, computed tomography; E, elective; HA, headache; HIE, hypoxic ischemic injury; ICP, intracranial pressure; MRA, magnetic resonance angiography; MRI, magnetic resonance imaging; MRS, magnetic resonance spectroscopy; MRV, magnetic resonance venography; PMRI, perfusion magnetic resonance imaging; ND, neurologic deficits; U, urgent.

edema, hemorrhage, and/or mass effect, which may preclude safe lumbar puncture (Fig. 24-54). CT is valuable for evaluation of intracranial fluid collections, and bone windows may reveal abnormalities of the calvarium (Fig. 24-55). In the setting of macrocephaly, ventricular size and extra-axial fluid or mass can be determined and bone windows allow assessment of the calvarium and sutures (Fig. 24-56). In addition to changes in ventricular size, shunt position or edema or hemorrhage can aid in evaluation of shunt function (Fig. 24-57). High-resolution images of the cranial vault and brain with 2D and 3D reconstructions allow detailed analysis of craniosynostosis or other cranial anomalies (see Chapter 22).

Contrast-enhanced CT of the Brain

Contrast-enhanced (CE) CT of the brain is becoming a relatively rare examination, as an unenhanced CT scan that is positive is usually followed by an MRI examination. And an unenhanced CT that is negative, but does not answer the clinical question, is also usually followed by an MRI examination.

In ordering a contrast-enhanced examination the patient's clinical history, history of allergies, renal function, hydration status, and medications should be known and reviewed. Allergic reactions to iodinated contrast are rare, but do occur, in the pediatric population.

Table 24-9	Density Characteristics of CNS Structures on Computed Tomography

DENSITY (HU)							
Gray Matter	**White Matter**	**CSF**	**Acute Blood**	**Calcification**	**Bone**	**Air**	**Fat**
30 to 40	20 to 30	0	55 to 75	100 to 400	1000	−1000	−100 to −40

CNS, central nervous system; CSF, cerebrospinal fluid; HU, Hounsfield unit.

Figure 24-54   Near drowning/cardiac arrest; diffuse cerebral edema. Unenhanced axial CT images of a patient after cardiac arrest from near drowning delineate effacement of the fourth ventricle (**A,** *arrow*), effacement of the perimesencephalic cisterns (**B,** *arrow*), ischemic changes in the basal ganglia (**C,** *arrow*), and partially effaced lateral ventricles (**D,** *arrow*). On each of the images there is loss of gray/white matter differentiation and sulcal effacement.

Systemic factors that may lead to nephrotoxicity from iodinated contrast include the following: dehydration, anuria, creatinine greater than 3 mg/dL, diabetes, hepatorenal syndrome, multiple myeloma, metformin (Glucophage) use.

If MRI is not readily available or feasible in a reasonable period of time, CE-CT imaging should be considered if infection or tumor is suspected. It is also an adjunct to PET imaging if concern for tumor exists. When a CSF leak is suspected, in complicated hydrocephalus, or in the presence of intracranial cysts concerning which questions of communication arise, the examination may require subarachnoid or intraventricular contrast for diagnosis.

Contraindications to CE-CT imaging include the following: allergy to iodinated contrast material, acute renal failure (chronic renal dysfunction may be a relative contraindication), and trauma with vascular injury. If vascular injury is suspected, an unenhanced CT scan should first be obtained because contrast may obscure hemorrhage (Fig. 24-58).

Intracranial and Extracranial CT Angiography and CT Venography

Computed tomography angiography (CTA) and computed tomography venography (CTV) provide detailed anatomic information about the cranial vasculature. This is particularly valuable in trauma to assess arterial and/or venous injury, and in evaluating acute neurologic deficits by examining the vasculature for stenosis, dissection, or vascular malformation (Fig. 24-59). Tumors involving intra- or extracranial sites or the skull base can be evaluated for their vascularity or their relationship to adjacent structures (Fig. 24-60). In patients with subarachnoid hemorrhage due to aneurysms, CT angiography may delineate aneurysms in patients who are poor candidates for traditional angiography or digital subtraction angiography (DSA), or direct the focus of subsequent DSA. Postoperative evaluation of patients with aneurysms or arterial venous malformations by CTA or CTV may be better than by MRI. CTA is also valuable in assessing intracranial infection with possible venous thrombosis (Fig. 24-61).

CT of the Paranasal Sinuses, Facial Bones, Skull Base, Orbits, Temporal Bones, Neck, and Spine

CT imaging of the skull and facial bones includes evaluation of the paranasal sinuses, particularly with acute or chronic sinus disease and in preparation for surgery with medically refractive sinus disease. Imaging usually does not include

Text continued on page 1007

Figure 24-55 **A,** Accidental head trauma. *Left:* Unenhanced axial CT image at the level of the lateral ventricles delineates a large right hyperdense epidural hematoma *(arrow)*, with midline shift/subfalcine herniation, right to left *(double-headed arrow)*, effacement of right lateral and third ventricles, and early obstruction of the left lateral ventricle. *Right:* Axial image at the same level on the bone window setting delineates a nondisplaced fracture of the right frontal bone *(arrow)*. **B,** Nonaccidental trauma. *Top left:* Unenhanced axial CT image at the level of the lateral ventricles delineates a left subdural hematoma *(top arrow)*, effacement of the left lateral ventricle, and superficial scalp hematoma *(bottom arrow)*. *Top right:* Axial CT image at the same level on the bone window setting delineates a nondisplaced right parietal fracture *(arrow)*. *Bottom left:* Three-dimensional reconstruction of the calvarium, viewed from the vertex, with the extent of the fracture well delineated. *Bottom right:* Three-dimensional reconstruction of the calvarium, viewed from the left lateral projection with delineation of the full extent of the fracture from the coronal to lambdoid suture. *Double-headed crooked arrow,* coronal suture; *straight arrow,* sagittal suture; *Z line,* lambdoid suture.

Figure 24-56 Macrocephaly noted at well-baby visit. Axial CT image at the level of the lateral ventricles delineates prominent lateral ventricles *(bold arrow)* and prominent anterior extraaxial spaces *(thin arrow)*. Typical appearance for benign extraaxial collections of infancy, a benign self-limiting process.

Figure 24-57 Patient with shunted hydrocephalus: Progressive hydrocephalus, probable shunt malfunction. **A,** Axial CT image at the level of the lateral ventricles delineates dilated lateral ventricles with shunt in the frontal horn of the left lateral ventricle *(short thick arrow)*. Sulci are visualized *(dashed arrows)*. **B,** Axial CT image at the same level several days later, showing enlarged lateral ventricles with shunt position unchanged *(short thick arrow)*, and effacement of sulci *(dashed arrows)*.

Figure 24-58 Patient presenting with seizure. **A,** Unenhanced CT at the level of the temporal horns of the lateral ventricles delineates a large, hyperdense, left frontal lobe intraparenchymal hematoma. Significant mass effect and dilatation of the right temporal horn/obstructive hydrocephalus are visible. **B,** Contrast-enhanced examination performed on the same day shows marked relative hypoattenuation of the hematoma.

Figure 24-59 Patient presenting with left upper extremity weakness, left facial droop, and difficulty speaking. **A,** Axial CT source image from computed tomography angiography (CTA); *arrow* points to flap/dissection *(thin gray line)* in the lumen of the right internal carotid artery. **B,** Axial image just below the dissection shows a relatively narrow caliber of the right internal carotid artery *(arrow)* when compared with the left internal carotid artery. **C,** Coronal reconstruction of CTA delineates flap/dissection *(arrow)* in right internal carotid artery. **D,** Coronal reconstruction indicating normal appearance of the left internal carotid artery.

Figure 24-60   Patient presenting with nasal speech and cranial nerve deficits. **A,** Axial contrast-enhanced CT on the soft tissue window setting, at the level of the skull base, delineates a large soft tissue mass *(arrows)* centered at the clivus and both anterior and posterior to it (i.e., intracranial extension). **B,** Axial image on the bone window setting delineates associated bone erosion *(solid arrows)* and invasion of the left jugular foramen *(dashed arrow).* **C,** Sagittal soft tissue reconstruction delineates extent of the mass both into the naso- and oropharynx as well as its intracranial extension *(arrows).* **D,** Sagittal reconstruction on the bone window setting delineates the extent of clival erosion *(arrows).*

Figure 24-61 Patient presenting with change in mental status with sinus thrombosis. **A,** Unenhanced CT delineates a hyperdense anterior portion of the superior sagittal sinus *(arrow)*, suggesting venous sinus thrombosis. **B,** Contrast-enhanced CT confirms lack of opacification of the anterior portion of the superior sagittal sinus *(arrow)* and associated areas of cortical hypodensity/ischemia *(diverging dotted arrows)*.

intravenous contrast. However, if intracranial or intraorbital extension is suspected, then a contrast-enhanced scan is indicated (see Chapter 23, Fig. 23-62). CT imaging is indicated for examination of the facial bones and skull base after trauma (Fig. 24-62), suspected infection (CE examination indicated), and facial anomalies (reconstruction with high-resolution 2D and 3D images) (Fig. 24-63). In the setting of a suspected mass, a CE examination should be performed. If a vascular or primary dental lesion is suspected, a targeted unenhanced image in the area of interest before intravenous contrast is recommended to assess for calcifications and/or bone matrix because prior administration of contrast may obscure these findings (e-Fig. 24-12).

Imaging of the orbits is indicated in trauma, congenital anomalies (Fig. 24-64), and infection (CE examination is indicated; see Chapter 23, Fig. 23-62). In the setting of leukocoria or suspected tumor, imaging before and after contrast to determine the presence of calcifications is important, particularly if retinoblastoma is suspected (Fig. 24-65). Proptosis, with or without possible infection, warrants CT imaging.

CT images of the temporal bones may be diagnostic after trauma (Fig. 24-66), infection (e-Fig. 24-13), hearing loss (e-Fig. 24-14), cranial nerve deficits, or if a temporal bone tumor is suspected (Fig. 24-67). CE examinations are indicated in infection and suspected tumor.

When swelling of the soft tissues of the neck is evaluated, a CE examination is indicated to examine for infection, lymphadenopathy, masses, or metastases (Fig. 24-68).

Indications for CT examination of the spine include trauma (e-Fig. 24-15) and complex spinal anomalies. CT imaging may be used as a complementary examination to MRI in evaluating anomalies (e-Fig. 24-16) and infection, to assess bone erosion and destruction, and posttreatment healing (Fig. 24-69). These studies of the spine are generally done without intravenous or intrathecal contrast. When MRI is not available, the only clinical indications for contrast-enhanced CT of the cervical spine are for suspected infarction, diskitis, abscess, or tumor (Fig. 24-70).

Intrathecal contrast imaging of the spine is indicated to evaluate the position and integrity of an intraspinal catheter, delineation and localization of a suspected thecal sac arachnoid cyst (complementary examination to MRI), and in patients in whom MRI studies are suboptimal with possible disk herniation or canal stenosis associated with radicular pain or who may have suspected arachnoiditis.

CURRENT ROLE OF MRI IN CNS IMAGING

MRI of the brain is now the modality of choice in almost all suspected nontraumatic intracranial pathology. In evaluation of the spine, head, and neck, it is equal to and often superior to CT in imaging many disease entities. In certain cases, a supplementary CT examination may be required for evaluation of the presence of calcifications, bone matrix, and bone remodeling or destruction, the appearance of which may allow a more definitive preoperative or pretreatment differential and/or diagnosis.

In ordering a contrast-enhanced MRI the patient's clinical history, history of allergies, renal function, hydration status, and medications should be known and reviewed. Allergic reactions to gadolinium-based contrast agents (GBCAs) are rare in the pediatric population. However, in patients with renal dysfunction or acute renal failure, contrast enhancement may place them at risk for the development of nephrogenic systemic fibrosis (NSF; see Nephrogenic Systemic Fibrosis in Children, earlier, and see e-Table 24-6).

Metallic objects often produce signal distortion and field distortion artifacts. This may render an examination suboptimal or possibly nondiagnostic. In the pediatric population the most common cause of suboptimal or nondiagnostic MRI examinations is dental braces and retainers; a diagnostic examination of the orbits, face, and sinuses or skull base is not possible in their presence. Intra- and extracranial MRA and MRV are also markedly degraded and often nondiagnostic. Routine sequences of the brain are variably compromised but

Figure 24-62 Trauma to the face: Naso-orbital ethmoidal complex fractures. **A,** Axial CT image on soft tissue window delineates extent of soft tissue injury to the orbit. *Arrow* points to a hematoma and displacement of the medial rectus muscle. **B,** Axial image on the bone window setting delineates complex, comminuted, and displaced fractures of the medial orbital walls/lamina papyracea *(posterior arrows)* and cribriform plate *(anterior arrows)*. **C,** Coronal reconstruction delineates the complex comminuted fractures, which also include the frontal sinuses and fovea ethmoidalis *(diverging arrows)* and left orbital roof *(upper arrow)*, and redemonstrates the extensive fracture of the medial orbital wall/lamina papyracea *(lower arrow)*. **D,** Lateral view of the 3D reconstruction demonstrates the marked posterior displacement of the nasoethmoidal complex *(long arrow)* in relation to the frontal sinus/frontal bone *(short arrow)*.

Figure 24-63 Newborn presenting with fusion of gums: Syngnathia. Three-dimensional reconstruction of the calvarium and face demonstrates lower facial hypoplasia due to maxillary and mandibular hypoplasia *(long arrows)* and their midline fusion *(short midline arrow)*.

Figure 24-64 Infant with right proptosis: Bilateral colobomas. Axial image through the orbits delineates a large right orbital cyst *(arrow)* with connection to a hypoplastic proptotic globe. On the left there is a small orbital cyst with a relatively normal-appearing globe *(arrow)*.

Figure 24-65 Patient with leukocoria/white eye reflex: Retinoblastoma. **A,** Unenhanced axial CT of the orbits demonstrates a calcified mass in the posterior aspect of the right globe *(arrow)*. **B,** Contrast-enhanced CT of the orbits demonstrates an enhancing soft tissue component to the mass.

Figure 24-66 Head injury with hemotympanum. Axial unenhanced CT image through the left temporal bone demonstrates a transverse fracture *(arrows)* with ossicular dislocation (note separation of the malleus and incus on the left in comparison with the right "ice cream scoop separated from cone"); fracture traverses through the expected tympanic course of the facial nerve *(dotted line)* and through the internal auditory canal/inner ear. Associated opacification of the left middle ear and mastoid and pneumocephalus are also seen.

Figure 24-67 Patient presenting with left facial palsy: Hemangioendothelioma at surgical resection. **A,** Axial CT through the temporal bone set on the bone window setting demonstrates a large destructive mass of the left petrous bone at the level of the geniculate ganglion/first turn of the facial nerve *(arrow)*. Opacification of the left middle ear and mastoid is related to extension of the mass into the eustachian tube. **B,** Contrast-enhanced CT on the soft tissue window setting at the same level delineates heterogeneous enhancement of the mass *(arrow)*.

Figure 24-68   Patient presenting with new neck mass: Thyroglossal duct cyst. **A,** Axial contrast-enhanced image through the neck just below the level of the hyoid demonstrates a discrete cystic mass, just to the right of midline, without a discernible wall or enhancement *(solid arrow)*. The mass is intimately associated with the adjacent strap muscles *(dotted arrow)*. **B,** Sagittal reconstruction delineates the mass at the level of the fiducial placed to localize the mass *(arrow)*.

usually diagnostic. Gradient echo and diffusion images are usually severely compromised.

In addition, there are metallic objects/implants that may pose a hazard either to the patient (e.g., aneurysm clips) or to the function of the implant (e.g., pacemakers or cochlear implants). MRI safety screening is performed on all patients and accompanying parents/family. It is imperative that in cases of prior surgery or interventional procedures and the possible presence of implants, information about the implants be available at the time of scheduling of the MRI examination. The prospective MRI compatibility and clearance of any implants can then be determined, and will preclude the MRI examination from being deferred or canceled on the patient's arrival.

Newer MRI Sequences and Their Utility

New, improved, and faster magnetic resonance imaging sequences and modalities have been developed for assessing anatomy, pathology, and function.

FLAIR—fluid attenuation inversion recovery sequence: By attenuating signal from CSF, sensitive delineation of foci of signal abnormality adjacent to the ventricles and subarachnoid space are better defined.

Figure 24-69   Patient presenting with back pain and neurologic deficits. At resection: Aneurysmal bone cyst. **A,** Axial contrast-enhanced image on a soft tissue window setting through the lower thoracic spine delineates a heterogeneous expansile destructive mass *(solid arrows)* involving the vertebral body and more extensively the posterior elements with intraspinal encroachment. Fluid–fluid levels *(dotted arrows)* are suggested within the mass. **B,** Same axial image on a bone window setting delineates bone expansion/remodeling and destruction. **C,** Sagittal reconstruction on a soft tissue window setting delineates the marked narrowing of the spinal canal and thecal sac *(arrows)* by the mass.

Figure 24-70 Patient, presenting with neck pain, *Fusobacterium necrophorum*–induced sepsis. **A,** Contrast-enhanced axial CT through the upper neck delineates a clot *(arrow)* in the right jugular vein. **B,** Axial contrast-enhanced image just below delineates right anterior rim, enhancing epidural fluid collection. The diagnosis was Lemierre disease with epidural abscess.

GRE (T_2*)—gradient echo sequence: By enhancing magnetic susceptibility, sensitive delineation of hemorrhage and vascular malformations, calcifications, and iron deposition is possible.

DWI/DTI—diffusion-weighted imaging and diffusion tensor imaging sequences: By using differences in the rates and direction of diffusion of water molecules in normal and abnormal tissues, diffusion imaging allows sensitive detection and evaluation of acute cerebral injury in ischemia/hypoxia, trauma, metabolic disorders, and infection. It allows more sensitive monitoring of markers of brain maturation in the neonatal period. It may also suggest the grade of intracranial tumors. Tensor imaging uses anisotropy/direction to map axonal tracts, allowing evaluation of their course; caliber; and assessment of possible disruption, displacement, or anomalous pathways. This supplementary information to anatomic MRI results in more sensitive and sophisticated assessment of neurologic deficits, and the preoperative localization of "eloquent" tracts, that is, important functional regions, in relation to tumors and other brain lesions.

3D GRE—high-resolution T_1-weighted gradient echo sequence: This technique provides sensitive delineation of brain injury in neonates, brain lesions and cortical dysplasias, and preoperative localization of tumors.

STIR—fat-suppressed short T_1 inversion recovery sequence: By suppressing the signal of fat, sensitive delineation of lesions in areas where fat/lipomatous tissue is present, such as in the orbits, face, skull base, neck, and spine, becomes possible.

MRA/MRV—magnetic resonance angiography and venography; examples include 3D and 2D time-of-flight (TOF) and phase-contrast (PC) angiography and 2D TOF and PC venography: These methods may be used to delineate areas of stenosis, luminal irregularity or occlusion, direction of flow, vascular malformations, and aneurysms.

MRS—magnetic resonance spectroscopy: MRS may be used to assess the distribution and quantification of naturally occurring molecules within the CNS. Various techniques are available. The most commonly used is the point-resolved spectroscopy sequence (PRESS). Both short T_E

(echo time) and long T_E acquisitions can be obtained. All provide sensitive noninvasive analysis of brain metabolites and cellular biochemical changes, used in assessing brain maturation, brain ischemia, injury, and encephalopathy. In these entities it may also provide prognostic information. In the diagnosis and characterization of inborn errors of metabolism, it may not be specific but may help to narrow the entities to be considered. Another indication is preoperative characterization and possible diagnosis of brain tumors as well as their postoperative and posttherapeutic assessment (Fig. 24-71).

PMRI—perfusion magnetic resonance imaging: Dynamic contrast-enhanced T_2* or unenhanced techniques such as arterial spin labeling (ASL) and blood oxygen level–dependent (BOLD) sequences are used. Sensitive delineation of relative cerebral blood flow with evaluation of cerebral blood volume (CBV), cerebral blood flow (CBF), and mean transit time (MTT) in targeted areas of the brain is possible. PMRI is used primarily in assessing ischemic areas of the brain. It can also be used in differentiating tumor progression from posttreatment changes.

fMRI—functional magnetic resonance imaging: fMRI localizes function to anatomic areas. The most widely used technique is the BOLD sequence. This relies on local changes in cerebral blood flow and changes in oxyhemoglobin and deoxyhemoglobin with targeted brain activation. Cortical activation by a focal task, or by a visual or auditory stimulus, results in local increased metabolic demand and hence an increase in local blood flow, which raises the concentration of oxyhemoglobin and decreases the concentration of deoxyhemoglobin. The decrease in deoxyhemoglobin results in an increase in signal intensity. Subtraction of pre- and postactivation images results in localization of the area of the brain activated by the task or stimulus. It can be used in preoperative delineation of "eloquent" areas before resection of brain tumors or vascular malformations as well as cortical dysplasias and other seizure foci. It is also used in assessing cognition, language, and motor skill acquisition and behavioral dysfunction.

Normal Brain Spectra

Figure 24-71   Normal brain spectra. Cr, creatine; Glu/Gln, glutamate/glutamine; ml, *myo*-inositol; LCModel, a program for the automatic quantitation of in vivo proton MR spectra; NAA, *N*-acetylaspartate; tCho, total choline.

RARE—rapid acquisition relaxation-enhanced technique, such as single-shot fast spin-echo (SSFSE) and half-Fourier acquired single-shot turbo spin-echo (HASTE), as well as other fast and ultrafast techniques: These allow rapid scanning of the entire pediatric brain. They are adequate for assessing ventricular size and shunt position in patients with shunted hydrocephalus. These sequences do not allow adequate delineation and diagnosis of other brain pathology. Table 24-10 shows signal characteristics of CNS tissues on various MRI sequences. e-Table 24-9 delineates the appearance of blood at various stages of hemorrhage. e-Table 24-10 lists metabolites detected in the brain by MR spectroscopy.

CLINICAL INDICATIONS FOR MRI IN CNS IMAGING

Unenhanced MRI of the Brain

Ultrafast, multiplanar targeted MRI can be used as an alternative to CT for routine follow-up of hydrocephalus, and evaluation of ventricular size and shunt position (Fig. 24-72).

In patients with stroke, MRI along with MRA, MRV, and PMRI can assess location/territory, size, area at risk, and underlying vascular disease or anomalies (Fig. 24-73). Addition of MRS to MRI may provide information as to the etiology of perinatal ischemia or seizures (Fig. 24-74) or prognostic information in severe traumatic brain injury (e-Fig. 24-17). Adrenoleukodystrophy (ALD) is one of the few entities for which a contrast examination may provide important information. Although MRS often is not specific, the pattern may be suggestive of a distinct group of entities (Fig. 24-75).

Contrast-enhanced MRI of the Brain

Contrast-enhanced magnetic resonance imaging (CE-MRI) can provide anatomic detail in a variety of disorders including phakomatoses such as neurofibromatosis, Sturge-Weber syndrome, tuberous sclerosis, and others (e-Fig. 24-18). CE-MRI can depict associated cerebritis or abscess, empyema, or parenchymal ischemia related to vascular involvement (e-Fig. 24-19). MRA and MRS may augment CE-MRI in the setting of vascular malformation (Fig. 24-76), brain tumors (particularly

Table 24-10	Signal Characteristics of CNS Tissues Examined by Various Magnetic Resonance Imaging Sequences				
	CSF	**Gray Matter**	**White Matter**	**Fat**	**Lesions**
T₁	Dark-hypointense	Rel dark-hypointense	Rel bright-hyperintense	Bright-hyperintense	Variable; majority dark-hypointense
T₂	Bright-hyperintense	Rel bright-hyperintense	Rel dark-hypointense	Bright-hyperintense	Variable; majority bright-hyperintense
FLAIR	Dark-hypointense	Rel bright-hyperintense	Rel dark-hypointense	Bright-hyperintense	Variable; majority bright-hyperintense
DWI	Dark-hypointense	Rel bright-hyperintense	Rel dark-hypointense	Dark-hypointense	Variable; majority bright-hyperintense
ADC	Bright-hyperintense	Rel bright-hyperintense	Dark-hypointense	Bright-hyperintense	Variable Bright-hyperintense: Vasogenic edema, low-grade tumor Dark-hypointense: Cytotoxic edema/ischemia and high-grade tumors
GRE	Bright-hyperintense	Rel bright-hyperintense	Rel dark-hypointense	Rel dark-hypointense	Variable Bright-hyperintense: Majority Dark-hypointense: If blood, fat, or calcium present
STIR	Bright-hyperintense	Rel bright-hyperintense	Rel dark-hypointense	Dark-hypointense	Variable; majority bright-hyperintense

ADC, apparent diffusion coefficient mapping; CSF, cerebrospinal fluid; DWI, diffusion-weighted imaging; FLAIR, fluid attenuation inversion recovery; GRE, gradient echo; Rel, relatively; STIR, short tau inversion recovery.

Figure 24-72 Patient presenting with possible shunt malfunction. **A,** Axial, and **B,** T₂ single-shot fast spin-echo (SSFSE) acquisitions, each taking less than 1 minute to run, suffice for assessing ventricular size and shunt position *(arrows)* without radiation.

Figure 24-73 Patient presenting with new-onset neurologic symptoms; rule out stroke. **A,** *Left:* Axial fluid attenuation inversion recovery (FLAIR) image at the level of the basal ganglia delineates relative hyperintensity in and swelling of the left basal ganglia and adjacent insular cortex *(arrows). Right, top and bottom:* Diffusion-weighted imaging (DWI) and apparent diffusion coefficient (ADC) images at the same level demonstrate hyper- and hypointensity, that is, restricted diffusion. Acute stroke. **B,** Two maps: Time to peak *(left)* and cerebral blood flow *(right),* from the perfusion study obtained. Note the asymmetry between the two cerebral hemispheres.

Figure 24-74   Patient presenting after profound perinatal hypoxia. **A,** Axial T₂ image at the level of the basal ganglia. Extensive hyper- and hypointensity in the basal ganglia and thalami are compatible with the clinical history and represent profound hypoxic ischemic injury. **B,** Magnetic resonance spectroscopy (MRS) delineating decreased *N*-acetylaspartate *(solid arrow),* elevated lactate *(dotted arrow),* and elevated lipid *(dash-dotted arrow)* compatible with cell death/apoptosis. **C,** Axial T₁ image with corresponding diffuse hyperintensity in the basal ganglia and thalami.

primary brain tumors) (Fig. 24-77), demyelinating or inflammatory disease, or acute change in mental status (Fig. 24-78).

Intracranial and Extracranial MR Angiography and MR Venography

MRA and MRV offer detailed information in a variety of clinical settings, including vascular relationships and integrity. These include, in part, stroke, vascular dissection, stenosis, luminal irregularity, occlusion, moyamoya disease, and vascular malformations (e-Figs. 24-20 and 24-21); vascular

relationships to tumors (Fig. 24-79); and vascular complications of infection (e-Fig. 24-22).

Additional Indications for MRI of the Head

The following examinations and clinical indications should be ordered as such, and not as an MRI of the brain with clinical indication provided. The majority are performed with contrast. Many entities will require CT as well for delineation of osseous involvement and the presence of calcifications.

Figure 24-75   Patient with developmental delay: Leukodystrophy of unknown etiology. **A,** Axial T₂ image at the level of the lateral ventricles delineates diffuse hyperintensity and relative paucity of white matter. Abnormally hypointense basal ganglia. **B,** Comparison image of the brain of a child of the same age with normally myelinated white matter, which is hypointense on a T₂ sequence. Normal signal characteristics of basal ganglia. Genetic testing and magnetic resonance spectroscopy (MRS) were nonspecific.

Figure 24-76 Neonate presenting with congestive heart failure. **A,** Axial T₂ MR image at the level of the lateral and third ventricles delineates marked dilatation of the vein of Galen/straight sinus *(black arrow)* and enlarged tortuous adjacent feeding vessels *(white arrows)* arising from both the anterior and posterior circulation. **B,** T₂ coronal image of the findings in **(A). C,** Coronal source image from magnetic resonance venography (MRV) delineates not only the intracranial findings but also the associated markedly dilated neck vessels *(arrows),* which account for the congestive heart failure. **D,** Lateral projection from the MRV reconstruction showing venous drainage into the superior sagittal sinus *(dashed arrow)* as well as transverse and sigmoid sinuses and jugular veins *(solid arrows).*

- MRI of the orbits for congenital anomalies, tumors, infection, pain, or proptosis: The latter evaluation should determine the extent (intra- or extracoronal) and possible etiologies of proptosis, such as thyroid orbitopathy, pseudotumor, or tumor.
- Temporal bone MRI: Indications include sensorineural hearing loss to assess inner ear structures for congenital anomalies, labyrinthitis ossificans, and lesions of the cochlear nerve (Fig. 24-80). MRI is valuable in assessing disorders causing facial nerve palsies, tinnitus and dizziness, and middle ear and mastoid infections, and particularly in evaluating for intracranial or neck extension or vascular complications.
- Examination of the skull base, face, and sinuses by MRI for tumors, cranial nerve palsy, and infection: Allows assessment of size and extent, perineural spread, and venous complications such as cavernous sinus involvement (e-Fig. 24-23).

MRI of the Pituitary and Hypothalamic Region

Neuroendocrine abnormalities with hypothalamic or pituitary dysfunction are amenable to evaluation by MRI, which can be used to assess pituitary size and anatomy, for example, the presence of the pituitary stalk and neurohypophysis, as well as adjacent structures (Fig. 24-81).

MRI of the Neck and Spine

Indications for MRI of the neck include palpable masses, suspected metastatic disease, pain, dysphagia, and hoarseness.

Unenhanced MRI of the spine is done to evaluate the spinal cord, canal, osseous elements, ligaments, and paravertebral muscles. Indications include trauma (Fig. 24-82), anomalies (e-Fig. 24-24), pain, radiculopathy, and marrow abnormalities.

Enhanced MRI of the spine should be performed if infection or inflammation is suspected (Fig. 24-83), or in the presence of a primary or metastatic tumor. Intraspinal, osseous, or paravertebral areas should be examined for involvement.

NUCLEAR MEDICINE IMAGING

Single-photon Emission Tomography

Single-photon emission computed tomography (SPECT) is done with a gamma camera mounted on a special gantry that can rotate a full 360 degrees around the patient, who has been

Figure 24-77 Infant presenting with increasing head size and change in mental status. **A,** Axial T$_2$ MR image at the level of the lateral and third ventricles delineates ventricular dilatation *(solid arrow)* and a large heterogeneous intraventricular mass *(dashed arrows)*. **B,** Axial fluid attenuation inversion recovery (FLAIR) image at the same level better delineates the adjacent hyperintense edema and transependymal flow of cerebrospinal fluid. **C,** Contrast-enhanced T$_1$ image delineates heterogeneous enhancement of solid and cystic components. **D,** Magnetic resonance spectroscopy (MRS) delineates elevated lactate and lipid peaks *(divergent arrows)*, decreased N-acetylaspartate peak *(long solid arrow)*, and elevated choline peak *(short solid arrow)*; all of which may be seen in many tumors. An elevated *myo*-inositol peak *(dashed arrow)* is present, strongly suggestive of choroid plexus papilloma, proven at pathology.

Figure 24-78 Previously well patient presenting with seizures and profound mental status change after an upper respiratory tract infection. **A,** Axial T_2 MR image at the level of the basal ganglia delineates marked swelling and hyperintensity in the thalami *(solid arrow)* and posterior cortex/occipital lobes *(dashed arrow)*. **B,** Coronal T_2 image delineates additional involvement of the brainstem *(solid arrow)* and the cerebellum *(dashed arrow)*. Other sequences also demonstrated restricted diffusion and petechial hemorrhage. The constellation and distribution of findings is most suggestive of acute necrotizing encephalopathy of childhood.

Figure 24-79 Patient presenting with syncope: Meningioma. **A,** Axial contrast-enhanced T_1 image at the level of the lateral ventricles delineates a large, avidly enhancing left frontal mass *(thick arrows)* abutting the sagittal sinus *(thin arrow)*. Note the significant mass effect on the lateral ventricles and subfalcine herniation. **B,** Coronal reconstruction of magnetic resonance angiography (MRA) indicates marked displacement and draping of the anterior cerebral artery and middle cerebral arteries about the mass *(solid thick arrows)*. *Thin arrow* points to the sagittal sinus and the *dashed arrow* indicates a draining vein.

Figure 24-80 Patient with sensorineural hearing loss and cochlear dysplasia on CT: Cochlear nerve aplasia. **A,** Oblique sagittal FIESTA (fast imaging employing steady-state acquisition) sequence through the internal auditory canals on the normal side. *Solid upper arrow* points to the facial nerve. *Solid horizontal arrow* points to the superior and inferior vestibular nerves. *Dashed arrow* points to the cochlear nerve. **B,** Side with cochlear dysplasia: *dashed arrow* points to the expected location of the cochlear nerve, which is not present.

Figure 24-81 Three-year-old patient presenting with pituitary dysfunction: Panhypopituitarism. Sagittal midline T_1 MR image delineates a "bright spot," the posterior pituitary/neurohypophysis, not in the posterior aspect of the sella as expected but just posterior to the chiasm at the expected location of the proximal stalk *(arrow)*. The stalk is absent and the pituitary gland is small, indicating ectopic posterior pituitary with interruption of the stalk. Thinning of the posterior aspect of the corpus callosum is related to periventricular leukomalacia in this patient, who was premature.

Figure 24-82 Trauma: Ligamentous flexion injury. **A,** Sagittal midline T_1 MR image of the cervical spine delineates marked reversal of cervical lordosis *(solid arrow)* and splaying of the spinous processes. **B,** Sagittal short tau inversion recovery (STIR) image at the same level better delineates the hyperintense prevertebral edema *(solid arrow)* and the hyperintense epidural hematoma *(dashed arrow)* that markedly compresses the cord. **C,** Axial T_1 image delineates the epidural hematoma and the compressed cord and thecal sac surrounded by the hypointense dura *(solid arrow)*. **D,** Axial T_2 image at same level delineates the hyperintense epidural hematoma *(solid arrows)* and compressed cord.

Figure 24-83 Patient presenting with back pain and fever: Osteomyelitis and epidural abscess. **A,** Sagittal midline T$_2$ MR image of the lumbar spine delineates relative hyperintensity in the L4 vertebral body *(solid arrow)* and an epidural collection *(dashed arrow)*. **B,** Sagittal T$_1$ image at the same level delineates corresponding hypointensity in the L4 vertebral body *(solid arrow)* and the epidural collection *(dashed arrow)*. **C,** Axial T$_2$ image at the level of L4 demonstrates an abnormal signal/hyperintensity in the vertebral body *(solid arrow)*. **D,** Contrast-enhanced T$_1$ fat-saturated image at the same level delineates enhancement of the L4 vertebral body *(solid arrow)* and enhancement of the epidural collection with a small central focus of fluid hypoattenuation *(dashed arrow)*.

injected with a gamma-emitting radioisotope (called a *radio-nuclide*); image acquisition is done at multiple angles. Using these data, SPECT images can be reconstructed and displayed as coronal, sagittal, or transverse slices. The major advantage of SPECT is its superior contrast and anatomic delineation compared with conventional planar imaging. SPECT/CT is a hybrid form of imaging modality combining SPECT with CT, which can provide better anatomic localization and attenuation correction.

Positron Emission Tomography

Positron emission tomography (PET) is a specialized modality used to image the high-energy photons of positron-emitting tracers such as ^{18}F, ^{11}C, ^{13}N, and ^{15}O. Positrons (positive electrons) travel a few millimeters into tissue before colliding with negative electrons. This colliding event (called *annihilation*) results in the creation of two 511-keV photons, which travel

away from each other at almost 180 degrees. Most PET systems have a dozen to several hundred detectors arranged in a circular or polygonal configuration. Only two coincident photons reaching two opposite detectors at the same time are registered in the system, ultimately resulting in an electrical current allowing image reconstruction. PET/CT is a hybrid imaging modality that provides better anatomic localization of findings on functional images and faster image acquisition than conventional PET alone.

Gamma Camera

The gamma camera, also called a scintillation camera or Anger camera, is an imaging device used to image gamma radiation–emitting radioisotopes. This technique is known as *scintigraphy* and is used to image and analyze the distribution of gamma-emitting radionuclides medically introduced into the human body. The gamma camera consists of a collimator, a crystal plane, and an array of photomultiplier tubes connected to a computer system. The collimator is typically a single plate of lead or tungsten with many holes through it; this allows only photons traveling parallel to the collimator holes to reach the crystal, which is located behind the collimator. Once photons reach the crystal, they are absorbed into the crystal and this absorbed energy is emitted as flashes of light, a process called *scintillation*. The brightness of light is proportional to the energy absorbed by the crystal. The light flashes are converted into an electronic signal that is ultimately processed to produce an image.

Radiopharmaceuticals

A radiopharmaceutical is a molecule (the pharmaceutical) incorporating a radioactive tracer (the radionuclide, or radio-isotope); it is designed to be used in the diagnosis of a physiologic or pathologic process and for the treatment of disease. Typically, radiopharmaceuticals do not elicit a physiologic or pharmacologic reaction and do not impact the physiologic process being measured.

Radioisotopes commonly used in nuclear medicine are either gamma or beta emitters. Gamma emitters are suitable for imaging because the gamma photons emitted travel a longer path and have a higher capacity to penetrate matter. Beta emitters are more suitable for treatment because the beta particles emitted have a shorter traveling path and less ability to penetrate matter.

A summary of radiation exposure from pediatric nuclear medicine procedures is given in Table 24-11.

Technetium-99m

The principal radioactive tracer in nuclear medicine is technetium-99m (^{99m}Tc; the "99" indicates the atomic weight and the "m" stands for *metastable*). Its availability, short half-life (6 hours), and ideal gamma energy emission make radiopharmaceuticals incorporating ^{99m}Tc suitable for standard gamma camera imaging.

PET Radiopharmaceuticals

PET radiopharmaceuticals have the same components of radioisotope atom and larger molecule as other radiopharmaceuticals, except that positron-emitting radioisotopes are used instead of gamma or beta emitters. Positron-emitting radionuclides include carbon-11 (^{11}C), oxygen-15 (^{15}O), and nitrogen-13 (^{13}N), and these can be combined with various biologic tracers to image physiologic or metabolic processes.

^{18}F-FDG (Fluorodeoxyglucose)

One of the most commonly used PET radiopharmaceuticals is fluorodeoxyglucose, commonly abbreviated ^{18}F-FDG or FDG, a glucose analog, with the positron-emitting radioactive isotope fluorine-18 taking the place of the normal hydroxyl group at the 2′ position in the glucose molecule. In the absence of this 2′ hydroxyl group, which is needed for glycolysis, FDG cannot be further metabolized in cells after phosphorylation.

| Table 24-11 | Radiation Exposure from Pediatric Nuclear Medicine Procedures |

			EFFECTIVE DOSE (MSV) AT AGE:				
	Procedure	**Dose Administered (mCi/kg)**	**1 Year (10 kg)**	**5 Years (20 kg)**	**10 Years (33 kg)**	**15 Years (57 kg)**	**Adult (70 kg)**
Cardiovascular	^{99m}Tc-sestamibi (rest)	0.15	3.9	3.1	3.3	3.8	3.3
	^{99m}Tc-sestamibi (stress)	0.35	6.7	6	6.8	7.4	5.8
	^{18}F-FDG viability	0.14	4.9	5.2	6.2	7.4	6.9
	^{99m}Tc-MUGA	0.26	14.4	7.8	5.2	4.9	4.7
Respiratory	^{99m}Tc-MAA perfusion	0.07	1.6	1.8	2	2.4	2
	^{99m}Tc-DTPA ventilation	Fixed dose: 40-60 mCi	2.4	1.3	0.9	0.6	0.5
	^{133}Xe ventilation	0.3	0.6	0.6	0.6	0.6	0.6
Genitourinary	^{99m}Tc-MAG3 renogram	0.15	1.2	1.3	2.2	2.8	2.7
	^{99m}Tc-DTPA renogram	0.1	0.6	0.7	1	1.3	1.3
	^{99m}Tc-DMSA	0.05	0.7	0.8	0.9	1.2	1.1
Gastrointestinal	Hepatobiliary ^{99m}Tc-IDA	0.05	1.9	1.7	1.8	2.2	2.2
	Liver/spleen ^{99m}Tc-sulfur colloid	0.05	0.9	1	1.1	1.3	1
	Spleen ^{99m}Tc-labeled denatured RBC	0.06	16.3	9.6	6.2	7	6.4
	GI bleeding ^{99m}Tc-labeled RBC	0.21	5.8	3.3	3.6	3.9	3.8
	^{99m}Tc-pertechnetate Meckel diverticulum scan	0.05	1.5	1.6	1.6	1.8	1.7
	^{99m}Tc-sulfur colloid gastric emptying	Fixed dose: 0.5 mCi	2.6	1.4	0.9	0.6	0.4
Infection	^{99m}Tc–HMPAO-labeled WBC	0.2	4.6	5	5.4	5.9	5.7
	^{111}In-labeled WBC	0.007	8.3	9.3	10.3	11.7	10.7
	^{67}Ga-citrate	0.05	23.7	12.2	12.2	13.7	13
Bone	^{99m}Tc-MDP	0.25	2.5	2.6	3.4	3.7	3.7
CNS	Brain SPECT ^{99m}Tc-ECD	0.29	14.8	8.1	5.6	6.1	5.7
	Brain SPECT ^{99m}Tc-HMPAO	0.29	18.1	10	6.3	6.7	7
	Brain ^{18}F-FDG PET	0.14	4.9	5.2	6.2	7.4	6.9
Endocrinology	^{123}I thyroid uptake scan	0.0033	3.7	2	1	1.2	0.9
	^{99m}Tc-pertechnetate thyroid scan	0.15	4.4	4.7	4.8	4.4	3.4
	^{99m}Tc-sestamibi parathyroid scan	0.32	27.5	14.5	9.3	8.1	7.5
Oncology	^{123}I-MIBG	0.14	3.5	3.8	4.4	5	4.7
	Body ^{18}F-FDG PET	0.14	4.9	5.2	6.2	7.4	6.9

Note: Dose is based on the recommendations included in the following: Gelfand MJ, Parisi MT, Treves ST; Pediatric Nuclear Medicine Dose Reduction Workgroup: Pediatric radiopharmaceutical administered doses: 2010 North American consensus guidelines, *J Nucl Med* 52:318-322, 2011; and Treves ST: *Pediatric nuclear medicine/PET*, ed 3, New York, 2006, Springer. *Note:* For comparison, in the United States, one receives about 3 mSv (300 mrem) of exposure from natural background radiation every year.

CNS, central nervous system; DMSA, dimercaptosuccinic acid; DTPA, diethylenetriaminepentaacetic acid; ECD, ethyl cysteinate dimer; FDG, fluorodeoxyglucose; GI, gastrointestinal; HMPAO, hexamethylpropyleneamine oxime; IDA, iminodiacetic acid; MAA, macroaggregated albumin; MAG3, mercaptoacetyltriglycine; MDP, methylene diphosphonate; MIBG, metaiodobenzylguanidine; MUGA, multigated acquisition; PET, positron emission tomography; RBC, red blood cell; SPECT, single-photon emission computed tomography; WBC, white blood cell.

Also, the phosphorylated FDG, ^{18}F-FDG-6-phosphate, cannot cross the cell membrane and therefore becomes trapped within the cell, thus representing the distribution of glucose use by metabolically active cells such as in inflammation or malignancy.

Cardiovascular System

Myocardial Perfusion Imaging, Using SPECT and PET

Myocardial perfusion images are used to evaluate coronary artery blood flow, based on the distribution of radioisotope extracted into the myocardium, which is proportional to myocardial perfusion. Combined rest with exercise or pharmacologic stress images allows detection of hemodynamically compromised coronary artery territories. During exercise, coronary vessels dilate to meet increased oxygen demand and there is a significant difference in the degree of dilation between normal and diseased vessels, creating a relative count deficiency in the myocardium supplied by diseased coronary vessels. Pharmacologic vasodilators (adenosine or dipyridamole) are used for those who have physical limitation; baseline ECG abnormalities such as left bundle branch block or Wolff-Parkinson-White syndrome; and permanent ventricular pacing. Inotropic agents (e.g., dobutamine) are also used for patients who cannot undergo exercise and for whom pharmacologic vasodilators are contraindicated (mainly those with bronchospastic airway disease). By the gating technique, wall motion and ejection fraction can be assessed, which increases diagnostic accuracy.

There are several types of radiopharmaceuticals used for myocardial perfusion SPECT imaging including thallium-201 chloride, technetium-99m sestamibi (Cardiolite), and technetium-99m tetrofosmin (Myoview), used for both exercise and pharmacologic stress tests. Rubidium-82 positron emitters are used for pharmacologic stress myocardial perfusion PET imaging. (PET is not used in exercise stress testing.) Rubidium-82 PET has the highest sensitivity among the myocardial perfusion imaging techniques.

Determining Whether a Myocardial Perfusion Scan Is Needed

To determine whether a myocardial perfusion scan is indicated, the clinician should do the following:

1. Evaluate specific signs or symptoms that are induced or aggravated by exercise

2. Assess or identify abnormal responses to exercise in children with cardiac, pulmonary, or other organ disorders, including the presence of myocardial ischemia and arrhythmias (Kawasaki disease, congenital left main ostial stenosis, ALCAPA [anomalous origin of the left coronary artery to pulmonary artery], hypertrophic cardiomyopathy, and cardiomyopathy in Duchenne progressive muscular dystrophy)

3. Assess the efficacy of specific medical or surgical treatments (post–arterial switch operation, tetralogy of Fallot repair, and cardiac transplantation)

4. Assess functional capacity for recreational, athletic, and vocational activities

5. Evaluate the prognosis, including both baseline and serial testing measurements

6. Establish baseline data for the institution of cardiac, pulmonary, or musculoskeletal rehabilitation

The rest images are usually acquired 30 to 60 minutes after intravenous injection of ^{99m}Tc-sestamibi/tetrofosmin. For stress images, the radiopharmaceutical is injected at peak stress, which is more than 85% of the maximal predicted heart rate on a treadmill for the exercise stress. For pharmacologic stress, the radiopharmaceutical is injected immediately after dipyridamole infusion and 2 to 3 minutes after the start of adenosine infusion. The stress images are acquired 10 to 20 minutes after the injection of radiopharmaceutical for exercise stress testing and 45 to 60 minutes after the injection of radiopharmaceutical for pharmacologic stress testing (Fig. 24-84).

Myocardial Viability, Using Thallium-201 SPECT and FDG PET

Viable myocardial cells metabolize fatty acid and glucose, and these physiologic characteristics can be used in the assessment of viable myocardium. ^{18}F-fluorodeoxyglucose (FDG) is a glucose analog and is transported from the blood to the myocardial cells, where it undergoes phosphorylation. Phosphorylated FDG becomes trapped inside the myocardial cells without being further metabolized in the tricarboxylic acid (TCA) cycle. Therefore, the distribution of FDG reflects glucose utilization by viable myocardial cells, because only viable myocardial cells with cellular metabolic integrity can use glucose.

One of the characteristics of ^{201}Tl is that it is continuously transported into and washed out of viable myocardial cells, a process resulting in *redistribution*. Therefore, thallium can be used to evaluate viable myocardial cells, and is especially helpful in confirming viable myocardium before planning a revascularization.

MUGA Scan or Gated Blood Pool Imaging

A multigated acquisition (MUGA) scan is considered the gold standard for calculation of the left ventricular ejection fraction with high reproducibility. The patient's autologous red blood cells (RBCs) are labeled with technetium-99m and reinjected into the patient. Images of radiolabeled blood within the cardiac chamber are acquired by gamma camera with ECG gating. A MUGA scan is done to determine the ejection fraction in patients receiving chemotherapy (some chemotherapy agents are harmful to the heart) and also to assess cardiac risk before surgery.

Pulmonary System

Ventilation/Perfusion Lung Scan

Lung perfusion images are acquired with ^{99m}Tc-macroaggregated albumin (MAA). Because the mean size of MAA particles (20 to 40 μm) is greater than that of the capillary, these become trapped in the first pulmonary arterial capillary bed they encounter after intravenous injection. Typically 200,000 to 500,000 particles (minimum, 60,000) are injected into adult patients, artificially causing embolization of less than 1% of the pulmonary capillaries. Pediatric patients, patients with pulmonary hypertension, and patients with right-to-left shunt should receive 100,000 particles because they have fewer pulmonary arterioles. For newborns, the number of particles should not exceed 50,000. Particles lodged in the capillary beds are degraded by enzymatic and macrophage activity within hours, restoring original perfusion. When there is a pulmonary embolus in a certain area, the perfusion to this region is decreased, causing decreased radioactivity on images.

For lung ventilation images, ^{99m}Tc-diethylenetriaminepentaacetic acid (DTPA) aerosol or ^{133}Xe gas is used. ^{99m}Tc-DTPA aerosol ventilation images can provide multiple projections but can image only the initial breath phase of the ventilation. On the other hand, ^{133}Xe gas ventilation images can provide only one projection of the lungs but can image all the

Figure 24-84   Myocardial perfusion imaging with exercise stress test in an 18-year-old female with Kawasaki disease and left anterior descending artery coronary aneurysm presenting with chest pain. The patient, exercised according to the Bruce protocol for 12 minutes, achieved 100% of the maximal, age-predicted heart rate. No scintigraphic evidence of stress-induced ischemia or prior myocardial infarction was found.

ventilation phases including the initial breath phase, equilibrium phase, and washout phase. Indications include the following: diagnosing acute pulmonary embolus, evaluating and follow-up of chronic pulmonary embolus, assessing quantitative perfusion and ventilation function for presurgical evaluation, and assessing quantitative perfusion and ventilation function for follow-up after surgery (Fig. 24-85).

Right-to-left Shunt Study

^{99m}Tc-MAA is the most commonly used radiopharmaceutical for the evaluation of right-to-left shunt. As in lung perfusion studies, all of the particles are trapped in the pulmonary arterial capillary bed in the absence of right-to-left shunt. With right-to-left shunt at any level, particles will enter the systemic circulation in proportion to the flow and become trapped in the capillary and precapillary beds of systemic organs. The percentage of right-to-left shunt is calculated as (whole body count—lung count)/whole body count × 100. Pruckmayer and colleagues (1999) demonstrated that lung perfusion scintigraphy detects more abnormal pulmonary flow patterns than contrast echocardiography and was able to uniquely quantify right-to-left shunt volume. The indications are to evaluate the

presence of right-to-left shunt and to quantify the degree of right-to-left shunt before and/or after a surgical procedure for congenital heart disease (Fig. 24-86).

Genitourinary System

Basic Renogram

The basic renogram consists of a series of images of the kidneys, taken as the radiotracer is delivered to the vasculature, removed from the blood into the renal cortex, transits the kidney, and is excreted to the collecting system and the bladder. Renogram curves are also generated, quantifying the radiotracer movement in each kidney.

Two radiopharmaceuticals are used: ^{99m}Tc-mercapto-acetyltriglycine (MAG3), which is extracted by tubular secretion, and ^{99m}Tc-DTPA, which is extracted by glomerular filtration. The most commonly used radiopharmaceutical is ^{99m}Tc-MAG3, because it has a higher extraction fraction than DTPA and fewer false positive or indeterminate study results, and therefore is a better diagnostic agent, especially in patients with impaired renal function and in neonates.

Figure 24-85 Ventilation and perfusion scan: Low-probability V/Q scan. *First row:* 99mTc-diethylenetriaminepentaacetic acid (DTPA) ventilation images demonstrate mildly heterogeneous distribution of the tracer distribution and central airway deposition without significant ventilation defects. *Second row:* 99mTc-macroaggregated albumin (MAA) perfusion images demonstrate mildly heterogeneous distribution of the tracer distribution, which is mismatched by the ventilation images.

Figure 24-86 Lung perfusion and right-to-left shunt study: A 6-month-old with tetralogy of Fallot, status after multiple pulmonary artery stent and pulmonary artery dilation. 99mTc-macroaggregated albumin (MAA) particles were injected intravenously and show asymmetrically decreased perfusion to the left lung and localization to kidneys and brain, indicating a right-to-left shunt.

Indications include the following: evaluating basic renal function in native kidneys; determining the relative quantitative function of each native kidney; evaluating arterial flow and function in transplanted kidneys; helping to diagnose rejection and acute tubular necrosis in transplanted kidneys; and detecting urinary leak, infarct, or outflow obstruction in transplanted kidneys.

Diuretic Renogram

Diuretic renography is the noninvasive equivalent of a Whitaker test. The Whitaker test (a pressure perfusion flow study) is an invasive and nonphysiologic study requiring percutaneous nephrostomy, and the diagnosis is based on an abnormal increase in pressure after perfusion of fluid directly into the dilated system. Diuretic renography is based on the endogenous urine flow rate after dieresis administration, and the diagnosis of obstruction is based on abnormally slow washout of radiotracer from a dilated collecting system. Other anatomic imaging techniques such as an intravenous pyelogram, CT, or ultrasound can evaluate structure without any information on urodynamics. Diuretic renography is done to diagnose functional urinary tract obstruction in the presence of clinical suspicion for urine outflow obstruction or incidental detection of dilated renal collecting system (Fig. 24-87).

Flow images   Functional images

Figure 24-87 Diuresis renogram: A 10-year-old with bilateral vesicoureteral reflux and left hydronephrosis. Posterior flow images obtained after intravenous injection of 99mTc-diethylenetriaminepentaacetic acid (DTPA) show decreased perfusion to the left kidney. The functional renogram shows a mildly dilated collecting system of the left kidney with prompt clearance after administration of diuretic, indicating no significant ureteropelvic junction obstruction.

Figure 24-88 Renal cortical scintigraphy: ^{99m}Tc-dimercaptosuccinic acid (DMSA) study with posterior and posterior oblique pinhole views of both kidneys. A normal DMSA study exhibits uniform uptake in the renal cortex with reduced uptake centrally in the medulla and collecting system. LPO, left posterior oblique; LT post, left posterior; RPO, right posterior oblique; RT post, right posterior.

RT Post Kidney

LT Post Kidney

RPO Kidneys

LPO Kidneys

Angiotensin-converting Enzyme Inhibitor Renogram

Renovascular hypertension is caused by renin secretion from the juxtaglomerular apparatus of the underperfused stenotic kidney, caused by afferent arteriole stenosis. Through the renin–angiotensin cascade, the final product, angiotensin II, causes vasoconstriction of the postglomerular (efferent) arteriole, and this can maintain the transglomerular pressure gradient and GFR in the presence of decreased perfusion pressure. However, angiotensin-converting enzyme (ACE) inhibitors reduce this compensatory mechanism by inhibiting vasoconstriction of the postglomerular (efferent) arteriole and therefore decreasing the transglomerular pressure gradient and GFR.

It is important to distinguish physiologically significant renal artery stenosis from anatomic renal artery stenosis. Because not all renal artery stenoses are the cause of renovascular hypertension, revascularization of a stenotic renal artery may not result in any improvement in blood pressure in as many as 30% to 40% of patients undergoing the procedure. An ACE inhibitor renogram has high predictive value in predicting the benefit from revascularization to relieve hypertension.

Renal Cortical Scintigraphy

A renal cortical scan is the most reliable and practical imaging technique for initial evaluation and monitoring of children with febrile urinary tract infection. It is more sensitive than ultrasound or intravenous urography in detecting pyelonephritis, with a sensitivity of 96% and specificity of 98% for detecting pyelonephritis. The radiopharmaceuticals used (^{99m}Tc-dimercaptosuccinic acid [DMSA] and ^{99m}Tc-glucoheptonate) preferentially bind to renal tubules, providing excellent anatomic information about the renal cortex. The primary indications are as follows: for early diagnosis and localization of acute pyelonephritis, to detect renal damage and to assess recovery or residual renal damage, and to measure relative function (percentage of the renal function contributed by each kidney in reference to total renal function) (Fig. 24-88).

VCUG

Conventional voiding cystourethrography (VCUG) with fluoroscopy is usually the first test done in males to evaluate the possibility of a posterior urethral valve and to grade the degree of reflux. If follow-up studies are needed, radionuclide cystography is preferable. A VCUG has the advantage of providing anatomic detail on the pelvicaliceal system, the ureters, and insertion of the ureters into the bladder. However, it has some limitations including relatively high gonadal radiation exposure and low temporal resolution, which can decrease sensitivity for detecting intermittent vesicoureteral reflux (VUR). On the other hand, radionuclide cystography has the advantages of low gonadal radiation exposure, high temporal resolution, high sensitivity, and lower cost although the anatomic resolution delineating the bladder and urethra is limited. Both studies can be complementary in some cases. A VCUG can be used to detect, quantitate, and monitor VUR; assess antireflux surgery; or diagnose familial VUR (asymptomatic sibling of children with reflux).

Two methods of radionuclide cystography can be employed. With direct radionuclide cystography, the bladder is catheterized and the study is performed by infusing saline mixed with radiopharmaceuticals directly into the bladder via a catheter. Imaging is performed continuously during filling of the bladder and voiding. The entire study can take about 30 to 60 minutes. Indirect radionuclide cystography, however, does not require bladder catheterization and images can be obtained from a basic renogram study.

Figure 24-89 Radionuclide cystography: An 8-year-old female with a history of reflux. Radionuclide cystography demonstrates moderate to severe vesicoureteral reflux on the right with pelvicaliceal dilation and mild to moderate vesicoureteral reflux on the left.

A patient receives an intravenous injection of radiopharmaceuticals (the same as are used in a renogram) and images of renal function, excretion of radiotracer into the bladder (bladder filling), voiding, and postvoiding are acquired. Although indirect radionuclide cystography allows bladder catheterization to be avoided, it is not as sensitive as direct radionuclide cystography for detecting reflux. The entire study can take about 30 to 60 minutes (Fig. 24-89).

Spleen and Hepatobiliary System

Hepatobiliary Scan

Using a bilirubin analog as radiopharmaceutical (^{99m}Tc-iminodiacetic acid [IDA]), the hepatobiliary scan allows visualization of the bilirubin pathway in the hepatobiliary system from uptake into the hepatocytes to excretion via the biliary system, gallbladder, common bile duct, and small bowel. Indications for the study include the following: diagnosing suspected acute cystic duct obstruction/cholecystitis, investigating possible biliary obstruction, diagnosing biliary dyskinesia and gallbladder ejection fraction, detecting bile leak, and differentiating biliary atresia from neonatal hepatitis.

^{99m}Tc-IDA is injected intravenously and serial images of the abdomen are acquired for 1 hour. If the duodenum and gallbladder are visualized by 1 hour, the study is complete. If the gallbladder is not visualized by 1 hour, 3- to 4-hour delay images or morphine sulfate (0.04 mg/kg) with additional image acquisition would be required to differentiate acute versus chronic cholecystitis. Morphine causes contraction of the sphincter of Oddi and redirects bile flow into the gallbladder with a patent cystic duct. When evaluation of the gallbladder ejection fraction is required and the gallbladder is visualized by 1 hour, cholecystokinin (CCK) is infused and additional images can be acquired during CCK infusion.

For differentiation of biliary atresia from neonatal hepatitis, initial 90-minute images, followed by 4-hour (and up to 24-hour) delay images are acquired (Figs. 24-90 and 24-91).

Liver/Spleen Scan

Because of advances in CT and MRI techniques, the liver/spleen scan is not frequently used. However, these radionuclide scans may be helpful to confirm the presence of an accessory spleen, to evaluate hepatosplenomegaly and hepatic function, and to characterize a suspected hepatic mass, that is, determine whether or not it is focal nodular hyperplasia. The radiopharmaceutical (^{99m}Tc-sulfur colloid) is injected intravenously and is phagocytized by the reticuloendothelial system and normally distributed in Kupffer cells of the liver (85%), macrophages of the spleen (10%), and bone marrow (5%). If there is any nonfunctioning lesion within the liver or spleen, it appears as a hypofunctioning, or "cold" defect.

Hemangioma Scan

A hemangioma, or tagged RBC, scan is highly accurate with high specificity (90% to 100%) and sensitivity (65% to 100%) depending on the size and location of the lesion and equipment used in scanning. This scan is particularly useful for characterizing a suspected hepatic mass on whether it may be a hemangioma.

Gastrointestinal System

GI Bleeding Scan

The advantage of a GI bleeding scan over angiography is its ability to localize the site of GI bleeding before angiographic intervention and to detect intermittent bleeding. Either ^{99m}Tc-labeled RBC scintigraphy or ^{99m}Tc-sulfur colloid scintigraphy can be used; each is approximately 10-fold more sensitive than

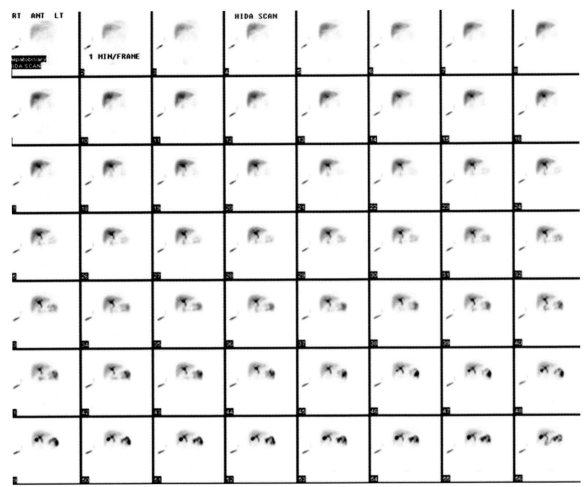

Figure 24-90 Hepatobiliary (HIDA) scan of a 17-year-old female with abdominal pain. This hepatobiliary study demonstrates visualization of the normal biliary duct, gallbladder, and bowel excretion.

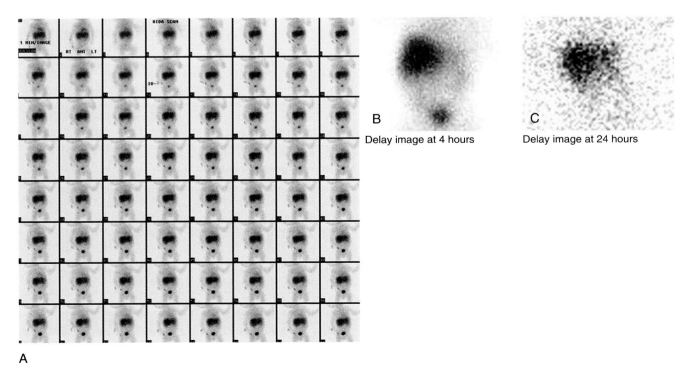

B Delay image at 4 hours

C Delay image at 24 hours

A

Figure 24-91 Hepatobiliary (HIDA) scan in biliary atresia: A 1-month-old with hyperbilirubinemia. ^{99m}Tc hepatobiliary scan shows no evidence of biliary excretion except for renal for the first 1 hour **(A)** and even at 24 hours **(C)**.

Figure 24-92 Gastrointestinal (GI) bleeding scan: Small intestinal bleeding. A focus *(arrow)* of activity initially appears in the proximal small intestine and subsequently moves both antegrade and retrograde from the site of bleeding.

angiography. The bleeding rate threshold for detection by ^{99m}Tc-labeled RBC scintigraphy is as low as 0.1 to 0.4 mL/minute, and 0.05 to 0.1 mL/minute for ^{99m}Tc-sulfur colloid scintigraphy, compared with 1 mL/minute for angiography. Colonoscopy has a low diagnostic yield for active bleeding and the small bowel is not successfully visualized by endoscopy. The main advantage of ^{99m}Tc-labeled RBC scintigraphy is its longer duration of imaging time to localize bleeding, which increases the rate of detection of intermittent bleeding. ^{99m}Tc-sulfur colloid scintigraphy is more sensitive and more widely used, although it has a smaller time window for imaging (20 minutes) due to rapid clearance by the reticuloendothelial system. Recent barium studies may obscure the site of bleeding (Fig. 24-92).

Meckel Diverticulum Scan

A Meckel diverticulum is an outgrowth of the ileum resulting from incomplete closure of the omphalomesenteric duct. In the Meckel diverticulum scan, ^{99m}Tc-pertechnetate localizes to the gastric mucosa and to ectopic gastric mucosa in the intestinal tract. The sensitivity and specificity of this study for the detection of ectopic gastric mucosa causing bleeding are approximately 85% and 95%, respectively (see Chapter 17, Fig. 17-61).

GI Motility Studies

GI motility scintigraphy provides more physiologic and functional information about GI motility, compared with a barium study, and objective assessment with quantification. The information is acquired as a dynamic image after oral administration of liquid labeled with ^{99m}Tc-DTPA or ^{111}In-DTPA, or a standardized solid meal labeled with ^{99m}Tc-sulfur colloid. Depending on the type of meal used, area of interest, and postimage processing, a GI motility study can be used to evaluate motility of the esophagus (esophageal transit), stomach (gastric emptying), and entire GI tract (panenteric transit study) or to evaluate gastroesophageal reflux or aspiration.

Esophageal transit: Esophageal manometry can also be used to assess esophageal peristalsis and pressure change at the upper or lower esophageal sphincter, with contrast radiography for anatomic evaluation and endoscopy for direct visualization and for biopsy. The advantage of esophageal scintigraphy is its noninvasive nature, quantification of data, and low radiation exposure.

Gastroesophageal reflux study: Twenty-four-hour pH monitoring is considered the gold standard for evaluation of gastroesophageal reflux. However, its disadvantages include false positive or negative results from contamination of the pH probe by gastric juice or neutral food content, and its invasiveness. It has been shown that a 1-hour gastroesophageal reflux study correlates well with 24-hour pH monitoring.

Aspiration study: Two scintigraphic studies (salivagram and milk scan) can be used for pulmonary aspiration.

The salivagram detects aspiration during swallowing (antegrade events) and the milk scan detects events associated with gastroesophageal reflux (retrograde events). The salivagram has been shown to be more sensitive than either a milk scan or video fluoroscopy in the detection of pulmonary aspiration.

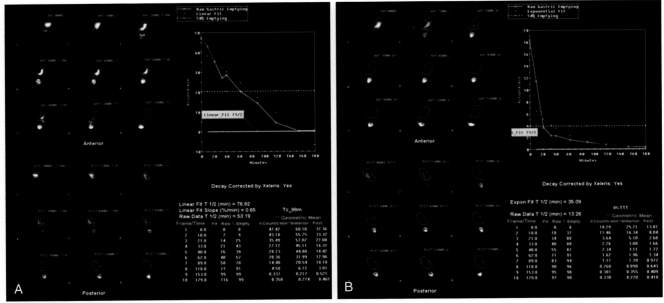

Solid gastric emptying   Liquid gastric emptying

Figure 24-93   Gastric emptying scan: Normal solid **(A)** and liquid **(B)** gastric emptying. Sequential images are shown with computer regions of interest around the stomach and small bowel. The regions of interest around the stomach have been used to generate time–activity curves and thus calculate the half-time for the radiotracer to leave the stomach.

An aspiration study is indicated to assess esophageal motility and reflux (esophageal transit) or gastric motility (gastric emptying), and to assess gastroesophageal reflux (pediatric milk study) or aspiration (pediatric milk study or salivagram).

Images are acquired for 1 to 4 hours after oral administration of radiolabeled solid and/or a liquid meal (for gastric emptying, esophageal transit study, and pediatric milk study). For a salivagram, images are acquired for 1 hour after administration of small drops of ^{99m}Tc-sulfur colloid liquid (Figs. 24-93 and 24-94).

Infection

^{111}In- or ^{99m}Tc-HMPAO–labeled Leukocyte Scan

An ^{111}In- or ^{99m}Tc-hexamethylpropyleneamine oxime (HMPAO)–labeled leukocyte scan localizes sites of soft tissue infection, inflammation, abscess, and osteomyelitis. These scans are used most often when there is suspicion for infection without any localizing sign or in the presence of negative or equivocal CT.

Although the three-phase bone scan has relatively good sensitivity (75% to 100%), the specificity (10% to 59%) is

Figure 24-94   Aspiration study: Radionuclide salivagrams positive for aspiration. There is intense continuous activity outlining the oropharynx, trachea, and right bronchus *(arrow)* on posterior views. Note that the last image is a cobalt flood source posterior to the patient, providing an outline of the form of the patient's body.

Anterior   Posterior

Figure 24-95 Leukocyte scan: Normal indium-labeled white blood cell scan. Anterior *(left)* and posterior *(right)* images demonstrate liver, spleen, and bone marrow activity.

low for diagnosing osteomyelitis. The radionuclide leukocyte scan has higher sensitivity and specificity than the three-phase bone scan in diagnosing osteomyelitis despite its poor resolution and lack of soft tissue and bony landmarks.

Indications include the following: diagnosing infection/abscess in soft tissues of the body, assessing the extent and severity of inflammatory bowel disease, diagnosing postoperative abscess in patients with fever and high clinical suspicion but inconclusive or negative CT scan, diagnosing infection in patients with known tumor and fever, diagnosing vascular graft infection, diagnosing osteomyelitis in diabetics with non-healing ulcers, and diagnosing osteomyelitis in patients with inconclusive three-phase bone scan or MRI (Fig. 24-95).

Gallium Scan

Gallium-67 (^{67}Ga)-citrate localizes to inflammatory tissues by forming complexes with circulating transferrin, which carries the radiolabel to sites of inflammation or tumor as well as other, normal tissues such as liver, spleen, bone marrow, gastrointestinal tract, and kidney; incorporates into leukocytes via lactoferrin; and is taken up by microorganisms through binding to siderophores, which are produced by bacteria.

Although combined bone/gallium scintigraphy has been replaced by labeled leukocyte imaging in the diagnosis of osteomyelitis, it remains the best way to evaluate vertebral osteomyelitis. Therefore, indications for a gallium scan are to diagnose osteomyelitis, especially vertebral osteomyelitis; to diagnose and evaluate the severity and extent of infection or inflammation in the lungs; and to determine the cause of fever of unknown origin, such as infection or occult tumor.

Gallium injection should be postponed at least 24 hours after blood transfusion or gadolinium-enhanced MRI (both can interfere with normal gallium biodistribution). After intravenous injection of ^{67}Ga-citrate, images can be obtained at 4, 24, or 48 hours with further delay images if needed (Fig. 24-96).

Three-phase Bone Scan for Infection

Although plain radiography is routinely performed as the initial imaging procedure for the diagnosis of osteomyelitis, it has relatively low sensitivity, ranging from 43% to 75%, and specificity, from 75% to 83%, and may not detect abnormality in the early phase. Osteomyelitis may take several days (approximately 10 days after the onset of infection) to become apparent. Therefore, plain radiography is helpful when positive; however, a negative study does not exclude osteomyelitis.

Bone scintigraphy is performed with ^{99m}Tc-labeled diphosphonates, usually methylene diphosphonate (MDP). Tracer uptake is dependent on blood flow and the osteoblastic activity for new bone formation. When osteomyelitis is suspected, a three-phase bone scan needs to be performed. Bone scintigraphy is widely available, relatively inexpensive, easily performed, and rapidly completed. The test is fairly sensitive and can be positive within 2 days of the onset of symptoms.

The three-phase bone scan includes the flow or perfusion phase, which is acquired immediately after radiopharmaceutical injection; followed immediately by imaging of the region of interest, that is, the blood pool or soft-tissue phase; and the third or bone phase, consisting of imaging performed 2 to 4 hours later.

CNS

Brain Perfusion SPECT Imaging

Two major types of radiopharmaceuticals are currently used for brain perfusion SPECT imaging: ^{99m}Tc-exametazime or HMPAO (Ceretec), and ^{99m}Tc-ethyl cysteinate dimer (ECD) (Neurolite). Both agents are injected intravenously and distribute in the brain proportional to blood flow. HMPAO is a lipophilic compound and thus may cross the blood–brain

Figure 24-96 Gallium scan: A 16-year-old with back pain with increased inflammatory marker. The scan demonstrates normal distribution in liver, bone, spleen, and lacrimal gland.

Ictal SPECT   Interictal SPECT

Figure 24-97   Ictal and interictal brain single-photon emission computed tomography (SPECT): An 11-year-old with intractable partial complex seizure and epileptogenic focus in the left temporal lobe. Ictal SPECT **(A)** demonstrates a focus of increased perfusion *(arrow)* in the left temporal lobe spreading to the left parietal lobe. Interictal SPECT **(B)** demonstrates a focus of decreased perfusion *(arrow)* in the left temporal lobe.

barrier into the brain, where it reacts with intracellular gluta-thione and is converted to a hydrophilic compound that pre-vents back diffusion out of the brain. Likewise, ECD has a lipophilic moiety that is converted to a hydrophilic compound by an unknown enzymatic reaction. Indications for brain per-fusion SPECT imaging are to identify seizure focus and to identify vascular spasm. The patient must lie still for the duration of the scan. If necessary, sedation is considered. For ictal brain SPECT, the radiopharmaceutical is injected as soon as possible after the onset of seizure activity detected during electroencephalogram (EEG) video monitoring (Fig. 24-97).

Brain Death Study

Administration of ^{99m}Tc-exametazime or HMPAO (Ceretec), and ^{99m}Tc-ethyl cysteinate dimer (ECD) (Neurolite) is one approach used to determine cerebral perfusion on the basis of cerebral uptake of radiopharmaceuticals. In the more tradi-tional approach, ^{99m}Tc-pertechnetate or ^{99m}Tc-DTPA is used to determine the presence of cerebral blood flow during the rapid angiographic flow phase right after bolus injection. Normally these radiopharmaceuticals do not cross the blood–brain barrier unless it is disrupted; they visualize only vascular structures.

Diamox Brain Stress SPECT

Acetazolamide (Diamox) is used to evaluate physiologically (hemodynamically) significant anatomic vascular lesions that can be masked and maintained by a compensatory mecha-nism. Acetazolamide, a carbonic anhydrase inhibitor, causes cerebral vasodilatation and increased cerebral blood flow in normal vessels, in contrast to high-grade stenotic vessels, which cannot dilate as much as normal vessels do. Therefore the regions of low flow reserve with relative hypoperfusion supplied by stenotic vessels become unmasked and visualized in contrast to areas supplied by normal vessels. The indication is to evaluate cerebral flow reserve.

^{18}F-FDG Brain PET

^{18}F-FDG is a glucose analog and is transported into viable cells, where it is phosphorylated and irreversibly trapped. A high-grade tumor uses more ^{18}F-FDG than do normal cells and appears as a "hot spot"; necrotic tissue has no uptake of ^{18}F-FDG, resulting in a "cold spot." ^{18}F-FDG can be used to identify a seizure focus, to differentiate recurrent tumor from radiation necrosis, and to assess the response of a high-grade brain tumor to treatment. For patients with seizures, EEG monitor-ing is needed.

CSF Flow Study (Radionuclide Cisternogram)

The radionuclide cisternogram visualizes CSF flow. This can differentiate communicating hydrocephalus (and normal pres-sure hydrocephalus) from nonobstructive causes of ventricu-lomegaly, such as atrophy. A lumbar puncture is performed by the clinician and ^{111}In-DTPA is injected intrathecally. Fluo-roscopic guidance can also be used. Images are obtained at 1 to 4 hours, 24 hours, and up to 72 hours depending on depart-ment protocol.

CSF Leak Study

CSF leakage can occur anywhere from the frontal sinus to the temporal bone (frequently at the cribriform plate) after trauma and can manifest as rhinorrhea or otorrhea. A nonresolving leak can cause meningitis, and often surgery is required to seal the leak. A presurgical radionuclide scan for CSF leakage is done to localize the leak and has greater sensitivity, espe-cially for intermittent leakage, compared with a CT myelo-gram, although anatomic detail cannot be provided.

Before the examination, the otolaryngologist places labeled cotton pledgets into the nasal cavity or ear. ^{111}In-DTPA is injected intrathecally after lumbar puncture. The patient lies supine or in the Trendelenburg position and performs the Valsalva maneuver until imaging at 1 to 4 hours to increase

CSF pressure and maximize the leak. Additional delay images up to 72 hours can also be obtained. When a leak is detected, or at 4 to 24 hours, the pledgets are withdrawn, weighed, and counted for radioactivity with further calculation of the pledget-to-plasma radioactivity ratio.

CSF Shunt Patency Study

A CSF shunt patency study is used to evaluate the patency of ventriculoperitoneal and ventriculoatrial CSF shunts and the Ommaya ventricular chemotherapy shunt. This test can provide images of CSF flow and evaluation of definitive shunt patency. The injection procedure should be arranged with a neurosurgeon or someone trained in this technique (Fig. 24-98).

Endocrine System

^{123}I Thyroid Uptake and Scan/^{99m}Tc-Pertechnetate Thyroid Scan

Iodine-123 (^{123}I) is an isotope that is absorbed readily by the intestine into the extrathyroidal iodine pool, actively transported into the follicular cells and oxidized, bound to tyrosine (organification), and subsequently incorporated into thyroid hormone, just like nonradioactive iodine. The ^{123}I scan demonstrates functioning thyroid tissue with both intact trapping and organification.

^{99m}Tc-pertechnetate is an anionic analog of iodine and is transported into the follicular cells without further

RT ANTERIOR LT

Figure 24-99 Thyroid scan: Diffuse goiter in a patient with Graves disease. The pinhole collimator image (^{123}I) demonstrates an enlarged thyroid gland with increased activity.

organification. The resulting images reflect exclusively the trapping capacity of the thyroid gland.

The scans may help to distinguish between Graves disease and hyperthyroidism caused by thyroiditis or factitious hyperthyroidism, to distinguish between Graves disease and multinodular goiter, to evaluate the functional status of a thyroid nodule, and to evaluate congenital thyroid anomaly (agenesis, sublingual thyroid) in a newborn (Fig. 24-99).

^{131}I Therapy for Hyperthyroidism

Radioactive ^{131}I therapy for hyperthyroidism has an approximately 80% success rate with single-dose treatment and presents minimal risk, although there is a likelihood of subsequent hypothyroidism. The treatment dose for Graves disease usually is calculated on the basis of the size of the gland, the 24-hour uptake, and the desired dose of radiation to be delivered to the gland. The indications for ^{131}I therapy are for the treatment of Graves disease and multinodular goiter.

Additional notes concerning ^{131}I therapy are as follows:

- A serum pregnancy test should be performed before ^{131}I injection for any female of reproductive age.
- Compounds that can affect iodine uptake need to be withheld (Box 24-1).
- After swallowing a ^{131}I capsule, the patient should follow, for 3 to 5 days posttherapy, the radiation safety instructions provided by the radiation safety office of the institution where treatment was received.

Post-thyroidectomy ^{123}I or ^{131}I Whole Body Scan for Thyroid Cancer

Please refer to ^{123}I Thyroid Uptake and Scan/^{99m}Tc-Pertechnetate Thyroid Scan, earlier. A post-thyroidectomy ^{123}I scan, or ^{131}I whole body scan, for thyroid cancer can be done to confirm the presence of postsurgical thyroid remnant, and to detect metastatic disease.

If the patient is a female of reproductive age, a pregnancy test should be performed; supplemental thyroid hormone is then discontinued until thyroid-stimulating hormone (TSH) exceeds 30 µU/mL. The patient should be on a low-iodine diet for 1 to 2 weeks before therapy and any exogenous iodine in the diet or medication that can decrease the uptake of

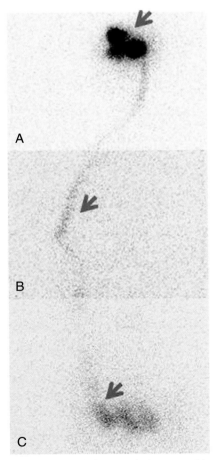

A

B

C

Figure 24-98 Ventriculoperitoneal shunt study: A 19-year-old male with a history of ventriculoperitoneal shunt placement presents with a headache. **A,** Lateral view of the head after injection into the shunt reservoir *(arrow)*. **B,** Lateral view over the chest shows activity progressing inferiorly *(arrow)*. **C,** Lateral view over the abdomen demonstrates activity at the end of the catheter *(arrow)*, diffusing throughout the abdomen, and collecting in the right and left paracolic gutters.

therapeutic ¹³¹I should be withheld (Fig. 24-100; and see Box 24-1).

¹³¹I Ablative Therapy for Thyroid Cancer

Some thyroid tissue remains after total thyroidectomy in 90% to 100% of patients, because of the risks of injury to the superior or recurrent laryngeal nerves and parathyroid glands. Also, 20% to 80% of papillary thyroid carcinoma and, to a lesser extent, follicular carcinoma can be multifocal and therefore a thyroid remnant after total thyroidectomy may still contain thyroid cancer. Treatment of patients with papillary thyroid carcinoma greater than 1.5 cm in size by a combination of thyroidectomy, ¹³¹I ablation, and thyroid hormone

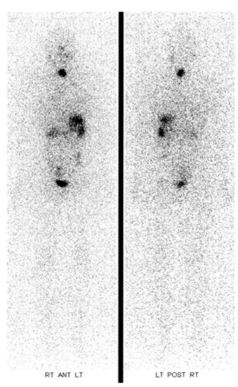

RT ANT LT   LT POST RT

Figure 24-100 Whole body iodine scan: A 16-year-old girl with a history of papillary thyroid cancer, status post–total thyroidectomy and lymph node dissection. Whole body iodine images demonstrate focal activity in the thyroid bed, indicating residual thyroid tissue or cancer, and normal distribution of tracer activity in the salivary gland, stomach, bowel, and bladder.

suppression results in a lower recurrence rate compared with surgery alone, surgery plus external radiation, or surgery plus thyroid hormone.

Once the thyroid is completely ablated, the patient undergoes periodic TSH-stimulated thyroglobulin testing, which is highly sensitive and specific for thyroid cancer follow-up; however, thyroid cancer metastases may be nonfunctional, that is, they may produce little or no thyroglobulin; because the anti-thyroglobulin antibody used to detect thyroglobulin does not recognize serum thyroglobulin in these patients, false negative results are produced. False negative results may also occur in patients with a high level of anti-thyroglobulin antibody. Therefore a diagnostic whole body iodine scan with ¹³¹I, which produces both gamma photons (for imaging) and beta particles (for therapy), is performed. Once ¹³¹I is trapped and organified by normal thyroid tissue or differentiated thyroid cancer, it decays inside the cells and emits beta particles, which disrupt the cellular DNA and further cell division, leading to cell death.

Parathyroid Scan

Parathyroid scans can help localize a hyperfunctioning parathyroid adenoma before surgery in patients with primary hyperparathyroidism and after parathyroid surgery in patients with persistent hyperparathyroidism. Two methods can be used.

Subtraction Technique

In the subtraction technique ⁹⁹ᵐTc-sestamibi/¹²³I or ⁹⁹ᵐTc-pertechnetate subtraction images are used. Both thyroid gland and hyperfunctioning parathyroid tissue take up ⁹⁹ᵐTc-sestamibi, whereas only the thyroid gland is visualized by ¹²³I or ⁹⁹ᵐTc-pertechnetate. By subtracting the ¹²³I results from those for ⁹⁹ᵐTc-sestamibi, hyperfunctioning parathyroid tissue can be localized.

Dual-phase Technique

⁹⁹ᵐTc-sestamibi is used in the dual-phase technique, which is based on the fact that there is a faster washout rate in normal thyroid tissue compared with abnormal parathyroid and adenoma or hyperplasia. It is easier to perform and less expensive than the subtraction technique, although less sensitive.

Various institutions may have different protocols through adopting either one of these or both techniques (Fig. 24-101).

Skeletal System

Bone Scan

Bone scintigraphy is performed with ⁹⁹ᵐTc-labeled diphosphonates, usually methylene diphosphonate (MDP). Tracer uptake is dependent on blood flow and the osteoblastic activity for new bone formation.

Indications include the following: detecting and follow-up for bone metastasis; determining the presence of fracture, stress fracture, or shin splint; evaluating skeletal abnormality as the cause of bone pain; evaluating avascular necrosis, reflex sympathetic dystrophy, and maturity of heterotopic ossification for surgical excision; follow-up of Paget disease; and evaluating the viability of a bone graft.

The three-phase bone scan consists of sequential flow images taken of one area of interest. Images of the first (or angiographic) phase are made immediately after intravenous injection of radiopharmaceutical. After a 10-minute delay the second-phase imaging (blood pool or soft tissue uptake) is done, and in the third phase, 3 to 4 hours later, delayed images are produced. A standard bone scan acquires images

Figure 24-101 Parathyroid scan: Parathyroid adenoma. A parathyroid adenoma (located at the inferior aspect of the left lobe of the thyroid; *arrow*) is revealed, by comparison of early and delayed images, as an area of increased activity relative to the thyroid.

Early image

Delayed Image

of the area of interest or the whole body 3 to 4 hours after intravenous injection of radiopharmaceutical (Fig. 24-102).

Oncology

123I-MIBG Scan

Meta-iodobenzylguanidine (MIBG) is a catecholamine precursor analog and represents a functional type 1 catecholamine. It is taken up into presynaptic nerve terminals of adrenergic origin by a type 1 catecholamine uptake mechanism, and concentrated within the secretory granules of catecholamine-producing cells. MIBG is concentrated in both the cytoplasm and norepinephrine storage granules of neuroblastoma cells, and particularly in the granules of pheochromocytoma cells. The sensitivity of 123I-MIBG scintigraphy for neuroblastoma ranges from 83% to 94%, with a specificity of nearly 100%, higher than that of 111In-DTPA-octreotide scintigraphy for somatostatin receptor (sensitivity of 55% to 70%) and other metabolic imaging techniques such as FDG PET. MIBG scintigraphy also has been used to assess treatment response and can provide prognostic value (Fig. 24-103).

18F-FDG PET

18F-FDG is a glucose analog, and FDG images represent glucose metabolism in suspected tumor cells, which have a high rate of glucose utilization compared with normal tissue. These scans are useful for initial staging, for assessment of treatment response, for disease monitoring after completion of therapy, to differentiate residual tumor from a scar or necrosis, and to assess prognosis.

18F-FDG PET scans have shown consistently superior diagnostic accuracy over other, more conventional imaging modalities and overall a 25% to 35% change in management plan may be contributed by FDG PET across all cancer types. PET/CT increases specificity even further by decreasing false

Planar bone scan

Bone SPECT transaxial view

Bone SPECT sagittal view

Figure 24-102 Bone scan and single-photon emission computed tomography (SPECT)/CT: A 10-year-old boy with a bilateral L5-S1 pars defect. **A,** Planar bone scan demonstrates focal activity in the fifth lumbar vertebra of the spine. **B** and **C,** Bone SPECT/CT and fusion images in transaxial **(B)** and sagittal **(C)** projections demonstrate focal activity in the bilateral pars interarticularis defect, indicating spondylolysis in L5.

RT ANT LT

LT POST RT

CT

SPECT

Fusion

A

Planar I-123 MIBG scan

I-123 MIBG SPECT

Figure 24-103 [123]I-*meta*-iodobenzylguanidine (MIBG) scan: An 11-month-old female with metastatic neuroblastoma. **A,** Planar ^{123}I-MIBG scan demonstrates an intensely MIBG-avid mass in the left upper abdominal region and pelvic masses, with multiple skeletal lesions. **B,** ^{123}I-MIBG single-photon emission computed tomography (SPECT) demonstrates an intensely MIBG-avid mass in the left upper abdomen.

positive findings and allowing more accurate anatomic localization. The utility of ^{18}F-FDG PET has been well established in lymphoma. Many previous studies have reported the superiority of ^{18}F-FDG PET in the assessment of tumor recurrence and distant metastasis of soft tissue sarcoma over other imaging modalities. Current experiences suggest a potential role for

^{18}F-FDG PET in monitoring treatment response, assessing the extent of Wilms tumor metastasis, and differentiating between nephrogenic rests and nephroblastomatosis, as well as in the staging and monitoring of treatment response and monitoring recurrence of primary bone tumor (osteosarcoma, Ewing sarcoma) and hepatoblastoma (Fig. 24-104 and Table 24-11).

PET

Fusion

CT

PET

Fusion

CT

Figure 24-104 Fluorodeoxyglucose positron emission tomography (^{18}F-FDG PET): An 18-year-old male with a history of recently diagnosed Hodgkin lymphoma. ^{18}F-FDG PET demonstrates multiple cervical, mediastinal, abdominal, and pelvic lymphadenopathies and splenic involvement.

Bibliography

American College of Radiology: *ACR appropriateness criteria* (website). http://www.acr.org/ac. Accessed October 2011.

American College of Radiology: *ACR manual on contrast media v7* (website). http://www.acr.org/secondarymainmenucategories/quality_safety/contrast_manual.aspx. Accessed October 2011.

Amis ES Jr, Butler PF, Applegate KE, et al: American College of Radiology white paper on radiation dose in medicine, *J Am Coll Radiol* 4:272–284, 2007.

Barkovich AJ: *Pediatric neuroimaging*, Philadelphia, 2005, Lippincott Williams & Wilkins.

Blickman JG, Parker BR, Barnes PD: *Pediatric radiology: The requisites*, Philadelphia, 2009, Mosby Elsevier.

Catanzano TM: *How to think like a radiologist: Ordering imaging studies*, Cambridge and New York, 2009, Cambridge University Press.

Gillard JH, Waldman AD, Barker PB: *Clinical MR neuroimaging: Diffusion, perfusion and spectroscopy*, Cambridge and New York, 2005, Cambridge University Press.

Haller JO, Slovis TL, Joshi A: *Pediatric radiology: an introduction for medical students, residents, and pediatric health care providers*, ed 3. Berlin, 2005, Springer.

Kanal E, Barkovich AJ, Bell C, et al: ACR guidance document for safe MR practices: 2007, *AJR Am J Roentgenol* 188:1447–1474, 2007.

National Cancer Institute: *Radiation risks and pediatric computed tomography (CT): A guide for health care providers* (website). http://www.cancer.gov/cancertopics/causes/radiation/radiation-risks-pediatric-CT. Accessed October 2011.

Osborn AG: *Diagnostic neuroradiology*, St. Louis, 1994, Mosby.

Panigrahy A, Nelson MD Jr, Bluml S: Magnetic resonance spectroscopy in pediatric neuroradiology: Clinical and research applications, *Pediatr Radiol* 40:3–30, 2010.

Pruckmayer M, Zacherl S, Salzer-Muhar U, et al: Scintigraphic assessment of pulmonary and whole-body blood flow patterns after surgical intervention in congenital heart disease, *J Nucl Med* 40:1477–1483, 1999.

Siegel MJ: *Pediatric sonography*, ed 4. Philadelphia, 2011, Lippincott Williams & Wilkins.

Slovis TL: *Caffey's pediatric diagnostic imaging*, ed 11. Philadelphia, 2008, Elsevier.

Swischuk LE: Emergency pediatric imaging: current status and update. *Semin Ultrasound CT MRI* 28:158–168, 2007.

Swartz JD: *Imaging of the temporal bone*, New York, 1986, Thieme.

INDEX

Page numbers followed by "f" indicate figures, "t" indicate tables, and "b" indicate boxes. Page numbers beginning with "e" indicate online-only material.